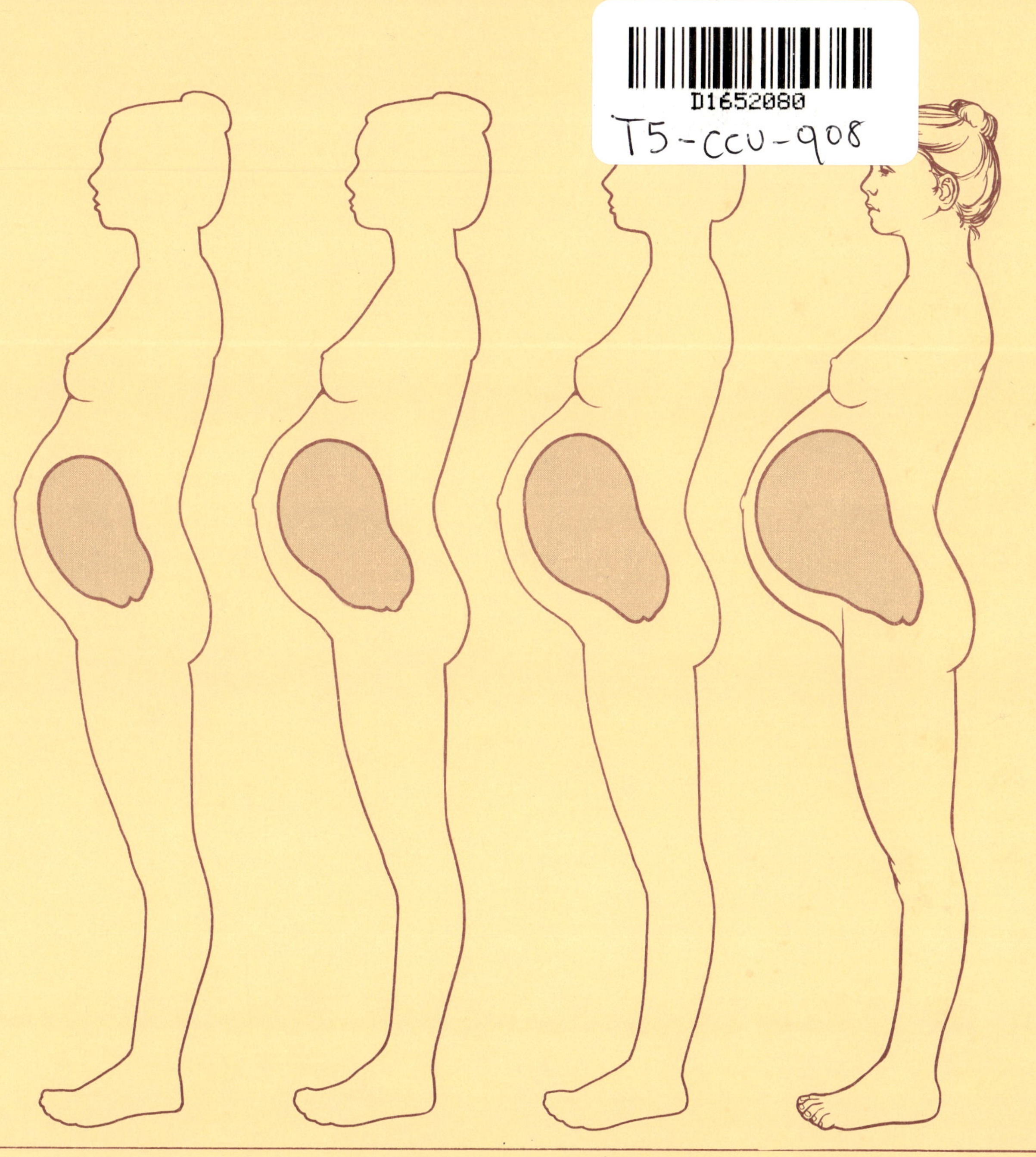

28 WEEKS | 32 WEEKS | 36 WEEKS | 40 WEEKS

MATERNITY NURSING

MATERNITY NURSING
THEORY TO PRACTICE

GLENDA FREGIA BUTNARESCU
Associate Professor
University of Texas Health Science Center
at San Antonio
School of Nursing
San Antonio, Texas

DELIGHT MOCAS TILLOTSON
Assistant Professor
Associate Dean
University of Texas Health Science Center
at San Antonio
School of Nursing
San Antonio, Texas

A WILEY MEDICAL PUBLICATION
JOHN WILEY & SONS
New York · Chichester · Brisbane · Toronto · Singapore

Cover designer: Wanda Lubelska
Copy editor: Harriet Serenkin
Editorial supervisor: Anita Wayne

The art program for the book was directed and supervised by Jo Ann Crow, Ph.D., Associate Professor, Coordinator, Curriculum Resource Center, The University of Texas Health Science Center at San Antonio, School of Nursing, San Antonio, Texas.

The line illustrations for the book were done by Mickey Senkarik, M.S., Morris and Senkarik Design Illustration, Helotes, Texas.

Library of Congress Cataloging in Publication Data:

Butnarescu, Glenda Fregia.
Maternity nursing.

Includes index.
1. Obstetrical nursing. I. Tillotson, Delight
Mocas. II. Title. [DNLM: 1. Obstetrical nursing.
2. Pregnancy—Nursing texts. WY 157 B987m]
RG951.B877 1983 610.73'678 82-17614
ISBN 0-471-07793-3

Printed in the United States of America

10 9 8 7 6 5 4 3 2 1

To ***Jo Ann Crow, Ph.D.,*** friend and colleague whose expertise in the field of educational media and graphic arts has helped teachers of nurses to improve their skills and expand their teaching repertoires.

Glenda Fregia Butnarescu
Delight Mocas Tillotson

To the memory of my parents, ***Demetrius Papanicolaou Mocas, M.D.,*** and ***Flora Coleman Mocas, R.N.,*** whose lives and commitment to quality in health care had a profound impact on my choice of profession and area of practice.

Delight Mocas Tillotson

CONTRIBUTORS

Jo Ann Crow, Ph.D.
Associate Professor
Coordinator, Curriculum Resource Center
The University of Texas Health Science Center at San Antonio
School of Nursing
San Antonio, Texas

Patricia A. Farrell, R.N., M.S.
Lt. Col. USAF (Ret.)
Member
Texas Genetics Advisory Committee
San Antonio, Texas
Chapter 24 Inheritance and Its Legacy

Jean A. Foster, R.N., M.S.N.
Clinician III: Nurseries
Medical Center Hospital
San Antonio, Texas
Chapter 23 Fetal–Neonatal Disorders

Judith A. Harris, R.N., M.S.N.
Director of Nurses: Maternal–Child Health
Medical Center Hospital
San Antonio, Texas
Chapter 11 Pregnancy: Fetal Perspective

Dona Pardo, R.N., M.S.N.
Formerly Assistant Professor
The University of Texas Health Science Center at San Antonio
School of Nursing
San Antonio, Texas
Chapter 15 Preparation for Childbirth

Linda G. Staurovsky, R.N., C.N.M., M.N.
Assistant Professor
The University of Texas Health Science Center at San Antonio
School of Nursing
San Antonio, Texas
Chapter 26 Health Maintenance for Women
Chapter 27 Reproductive Related Health Care Problems of Women

Patricia P. Villarreal, R.N., M.S.
Associate Professor
Coordinator, Junior Year
The University of Texas Health Science Center at San Antonio
School of Nursing
San Antonio, Texas
Chapter 18 Parenthood

PREFACE

Contemporary maternity nursing is part of a rapidly changing health care delivery system that reflects use of a burgeoning scientific knowledge base, sophisticated technology, professional role change, and consumerism. Today's maternity nurse is a prominent contributing member of this system, and, as such, the maternity nurse must be prepared to demonstrate the best that professional nursing has to offer through the sound use of knowledge, judgment, and skill.

This text, written by two experienced nurse-teachers, is an effort to present maternity nursing content in an interesting way that facilitates learning. Much basic information from nursing and related disciplines is included. Information is presented that is not available in current maternity nursing texts, such as women's health maintenance and the battered pregnant woman. However, no effort is made to repeat the content from pertinent disciplines that is readily available to the nurse in other published writings.

The content, readability, and organization will make this book useful for all levels of professional nursing programs. There has been a conscious effort to avoid the redundancy so common to many basic texts. Practicing nurses and graduate students will find the book useful as a reference. The book is also written with the maternity nursing teacher in mind. A separate teacher's manual is available for use with the text.

The focus of this book is the pregnant woman and neonate within the context of the family. We strongly believe that reproduction and related events are family experiences.

The book is divided into six units. Although each unit is dependent to some extent on the one preceding it, each can be used independently.

Unit One, "Maternity Nursing in Today's World," looks at today's nursing practice for families experiencing reproduction-related events. It focuses on the practice of and the teaching–learning process of maternity nursing and provides a framework for examining selected issues that may confront today's maternity nurse.

Unit Two, "Developmental Readiness for Pregnancy and Parenthood," attends to both physical and psychosocial developments. The unit presents a detailed discussion of the scientific basis for human reproduction. Adolescence as a period of personal bio-psycho-social synthesis and the role of the nurse in assessing reproductive readiness are emphasized.

Unit Three, "Pregnancy," examines pregnancy from three vantage points—the pregnant woman, the fetus, and the family. Sexuality is discussed, including the reasons why nurses must be particularly understanding in conversations on this still sensitive subject. Education for pregnancy and parenthood is also addressed.

Unit Four, "Childbirth, Recovery, and Early Parenthood," emphasizes the knowledge and skill needed by the nurse to assess the pregnant woman's and her family's progress and to help the woman through labor and recovery. The unit includes the adaptation of the neonate to extrauterine life and the early adjustment of the family to parenthood. Parenting and the various categories of parents are discussed in detail.

Unit Five, "Reproductive Risk," deals with a major contemporary health problem. The scope and characteristics of threats to healthy reproductive outcome are covered. Assessment of reproductive risk and selected maternal risk conditions that can occur during pregnancy, labor, and recovery are addressed. A look at the impact of reproductive risk on the individual, family, and society is included. Fetal–neonatal disorders are discussed from both pathophysiologic and genetic perspectives.

Unit Six, "Women's Health," includes material needed by nurses to promote the health of women during their childbearing years. Emphasis is given to gynecologic examination and family planning. Induced abortion and reproduction-related health care problems of women are also discussed.

The book closes with an Epilogue (Chapter 28), six appendixes, and a glossary. Chapter 28 analyzes the status, direction, and potential of maternity nursing and addresses selected issues and changes in the role and function of the nurse and of the health care delivery system. Appendix A contains *The Pregnant Patient's Bill of Rights* and *The Pregnant Patient's Responsibilities.* Appendixes B and C include two guides for mastering text material and assessing study habits. Forms used for patient and hospital records are included in Appendixes D and E. Appendix F, "Assessment Tools," includes a chart for determining adequate nutrition during pregnancy, a summary of the information that might be contained in a health history, and graphs showing growth rates for infants.

The glossary contains definitions of terms specific to obstetric and gynecologic nursing, as well as some related terms from other disciplines and common words that have specific applications in the field of maternity nursing.

Glenda Fregia Butnarescu
Delight Mocas Tillotson

ACKNOWLEDGMENTS

Smiles come easily when the manuscript is completed and the body and brain are beginning to recover from the demands of library research and writing and rewriting. Writing, however, is much like childbirth—memory of the stresses are diminished by the joy and pleasure with the product. Completion of a book of this magnitude affords us the opportunity to recall some of the experiences that enabled the project to be finished and to realize that while writing a book may, at times, be a lonely experience, it is not experienced alone. Many people give of themselves in numerous ways to make the finished product possible. We would like to recognize by name each person who contributed in both small and large ways to the completion of so personal a project as this book. However, this is neither practical nor possible. We would like to recognize some of those people who worked most closely with us or who were most affected by the writing of this book and to assure them that their contributions were appreciated.

First and foremost, to Leoda Harmon and David Tillotson, Jr., go both love and many thanks for the support they gave in so many ways. Mothers and husbands are supposed to give encouragement, to listen, and to lend a shoulder at times, but these two people far exceeded the usual demands for such help. We could not have completed the project without them and their sustained support through words of encouragement, periods of silence, and tolerance of erratic demands and disrupted life-styles.

We give sincere gratitude to Tamara Palm, photographer and friend, who covered many miles in the name of this project, and to Wendy Tillotson-Worcester and Mark Tillotson, who took some special photographs for the book. Thanks also go to Janice, Frank, and Jonathan Spikes; Judy, John, Terry, and Marcus Rennick; Luci, Douglas, Courtney, and Jonathan Coffey; Patty, Richard, and Valerie Villarreal; Betty, Edmon, and Shannan Marcontell; and Alfred, Carolyn, and Denise Smith, all of whom opened family photograph albums to us and/or served as models for some pictures. Our appreciation also goes to Cindy Kaufman and the nurse-midwives of the Nurse-Midwifery Birthing Service, Eugene, Oregon, and their clients who permitted our use of their photographs.

Colleagues and students from The University of Texas Health Science Center at San Antonio have our deepest gratitude and respect for their support; they offered encouragement and critical comment throughout the project. Special acknowledgments are given to Dr. Patty L. Hawken, Dean of the School of Nursing, who served as our educational consultant and critically reviewed the content on teaching and learning, and to Dr. Jo Ann Crow, Associate Professor, who directed the art program for the book. Others associated with the Health Science Center who facilitated our efforts and supported our work include Sandra Lynch, Amy Perkins, and Diana Cutshaw, Nurse Clinical Specialists, who allowed us to invade the Brady/Green Hospital Nurse Directed Prenatal Clinic with our questions and camera; Judy Harris, Director of Maternal Child Nursing; and Fran West and Marlene Upright, Clinician III, Medical Center Hospital, who shared of themselves and their time as well as cleared the pathway for our cameras. A special thank you to Virginia Mousseau, Associate Administrator of Nursing, Medical Center Hospital, who aided us in our use of numerous forms from that hospital.

Manuscript support was provided on the spot and without complaint by Betty Clutts and Kathleen Boehm of the School of Nursing. A very special thank you to Anne Morrison who typed most of the manuscript. Not only did Anne type our words, but, to paraphrase Kipling, she kept her head when those around her were losing theirs. Thank you to Brenda Moylan who helped Anne with typing in the final days of manuscript preparation.

Our association with John Wiley & Sons predates this work, and their pattern of support, encouragement, and quality production has done much to enable us first to become interested in doing the project and then to see it through. Wiley has on its staff many highly qualified people. We were privileged to work closely with some of these people and indirectly with others. The people who deserve much more than verbal recognition are Cathy Somer, former Editor for Nursing and Allied Health, who initiated the project, and Andrea Stingelin, present Editor for Nursing and Allied Health, and her staff, who supported the project through to completion. Andrea's optimism, experienced help, knowledge, and sense of humor were major support resources for us and kept the project on its course.

Glenda Fregia Butnarescu
Delight Mocas Tillotson

GENERAL CONTENTS

UNIT ONE MATERNITY NURSING IN TODAY'S WORLD

UNIT TWO DEVELOPMENTAL READINESS FOR PREGNANCY AND PARENTHOOD

UNIT THREE PREGNANCY

UNIT SIX
WOMEN'S HEALTH

EPILOGUE

DETAILED CONTENTS

15 PREPARATION FOR CHILDBIRTH → 283

UNIT FOUR CHILDBIRTH, RECOVERY, AND EARLY PARENTHOOD

16 LABOR → 305

UNIT ONE

MATERNITY NURSING IN TODAY'S WORLD

INTRODUCTION

Maternity nursing practice today is a blend of the humanistic and scientific aspects of health care that are designed to promote health and to prevent disease and disorders, as well as to enhance the treatment of illness states. The focus of maternity nursing is the woman during pregnancy, childbirth, and recovery; her unborn/newborn child; and her family. Maternity nursing is also concerned with the periods preceding and between pregnancies, with special interest in family planning, preparation for pregnancy and parenthood, and intergestational health maintenance for women.

Unit One is designed to help you visualize the scope of maternity nursing and begin to understand its strengths and weaknesses, as well as its past and its potential for the future. This unit will also help you to develop an appreciation for the study of maternity nursing as a specialty area of professional nursing.

Chapter 1, "A Commentary on Contemporary Maternity Nursing," represents our perceptions of contemporary maternity nursing. The chapter discusses the scope of maternity nursing, its unique characteristics, and its evolution, with attention to historical events important to the maternity nurse.

Chapter 2, "The Roles of the Teacher and Learner in Maternity Nursing," sets the stage for the study of maternity nursing. The teaching–learning process is discussed, with emphasis on the respective roles of the teacher and the learner. General beliefs and characteristics of learning and the relationship of the teaching–learning process to the nursing process are described.

In Chapter 3, "Issues in Reproductive Health Care," concerns of nurses are discussed, with emphasis on the identification of important issues for maternity nurses, analysis of such issues, and clarification of personal values concerning issues. The broad issue of consumer rights is used to demonstrate one way in which issues are generated from broader societal concerns. Selected issues are discussed briefly, and you are directed to the sections of the book where these issues are dealt with more completely.

Unit One provides some useful information, but its principal purpose is to help you gain a feeling for and a conceptual approach to the study of maternity nursing.

BEHAVIORAL OUTCOMES

Upon completion of the study of this unit you should be able to:

- ▲ Describe the scope of contemporary maternity nursing
- ▲ Describe the evolution of maternity nursing
- ▲ Define teaching and learning
- ▲ List five beliefs about learning
- ▲ Describe the roles of the teacher and the learner in the study of maternity nursing
- ▲ Explain three domains of learning
- ▲ Compare the teaching–learning process to the nursing process
- ▲ Identify five issues of concern to maternity nurses
- ▲ Explain the significance of selected types of statistics to maternity nursing
- ▲ Examine personal beliefs about human reproduction and the issues affecting it

1

A COMMENTARY ON CONTEMPORARY MATERNITY NURSING

Maternity nursing brings the nurse into contact with the most intimate aspects of the physical, social, and emotional domains of individual and family life. It recognizes pregnancy and childbirth as a many faceted experience: as a desired, fulfilling time for the pregnant woman and her family; as a period of growth and development in which the parents relinquish their childhood and adolescence and take on the role of adult with responsibility for another human life; as a period of crisis or potential for crisis in which anxieties, fears, and frustrations are often present; as a period of energy expenditure, both physical and emotional; and as a time of coming together as a family instead of being two separate people. For most it is a healthy and satisfying event; for some it is a time of stress and even loss. Maternity nurses provide care for people during all of these moments. As such, they are privileged care givers in this most personal experience and share daily in the human efforts to maintain the species.

The goals of maternity nursing are the promotion and maintenance of the optimum health possible for a woman, her unborn or newborn infant, and her family, all within the context of personal and societal values concerning sexual behavior, pregnancy, childbirth, and parenthood. In other words, maternity nursing is concerned with the maintenance of individual and family well-being in conjunction with the epitome of creativity—the reproduction of another human being.

The capacity for human reproduction is present in healthy men and women for an extended time span beginning with puberty and ending, for the woman, with menopause. The nurse will encounter women whose ages range from early adolescence through the late forties, or even the early fifties, and men at any postpubertal age with the preponderance of people falling somewhere in the young adult or mature age category.

The reproductive experience is cyclic in nature; it is a series of regularly occurring events that are rhythmic in character and interrelated in such a way that there is no clear distinction between them. The health and characteristics of the parents are closely intertwined with that of their offspring, for the traits of parents are often repeated in their children and the health of parents have an impact on the health of their children and their grandchildren (Fig. 1.1). This cyclicity and continuity associated with reproduction requires the nurse to use a broad range of theory and skill in caring for expectant and young women—to help them recall the past in order to understand the requirements of the pregnancy and to look beyond the present in

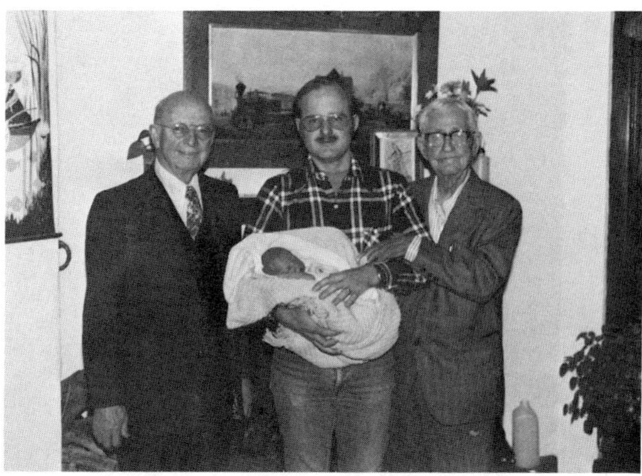

Figure 1.1
The species is maintained from generation to generation.

anticipation of the future. In order to recognize and comprehend the needs of the family regardless of where they are appearing in the cycle or developmental continuum, the nurse must be knowledgeable about the physiology and psychosociology of reproduction, as well as have an understanding about growth and development.

Maternity nursing also brings nurses into face-to-face confrontation with their own beliefs, values, and attitudes about life and human reproduction, requiring careful examination of self in order to provide personalized care for others. Personal and professional demands, which are similar to, yet different from, those experienced in other areas of nursing practice, are often made on the nurse. For example, the maternity nurse must grapple with issues like elective abortion and the right to life of an unborn fetus.

Maternity nursing is concerned with all aspects of the reproductive experience: the physical and psychosocial foundations that prepare the species to reproduce itself; the experiences of pregnancy, childbirth, and recovery; parenthood, particularly the early period of parenthood; aberrations associated with reproduction; and the period between pregnancies, especially those events concerning the health of the woman. In order to attend to needs and concerns of the woman and her family, the maternity nurse must be able to assume a variety of roles, such as care giver, teacher, and counselor, that will be discussed throughout this book, and to apply knowledge and data to consumer needs in a goal-directed, reasonable, and safe manner.

This chapter addresses maternity nursing from a contemporary vantage point examining both the scope of maternity nursing practice and the historical antecedents to today's nursing practice.

SCOPE OF MATERNITY NURSING

"Maternity," like "obstetrics," is an inadequate and misleading term for describing the scope of the nursing practice to which it refers. *Maternity* refers to motherhood, and the care of women in the early stages of motherhood is certainly an aspect of nursing during the reproductive experience. *Obstetrics* is used to describe the care given to women during a specified period of time, that of pregnancy, childbirth, and recovery from childbirth. Both concepts are integral parts of reproductive health care, but they are only parts. Maternity nursing is the most commonly encountered contemporary term, but you will also come across obstetric nursing, maternal/-newborn nursing, maternal–child health nursing, perinatal nursing, and many other variations. While each term refers to something somewhat different, they are all derived essentially from the same theory and skill base. All are concerned with health care for families who are, or have the potential to become, pregnant and include the periods preceding conception and during pregnancy, childbirth, and recovery, with particular attention to the pregnant woman and her fetus/neonate. Maternity or obstetric nursing practice is closely aligned, conceptually, with *gynecologic nursing,* the specialty that attends to the health problems and reproductive-related diseases or disorders of women and to the health maintenance or promotion of women during the childbearing years. *Maternity nursing* is used repeatedly throughout this book in its broad, contemporary sense and is defined as the provision of nursing services to a woman and her family in anticipation of or during the periods of pregnancy, childbirth, and early parenthood. It is, further, the provision of care to her newborn infant during the first four weeks of life. Maternity nursing is characterized by the following: the deliberative use of patient data in concert with an accurate and relevant theory base; commitment to concern for the care of the family during the reproductive experiences; consistency of safe nursing care services; and accountability for actions. Maternity nursing is demonstrated through direct and indirect nursing services that are responsive to consumer needs and that are provided in both institutional and community settings. It is predicated on beliefs about life/death and wellness/illness, as much as on beliefs and values about professional nursing. Some such beliefs are as follows:

▲ Every individual has the *right* to be born healthy.

▲ The reproductive experience is influenced by intradynamic and extradynamic forces that both precede and accompany conception, pregnancy, childbirth, and the early parenting period.

▲ Pregnancy occurs as part of a developmental continuum and constitutes, for most, a maturational crisis.

▲ *Beliefs, values,* and *attitudes* held by pregnant families are the result of a combination of life experiences and are often closely aligned with those of the family from which the partners come and the peer groups with whom they are associated, as well as the culture and society of which they are a part.

▲ Maternity nursing is a specialized component of professional nursing.

▲ Nursing care is delivered through an interdependent and collaborative relationship with the consumer and other health care providers.

▲ Nursing care that is responsive to consumer needs and that uses a sound theory base can facilitate a healthy reproductive outcome.

▲ The principal role of the maternity nurse is that of provider of goal-directed, family-centered nursing care in whatever setting it is required.

Maternity nursing is about people. Its practice involves not only the woman seeking health care services, but the family from which she comes and, indirectly, the support network (friends, extended family) upon which she relies. The health care professionals providing care to the woman and her family during the period of reproductive-related events include, most directly, the physician(s) and nurse(s) (Fig. 1.2). However, people from other

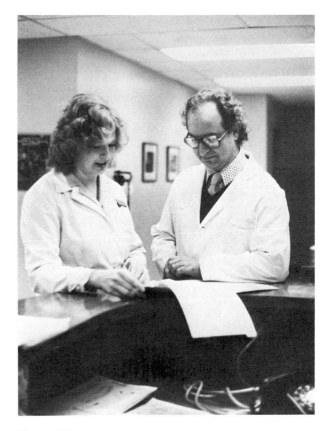

Figure 1.2
The physician and nurse are the two health providers with whom the woman has the most contact during pregnancy.

health-related disciplines are also involved, often in a transitory manner, and include the nutritionist, the social worker, and personnel from the institution's support services such as laboratory and radiology. The number of people with whom the woman and nurse comes into contact during the weeks and months of pregnancy and the periods preceding and following it are many (Fig. 1.3). While these people are known and relied upon by the nurse and the physician, they are often only a collage of unknown and sometimes even frightening faces to the woman. Since many of the services nurses deliver are necessary to ensure optimal health care, they are in a prime position to coordinate services and collaborate with others in such a way that the woman will view them in a helpful rather than hurtful sense and that they, in turn, will view the woman as a person with feelings as well as needs. The tone of maternity nursing can be warm and caring or it can be cold and impersonal. The nurse often makes the difference.

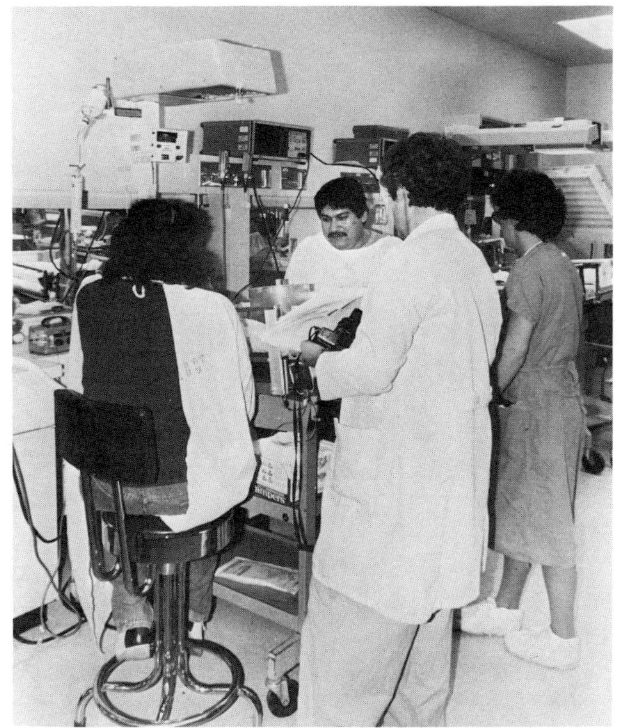

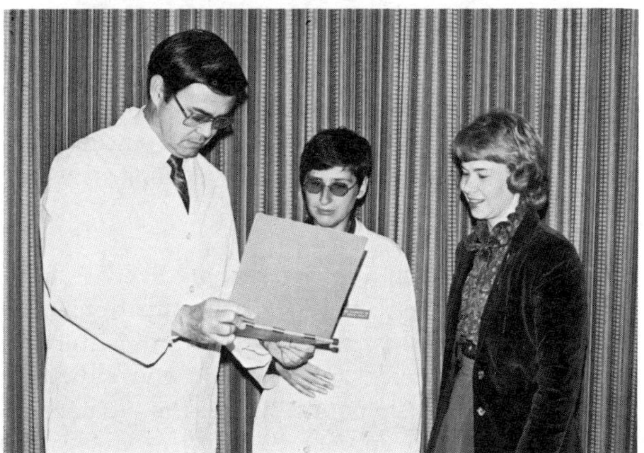

Figure 1.3
Other health care personnel, such as laboratory and radiology technicians, social workers, nutritionists, and nurses' aides participate in the care of the pregnant woman and her family.

The Consumer

The focus of health care during pregnancy, childbirth, and recovery is the woman, her unborn fetus, and later her newborn infant. However, she is cared for as a total self—a self that is part of her past, concerned with her present, and anticipating her future—that of mother. She is also cared for as part of a family unit and, in most cases, as part of a pregnant couple. The events associated with pregnancy and childbirth are those of becoming parents, for both the woman and her partner—a role that is new to many couples. Even those couples who have had children often approach each pregnancy with new or different expectations, hopes, and fears.

The *family* is the basic unit from which the pregnant couple comes and as such should be considered in any care plan developed with and for the client. Family-centered maternity care emerged during the late 1950s and 1960s. This concept has influenced the practice of maternity nursing for almost a quarter of a century. It is the basis for many of the changes made in the health care delivery system relative to pregnancy and childbearing (Fig. 1.4). Practices such as *rooming-in,* visitation rights for children, fathers in the labor and delivery rooms, and alternative birthing units or centers all evolved because of consumer needs and professional or lay responses to the philosophy of including the family in the care of the woman during pregnancy, as well as emerging

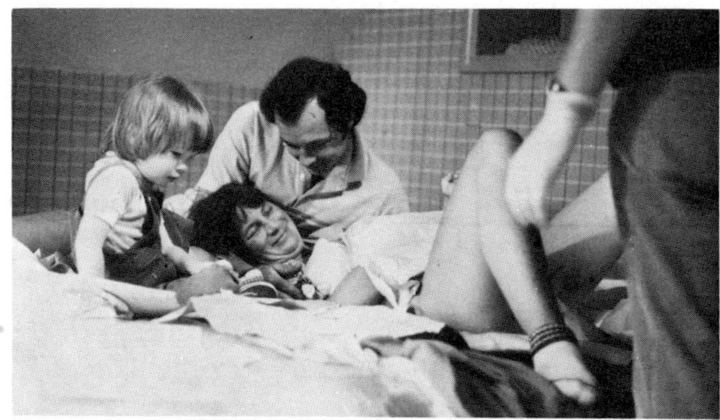

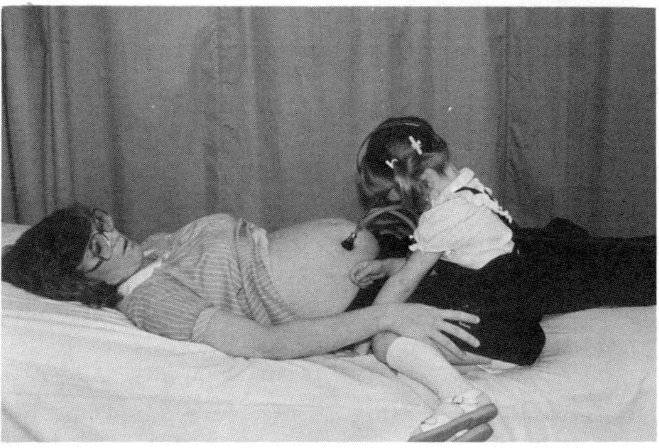

Figure 1.4
Some families include their other children in the childbirth experience today.

new concepts and theories for social and medical sciences. A major proponent of family-centered maternity care is Ernestine Weidenbach who wrote:

> *The nurse who practices family-centered maternity nursing regards childbirth not merely as a natural physiologic experience but as a socially significant process, essential for creation, growth and development of the family, the unit structure of our society . . .*
>
> 1967, p. 17

She went on to say:

> *The strength of the family is enhanced by the bonds of love and understanding of its members. Such bonds have their roots in deep, shared, meaningful experience of which childbearing can be one.*
>
> 1967, p. 17

Recognizing that the consumer is a person coming from some type of family unit experiencing pregnancy and childbirth within the context of that unit and the society of which that family unit is a part is important for the maternity nurse. Perhaps even more important, is the realization bý the nurse that the consumer and family are not a stereotypical "ideal" family. Instead, the consumer wears many faces (Fig. 1.5). The American ideal and the joy of the nurse is the healthy, married, middle-income couple who have planned and are joyfully anticipating the arrival of the new child. Large numbers of consumers fit this image. However, a significant number seeking reproductive health care do not. Not all couples are married. Some are single expectant parents; others are couples who have established a caring relationship but choose not to marry. Not all pregnancies are planned; many are "accidents" due to lack of knowledge about family planning or, occasionally, contraceptive failures. An unplanned pregnancy is not necessarily an unwanted pregnancy or an unwanted child. Not all consumers are healthy. Some are at risk for reproductive-related or other reasons. All babies are not healthy at birth. Some have diseases or disorders that result in disabilities or death. Some babies will die in utero and be *aborted;* some will be *stillborn,* in which case the family will need supportive, as well as physical, nursing care to help it cope with its feelings of grief, loss, and even failure. Not all expectant families are financially solvent. Many have inadequate economic resources for supporting the needs of the pregnancy and, later, the child. Occasionally, a pregnant woman or her newborn infant will require long-term hospitalization, placing even further strain on limited finances. Most, but not all, parents will be "good" parents. Some parents are inadequately prepared to receive and parent their child. Most new parents need some assistance with their new role. Most make the adjustment to parenthood in a healthy fashion; others require much assistance; and some are unable to assume a healthy and safe parenting role. There are increasing cases of reported parent abuse of children, sibling abuse of sibling, and spouse abuse of spouse. A large number of family units are intact with both parents present and a supportive extended family available. However, some pregnant women come from broken homes and may face the parenting role without the support of a partner or family.

Maternity nursing practice brings the nurse into contact with all of these consumers, as well as others not mentioned here. Whatever the characteristics and needs of the woman and her family the nurse is a key health professional with the knowledge and skill to assist them during these periods by providing concerned nursing care, including education, referral, and consultation.

The Nurse

Today's maternity nurse, like the consumer, wears many faces (Fig. 1.6). No longer is the pronoun "she" appropriate for reference to the nurse, for increasing numbers of men are selecting nursing as their profession, and some of these men practice maternity nursing. The hospital is still the single largest employer of maternity nurses, and of nurses generally, for much of reproductive health care is still delivered in an institutional setting. But maternity nurses also practice in community settings, such as community health clinics, physician's offices, birthing centers, and educational settings (Fig. 1.7). Maternity nursing is not bound by any physical setting; it is appropriate wherever the needs of the consumer abound and wherever the nurse can safely and legally practice.

Maternity nurses assume many and varied roles in their practice. The nurse may practice as a staff nurse or as a team leader in a separate area of maternity nursing, such as the *antepartal* (during preg-

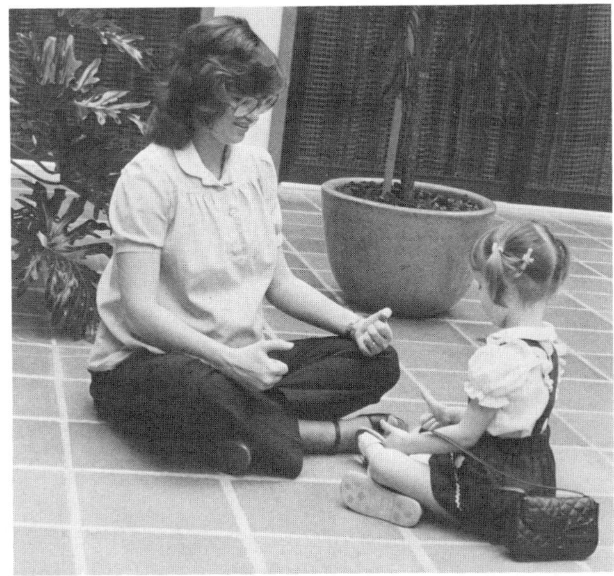

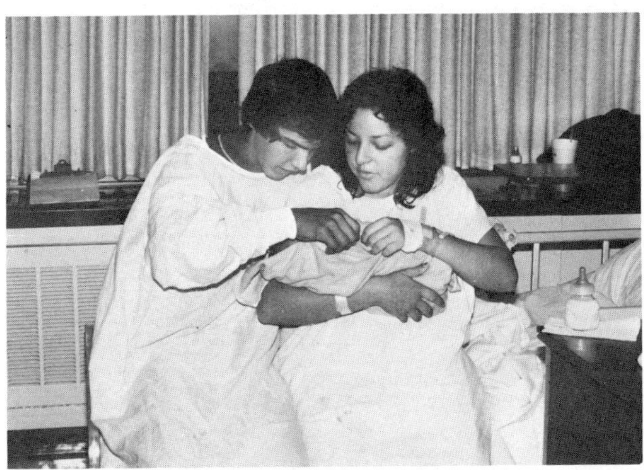

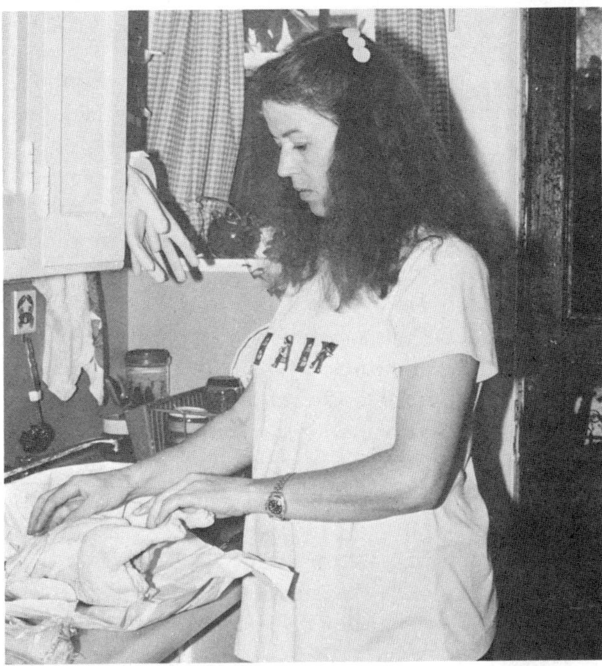

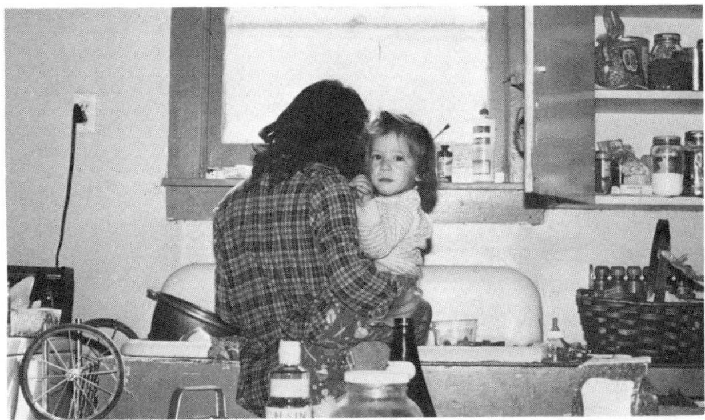

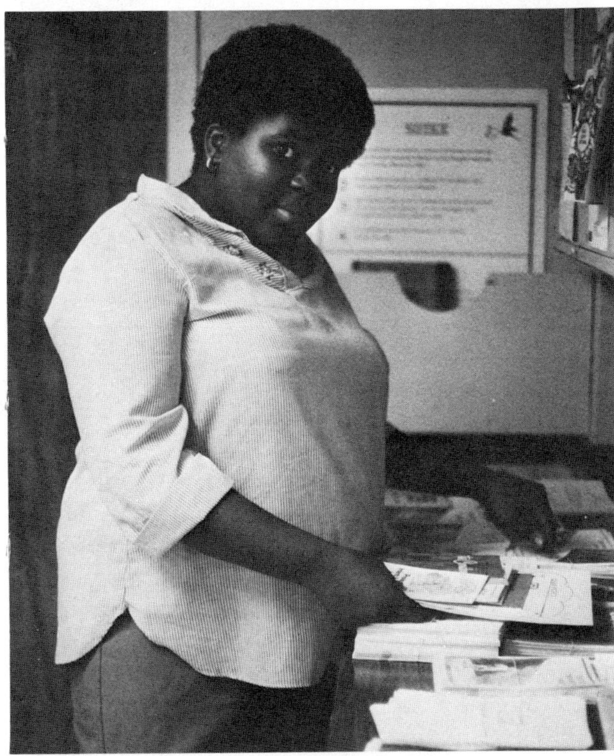

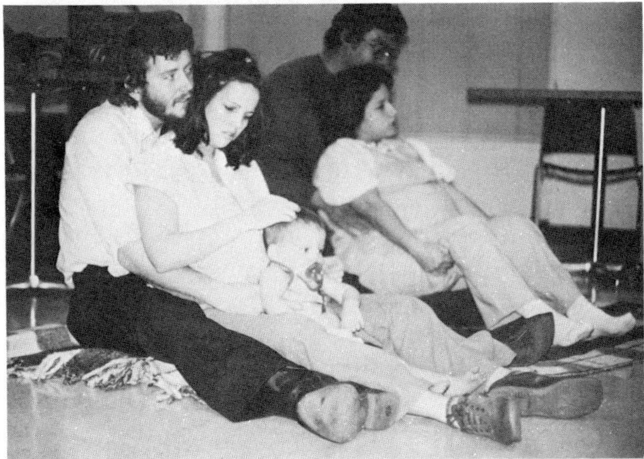

Figure 1.5
The consumer of maternity services represents a wide range of ages, socioeconomic strata, and cultural backgrounds.

nancy), *intrapartal* (during labor), *postpartal* (following delivery), or nursery areas. With advanced training and education, nurses may take on the roles of practitioner, clinical specialist, *nurse-midwife,* parent-educator, nurse administrator, or nurse educator. Some nurses will continue through doctoral study and prepare for leadership roles in all of these areas or become involved in research of reproductive-related nursing questions and problems.

Because the maternity nurse is a member of the nursing profession, many of the characteristics are closely aligned with the profile of professional nursing in regard to age, sex, and numbers in the various practice settings, as well as the commitment to standards of care developed and supported by the American Nurses' Association, the Nurses Association of the American College of Obstetrics and Gynecology, The American College of Nurse-Midwives, and subsections of these organizations. One important characteristic of professional nurses is that they care about the patients for whom they provide nursing services. In this era of concern with self, nurses remain the health care professional in close, consistent contact with the consumer. The period of this sustained contact is even more pronounced during the long months of pregnancy and childbirth. Too many of the settings within the health care delivery system are not designed to communicate a climate of caring for the consumer, making it even more important that the nurse be able to demonstrate the humanistic components of health care services.

> *It's the essential graciousness and the comforting skills that are really the heart of nursing, and I think people appreciate nurses for these qualities.*
>
> *Rubin, 1976, p. 149*

The maternity nurse, however, does more than demonstrate caring. Maternity nursing practice requires that a nurse be well educated, with knowledge of social sciences, as well as of biophysical and medical sciences, and be skilled in basic as well as newer modalities of patient care. Each day the nurse is called upon repeatedly to make sound, informed judgments about the needs of the consumers and to stand accountable both professionally and legally for the judgments made and the skills practiced.

The maternity nurse is a member of the health team and as such must be adept in both communication and interpersonal skills; such skills are used in daily contact with other team members, as well as with the consumer for whom the team is caring. The nurse is often the link between the consumer and other members of the team—a link that is important in any area of nursing practice, but especially so in the intimate facets of reproductive health care.

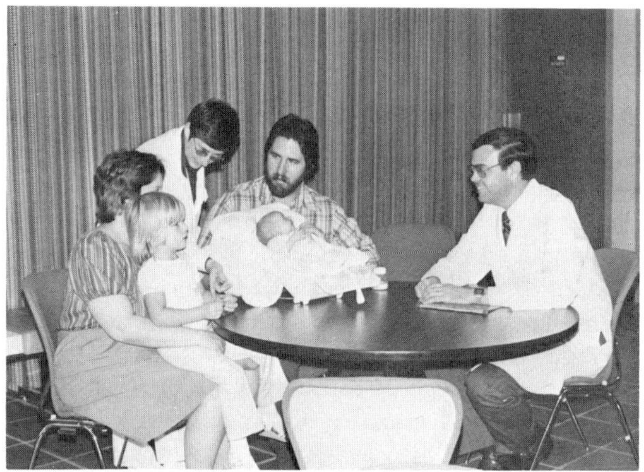

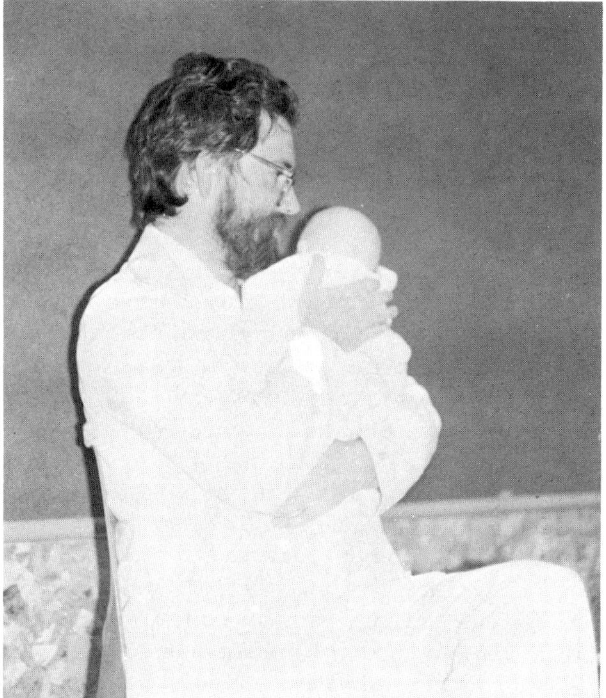

Figure 1.6
Both men and women may choose to practice maternity nursing.

The maternity nurse is also a person who, like the consumer, reflects the values, beliefs, and attitudes of the family, culture, and society from which he or she comes (Fig. 1.7). Because of this individuality, the nurse is often faced with conflicts in values when caring for consumers whose backgrounds are different from that of the nurse or when participating in a health care system whose demands and practices differ from those of the consumer, the nurse, or both. Maternity nursing students need to realize that it is all right to be themselves and that it is healthy to reflect their heritage and position in society. But they must also recognize and respect those who are different from themselves and must provide nursing care that represents the best of themselves, while attending to the unique characteristics of the consumer. They must work within the demands of the system or toward the change of those practices that they cannot in good conscience accept for the consumer or themselves.

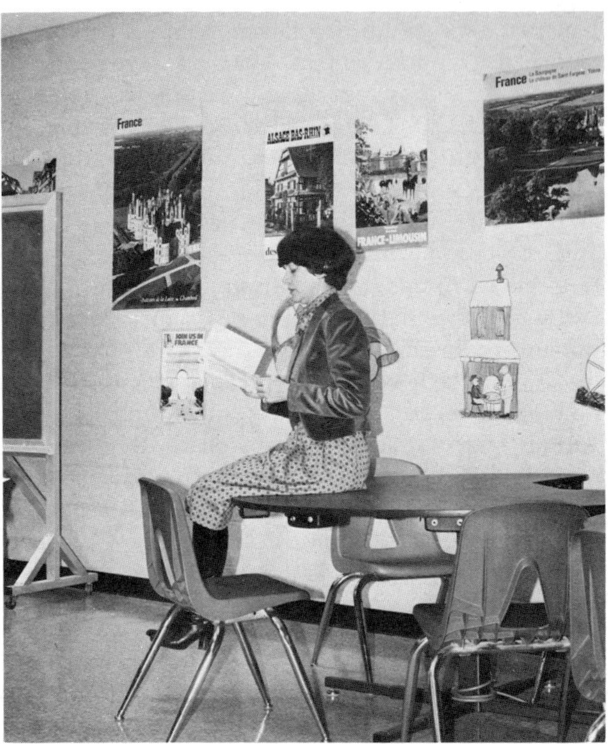

Figure 1.7
The maternity nurse is a member of a health care profession, but the nurse is also an individual with unique personal characteristics.

The Health Care Delivery System

Health care in the United States can be viewed from two perspectives. First, medical care has as its primary focus the care of people who are sick in order to restore them to a healthy state. Second, there is the broader concept of health care in which the concern is with promoting and maintaining health as well as restoring it. Medical and health care are often used synonymously, and the *health care delivery system* is used to refer to both curative and preventive aspects of health care. Consumers of *reproductive health care* services fall into both categories since normal pregnancy and childbirth are not illness states, yet a significant number of consumers are at *reproductive risk* because of disease or disorder that requires diagnostic and therapeutic services (Fig. 1.8).

The health care delivery system is composed of several parts.

- ▲ Private and public institutions such as hospitals, which are the most easily recognized or visible component of the system. Hospitals are also the most costly unit of the health care delivery system, and they are the single largest employer of nurses. Most pregnant women deliver their babies in a hospital setting.
- ▲ Most ambulatory services are provided on an outpatient basis, although some are associated with hospitals and include service settings such as public health agencies and clinics, private clinics, and individual and group practice by health professionals, the majority of whom are physicians.
- ▲ Support services such as laboratory, radiology, and pharmacy may either be a part of a hospital or community based.
- ▲ Third-party payers are national and state government programs and private insurance companies.

Characteristics of the health care delivery system include:

- ▲ ***Size.*** The system is large and getting larger.

> *Since the beginning of the Industrial Revolution there has been a tremendous increase in the mass of knowledge (science) and in the development of new products and methods (technology). These changes have resulted in the most expensive medical tradition —and with the possible exception of Sweden, the most advanced medical technology in the world.*
> *Oatman, 1978, p. 23*

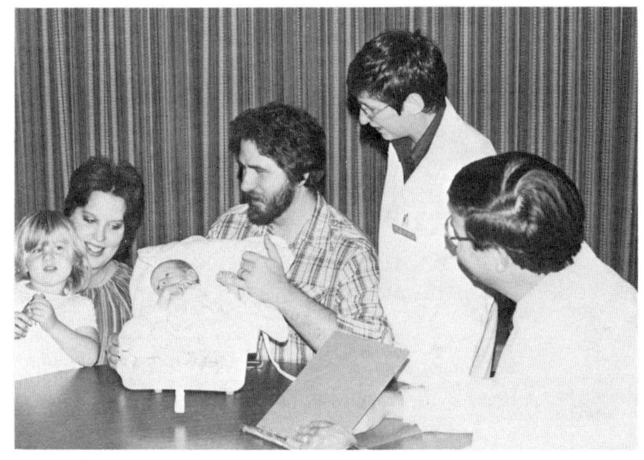

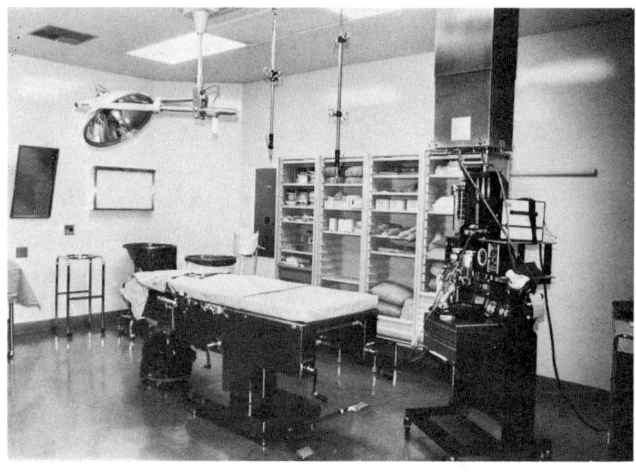

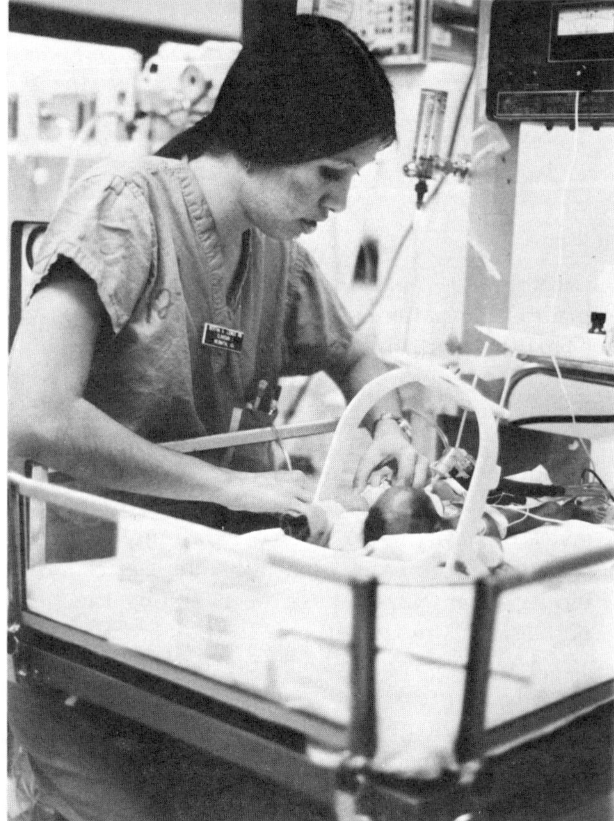

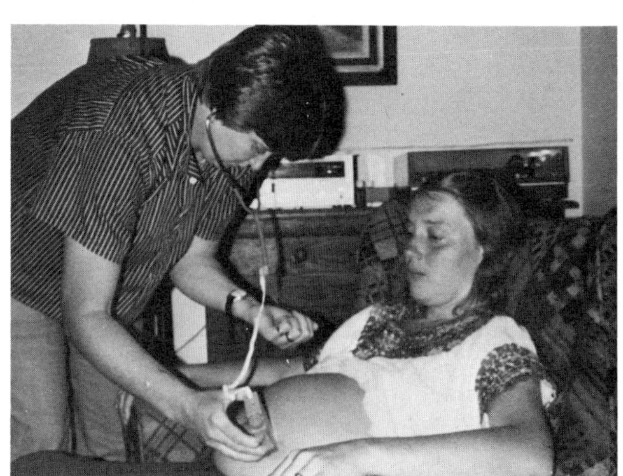

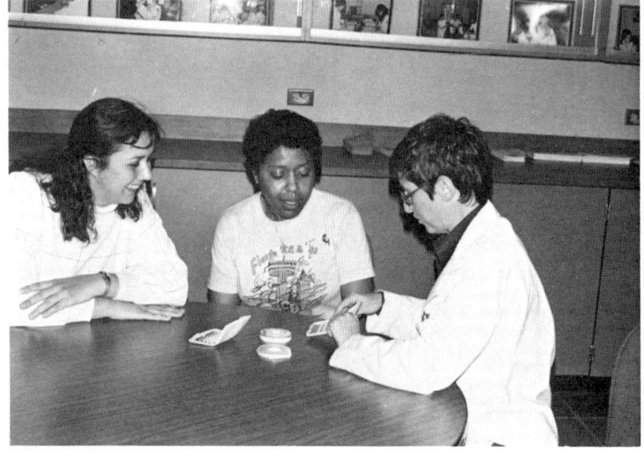

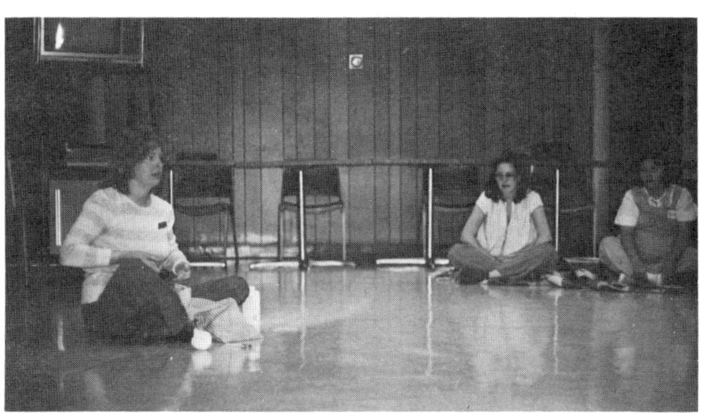

Figure 1.8
Maternity nurses may practice their specialty in a variety of settings.

The United States however, has consistently lagged behind the other developed countries of the industrialized Western world, as evidenced by the major health indices such as mortality and morbidity statistics. Maternal–child health, particularly, has failed to keep pace with other countries in regard to fetal and neonatal mortality reports.

- ▲ ***Cost.*** Health care in the United States is expensive; the average cost per person (regardless of sex) per year was $564 in 1975 and more than double that figure in 1980. The United States government spends 12 cents of every tax dollar for health care programs such as Medicaid and Medicare. Private insurance rates have been soaring over the past 20 years. Only recently have individual private insurance companies provided any semblance of comprehensive care for maternity cases (pregnancy has been considered predictable and therefore not covered). The federal government provides little assistance to the middle-income family and inadequate assistance to the indigent population in spite of federal programs that underwrite some of the costs associated with the birth of an infant.
- ▲ ***Location of Services.*** Health care services are available, but they are not distributed evenly either in regard to the number of services or the quality of those services. Medical centers tend to be located in large, urban areas leaving the suburban and rural areas with services of a more limited scope. In spite of the availability of medical center services, the citizens of the inner city with their rural counterparts often have to make do with lesser quality health care. Further, high-quality health care may not be available even when a citizen can afford it.
- ▲ ***Personnel.*** Personnel, like services, are unevenly distributed throughout the United States, again with the inner cities and the rural areas hurting the most. There is a greater shortage of nursing personnel in the slum areas and the more remote rural areas. Nationally, there is a functional, if not literal, shortage of professional nurses. This is seen in maternity nursing as in nursing generally, leaving much of the health care for expectant families in the hands of lesser prepared personnel such as vocational nurses and trained attendants.
- ▲ ***Quality of Care.*** Diagnostic and curative health care services, when they are available, are superior in the United States in comparison to most other Western countries. Even available services, however, are too often depersonalized with too much attention to the task and too little attention to the person.

> *I worked in one antepartum service which was the epitome of depersonalization. First . . . everyone had to sit on benches. There was one toilet, and personnel used that. Patients didn't have one of their own; they had to use the same one. And there were no restrooms for their husbands at all. When you look at these factors, you can see an awful lot about how the patient's feeling of being an individual is reduced. The patients in this service for pregnant women were crowded and herded and called by numbers, not names.*
>
> *Rubin, 1976, p. 149*

Rubin goes on to describe changes that were made. One patient's response to the changes was: "This is beautiful. It's as though what you're doing is really important" (Rubin, 1976, p. 149). Many health care centers have made just such changes over the past several years in efforts to improve the quality of care and to make the environment more caring. Consumer pressure and professional concern have been two of the motivators for readjusting the focus of health care, especially maternity care. Nurses have been among the health professionals most sensitive to the need for change and have been actively involved in consumer efforts to improve the quality of health care and make it more personalized and humane. Alternatives to routine hospital care are available today through *birthing centers* outside of the hospitals and *birthing rooms* or units attached to or within the hospitals (see Chapter 28). Most of the care for healthy pregnant families is still provided through the community hospital and the physician in private practice in the towns and communities.

- ▲ ***Focus of Care.*** Reproductive health care today, like health care generally, is essentially diagnostic and curative rather than preventive of disease and disorder. Much obstetric care, however, is designed to promote healthy reproductive outcomes through early and sustained prenatal supervision and careful medical and nursing management during the labor and recovery periods. Large medical centers—often where the more specialized physicians practice and the better educated nurses work—still tend to operate as centers for the management of the consumer at reproductive risk. Such a focus of care is not inappropriate, but it is often inadequate for the health care needs of the consumer, both in scope and quality. Increasingly, nurses are assuming greater responsibility for the care of the healthy expectant families. Further, nurses are the principal health educators among health professionals providing care to expectant families.

The health care delivery system is paradoxical in nature. Theoretically, it has the scientific capability for providing high-quality health care for all citizens, yet there are gaps and inequities. Realistically, there are many issues that derive from the system. Some of these issues, along with issues arising from the consumer and the nursing profession, are discussed in Chapter 3. Whatever the environment or the issue, nurses work within the framework that is the health care delivery system, in fact, they comprise the single largest group of health personnel providing care to the consumer today.

EVOLUTION OF MATERNITY NURSING

Contemporary maternity nursing, as it is conceptualized here, did not just occur. Rather, it evolved over a period of years in response to social forces and events that have influenced the nation itself and the provision of health care in the United States, particularly, maternal–child health care. The forces and events predated the early settlement of the United States and reflected the approaches to health care practiced in England and Europe that relied upon the limited understanding of both the world and the human body from the post-Renaissance period. The health care that people practiced in the new country was a combination of the medicine from their homelands and native American folk practices, both of which were heavily influenced by religious beliefs and spiritualism. The goal of health care during this period was the prevention of illness in order to ensure survival. However, the knowledge and techniques needed to accomplish this goal were far less sophisticated than those seen today, and therapeutic medicine was almost nonexistent by today's standards. Maternal and infant mortality was high, and much of obstetric care was in the hands of uneducated *midwives,* the women of the community, or both.

The early exploration of the United States, followed by the arrival of many different racial and ethnic groups and their settlement of the country, the expansion of the new nation from coast to coast, and the classical liberal ideology that became the American creed during the early agrarian society—with its decentralized government, value of individualism, and right to self-choice and equality—did much to set the stage for the beliefs, values, and attitudes that are seen today as part of the contemporary health care scene. The rise of industrialization in the late nineteenth century laid the groundwork for the technological revolution from which health care draws much of its methodology and knowledge and led to a higher standard of living for many citizens. The American middle class emerged as an economic by-product of this industrial movement, as did the reinforcement of the economic extremes of the poor and the wealthy. Industrialization further distorted the potential for pragmatic liberalism in that it provoked increased government control of industry (and eventually government control of many health care services). It also provided money for education and research that has resulted in more and improved technology that has benefitted many areas of society, including the health sciences.

The rise of special interest groups beginning in the late nineteenth and early twentieth centuries and the active political involvement of such interest groups as the American Medical Association and, more recently, the American Nurses' Association; the Great Depression and its social welfare programs of which the Social Security Act of 1935 and subsequent amendments provided the basis for governmental intervention into what had been free enterprise health care; the two great wars, both of which have had a major influence on the development and expansion of technology, which benefitted the health sciences; the post-World War II era of consumerism with the augmentation of consumer demands about health care services and costs (e.g., the parent education movement); and the space program with its sophisticated technology that provided new and better diagnostic and therapeutic modalities for use by health professionals (electronic monitoring, sonography, and others) have all further influenced the way in which health care is conceptualized and practiced in the United States. The women's rights movement has had a particular impact on the status of women and the issues affecting the health care of women and children. Since the preponderance of nurses are women, this movement has also influenced the practice of professional nurses, including their role and status.

Specific events that are of relevance or importance to maternity nursing and maternal–child health care are included here. Some of these events are discussed; others are listed in Table 1.1, where their significance is briefly noted.

Attitudes and practices concerning women's position in society and health care for pregnant women and their offspring at any given time in history have reflected the values and beliefs prevalent during that era. Two themes thread throughout the ages, however. Women have been valued and revered for their sexual and procreative functions. They have also been feared, avoided or isolated, and viewed as unclean during the periods of menstruation and recovery from childbirth, all because of this same procreative function. Further, they have challenged the ingenuity of physicians throughout time, physicians who, for the most part, avoided the study of obstetric-related problems for fear of scorn by their peers. Health care during pregnancy and childbirth was the responsibility of the woman herself, of other women of her household or community, or of untrained midwives. Much of what is known about pregnancy, childbirth, and health care was derived from religious writings such as the Bible and the sacred books of Eastern religions such as Hinduism.

The sixteenth and seventeenth centuries in Europe ushered into being the "modern" specialties of obstetrics and gynecology with greater numbers of physicians concerning themselves with pregnancy and childbirth, particularly those cases where there was disease or disorder. The untrained midwives continued to supervise and assist with normal pregnancy and childbirth. However, programs for the training of midwives began during this era, with the first school for midwives at Hotel Dieu, Paris. Most of this training was associated with the development of lying-in wards in Europe that were first established in the early sixteenth century for the delivery of pregnant women who were indigent or outcasts.

The nineteenth century saw the emergence of the work of Semmelweiss (1847) that was directed toward the control of puerperal infection; Pasteur (1850) that led to the process of pasteurization of milk; Simpson (1853) who first used chloroform for relief of pain during labor and surgery; and Credé (1884) who pioneered Credé's method and the use of a 2% solution of silver nitrate for the prevention of *ophthalmia neonatorum,* the gonorrheal infection of the newborn's eyes that results in blindness.

Increased attention to the health of pregnant women during the sixteenth through the nineteenth centuries did not erase the attitude that the woman was expendable; the child, rather than the mother, was to continue for years to be the celebrant. As the status of women began to change for the better, attitudes and obstetric practices tended to change also.

During the early colonization of North America there were few women among the intrepid explorers and, hence, few instances of pregnancy and childbirth. The only cases were among the few settlers and the natives, about which there is little recorded. The first recorded birth of a child born to English settlers in the New World was Virginia Dare in 1587 at Roanoke, Virginia. History does not reveal the nature of her mother's prenatal care, labor, and delivery. Likewise, little is known about the childbearing practices of the native Indians.

The young United States was an agrarian society with large, intact family units settled along the eastern seaboard. Childbirth took place in the home with the women of the family or the neighborhood helping each other. Occasionally, the physician—if there was one available—attended a complicated birth. Each child born was a highly valued addition to the sparse work force that was needed to clear and till the lands and harvest the crops.

During the eighteenth and nineteenth centuries, American settlers dispersed to all corners of the United States. Women were as scarce during this period as they were in the earlier years. Repeated childbearing without the sophisticated health care that is available today shortened the lives of these pioneer women. The major killers then, as now, were hemorrhage and infection. As the country matured, so did obstetric care. The middle of the nineteenth century began the period of industrialization in the United States. Families began to congregate around urban centers. Hospitals were built,

TABLE 1.1
HISTORICAL BASIS FOR MATERNITY NURSING

Year/Place	*Event*	*Significance*
Circa 1550 B.C. (Egypt)	Recording of Eber's *Papyrus.*	Provided the first record of medical interest about and concern with women's conditions and diseases. Described practices regarding women's diseases, menstruation, labor, abortion.
Circa A.D. 2 (Rome)	Writings of Soranus (Greek physician) on obstetrics. Two writings in particular: *On the Obstetric Art* and *Acute and Chronic Diseases.*	First record of a physician specializing in obstetrics and gynecology. Description of practices during that historical period.
1500s (France)	First lying-in wards were opened in hospitals in Europe.	These were places established for the delivery of the indigent and outcast women, particularly those with diseases or disorders.
1514–1564 (Belgium)	André Vesalius, anatomist and physician, wrote *Seven Books on the Structure of the Human Body.*	Comprehensive study of the anatomy of the human body. First major text in anatomy.
1560–1631 (England)	Peter Chamberlen, inventor of the obstetric forceps.	Introduced the idea of instrumentation in obstetrics. Precurser to modern obstetric forceps.
1578–1657 (England)	William Harvey, physician who discovered the circulation of blood.	Led to the study of circulation in the human. He also developed the science of embryology. A supporter and innovator in midwifery education.
1637–1709 (France)	Francois Mauriceau, French obstetrician.	Contributed important information about the practice of obstetrics. Introduced delivery in bed, mechanism for breech extraction. Described the contagious nature of puerperal infection. Introduced suturing of lacerations as a result of birth trauma.
1651–1724 (Holland)	Hendrik van Deventer, Dutch physician who studied the pelvis and wrote on midwifery.	Described the relationship among the pelvic morphology, position, and birth.
1697–1793 (England)	William Smellie, physician.	Described the mechanisms of labor.
1762 (United States)	William Shippen. Established first co-educational midwifery school in the United States in Philadelphia.	Set the stage for the practice of obstetrics by men in the United States.
1819–1892 (Germany)	Karl Sigmund Credé, German gynecologist. Wrote *The Prophylactic Treatment of Ophthalmia Neonatorum.*	Developed a method of placental expression known today as the Credé's method. Advocated the use of a 2% solution of silver nitrate in the eyes of newborn infants to prevent ophthalmia neonatorum.

TABLE 1.1 (continued)

Year/Place	*Event*	*Significance*
1820–1910 (England)	Florence Nightingale, pioneer in professional nursing.	Advocated and practiced the tenets that are the basis for professional nursing practice.
1843 (United States)	Oliver Wendell Holmes, physician. Advocated the use of aseptic technic in obstetrics.	This later became accepted as a standard for widespread use in medical practice.
1847 (Hungary)	Semmelweis, 1818–1865. First introduced handwashing in chloride of lime before examining women in labor.	Provided a mechanism for decreasing puerperal infection.
1853 (England)	Introduction of use of chloroform anesthesia in obstetrics by Dr. Jonas Y. Simpson (1811–1870).	Introduced relief of pain during childbirth and aid during delivery.
1860s (United States)	Establishment of local societies of obstetrics and gynecology.	Organized improved medical care for pregnant women, primarily to prevent maternal mortality. Led to the establishment of The American College of Obstetrics and Gynecology, a national organization with state and local bodies.
1869 (United States)	State board of health was established in Massachusetts.	Primarily for control of communicable disease. There is a state board of health in all 50 states.
1893 (United States)	Establishment of infant milk depots in New York City.	Helped to meet the nutritional needs of infants. No longer in existence, although other types of federal and state food subsidies are available.
1897 (United States)	In Minnesota, first appropriation by a state for care of handicapped children.	Provided assistance to families with handicapped children. Federal and state funds are provided for this and many other services to both the families and the children.
1900 (United States)	Introduction of the concept of "prenatal care" and the development of prenatal clinics in the United States by physicians concerned with obstetric care.	An effort to decrease complications of pregnancy and birth through early supervision and teaching, as well as by early assessment and detection of problems.
1901 (United States)	Affiliation by the Instructive District Nursing Association of Boston with the South End Branch of Boston Lying-In Hospital.	Used nurses to provide prenatal instruction, as well as to do assessment and detection and to report problem cases to physicians. Nurses are still providing a large part of the prenatal instruction in the United States today.
1903 (United States)	First full-time school nurse (Lina S. Rogers) from the Henry Street Visiting Nurse Service was assigned to the New York City Health Department.	Provided a mechanism to teach parents and children about prevention of illness and malnutrition. To do health screening and case finding, as well.

Year/Place	*Event*	*Significance*
1906 (United States)	Introduction of a bill in the United States Congress to establish the Children's Bureau.	Effort to provide study for the cause and prevention of infant mortality. Bill failed to pass in Congress.
1907 (United States)	Association for improving the conditions of the poor in New York City employed two nurse-teachers.	Visited pregnant women in families receiving care from this association and provided prenatal care and teaching. Formalized the involvement of nurses in prenatal care.
1909 (United States)	Establishment of the American Society for the Study and Prevention of Infant Mortality.	Organized the study of causes and extent of infant mortality. Functions have been absorbed by other organizations, both federal and professional, as well as at state and local levels.
1909 (United States)	First White House Conference called by President Theodore Roosevelt.	National effort to identify and discuss the problems and care of dependent children. Still being held every 10 years.
1912 (United States)	Children's Bureau established.	"To investigate and report on all matters affecting children and child life." Charter of the Children's Bureau.
1914 (United States)	Publication of the first edition of *Infant Care—Care of Children by the Children's Bureau.*	First federal effort to educate parents through inexpensive publication.
1915 (United States)	First Birth Registration Office established.	Promoted completeness and accuracy of data concerning birth. Functions absorbed by the Bureau of Vital Statistics on the national level; state and local departments also exist to collect this information
1917 (United States)	Metropolitan Life Insurance Company contracted to pay the Visiting Nurse Service for two prenatal visits to maternity patients having their policy.	Effort to decrease infant and maternal mortality and morbidity, thereby decreasing cost to the insurance company for payments in these areas.
1917 (United States)	Establishment of the Women's City Club in New York City, the first maternity center, later to become Maternity Center Association.	Provided medical supervision and nursing care throughout pregnancy to four weeks postpartal. Still in existence, offering these as well as other services to pregnant families.
1917 (United States)	Visiting Nurse Service of Henry Street Settlement in New York City established the first 24-hour-delivery nursing service. This was the first complete maternity nursing service to be provided.	Provided prenatal, intrapartal, and postpartal nursing for private and clinic patients. Served as a field for clinical experience for students enrolled at the Manhattan Maternity Hospital.
1921 (United States)	Congress passed the Sheppard–Towner Act, the first maternity and infancy act.	Provided funds to states to enable them to develop health services for mothers and children. Repealed in 1929, through major efforts of the American Medical Association, because of the implication of socialized medicine. The American Pediatric Society dissented.

TABLE 1.1 (continued)

Year/Place	*Event*	*Significance*
1921 (United States)	American Birth Control League was founded.	Provided information and help to families desiring birth control. To help repeal laws preventing the dissemination of such information and birth control devices.
1924 (United States)	Bill to remove prohibition against sale of contraceptives and dissemination of information about birth control introduced in Congress.	Aided in the provision of birth control information and services to those families desiring them. Bill failed to pass in Congress.
1925 (United States)	Frontier Nursing Service established by Mary Breckinridge in Kentucky. Introduced nurse-midwifery in United States.	Provided health care services to the indigent living in the remote mountain areas of Kentucky. Included in these services were home delivery, general public health nursing, maternity care, and promotion of family health.
1929 (United States)	Development of the Children's Bureau's plan for Children's Health and Welfare Programs.	Provided aid to dependent children money for maternal–child health (MCH) services; aid for child welfare services; aid to states for MCH demonstration projects; grants to extend and strengthen child welfare services. Became the basis for the child health and welfare sections of the Social Security Act and later amendments to the Social Security Act.
1930 (United States)	Publication of the Children's Charter out of a White House Conference on Child Health and Protection.	Identified specific rights of children in terms of health care and protection. Exists today and has given direction to the development of programs to guarantee these rights.
1932 (United States)	Establishment of the Lobenstein Midwifery Clinic by the Association for the Promotion and Standardization of Mid-wifery.	Provided comprehensive health care to pregnant families by nurse-midwives. In 1935, it became part of the Maternity Center Association in New York City and took on the responsibility for the training and education of nurse-midwives, as well as patient care.
1933 (United States)	Publication of *Natural Childbirth* by Dr. Grantly Dick Read, an English obstetrician. In 1944, this same idea was presented in another volume, *Childbirth Without Fear,* published in the United States and aimed at the consumer rather than the professional.	Effort to convince physicians providing care to pregnant women that childbirth was a natural phenomenon and should be treated as such and that pain in labor was the result of tension resulting from fear. To present this concept to consumers to provide them with a better understanding of their childbirth. Widespread controversy among the medical profession with subsequent impact on the change in attitude among professionals about the management and preparation of pregnant families. Became the foundation for the early childbirth preparation programs.

Year/Place	Event	Significance
1934 (United States)	Publication of the *Complete Study on Maternal Mortality in Fifteen States,* by the Children's Bureau.	Informed and reported the situation concerning the extent and cause of maternal mortality in the United States. Many states followed this study with efforts to study the problem as it existed at the state level. Programs of concerted efforts to decrease maternal mortality grew out of this study.
1939 (United States)	Establishment of a school for nurse-midwives at Frontier Nursing Service in Kentucky.	Provided education and training of nurse-midwives to improve delivery of health care to a rural population in order to promote health and decrease maternal and infant mortality and morbidity. Made an impact on the health care of the women and children in this area. Along with the Maternity Center Association in New York City, laid the foundation for acceptance of nurse-midwifery.
1941 (United States)	Mothers' charter adopted by the American Committee for Maternal Welfare.	Corollary to the Children's Charter to specify rights each mother has to quality health care. Exists today and has influenced the development of programs to guarantee these rights.
1942 (United States)	Cornelion Corner organized in Detroit. This was an effort by a group of psychiatrists, a pediatrician, an obstetrician, and a nurse plus allied health care workers.	Promoted research in child development and family life. Education for child development and family life. Promotion of demand feeding in infants. Stimulated interest by the professionals and consumers in these areas. Contributions to knowledge in the areas of child development and family life.
1943 (United States)	Introduction of the concept of rooming-in by Dr. Arnold Gesell and Dr. Frances Ilg in their book, *Infant and Child in the Culture of Today.*	Promoted maternal–infant relationships. Parent teaching regarding parenting and care giving. Influenced attitudes and actions concerning approaches to hospital care of mothers and infants following delivery. Laid the foundations for the movement toward rooming-in units in hospitals.
1954 (United States)	American Academy of Pediatrics published *Standards and Recommendations for Hospital Care of Newborn Infants—Full Term and Premature.*	Provided guidelines for hospitals and staff to provide care to newborn infants. Standards for evaluating care were intended to ensure basic kinds of care for all infants and to upgrade existing care services.
1955 (United States)	Establishment of the American College of Nurse-Midwifery.	Promoted the organization of nurses prepared in nurse-midwifery. Established guidelines and standards for the practice of nurse-midwifery. Promoted the practice of nurse-midwifery.

TABLE 1.1 (continued)

Year/Place	*Event*	*Significance*
1956 (United States)	Establishment of La Leche League by consumers.	Promoted breast-feeding as a natural and preferred way of feeding a newborn infant. Supported and encouraged parents. Educated parents about breast-feeding. This organization has served a large number of parents wishing to breast-feed their infants. Consultant services have been offered to both consumers and professionals. Publication of materials such as the *Womanly Art of Breast Feeding.* Increased consumer and professional awareness of breast-feeding as a natural way of feeding an infant.
1960 (United States)	Introduction in the United States of the LaMaze method of preparation for childbirth by Dr. Clement Yahia. This method was first introduced in France by Dr. Fernand LaMaze in 1951.	Promoted preparation for the childbirth experience through the use of education and physical preparation, which coordinated the mind and the body in order to function efficiently during labor, thereby increasing individual control of labor and reducing discomfort.
1960 (United States)	Establishment of local preparation for childbirth groups in the United States, mostly through the efforts of lay couples. Out of this effort grew the International Childbirth Education Association (ICEA).	Promoted preparation for childbirth through the offering of consumer-planned and taught courses using primarily the concepts by Dr. LaMaze. Helped facilitate the nationwide organization of such courses and programs. Increased consumer involvement in preparation for childbirth efforts. Increased the options for preparation for child birth programs available to the consumer.
1960 (United States)	Establishment of the American Society for Psychoprophylaxis in Obstetrics (ASPO) through the efforts of physicians, nurses, physiotherapists, and parents.	Promoted professional interest and responsibility for preparation for childbirth education, using the concepts introduced by Dr. LaMaze to better prepare the consumer for the experience of childbirth in as natural a sense as possible. Helped facilitate the nationwide organization of such courses and programs. Increased the options for preparation for childbirth programs available to the consumer.
1961 (United States)	Establishment of the National Institute of Child Health and Human Development.	Provided a national center for basic research in child health and human development. Has conducted research in the areas of child health and human development. The center has organized and held conferences on issues related to health care for mothers and children.

Year/Place	*Event*	*Significance*
1963 (United States)	Authorization for grants for comprehensive maternity and infant care projects.	Provided monies to large and middle-sized cities to help provide adequate health care to mothers and infants at risk. In 1975, there were 56 sites in operation in 34 states, the District of Columbia, and Puerto Rico.
1965 (United States)	Amendments to the Social Security Act for the provision of comprehensive health care for children and youth. Section 509, Title V, Social Security Act.	Provided comprehensive health care services to children and youth from low-income families. In 1971, there were 65 projects in operation, providing care to 335,000 children and youth annually.
1967 (United States)	Reorganization of the Department of Health, Education and Welfare with dismemberment of the Children's Bureau, by executive order.	Intended to provide more efficient administration of programs by separating health and welfare and placing them under departments or agencies handling concerns specific to each of these areas.
1969 (United States)	Establishment of an Office of Child Development by executive order.	Assumed responsibility for functions of the Children's Bureau delineated in the Act of 1912 and not delegated to education or welfare in the reorganization of the Department of Health, Education and Welfare in 1967.
1969 (United States)	Establishment of the Nurses Association of the American College of Obstetricians and Gynecologists (NAACOG).	"To promote highest standards of obstetric and gynecologic and neonatal nursing practice and education. Cooperation with qualified physicians and nurses. Stimulation of interest in Obstetric, Gynecologic and Neonatal Nursing." Charter of NAACOG. Conferences planned jointly by nurses and physicians have been held, presenting current topics and issues. Development and administration of certification procedures for nursing in the area of obstetric, gynecologic, and neonatal nursing. Publication of a journal dealing with subjects relevant to obstetric, gynecologic, and neonatal nursing practice, the *Journal of Obstetric, Gynecological, Neonatal Nursing.*
1971 (United States)	Adoption of a statement by the American Medical Association supporting centralized community or regional perinatal intensive care centers.	Directed attention to the development and operation of centralized special care facilities. Supported increased efforts toward early assessment, detection and treatment of risk pregnancy. Promoted an interdisciplinary approach to perinatal health care. Position endorsed by the Committee on Fetus and Newborn and the Executive Board of the American Academy of Pediatrics. Endorsed by the Executive Board of the American College of

TABLE 1.1 (continued)

Year/Place	***Event***	***Significance***
		Obstetrics and Gynecology in principle. Centers have been developed and are operating in some parts of the country. Efforts to establish more centers are underway in other parts of the country.
1972 (United States)	Twenty-seventh Amendment to the Constitution proposed March 22, 1972.	"Equality of rights under the law shall not be abridged by the United States or by any state on account of sex." Amendment failed in 1982.
1973 (United States)	Publication of *Standards for Maternal–Child Health Practice* by the Division of Maternal–Child Health Nursing of the American Nurses' Association.	Provided standards and guidelines for improving the practice of maternal–child health nursing, the education of the professional nurse, evaluation of nursing practice and patient care.
1973 (United States)	The Supreme Court of the United States ruled as unconstitutional all laws prohibiting or restricting a woman's right to obtain an abortion during the first 90 days of pregnancy.	Gave women the right to have greater control over their own reproductive destiny. Intended to decrease maternal casualty from the increasing use of illegal abortion facilities.
1974 (United States)	Congress passed the National Planning and Resources Development Act (PL 93-641).	Proposed restructure of the health services delivery system in the United States in order to meet national health priorities. Shifted the focus of health care programs from categorical to community–family health.
1974 (United States)	Publication of *Obstetric, Gynecologic and Neonatal Nursing Functions and Standards* by NAACOG.	Established guidelines for gynecologic and neonatal nursing policies and procedures and appropriate functions in order to provide standards to facilitate quality nursing care.
1978 (United States)	United States Congress passed the Hyde Amendment that addressed the use of federal funds to pay for abortion.	Established three conditions under which abortion will be paid for by the federal government for women receiving Medicaid. (1) Continuation of the pregnancy will endanger the life of the woman. (2) Agreement by two physicians that continuation of the pregnancy will cause severe or extensive damage to the physical well-being of the woman. (3) Confirmation that the pregnancy was due to rape or incest and that it was reported to an official agency.
1979 (United States)	United States Supreme Court overturned a Massachusetts abortion law that required	Established the right of a minor who is pregnant to have a voice in decisions

Year/Place	Event	Significance
	judicial approval for an abortion to be performed on a girl who was under 18 years of age when her parents did not give consent for the abortion.	made concerning termination of her pregnancy.
1980 (United States)	United States Supreme Court decision upholding the constitutionality of the Hyde Amendment of 1978.	This decision came about in response to a class action suit filed following the passage of the 1978 Hyde Amendment. The long-range effects of this decision are not yet known. It did establish the right of Congress to set conditions on the use of federal funds for health programs provided by the federal government.

Source: Adapted from Butnarescu, G. F. *Perinatal Nursing, Volume I—Reproductive Health.* New York: John Wiley & Sons, 1978, pp. 30–38. Used with permission.

and the medical specialties of obstetrics and pediatrics were organized and gained recognition. The idea of health care during pregnancy was introduced as a way of preventing complications during delivery, and the concept of prenatal care came into being around the turn of the century through the efforts of Florence Nightingale in England and Clara Barton and others in the United States. By the turn of the century, American nurses such as Lina Rogers were undertaking the teaching of parents and children and Margaret Sanger was fighting for the right of women to control their reproductive destiny through the *birth control* movement. Nurses began to be viewed as interested, informed, and capable of speaking for the needs of expectant and young parents—a trend that continues to the present. It is quite likely that these nurses were successful for a variety of reasons, of which concern and persistence were uppermost.

As the twentieth century matured, nurses, along with others, continued to be a force in the movement toward better health care for pregnant women and their children. The first half of the twentieth century saw the establishment of the American Birth Control League, the Frontier Nursing Service in Kentucky, and the Lobenstein Midwifery Clinic in New York City. Parent education gained momentum through written publications from the Children's Bureau and the Visiting Nurse Service of Henry Street Settlement in New York City, which set the example for nurse-provided health care during pregnancy. Physicians, who have always been in the forefront of efforts for improved maternal–child health, came forth with concepts like *rooming-in* and natural childbirth.

The second half of the twentieth century has witnessed the establishment of standards for care in hospital nurseries and for nursing practice. The Social Security Act has been amended to provide for maternal–child health services through programs such as Medicaid and Maternity and Infant Care Projects. Specific organizations reflecting specialized practice groups in maternity nursing, such as the American College of Nurse-Midwifery, Maternal–Child Nursing Section of the American Nurses' Association, and the Nurses Association of the American College of Obstetricians and Gynecologists have been created. Elective abortion has been legalized by the Supreme Court but has since been placed in an equivocal position regarding the use of federal money for such procedures.

The list of events and efforts that have led to maternity nursing as it is envisioned and often practiced today is extensive. Nurses should take pride in their contributions toward the improvement of health care for pregnant women and newborn infants and for their recognition of the family as a part of this reproductive experience. They must also carefully examine the problems and issues arising from and surrounding this category of health care and nursing practice and anticipate the directions in which such care and practice must go to keep abreast of a burgeoning technology and changing needs of the consumer, the nurse, and the system.

SUMMARY

Contemporary maternity nursing was discussed as a specialized area of practice within the broad scope of professional nursing. The concern of maternity nursing is the health care of women and their families, whose needs emanate from events associated with human reproduction. Its primary focus is the care of the pregnant woman and her unborn infant.

Maternity nursing uses an extensive knowledge base that is drawn from the social, biologic, and health sciences. Its practice base comes from nursing, as well as from the medical specialty of obstetrics and gynecology.

The scope of maternity nursing includes the consumer, who comes from all social and economic strata and who represents all developmental stages within the reproductive years; the nurse, who is an individual person, as well as a professional who presents in a variety of roles and practices in institutional and community settings; and the health care delivery system, which is described in terms of its composition and characteristics.

The chapter closed with a discussion of the evolution of maternity nursing as a result of the forces that have molded maternal–child health care in the United States. People and historical events that have influenced both maternity nursing and maternal–child health care were discussed or cited.

REFERENCES AND READINGS

Oatman, E. F. (Ed.). *Medical Care in the United States.* New York: H. W. Wilson, 1978.

Rubin, R. Stop and Think . . . What Are We Doing? *Am J MCN* 1(3):146, 1976.

Weidenbach, E. *Family-Centered Maternity Nursing.* New York: G. P. Putnam's Sons, 1967.

2

THE ROLES OF THE TEACHER AND LEARNER IN MATERNITY NURSING

Teaching is the art of helping a person acquire new knowledge and skills. Teaching involves planning materials and content, providing feedback, and making an evaluation. *Learning* is a change in behavior as a result of teaching. Actually, teaching and learning cannot be separated since teachers and learners teach and learn from each other simultaneously. Teaching and learning are discussed separately to explore the processes and to assist you in becoming better teachers and more satisfied learners. This chapter discusses the teaching–learning process, including the roles of the teacher and the learner, beliefs about learning, the domains of learning, behavioral objectives, and the relationship of the teaching–learning process to the nursing process.

Each unit of this text has a list of outcomes for you, the learner, as well as tools for evaluation. This chapter provides a foundation for the rest of the text, as well as for the practice of professional nursing.

THE TEACHING–LEARNING PROCESS

The teaching–learning process encompasses other processes that you will encounter in nursing, for example, problem solving and communication. Moreover, patient teaching is a basic nursing skill and is an essential part of the professional nursing role. In order to teach, you must understand how learning takes place. If it were known exactly how each person learned or if everyone learned in the same way, teaching would be quick, simple, and efficient. The fact is that each of us learns in many ways and, perhaps, more efficiently in one way than another. For example, some of us prefer lectures, others independent study; some of us learn by watching, others by doing; some by reading, others by listening. We also know that learning does not take place only in the formal classroom but occurs in many settings and is a lifelong process.

In the past the teaching–learning process focused on teaching, that is, on how content and materials were presented to students, not on outcomes. Then along came the focus on accountability: schools became accountable to consumers and administrators, and teachers became accountable to students. The focus shifted to learning outcomes, which led to learning objectives or outcomes that are clearly stated and measurable—behavioral objectives. Much of education today is based on teaching by objectives, a process that can ultimately measure the behavioral changes that have occurred in the learner. The basic premise of the teaching–learning process, however, is that each learner is unique and each learning situation is different. Successful teaching depends on applying appropriate principles of learning to a specific situation.

ROLE OF THE TEACHER

The role of the teacher is to help people learn, and this chapter focuses on the deliberate efforts of a *person* to assist learning. It is well documented that people learn via media, films, videotapes, textbooks, and computers, but the *person* who teaches, that is, assists the learner in acquiring new knowledge and skills, is most often a key factor. Teaching does not have to involve a long period of time or a complex skill. It is done in response to a need for knowledge and may require a lengthy lecture or a brief response.

It is our basic premise that teaching is a part of the care of every client and, therefore, a nurse's responsibility. It is also true that the teaching and learning roles of a person are constantly shifting and intertwining throughout life. It is possible, therefore, that you may be the learner at one point in your professional career and the teacher at another point.

The role of the teacher includes many important characteristics, such as knowledge, motivation, optimism, interpersonal and communication skills, and a sense of humor. The teacher must have knowledge and skill related to the subject matter and a positive attitude toward the subject and the learner. An effective teacher must be motivated to teach and realizes that the reward is seeing students learn and achieve. The demonstration of new knowledge seen by behavioral changes in the learner is the measure of success. For example, the learner can say, "I understand" or "I know," but until the knowledge is demonstrated behaviorally, the evaluation cannot take place. Johnny says, "I know how to throw the ball overhand," but when you see Johnny throw the ball, you can evaluate his learning.

The role of the teacher requires remembering that people, *not* classes, are taught. Individual learners differ in their speed, attitude, and interest; the challenge for the teacher is to reach the *person.* The teacher's success requires both interpersonal and communication skills. Methods for teaching are the teacher's responsibility and are part of the plan. Whether it is large or small group discussions, lecture, role playing, or demonstration, the teacher selects those methods that will be effective for the learner. Success for the teacher is not a straight line but is very uneven, characterized by peaks and valleys, and an appropriate sense of humor can frequently keep learning on a more direct road. When small disasters occur, the skilled teacher with a sense of humor can often salvage the situation so that learning can continue (Fig. 2.1). Humor carried to extreme, however, can become sarcastic or abrasive. In summary, a good teacher needs to be intelligent, sincere, knowledgeable, and a good communicator; needs a sense of humor; and needs to be able to see and accept people as they are.

ROLE OF THE LEARNER

The role of the learner is that of an active participant or shared partner, each of which reflects the truism that learning is a two-way communication process. Ideally, the learning goal is mutually determined by the teacher and the learner, but in some cases in education and in patient teaching the goal—the thing that is to be learned—is defined solely by the teacher. For example, as a nursing teacher, I *know* you must learn to take a blood pressure accurately. As a nurse, you *know* that the new diabetic needs to learn how to administer his or her insulin. These are teacher-determined goals, but many other goals will be mutually determined by teacher and learner. For example, if you, the learner, are to visit the home of a mother and new infant in order to help with the baby's bath, you will most likely select the strategies for teaching with the assistance of your teacher.

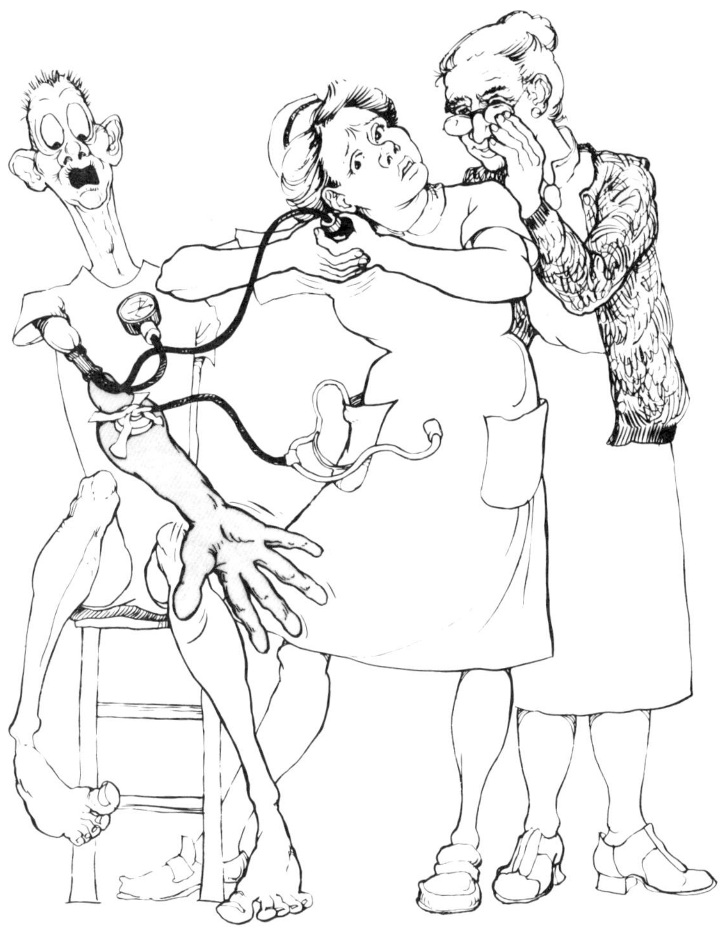

Figure 2.1
The teacher supports, encourages, and corrects; both student and client *do* survive learning.

The learner is responsible for achieving the behavioral or learning objective. If the learner is unsuccessful, the teacher is responsible for investigating what factors are inhibiting learning and for facilitating successful achievement of the learning objective. In summary, the learner is the achiever; the teacher is the facilitator and evaluator.

Characteristics of the Learner

Characteristics of the learner in maternity nursing today are as varied as the people in the nursing profession. The age range of students in nursing programs is from 21 to 60. Academic backgrounds of students vary from high school graduates to those with doctorates in other fields. As with adult learners in other fields, people choosing a career later in life or choosing a second career are, in general, highly motivated. It is true that you need to like people and be empathetic to be a nurse, but other characteristics, including intelligence, understanding, and diligence, also make for success.

LEARNING BELIEFS AND PRINCIPLES

There are some generally accepted beliefs and characteristics of learning, sometimes referred to as *principles of learning,* which are important to the practice of nursing.

Perception Is Necessary for Learning

Perception, which is necessary for learning to occur, can be analyzed in three steps: (1) Sense organs receive a message, (2) the afferent nervous system transfers the impulse to a sensory area in the brain, and (3) the brain interprets—sight, sound, taste, smell—and sends the message back. This principle of learning has many applications to nursing. For example, it is known that hearing ability decreases as age increases. If you were involved in health teaching with elderly patients, it would be important to know that perception was affected.

It is also generally believed that if the learner perceives the new information to be significant or relevant, learning is more likely to occur.

Conditioned Response Is a Method of Learning

The term *conditioned response* is best remembered from Pavlov's experiments with dogs. An example in nursing is an ill child who has had an uncomfortable procedure done by a doctor in a white coat who then begins to cry as soon as he sees someone in white. There are many examples of learning by conditioned response in life: answering the phone, stopping at a red light, or putting on a sweater when you are cold, are a few.

Trial and Error Promotes Learning

Trial and error is a self-explanatory mode of learning; riding a bicycle is a classic example. In health care, teaching done by repeated demonstrations often reflects this learning principle.

Imitation Is Basic to Learning

Learning frequently occurs by *imitation;* for example, the child who copies her mother or father in eating, dressing, or combing her hair. In nursing, by practicing good health habits, such as handwashing, patients will learn by imitation.

Conceptualization Enhances Learning

Concept formation is an extremely useful principle of learning. When you conceptualize, you have a general notion or idea about something, you are able to understand similarities, differences, and relationships, you have a mental picture of the concept. An example is the word "dog." The word "dog" conjures up four legs, a tail, ears, a bark, and, depending on your particular experience, may lead you to a specific mental picture such as a Doberman pinscher or a collie. The point is you have a concept of dog or what "dogness" is. Many words are concepts—health, illness, joy, pain, just to name a few. The importance of conceptual learning is that it allows you to integrate and generalize information more efficiently. With the knowledge expansion of the 1970s and the 1980s, it is impossible for anyone to learn all the facts about a particular subject. But to have a concept, a meaningful idea, or a mental picture, allows you to proceed more quickly to the explicit knowledge you need. When you conceptualize, the process includes perception, verbal symbols, integration, generalization, and abstraction. To go back to the dog example, when you conceptualize "dog," you are able to conceptualize the idea without reference to any particular dog, that is, only in relation to those features that are common to all dogs.

Motivation Is Crucial for Learning

Motivation is a critical principle of learning. A person must be motivated to learn. Motivation is the drive that causes action. A simple example is when you are hungry, you eat. In health care teaching, it is sometimes necessary to motivate the client, in other words, to help the person see the need or importance for the behavior. Conversely, if the teacher sees no interest or motivation in the learner, this situation must be assessed.

Physical and Mental Readiness Are Basic to Learning

Physical and mental readiness is necessary for learning to take place. A classic example is toilet training young children. Until musculoskeletal and neurologic development have progressed to the readiness point, the infant cannot be successfully toilet trained. The teacher has the responsibility of differentiating between lack of physical or mental readiness, and lack of motivation.

Active Participation Enhances Learning

Effective learning requires *active participation.* Whether it is playing the piano or taking a blood pressure, active participation is essential. It is important to remember that much significant learning takes place through doing. Moreover, if learners have the opportunity to choose their own direction and decide their own course of action, learning is maximized. Evidence from industry as well as education demonstrates that active learning is more effective than passive learning.

New Learning Builds on Past Experience

New learning is effective when based on *previous knowledge and experience.* This is probably one of the most significant principles in adult education. The student who has given birth to a child brings different knowledge and experience to the study of maternity nursing than the one who has not. In a more general sense, nursing programs are designed to build on knowledge introduced in the first semester as the student proceeds through subsequent semesters.

Emotional Climate Affects Learning

Is the learner afraid or excited? What is going on in the family, with co-workers, or in the classroom? All of these factors may affect learning and frequently need to be assessed. Another facet of this belief is that when the threat to self is low, learning proceeds easily. For example, children learn new rules fairly easily, but if ridicule, scorn, and threats are used, it will affect the child's perception of self and learning will be more difficult.

Repetition Enhances Learning

Repetition strengthens learning and frequently leads to habit formation. Being served and eating balanced nutritious meals lead to good eating habits in most instances. Many complex interpersonal or physical skills are frequently improved by repetition.

Satisfaction Reinforces Learning

A *sense of accomplishment* promotes a sense of well-being and learning flourishes. Giving someone a task the nurse knows the person can accomplish leads to satisfaction and lays the groundwork for further learning.

Receptivity Enhances Learning

The person who is *open* to new experiences and listens attentively learns more easily. In a society such as ours where change is a way of life, those people who continue to be receptive to new experiences are lifelong learners and undoubtedly live life more fully.

The beliefs about learning just described have been taken from a variety of teaching–learning theorists. Many of these principles are not new, but focusing on them in relation to nursing and patient teaching is important. Successful teaching depends on applying the appropriate principles to a specific situation, remembering that each learner is unique and each learning situation is different.

DOMAINS OF LEARNING

Categories or domains of learning are defined as cognitive, psychomotor or affective and are classified by Benjamin Bloom in *The Taxonomy of Educational Objectives. Cognitive behaviors* involve the recall of information and range in complexity from knowledge through comprehension, application, and analysis to the highest cognitive activities of synthesis and evaluation. *Psychomotor behaviors* are those requiring neuromuscular coordination and also can range from simple to complex. The three steps in the psychomotor domain are integration, application, and acquisition. *Affective behaviors* are those that may be hidden from observation but are evident by values placed on learning or attitudes toward people or things. Often, affective behaviors are the direct result of learned cognitive or psychomotor behaviors. Beginning levels of affective behaviors involve activities such as valuing, responding, and receiving. Higher levels involve organizing and internalizing at which point the person demonstrates consistent automatic responses to situations affectively. For example, people who have internalized right and wrong in their personal value systems will reflect that in interactions with others.

Nursing skills may be either cognitive or psychomotor. A psychomotor skill involves making complex motor responses without conscious thought; a cognitive skill is complex mental responses without conscious thought. An example of the former is riding a bicycle; of the latter is doing multiplication tables. In nursing, often all three types of learning (cognitive, psychomotor, and affective) are necessary to perform a task competently.

BEHAVIORAL OBJECTIVES

A *behavioral objective* is a statement that clearly indicates how well a learner must do an action or behavior under particular conditions. Behavioral objectives include three things: (1) the *behavior*—what the learner should do; (2) the *criteria*—how well the learner should do it; and (3) the *condition*—under what conditions the behavior should be performed. Behavioral objectives are guides used by teachers to direct learning and to evaluate that learning has taken place.

The four steps used in writing behavioral objectives are as follows:

- ▲ Describe the expected behavior of the learner. The teacher selects the verb to describe the action and level of the dominant domain.
- ▲ State the result of the performance or that which will be evaluated to determine if the objective has been achieved.
- ▲ State the conditions under which the learner will be placed during the time he or she is performing the behavior or being evaluated.
- ▲ Decide on the criterion or standard for evaluating an acceptable performance of the behavior.

For example, a behavioral objective in the cognitive domain might read: *At the end of the lecture, list at least three of the six symptoms of the common cold.* The choice of the verb or action term should convey what is expected of the learner, in other words, the verb is the key to the performance the learner must demonstrate. In the above example, it is clear that listing symptoms is what is required.

An example in the psychomotor domain might be: *At the end of the learning laboratory experience, demonstrate the correct procedure for taking an oral temperature.* It is clear that the learner must do the procedure correctly since that is how the learner will be evaluated as having learned the skill.

Some behavioral objectives may include two domains although one is clearly dominant. For example: *In three successive demonstrations, read the patient's oral thermometer within 0.2 degrees of the instructor's reading.* The above implies that the learner knows how to take an oral temperature and focuses on the cognitive skill of reading accurately. This also infers that the learner understands the scale on the thermometer so that the objective is a higher level of cognition and recall of facts.

The affective domain includes feelings, attitudes, and appreciation. Cognitive and psychomotor behaviors are frequently accompanied by affective behaviors. An example of a high-level affective behavioral objective is: *Consistently exhibit interpersonal skills of listening, reflecting, and clarifying when questioning clients about their pain.* Achievement of the above objective would demonstrate high-level affective behaviors indicating that the learner is aware of feelings, values, and emotions.

EVALUATION OF THE LEARNER BY OBJECTIVES

Evaluation, a familiar term to both learners and teachers, implies measurement. The purpose of evaluation is to determine how much the learner has achieved. It includes feedback, which is information given to students about their progress toward achieving the behavioral objectives. If the goals—behavioral objectives—are specific and stated in terms of observable behaviors, the decisions are easy and evaluation is clear. Evaluation of a behavioral objective can be judged by seeing the performance or the behavior. The learning objective can also be evaluated using a paper-and-pencil test. The learner can be asked to respond in writing to a test question that directly relates to the objective. An example of a *performance objective* would be: *Select four medications from the medicine cabinet that are used to treat pneumonia.* The objective is evaluated by observing the student select the appropriate medications, but it could also be evaluated from a written response on a paper and pencil test. Behavioral objectives are an essential ingredient in the teaching–learning process.

THE RELATIONSHIP OF THE TEACHING–LEARNING PROCESS TO THE NURSING PROCESS

The *nursing process* is an organized or systematic way to plan professional nursing activities with or for the client. The nursing process is a sequence of cognitive steps based on data about the person to promote the well-being of the person and to guide the deliberative actions of the nurse in providing quality nursing care. The nursing process incorporates the art and science of nursing into a logical methodology that results in the intelligent, empathetic, and caring actions of the professional nurse. It is scientific validation of behaviors, including objective and subjective data collection, that substantiates nursing actions and results in what is frequently described as *intuitive nursing.* In other words, the collection of data about the client combined with the psychosocial and physiological knowledge base of the nurse leads to nursing actions that may appear intuitive but are not and, in fact, are based on data that are collected and plans that are thoughtfully carried out. We subscribe to the belief that all behavior has meaning and the logical processing of client data is the basis of professional nursing practice.

NURSING PROCESS

There are many descriptions of the nursing process and a variety of terms to identify the steps of the process in the literature (Fig. 2.2). Some nursing processes outline five steps, others seven or eight, but basically most processes describe five steps similar to the ones here.

Assessment

Assessment is the data-collection phase in which the nurse collects all the information about the client. Of course, the best source of data is the person; other sources are the records, other nurses or health care workers, family members, and reference materials.

The terms objective and subjective data are frequently used to classify data. *Objective data* are what the nurse sees, hears, or measures during the exami-

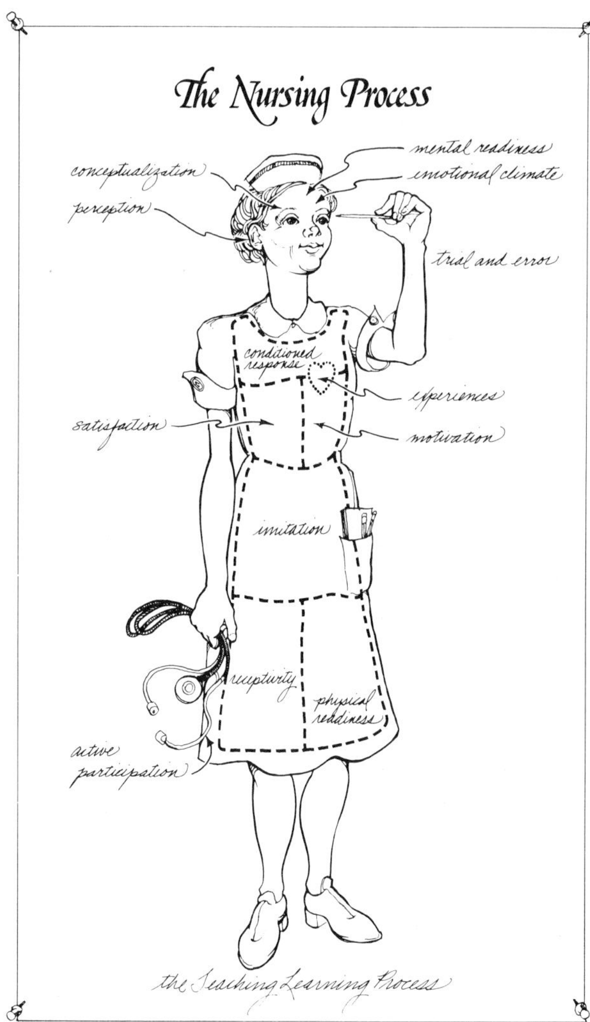

Figure 2.2
Readiness to practice maternity nursing.

nation. *Subjective data* are what the person describes and tells the nurse. It is important to remember that data can always be validated, that is, if there were two people assessing the person, both could hear, see, and collect the same thing—data. During assessment, the nurse frequently collects more data than is needed for a given situation. If a woman is in labor, it is important to monitor her vital signs and assess her behavior as well as collect information about the fetus; but it probably is not important to know that the mother did not finished painting the baby's crib before coming to the hospital. Yet this information might be very important to know after the baby arrives.

Nursing Diagnosis

Nursing diagnosis of the client is made after data are collected. This is different than the medical diagnosis that the physician makes since that is usually about a disease or condition. A nursing diagnosis integrates the information he or she has collected and lays the foundation for the next step, which is planning. Nursing diagnosis is frequently an indication of adaptation or need to adapt. To go back to the example of the laboring woman, if her vital signs were normal and there was no evidence of abnormal psychological or physical stress in mother or fetus, the diagnosis might be that labor was progressing normally.

Planning

Planning is dependent on accurate data collection and nursing diagnosis. During this phase, the nurse makes plans to meet the needs of the client. In other words, the nurse establishes goals or objectives for the client. It is hoped that this can be done with input from the person, as she or he should be involved in planning for her or his own care. In establishing objectives, it is essential that outcome criteria be stated in terms of expected measurable behaviors. This builds the foundation for evaluation.

Implementation

Implementation, or the intervention step, puts the plan established in the preceding phase into action. Outcome criteria have been set, the plan is clear, and the nurse can proceed toward accomplishing the goal. If the nurse is not initially successful, it may be necessary to modify the intervention to achieve the desired outcome.

Evaluation

The *evaluation* step is where the nurse determines the success and effectiveness of the nursing care and evaluates the diagnosis, plan, and intervention. Were the actual outcomes the same as the desired outcomes? If not, why? Was the original data collection incomplete? Was the diagnosis theoretically sound or was the goal or plan unrealistic for this client at this time? An inaccurately based assessment will lead to ineffective nursing care. Unfortunately, the opposite is not always true. In other words, a good or sound assessment does not automatically lead to effective nursing care. There are variables during the process that can adversely affect a well thought-out plan. In such situations the nurse must repeat the process and modify his or her actions. Repeated experience with nursing process steps increases success, and the nurse operating from a solid knowledge and theoretical base can consistently plan, implement, and evaluate effective nursing care efficiently. In fact, once the steps are well integrated, the process is not time consuming. It is because the process has been mastered that the nurse appears to function spontaneously or intuitively.

The similarities between the teaching–learning and the nursing processes should simplify the understanding of both processes. In the teaching–learning process, the teacher collects information about the learner, individually or mutually selects a goal, which is stated behaviorally, and then plans for the teaching. In the nursing process, the implementation phase includes all the activity involved in teaching, including feedback and rewards. Evaluation requires that a deliberative evaluation of the goal be made. Was the desired outcome reached? If you can remember that each process involves assessment or data collection, goal setting, planning, intervention or action, and evaluation, and teach yourself to use these steps at each opportunity, you will make giant strides on the road to professional nursing practice.

SUMMARY

Teaching and learning were defined; processes of teaching and learning were discussed. Roles of the teacher and learner were explored, acknowledging that teaching and learning are complex activities. Characteristics of effective teachers were described and the point was made that successful teaching includes use of interpersonal and communication skills. The fact that each individual learner is unique and each learning situation is different was stressed. The mutuality of learning between learner and teacher was explored, and its importance analyzed. Active participation on the part of the learner was acknowledged as significant. The fact that learning or content that is relevant to the learner enhances success was also acknowledged.

Beliefs from the literature about learning were summarized. Such factors as perception, conditioned response, trial and error, imitation, conceptualization, motivation, physical and mental readiness, and satisfaction were explored. The idea that principles of learning from the behavioral and natural sciences lay the foundation for effective teaching and the subsequent implications for client teaching in nursing situations were clarified.

Categories of learning and the use of behavioral objectives were explored in the section "Domains of Learning." Definitions of cognitive, psychomotor, and affective domains were presented. Steps and criteria for writing behavioral objectives were described, and examples of cognitive, psychomotor, and affective objectives were given. Evaluation, the final step in the teaching–learning process, and the relationship of evaluation to behavioral objectives were emphasized.

The final topic was the nursing process. The point was made that although many authors describe nursing process, basically all nursing processes have five steps, which are assessment, nursing diagnosis, planning, implementation, and evaluation, even though the terminology may vary. Each step of the nursing process was discussed, and the importance of nursing process to professional nursing practice was stressed. The final point was the parallel between the teaching–learning and nursing processes, realizing that an understanding of both is basic to professional nursing practice.

REFERENCES AND READINGS

Beland, I., Passos, J. Y. *Clinical Nursing—Pathophysiological and Psychological Approaches* (4th ed.). New York: Macmillan, 1981.

Bevis, E. O. *Curriculum Building in Nursing, A Process.* St. Louis: C. V. Mosby, 1973.

Bloom, B. S. *Taxonomy of Educational Objectives, Handbook I: Cognitive Domain.* New York: David McKay, 1956.

Bloom, B. et al. *Handbook on Formative and Summative Evaluation of Student Learning.* New York: McGraw-Hill, 1971.

Carruth, B. F. Modifying Behavior through Social Learning. *Am J Nurs* 76:1804, 1976.

Ginott, H. G. New Ways of Praise and Criticism, in *Between Parent and Child.* New York: Macmillan, 1965, Chap. 2.

Gronlund, N. E. *Determining Accountability for Classroom Instruction.* New York: Macmillan, 1974.

Gronlund, N. E. *Measurement and Evaluation in Teaching, Instructor's Manual* (2nd ed.). New York: Macmillan, 1971.

Gronlund, N. E. *Stating Behavioral Objectives for Classroom Instruction.* New York: Macmillan, 1970.

Guinee, K. K. *Teaching and Learning in Nursing.* New York: Macmillan, 1978.

Guinee, K. K. *The Professional Nurse: Orientation, Roles, and Responsibilities.* New York: Macmillan, 1970.

Havighurst, R. J. *Developmental Tasks and Education* (3rd ed.). New York: David McKay, 1972.

Kramer, M., Schmalenberg, C. Constructive Feedback. *Nurs '77* 7:102 1977.

Krathwohl, D. R. et. al. *Taxonomy of Educational Objectives, Handbook II: Affective Domain.* New York: David McKay, 1964.

Luckmann, J., Sorenson K. C. Man Struggles to Maintain a State of Balance, in *Medical-Surgical Nursing—A Phychophysiologic Approach.* Philadelphia: W. B. Saunders, 1974, Chap. 3.

Mager, R. F. *Developing Attitudes Toward Learning.* Belmont, Calif.: Fearon, 1968.

Mager, R. F. *Goal Analysis.* Belmont, Calif.: Fearon, 1972.

Mager, R. F. *Preparing Instructional Objectives.* Belmont, Calif.: Fearon, 1962.

Murray, R., Zentner, J. Guidelines for More Effective Health Teaching. *Nursing '76* 6:44, 1976.

Narrow, B. *Patient Teaching in Nursing Practice.* New York: John Wiley & Sons, 1979.

Redman, B. K. *The Process of Patient Teaching in Nursing* (3rd ed.). St. Louis: C. V. Mosby, 1976.

Reilly, D. E. *Behavioral Objectives in Nursing Evaluation of Learner Attainment.* New York: Appleton-Century-Crofts, 1975.

Rogers, C. R. *Freedom to Learn.* Columbus, Ohio: Charles E. Merrill, 1969.

Schweer, J. E. Teaching Student to Teach Health Care to Others. *Nurs Clin North Am* 6(4):679, 1971.

Skinner, B. F. *The Technology of Teaching.* New York: Appleton-Century-Crofts, 1968.

Sturdevant, B. Why Don't Adult Parents Learn? *Superv Nurs* 8:44, 1977.

Travers, R. M. W. *Essentials of Learning.* New York: Macmillan, 1967.

Tyler, R. Behavioral Objectives. *Today's Education* 64(a):41, 1975.

3

ISSUES IN REPRODUCTIVE HEALTH CARE

Health care in the United States is a composite of systems and subsystems that derives its form of organization and operation from a number of sources: a diverse consumer population; health care providers, including professional and nonprofessional people; local, state, and national governments; health science educators and institutions; professional organizations, special interest groups, and private industry—each bringing its particular beliefs, values, attitudes, and demands to form what is, perhaps, the most complex health care delivery system ever devised. It is not surprising that this system is the focus of, or source for, the generation of multiple areas of general or specific public interest. In a large number of these areas, disagreement among different factions of the nation have arisen, and many of the areas have promoted considerable discussion and attention by newspapers and television. Such areas of widespread concern, dispute, or disagreement are known as *issues.* There are hundreds of issues that arise from health-related concerns. These issues have different degrees of importance to different people; they also affect people in different ways.

Conflict is an integral part of most issues and may take the form of personal conflict that arises from unclear or dissonant values and beliefs. For example, the nurse whose values do not permit acceptance of *elective abortion* as a choice for dealing with an unwanted pregnancy or whose feelings about abortion are not clear will have personal conflict when working in a situation where nursing is required for a woman having or recovering from an abortion. Another form of conflict is open disharmony between opposing factions in which the legal system becomes the arena for contest, for example, a law suit against a hospital for denying an expectant father the right to attend the delivery of his child.

The nurse is often caught in the middle of reproductive health care issues. This is especially true when the dispute is between the consumer and the system. The nurse may respond to such a position with increased levels of frustration and conflict since most nurses cannot dissociate themselves from issues that affect the client, the system, or persons within the system. To do so requires a detachment that denies personal feelings which are frequently unclear or ambivalent.

Nurses need to be sensitive to issues affecting themselves, the person toward whom their care is directed, and the system within which they work. But nurses also need to be able to identify clearly the issue under dispute and to confront it through careful analysis of its characteristics, as well as through clarification of their personal values concerning that issue.

This chapter discusses ways for maternity nurses to attend to issues that are of special importance to their nursing practice, issues such as increased use of technological modalities for the management of healthy pregnancy and childbirth, elective abortion, poor pregnancy outcome, and expanded role practice for nurses. Discussion of these and other issues appears in sections throughout this book where they are viewed as an integral part of maternity nursing practice. This chapter discusses generation of issues, using biostatistical information as one way of generating issues and consumer rights as another, and ways of dealing with issues, including issue analysis and values clarification. The chapter ends with some of the issues to which you should attend as you read this text.

IDENTIFICATION OF ISSUES

Two ways of issue generation are discussed here. First, the official reporting of *vital statistics* provides information about the scope and incidence of certain events like birth and death. Such written reports provide the information against which a desired goal or state can be compared. Is the birthrate higher or lower than that desired by the nation? Does the incidence of maternal or infant mortality require that measures be undertaken to combat the problem? Second, issues are often born of other issues of a more global nature. For example, the issue of human rights has generated disputes about a number of personal rights concerning health care, such as the right of women to control their reproductive destiny through birth control and elective abortion.

Issues reach public attention and prominence by the way in which they are presented to the people and to official groups. If an issue is picked up by the media and given widespread attention, it will gain the interest of larger numbers of people than if it is ignored by the media or confined to state or local audiences. The larger the area of interest, the greater the chance that some official or nonofficial action will be taken to resolve the issue under dispute.

Selected Reproductive Biostatistics

One way of quickly gaining a view of the scope or incidence of an issue or event is to look at the statistics reported about that topic. Statistics is the mathematical representation of numerical data. *Biostatistics* is the category of statistics that addresses data concerning human mortality, morbidity, birth, and general characteristics of a human population. In 1915, the first birth registration office was established in the United States for the purpose of collecting accurate data about birth in this country. Today, national biostatistic data are reported out of the Bureau of Vital Statistics in Washington, D.C. State and local health departments collect and report similar information as it relates to a particular locality or state. Nurses collect data about vital statistics each time they ask a client's age or place of birth or take the person's height or weight, or note the sex. Nurses also use statistics to help them understand the magnitude of an event (e.g., the birthrate is decreasing nationally) and to help them set priorities for care among people with illness states (e.g., hemorrhage takes the life of more pregnant women than does malnutrition).

Biostatistics are usually reported as measurement of a part of a total picture. *Rate* is used to describe the proportional relationship between two numerical values. Several categories of biostatistics are of special importance to the maternity nurse and are discussed here briefly. These same categories are discussed in more detail in the chapters that attend to conditions or problems where these statistics are relevant.

BIRTHRATE

The *birthrate,* as generally reported and referred to by most people, is called the *crude birthrate;* it is the relationship of the number of births to the general population in a specified year. Birthrates tend to vary from year to year, as does the total population. The number of births may have increased during a year, yet the birthrate may have decreased. This discrepancy is because of the relationship of the birth figures to the total population figures. Factors such as the death rate, immigration, and emigration affect these biostatistics. This often confuses people who rarely use biostatistical information. The crude birthrate in the United States has declined over the past 25 years, but there is now an upward trend. (Fig. 3.1).

Birthrate may be reported in more specific terms such as the *refined birthrate*—the ratio of births to the female population—or the *true birthrate*—the ratio of births to the female population of childbearing age.

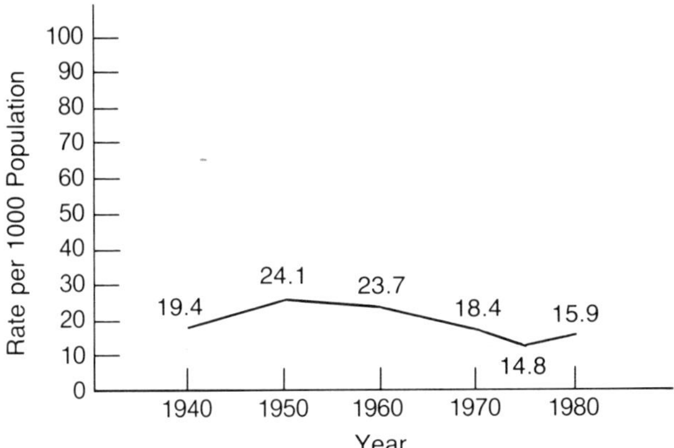

Figure 3.1
The crude birth rate in the United States, 1940–1980.

The nurse must understand the type of data being reported if the data are to be useful in nursing practice.

Birthrates are important figures since they provide information from which health planning groups can estimate future health care needs. They also provide a basis for comparison of population figures between the United States and other countries, and they help people to understand local, national, and worldwide trends in childbearing.

MATERNAL MORTALITY

Maternal mortality refers to the death of a woman during pregnancy, childbirth, or the 6-week period following birth. Since 1960 the *maternal mortality rate* has been defined as the number of maternal deaths per 100,000 live births. Before 1960, it was defined as the number of maternal deaths per 10,000 live births. This change is important for the nurse to know in order to comprehend the figures being reported, particularly if the reference predates 1960. Recently, maternal deaths may be reported only in regard to the presenting obstetric cause, giving a more precise correlation between maternal death and its cause. Emphasis must be placed on how important it is for the nurse to notice the nature of the statistics being reported in order to understand fully and accurately what is being read.

Maternal mortality rates have shown a striking decrease over the past 60 years. This decrease is especially apparent from 1940 to 1980 (Fig. 3.2), with the rates of 376.0 maternal deaths per 100,000 live births in 1940 dropping to a low of 6.9 per 100,000 in 1980. The early years of reporting maternal mortality show a sordid picture of the loss of life among young women during pregnancy and the periods following it. The marked improvement during the past four decades can be attributed to a combination of factors, including the use of blood transfusions and antibiotics. Many of the earlier maternal deaths were from hemorrhage or puerperal infection. Women today still die of these causes. But death is often more likely a result of contributing factors over which the health care provider has little or no control, such as failure of the woman to seek early and adequate health care. Prenatal care that provides the pregnant woman with improved health supervision during pregnancy, as well as with adequate education about pregnancy and childbirth, contributes to improved prognosis for many pregnant women today, especially those prone to reproductive risk conditions such as hypertensive disorders (see Chapter 21). Improved technology that enables early diagnosis and treatment of disorders that predispose to maternal risk and subsequent death has also been a factor in decreasing maternal death. Another, somewhat more controversial, factor has been the association between hospitalization for delivery and decreased maternal death rate. Few would argue that since women have been hospitalized for the delivery of their infants and kept in the hospital for a period of time following delivery, a lower maternal death rate has been reported. What is not clearly established is the cause–effect relationship between

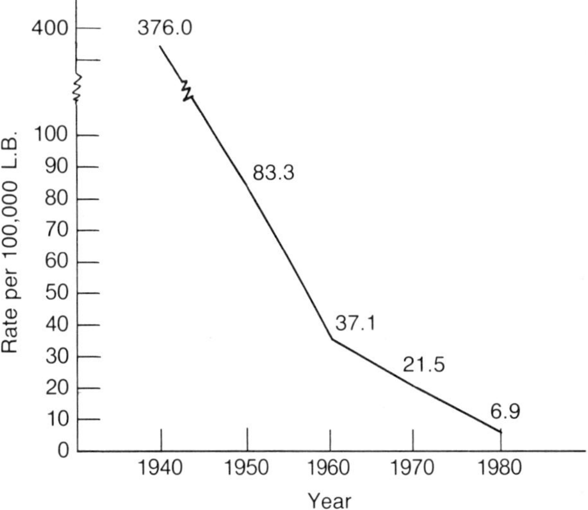

Figure 3.2
Maternal mortality, 1940–1980.

the two variables. Maternal mortality is a complex issue and is not usually associated with a single cause, but rather with a combination of factors, many of which are preventable. Much progress has been made toward saving the lives of pregnant women and young mothers; however, the goal is to decrease this mortality even more and ultimately to erase it. The 1980 mortality rate can only be viewed as encouragment toward reaching such a goal.

PERINATAL MORTALITY

Perinatal mortality refers to *fetal mortality*—those deaths occurring during pregnancy and before birth —and *neonatal mortality*—deaths occurring during the first four weeks of life (see Chapters 21–23). The definitions of the three rates are as follows:

perinatal mortality rate—combined number of fetal and neonatal deaths per 1,000 live births.
fetal mortality rate—number of fetal deaths per 1,000 live births. State laws vary according to what is considered a fetal death. Many states require that a fetus must have reached the point of *viability,* ability to live outside of the uterus following birth, before the death can be considered a fetal death. In some states, fetal death is recorded only if it occurs past the twentieth week of gestation.
neonatal mortality rate—number of neonatal deaths per 1,000 live births.

The causes of fetal and neonatal death are frequently interrelated. Combining them under the classification of perinatal mortality reflects this interrelationship. The combined classification makes access to the information more readily available to interested people. It also helps conceptually to bridge the separation between fetal and neonatal life that is caused by birth. The perinatal period represents a time of increased vulnerability of the fetus and neonate to different stresses. The perinatal mortality rate in the United States is far higher than that acceptable to a nation with such advanced medical technology. Perinatal mortality represents a significant loss of potential human lives and is one of the blights on health care in this country.

INFANT MORTALITY

Infant mortality is the death of a child during the first year of life.

infant mortality rate—number of deaths during the first year of life per 1,000 live births.

The infant mortality rate began a downward trend in the late 1950s that continues to the present, showing a decrease in infant mortality rate from 47.0 in 1940 to 12.5 in 1980, the lowest rate ever recorded (Fig. 3.3).

In spite of progress made toward decreasing infant deaths, both in the United States and worldwide, the United States continues to have an infant mortality rate—like its perinatal mortality rate—that is incompatible with its medical capability to prevent infant death. Infant death and perinatal and maternal mortality represent social problems of significant dimensions. The incidence of high-risk pregnancy and its concommittant poor outcome for mother and infant is greater among the indigent, nonwhite population. Infant mortality of nonwhite infants is almost double that of white infants. Maternal mortality is almost four times higher among nonwhite women. These figures are a result of many different factors, some of which are unknown. What is known, however, shows great inequities between health care services available to the poor and those available to the affluent; many nonwhite citizens are classified as poor. Inequities in health care are not solely related to socioeconomic strata but are, in part, a result of maldistribution of health care services, with fewer and poorer quality health care services available in the rural and inner city areas, the residence of many low-income citizens.

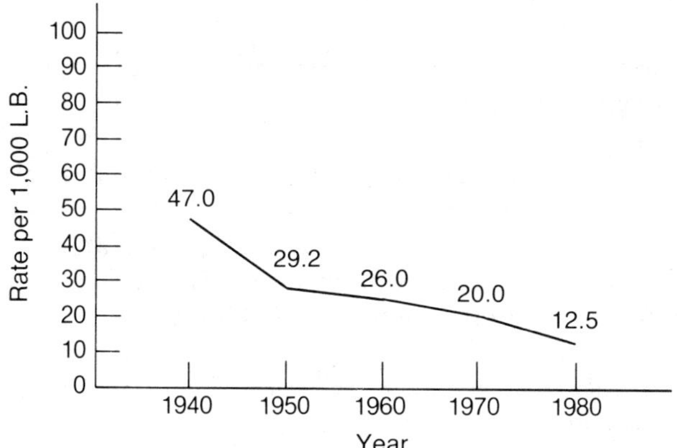

Figure 3.3
Infant mortality, 1940–1980.

Statistics present only a partial picture of the incidence of events associated with maternal–infant health. Statistics, do, however, provide a baseline for further investigation of certain areas of concern, a way of comparing different categories of health-related events, and a framework for looking at the scope of maternal–infant health. Statistical references will be used throughout this book.

Consumer Rights

A *right* is something due to a person in "accordance with or conformable to justice, law, morality or another standard" (Morris, 1976, p.1118). It is a reasonable personal or collective demand for something that people believe to be due them. Human rights have been a cornerstone of the American democratic system, and protection of human rights has been a goal for all nations of the free world. Today, human rights is a major international issue.

The American public has always been interested in and concerned with its rights. The surge of industrialization in the United States in the latter half of the nineteenth century brought another classification of human rights into prominence—*consumer rights.* Interest in consumer rights in regard to commercial products and health care did not emerge in an organized way until the post-World War II period of consumerism, although selective individual concerns were apparent years before. *Consumerism* is a social movement that seeks to protect the rights of the consumer, primarily in regard to fair practice laws in the areas of commercial products, and reflects concerns, such as honest labeling and advertising, packaging, fair pricing, and maintaining safety standards. Concerns about merchandizing techniques first met with resistance from industry, but later success was possible in several areas, such as automobile safety and accurate labeling of products. Consumerism has touched the health care industry as well, and the application of consumer rights to quality health care has become an issue of significant proportions.

Consumers' concerns about their rights to quality health care, in concert with concerns by many health care service providers, have given rise to a number of health care issues, such as the view that women have the right to determine whether or not they will have children, the number of children families will have, and the interval between pregnancies. Dissemination of birth control information without legal constraint and the option of elective abortion have also derived from consumers' concerns with the right to control pregnancy and childbirth. The right of women and their families to have a voice in health care decisions made about them and their unborn child, the right of families to participate in the childbirth experience, the right to life of the unborn fetus or the newborn child have all derived, in part, from the initial issue. Consumer rights impact greatly on the practice of professional nursing, creating conflict with existing practices and concern with changing those practices that do not recognize the rights of the people receiving health care.

The consumer issue of women having the right to control their reproductive destiny became apparent around the turn of the century through the efforts of a nurse, Margaret Sanger, to bring about repeal of birth control laws that prohibited the legal sale and use of contraceptives. Margaret Sanger and her supporters persisted in spite of much organized resistence and laid the groundwork for the general provision of birth control information and devices.

The work that began in the early 1900s to provide women with the right to make a decision concerning whether or not they would become pregnant reached a high point in 1973 with the Supreme Court decision concerning the legalization of elective abortion for women during the first trimester of pregnancy. This issue is far from resolved; however, the decision did give legal force to the right of women to go beyond the decision of whether or not to become pregnant to the decision of whether or not to carry a pregnancy to its completion. The 1973 Supreme Court decision was received amid mixed responses, ranging from the belief that it was a major event in giving women equality to the view that it was further impetus for the deterioration of American morality.

The right of women and their families to have a voice in health care decisions made about themselves and their unborn children is another issue that has arisen from the issue of consumer rights. Much of what is obstetric medical practice today consists of tasks and procedures performed on the consumer, often without clear explanation of the purpose or the necessity for such procedures. It is this type of health care against which many consumers and health care providers alike take issue and for which they seek change.

Procedures such as *episiotomy,* the performance of a surgical incision to enlarge the vaginal opening during childbirth, have been questioned as being necessary for *every* woman at the time of delivery. The widespread use of drugs during labor without full explanation of their effect on the mother and her unborn child is another area of concern. Many women believe that childbirth has been moved out of the realm of a natural, normal event and has been placed into a hospital environment where it is treated as though it requires extensive medical and surgical management. Management that is often performed without consultation with the woman or her family is another sensitive issue.

Advances in medical science over the past years have brought techniques and approaches that provide for sophisticated diagnosis and treatment of problems associated with reproductive risk. Many of these procedures, such as biochemical studies of the amniotic fluid and electronic and sonographic monitoring for all pregnant women during labor, have become usual practice, in some areas, for all pregnant women regardless of their health or risk classification. Often the woman is not consulted about the use of these modalities but must accept the stress associated with the procedures, as well as pay the bills for their use. A number of related issues has been generated from the use of such technology. For example: Should all pregnant women be managed the same way during pregnancy? Is such technology needed for the healthy pregnant patient? What effect does the use of this technology have on the fetus and, later, the neonate?

The right of families to participate in the childbirth experience has been the impetus for some women to insist that their child be born in the home rather than in the hospital. For a number of years, hospitals refused to allow the husband or partner to participate in the woman's labor and delivery. Children were not permitted to visit their mothers who were hospitalized for childbirth. Some institutions still retain these restrictions in spite of efforts by consumer and professional groups to permit family support and access to the pregnant woman during childbirth. In theory, few argue that childbirth is a family experience, but many arguments are frequently mounted to explain why involvement of the family, in a direct way, is not a desired or even healthy practice. This issue has spawned other issues, such as home birth, alternatives to hospital delivery, and early discharge.

Does the unborn fetus have any rights? What rights does a newborn infant have? These questions are part of the issue of fetal–neonatal rights, an issue that is far from resolved in today's reproductive health care world. When the United States Supreme Court ruled on the abortion question in 1973, and again in 1979, in regard to the use of federal monies to pay for elective abortion for the indigent woman, the Court did not deal with the question of the right of the unborn fetus to life. Groups on both sides of the issue have come forth pushing for clarification of the issue of when life begins, another subissue of the right of the fetus.

There is no easy or quick answer to any of the issues associated with consumer rights, as there is rarely an easy solution for most issues. The issues are real, however, and the maternity nurse is likely to encounter questions about any or all of these issues in any given day, in any job, in any given location.

The issue of consumer rights has been presented here to help you see how issues are generated from other issues and how complex is the question of human rights. Another issue could have served the same purpose. Many of these questions or issues will reappear throughout the book since maternity nurses need to be aware of and responsive to consumer rights. Nurses are seen by some people as the ones who speak out for the right of the consumer to quality health care. You will generate other issues in your mind as you study and practice maternity nursing.

DEALING WITH AN ISSUE

The nurse must deal with issues in order to practice nursing effectively. The nurse may approach an issue from either of two extremes: one is to ignore the issue, the other is to confront the issue openly in a public arena, such as by giving testimony or participating in action groups that are working to resolve some aspect of the issue. Most nurses find themselves somewhere between these two extremes. Two examples are by continuing to practice, while regarding the issue in a somewhat distant, disinterested posture, insisting to themselves that the issue should not be of concern to nursing and that nurses should not become involved, or by attempting to resolve the issue in a way that is satisfactory to them, their client, and their profession.

Two ways of dealing with reproductive health care issues are suggested here: careful analysis of the characteristics of the issue and clarification of personal values concerning the issue.

Analysis of an Issue

Analysis is a cognitive function through which a person is able to examine distinct parts of something—in this case an issue—and to note the relationship of the parts to each other and to the whole. Analysis permits the sectioning of an abstract phenomenon into small discrete units, which then enables the thinker to deal with these units through the use of a more limited scope of cognitive operation such as identification, description, and explanation. This breakdown can be accomplished through formulation of questions that will redirect thinking.

- ▲ Where did the issue originate? That is, who first became concerned with the subject and why?
- ▲ What is the nature of the dispute? What are the opposing positions taken and who are the participants in the dispute?
- ▲ Who, or what, does the issue affect and in what way is its effect apparent? Who is helped or who is harmed by the anticipated outcome according to the opposing positions?
- ▲ Where does nursing fit into the picture? Has a position been taken by an official nursing group? If so, what is that position and is it compatible with your personal position regarding the issue?
- ▲ How can the issue be resolved? What options are available and what role can the nurse play in resolution of this particular issue?

Examination of an issue through analysis enables nurses to comprehend it more completely and accurately, as well as to identify and clarify their own feelings and positions concerning the issue and to interpret the nature of the issue to colleagues and consumers within and outside of the health care system.

Values Clarification

Clarification of your values is an introspective process that enables you to confront personal beliefs about concepts such as life/death, love/hate, action/inaction, and morality/immorality. Introspection provides for the holding of a mirror to your life and seeing the reflection. Many nurses find, when looking at their own opinions and attitudes, that sitting astride the fence may be the more comfortable position, but it may not serve to clarify their nursing practice regarding sensitive issues nor help them to understand the needs of the client who is their area of focus.

Capability for clarifying your values is tied closely to your stage of cognitive development (see Chapters 7 and 8). Most adults are capable of performing the more formal, abstract operations that are indicative of mature cognitive functioning. Some of you, however, may have never used these operations to examine yourselves in regard to the types of issues the maternity nurse is likely to encounter. In a nursing program you may question the wisdom of your teacher in assigning you to write your philosophy of life or nursing, insisting that such an exercise has little practical value for care of people—the real reason that you came into nursing. The written statement of your philosophy may be the first formal mechanism you have encountered that directs you to look at your beliefs and opinions and how those beliefs affect your values—the things you think are important or hold dear—or your attitudes—your overt representation of feelings, opinions, and values. Before writing a personal philosophy, you must examine what you *think* or *believe* about a particular area of concern. One of the pitfalls of doing such an introspective analysis is the tendency to overpersonalize an issue or idea. "I could never have an abortion," or "I want to have all of my babies by natural childbirth because that is what God intended," or "She is foolish to have her baby at home." Analysis of personal values will enable you to be comfortable with yourself and your beliefs, and in turn, to be more accepting and objective about the values of other people.

Another way of examining your values is through dialogue with other people you respect and trust. This sharing and comparing of beliefs and values may help you to acquire a clearer view about yourself. More formalized ways of examining personal values are also available. (See the reading lists at end of this chapter.)

SELECTED ISSUES OF IMPORTANCE TO MATERNITY NURSING

Three categories of issues are of importance to the practice of maternity nursing: client-centered issues, system-centered issues, and profession-centered issues. These issues are not discussed in detail here but are dealt with in the maternity nursing topic to which they are most relevant.

Client-Centered Issues

Client-centered issues are those issues that derive from consumer concerns or affect the consumer directly. One such issue, discussed earlier in this chapter, is *consumer rights.* Consumer rights directs the nurse toward the areas of concern and interest of the people for whom care is being provided.

Elective abortion is another consumer-centered issue with which the nurse is concerned. *Elective abortion* is the voluntary termination of a pregnancy when the continuation of the pregnancy poses no threat to the health of the expectant mother or her unborn child. Abortion is discussed in more detail, both as a procedure and as an issue, in Chapter 26.

Reproductive risk to the pregnant woman or her unborn child often results in a poor pregnancy outcome. It is an issue of considerable magnitude in the United States today, not only in terms of the disparities in health care that often contribute to the problem, but as a health problem of serious dimensions to many families. The six chapters in Unit Five that are devoted to reproductive risk reflect the importance of this problem for the maternity nurse today.

Another client-centered issue is *consumer dissatisfaction with the present health care delivery system for pregnant families.* This issue has resulted in opposing arguments concerning alternatives to hospital delivery, as well as changes in the ways in which health care needs during labor and delivery are attended to both within and outside of the usual institutional setting. *Alternatives to hospital delivery* are discussed in Chapter 28 together with the issue of *depersonalization of health care services for pregnant families.*

Health Care System-Centered Issues

One of the health care system-centered issues that is of great dispute today is that of the *cost of health care services,* specifically, reproductive risk health care. Over the past several decades, the cost of health care has soared bringing health care into a luxury category for many people. This issue is a complex one and involves the total health care industry, including the federal government and the insurance industry. The United States has been accused of being a country of haves and have nots economically, and increasingly this is becoming the case in regard to the purchase of health care. Cost of health care is discussed in Chapter 20.

Another issue generated by the health care delivery system, and mentioned earlier, is that of the increased use of *medical technology for families experiencing normal pregnancy.* While improved medical technology has given the health sciences increased and improved capability for providing health care of a diagnostic and therapeutic nature to large numbers of people, some health care providers, like consumers, contend that this technology has been used unnecessarily and inappropriately for healthy families.

Inequities in health care delivery for different groups of people in different locations in the nation have led to concern with the issue of *what are the appropriate models for health care delivery.* Reproductive health care services are costly; as with other health care services, there is overlap and duplication of many services and lack of availability of other services. The past several years have seen the emergence of models of perinatal health care that were built upon the concepts of consolidation of services within one institution in a city or region in order to decrease both duplication and omission of services. The movement toward consolidation and regionalization has transferred some reproductive health care services from local communities to the larger urban areas, often in medical center complexes. Access to these services necessitates travel on the part of the consumer, and, in the event of long-term hospitalization, may result in separation of families for long periods of time. This is particularly true in regard to the pregnancy that is at reproductive risk. Both the concept and the cost of such changes in models of patient care have become issues that have generated much discussion.

Profession-Centered Issues

There are several issues that have special relevance to maternity nursing that derive from changes occurring in the nursing profession (see Chapter 28). One such issue is the *expanded role of the nurse.* Over the past two or more decades, professional nursing has undergone considerable change in regard to the scope of its practice. These changes have included both reorganization of existing roles and the emergence of new roles for nurses, such as the nurse-practitioner and the nurse-midwife. Although the contributions of maternity nurses in such roles have been demonstrated, the future of these and other roles for maternity nurses is not certain.

Standards of care is another issue of professional concern. In 1973, the American Nurses' Association established standards of care in the various specialty areas of nursing practice. These standards were intended to serve as guidelines for quality nursing practice. Maternal–child nursing was one such area. Since that time, other organizations, such as The Nurses Association of the American College of Obstetricians and Gynecologists and the American College of Nurse Midwives, have added to these standards. Maintenance of nursing standards and assurance of the quality of nursing practice are concerns of all nurses. In addition, there are areas of specific concern unique to each specialty.

Professional rights is another issue. Much attention has been given to consumer rights, but professional health care providers also have rights, including the right to make sound judgments about the care of their clients, the right to clear delineation of their professional responsibilities, and the right to compensation for services provided.

The *legal parameters* of professional nursing have come into question as an issue in regard to changing roles among health professionals, particularly role expansion in nursing. There are a number of issues that derive from concern with the legal limits of professional nursing practice and with the ways in which these vary from state to state.

There are also *ethical concerns* that affect, in some way, the client, the system, and the profession. Ethical concerns, as such, are not singled out for discussion but are dealt with in association with the topic being discussed. For example, decisions concerning whether to continue or to stop care for an infant whose prognosis is poor and whose family requests such an action are discussed when management of the critically ill infant is explained.

SUMMARY

This chapter addressed the issues in reproductive health care and the importance of these issues to the maternity nurse. An issue was defined as a point of dispute or disagreement among people or a topic of widespread concern to the general public. Two ways of generating issues were presented; the use of biostatistics to describe the scope and incidence of selected issues and events and the generation of issues from a broader area of concern such as consumer rights. Two methods for attending to issues were discussed briefly: analysis of the issue and clarification of personal values concerning the issue. The chapter ended with identification of three categories of issues that are of particular importance to the maternity nurse and which are attended to in other sections of the book: client-centered issues, system-centered issues, and profession-centered issues.

REFERENCES AND READINGS

American Nurses' Association. *Standards of Maternal Child Health Nursing Practice.* Kansas City: American Nurses' Association, 1973.

Butnarescu, G. F. *Perinatal Nursing, Volume 1—Reproductive Health.* New York: John Wiley & Sons, 1978.

Chase, H. C. Perinatal Mortality: Overview and Current Trends. *Clin Perinatol* 1:3, 1974.

Dispel, H. The Fetus as a Person: Possible Legal Consequences of the Hogan–Helm Amendment. *Fam Plann Perspect* 6:6, 1974.

Haire, D. *The Cultural Warping of Childbirth.* Hillside, N.J.: International Childbirth Education Association, 1972.

Harper, M. W., Marcom, B. R., and Wall, V. D. Abortion: Do Attitudes of Nursing Personnel Affect the Patient's Perception of Care? *Nurs Res* 21:327, 1972.

Lader, L. *Abortion II.* Boston: Beacon Press, 1973.

Miller, C. A. Health Care of Children and Youth in America. *Am J Public Health* 65:355, 1975.

Morris, W. (Ed.). *The American Heritage Dictionary of the English Language.* Boston: Houghton Mifflin, 1976.

Summary of Births, Deaths, Marriages and Divorces in the United States—1980. *Monthly Vital Statistics Report.* September 17, 1981.

Wallace, H. F., Gold E., (Eds). and Lis, E., (Eds). *Maternal and Child Health Practices.* Springfield: Charles C. Thomas, 1973.

World Health Organization. *Improvement in Infant and Perinatal Mortality in the United States, 1965–1973.* Washington, D.C.: U.S. Department of Health, Education and Welfare, 1976.

UNIT TWO

DEVELOPMENTAL READINESS FOR PREGNANCY AND PARENTHOOD

INTRODUCTION

Developmental readiness for pregnancy and parenthood is broadly defined here as the physical and psychosocial capability of people and families to cope with the demands and complete the tasks of pregnancy, childbirth, and early parenthood.

Readiness to undertake any task or to accomplish any goal is highly personalized; it is often difficult to determine just where on a developmental continuum a person or family should be placed. There are general guidelines that can provide some indication of the reproductive maturation of a person and the ability of that person's family to see pregnancy in a healthy way and embark upon the tasks of parenthood with an awareness of the scope of these tasks and preparation for dealing with them. These guidelines are arbitrarily called *characteristics* of developmental readiness for reproduction. They will be addressed extensively in Chapters 4 to 9, as well as throughout this book.

The following list defines the characteristics of developmental readiness.

- ▲ Physical development of the male and female is adequate to support conception.
- ▲ Physical development of the female is capable of accommodating the processes necessary for completion of pregnancy, childbirth, and recovery.
- ▲ Genetic characteristics for producing healthy offspring are believed to be present.
- ▲ Capacity for establishing and maintaining intimate relationships with others exists.
- ▲ Evidence of the potential for giving to and caring for another human being is seen.
- ▲ Capacity for adaptation and coping exists.
- ▲ Healthy motivation for becoming pregnant is apparent.
- ▲ Learning capacity is present.
- ▲ Communication capability skill is apparent.
- ▲ Sexual identification and potential for sexual response are present.

Rudimentary assessment of the presence or absence of these characteristics is within the scope of professional nursing practice. Precise diagnosis of degree of development and readiness for reproduction may depend upon more sophisticated assessment modalities than the professional nurse has the knowledge and skill to use. However, careful use of data collection strategies and a sound theory base should result in general inferential judgments about whether or not a person or couple is ready to undertake, with minimal difficulty, the events of pregnancy, childbirth, and early parenthood. This assessment also helps the nurse to make judgments about referral to other health care providers.

Human reproduction requires input from both the male and the female. The heritage of the child comes from both parents. The importance of the female in human reproduction is not diminished by attention to the male as well. The primary role of the female in the reproductive process is fully recognized for she both nurtures and gives birth to the fetus. The text and graphics in this unit are arranged to enable you to compare the male and female reproductive systems to understand their similarities and differences, as well as their structure and function, and their social, as well as their physical development.

This unit consists of six chapters: Chapter 4, "Physical Development: Anatomy and Physiology," addresses physical development with attention to male and female reproductive anatomy and physiology. In Chapter 5, "Endocrine Control of Reproductive Readiness," the interrelationship of the central nervous system, the pituitary, and the male and female gonads is discussed in detail with particular attention given to the menstrual cycle. Chapter 6, "Genetic Basis for Reproduction," explores chromosomes, their role in human reproduction, the cellular processes of mitosis and meiosis, and gametogenesis. Chapter 7, "Psychosocial Development," focuses on selected theories of development, as well as the establishment and maintenance of relationships with others, particularly the opposite sex. Chapter 8, "Adolescence: A Period of Integration," looks at puberty and adolescence as the biophysical and psychosocial "coming together" of male and female human systems, making reproduction possible. Unit Two closes with Chapter 9, "Assessment of Reproductive Readiness." The areas relevant to assessment of reproductive readiness, as well as selected strategies and skills needed for the nurse to perform such procedures, are covered.

Unit Two provides the basis upon which much of the content in subsequent units depends.

BEHAVIORAL OUTCOMES

Upon completion of the study of this unit, you should be able to:

- ▲ Define developmental readiness for pregnancy and parenthood
- ▲ Identify the characteristics of developmental readiness for reproduction
- ▲ Explain key concepts from selected theories of human development, biology, genetics, psychology, and sociology and their relevance to reproductive readiness
- ▲ Explain the characteristics of major conceptual frameworks for preparation for pregnancy, childbirth, and early parenthood
- ▲ Identify skills and processes appropriate for determining developmental readiness for the reproductive events
- ▲ Explain the theoretical basis for the skills and processes used to determine developmental readiness for reproduction
- ▲ Apply understandings about concepts and theory drawn from nursing and related disciplines to the assessment and preparation of people and families for pregnancy, childbirth, and early parenthood

4

PHYSICAL DEVELOPMENT: ANATOMY AND PHYSIOLOGY

Maternity nursing relies greatly upon concepts and theories drawn from the biomedical sciences to help direct its clinical practice. Maternity nurses use this information to determine client need and to provide both direct and indirect nursing care. Assessment of physical readiness and interpretation of the data collected can only be done if the nurse is knowledgeable about physical development. Making appropriate nursing judgments about the care of pregnant families is dependent upon knowing the normal physical development since family planning technology is based upon this information and adaptation to and physiologic need during pregnancy derives in part from physical status and potential. Maternity nurses use this knowledge base not only in daily practice, but also to support and give credence to their teaching role in providing health education related to sexuality, pregnancy, childbirth, and recovery. They are the primary teachers of expectant parents, and the role models and teachers for other nurses, students of nursing, and people from other health-related disciplines. Maternity nurses are often the primary consultants to teachers who are responsible for family life education, in both the public and private school systems, as well as consultants to the parents of the children being taught. As with other nurses working in specialty areas, maternity nurses serve as consultants to their peers, people in other disciplines, and to individual and group consumers. Many of the activities arising from these roles necessitate the need for understanding the physical development underlying reproduction.

As a student of maternity nursing, you may have prior knowledge about physical development. Physical development is included in this book as well, however, so that you can acquire a basis for ready retrieval and be able to see its clinical relevance to maternity nursing. Since this is not a complete anatomy and physiology text, much of what is presented has been carefully selected for maternity nursing students.

The male and female reproductive organs (internal and external genitalia) are the primary focus of this section (Fig. 4.1). These organs develop after fertilization from undifferentiated (similar) embryonic tissue early in prenatal life. Although the structure and appearance of the male and female systems be-

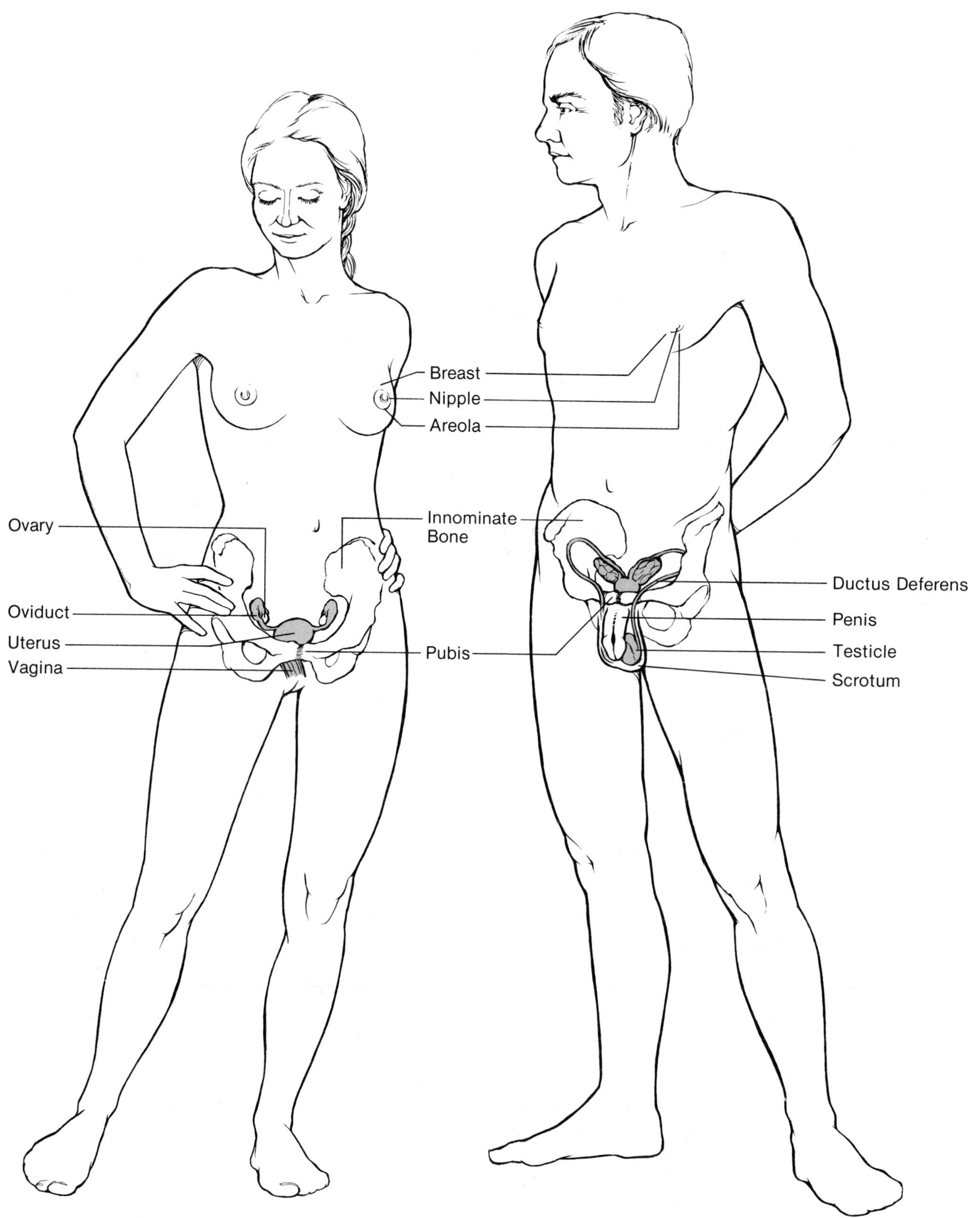

Figure 4.1
Frontal view of the adult male and female reproductive organs shown in a standing posture. *Left:* female; *right:* male.

come increasingly different as they grow and mature, they remain functionally quite similar. For a complete picture of the biologic basis for human reproduction, understanding of both the structure and function of these organs is necessary. A second focus of this chapter is the supportive or accessory structures to human reproduction—the pelvic bones, ligaments, and muscles (essentially those of the female)—and the breasts.

GONADS

The key to human reproduction is found in the male and female gonads. The *gonads,* whose development results initially from the genotype provided by the parent gametes at the time of *fertilization (conception),* are endocrine organs that work in concert with the central nervous system, particularly the hypothalamus, and the anterior pituitary gland to control the reproductive function in the human. They do this through a reciprocal relationship that includes the initiation and inhibition of gonadotrophin and steroid hormones. These hormones play a major role in initiating, supporting, and controling the process of *gametogenesis* (the maturation of the immature male and female germ cells). The gonadal steroid hormones also provide for the development of the male and female secondary sexual characteristics. This hypothalamic–pituitary–gonadal relationship is discussed in more detail in Chapter 5.

In early embryonic life, the structures that become the male and female gonads are indistinct, undeveloped tissue. These structures are present by the twenty-ninth day after fertilization but cannot be recognized as an *ovary* or a *testicle.* The female reproductive system tends to develop somewhat more slowly than does that of the male. The factors that control, cause, and regulate gonadal and accessory reproductive organ development along sex lines are not completely known. It has been believed for several years that the male sex chromosome (the Y chromosome) is the factor that initiates this differentiation, and it is known that the male testes produce androgenic hormones soon after their early embryonic differentiation. These hormones are believed to influence the sex line development since, in the absence of the testes, development always follows female lines. Recently, however, there has been evidence that a substance called the H–Y antigen is present on the cell surface of the male mammals, which seems to correlate closer with differentiation of these testes than does the Y chromosome (Wachtel et al., 1975). Further study has reinforced this idea and has suggested that the H–Y antigen, located on the surface of the *Sertoli cells,* may very likely be the regulator of early testicular differentiation (Ciccarese & Ohno, 1978). Both the Sertoli cells that later line the seminiferous tubules in the testes and *Leydig's cells,* the hormone-producing cells of the testes, are present in early embryonic life.

Ovaries

The female gonad is known as the *ovary.* Each anatomically normal female has two ovaries nestled in the soft tissue of the pelvis, one on each side of the uterus (womb) at about the level of the pelvic brim, the upper margin of the cylindrical part of the pelvis. The ovaries are often compared to an unshelled almond in size and shape. During the reproductive years (*puberty* to menopause), each ovary measures about 2.5–5.0 cm long, 1.5–3.0 cm wide, and 0.6–1.5 cm thick and weighs 5.0–8.0 gm. Their sizes vary according to age, with all dimensions decreasing slightly after *menopause,* the functional end of the female reproductive years. Clear, fluid-filled cysts can be seen on the surface of the ovary. These cysts represent the female germ cell follicles in different stages of development. The shell of a ruptured follicle that has released a female germ cell, *ovum,* can also be seen as a small yellow structure called the *corpus luteum* (yellow body). The presence of these follicles give the ovary a slightly uneven surface. As the woman grows older, the ovarian surface becomes more nodular, resembling somewhat the texture of an English walnut.

The ovary (Fig. 4.2) is composed of two parts—the thicker outer aspect or layer called the *cortex* and the central section called the *medulla.* The entire ovary is covered by a thin epithelium. The cortex of the ovary contains numerous follicles dispersed throughout the connective tissue cells and fibers. These follicles were provided during prenatal life in the form of primitive germ cells called *oogonia.* These germ cells are present in the ovary by the twentieth to twenty-second week of gestation, undergo partial maturation by the time of birth, and then remain in a quasidormant functional state until puberty, by which time many of them have degenerated. From

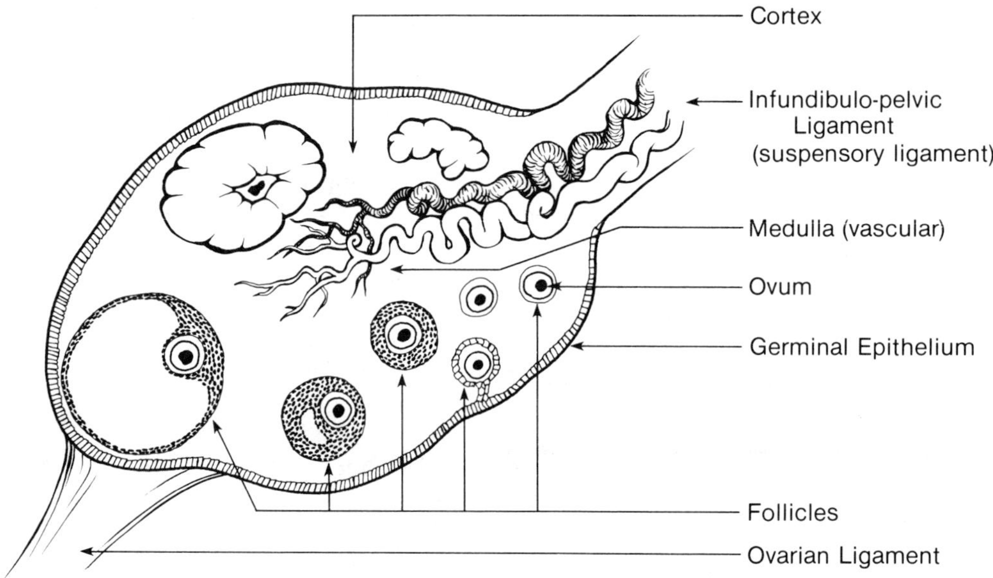

Figure 4.2
Section of ovary showing stroma, vascular structures, follicles, and ligaments.

puberty throughout the reproductive years, these follicles range in development from immature primordial follicles to mature follicles known as the *Graafian follicles.* The follicles contain a female germ cell *(oocyte)* that is surrounded as it matures by increasing numbers of *granulosa* cells. The granulosa cells are embraced by *theca externa* and *theca interna* cells. These cells produce steroid hormones necessary for ovulation (see Chapter 5, section on the menstrual cycle). The outer tissue area of the cortex is called the *tunica albuginea* and is dull white because of its transparent epithelial covering. The medulla is the middle part of the ovary and is made up of loose connective tissue, arteries, and veins. It also contains a small number of smooth muscle fibers.

Three ligaments anchor the ovaries in the pelvis. They are held to the posterior part of the pelvis by the *broad ligament;* to the wall of the pelvis by the *infundibulopelvic* (or *suspensory*) ligament; and to the uterus by the *utero-ovarian* ligament. The ovaries are moveable and their position can be affected by several things.

▲ ***Posture.*** If a woman stands erect, the ovaries are in an almost vertical position; when she lies down on her back, the ovaries shift to a more horizontal position.

▲ ***Pregnancy.*** As the uterus increases in size during pregnancy, the ovaries are shifted slightly upward in the pelvis.

▲ ***Pelvic Pathology.*** Uterine or ovarian tumor growth will also alter the position of the ovary or ovaries.

The ovaries are supported by a rich vascular supply, primarily from the ovarian artery and vein. Nerves from both the sympathetic and parasympathetic systems service the ovaries. Lymphatic vessels and nodes are abundant in the pelvis and furnish support for all structures there.

Two essential functions for human reproduction are provided by the ovaries: they produce and release the mature female germ cell, the ovum, on a cyclic schedule beginning after puberty and continuing through menopause, and they secrete the steroid hormones *estrogen* and *progesterone.* (See Chapter 5.)

Testes

The two male gonads, the *testes,* are morphologically similar to the ovaries. They are ovoid, slightly flattened, and somewhat larger than the ovaries. The testes develop inside of the body cavity during prenatal life. In most cases, during the last two months of gestation they descend into a two-chambered pouch called the *scrotum* (or *scrotal sac*), located outside of the body cavity. Infants are sometimes born with undescended testes. Testicular descent is necessary, however, for *spermatogenesis* (production and maturation of the male germ cell) to occur because of the sensitivity of *spermatozoa* (sperm) to temperature extremes, especially high temperatures. Normal body temperature may interfere with spermatogenesis.

The testes contain an outer layer (similar to that of the female cortex) also called the tunica albuginea. This structure is made up of fibroelastic connective tissue with scattered smooth muscle cells. Each testicle is divided into approximately 250 wedge-shaped lobes, each containing one to three coiled tubes about 2–3 ft long, 60–90 cm, the *seminiferous tubules* (Fig. 4.3). These tubules are lined with *germinal epithelium* and *spermatogenic cells.* The lobes are separated by a septum. In addition, the testes also contain the Sertoli cells located in the seminiferous tubules. The Sertoli cells are elongated and are believed to furnish a nutritive substance for the *spermatids* (immature sperm) during their maturation. Leydig's or interstitial, cells are also present in the interstices of the tubules; these cells

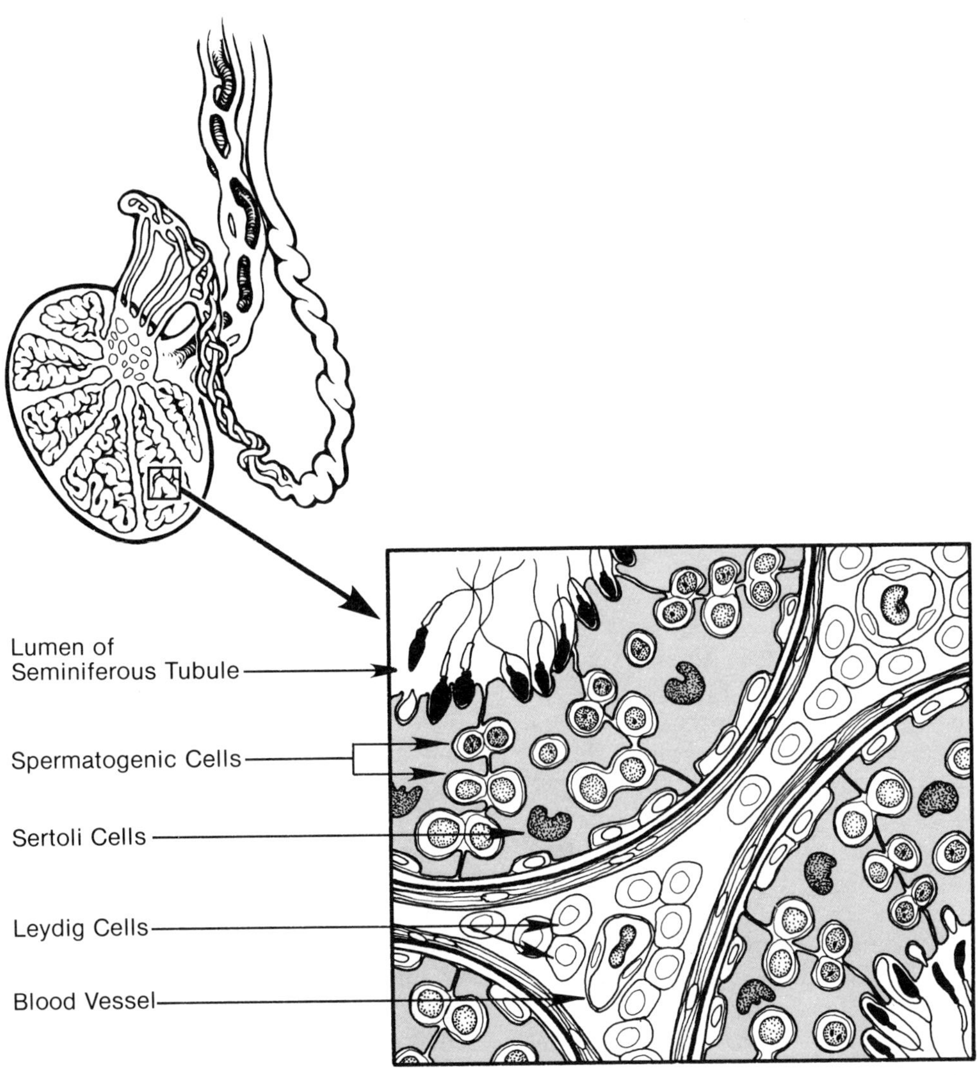

Figure 4.3
Testicle with inset showing a section of one lobe.

secrete the male androgenic hormones, particularly *testosterone* (see Chapter 5).

The testes, like the ovaries, serve two functions. They secrete steroid hormones beginning in early prenatal life when the embryonic testes produce testosterone as well as a nonsteroid hormone that is believed to cause regression of some fetal tissues. The androgenic hormones, essentially testosterone, are responsible for the development of male secondary sex characteristics (see Chapter 8). Under the stimulation of testosterone, the testes produces the male gametes, the spermatozoa.

Unlike the ovaries, the testes do not produce germ cells during the prenatal period. With the onset of puberty, the male gametes are produced and matured on a continuous rather than cyclic schedule throughout the remainder of a man's life. Although male gametogenesis is known to decrease as a man ages, there is no definitive termination of his reproductive capability, such as menopause. A comparison of basic characteristics of the male and female gonads is found in Table 4.1.

DUCTILE SYSTEM

In early embryonic life, the two primordial, undifferentiated ducts, the mesonephric (wolffian) and paramesonephric (mullerian), are present in the developing organism. About the seventh week (forty-seventh day) of prenatal life, these two ducts begin to differentiate with the mesonephric duct developing into the male urogenital system and the paramesonephric duct developing into the female urogenital system (Fig. 4.4). With this differentiation in the male, the urinary and genital systems are closely interrelated, whereas in the female there is a clearer distinction.

The ductile structures having reproductive significance are the female oviducts (fallopian tubes), the uterus, and the vagina. These structures, along with the ovaries, are frequently referred to as the internal female genitalia or reproductive organs (Figs. 4.5 and 4.6). The male ductile system includes the *epididymides,* the *ductus deferens (vas deferens),* the *seminal vesicles,* and the *ejaculatory ducts* (Fig. 4.7). Although these structures may be referred to as the male internal reproductive organs, they are external to the pelvic and abdominal cavities after birth.

Female Ductile System

Female oviducts are two tubular structures attached bilaterally to the uterine corpus at one end and approaching, but not attaching to, the ovaries at the distal end. They are about 8–14 cm long. Unlike the picture presented in many drawings of the fallopian tubes and uterus, the oviducts do not extend directly out laterally from the uterus but, rather, curve outward in an embracing fashion upward from the uterus and slightly toward the back and are suspended by the *mesosalpinx,* a fold of the *broad ligament.* Fingerlike projections called *fimbrae* are found at their distal end. These "fingers" reach toward the ovary to guide the extruded ovum into the oviduct, where it will either travel on through the patent lumen, a distance of about one-third to one-half the length of the tube, and be fertilized, or travel on toward the uterus where it will die. It is possible for the ovum to move through the oviduct because of the sweeping motion of ciliated cells lining the lumen and the peristaltic movements of the muscular tube.

The oviduct is composed of four parts or segments. The funnel-shaped portion near the ovary, containing the fimbrae, is called the *infundibulum* and is similar to a trumpet in appearance. The *ampulla* is the outer one-third to one-half of the tube. The *isthmus,* somewhat firmer in consistency than the ampulla, is located between the ampulla and the uterus. The *interstitial part* is the portion that passes through the uterine muscle and opens into the uterine cavity. The lumen of the tube is narrower at the uterine end.

The oviduct is made up of three layers of tissue: the *mucous membrane,* composed of ciliated and secretory columnar epithelium; the *musculature,* in which the inner layer is a circular arrangement of fibers and the outer layer is a longitudinal arrangement of cells; and the *serous layer,* which is covered with peritoneum.

The fallopian tubes provide the only connection between the uterus and the overies. Their primary function is ovum transport after ovulation and fertilization. Occasionally, the oviducts will become blocked or occluded because of infection, trauma, or abnormality. In such an event, infertility is likely to result because of the inability of the sperm and ovum to meet (see Chapter 27). The fallopian tubes are sometimes "tied" as a sterilization procedure (see Chapter 26).

The *uterus,* or womb, is a muscular organ whose size and shape in the nonpregnant state are similar

TABLE 4.1
A COMPARISON OF MALE AND FEMALE GONADS

Characteristics	*Female: Ovary*	*Male: Testes*
Appearance	Two slightly flattened, ovoid structures. Size varies: 2.5–5.0 cm long; 1.5–3.0 cm wide; 0.6–1.5 cm thick. Weighs 5–8 gm. Dull, white color; surface is somewhat nodular rather than smooth.	Two slightly flattened, ovoid shaped, structures. Approximately 5 cm long.
Location	Upper pelvic cavity; attached bilaterally to the pelvic wall by infundibulopelvic ligament and to the uterus by utero-ovarian ligament. Posteriorally it is attached by broad ligament.	Contained in the scrotum, a two-chambered pouch, located outside of the male pelvic cavity.
Histology	Consists of two sections: the *cortex,* or outer layer, contains ova surrounded by granulosa cells encompassed by theca interna and theca externa cells. Granulosa and theca interna cells produce ovarian hormones. The cortex also contains connective tissue cells and fibers. Thin, epithelium covering. The *medulla* (central portion) is made up of loose connective tissue, arteries, and veins; small number of smooth muscle fibers. Cells (hilus) similar to the interstitial cells of the testes, have been described. Blood supply is essentially from the ovarian vein and artery. Both sympathetic and parasympathetic nerves service the ovary.	Contains several different types of tissue to support production of sperm and of hormones. *Interstitial (Leydig's) cells* produce testosterone, necessary for spermatogenesis and male sexual capability and function. *Sertoli* cells line the seminiferous tubules; they are supportive cells and provide some nutrition for sperm. *Germinal epithelium* or *spermatogenic cells* line approximately 750 ft of seminiferous tubules. These cells produce sperm in an immature state.
Function	Production of ova (usually one mature ovum is released each menstrual cycle). Secretes two steroid hormones: *estrogen* and *progesterone.*	Production of spermatozoa. Millions of sperm are released with each male ejaculation. Secretes the male androgenic hormone, principally *testosterone.*

to a pear. The approximate dimensions of the uterus of a woman who has not been pregnant, a *nulligravida,* are 5.5–8.0 cm long, 3.5–4.0 cm wide at the top, and 2.0–2.5 cm thick; it weighs about 45–70 gm. The uterus of a nonpregnant woman who has borne a child, a *multigravida,* measures approximately 9.0–9.5 cm long, 5.5–6.0 cm wide, and 3.0–3.5 cm thick; it weighs about 50–80 gms. For a comparison of uterine sizes, see Figure 4.8.

The uterus contains a triangular-shaped cavity that is able to be distended. In nulligravidas, the anterior and posterior walls of the uterus bulge slightly inward almost touching, decreasing the uterine cavity to a narrow cleft. The cavity is larger in multigravidas.

The uterus is divided into two distinct parts: the *corpus,* or body, and the *cervix,* or neck. The corpus is often further divided into the *fundus,* or rounded upper top part of the uterus, located between the insertion of the fallopian tubes, the *main body,* which is between the oviduct insertions and the cervix, and the *isthmus,* the lowest part of the corpus just above the cervix. Clinically, these subdivisions, particularly the fundus and isthmus, have relevance during labor. The cervix is an elongated lower one-third of the uterus made up of connective tissue, some

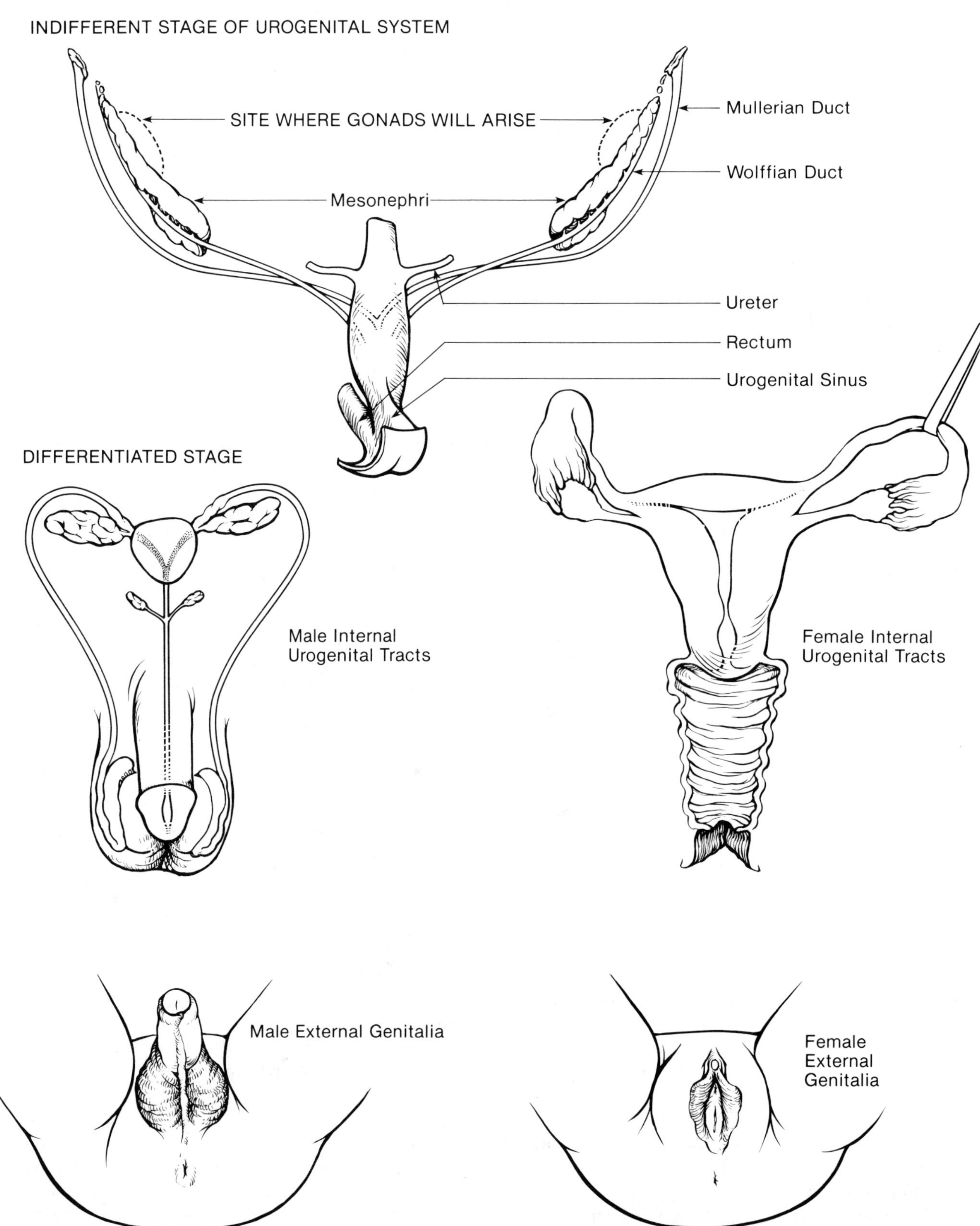

Figure 4.4
Differentiation of male and female genitalia during embryologic development.

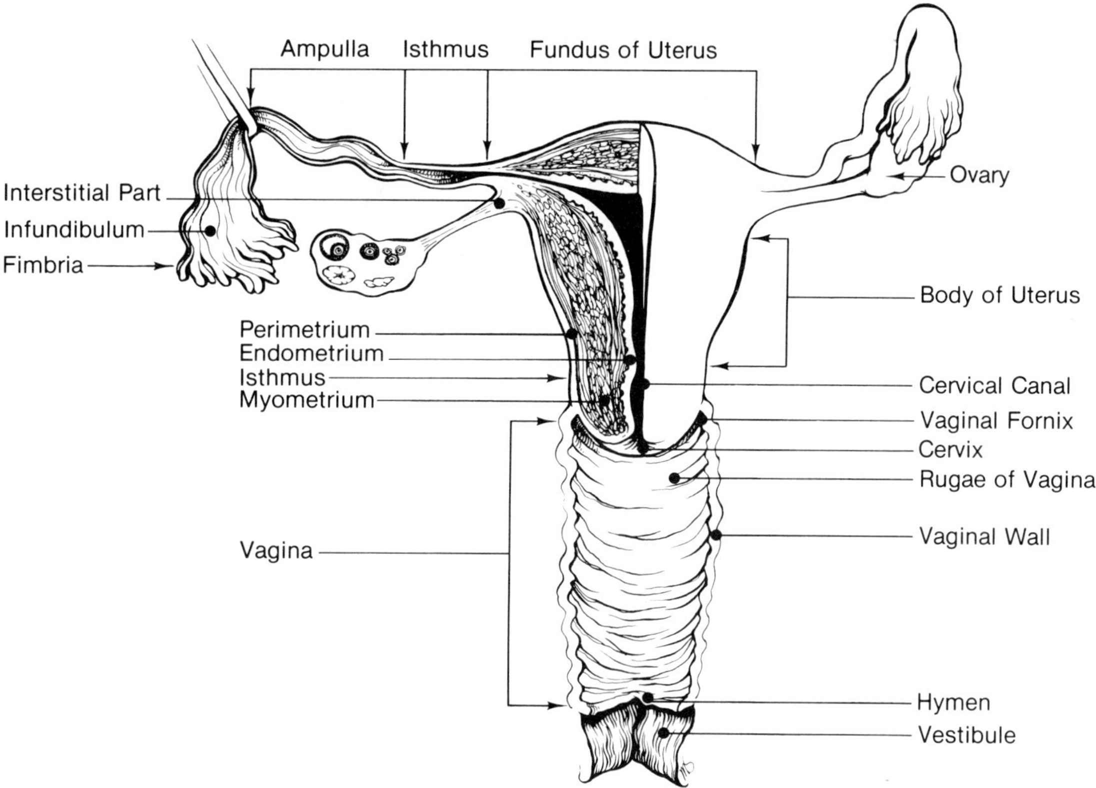

Figure 4.5
Frontal view of female internal reproductive system.

smooth muscle, large numbers of blood vessels, elastic tissue, and cervical mucosa composed of columnar epithelial and glandular cells. The columnar cells are mucoid secretory cells, and the squamous epithelium covers the cervix. The cervix has a pencil-slim canal that runs through its center and provides an opening to the vagina below and the corpus of the uterus above. The cervical canal has an external and internal os that can be differentiated only by its histology. The external os can be visualized by speculum exam through the vagina. The cervix is capable of effacing (thinning out) and dilating (opening) sufficiently to accommodate the body of a term infant.

Although the uterus is a pelvic organ, it connects with the peritoneal cavity through the lumina of the oviducts and with the distal end of the vagina through the cervix. The fundus is situated in the pelvic cavity in a slightly anteflexed position (bent forward) above the bladder and the corpus posteriorally. The rectum is posterior to the uterus.

Stability of the uterine position is possible because of direct and indirect soft tissue support provided by the pelvic ligaments and muscles. The ligaments directly supporting the uterus are the *broad ligaments,* the *round ligaments,* and a group of ligaments arising from connective tissue and fascia called the *pubocervical ligaments,* the *uterosacral ligaments,* and the *transverse ligaments of the cervix.* Muscular support comes from the *levator ani* and *coccygeus muscles,* the *urogenital diaphragm,* and the *perineal body.* (See the discussion on muscles and ligaments later in this chapter.)

The tissue layers of the uterus are similar to those of the oviducts. The serosal, or outer layer, essentially is made up of connective tissue covered with serosal cells and is called the *perimetrium* (not to be confused with the peritoneum, which covers the anterior and posterior parts of the uterus but is not a part of its structure). The muscle layer, or *myometrium,* contains smooth muscle cells interlaced in bundles. The inner layer, or *endometrium,* is a vascular layer that varies with cyclic changes during the menstrual cycle (see Chapter 5).

The uterus serves several purposes. During pregnancy, through cell hypertrophy and some hyperplasia, it can grow to a size that is adequate for the

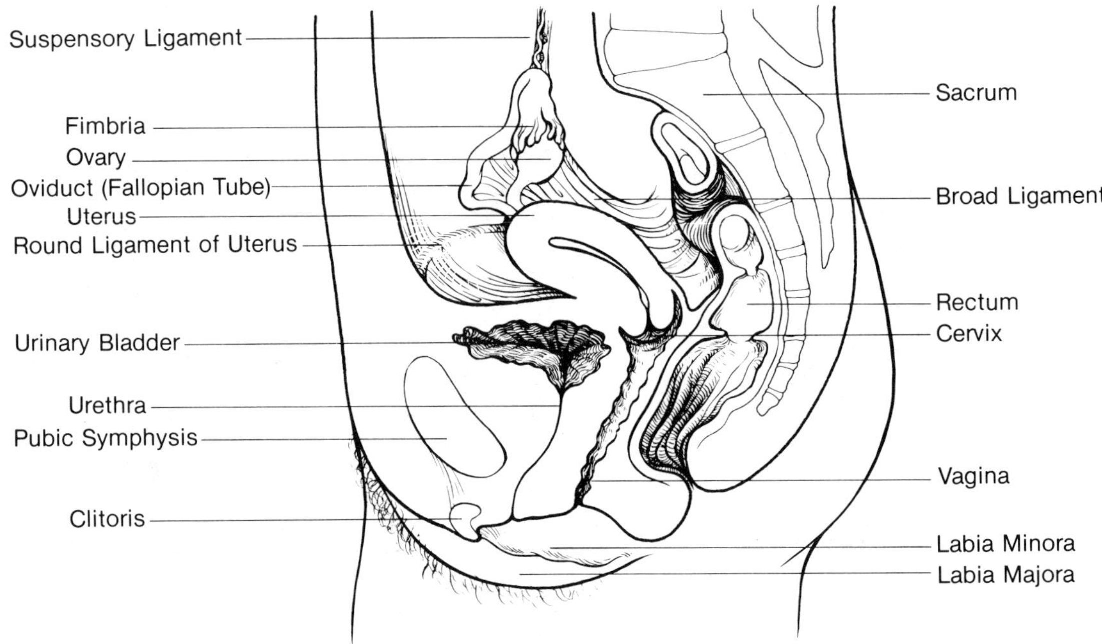

Figure 4.6
Sagittal view of the female reproductive system.

growing fetus. The uterine myometrium can contract with enough intensity to dilate and efface the cervix and, with the aid of the abdominal muscles, expel the fetus and placenta (afterbirth) during labor. It is the organ of *menstruation,* the cyclic shedding of the endometrium when fertilization has not occurred.

The *vagina* is a tubular structure with *rugae,* corrugated folds of tissue, enabling it to distend. Its anterior wall measures 6–8 cm, and its longer posterior wall is about 7–10 cm. The vagina is an integral organ linking the uterus with the vulva through an opening called the vaginal orifice. It lies between the bladder and the rectum. The end of the vagina near the uterus is a blind vault containing the lower part of the cervix. This distal end of the vagina, the *vaginal fornix,* has thin anterior and posterior walls that separate it from the peritoneal cavity.

The vagina is lined with stratified squamous epithelium. It contains large, flat surface cells with small nuclei and basal cells with large vesicular nuclei. The vagina is sensitive to stimulation by estrogen. The number of cells varies cyclically with the amount of estrogen produced by the ovaries.

Because of its distensibility, the vagina can enlarge to many times its original size, enabling it to serve as the birth canal for exit of the fetus during labor; it is the female copulatory organ, capable of receiving the penis in an erectile state; and it can tolerate the introduction of an instrument such as the vaginal speculum used during pelvic examination of the cervix. During the menstrual period, the vagina is the passage for release of menstrual blood.

There is an extensive vascular, lymphatic, and nerve supply to the female pelvic organs and structures. Major blood vessels abound; lymphatic vessels are readily available and are interspersed with lymph nodes. There is an abundant supply of both afferent and efferent autonomic nerves. The venous and lymphatic supply follows similar patterns.

Male Ductile System

The *epididymides* are narrow, oblong structures located along the superior posterior parts of each testicle. They appear as coiled tubes about 480 cm long with three distinct parts that differ in shape. The *globus majus,* or head, is the largest part; the *midportion* is a long narrow body; and the *globus minor,* or tail, appears as a pointed end. The tail lies

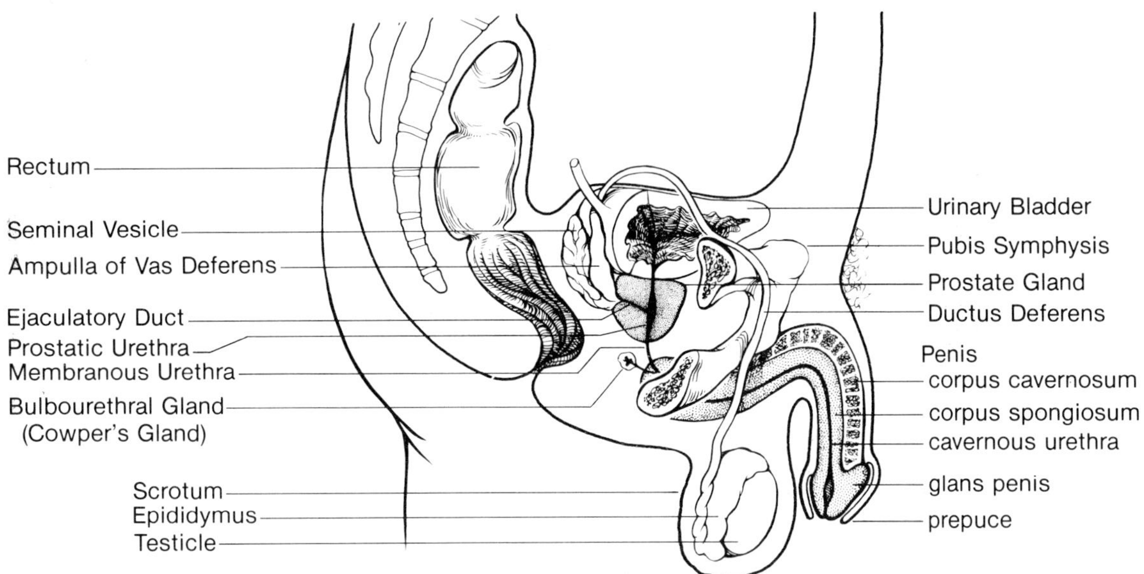

Figure 4.7
Sagittal view of male internal reproductive system.

alongside of the ductus deferens, while the head is attached to the testicle by 10–15 efferent ductules, connective tissue, and the tunica vaginalis that covers the testes and the epididymides. Pseudostratified epithelium lines the epididymides. The epididymides also contain smooth muscle and a rich vascular supply. Their function is the storage of spermatozoa before ejaculation. The environment provided by these structures can either encourage or deter the reproductive potential of the spermatozoa.

The *ductus deferens* (vas deferens) are the excretory ducts of the testes. These ducts are bilateral tubes approximately 35–45 cm long. They reach from the top of the epididymides to the seminal vesicles, look like elongated cylinders that are slightly larger at the inner end, and connect with the neck portion of the seminal vesicles forming the ejaculatory duct. The ductus deferens have an inner mucous layer, a muscular layer in the middle, and a fibrous outer layer. The part of the ductus known as the *ampulla* contains epithelial cells that have secretory capability, giving it a glandular function. The ductus deferens combines with blood and lymph vessels, as well as nerves, to form the spermatic cord. The principle functions of the ductus deferens are the storage and transport of the spermatozoa.

The *seminal vesicles* are two lobulated pouches of membrane. They each contain a coiled tube having several irregular diverticula. The proximal part of the tube merges with the ductus deferens, as mentioned earlier, to form the ejaculatory duct. The vesicles are made up of columnar epithelium and smooth muscle fibers. They secrete a thick fluid (*seminal fluid*) that is composed of fructose, ascorbic acid, potassium, bicarbonate, and a few proteins. Seminal fluid plays a role in nourishing the sperm and in aiding sperm transport. *Prostaglandins,* a derivative of long-chain polyunsaturated fatty acids, are also found in seminal fluid. Although the precise role of prostaglandins is not clear, they may play a role in penile erection, ejaculation, and sperm transport. They are also thought to play a role in the initiation of labor (see Chapter 16).

The *ejaculatory ducts* are two short tubes, about 2.5 cm long, that form a canal between the ductus deferens and the seminal vesicles. They penetrate the base of the prostate gland, descend through its lobes, and open into the urethra. The function of these ducts is to eject *semen*—a thick whitish fluid containing spermatozoa, nutrients, glandular secretions, and some epithelial cells—into the male urethra. The ejaculatory ducts form another section of the sperm transport mechanism, which aids the sperm in reaching its goal, the ovum.

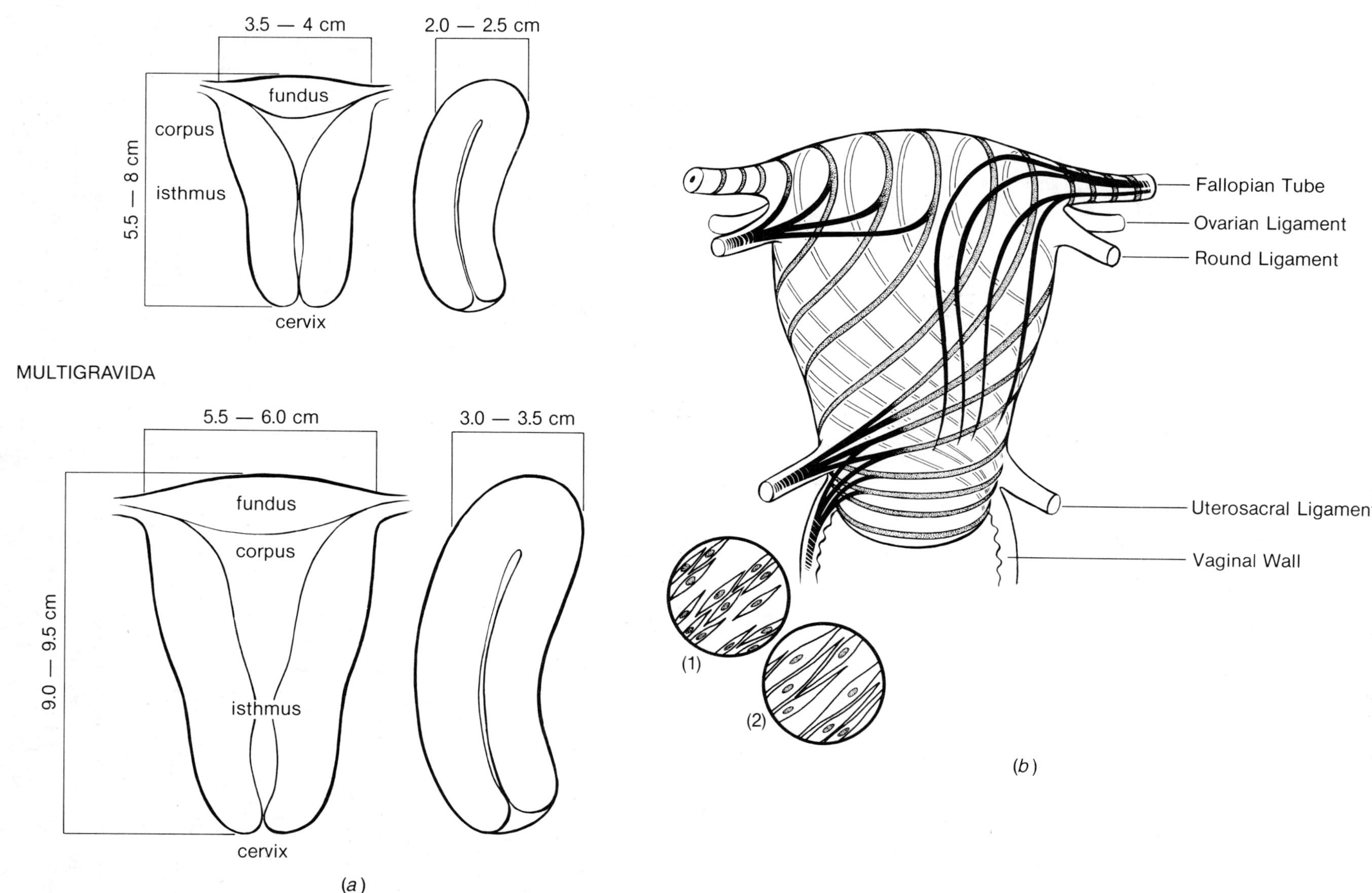

Figure 4.8
The uterus. *(a)* Comparison of nulligravid and multigravid uteri. *(b)* Uterine musculature and ligaments: (1) nonpregnant muscle cell; (2) muscle cell during pregnancy.

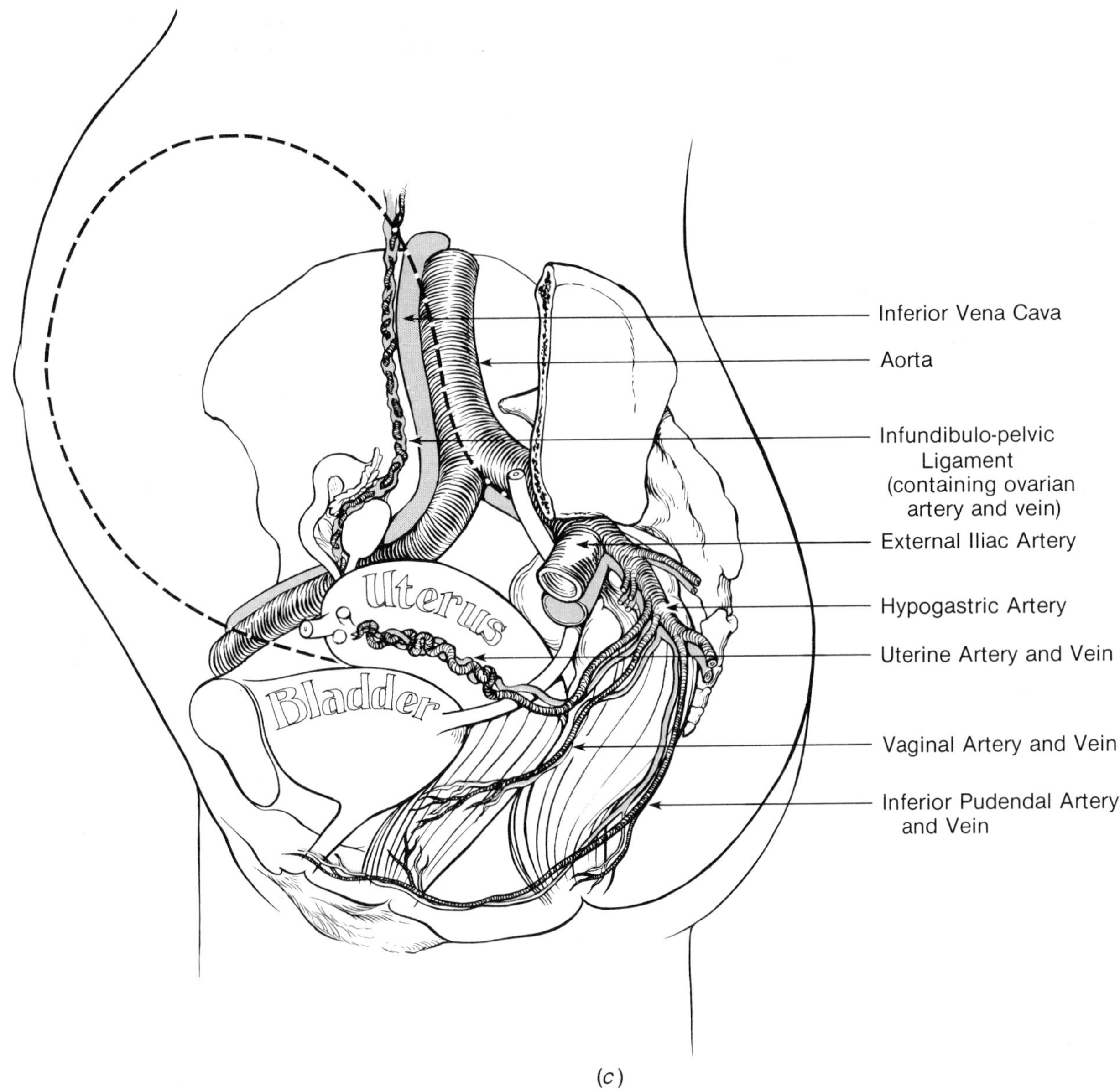

Figure 4.8 (continued)
(c) Blood supply to uterus.

GLANDULAR STRUCTURES

Both the male and female reproductive systems contain glandular structures, some serving an unclear function and others relating directly or indirectly to the reproductive process.

Female Glands

There are two types of glands in the female vulva. Two small *paraurethral ducts (Skene's glands)* are located near the urinary meatus. Skene's glands have a diameter of about 0.5 mm. They usually open via a duct on the vestibule on the sides of the urethra and occasionally open onto the posterior wall of the urethra just inside the urethral orifice. They serve no definitive purpose but may help control bacterial entry into the urethra and sometimes harbor gonococci. Skene's glands are the homologues of the male prostate gland.

Bartholoin's glands are located in the vestibule of the female vulva and lie in perineal tissue on each side of the vaginal opening (see the section, External Genitalia, in this chapter). They secrete a mucoid fluid that moistens the inner surface of the labia. These secretions increase during sexual excitement and lubricate the vaginal introitus, aiding the entry of the erect penis during *sexual intercourse.* Bartholin's glands are the homologues of the male bulbourethral glands.

Male Glands

The male has several sets of glands. The *prostate gland* is about the size of a chestnut, weighs about 20 gm, and contains one median and two lateral lobes. It is a musculoglandular organ, is located below the bladder, and encloses the urethra, which passes through its upper surface near the anterior border and exits near the apex. The prostate is penetrated by the two ejaculatory ducts. There are within it 30–50 tubuloalveolar glands that secrete a thin fluid that is added to the seminal fluid, diluting its viscosity and aiding sperm transport. This fluid is acidic and contains zinc, proteolytic enzymes, citric acid, and acid phosphotase. Fifteen to 30 ducts open from the prostate gland into the urethra.

The *bulbourethral glands (Cowper's)* look very much like two small brownish-yellow peas. They are located bilateral to the urethra and below the prostate gland. Their execretory duct runs alongside of the urethra (about 3–4 cm) and opens into it. The fluid secreted by these glands is alkaline, made up essentially of mucoproteins. This alkalinity may help to neutralize the acid secretions of the vagina, aiding sperm viability since an acid medium is lethal to the spermatozoa.

The male genital tract contains two other glands: the *urethral glands (Littre's),* which are multiple mucosal glands that open into the cavernous portion of the urethra, and the *preputial glands (Tyson's),* which are scattered over the prepuce of the penis, particularly in the region of the neck of the penis, and are similar in structure to the sebaceous glands of the skin. Neither the urethral glands nor the preputial glands have a known reproductive relevance.

EXTERNAL GENITALIA

The male and female external genitalia may be more familiar to you than are some of the other structures of the reproductive system. Therefore, they are presented here graphically with minimal discussion.

Female External Genitalia

The female external reproductive organs are often referred to as the *vulva,* a nonspecific structure that includes the mons pubis (also called the *mons veneris*), the labia majora and minora, the clitoris, and the vestibule, a triangular-shaped area that contains the urinary meatus, the paraurethral and vestibular glands, the vaginal orifice and the hymen (Fig. 4.9).

The *mons pubis* is the most anterior of the structures mentioned above. It is a soft, rounded mound of adipose tissue lying over the bony pubis symphysis, and covered with skin. Beginning with puberty, the mons pubis is first covered by a fine, sparse, straight hair, which then changes into coarse, kinky hair, increasing in amount and assuming the adult pubic distribution (see Chapter 8). The amount of hair decreases slightly after menopause. The mons pubis area contains sebaceous and sweat glands. It is not uncommon for women to develop infections of the hair follicles and glands in the mons pubis. This fatty mound is not found in males because of the absence of the hormone estrogen.

The labia contain two parts. The larger *labia majora* appear as two folds of fatty tissue covered with skin and hair and extend downward from the mons pubis to cover the labia minora and part of the vestibule. The edges of a labia majora may approach each other in the nulliparous adult, but they rarely do so in women who have borne a child. They are joined anteriorally but are separate posteriorally. Their male homologue is the scrotum. The *labia minora* are two smaller folds of connective tissue with numerous blood vessels and, unlike the labia majora, they are not covered with hair. They surround and partially cover the vestibular area. The labia minora join at the top, just above the clitoris, and form a structure called the *prepuce.*

The *clitoris* is the homologue to the male penis. It is a small projection shaped somewhat like a pea and forms the anterior apex of the vestibule. The clitoris is made up of erectile tissue and is greatly sensitive to tactile stimulation.

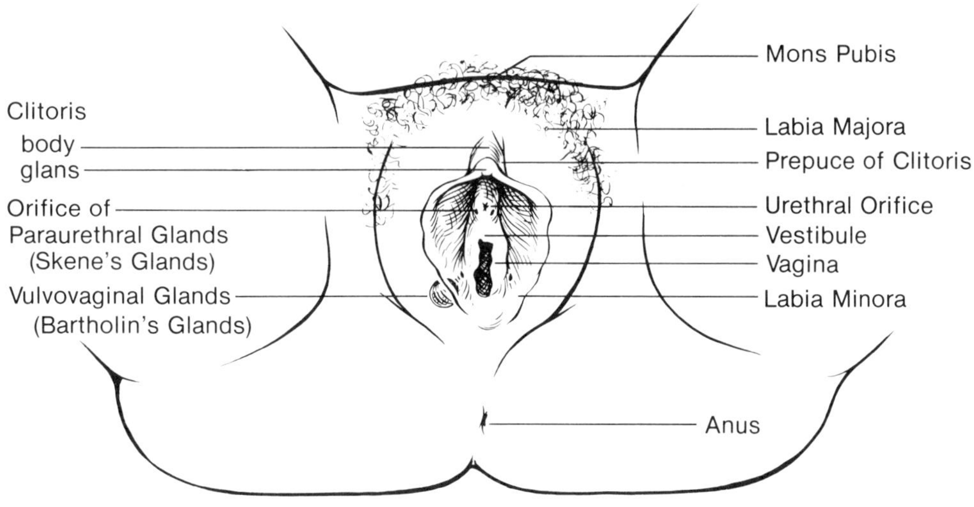

Figure 4.9
Female external genitalia.

The *vestibule* is a designated area in which the urinary and vaginal openings are located. The glandular structures adjacent to these openings are also included in the vestibule. The *vaginal orifice,* also called the *vaginal introitus,* is partially occluded by the *hymen,* a thin, sometimes tough fold of mucous membrane that is composed mostly of connective and elastic tissue and collagens. At one time the hymen was closely associated with the virgin state and was believed to be present in all women who had not experienced sexual intercourse. This has been found to be incorrect since it is absent in some virgin women as well. On occasion, the hymen may partially or totally occlude the vaginal opening. If the introitus is completely covered, the hymen is called an *imperforate hymen.* In such cases, the hymen must be surgically removed at or before puberty in order for menstrual flow to pass and for sexual intercourse to take place.

The *perineum* is the area bordered by the mons veneris anteriorally, the buttocks posteriorally, and the thighs laterally. The perineal soft tissues may be damaged during childbirth through abrasion or laceration.

Male External Genitalia

There are two external male reproductive organs, the scrotum and the penis. The *scrotum,* sometimes referred to as the *scrotal sac,* is a pouch that is suspended from the pubis and hangs behind the penis (Fig. 1.1). It is divided into two sections, with each compartment usually containing one testicle, epididymus, and part of one ductus deferens. During puberty, the scrotum, like the female labia majora, begins to be covered with fine, sparsely distributed hair. Its pigmentation increases and becomes darker than the rest of the skin. The scrotum is composed of subcutaneous tissue with some smooth muscle cells. In a relaxed state, its surface appears smooth; however, in a state of contraction, it takes on a wrinkled appearance. This contractile capability is present in order to protect the temperature-sensitive gonads and other structures from trauma. When the scrotum is exposed to low temperatures, the contraction pulls the sac and its contents closer to the body in order to warm it; when it is exposed to normal or increased body temperature, the tissue relaxes allowing the scrotal sac to hang away from the body. In addition to temperature, the scrotum and its contents are vulnerable to external trauma and pain from blows to the groin area.

The *penis* is an elongated, erectile organ suspended from the *urogenital diaphragm* (muscles of the male pelvic floor) and the anterior and lateral walls of the pubic arch (Fig. 4.10). It hangs just in front of the scrotum and is composed of three sections: the *root,* or proximal part attached to the pelvis; the *body,* an elongated structure containing three cylindrical parts (a paired *corpora cavernosa* and a single *corpus spongiosum*) encased in a fibrous capsule and bound to-

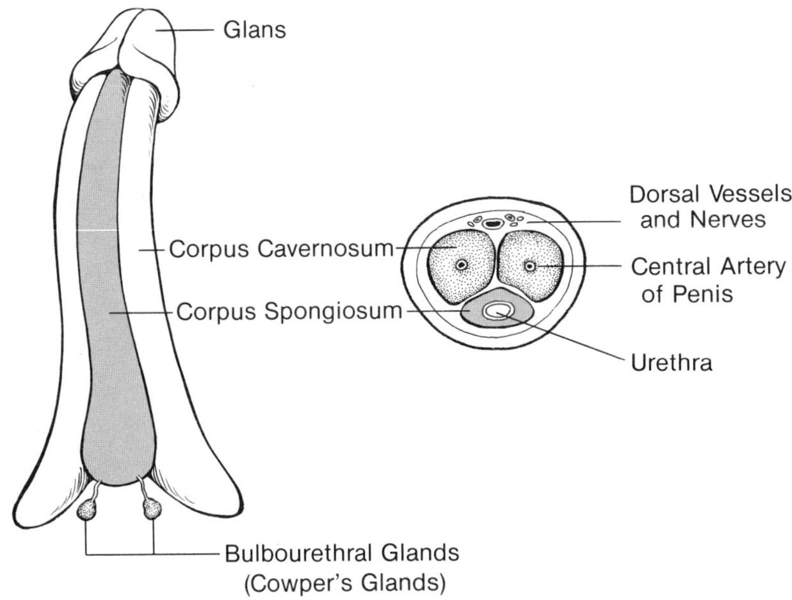

Figure 4.10
Sectional view of the penis.

gether by a sheath of connective tissue; and the *glans penis,* or distal tip of the penis. The penis is covered with skin.

The penis is composed essentially of erectile tissue, populated with multiple cavernous, vascular spaces. The corpora cavernosa is the most erectile tissue in the penis. During sexual excitement, the spaces become engorged with blood, enabling the penis to become turgid and erect. When the vascular spaces are filled, the blood causes them to expand and put pressure on the veins, constricting their lumen and preventing venous return, thus "trapping" or retaining the blood in the penis and keeping it in an erectile state. With decreased sexual excitement or release, the arteries constrict temporarily, preventing the entry of more blood, while the blood-filled cavities empty and the penis once more regains its flaccid state. Penile erection primarily is stimulated by the parasympathetic nerves and is inhibited by the sympathetic nervous system.

The *corpus spongiosum,* also called the *corpus cavernosum urethra,* lies between the two corpora cavernosa and somewhat toward the front of the penis. The male urethra is contained within the center of this structure and serves as a conduit for urine and semen.

The *glans penis* is made up of highly sensitive tissue similar to that of the clitoris. It is partly covered at birth by a fold of tissue, the foreskin or prepuce. In the normal state, this foreskin does not occlude the urinary meatus. If the opening of the foreskin is small and the tissue cannot be easily retracted over the glans, it is considered to be a condition called *phimosis. Circumcision,* surgical removal of part of the foreskin, is necessary when phimosis occurs in order to permit urination, allow for cleansing of the glans, and prevent infection. The glans contains the multiple preputial glands mentioned earlier. The secretions from these glands collect around and beneath the foreskin.

The penis has a dual function. It is the male copulatory organ, capable of erection and ejaculation of semen containing spermatozoa into the female vagina during sexual intercourse, and it is the male excretory organ for the elimination of urine.

ACCESSORY STRUCTURES

The Pelvis

Both the male and female pelves serve a supportive and protective role in regard to the reproductive organs. The male pelvis is not directly related to the reproductive process; it is discussed briefly in this section only to show a comparison to the female pelvis. The female pelvis, on the other hand, is of great significance to childbirth.

The adult bony pelvis is an articulated structure formed by four bones. Two *innominate bones* are located on each side of the pelvis and are joined, but not fused, in the front, creating the pubic arch (in childhood, the innominate bone was two separate bones, the *ilium* and the *ischium,* which fuse as physical maturity is reached), the coccyx, and the sacrum, which are found in the posterior portion of the pelvis. The pelvis is usually described as having two distinct parts—the upper, flared portion of the right and left innominate bones that creates the appearance of a basin or cradle and supports the abdominal organs, and the lower part, or cavity, that resembles a tube or cylinder.

COMPARISON OF THE MALE AND FEMALE PELVES

The male and female pelves differ in a number of ways (Fig. 4.11). The male pelvis is designed to support the greater weight of the male body. Its bones are heavier and more compact. There is less flaring of the tops of the innominate bones. The pelvic cavity and outlet (bottom) dimensions are less than that

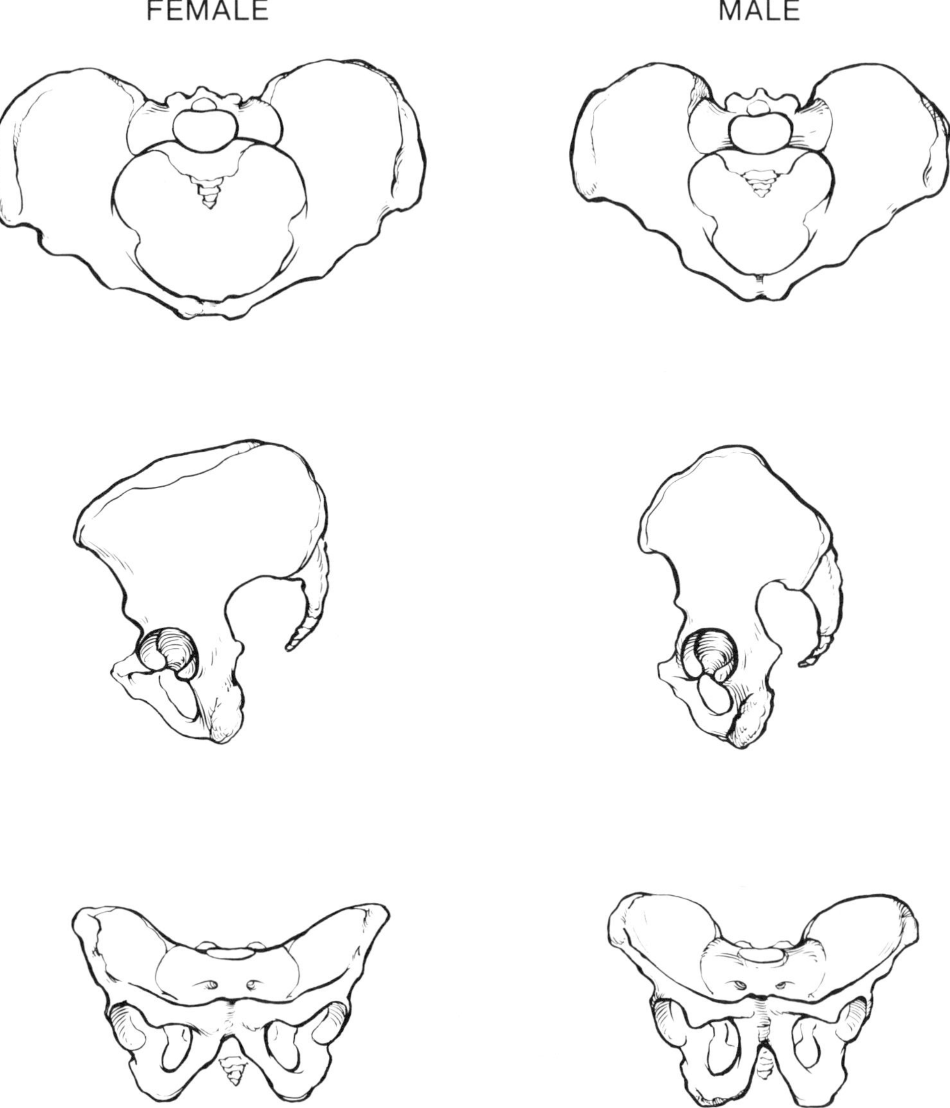

Figure 4.11
Comparison of male and female pelves—*top:* superior; *middle:* lateral; and *bottom:* frontal views.

of the female. The pubic arch is narrow. The sacrum is flatter, and the coccyx is less moveable. Its overall dimensions are less than those of the female pelvis.

The female pelvis, although it generally has larger overall dimensions than the male pelvis, weighs less, as do most of the bones in the female body. The upper parts of the innominate bones are more flared than those of the male pelvis; the pelvic inlet and cavity are larger; the pubic arch is wider; the curve of the sacrum is deeper; and the coccyx is moveable, thereby increasing the space at the pelvic outlet.

Functionally, the female pelvis is divided into two sections: The upper part is referred to as the *false pelvis* because it serves no obstetric purpose other than that of support of the gravid uterus. The lower part is referred to as the *true pelvis,* or obstetric pelvis, and is the birth canal through which the fetus must descend to be born (Fig. 4.12). The true and false pelves are separated by the upper pelvic brim, composed of the *linea terminalis,* the name given to the superior aspect of the pubis, and the sacral promontary. The cylindrical part of the female pelvis is the most important. This passageway must be compatible with the dimensions of the fetus if birth is to occur without complications. The flaring of the bones of the false pelvis and the tunnel appearance of the true pelvis make the pelvis resemble a funnel.

CHARACTERISTICS OF THE OBSTETRIC PELVIS

The *obstetric pelvis* is divided into three principle planes: the *pelvic brim,* or *inlet,* which is the uppermost part of the cylinder; the *cavity,* or *midplane;* and the *outlet* (see Figure 4.13 and Table 4.2). The pelvic inlet is significant because it is the point of entry of the fetus into the pelvic cavity. If for some reason the fetus cannot descend through this part, the birth canal cannot be negotiated, and the fetus must be delivered by a surgical procedure called *cesarean section* (see Chapter 22). The midplane of the pelvis is located about halfway down the cylinder at the level of two bony prominences called the *ischial spines.* The walls of the obstetric pelvis are almost straight; however, there is a slight convergence of the walls near where the ischial spines are located on each side of the pelvis. The spines jut out into the pelvic cavity, decreasing the dimensions of the pelvis. The pelvic outlet is the lowest part of the pelvis

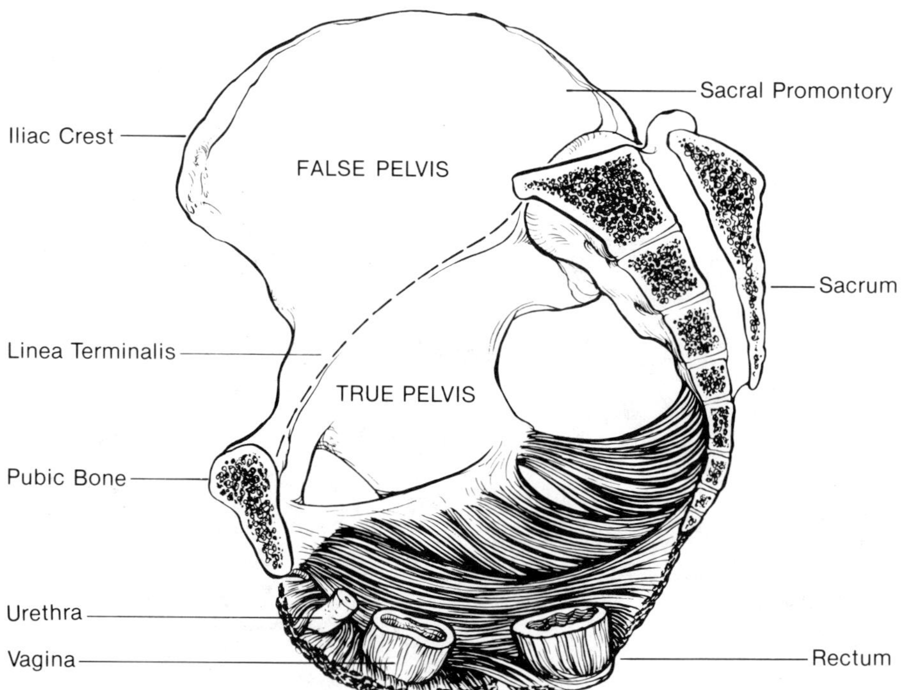

Figure 4.12
Female *true* and *false* pelves (saggittal view).

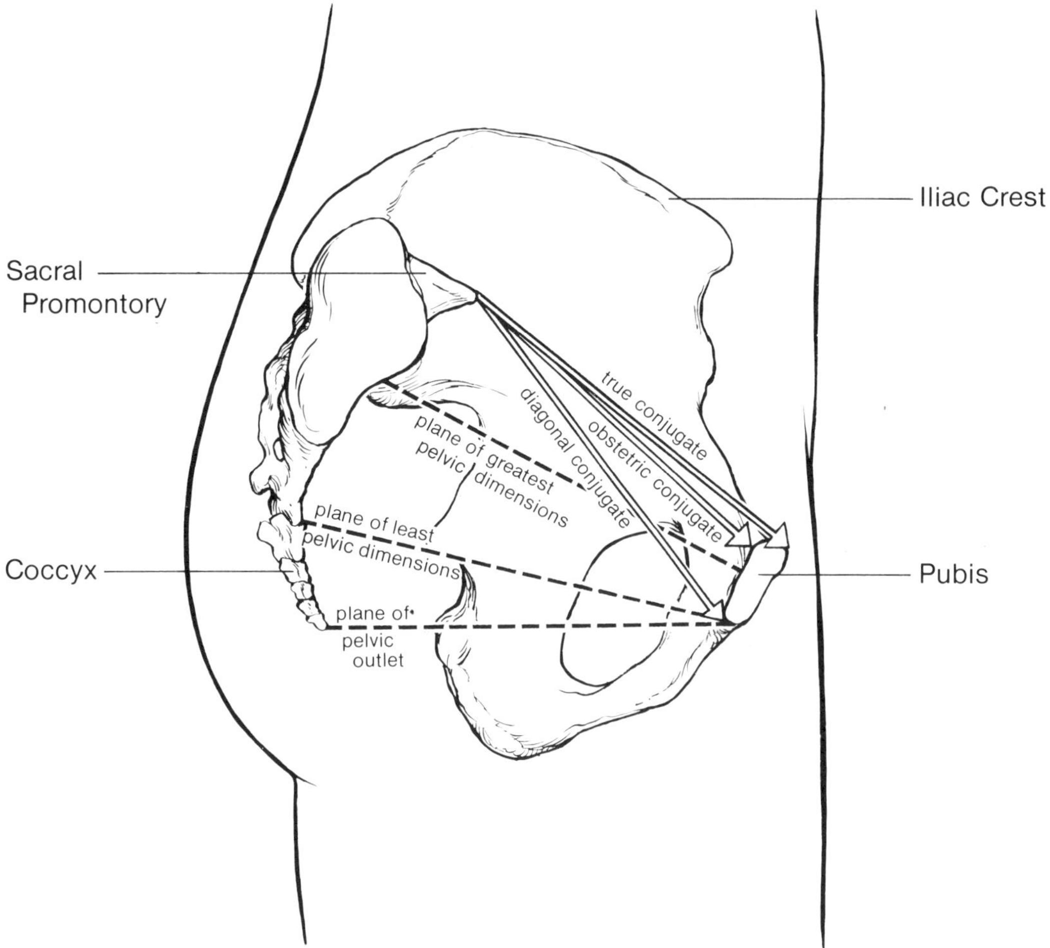

Figure 4.13
Planes of the female pelvis (saggittal view).

and has as its boundaries the pubic arch, anteriorally, the ischial tuberosities, laterally, and the sacrum and coccyx, posteriorally.

The shape of the pelvic inlet has led to distinct categories of classification of the female pelvis. The four basic classifications of the pelvis are the gynecoid (female type), the anthropoid (the name is derived from the anthropoid ape), the platypelloid (a flattened oval, named for the platypus), and the android (malelike) pelvis (Fig. 4.14). There are numerous variations of these pelvic types because of a multiplicity of factors such as sex, race, and general body size. The gynecoid pelvic shape is considered to be the "normal" shape of the female pelvis.

The classical *gynecoid* pelvic inlet is rounded in appearance when viewing it from the top of the pelvic cylinder. Its anterior–posterior diameter measures somewhat less than its transverse diameter. The walls of the pelvic cavity are essentially straight with some narrowing at the midplane. It has a deeply curved sacrum and an easily movable coccyx. The angle of the subpubic arch is wide, averaging 85 degrees. (See Fig. 4.15 for comparison of the angles of the male and female pubic arches.)

The *anthropoid* pelvic inlet appears more ovoid in shape. Its anterior–posterior dimension is slightly larger than its transverse diameter. Its side walls are essentially straight, and it is often narrow at the midplane, with the ischial spines prominent. The sacrum is straighter, longer, and narrower. The subpubic arch is more acute than in the gynecoid pelvis, usually less than an 85 degree angle.

The *platypelloid* pelvis looks like an elongated oval with a longer transverse diameter and a decreased

TABLE 4.2
FEMALE PELVIC PLANES

Pelvic Plane	*Description*	*Dimensions*	*Clinical Significance*
Plane of pelvic inlet: superior strait	Margins comprise upper boundary of true pelvis. Usually described as round with ovoid tendencies when looking into pelvic inlet from above. Four diameters considered to be significant.		Plane of pelvic inlet has obstetric significance because it is the entry point of the fetus into the true pelvis.
	ANTERIOR–POSTERIOR (AP) *Conjugata vera* uppermost AP measurement, but not narrowest. Measured from sacral promontory to center of top margin of symphysis pubis.	11.0 cm	Cannot be measured clinically. Becomes of clinical concern when the fetal presenting part fails to descend beyond this point. Can be measured by X-ray.
	Obstetric conjugate, mid-AP measurement. Measured form sacral promontory to greatest projection inward of midpoint of pubic bone.	10.6 cm	Smallest diameter of AP of pelvic inlet. Can be measured on X-ray, but its diameter can be roughly inferred by subtracting 1.5–2.0 cm from diagonal conjugate measurement.
	Diagonal conjugate, lowest AP diameter of inlet. Measured from sacral promontory in the posterior to the lowest margin of the junction of the pubic bones anteriorally.	12.5 cm	Can be estimated by manual pelvic examination and used to infer obstetric conjugate.
	TRANSVERSE Distance between lateral margins of pelvic inlet (linea terminalis).	13.5 cm	
	OBLIQUES (right and left) Distance between sacroiliac synchrondosis (posterior) to ileopectineal eminence diagonally to other side of pelvis.	12.75 cm	The diameters that usually accommodate fetal entry into pelvic inlet prior to internal rotation. Can be measured by X-ray.
Plane of midpelvis	Smallest plane of pelvis.		
	ANTERIOR–POSTERIOR Extends from the lower margin of the midpoint of the symphysis pubis to the fourth sacral vertebrae.	11.5 cm	
	TRANSVERSE Also called *bispinous* and *interspinous* diameters. Diameter estimated from one ischial spine across to ischial spine on opposite side of midpelvis.	10.0 cm	Smallest single diameter of the pelvis through which fetus must pass. Usual point of midplane arrest of fetal descent. Can be estimated on manual pelvic examination by describing characteristics of spines in terms of size, bluntness, or sharpness.
	POSTERIOR SAGITTAL Diameter is measured by estimating distance from imaginary point midway between ischial spines back to fourth to fifth sacral vertebrae.		Provides information about depth of posterior one-half of pelvic midplane.

Pelvic Plane	*Description*	*Dimensions*	*Clinical Significance*
Plane of greatest dimensions	Considered roomiest part of true pelvis. ANTERIOR–POSTERIOR Diameter from midpoint of pubic bone to junction of second and third sacral vertebrae. Other dimensions are not usually estimated.	12.5 cm	None.
Plane of pelvic outlet	Lower part of the true pelvis. ANTERIOR–POSTERIOR Diameter from inferior aspect of symphysis to tip of coccyx (anatomic AP).	9.5 cm	Significance of pelvic outlet is controversial because there are only a few cases of arrested fetal descent at this point. Soft tissue dystocia and/or a fractured coccyx may occur.
	Diameter from inferior aspect of symphysis to junction of sacrum and coccyx (obstetric AP).	11.5 cm	These measurements can easily be estimated clinically.
	TRANSVERSE Diameter between inner aspects of ischial tuberosities (bilateral).	11.0 cm	Combined measurements of transverse and posterior sagittal are sometimes considered to be of clinical importance, with any combined measurement of less than 15 cm being reason for concern.
	POSTERIOR SAGITTAL Diameter from imaginary midpoint of transverse to junction between sacrum and coccyx (obstetric) or tip of sacrum if movable (anatomic).	9.5 cm 7.5 cm	

Source: Adapted from Butnarescu, G. F. *Perinatal Nursing, Vol. I—Reproductive Health.* New York: John Wiley & Sons, 1978, pp. 95–96. Used with permission.

anterior–posterior measurement. The anterior–posterior margins appear to have been pushed together somewhat. It has shorter but straighter side walls, with a wide transverse diameter of the midplane. Ischial spines are less prominent, even blunt. The pubic arch is wide (the angle is much greater than 90 degrees), and the sacrum is wide with a deep curve.

The *android* pelvis has a narrow anterior–posterior diameter as well as a decreased transverse diameter. Its overall inlet measurements are less than the other types. It has a pronounced sacral promontory, and the narrow transverse diameter comes together to form a pseudoapex at the superior part of the midpubis, giving the inlet the appearance of a heart. Its cavity has deep side walls that converge at the midplane, where prominent ischial spines contribute to decreasing this already smaller bispinous diameter. The subpubic arch is narrow with an average measurement of 53 degrees. The sacrum tends to be flat, and the coccyx is less movable.

The shape of a pelvis is usually consistent in all of its planes. For example, the gynecoid pelvis is more likely to have adequate dimensions throughout, whereas the android pelvis will tend to be inadequate at all planes. Occasionally one plane will be contracted and the other dimensions adequate. The most common point of pelvic contraction is in the midplane of the pelvic cavity. Knowledge of pelvic morphology is not a precise predictor of labor outcome, but it provides some general guidelines for planning. The landmarks of the bony pelvis also provide help in evaluating fetal descent during labor.

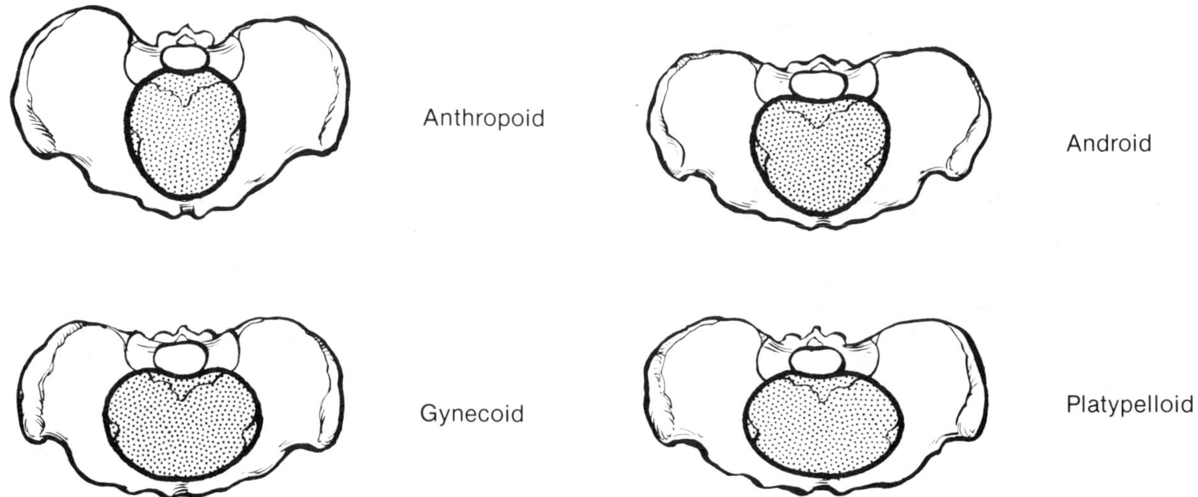

Figure 4.14
Classification of female pelvis by inlet shape.

The pelvis accounts for some of the minor birth traumas to the infant.

PELVIC SOFT TISSUE

There are numerous muscles and ligaments that are the soft tissues of the female pelvis (Figs. 4.16–4.18). These tissues not only serve as a support for the pelvic viscera, but they also anchor the internal female reproductive organs in the pelvis, soften the bony surface of the pelvis as the fetus travels through the birth canal, and aid or impede the process of labor. The most important of these structures are presented in Tables 4.3 and 4.4, with comments about their reproductive relevance.

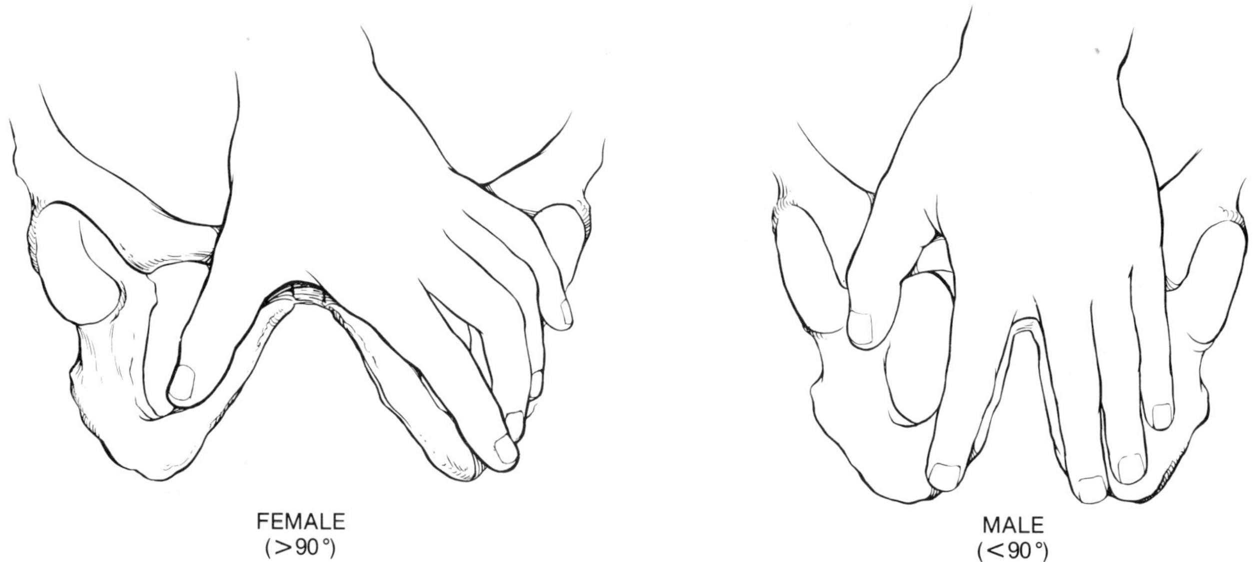

Figure 4.15
Comparison of angle of female and male pubic arches. Adapted from Smout, C. F. V, and F. Jacoby. *Gynaecological and Obstetrical Anatomy and Functional Histology.* Baltimore: Williams & Wilkins, 1953, 3rd ed.

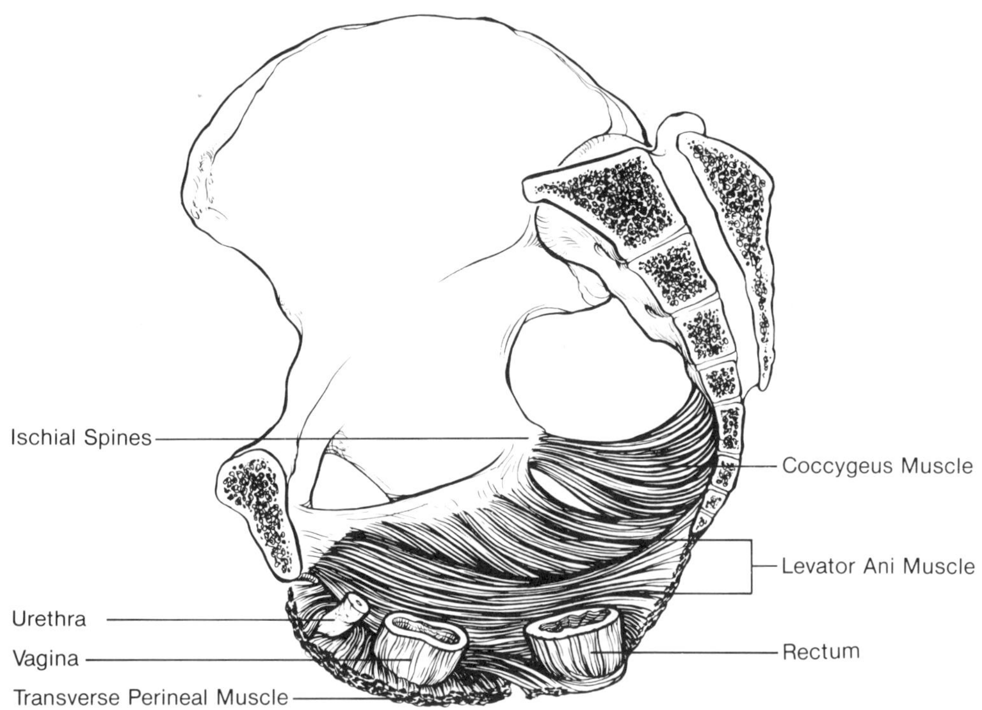

Figure 4.16
Sagittal view of female pelvis showing innominate bone and muscles.

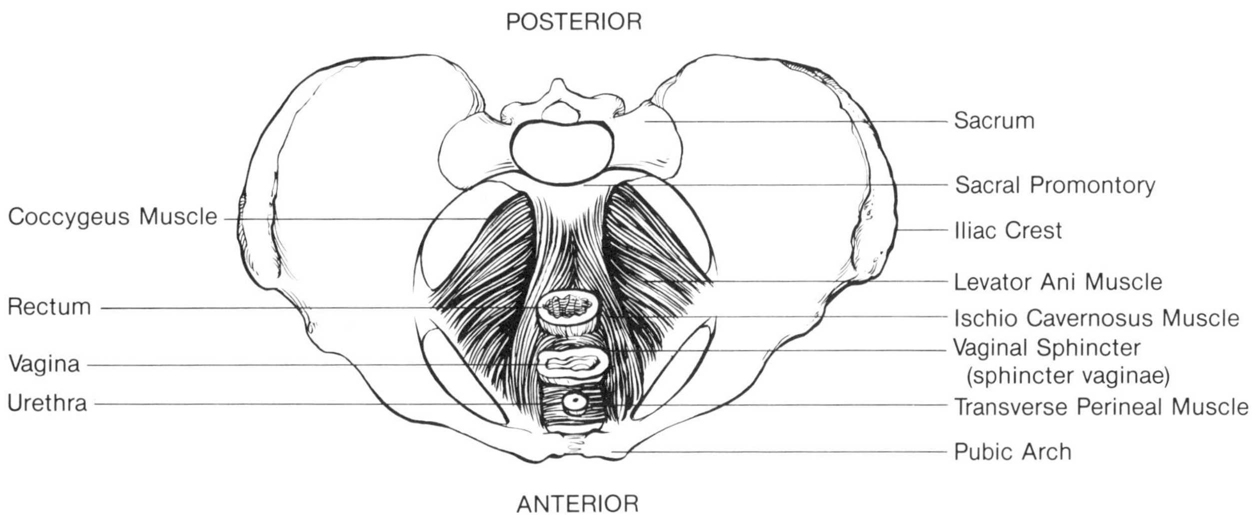

Figure 4.17
Superior view of female pelvis with pelvic floor muscles.

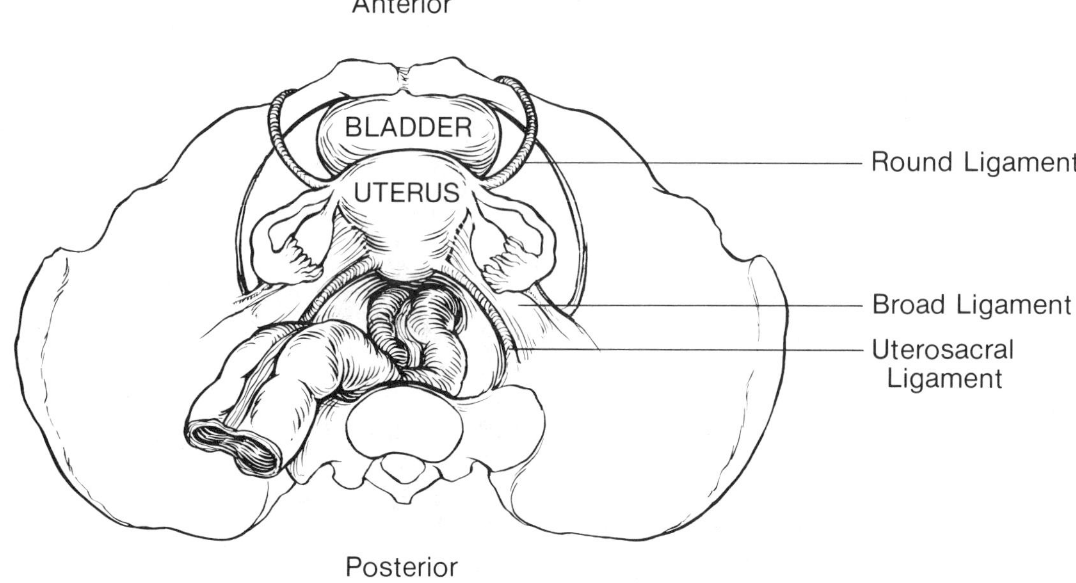

Figure 4.18
Ligaments of the female pelvis (superior view).

The Mammary Glands

The *mammary glands,* or *breasts,* are present in both the male and female. They derive from the embryonic ectoderm and appear in primitive form as early as the sixth or seventh week of prenatal life. Although they continue to develop during the fetal period and appear at birth as small breast buds and nipples, the breasts remain in a rudimentary stage of development throughout childhood. Both the male and female mammary glands will mature under hormonal stimulation; however, adequate internal stimulation is absent in the normal adolescent and adult man. The male breasts remain as nonfunctional organs throughout life. At puberty there is adequate endocrine support for the development of the female mammary glands. During this period, the breasts take on adult female characteristics. The breasts are considered to be accessory reproductive organs since they serve no direct reproductive function. Only the adult female mammary glands are discussed here.

The breasts appear externally as two convex structures arising bilaterally from the chest, anterior to the pectoral muscle (Fig. 4.19). Each breast extends from the right or left margin of the sternum laterally to the anterior border of the axilla. Each is covered by soft, smooth skin except for its center, where two areas of darker pigmented skin are found. The outer area of the center portion is called the *areola;* it is a circular area that contains numerous small nodular protrusions, which in turn contain *sebaceous glands,* called *Montgomery's tubercles.* The areola, which varies in size with each person, has an diameter of 2.5 in. The nipple rises from the center of the areola. It contains some smooth muscle and is capable of erection when stimulated. The nipple also has many nerve endings that transmit impulses to the hypothalamus and to the posterior pituitary gland causing it to release a hormone called *oxytocin.* This hormone is important for lactation since it causes the myoepithelial cells of the breast to contract and release milk. There are 15–20 small openings in the nipple through which milk is excreted during lactation.

Internally, each breast is made up of 15–20 lobes of glandular tissue surrounded by fatty and connective tissues. These lobes lie radially within the breast converging toward its center. Each lobe has a duct, the *lacteriferous duct,* that is lined with milk-producing epithelial cells called *acini cells.* This duct enlarges just beneath the areola and forms a milk-collecting sinus or reservoir called *ampulla.* Each ampulla connects with an opening in the nipple, completing the excretory route for the milk produced during lactation (Fig. 4.20).

TABLE 4.3
MUSCULATURE OF THE FEMALE PELVIS

	Characteristics				
Structure	*Description*	*Muscle and Origin*	*Insertion*	*Innervation*	*Reproductive Relevance*
Pelvic diaphragm	Usually described as resembling a sling because of its appearance when viewed from above. Contains pubic and iliac portions. Pubic portion encircles rectum and part of vagina; iliac portion arises on either side of pelvis. In most places, 3–5 mm thick.	LEVATOR ANI From pelvic surface of ischial spines and internal obturator fascia.	Midpoint of perineum anococcygeal, and coccyx.	Fourth sacral nerve; pudendal nerve.	Supports pelvic organs and gravid uterus.
		ILIOCOCCYGEAL Posterior part of levator ani, forward to obturator canal.	Lateral to coccyx and anococcygeal body.	Femoral nerve.	Supports and protects vagina, rectum, and urethra.
		PUBOCOCCYGEAL Anterior part of levator ani, in front of obturator canal.	Anococcygeal body and side of coccyx.		Constricts vagina and rectum forming a functional rectal sphincter. Can be lacerated during labor.
		PUBORECTALIS Part of pubococcygeus but with more lateral origin from pubic bone.	Posterior with corresponding muscles on opposite side.		
		COCCYGEUS Ischial spines and lesser sacrosciatic ligament.	Side border of lower sacrum and upper coccyx.	Third and fourth sacral nerves.	
Urogenital diaphragm	Usually described as a triangle lying between pubic arch and a line contiguous with ischial tuberosities.	DEEP TRANSVERSE PERINEAL Ischium; inferior ramus.	Medium raphe of perineum.	Pudendal nerve.	Supports upper part of urethra; aids in promoting urinary continence; often the site of trauma during childbirth leading to urinary retention because of edema immediately following delivery; weakening of musculature resulting in stress, incontinence or urethrocele.

TABLE 4.3 (continued)

Structure	Characteristics: Description	Characteristics: Muscle and Origin	Characteristics: Insertion	Characteristics: Innervation	Reproductive Relevance
Perineal body	Base of pelvis at which bulbo-cavernosus, superficial, transverse and external anal sphincter converge.	BULBOCAVERNOSUS Midpoint of perineum.	Fascia of clitoris.	Pudendal nerve.	Force of resistance during labor. Often lacerated at time of delivery of fetus.
		SUPERFICIAL TRANSVERSE PERINEAL Ischial tuberosity.	Central tendon of perineum.	Pudendal nerve—perineal branch.	
		EXTERNAL ANAL SPHINCTER Tip of coccyx.	Center of perineal tendon.	Fourth sacral nerve. Inferior hemorrhoidal nerve.	

Source: Butnarescu, G. F. *Perinatal Nursing, Vol. I—Reproductive Health.* New York: John Wiley & Sons, 1978, pp. 92–93. Used with permission.

TABLE 4.4
LIGAMENTS OF THE FEMALE PELVIC

Structure	Characteristics: Description	Characteristics: Function	Reproductive Relevance
Broad ligaments	Two large folds of peritoneum resembling wings that are attached bilaterally to uterus and extend to the pelvic wall. Margins of the broad ligaments are as follows:		None
	▲ ***Sides.*** Peritoneum.		
	▲ ***Base.*** Parallels the pelvic floor connective tissue.		
	▲ ***Midportion.*** Cardinal ligament is fixed to supravaginal portion of cervix and side of uterus.		
	▲ ***Inner Aspects.*** Superior two-thirds from mesosalpinx and is attached to fallopian tube, surrounds lower part of ureters and uterine vessels.		
	▲ ***Outer Aspects.*** Infundibulopelvic (suspensory) ligament extends from ovarian end of tube to pelvic wall. Layers of peritoneum with loose connective tissue in small amounts. Vessels. Parovarium with tubules (vertical). Lined with ciliated epithelium.	Anchors and stabilizes ovary. Carries the ovarian vessels to the ovary.	
Round ligaments	Bilateral ligaments located on each side of uterus just below insertion of fallopian tubes. Parallels broad ligament upward toward inguinal canal. Terminates in upper portion of the labia majora. Diameter is 3–5 mm. Composed of smooth muscle and connective tissue.	Positions and stabilizes uterus in antiflexed position.	May play a part in alignment of uterus for descent of fetus. Hypertrophy during pregnancy. Sometimes the site of "side" pain felt during pregnancy.
Uterosacral ligaments	Bilateral ligaments that originate in posterior and upper portion of cervix and vagina and around rectum, and inserts at second and third sacral vertebrae. Lateral boundaries for the cul-de-sac of Douglas.	Exerts traction on the uterus to help position it.	None

TABLE 4.4 (continued)

Structure	Characteristics: Description	Characteristics: Function	Reproductive Relevance
Sacrosciatic ligament	Bilateral ligaments extending from sacrum to ischium. Anterior or lesser is called sacrospinous ligament.		Serves as landmark for determining depth of posterior saggital of midpelvis. Can be felt on bimanual pelvic exam. *Pudendal block* is done in relation to this ligament.

Source: Adapted from Butnarescu, G. F. *Perinatal Nursing, Vol. I—Reproductive Health.* New York: John Wiley & Sons, 1978, p. 94. Used with permission.

The breasts remain essentially unchanged in the absence of pregnancy or exogenous hormonal stimulation. There are some changes associated with the menstrual cycle such as a slight increase in size just before menstruation and feelings of tightness, fullness, tenderness, or pain. These changes are associated with the high levels of estrogen and progesterone that promote the limited development of the ductile and glandular systems, respectively, during each cycle. Edema of the connective tissue, possibly as a result of influence of the hormone progesterone, has been noted. These cyclic changes regress after menstruation (see Chapter 5).

The breasts undergo great change during pregnancy in preparation for the production and release of milk to nourish the newborn infant. (See Chapter 19 for a discussion of lactation.) Pathophysiology affecting the endocrine function of the body will affect the breasts, and the breasts are a site for cancer (see Chapter 27).

SUMMARY

The physical basis for developmental readiness for reproduction was discussed using selected material from reproductive anatomy and physiology to compare the similarities and differences in the reproductive capability of the male and female. Special attention was given to the male and female internal and external reproductive organs and to accessory structures such as the pelvis and the breasts. This information is used by the maternity nurse in cooperation with other health care providers to assess physical readiness of men and women for their reproductive functions. It also provides the foundation for much of the health care appropriate during pregnancy, childbirth, and recovery.

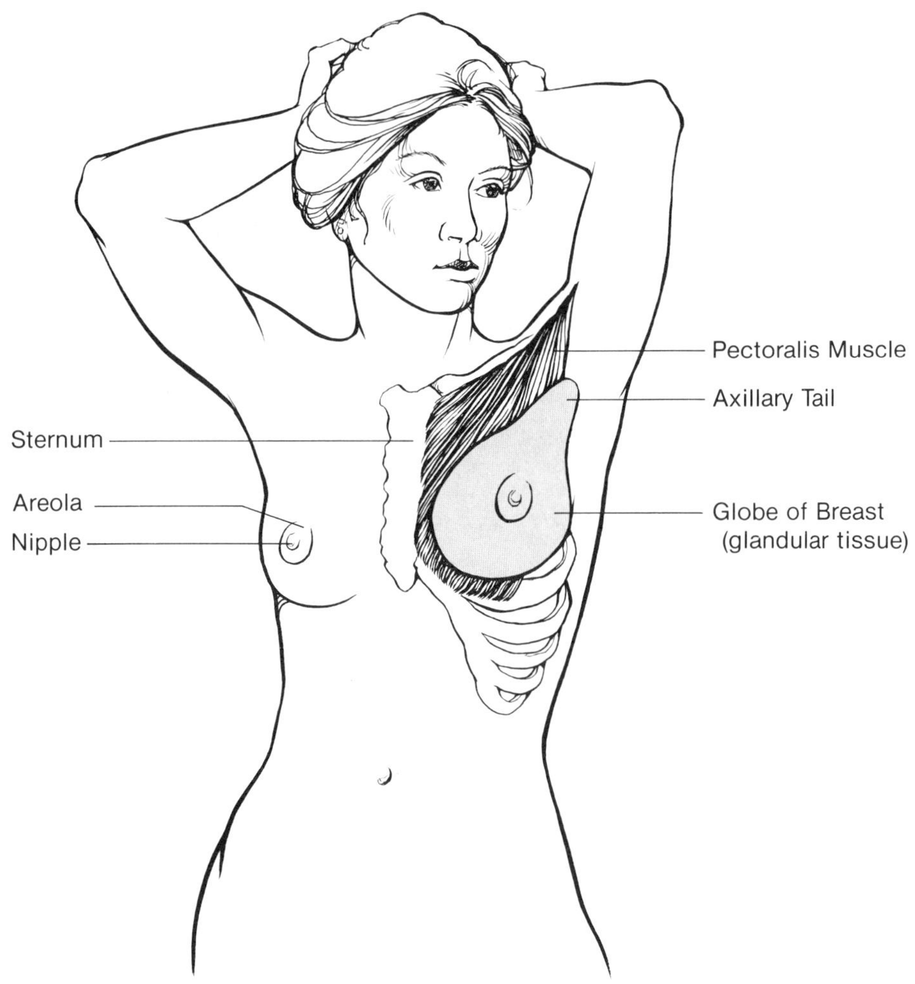

Figure 4.19
Frontal view of breast.

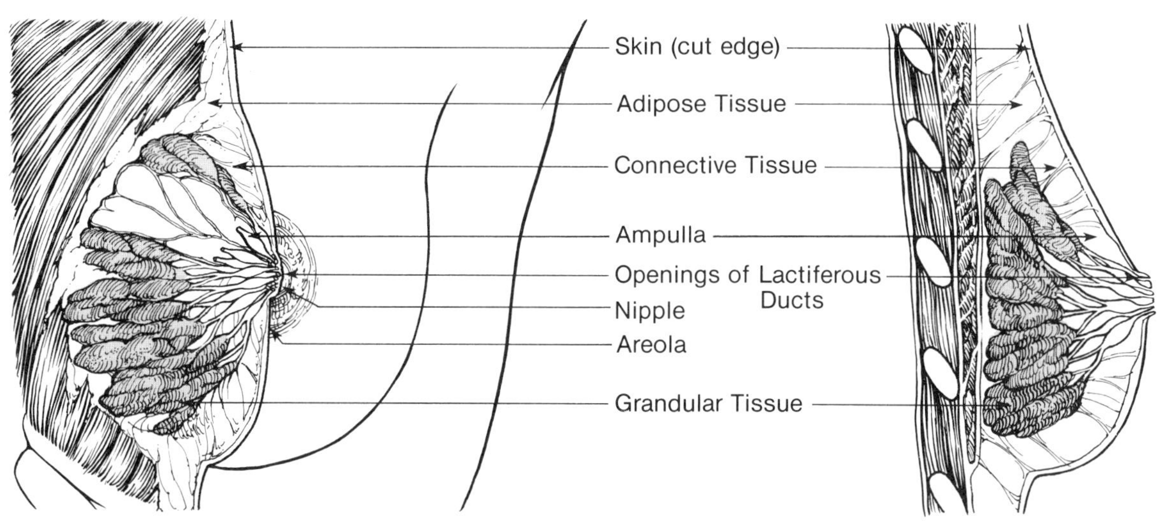

Figure 4.20
Cross section of breast. *Left:* frontal view; *right:* saggital view.

REFERENCES AND READINGS

Allen, E., Pratt, J. P., Newell, U. U., Bland, L. J. Human Tubal Ova; Related Early Corpora Lutea and Uterine Tubes. *Contrib Embryol* 22:45, 1930.

Baker, T. G. A Quantitative and Cytologic Study of Germ Cells in Human Ovaries. *Proc R Soc Lond (Biol.)* 1958:417, 1963.

Butnarescu, G. F. *Perinatal Nursing, Volume I—Reproductive Health.* New York: John Wiley & Sons, 1978.

Ciccarese, S., Ohno, S. Two Plasma Membrane Antigens of Testicular Sertoli Cells and H-2 Restricted Vs. Unrestricted Lysis by Female T Cells. *Cell* 13:643, 1978.

Grollman, S. *The Human Body: Its Structure and Function* (4th ed.). New York: MacMillan, 1978.

Guyton, A. C. *Textbook of Medical Physiology* (5th ed.). Philadelphia: W. B. Saunders, 1976.

Huff, R. W., Pauerstein, C. J. *Human Reproduction, Physiology and Pathophysiology.* New York: John Wiley & Sons, 1977.

Jacob, S. W., Francone, C. A., Lossow, W. W. *Structure and Function in Man* (4th ed.). Philadelphia: W. B. Saunders, 1978.

Ohno, S. Major Regulatory Genes for Mammalian Sexual Development. *Cell* 7:315, 1976.

Page, E. W., Villee, C. A., Villee, D. B. *Human Reproduction—The Core Content of Obstetrics, Gynecology and Perinatal Medicine* (2nd ed.). Philadelphia: W. B. Saunders, 1976.

Pritchard, J. A., MacDonald, P. C. *Williams Obstetrics* (16th ed.). New York: Appleton-Century-Crofts, 1980.

Smout, C. F. V., Jacoby, F., Lillie, W. W. *Gynecologic and Obstetric Anatomy: Descriptive and Applied* (4th ed.). Baltimore: Williams & Wilkins, 1969.

Spence, A. P., Mason, E. B. *Human Anatomy and Physiology.* Menlo Park, Calif.: Benjamin/Cummings, 1979.

Steinberger, A., Steinberger, E. *Testicular Development: Structure and Function.* New York: Raven Press, 1979.

Vander, A. J., Sherman, J. H., Luciano, D. *Human Physiology—The Mechanisms of Body Function* (2nd ed.). New York: McGraw-Hill, 1975.

Wachtel, S. S., Ohno, S., Koo, G. C., Boyce, E. A. Possible Role for the H-Y Antigen in the Primary Determination of Sex. *Nature* 257:235, 1975.

5

ENDOCRINE CONTROL OF REPRODUCTIVE READINESS

Mature reproductive endocrine function manifests itself at puberty, the developmental point in time at which a person becomes capable of producing offspring. As previously discussed, there is some endocrine function demonstrated during intrauterine life associated with the sexual differentiation of the male and female reproductive systems. From birth throughout childhood, changes in the reproductive systems of both the male and female are minimal or absent, most likely because the endocrine physiology that supports the reproductive processes is also minimal or absent. Before the clinical manifestations of puberty, endocrine changes that involve one of the most intricate communication networks in the human body begin to occur. This communication network is the interaction among the hypothalamus, the anterior pituitary gland, and the male and female gonads. It is this interplay that governs the reproductive function of the woman through menopause and of the man throughout his adult lifetime.

HYPOTHALAMUS–PITUITARY–GONADAL AXIS

Hypothalamic Hormones

The hypothalamus is located in the lower part of the brain and forms the floor and a section of the lateral wall of the third ventricle. The lowest part of the hypothalamus, the base that lies in closest proximity to the pituitary gland, is called the *median eminence.* In the 1940s, it was found that the hypothalamus contained a group of specialized neurosecretory cells that synthesized and secreted hormones. These hormones, called releasing factors (RF), have a stimulatory or inhibitory effect on the anterior pituitary gland. They are discharged in the median eminence and picked up by an extensive capillary network that empties into the *hypothalamic–hypophyseal portal vascular system.* The portal vessels pass through the pituitary stalk connecting the base of the hypothalamus to the pituitary gland (Fig. 5.1). This short circulatory connection is one of the most important transport mechanisms in the body. The releasing factors stimulate the anterior pituitary gland to secrete a number of tropic hormones that act on other body structures or organs (Fig. 5.2). You are already familiar with hormones, such as the thyroid stimulating hormone (TSH), which provokes the thyroid gland to secrete thyroxin; the adrenocortocotrophic hormone (ACTH), which is the impetus for the adrenal cortex to produce cortisol; and the growth hormone (GH), also called somatotropic hormone (SH), which is well known for its effect on the development and function of many body organs and tissues. Less familiar, however, may be three other major anterior pituitary hormones—the gonadotrophic hormones; which are *follicle stimulating hormone (FSH), luteinizing hormone (LH),* and *prolactin.* A releasing factor has been identified for each of the major anterior pituitary hormones except gonadotrophins. A single releasing factor, *gonadotrophin releasing factor (GnRF),* also called *luteinizing hormone releasing hormone (LHRH)* and *luteinizing releasing factor (LRF),* is believed to stimulate the production of both FSH and LH.

The hypothalamic hormones are controlled both by internal and external factors. Internally, they are monitored by the central nervous system through the mechanisms that arise in other parts of the brain and that stimulate and inhibit them. Externally, they are influenced by the steroid hormones produced by the gonads, which have an inhibitory feedback effect upon the brain. This stimulatory–inhibitory check and balance is cyclic for the female and is sustained in the male. The mechanisms for the synthesis and release of hypothalamic hormones is highly sensitive to many factors. Disruption at any point will affect the total interrelationship. For example, if there is an interruption in the production of gonadal steroid hormones, there will be decreased inhibitory feedback to the brain. Central nervous system pathophysiology or trauma will also affect this mechanism. Extreme stress associated with emotional or physical upheaval will interfere with this precise interaction. And, of course, the events of conception and pregnancy reorder the functioning of this system.

Pituitary Hormones

The pituitary gland, called the *hypophysis,* is a small but powerful organ located just below the hypothalamus at the base of the brain. It is approximately 1 cm in diameter, weighs about 0.5 gm, and is divided by the *pars intermedia* into two separate lobes, the *adenohypophysis,* or anterior lobe, and the *neurohypophysis,* or posterior lobe. The adenohypophysis secretes the three gonadotrophic hormones mentioned earlier: FSH, LH, and prolactin.

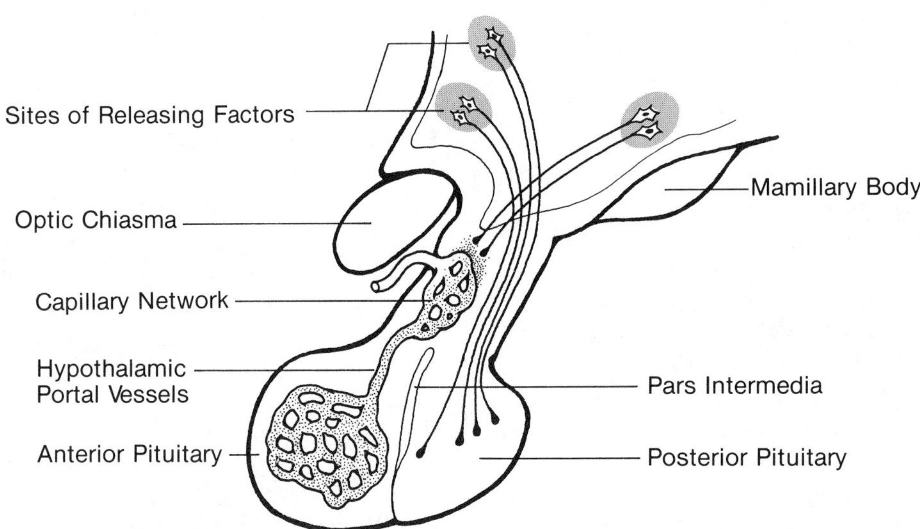

Figure 5.1
The anterior and posterior pituitary glands and hypothalamus.

Although the posterior lobe also secretes hormones, their function is different from those of the anterior pituitary and are not a significant part of the hypothalamus–pituitary–gonadal interplay.

The FSH is a glycoprotein similar in structure to the TSH. It also resembles, structurally and chemically, a hormone synthesized and secreted by the placenta during pregnancy, *human chorionic gonadotrophin (HCG).* FSH is first secreted by the pituitary gland when a person is about 8 years old. Its absence before then is believed to be one of the reasons why the male and female gonads remain essentially inactive during childhood. In the female, FSH acts upon the ovary to stimulate the development of the primordial (primary) ovarian follicles. Each ovarian follicle contains an immature ovum (oocyte). Usually, only one of these follicles is stimulated to develop each month, resulting in *oogenesis,* the origin and maturation of a female germ cell. As the follicle matures, cells within it secrete steroid hormones. FSH acts on the male gonad, the testes, to stimulate production and development of spermatozoa called *spermatogenesis.*

Luteinizing hormone is structurally and chemically similar to FSH. It is necessary for the final maturation of the gametes, particularly the ova, and it stimulates *ovulation,* which is the extrusion of the ovum from the mature follicle (graafian follicle). In the male, LH is also called the *interstitial cell stimulating hormone (ICSH)* because of its influence on the interstitial cells in the testes to produce the male steroid hormone testerone.

The third anterior pituitary hormone, prolactin, believed to have a gonadotropic effect, is a protein hormone much like the GH and another hormone produced by the placenta during pregnancy, *human chorionic somatomammotrophin (HCS)* also known as *human placental lactogen (HPL).* Prolactin is produced by the acidophilic cells of the anterior pituitary. In the absence of pregnancy or pituitary pathology, the levels of prolactin are quite low. Although the precise reason for this is not known, it is known that prolactin is responsive to inhibition by the neurotransmitter substance dopamine, which may be triggered by a prolactin inhibitory factor (PIF). Prolactin is necessary for preparing the female

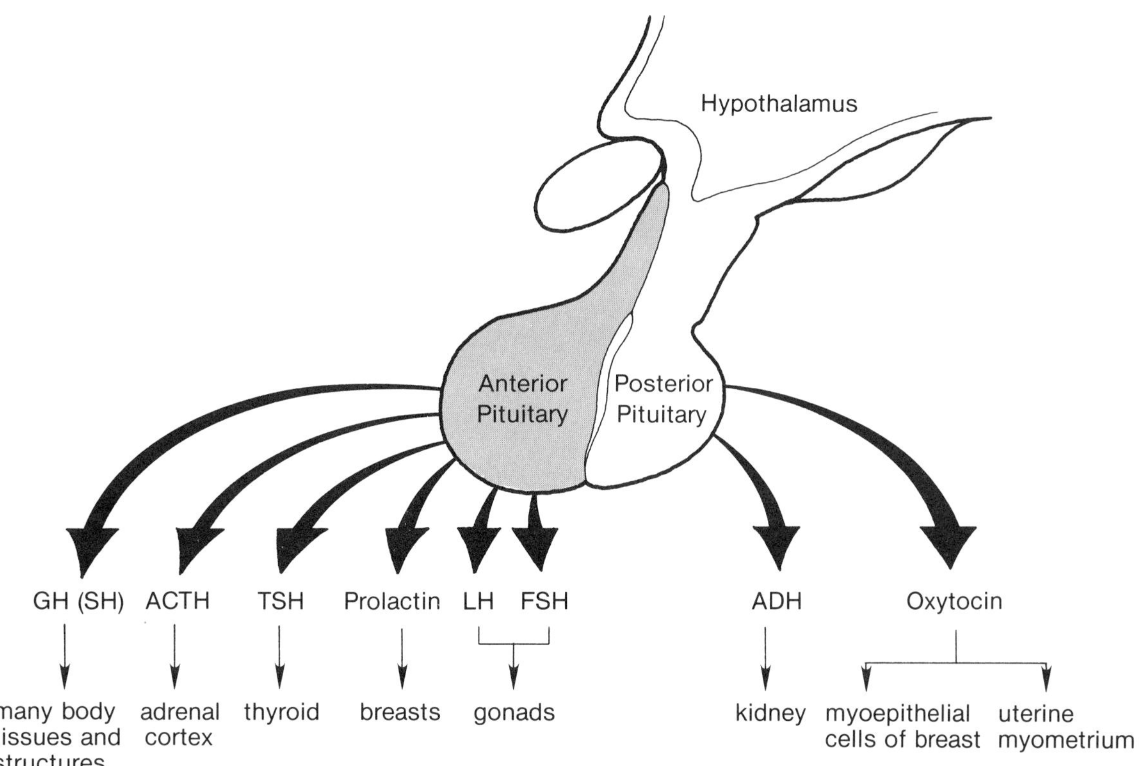

Figure 5.2
Pituitary hormone target areas.

breasts for lactation, as well for sustaining lactation once it is established.

Although the neurohypophysis is considered to be a section of the pituitary gland, it is really an extension of the hypothalamus and is comprised of neural tissue. Where the anterior pituitary lobe connects with the hypothalamus by a portal vascular system, the posterior pituitary lobe communicates via nerve fibers from the hypothalamic neurons. The neurohypophysis stores and releases two peptide hormones, *oxytocin* and *antidiuretic hormone (ADH).* These hormones are believed to be synthesized in the supraoptic and paraventricular nuclei of the hypothalamus and then travel to the pituitary for storage and ultimate release.

Oxytocin acts on smooth muscle tissue, particularly the uterine myometrium, causing it to contract. It also stimulates contraction of the myoepithelial cells found surrounding the alevoli of the breasts. This contractile effect of oxytocin may play a role in initiating and sustaining labor (see Chapter 16). It also provides for release of milk from the breasts during lactation (see Chapter 19). In addition, oxytocin is believed to be released in the female during sexual excitement and may be responsible for uterine contractility associated with female orgasm. The role of oxytocin in the male is not established.

Antidiuretic hormone facilitates reabsorption of water from the kidneys and enables the body to retain fluid. Large amounts of ADH are known to cause constriction of the arteriolar blood vessels, as well as to cause contraction of most smooth muscle tissue in the body, including the uterus; however, the contractile properties of ADH are much less than those of oxytocin. Figure 5.2 shows the interrelationship between hypothalamus, pituitary gland, and pituitary hormone target areas.

Gonadal Hormones

The gonads synthesize and release a number of hormones. The ovaries produce the principle female steroid hormones, *estrogen* and *progesterone,* as well as the androgenic hormone, testosterone, and androstenidione in smaller amounts. The testes produce the androgenic steroid, testosterone, dihydrotestosterone, and small amounts of estrogen. Other gonadal hormones are thought to exist but have not been identified and described completely.

There are three estrogens produced in the female: *estrone* (E_1), *estradiol* (E_2), and *estriol* (E_3). The estrogen produced in the greatest amount by the ovary is estradiol. This is the hormone usually meant when the term estrogen is used informally. Estrone is produced by the ovary, in much smaller amounts, and estriol is found in the liver as a by-product of estradiol and estrone. During pregnancy, the estrogens are markedly increased with the addition of the *placenta* (afterbirth) as an endocrine organ. Estrone increases 100 times its usual amount during pregnancy while estriol reaches levels almost 1,000 times that in the nonpregnant female (Liggins, 1972; Cohen, 1976).

Under the stimulation of the FSH of the anterior pituitary, target cells in the ovary produce the steroid hormones on a cyclic schedule often referred to as the menstrual cycle. The pituitary luteinizing hormone helps to change the structure of some of these cells just prior to and following ovulation and enables them to produce both estrogen and progesterone. The steroid hormones, particularly estrogen, inhibit the hypothalamus and the anterior pituitary gland, causing them to suppress the releasing factors, or the pituitary gonadotrophin hormones, or both (Fig. 5.3 *top*). This process is maintained throughout the female reproductive years in the absence of pregnancy, pathophysiology, psychopathology, or *oophorectomy* (surgical removal of the ovaries).

The male steroid hormone, testosterone, is secreted in large amounts by the interstitial cells of the testes (Leydig's cells) as a result of the gonadotrophin influence of the luteinizing hormone. The cells of Leydig constitute about 20% of the total mass of the testes in the adult male. Although spermatogenesis is initiated by both FSH and LH, testosterone is necessary for sperm maturation to take place. Testosterone deficiency usually results in male sterility or infertility.

Unlike the female gonadal hormones, male hormones are produced on a continuing (rather than cyclic) basis throughout a man's lifetime after puberty. Although there is a slow decrease in hormone production accompanying the aging process of the man, his fertility spans a much longer period than does that of the woman.

Testosterone inhibits the hypothalamus and anterior pituitary glands. It is known to suppress LH, but its action upon FSH is still unclear (Fig. 5.3 *bottom*).

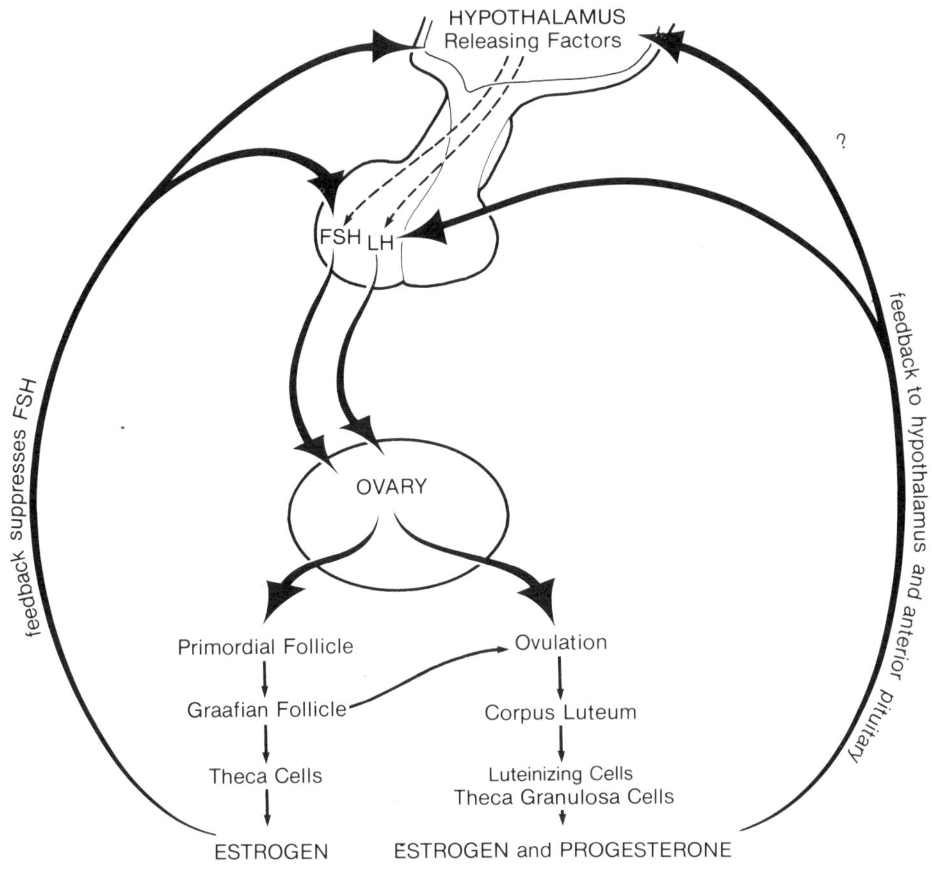

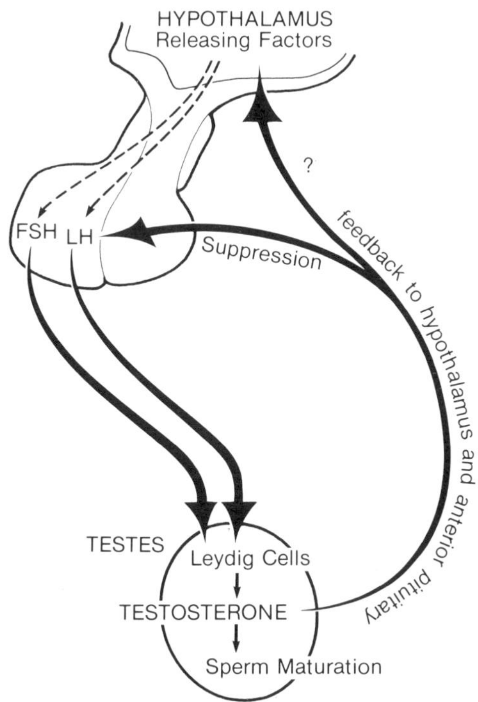

Figure 5.3
The stimulatory–inhibitory nature of the hypothalamus–pituitary relationship. *Top:* Female; *bottom:* male.

THE MENSTRUAL CYCLE

The female sexual cycle takes its name, *menstrual cycle,* from the periodic bleeding that occurs with the release and expulsion of the rich vascular inner lining of the uterus, called the *endometrium.* The onset of menstruation, *menarche,* occurs on the average between the ages of 10.5 and 15.5 and terminates with *menopause,* cessation of menstruation, about 35 years later. The primary purpose of the menstrual cycle is to provide for female germ cell maturation that results in extrusion of the mature egg from the ovarian follicle, the *graafian follicle.* This release of the ovum from the ovary into the peritoneal cavity is called *ovulation.*

The menstrual cycle is essentially controlled by the hypothalamic–pituitary–gonadal axis just discussed. This precise cycle is sensitive to a number of external as well as internal influences that may disrupt the endocrine balance necessary for its rhythm, for example, general health, race, and genetic and environmental factors, as well as physiologic, pathophysiologic, and emotional stresses. The menstrual cycle occurs with periodic regularity every 21 to 45 days in the absence of pregnancy or factors that disrupt or distort health. The average menstrual cycle is 28 days, beginning with the first day of bleeding and ending with the day preceding the next bleeding.

Ovulation occurs approximately 14 days before the onset of the next cycle. This is day 14 of a 28-day cycle, the midpoint. The coincidence that ovulation occurs at midpoint of this average cycle has been the cause of misunderstanding by health providers and consumers alike. *Ovulation does not occur at the midpoint of every woman's menstrual cycle.* If the cycle is 21 days, ovulation occurs on or about day 7; if the cycle is 35 days, ovulation occurs on about day 21.

The menstrual cycle can be divided into phases relating to either endocrine or physiologic activities (Fig. 5.4). The *endocrine cycle,* or *ovarian cycle,* consists of two phases: the *follicular,* or *preovulatory phase,* and the *luteal,* or *postovulatory phase.* The *physiologic cycle,* also called the *uterine* or *endometrial cycle,* consists of three distinct yet somewhat overlapping phases: the *menstrual phase,* the *proliferative phase,* and the *secretory phase.* The follicular phase of the ovarian cycle corresponds to the proliferative phase of the uterine cycle; the luteal phase corresponds to the secretory phase.

The ovarian cycle begins with the stimulation of the ovaries by the pituitary gonadotrophic FSH to promote the growth of about 20 of the thousands of immature ovarian follicles called *primary,* or *primordial, follicles* that were laid down in prenatal life. Each follicle usually contains one undeveloped egg called an *oocyte* (Fig. 5.5 *top*). During the follicular phase, the follicles and their eggs increase in size until one follicle reaches maturity and the egg, now called an *ovum,* is expelled from the follicle (Fig. 5.5 *bottom*). During this period of growth, the oocyte is surrounded by layers of granulosa cells that are, in turn, covered by layers of theca cells. These theca cells derive from the ovarian stroma or connective tissue forming the framework of the ovary. This inner cell mass, called the *theca interna cells,* is encased by a layer of connective tissue, called *theca externa,* and forms a capsule containing the oocyte, that is, the capsule of the developing follicle. As this capsule increases in size through growth of the oocyte and proliferation of the cells, the cells surrounding the ovum secrete a fluid that is important for several reasons:

- ▲ It contains large amounts of estrogen, essentially estradiol.
- ▲ The pressure from the fluid causes most of the theca and granulosa cells to shift to one side of the follicle, leaving a fluid-filled cavity in the follicle, called an *antrum.* The ovum resides in the middle of this cell mass near the surface of the follicle.
- ▲ The increased pressure inside the follicle (as a result of the fluid and growth of the egg) plays a role in the rupture of the follicle and the release of the egg.

Several days before ovulation, the other follicles that have been developing under the stimulation of FSH cease to grow and, usually, only one follicle reaches maturity. This follicle is now called the *graafian follicle.* As the follicle matures, estrogen is produced in increasing amounts. Estrogen has an inhibitory effect on the production of FSH, causing this hormone to decrease as the levels of estrogen increase. About 48 hours before ovulation, LH is released from the anterior pituitary gland and FSH increases again briefly. FSH and LH apparently act together to bring about the conditions necessary for ovulation to occur. These conditions are summarized as follows:

- ▲ There is a rapid increase in the size of the egg

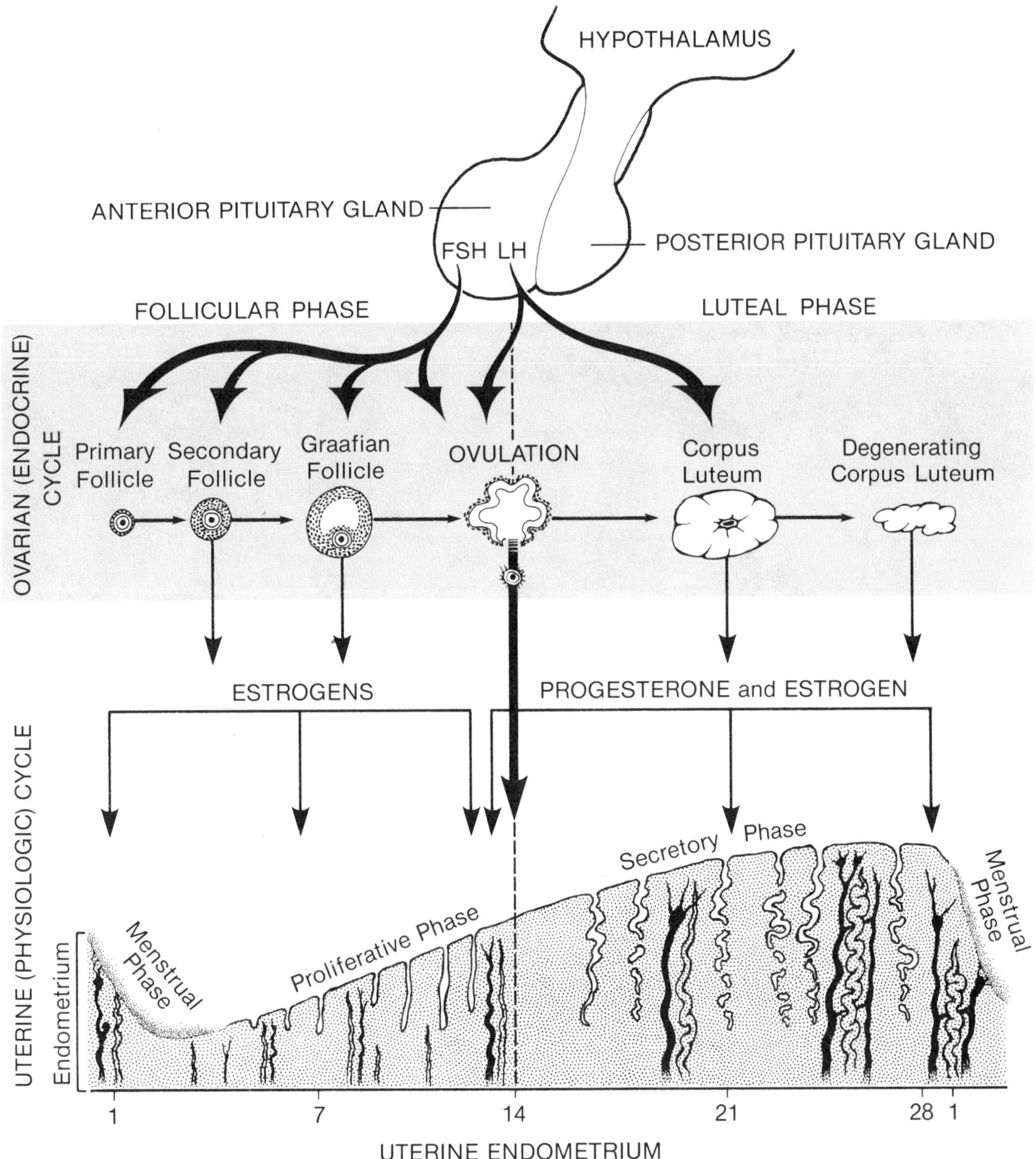

Figure 5.4
The menstrual cycle according to endocrine and physiologic activities.

and the follicle containing it to a mature follicle measuring about 1–1.5 cm.

- ▲ The theca, granulosa, and germ cells realign themselves to a location near the surface of the follicle.
- ▲ There is a transitory increase in FSH in association with a surge of LH. The presence of LH facilitates the conversion of the theca and granulosa cells to a different structure and appearance. These cells, now called lutein cells, produce estrogen and progesterone.
- ▲ There is action of the proteolytic enzymes on the capsule wall causing it to weaken. With the weakened follicle wall and the increased

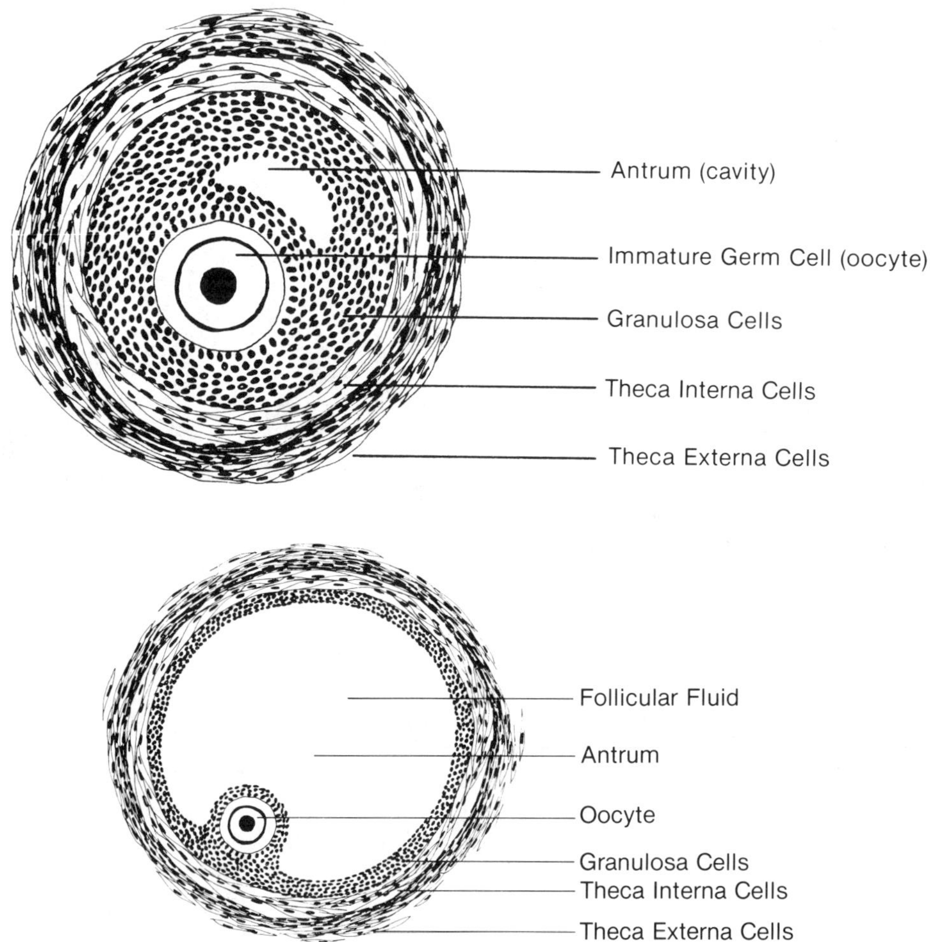

Figure 5.5
The ovarian follicle containing an immature germ cell (oocyte). *Top:* In an early stage of development; *bottom:* nearing ovulation.

follicle pressure, the follicle ruptures and releases the ovum into the peritoneal cavity near the fimbriated end of the oviducts.

Some of the granulosa cells adhere to the ovum as it matures and is extruded, creating a crownlike structure, called the *corona radiata,* that surrounds the ovum. Another layer, the gelatinous *zona pellucida,* also surrounds the ovum. These two layers form a barrier that the spermatozoa must penetrate in order to fertilize the ovum.

The presence of LH just before ovulation and the initiation of the follicle cell change process of *luteinization* introduces the second phase of the endocrine cycle, the *luteal phase.* This phase takes its name from the presence of the luteinizing hormone. After ovulation, the theca cells remaining in the ruptured follicle are converted into large, yellow lipid-filled cells. They have a well-developed blood supply and secrete large amounts of the steroid hormone, progesterone, and some estrogen. This shell of the follicle is now known as the *corpus luteum* (yellow body). The corpus luteum has a life span of 8–12 days under the stimulation of LH if conception does not occur. If the ovum is fertilized, the corpus luteum becomes known as the *corpus luteum of pregnancy* (see Chapter 10). In the absence of pregnancy, the corpus luteum degenerates about day 26 of a 28-day menstrual cycle. Its demise leads to a decrease in estrogen and progesterone, thus removing the gonadotrophin inhibitory influence of the ovarian steroids on the hypothalamus and pituitary gland and enabling FSH to increase once more. The decrease of progesterone and estrogen, particularly estradiol, also leads to the shedding of the endometrium (menstruation). The menstrual cycle begins again. The ovary containing follicles in various stages of development through ovulation is shown in Figure 5.6.

The physiologic or uterine cycle is so named because of the major physiologic changes that occur in the uterus and in the other internal reproductive organs as a result of the stimulation of the ovarian hormones (Table 5.1). These cyclic changes are preparatory for fertilization and the reception by the endometrium of the fertilized ovum.

Estrogen is produced in increasing amounts during the proliferative phase and stimulates the internal reproductive organs in a way different from yet complementary to that of progesterone. Estrogen is responsible for the proliferation of the glands, blood vessels, and stromal and epithelial cells of the endometrium. This rapid growth increases the thickness of the endometrium from 1–2 mm to 2–3 mm. Estrogen also promotes increases in sensitivity of the endometrium to progesterone. Estrogen stimulates growth of the myometrium. In the absence of pregnancy, this growth is insignificant; however, during pregnancy, it is profound (see Chapter 12). The cervical glands are stimulated to grow and to increase their secretions. These secretions undergo changes that promote the entry of the spermatozoa into the uterus and support their survival. The cervical mucous becomes thin, clear, and more alkaline in pH. The spermatozoa can more easily penetrate it; the increased pH is less hostile to the sperm and enables them to live longer in the vagina.

Estrogen-primed vaginal changes are designed to support rather than impede conception. The vaginal mucosa begins to prepare for pregnancy by *cornification,* or layering, of cells of the vaginal epithelium. Vaginal secretions become more alkaline and contain increased amounts of glycogen. In addition to acting on the internal reproductive organs, estrogen acts on the breasts to promote development of the ductile system.

Ovulation begins the *secretory phase* of the physiologic cycle. The changes that occur during this period are primarily the result of the influence of progesterone. Both estrogen and progesterone are present, however, and work together during this time. The endometrium that has been primed and readied by estrogen undergoes further change. The endometrial glands enlarge further and take on a serrated appearance. They are rich in glycogen. There is some edema of the glandular stroma and increased hypertrophy of the endometrial cells with a significant increase in cytoplasm. The endometrium appears as a rich, succlent, vascular bed ready to receive and initially nourish the fertilized ovum. Progesterone decreases uterine muscle contractions and makes it less sensitive to internal and external stimuli. This quiescent state helps to maintain the endometrium in anticipation of pregnancy and to retain the uterine contents following *nidation* (implantation of the fertilized ovum in the endometrium). Progesterone also affects cervical secretions, changing these secretions from a thin, clear, alkaline secretion to a thick, opaque, highly viscous, acid secretion that is lethal to the spermatozoa and difficult to penetrate. This tenacious substance literally

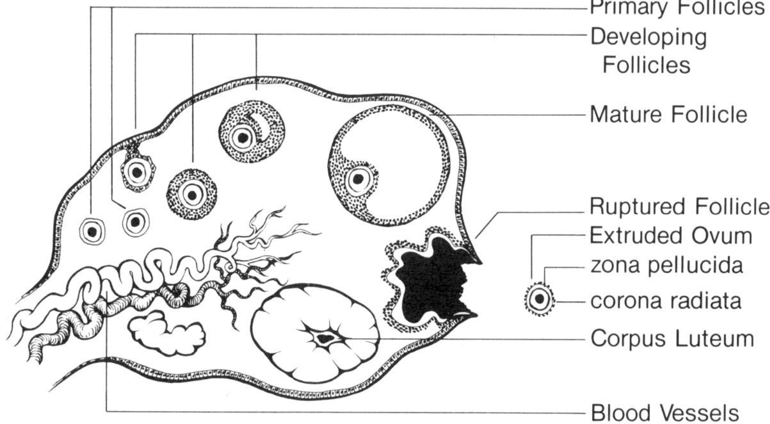

Figure 5.6
The ovary showing vascular structures and ovarian follicles at various stages of development and ovulation.

TABLE 5.1
A COMPARISON OF THE ACTIONS OF ESTROGEN AND PROGESTERONE

Target Organ	*Estrogen*	*Progesterone*
Uterus myometrium	Promotes growth of the myometrium. Increases myometrial sensitivity to oxytocin. Promotes myometrial sensitivity to influence of progesterone.	Decreases myometrial excitability, making muscle less sensitive to oxytocin and other substances. Decreases uterine contractions.
endometrium	Causes proliferation of the endometrium by stimulating glandular and stromal growth and promoting growth of spiral arteries. Increases endometrial sensitivity to progesterone.	Changes the endometrial glands from thin tubules to thick large serrated glands rich in glycogen. Causes edema of the glandular stroma. Causes the cells to hypertrophy and increases cytoplasm content.
Cervix	Promotes growth and secretion of the cervical glands. Decreases viscosity of cervical secretions. Increases pH of cervical secretions.	Changes cervical secretions from thin clear characteristics associated with estrogen to a thick, tenacous, viscous yellow-opaque color. Decreases pH.
Vagina	Causes vaginal cornification (layering of cells), that is, changes the vaginal epithelium into a stratified squamous epithelium with increased cell density. The degree of change correlates with amount of estrogen produced. This increase in cell density equals increased vaginal epithelial thickness. Increases glycogen content in vaginal secretions.	Decreases vaginal cornification.
Ovary	Acts locally to stimulate some follicle growth in the absence of FSH. Increases ovarian response to gonadotrophins. Promotes growth of ovaries.	No specific effect.
Oviducts	Increases size of oviducts. May aid in ovum transport by increasing peristaltic and ciliary activity of the tube.	Decreases secretory activity of the tubal mucosa. Increases glycogen and ascorbic acid. Decreases peristaltic and ciliary activity of the tube.
Breasts	Promotes development of the ductile system.	Promotes development of the lobular system. Inhibits effects of prolactin on the breasts.
Reproductive tract generally	Promotes growth and maintenance of smooth muscle and epithelium.	
External genitalia	Promotes growth and development. Responsible in part for pubic hair pattern.	
Body	Responsible for development and realignment of body shape associated with the female. Stimulates sebaceous gland secretions (see Chapter 8).	Elevation of body temperature.

Target Organ	*Estrogen*	*Progesterone*
Cardiovascular	Decreased estrogen causes hot flashes and flushes. Decreases body cholesterol.	
Hypothalamus and pituitary	Inhibitory feedback.	Inhibitory feedback.

closes the uterine door to the spermatozoa. Progesterone is believed to decrease the peristaltic and ciliary activity of the oviduct. Like estrogen, it also affects the breasts by promoting the development of the lobular system. It also inhibits the action of anterior pituitary hormone prolactin on the breasts.

The *menstrual phase,* or period of bleeding, has been described poetically as "the weeping of a disappointed uterus" when fertilization does not occur. Menstruation signifies the physiologic completion of one cycle and the beginning of the next. Menstruation occurs because of a combination of factors. With the degeneration of the corpus luteum, hormonal support is withdrawn and with it the endocrine stimulation to the endometrium. Vasoconstriction of the endometrial vessels follows shortly, possibly because of the absence of the vasodilatory effect of estrogen. Vasospasm leads to decreased oxygenation of the endometrial tissues with resulting necrosis, particularly of the blood vessels. This tissue destruction allows for seepage of blood into the vascular layer of the endometrium. With increasing necrosis, there are increasing hemorrhage sites until, finally, the entire endometrium is sloughed off into the uterine cavity. The presence of most foreign substances in the uterus will stimulate it to contract. Thus, with the release of the endometrium and the decrease in progesterone, the uterus contracts and expels the endometrium from the uterus. This released blood is called menstrual blood, or menstrual flow. Bleeding lasts 3–7 days in most instances. There is a loss of approximately 70–75 ml of blood and serum in almost equal amounts. Menstruation may be associated with varying degrees of discomfort, *dysmenorrhea,* or be free of pain (see Chapter 27). Menstrual blood does not usually clot because of the presence of a fibrinolysin. On occasion, excess bleeding may result in depletion of this clotting factor and blood clots will be present. Menstruation denudes most of the endometrium and necessitates the rebuilding of this lining through repetition of the cycle.

MALE REPRODUCTIVE ENDOCRINE PHYSIOLOGY

The male reproductive function, like that of the female, is under the direction and control of the hypothalamus, pituitary gland, and male gonads. This interrelationship was discussed earlier in this section. There is a relatively steady interplay among these endocrine structures that provides for the continuous production of male gonadal hormones and gametes, the spermatozoa (sperm). This differs from the cyclic sexual pattern seen in the female.

The anterior pituitary gonadotrophin hormones, the luteinizing hormone, and the follicle stimulating hormone, are the same in both the male and the female. These hormones are initiated by the gonadotrophin releasing factors in the hypothalamus. The gonadotrophin hormones then act on the testes as their male target organ, stimulating cells within the testes to produce androgenic (masculinizing) hormones and to bring to maturity the male germ cells.

LH stimulates Leydig's cells, found in the interstitial spaces between the seminiferous tubules of the testes, to produce testosterone, one of several androgens secreted in the male. Testosterone is the androgen produced in the largest quantities and is the most important male reproductive hormone. It has a number of actions that are not directly associated with the reproductive function (Table 5.2), but its most important functions related to procreation are the promotion of growth of the male genital organs and the support of spermatogenesis.

FSH is sometimes called the spermatogenic hormone because it is responsible for the initiation of spermatogenesis during which the undifferentiated male germ cells, *spermatogonia,* which are found in the germinal epithelium lining the seminiferous tubules of the testes, undergo a series of changes through which they acquire the capacities for rapid movement and fertilization of the ovum. FSH alone cannot complete this process but requires the help of LH

TABLE 5.2
ACTIONS OF TESTOSTERONE

Source	*General Actions*	*Specific Actions*
Leydig's cells of the testes	Stimulates development of the male genital tract.	Believed to play a major role in the early embryologic sex differentiation of male and female embryos. Stimulates the development of the male genitalia just prior to and during puberty.
	Promotes development of secondary sex characteristics in the male. (See Chapter 8.)	Responsible for stimulating the development of: ▲ The male skeletal system (height, size, and weight of bones) ▲ Muscular system (size and weight of muscles in the man) Promotes enlargement of the larynx and vocal cords (low voice pitch). Male hair distribution.
	Acts on the developing male gamete.	Promotes sperm maturation.

to stimulate the secretion of testosterone that, in turn, aids in the maturing of the immature spermatozoa, the *spermatocytes* (see Chapter 6, section on gametogenesis).

SUMMARY

Human reproductive endocrinology was discussed as the basis for the events that enable fertilization, pregnancy, and childbirth to take place. The physiologic basis for many of the methods and techniques available for family planning were also included. Nurses use this information not only in the planning for and providing of care for women during their pregnancy, labor, and recovery, but also as the basis for consumer education about family planning, pregnancy, and related events.

The endocrine basis for readiness for human reproduction was presented as an overview of the major events that prepare the male and female to undertake the tasks related to sexual function and pregnancy. Attention was given to the relationship between the central nervous system, particularly the hypothalamus, the anterior and posterior pituitary glands, and the male and female gonads—the testes and the ovaries, respectively. Major pituitary hormones were included along with the hormones produced by the gonads.

The female sexual cycle, the menstrual cycle, was discussed in some detail as the physiologic basis for fertilization. The chapter closed with a brief summary of the male reproductive endocrine function.

REFERENCES AND READINGS

Cohen, S. L. Estrogen in Pregnancy, in Goodwin, J. W., Godden, J. O., Chance, G. W. (Eds.), *Perinatal Medicine.* Baltimore: Williams & Wilkins, 1976.

Grollman, S. *The Human Body: Its Structure and Physiology* (4th ed.). New York: MacMillan, 1978.

Guyton, A. C. *Textbook of Medical Physiology* (6th ed.). Philadelphia: W. B. Saunders, 1981.

Hartman, C. G. How Large is the Mammalian Egg? *Rev. Biol* 4:373, 1929.

Huff, R. W., Pauerstein, C. J. *Human Reproduction, Physiology and Pathophysiology.* New York: John Wiley & Sons, 1977.

Hurteau, G. D. Gametogenesis to Implantation, in Goodwin, J. W., Godden, J. O., Chance, G. W. (Eds.), *Perinatal Medicine.* Baltimore: Williams & Wilkins, 1976.

Liggins, G. C. Endocrinology of the Foeto-Maternal Unit, in Shearman, R. P. (Ed.), *Human Reproductive Physiology.* London: Blackwell Scientific Publications, 1972.

Page, E. W., Villee, C. A., Villee, D. B. *Human Reproduction* (2nd ed.). Philadelphia: W. B. Saunders, 1976.

Schottelius, B. A., Schottelius, D. D. *Textbook of Physiology.* St. Louis: C. V. Mosby, 1970.

Younglai, E. V., Ruf, K. B. Ovulation, in Goodwin, J. W., Godden, J. O., Chance, G. W. (Eds.), *Perinatal Medicine.* Baltimore: Williams & Wilkins, 1976.

6

GENETIC BASIS FOR REPRODUCTION

Human reproduction is cyclic: the beginning of life has its basis in the past, and the developing human being will reflect its ancestry through the projection of its offspring. Fertilization initiates the life stages of a person, which eventually results once more in fertilization. Fertilization leads to embryologic and fetal development, which culminates in the birth of an infant. After birth the new life progresses through the years of childhood and then reaches adolescence. During adolescence the boy and girl undergo changes associated with puberty. Puberty activates the physical reproductive capability in the boy/man, girl/woman, and fertilization is once more possible and likely. This cyclic nature of reproduction (Fig. 6.1) assures the immortality of the human species through the transfer of traits from generation to generation. These genetic determinants endow each human conceptus with the developmental capability for being and becoming. Science has shown for a long time that the genetic endowment is not the only determinant of what the new life will ultimately become, but it is the primary one and, for some, the principal one.

This chapter provides an overview of some of the concepts necessary for understanding the genetic basis for human reproduction. These concepts, like those in preceding chapters, are needed to comprehend the processes associated with reproduction that are discussed in subsequent chapters of this book. Three areas have been selected in order to show their relevance to the study of human reproduction and particularly to maternity nursing: (1) the structure, function, and classification of human chromosomes, (2) the processes of cellular division, and (3) *gametogenesis,* the mechanism through which the male and female germ cells become mature and ready for fertilization. Disorders of genetic origin are discussed in Chapter 24.

HUMAN CHROMOSOMES

Propagation of life is possible because of the ability of cells to divide and replicate themselves, as well as to transfer certain characteristics from the parent cell to the new cell (daughter cell). The principles of human genetics were derived essentially from the work of Mendel in the late 1800s, published in 1866, and rediscovered in 1900. Since that time, particularly in the post-World War II years, the scientific world has been the progenitor of much new and far more sophisticated information concerning genetics and related disorders. Much of that work has centered around the characteristics and functions of the chromosome.

A *chromosome* is a rod-shaped structure found in the nuclei of cells. It derives from an amorphic substance, chromatin, which organizes itself into an identifiable shape. Chromatin is clear and transpar-

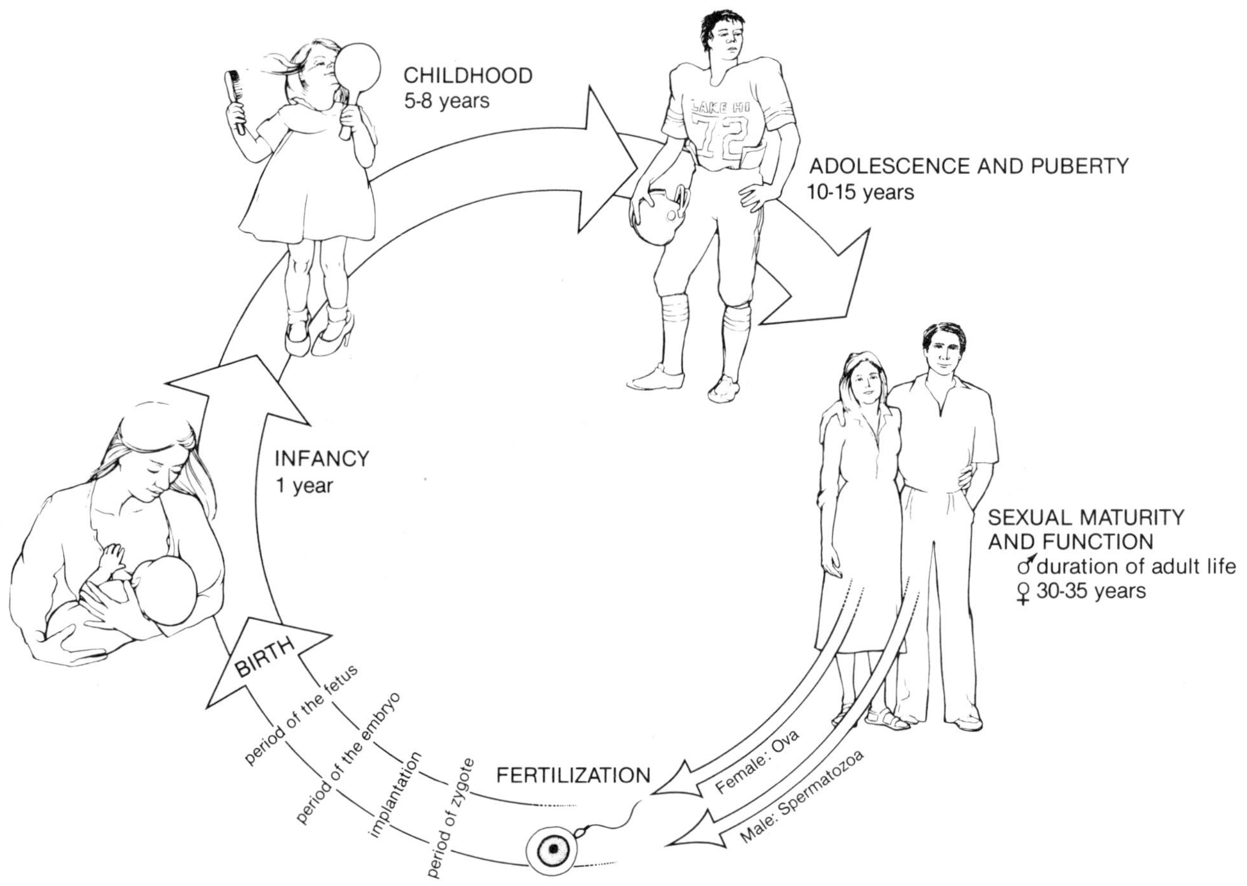

Figure 6.1
The cyclic nature of reproduction.

ent; however, it can be stained through the use of certain biologic materials giving the chromosome its name, *chromo,* meaning color, and *soma,* meaning body. The diameter of a cell nucleus is about one-thousandth of an inch, so the chromosomes contained within it are quite small. Each normal human cell contains a total of 46 chromosomes, 22 homologous (matched) pairs called *autosomes,* and two sex chromosomes—XX in the female and XY in the male. In turn, each chromosome contains *genes,* which are the molecular units that carry the genetic information peculiar to that person.

Chromosomal classification was first conceived at a meeting of cytogeneticists held in Denver, Colorado, in 1960. A seven-category classification was devised based on two features of the chromosome: its overall length and the location of its narrowest point of constriction, called the *centromere.* This was possible since all chromosomes have essentially one of three shapes: *metacentric,* where the centromere is located approximately in the center of the chromosome; *submetacentric,* where the centromere is located near the center but closer to one end than the other; and *acrocentric,* where the centromere is near one end of the chromosome. The acrocentric chromosomes often have additional bits of chromatin attached to their arms, called satellites (Fig. 6.2). The Denver classification matched like chromosomes according to shape and size and assigned them to seven groups categorized as A through G in order of decreasing size. For example, the largest chromosomes that were similar were placed in group A, the smallest chromosomes that were similar, in group G. (See Table 6.1.) This classification allowed for microphotography of the chromosomes, which provided the geneticist with pictures that could be cut, matched, and grouped according to size and morphology to form a genetic portrait of an individual—a *karyotype.* Later, a *chromosomal banding technique* was devised, permitting a more precise matching of

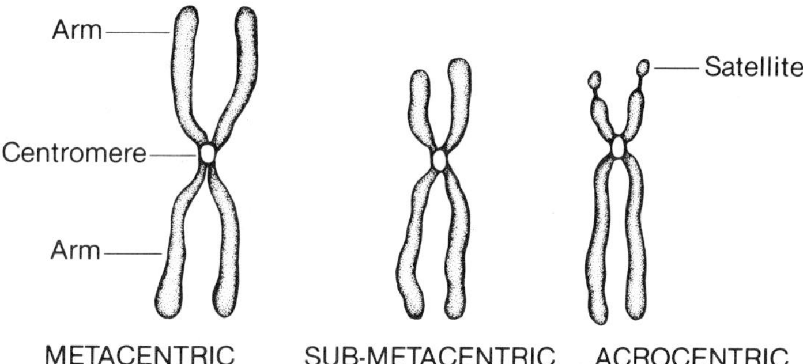

Figure 6.2
Chromosome morphology.

chromosomal pairs. This classification by a banding technique was derived from a conference of geneticists held in Paris in 1971 (Fig. 6.3). The karyotype has provided the *cytogeneticist* a tool for clearly identifying the genetic basis for many inherited disorders.

DNA/RNA

As early as 1928, evidence began to emerge showing that a substance called deoxyribonucleic acid (DNA) was the principle genetic material (Griffith, 1928). In the 1940s it was clearly established that this genetic information was encoded in DNA (Avery et al., 1944). Since that time, the study of molecular genetics has been an integral part of the field of genetics.

The DNA molecule contains one type of nucleic acid, which is composed of nucleotides, mixed with basic protein substances, *histones* and nonhistones, in approximately equal amounts. The DNA molecule looks like two coiled polynucleotide chains intertwined to form a double helix—a spiral-shaped structure (Fig. 6.4). The description of this helix in 1953 constituted a major contribution to the study of genetics (Watson & Crick, 1953). The two chains or strands are made up of phosphoric acid and deoxyribose, a sugar. These strands enclose four nitrogenous bases. The bases are comprised of two purines, adenine and guanine, and two pyrimidines, thymine and cytosine. These bases form the "glue" that holds the structure together. If the DNA molecule is pulled apart, portions of the bases can be seen to project into the two strands. These projections are believed to contain the substances that form a genetic code or blueprint for the developing life.

The *genetic code* directs the order or sequence of amino acids, the structural units of the protein molecule. For example, DNA directs the arrangement of amino acids in a sequential order (polypeptides). These amino acids are joined together by a peptide and form a polypeptide chain. The properties of the protein molecule rely upon the sequences of amino acid arrangement in the polypeptide chains. Since proteins are the basic building blocks of life, the genetic code can be said to direct the unique biologic development of each human being. This code is

TABEL 6.1
DENVER CLASSIFICATION OF CHROMOSOMES ACCORDING TO MORPHOLOGY AND SIZE

Group[a]	*Chromosomes by Pairs*[b]
A	1,2,3
B	4,5
C	6,7,8,9,10,11,12, plus X
D	13, 14, 15 (large acrocentrics)
E	16, 17, 18
F	19, 20
G	21, 22 (small acrocentrics), plus Y

[a] The letter categories are according to size in decreasing order: A = largest chromosomes; G = smallest chromosomes.

[b] Numbers refer to 22 matched pairs of chromosomes. X = female sex chromosome (only in group C); Y = male sex chromosome (only in group G).

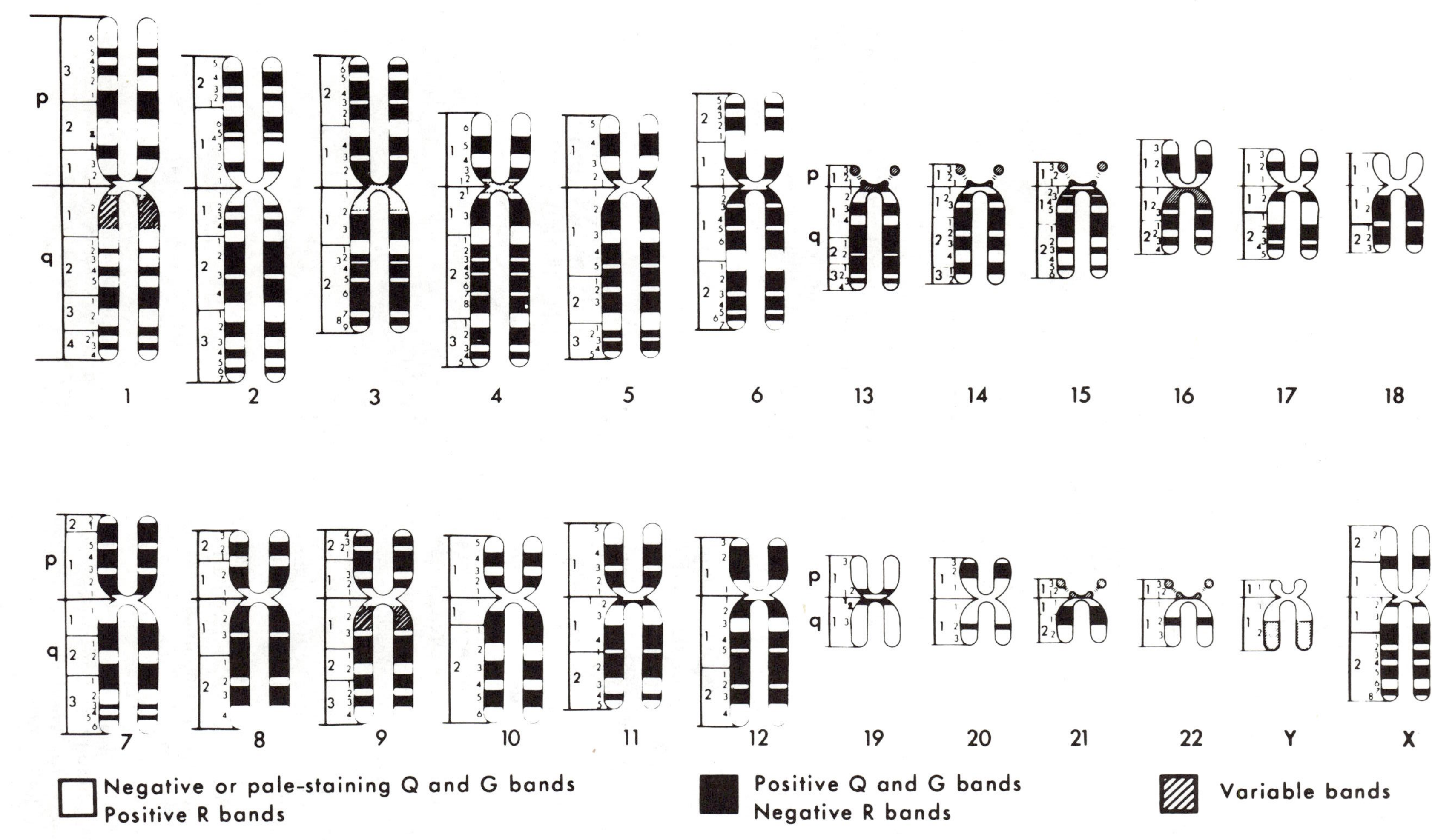

Figure 6.3
The chromosomal basis of heredity. Chromosome classification by a banding technique.
Source: Thompson, J. S. Thompson, M. W. *Genetics in Medicine.* Philadelphia: W. B. Saunders, 1980. Used with permission.

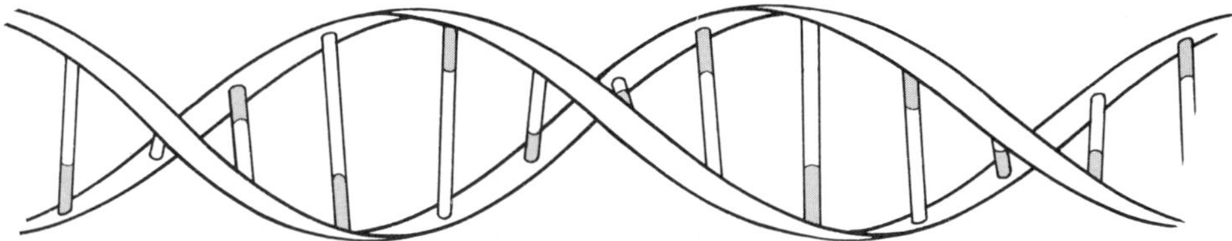

Figure 6.4
The DNA molecule.

based upon complex biochemical processes and is not described in detail here. However, it is important for you to be aware of its existence and some of its functions. The relevance of the genetic code to nursing practice is established in Chapter 24, which deals with genetic disorders.

The principle role of DNA, the encoding and transmission of genetic information from one generation to another, is considered to be the primary basis for molecular genetics. This process of transfer involves, in most cases, the following sequence:

- ▲ DNA encodes genetic information.
- ▲ DNA is then transcribed into another nucleic acid, *ribonucleic acid (RNA),* contained in the cytoplasm of the cell.
- ▲ RNA is translated into protein.

Recently, it has been found that this process is not constant in all cases. DNA may not be totally transcribed into RNA, nor all of RNA into protein. In some cases, the transcript process may even be reversed by an enzyme called *reverse transcriptase* (Thompson & Thompson, 1980, p. 32).

CELLULAR DIVISION

The cell divides by two mechanisms, or processes. *Mitosis* is a multiplication division in which the parent cell with its full genetic complement is replicated in the daughter cell, that is one cell divides into two, two cells into four identical cells, and so on. Body growth is possible because of mitosis; body tissue repairs itself through the mitotic process; the fertilized ovum becomes an embryo–fetus–infant–child–adult through mitosis.

A special cell division called *meiosis* occurs only in germ cells. This two-step process is necessary in order to provide each gamete with a haploid number of chromosomes (22 autosomes plus 1 sex chromosome) representative of the genetic characteristics of the parent cell. The first step of this process is called meiosis I. It is often referred to as the reduction division of meiosis since it is during this period that the 44 paired autosomes and the two sex chromosomes are divided and reduced to 23 chromosomes in each germ cell. An abbreviated description of mitosis and meiosis is included here for easy reference; for a more extensive discussion of these processes, see a genetics or physiology textbook.

Mitosis

Mitosis consists of five phases during which the parent cell replicates itself to form identical cells, called daughter cells (Fig. 6.5). Even though these steps are discussed separately, they are part of a continuous process and should not be viewed as distinct units.

The first step in mitosis is called *prophase.* During this phase, the centrioles become polarized; the nuclear capsule disintegrates; the neucleolus disappears, and the genetic material, chromatin, assumes a spiral shape and can be stained and identified as chromosomes containing two coiled threads of DNA that are called *chromatids.* These chromatids are joined together by a *centromere.* Upon completion of the prophase, the centrioles have moved to opposite *poles* in the cell. The chromosomes have located around the midsection or *equator* of the cell. Microtubules, thin fibers, extend from the centrioles and give rise to a spindlelike structure called the *mitotic spindle.*

The period during which the chromosomes attach to the microtubules by their centromere is called *metaphase.* Near the end of metaphase, the centromeres divide, and each original chromatid

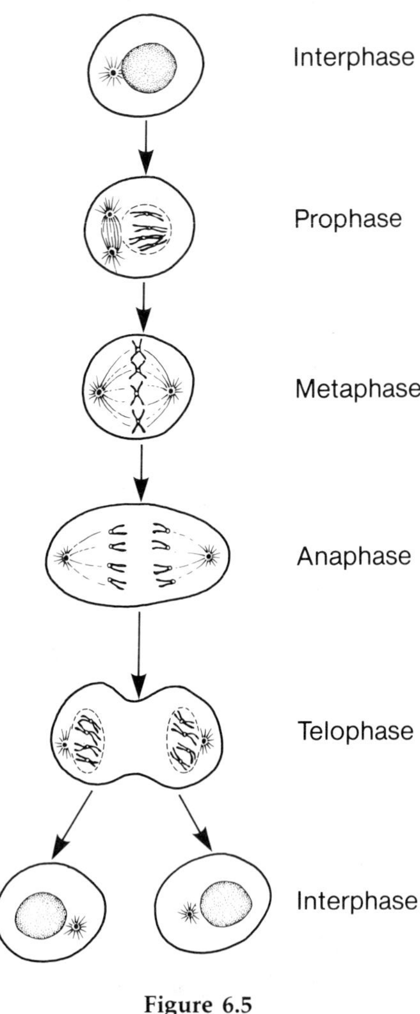

Figure 6.5
Mitosis.

becomes a separate chromosome. This process overlaps somewhat with the next phase and is sometimes discussed as part of anaphase. No nucleolus nor nuclear membrane is present.

The chromosomes become separate, single strands during *anaphase.* They move away from their equatorial location and position themselves at opposite poles. One chromatid from each chromosome goes to each pole. There is no nucleolus nor nuclear membrane present.

The reappearance of the nuclear membrane forming a new capsule occurs in *telophase.* The membrane becomes pinched or constricted and separates into two parts with each part encasing one of the polar areas. The nucleolus reappears, and the centrioles are replicated. The chromosomes return to a more central location and are no longer as distinct, but they more closely resemble their earlier uncoiled threadlike appearance. These daughter cells are identical with the parent cell.

Interphase, the period between mitotic cell divisions, provides a rest period for the new cell. It is characterized by the appearance of indistinct chromatin threads located in the cell nucleus. Although it is considered to be a resting period, it is not a completely dormant time; during this phase DNA is synthesized and replicated.

Meiosis

Meiotic cell division is specific to male and female germ cells. It enables these unique cells to undergo changes that provide for the transfer of genetic materials from both the male and female to occur at the time of fertilization. It is a result of the provisions made during the first meiotic division that the genetic foundations for inheritance first described by Mendel are possible. Meiosis occurs in two relatively continuous stages: meiosis I, the reduction division, and meiosis II, which closely follows mitotic cellular division.

MEIOSIS I (*Reduction Division*)

The first stage of meiosis I, as in mitosis, is called *prophase* and represents a complicated process with major differences from the mitotic prophase. A number of stages within this phase have been described: leptotene, zygotene, pachytene, and diplotene.

Leptotene derives its name from the prefix *lepto,* meaning slender or delicate. The chromosomes are seen as thin threads. They differ from the chromosomes seen at this period of mitosis in that they have alternating thicker and thinner areas instead of a smooth outline. The thicker parts of the chromosome are called *chromomeres.*

The yoked or joined stage is called *zygotene.* At this time the chromosomes that are alike unite to form homologous pairs called *bivalents.* The female sex chromosomes (X) are alike and can pair; however, the male sex chromosomes (X and Y) can join only at the tips of their arms.

The chromosomes thicken in the *pachytene* stage (prefix *pachy,* thick), are more visible, and can be stained. Two chromatids for each chromosome are seen, appearing as quadrivalent structures containing four strands of genetic material. During this

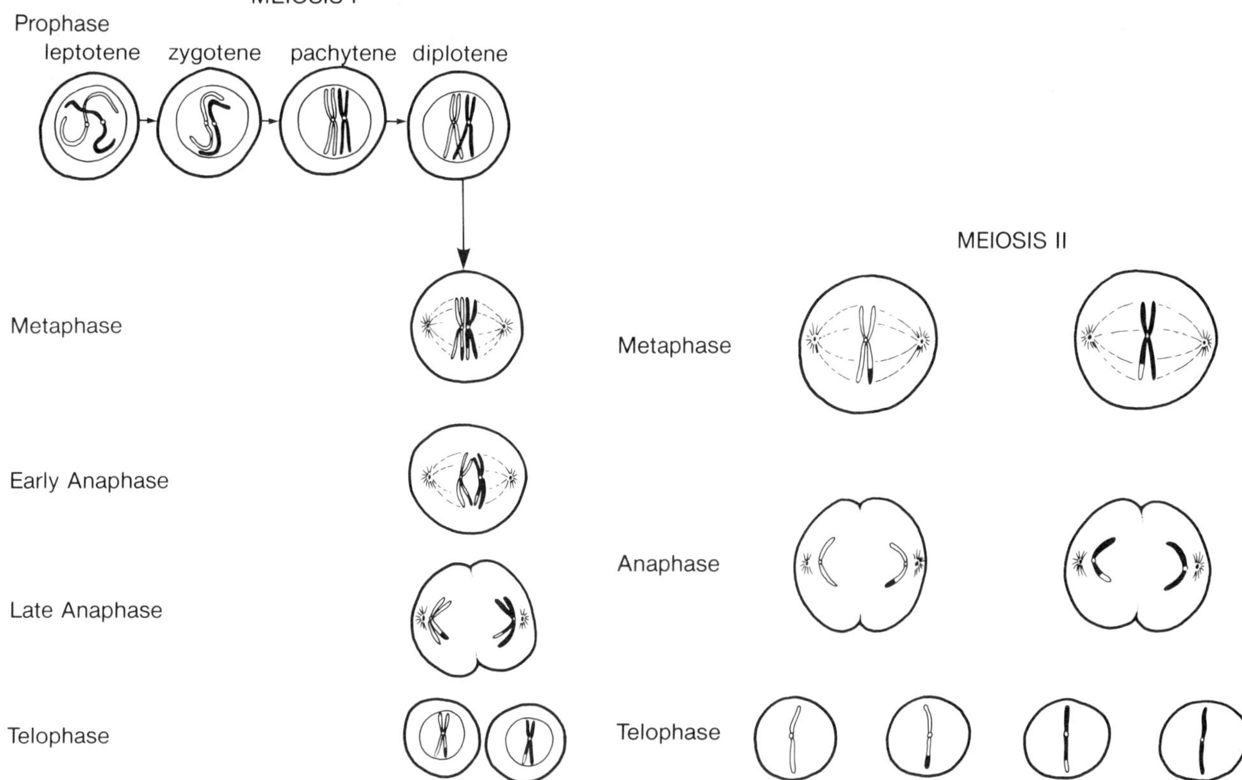

Figure 6.6
Left: Meiosis I (Reduction Division). *Right:* Meiosis II.

stage, the forces that have attracted the chromosomes to each other start to weaken, and the pairs begin to separate from each other.

The *diplotene* stage finds a longitudinal separation of the part of each bivalent chromosome. However, the chromatids remain joined at the midsection, or centromere, creating a chiasma, or X-shaped junction. This point of union probably provides for genetic material to be exchanged.

The remaining phases of meiosis I follow a pattern similar to that found in mitosis. *Metaphase I* is comparable to the mitosis metaphase. There is a difference between mitotic *anaphase* and meiotic *anaphase I* in that in anaphase I the centromere uniting each homologous pair does not divide. This enables each bivalent to move as a unit. The paired bivalent units, however, do separate from their quadrivalent alignment, and the bivalents randomly sort themselves out and move toward opposite poles with a representative of each pair of chromosomes. *Telophase* is essentially the same as in mitosis. The cells separate, and two daughter cells are formed with each having half of the chromosomes of the parent cell, 22 single autosomes and one sex chromosome. There is a shortened version of the interphase between Meiosis I and II (Interkinesis). There is, however, no synthesis nor replication of genetic material. This interphase is not distinct and Telophase of Meiosis I may appear to merge into Prophase of Meiosis II.

MEIOSIS II

Meiosis II also closely follows mitotic cellular division. There is replication of the germ cell with its reduced chromosome count in *prophase II*. Each centromere divides longitudinally, allowing the chromatids to separate. *Anaphase II* finds four gametes with each one usually having an identical haploid chromosome number. These cells become the male or female gametes. The functional capabilities of these four gametes differ in the male and female and are described in the following section, Gametogenesis.

GAMETOGENESIS

Gametogenesis is a precise process through which the primitive male and female germ cells are changed into mature gametes (Fig. 6.7). The process is similar in the male and female since it relies upon the mitotic cell division of mitosis. Gametogenesis does, however, require the cellular division unique to germ cells, called meiosis, during which the usual chromosome number of 46 is divided equally so that each mature gamete contains 23 chromosomes, or half of the genetic complement required to complete the whole, at the time of fertilization. The union of the sperm and ovum literally brings together two genetic halves from the parents.

Oogenesis

Oogenesis, the maturation of the female germ cells, covers a span of years, beginning with the prenatal period and reaching functional maturity with puberty. It can arbitrarily be divided into three time periods: the prenatal period, the period of the follicle, and the postovulatory period.

Prenatal period. During the *prenatal period,* the primitive germ cells, *oogonia,* are derived from the germinal epithelium found on the surface of the fetal ovaries. This germinal epithelium grows inward into the connective framework of the ovary and multiplies thousands of primordial ova. The oogonia then divide by mitosis to create daughter cells containing a full genetic endowment of 44 autosomes and two X sex chromosomes. The oogonia are now called *primary oocytes.*

The primary oocytes become the reservoir from which one ovum will be produced each month during the female reproductive life span. As many as 6.8 million germ cells have been reported to be present in the fetal female (Baker, 1963). At birth, as many as 750,000 of these cells are present in the two neonatal ovaries. Many of these cells will degenerate before puberty leaving approximately 200,000–500,000 available to reach maturity. Far fewer of these cells actually do become mature, and even fewer are fertilized. Some of the primary oocytes enter but do not complete the prophase of the first meiotic division before birth. They must wait for puberty, a span of 10–15 years, before they progress further toward maturation.

Period of the follicle. The *period of the follicle* begins with the onset of puberty and resumes the process

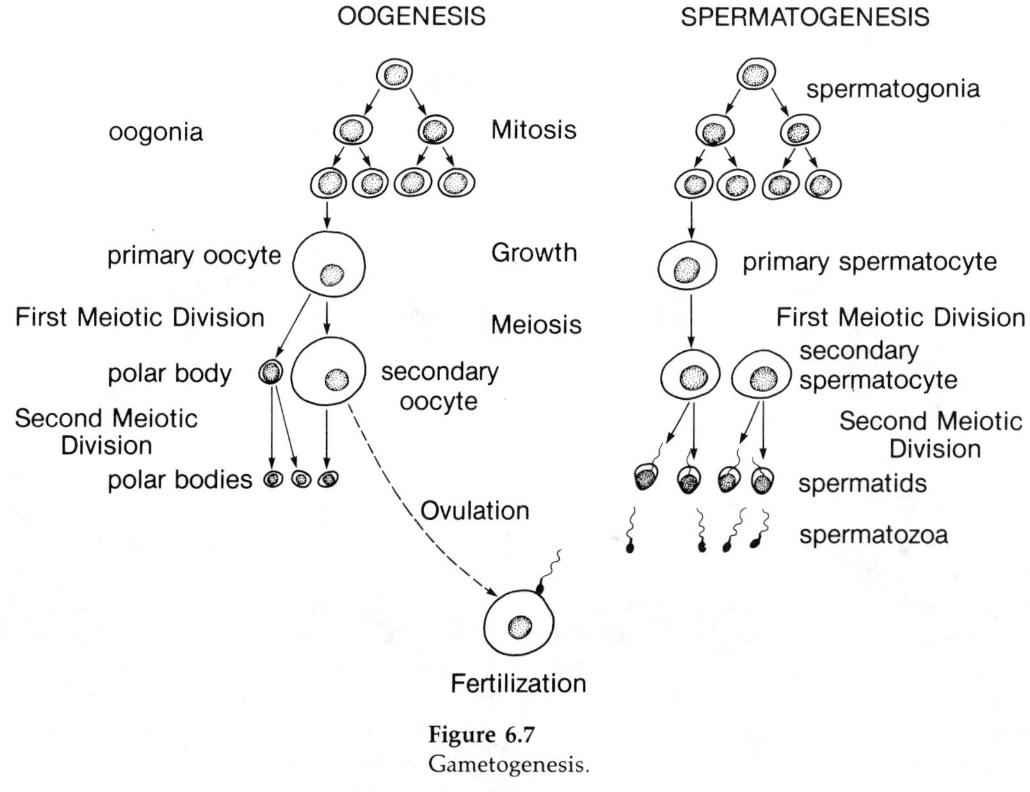

Figure 6.7
Gametogenesis.

of female germ cell maturation (see female sexual cycle in Chapter 5). During this period, some of the primary oocytes will complete the meiotic division. Each month about 20 immature follicles, each containing a primary oocyte, will be stimulated by FSH to grow during the follicular phase of the ovarian cycle. Only one of these follicles with its egg usually will reach maturity. The primary oocyte will divide during meiosis I, producing two cells. These cells are not identical; rather, they are quite unequal in size. The genetic material is equally dispersed between the two cells; however, one of the cells contains most of the cytoplasm. The larger cell is now called the *secondary oocyte,* while the smaller cell is called the *first polar body.* This begins the second meiotic division during which the secondary oocyte reaches metaphase.

Postovulatory period. The second meiotic division occurs during the *postovulatory period,* but is believed to be incomplete unless fertilization occurs, after which it is rapidly completed. During the second meiotic division, a large mature ovum that contains almost all of the cytoplasm is produced with a second polar body. The cytoplasm is believed to be needed for nutrition of the zygote immediately following fertilization. Like the first meiotic division, the polar body is small and contains equal parts of the genetic material but little of the cytoplasm. Sometimes the first polar body will divide in meiosis II and produce two more polar bodies. The polar bodies usually degenerate and serve no reproductive purpose other than to become a receptacle for the discard of genetic materials not needed. In rare cases, however, they may develop embryos. Each primary oocyte that undergoes maturation will produce one ovum—a haploid cell containing the X sex chromosome and 22 single autosomes—and two or possibly three polar bodies.

Spermatogenesis

Spermatogenesis occurs in three stages and requires approximately 64 days for completion. These stages are proliferation of the spermatogonia, reduction division of the spermatocytes, and spermiogenesis.

Proliferation of the spermatogonia. During this stage, the spermatogonia undergo a mitotic cellular division during which part of the germ cells increase and grow to reach their first level of maturity. They are then known as *primary spermatocytes.* The remainder of the spermatogonia remain for later development. Each primary spermatocyte has a full genetic complement of 46 chromosomes.

Reduction division of the spermatocytes. The spermatocytes undergo meiosis I during which each spermatocyte divides into two separate bodies containing one-half of the genetic materials of the parent cell—22 autosomes and one X or Y sex chromosome. They are now called *secondary spermatocytes.* Through meiosis II, each spermatocyte reproduces itself and forms two structures called *spermatids* containing 23 unpaired chromosomes. The sex chromosomes are usually divided evenly between the spermatids. The appearance of the spermatid structure is still quite like that of the germinal epithelial cell, and the spermatids must undergo further development to take on the characteristic appearance of the mature sperm.

Spermiogenesis. During this period, the spermatids retain their attachment to the Sertoli cells in the seminiferous tubules, probably because of the nutrients the cells are believed to provide, as well as their possible contribution of other substances that influence the changes in the structure of the sperm. The epitheloid characteristics of the sperm change to those of a mature spermatozoa comprised of a large ovoid head, a neck, a body, and a tail (Fig. 6.8). The sperm head contains the germ cell nucleus with its genetic materials. It also has a caplike area at the front of the head called the *acrosome.* The acrosome is believed to contain proteolytic enzymes that help erode the covering of the ovum, enabling the sperm head to penetrate and fertilize the ovum. The neck contains the centrioles; the body houses the mitochondria, probably the sperm's energy source, and cytoplasm. The tail is an elongated structure containing contractile filaments that enable the mature sperm to move forward through a lashing motion.

After their development, the spermatozoa are released from the Sertoli cells and stored in the epididymides where they acquire the motility just mentioned and the capacity for fertilization. This maturing phase requires about 10–14 days. Exactly how the epididymides contribute to the maturation of the sperm is not clearly understood. Some suggested ways are that the contribution of a fluid filled with nutrients, enzymes, and hormones facilitates its maturity or that this storage period provides the time for the aging required to reach maturity.

The mature spermatozoa are capable of rapid forward movement in a straight line. They can

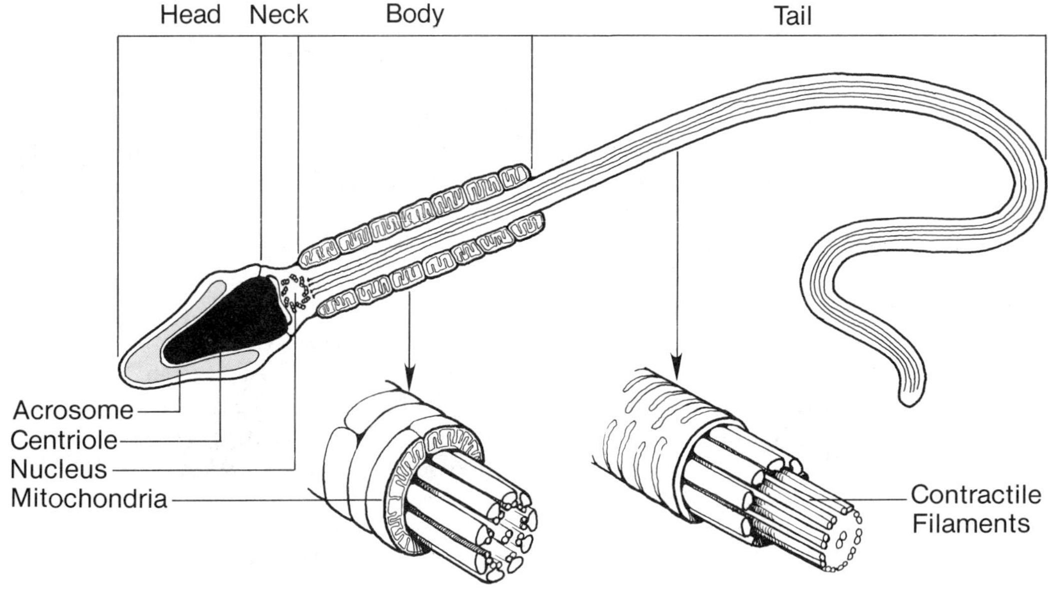

Figure 6.8
Cross-sectional and sagittal views of a mature spermatozoon.

travel at a speed as great as 20 cm/hr following ejaculation into the female genital tract. The life expectancy of the sperm following release from the penis in semen of normal amount and temperature is about 24–72 hours.

Each primary oocyte that undergoes maturation will produce one ovum—a haploid cell containing the X sex chromosome and 22 single autosomes—and two or possibly three polar bodies. However, each spermatocyte will yield four spermatozoa.

The ovum and spermatozoon differ in a number of ways. The ovum is large when compared with the sperm and if it is placed on a dark background with bright light, can sometimes be seen without the aid of magnification. At maturity, the ovum measures approximately 0.133–0.140 mm in diameter (Hartman, 1929; Allen et al., 1930). The mature graafian follicle measures about 6–12 mm in diameter. In contrast, the sperm is much smaller and requires the use of a microscope in order to be seen. Its total length is about 0.06 mm. The ovum is nonmotile; the sperm is highly motile. The nucleus of the ovum is surrounded by nutritive-rich cytoplasm containing yolk granules; the sperm nucleus is located in the head and does not have cytoplasmic support. Ovum maturation is complete following fertilization; sperm maturation is complete before fertilization. The life of the unfertilized ovum is approximately 24 hours; the life of the spermatozoon may be 48–72 hours in the female genital tract.

SUMMARY

Basic content essential for understanding the genetic foundations for human reproduction was presented. Genetic principles form the basis for the transfer of human traits and characteristics from one generation to the next, creating the cyclic nature of reproduction. Characteristics and functions of chromosomes were briefly described, including the roles of DNA and RNA. Mitotic and meiotic cellular division were reviewed to lay the foundation for understanding the ensuing discussion of gametogenesis—male and female germ cell maturation.

REFERENCES AND READINGS

Allen, E., Pratt, J. P., Newell, U. U., Bland, L. J. Human Tubal Ova; Related Early Corpora Lutea and Uterine Tubes. *Contrib Enbryol* 22:45, 1930.

Avery, O. T., MacLeod, C. M., McCarty, M. Studies on Chemical Nature of Substance Inducing Transformation of Pneumococcal Types: Induction of Transformation by Deoxyribonucleic Acid Fraction Isolated from Pneumococcus Type III. *J Exp Med* 79:139, 1944.

Bodmer, W. F., Cavalli-Sforza, L. L. *Genetics, Evolution and Man.* San Francisco: W. H. Freeman, 1976.

Fraser, F. C., Nora, J. *Genetics of Man.* Philadelphia: Lea & Febiger, 1975.

Griffith, F. The Significance of Pneumococcal Types. *J Hyg* 27:113, 1928.

Hamerton, J. L. *Human Cytogenetics. Vol. I, General Cytogenetics; Vol. 2, Clinical Cytogenetics.* New York: Academic Press, 1971.

Hartman, C. G. How Large Is the Mammalian Egg? *Rev Biol* 4:373, 1929.

Paris Conference (1971). *Birth Defects* 11(9), 1975 (Suppl.) Reprinted in *Cytogenet Cell Genet* 15:201, 1975.

Paris Conference. Standardization in Human Cytogenetics. *Birth Defects* 8(7), 1972.

Thompson, J. S., Thompson, M. W. *Genetics in Medicine.* (3rd ed.), Philadelphia: W. B. Saunders, 1980.

Watson, J. D., Crick, F. H. Molecular Structure of Nucleic Acids; A Structure for the Deoxyribonucleic Acid. *Nature* 171 (April 25):737, 1953.

Yunis, J. J. (Ed.). *Molecular Structure of Human Chromosomes.* New York: Academic Press, 1977.

7

PSYCHOSOCIAL DEVELOPMENT

The maturing of mental processes, such as thought, perception, and feeling, and sociologic development, particularly the establishment and maintenance of interpersonal relationships, the assumption of roles, and the acquisition of sexual identity, are so intimately related that they are often informally referred to as *psychosocial development.* Strictly speaking, the person only develops physically and psychologically—the body and the mind. This development occurs, however, within the context of a personal and social environment in which the person thrives or fails to thrive, and which provides the societal, cultural, and ethnic influences that contribute to the uniqueness of each person. This chapter addresses selected theories of human development, affectional relationships, and sexual development within the context of developmental readiness for pregnancy, childbirth, and parenthood.

> *The infant is born with two endowments . . . he [or she] possesses at birth a genetically determined endowment which is common to all [humans] and also uniquely individual and which has been modified by interaction with the intrauterine environment. [The child] will grow into and assimilate a cultural heritage that is a product of the cumulative experiences of the particular ethnic group into which he [or she] is born, but which also will be somewhat different for him [or her] than any other individual. The two will be inextricably intertwined as the child matures and develops.*
>
> *Lidz, 1968, p. 5*

Figure 7.1 illustrates the developing child as an integral part of a family and society.

Psychosocial readiness is the ability of the man and woman to make sensible judgments concerning their participation in events associated with human reproduction and to undergo the experiences of pregnancy, childbirth, and parenthood. Psychosocial readiness relies upon the maturing of mental processes within a social context that enables the person to establish and maintain affectional relationships, acquire a sexual identity, and develop the ability to function as a sexual partner.

SELECTED THEORIES OF HUMAN DEVELOPMENT

In 1759, Wolff introduced the principle of epigenesis (*epi,* upon + *genesis,* beginning), which states that development occurs through an orderly process that begins with a structureless cell and continues with a series of sequential events, each event being derived from the one preceding it. This biologic principle of development was first used by Freud and later by others to explain the psychology of development. It has formed the nucleus for much of what is believed today about human development as a progression

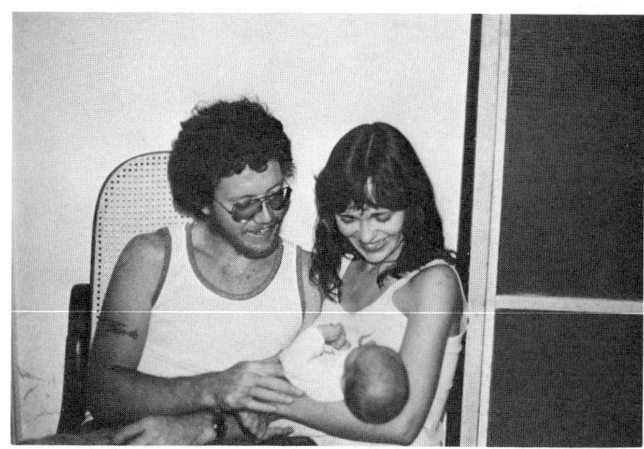

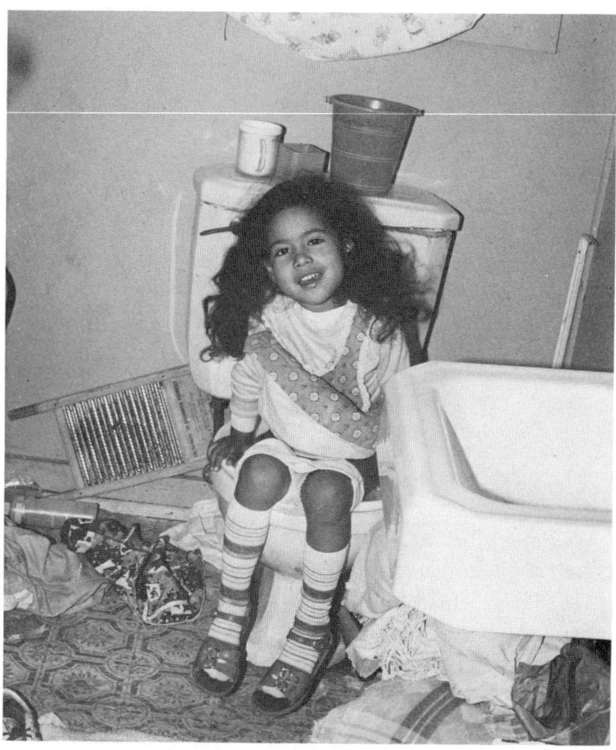

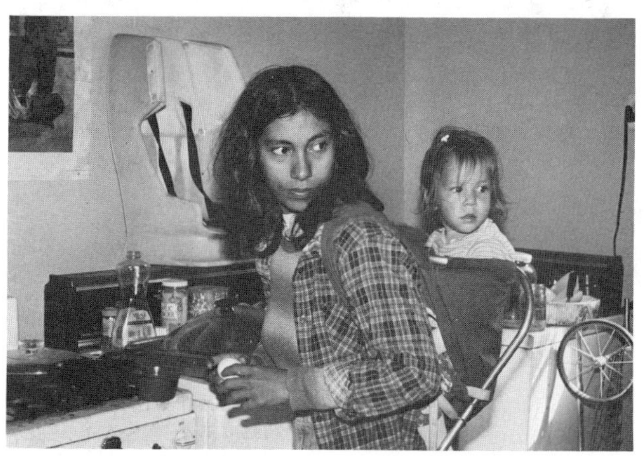

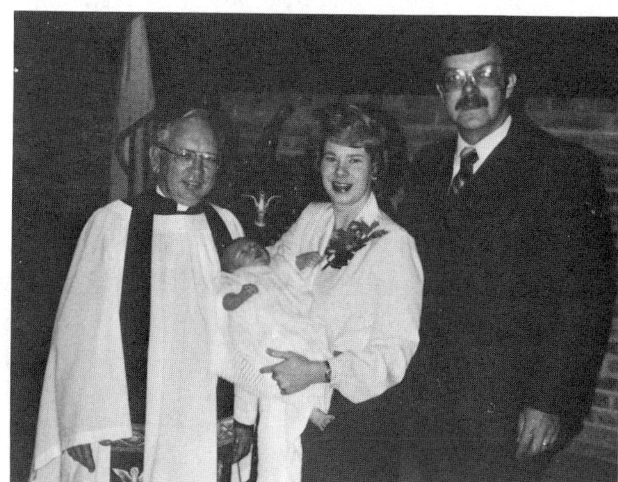

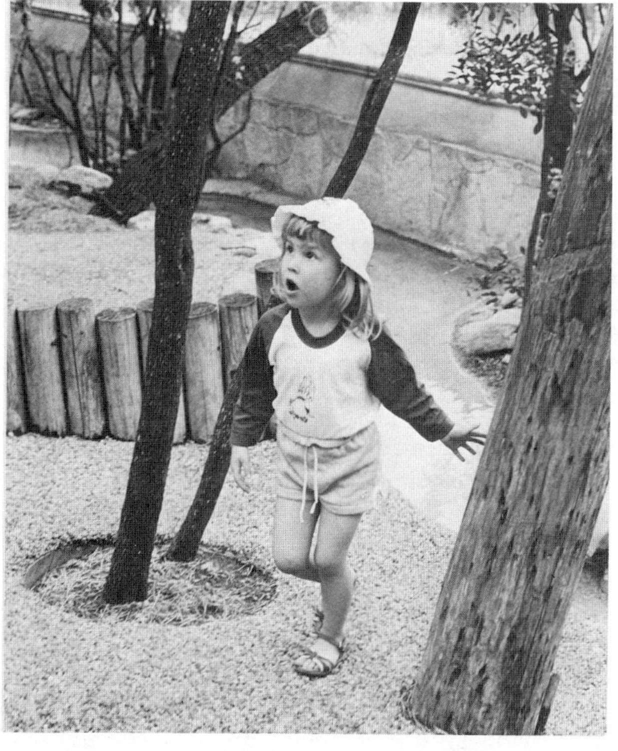

Figure 7.1
The developing child is an integral part of a family and of the society and culture to which that family belongs.

from the simple to the complex, from earlier to later, from immature to mature.

Psychologic development has been studied by many different theorists and from both complementary and contradictory points of view. There is no one theory of psychologic development. Particular theorists or developmental schools of thought have dominated thinking during different or concurrent periods of time. The major schools of developmental psychology include *Psychoanalytic Theory,* which was fathered by Sigmund Freud and dominated much of the later nineteenth and early twentieth centuries; *Social Psychology,* which arose in concert with the disciplines of anthropology and sociology in the late nineteenth and early twentieth centuries and in part in revolt against the views of the Freudian psychologists; *Humanistic Psychology,* which was also a statement against what was preceived as the narrow instinctual views of the Freudian school; and the *Organismic,* or holistic, point of view, which was introduced in the post-World War I era.

There is often overlap among these schools of psychologic thought, and, at times, it is difficult to assign a particular theorist to one theoretic stance. In the discussion that follows, we have placed theorists in the schools from which most of their ideas appear to derive with recognition that authorities in the various fields are likely to take issue with the assignment of some of these theorists.

Other points of view about developmental psychology have been expressed, many of which were derived from or are closely associated with the schools of thought just mentioned. Though theorists such as Alfred Adler, Carl Rogers, and B. F. Skinner are not discussed here, you are encouraged to explore their writings, as well as the writings of those theorists discussed in this chapter.

Psychoanalytic Theory

The *psychoanalytic school* of developmental thought was founded by Sigmund Freud (1856–1939) in the late nineteenth century. Before the work of Freud, efforts to study the human mind were restricted to observation and analysis of the conscious mind—information that could be reported by the person and behavior that could be observed by others. Freud believed that the conscious mind was only one small part of the total mental processes; below or underlying this consciousness lay the essential mental processes, ideas, thoughts, feelings, urges, perceptions, and passions that directed or controlled human behavior and thought. He insisted that understanding of the total mind was dependent upon tapping and analyzing the unconscious mind. Freud first attempted this "psychoanalysis" through the use of hypnosis, but he abandoned this method early in his work and relied instead upon the method of free association in which the client talked without restriction about personal thoughts, symptoms, needs, and so on. For over 40 years, Freud amassed much information about personal thought and behavior. From this information obtained through free association, Freud formulated his theory of human psychologic development. His ideas have had a profound impact on developmental psychology.

Freud believed that the personality is made up of three major separate, but related, systems: the *id,* the true unconscious in which the instinctive impulses reside; the *ego,* the conscious part of the mind; and the *superego,* the conscious monitor of the ego. Psychoanalytic theory postulates the following.

▲ Human functioning is possible because of instinctual energy wishes or drives that arise from sources of excitation located in body regions and whose purpose it is to satisfy the excitement. Freud saw the sexual drive, which he viewed in a broader context than it is often used today, along with the death wish, *thanatos,* as the major instincts that influence a person's behavior.

▲ These instinctual drives are directed toward maximum gratification of a person's wishes or needs (Fig. 7.2).

▲ There is a mechanism or system that monitors, controls, or sets limits on indiscriminate gratification of the instinctual drives (the superego).

▲ There is a process (probably unconscious) through which ideas reach the conscious level and are acted out. The concentration of psychic or emotional energy upon an idea or object (cathexis) facilitates the rise of that idea to the conscious level. In the normal person and under normal conditions, only conscious ideas are converted into behavior; in the presence of serious psychopathology, unconscious ideas are acted out.

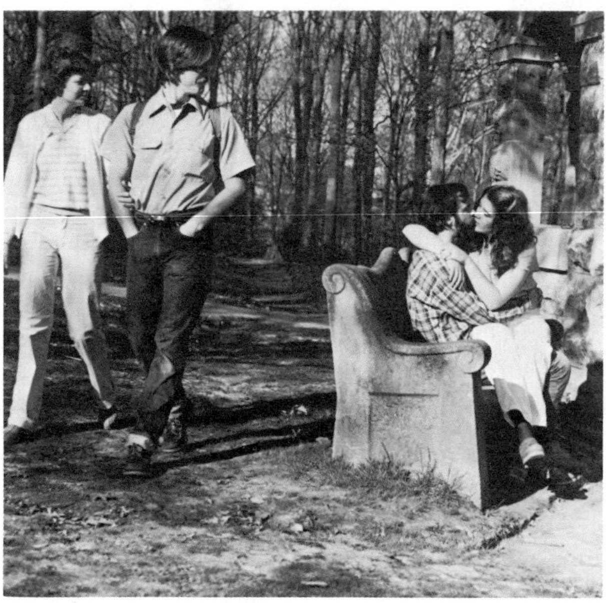

Figure 7.2
Psychoanalytic theory proposes that much of human behavior is intrinsically determined by instinctual drives that gratify a person's wishes or needs. Sexual drive is seen as a principle force, along with motives such as hunger and thirst. Source: Lion, E. M. *Human Sexuality in Nursing Process.* New York, John Wiley & Sons, 1982, used with permission.

Freud described stages of development from infancy through adolescence that were motivated or dominated by instinctual drives. Table 7.1 presents a comparison of Freud's perception of human development with that of other theorists.

There is probably no theorist who has made so profound an impact upon the understanding of the psychology of human development and yet has been so widely and severely criticized as Freud. Today his ideas still form the basis for much of what is believed about human behavior. To a large extent, insight into pregnancy has been gained from people who represent the psychoanalytic school of thought. Helene Deutsch (1945) and Gerald Caplan (1959, 1961, 1973) are two such people whose works are discussed later in this book.

Social Psychology

During the late nineteenth century, the disciplines of sociology and anthropology were gaining increased prominence. The person was more and more being viewed as part of a social system that influenced what the person became, as the person in turn affected the composition and function of the group (Fig. 7.3). As mentioned earlier, some social psychologists developed their ideas in opposition to the views of Freud, while others used those same ideas to look at the person within the context of the society of which he or she was a part. A number of theorists have been identified with the school of *social psychologic* thought, such as Alfred Adler, Karen Horney, Erik Erikson, Harry S. Sullivan, and Eric Fromm. All made a major contribution to viewing psychologic development within the social context. Erik Erikson and Harry S. Sullivan are discussed here, primarily because of their focus on human development.

Sullivan (1892–1949) came from the psychoanalytic school, but he viewed personality and behavior as occurring within the context of interpersonal relationships, using descriptive data obtained through the use of strategies and skills basic to psychoanalysis. He is categorized as a neo-Freudian because of his reliance upon Freud's approach to periods or levels of development. He also adopted Freud's idea of the importance of the mother in influencing the development of her child. Sullivan believed that security is the goal of personal development and that anxiety that arose within the framework of interpersonal relationships is a developmental motivator.

Sullivan's *Interpersonal Theory of Psychiatry* (1953) is strongly allied with the tenets of social psychology and includes the following central ideas:

- ▲ The person does not exist apart from interactions and relationships with other persons.
- ▲ Human life is characterized by a pattern of interpersonal relationships that begin with birth and recur throughout a lifetime.
- ▲ The human being passes through clearly definable stages or periods of development beginning with birth and going through adolescence.
- ▲ Behavior is learned through interactions with other persons and is not the result of instinctual drives.

Sullivan recognized the importance of heredity and biology on development. However, in his writings he subordinates biologic factors to interpersonal experiences.

Interpersonal theory is relevant to the study of maternity nursing. The interpersonal relationships of the expectant parents with each other, their families, and others are likely to be influenced by what each brings to the pregnancy and are likely to affect their attitudes toward and their expectations of pregnancy. Often interpersonal relationships determine how people will respond to and cope with pregnancy, childbirth, and parenthood.

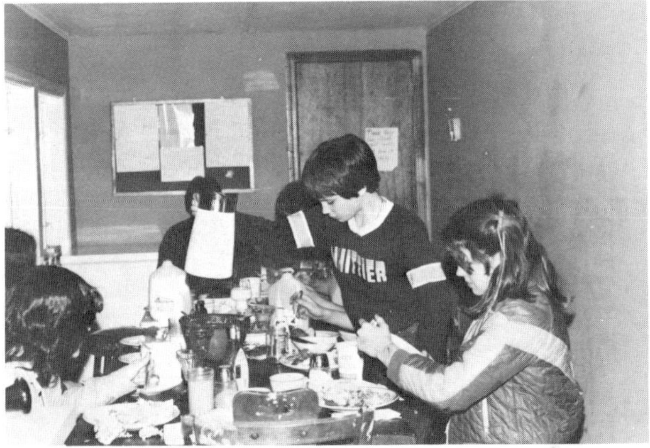

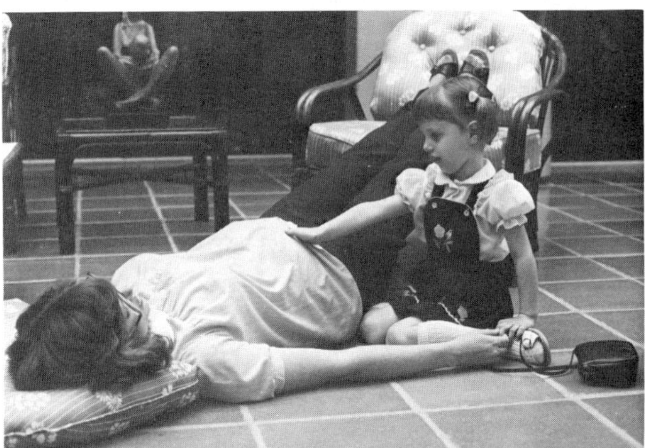

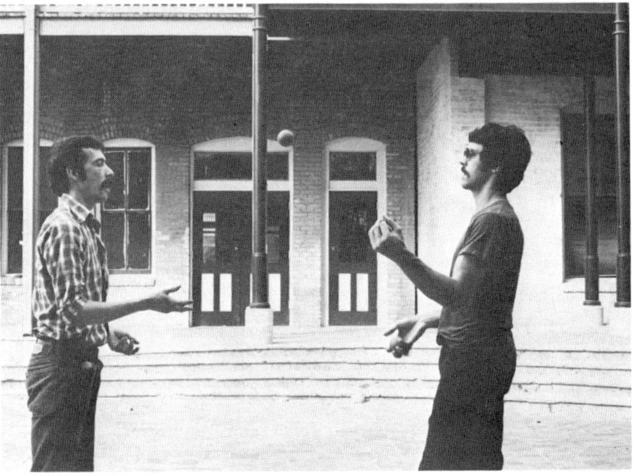

Figure 7.3
Social psychology views the person as developing within the context of a social system, predominately through interactions with others within that system. The influence of the environment, particularly social, on the person is viewed as significant to development.

Stage Developmental Theory was introduced by Erik Erikson (1902–), a social psychoanalyst, who applied the theory of psychoanalysis to social and anthropologic study. He identified Eight Ages of Man, attempting to explain human development according to clearly identifiable periods during which the foundations for certain behaviors were laid down (Erikson, 1950) (Fig. 7.4). His emphasis is on a person's view of him or herself as a social being rather than as someone controlled by psychosexual motives. Erikson did not originate the concept of *developmental task,* but his Eight Ages of Man provide a framework for using the concept to specify needs or activities associated with these periods of development (Havighurst, 1953). Developmental task has been used by others to describe activities that must be carried out during pregnancy (Duvall, 1957, 1977; Rubin, 1961, 1967, 1977; Tanner, 1969; Clark, 1979). These tasks have not emerged by the application of a developmental theoretic framework to the study of pregnancy, but rather through the use of reported descriptive data or collected inductive data.

Humanistic Psychology

Humanistic psychology was the result of efforts of people such as Gordon Allport, Carl Rogers, and Abraham Maslow who could not support the psychoanalytic school of development. These men viewed human development as motivation that arose from an innate source and growth as a basic human drive with the ultimate goal being the realization of the meaning of one's existence.

Abraham Maslow (1908–1970) recognized that much of psychologic study derived from the analysis of people with emotional or mental disease or disorder. He believed that the strongest (healthiest) not the weakest (sickest) representatives of society should be the focus of study. Much of his work was a retrospective analysis of successful figures in history. Maslow saw development and health as springing from the satisfaction of five categories of human need, each dependent upon the one preceding it for healthy achievement (Fig. 7.5). These five

TABLE 7.1
COMPARISON OF SELECTED HUMAN DEVELOPMENTAL THEORIES (BIRTH THROUGH YOUNG ADULT)

	S. Freud	*H. S. Sullivan*	*E. H. Erikson*[a]
BACKGROUND	1856–1939 Country: Austria Psychoanalytic School	1892–1949 Country: United States Interpersonal School	1902– Country: United States Social Psychoanalyst
THEORETICAL FOCUS	PSYCHOANALYTIC Intrapsychic behavior is a product of the interaction among the id (unconscious), ego (conscious), and superego (conscience).	INTERPERSONAL Personality and development are viewed in the interpersonal framework. Grew out of Freud's theory of psychoanalysis in association with theories drawn from sociology.	PHYCHOSOCIAL Application of psychoanalytic theory to the child in culture and society. Grew out of the Freudian school of thought. Identified developmental ages.
DEVELOPMENTAL FOCUS	INFANCY: 0–1½ yr, oral sensory stage Primary source of pleasure is the mouth.	INFANCY: 0–2½ yrs Important concepts are empathy, anxiety, and the self-system. Chief interpersonal need is for tenderness.	BASIC TRUST VS. MISTRUST: 0–1 yr Development of trust, which is seen as basic to the development of a healthy personality. Emphasizes the importance of the mother–infant relationship. Supports consistency of sensitive care. Discontinuity of care believed to be the basis for mistrust in later developmental periods. Acquisition of *hope* is crucial to this stage.
	TODDLER: 1½–3 yr, anal period Elimination and retention constitute primary sources of pleasure. Child's first encounter with limit setting and discipline, e.g., toilet training. Development of object relationships.	CHILDHOOD: 2½-4 yr . Further development of the self-system occurs. Increased interaction with peers and use of consensual validation. Chief interpersonal need is for adult participation.	AUTONOMY VS. SHAME, DOUBT: 1½–3 yr Anal needs dominate. Father becomes important figure. Increased sense of self-control without loss of self-esteem promotes sense of goodwill, pride, autonomy. Develops appreciation of limits while knowing security within the limits. Develops a sense of dignity and lawful independence of the adults around. In the absence of autonomy, a sense of loss of control

J. Piaget	H. Werner	T. Parsons and R. F. Bales
1896–1982 Country: Switzerland Cognitive School of Developmental Theory	Country: United States Organismic Developmental Psychology	Country: United States Sociological Perspective
INTELLECTUAL Examines the nature and processes of the child's thought and language.	ORGANISMIC Emphasizes that human development is based upon inherent structure of the individual. Views the person in a holistic sense. Uses biologic principles to direct analogies to psychologic development. Considered by some to be the most completely developmental of any theorist.	SOCIOLOGIC Views the child's personality development as being determined by interactions within the family as a social system that fosters socialization of the child to family and societal expectations. Derived from Freud's psychoanalytic theory. Parsons and Bales' phases of socialization correspond to Freud's stages of psychosexual development. Views the infant as a "deviant" whose behavior must be changed through socialization to conform.
SENSORIMOTOR: 0–2 yr, assimilation vs. accommodation During this period the child learns to coordinate actions with perceptions, e.g., child can follow an object with eyes; grasp it; rattle it; suck it. Begins to learn that objects are permanent and exist even out of sight (peek-a-boo). Achieves a rudimentary understanding of some relationships in space, causality, and time. Evolution of abilities necessary to construct and reconstruct objects. Period of experimentation and exploration. Reasoning is by means of mental image. All animate and inaminate objects are designated alive.	Does not specifically address "stages" of development. Believes that human development proceeds from the undifferentiated general state to that of the differentiated, articulated state (principle of orthogenesis). Parallel between the complete developmental history of the individual organizm and cultural growth. Studies primitive societies and compares them with technological societies. Lists five aspects of the developmental process; however, these are not truly analogous to developmental stages as perceived by other theorists. SYNCRETIC VS. DISCRETE *Syncrecis* is the fusion of qualities at a later developmental stage that are discrete or separate at an earlier stage, e.g., color and sound may be so closely related in a child's mind that they are perceived as one. In the adult they may be seen as related, but they can be recognized as distinct. DIFFUSE VS. ARTICULATED Parts may be perceived as separate rather than incorporated or articulated with the whole. The child often views objects in a more segregated than related way, e.g., a tree is seen as a tree not as a composit of leaves, branches, and trunk.	PHASES OF SOCIALIZATION ORAL DEPENDENCY: 0–2 yr First social system is the mother and child. This dyadic social system occurs only in a de facto sense as the child does not see self as an active part of the system. Child is dependent upon mother for need satisfaction; all of her activities that are directed toward child are important, e.g., closeness, withdrawal. Child's welfare takes precedence over mother's own comfort. Mother assumes all roles associated with decision making, power, initiation, and leadership; child is the recipient.

TABLE 7.1 (continued)

	S. Freud	*H. S. Sullivan*	*E. H. Erikson*[a]
			and of foreign overcontrol leads to a lasting propensity for doubt and shame. Acquires will.
	PRESCHOOL: 3–6 yr, phallic period (locomotor genital) Genitals provide the primary source of pleasure. Emergence of the Oedipus complex.	JUVENILE: 4–8 yr Socialization of the child as competition, cooperation, and compromise are learned. Chief interpersonal need is association with people of the same sex who are "like him or her."	INITIATIVE VS. GUILT: 3–6 yr Highlights the free possession of surplus energy for planning and for attacking or solving problems. Task of sex role identification. Opportunity for development of superego (conscience). Period of readiness for rapid learning and cooperation. Acquires purpose.
	LATENCY: 6–12 yr Sexual drives are normally dormant. Expanding peer relationships.	PREADOLESCENCE: 8–12 yr First intimate interpersonal relationship occurs with a peer of the same sex.	INDUSTRY VS. INFERIORITY: 6–12 yr Active period of socialization, particularly with peer group. Learns to win recognition by producing things and solving problems or completing tasks. Develops fundamental skills of technology. Vulnerable to development of a sense of inadequacy and inferiority. Acquires competence.
	PUBERTY AND ADOLESCENCE: 12 + yr Sexual desires and urges become prominent and the person seeks fulfillment of them. Resurgence of Oedipal complex; family triangle conflict and resolution.	LATE ADOLESCENCE: 12 + yr The person experiences needs for personal security, intimacy, and lust. Marks the establishment of a love relationship and the ability to live and share homosexuality. Limits choices; makes vocational choice and begins preparation.	IDENTITY VS. IDENTITY DIFFUSION: 13 + yr Search for self-identity with the ego's ability to integrate all identifications. Period of rapid physiological and psychological revolutions. Emancipation from parents and family. Evaluates own limits and powers. Period of heterosexual relationships. Achieves socially responsible behavior and learns to cope with emotions. Develops an ideology and philosophy of life. High risk of role confusion, linked with previous

J. Piaget	*H. Werner*	*T. Parsons and R. F. Bales*
PREOPERATIONAL THOUGHT: 0–7 yr PRECONCEPTUAL STAGE: 2–4 yr Egoentric, understands only own point of view. Experimentation with language, thought, and active learning continues. Establishes relationship between experience and action and begins to manipulate environment through action. Develops a symbolic thinking. Plays symbolic games. Reorganizes picture of the world through imaginative play, but lacks concept of reversibility. Cannot readily classify objects that vary in more than one characteristic. Indulges in animistic thinking, e.g., inanimate objects have powers and abilities. PERCEPTUAL OR INTUITIVE STAGE: 4–7 yr Able to visualize mentally only that which has been seen. Initiative play gradually replaces symbolic play. Imitates reality but enriches it with imagination, e.g., playing house, assuming roles. CONCRETE OPERATION: 7–12 yr Not egocentric. Believes own reasoning should agree with the reasoning of others. Begins to understand cause and effect in concrete immediate situations but cannot yet deduce hypothetically. Can carry out actions mentally without carrying them out physically. Animate and remote inanimate objects	RIGID VS. FLEXIBLE AND LABILE VS. STABLE This refers to function of an organization. Child's behavior tends to be rigid and repetitive. Lower animals exhibit repetitive rigid behaviors. Believed there was a similarity between the repetitive, ritualistic, inflexible behavior of primitive societies and the lower stages of human development. Similar differences between primitive societies and advanced societies as those between child and adult. MENTAL FUNCTIONING Mental functioning could be analyzed into a number of different functions, with some of these functions at lower levels than others. Lower functions are subordinated to the higher ones. Different functions may obtain same objective. Primordial (primitive) functions may develop to a greater extent in some people than in others. Whatever the level of functioning, it tends to stabilize and become rigid in adaptation to the environment. Crisis initiates the need to find a new level of functioning. It could cause some organisms to return to a lower level of functioning. Introduced the concept of "microgenesis," which postulates that something as rapid as the seconds needed to perceive an object, went through the processes needed to move from undifferentiated perception to a differentiated and articulated level of perception.	LOVE DEPENDENT PERSONALITY: 2–3 yr Primary relationship is with mother. Learns proper balance between autonomy and conformity, e.g., toilet training. Child begins to become a separate entity in the mother–child dyad. Mother is the superior being in terms of power and activity (instrumental role, viewed as concerned with external problem solving); child is the weaker member and is seen in an expressive role, (activities concerned with or centered around expression of feelings). Child begins to acquire patterns of behavior compatible with family social system. Begins to demonstrate some autonomy. Too much autonomy may lead to disapproval by mother. Child encouraged to take on new tasks; rewards given for success. Child begins to expect approval. POSTOEDIPAL STAGE OF PERSONALITY STRUCTURE: 3–12 yr Child moves from dyadic relationship with mother to a more differentiated four-member family system that includes mother, father, child, and sibling(s) of the opposite sex. Father emerges as a dominant figure imposing new and different demands on child; mother assumes a conciliatory role. Child's relationship with father is achievement oriented, with rewards for performance given in terms of whether or not they are deserved. Parsons sees this as being the possible basis for the competitive, hostile relationship sometimes seen between father and son. For the boy, sex role identification with father occurs. (Girl's sex role identification coincides with preoedipal period.) Child develops self-esteem and self-control capability; becomes capable of giving and receiving.

TABLE 7.1 (continued)

	S. Freud	*H. S. Sullivan*	*E. H. Erikson*[a]
			doubts as to sexual identity. Acquires fidelity.
	YOUNG ADULTHOOD Freud did not address this period, but believed that the structure of the personality was well established prior to this time.	MATURITY Characterized by interpersonal growth of the person who has capacity for happiness, self-awareness, and self-respect.	INTIMACY VS. ISOLATION Characterized by the increasing importance of human closeness and sexual fulfillment. Intimacy requires the capacity to commit yourself to concrete affiliations and partnerships and to develop the ethical strength to abide by such commitments, even though they may call for significant sacrifices and compromises. Forms a durable heterosexual relationship, mutually regulating work, procreation and recreation. Arrives at a working philosophy of life. Tolerant, self-objective, has mastered the environment. Ego dominant factor in personality and has developed capacity for self-realization. Capable of collaborating with others. Avoidance of intimacy leads to a sense of isolation and consequent self-absorption.

J. Piaget	H. Werner	T. Parsons and R. F. Bales
have life, e.g., sun, moon, planets.		
FORMAL OPERATIONS: 11–16 yr Develops capacity to make free use of hypothetical reasoning and considers all possible solutions to problems. Capable of conceptualizing, thinking propositionally, and using abstract reasoning. Can philosophize, idealize, conceive of many possible ways the world could operate and many alternative ways in which it would be better. Has difficulty reconciling idealistic hopes with practical possibilities. Only plants, animals, and human beings have life.		FURTHER DIFFERENTIATION OF PERSONALITY: 12 + yr Child becomes fully a part of the nuclear family with its roles, attitudes, and values. Explores emotional involvements outside of the home; peer relationships become important and influential. Has a clearly developed male or female sex role. (Note: Parsons and Bales view the phases of socialization of the child as having a branching effect, moving from a single undifferentiated focus—oral dependency—to increased number and complexity as the child develops.)
YOUNG ADULTHOOD Thinking takes on more objectivity and person is increasingly able to see the viewpoints of others. (Flavell, 1963)		

[a] Erikson's Eight Stages of Man takes into account the development of the mature person and includes the stages of Generativity vs. Stagnation and Ego Integrity vs. Despair. These stages are not included here in order to facilitate a more useful comparison with those theorists whose work goes only through the young adult stages. Theorists in the text who do not address specific developmental periods are also omitted from this chart.

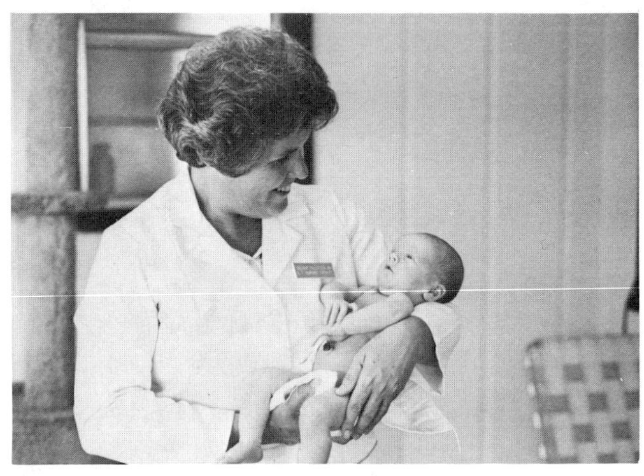

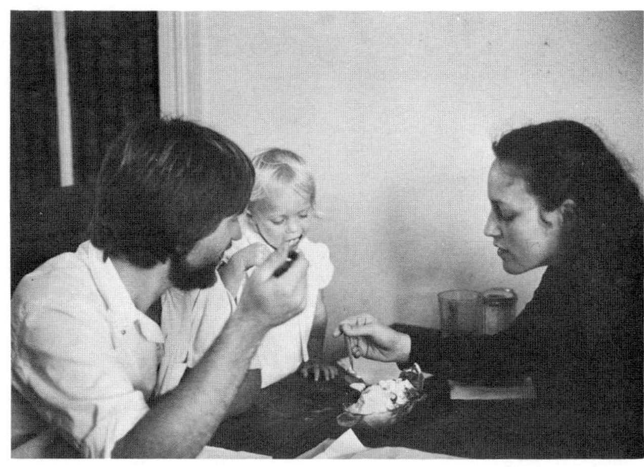

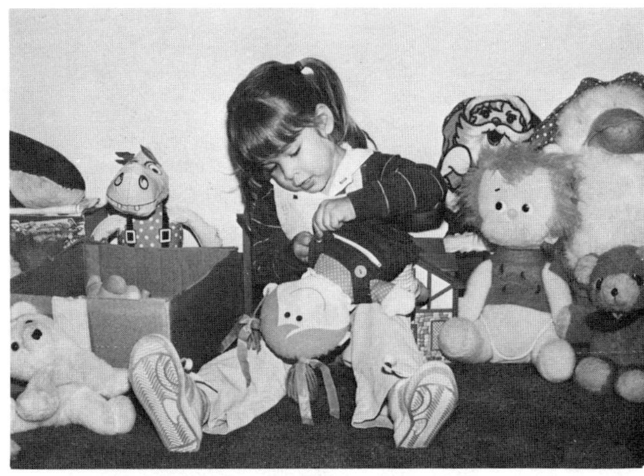

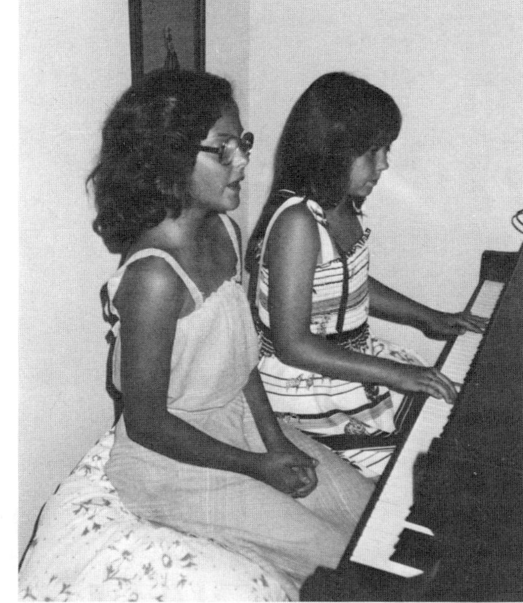

Figure 7.4
Erikson saw human development as occurring through eight sequential life stages.

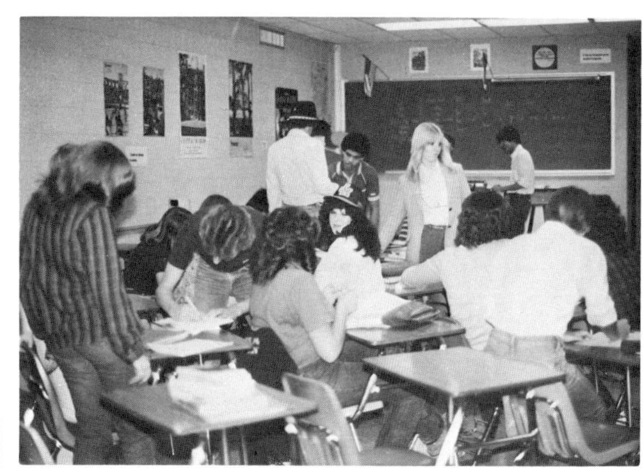

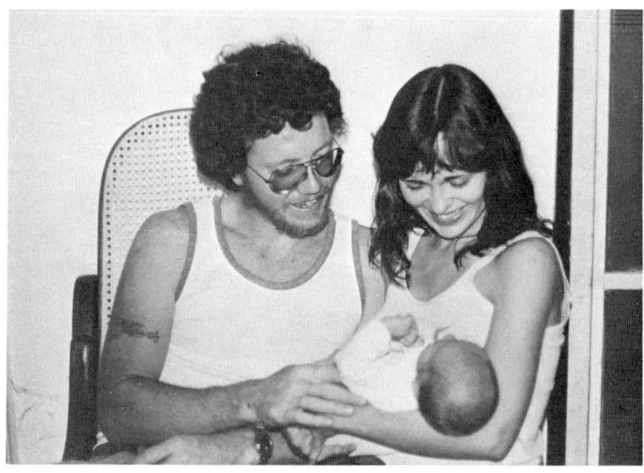

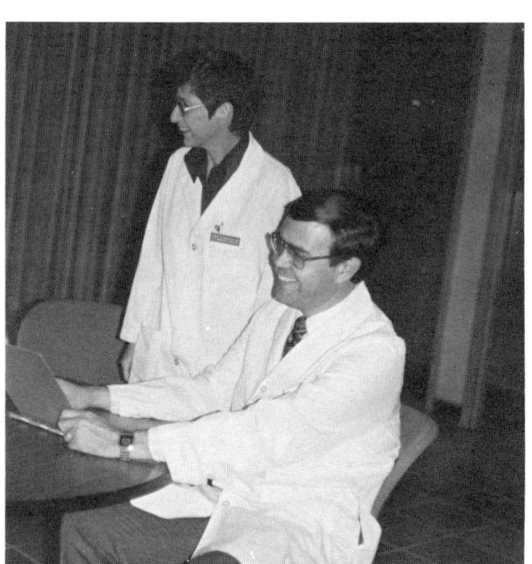

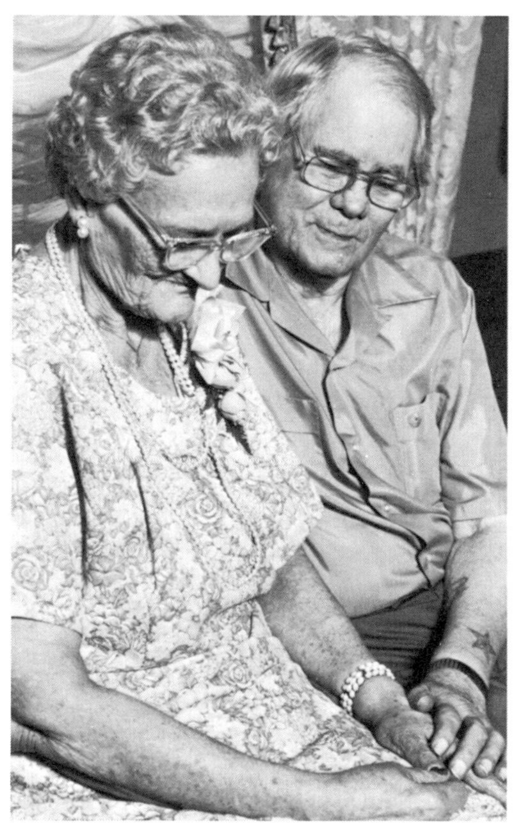

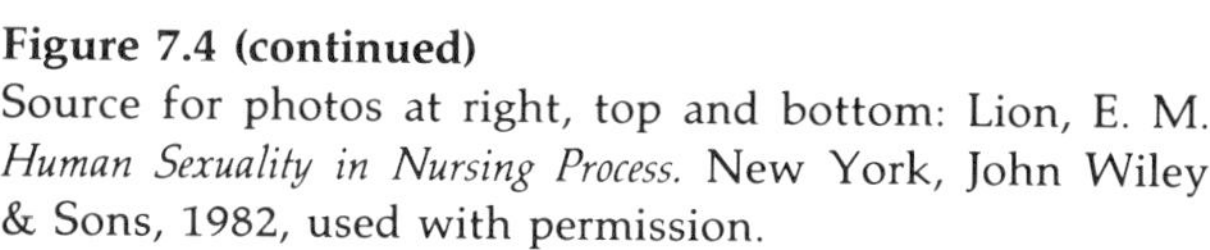

Figure 7.4 (continued)
Source for photos at right, top and bottom: Lion, E. M. *Human Sexuality in Nursing Process.* New York, John Wiley & Sons, 1982, used with permission.

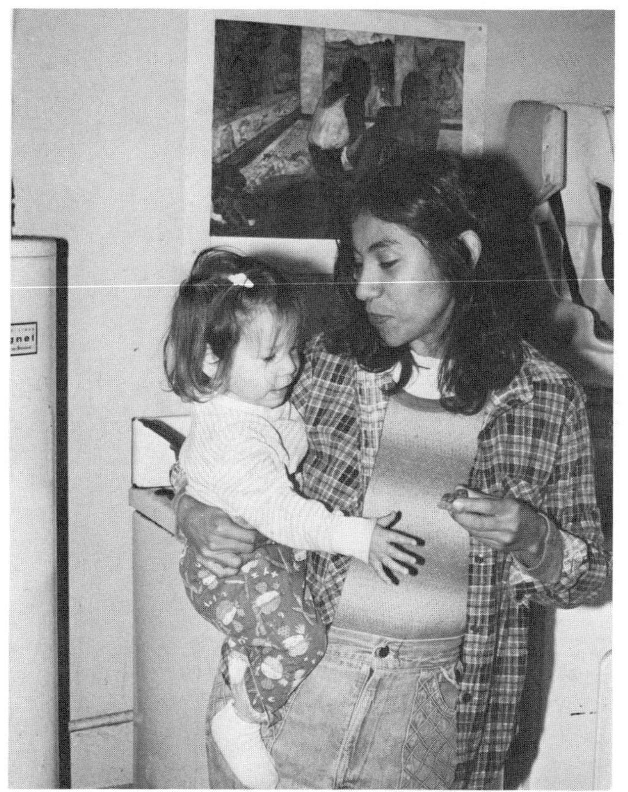
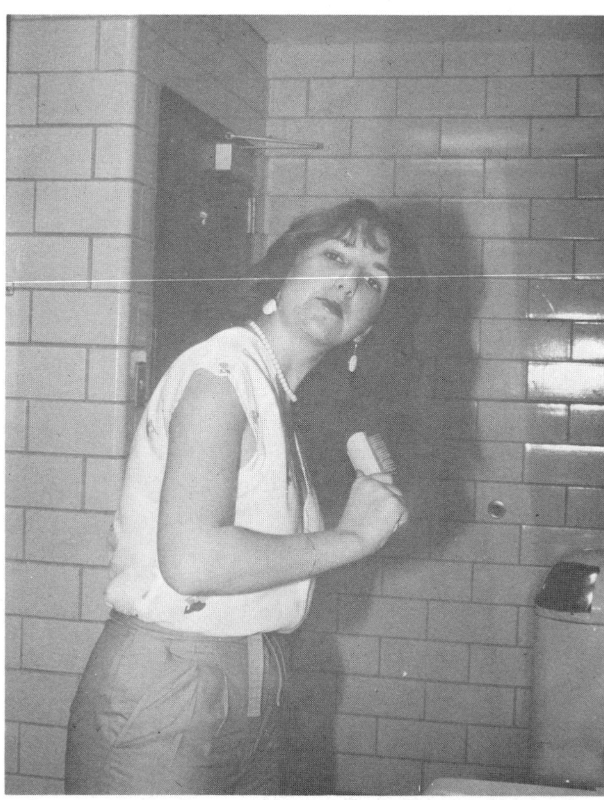
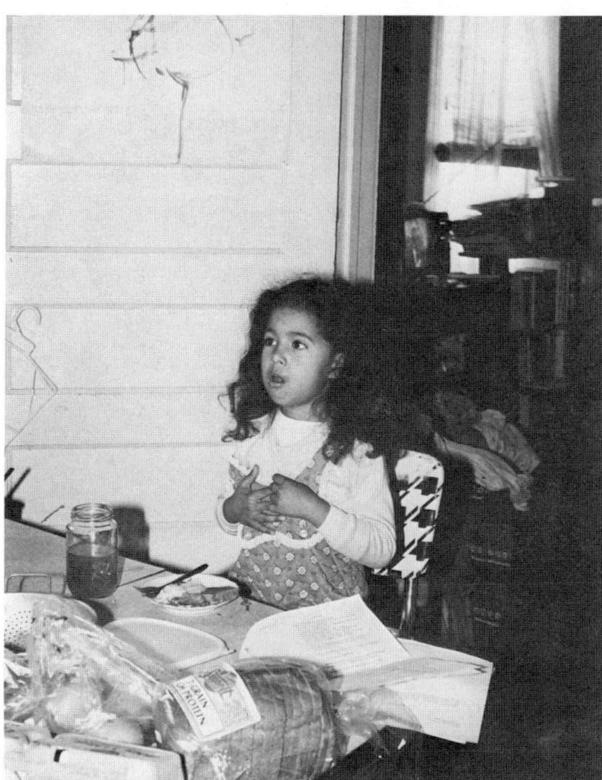
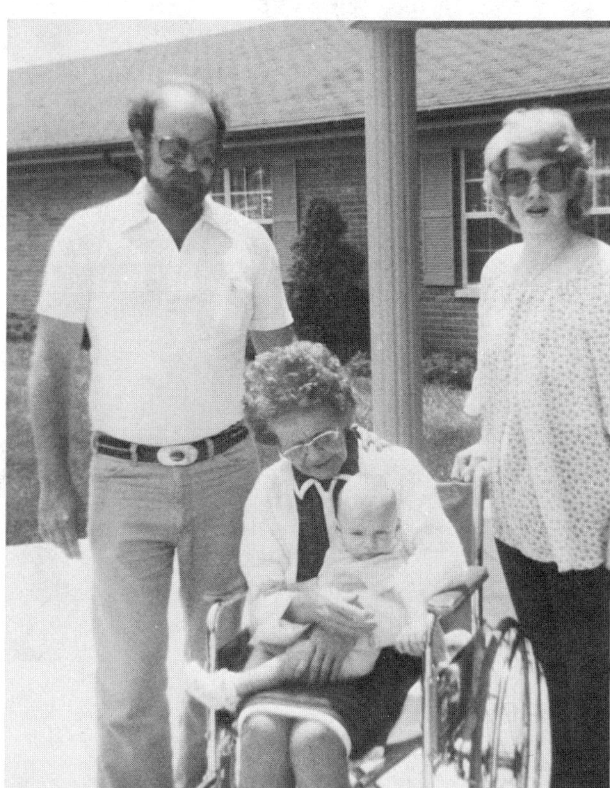

Figure 7.5
According to Maslow, human development and health occur through the satisfaction of a needs hierarchy that moved from basic needs for survival through needs associated with realization of a person's full potential.

categories are physiologic needs, love, belongingness, and self-esteem needs and self-actualization. He believed that achievement of the basic needs (physiologic and love) were of great importance during early childhood development periods, particularly the first 2 years of life. Achievement of the remaining needs were greatly affected by the meeting of these first two. Self-actualization was the ultimate accomplishment, developmentally, but Maslow did not believe that all people will reach this goal.

Maslow believed that the encouragement of curiosity in childhood was a necessary mechanism for promoting learning and healthy personality development. His contribution to human development theory was essentially through the encouragement of study of people from a healthy rather than ill point of view. He has been criticized for his research methods; however, Maslow's work has been accepted by a large number of people, possibly because of its pragmatic usefulness.

The Cognitive View

Jean Piaget (1896–1982), was a developmental psychologist who reported most of his work from Geneva, Switzerland, beginning in the 1920s (Piaget, 1954, 1963). Piaget examined the processes and nature of the thought and language of children—to a great extent, his own children. Cognitive development, according to Piaget, is illustrated in Figure 7.6.

Piaget wrote and published a great deal about his thoughts and observations. Flavell translated Piaget's work into English; interest in his work in the United States began in the 1930s, decreased somewhat, and was rekindled in the 1950s. Today, Piaget's work is the catalyst for the study of cognitive functioning by developmental theorists in this country and in others. His studies center around the child and make no clear transfer of his findings to the adult, particularly, the pregnant woman.

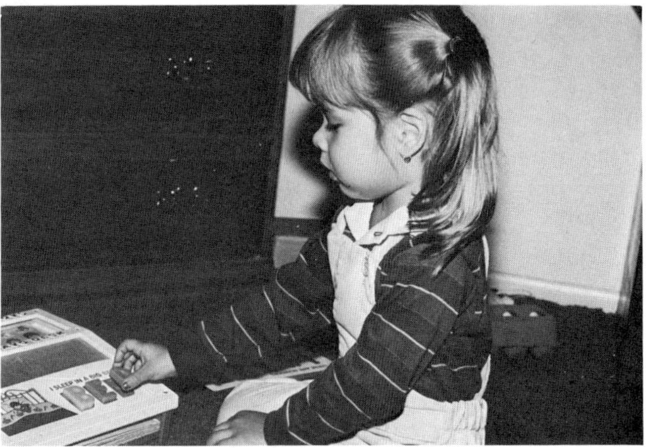

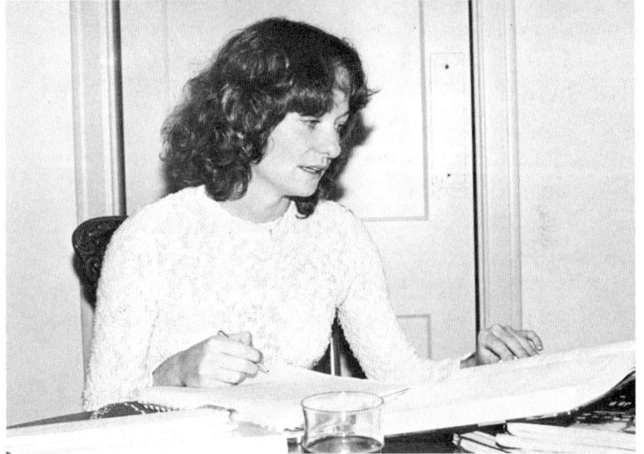

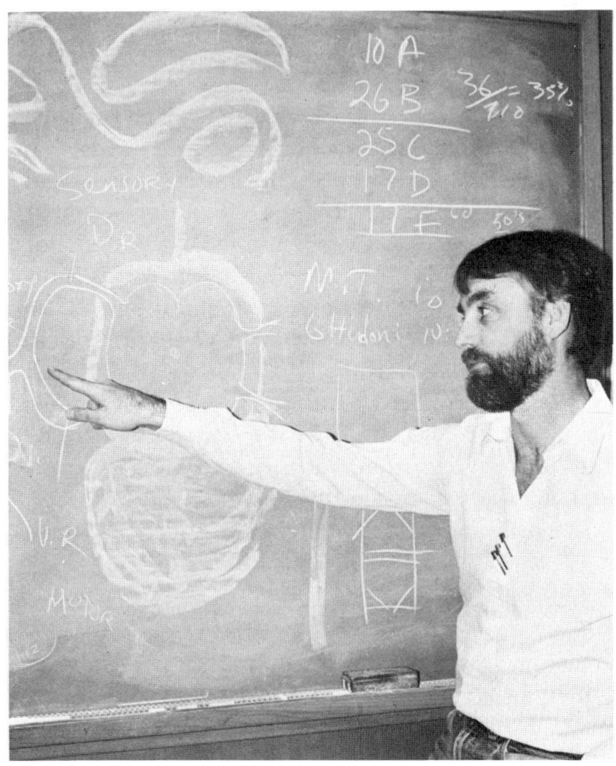

Figure 7.6
Cognition is a part of human development. Piaget saw cognitive development as proceeding from the ability of the young child to learn to coordinate actions with perceptions (sensorimotor) through the stages of perceptual or intuitive thought to mature cognitive functioning that enabled the person to attend to abstract formal cognitive operations, such as analysis and introspection.

Organismic Psychology

After World War II, Heinze Werner immigrated to the United States from Germany, and his theory of *Organismic Developmental Psychology* began to gain recognition (Fig. 7.7). Werner is believed by some to be the most "completely developmental" in orientation of any developmental psychology theorist today (Baldwin, 1968, p. 495).

Organismic developmental theory proposes that "all behavior and all responses are reactions of the total organism to the total stimulus situation" (Baldwin, 1968, p. 521). *Holism,* or *holistic organismic response,* is one of the major concepts supporting Werner's theory. Werner, whose background was in biology, particularly embryology and neurology, believed that there was an analogy to be drawn between biologic and psychologic developmental processes. He applied his knowledge of biologic development to the study of psychosocial development. Responses to his studies have included both rejection of and support for his ideas. He is one of the few developmental theorists who has attempted to describe a bio–psycho–social–cognitive parallelism in human development.

Sociologic Perspective

Talcott Parsons and Robert Bales present a *sociologic view* of a child's personality development. Although they derived some of their thinking from Freud, they see the personality of the child as being greatly influenced by the interactions within the family social system. Their theory of personality development views development as occurring through phases of socialization that correspond closely to Freud's stages of psychosexual development. Although the work of Parsons and Bales has not been as widely accepted as that of some of the other theorists, it does seem to partially support some of the contemporary ideas concerning early mother–child relationships and the importance of the family to the development of a psychosocially healthy person.

The usefulness of developmental theory to nurs-

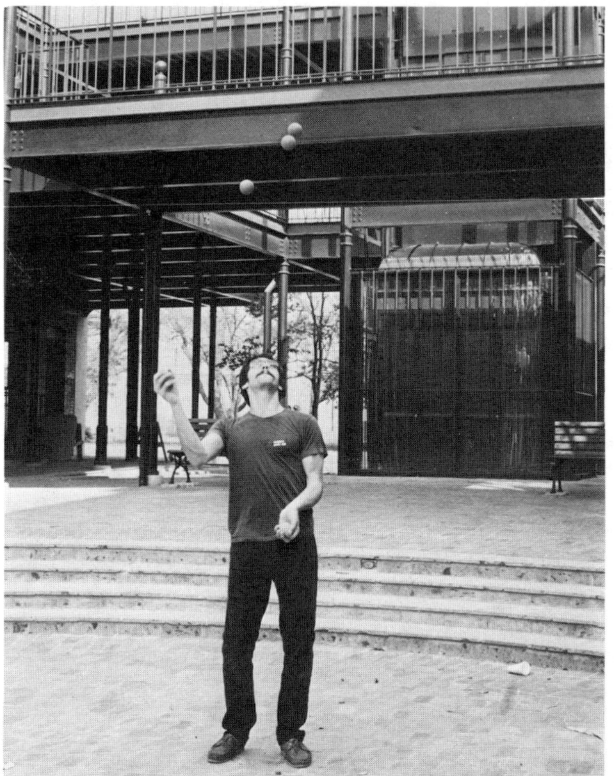

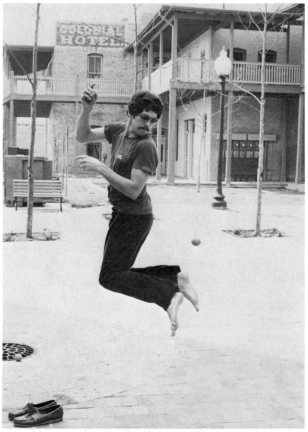

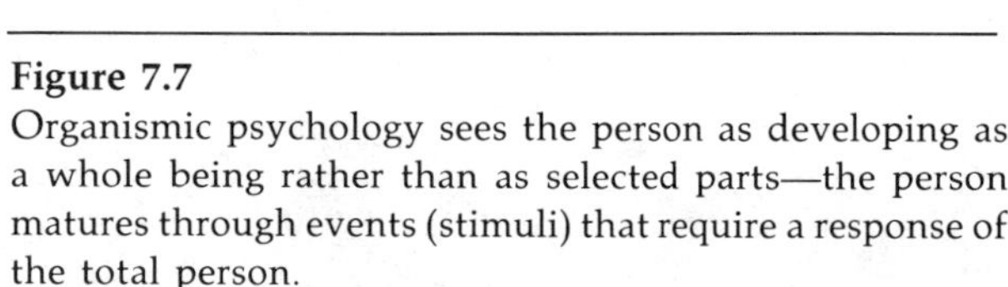

Figure 7.7
Organismic psychology sees the person as developing as a whole being rather than as selected parts—the person matures through events (stimuli) that require a response of the total person.

ing practice relies, to a great extent, on the nurse's understanding and acceptance of the theorist's point of view. Much of the basis for nursing care today reflects the selective use of particular parts of several different theories. Few would argue that developmental theory has given nurses, as well as other health care providers, a wealth of ideas from which they can better comprehend human growth and behavior.

SEXUAL IDENTIFICATION AND RESPONSE

Affectional Relationships

Relationships with other people are an integral part of living, and, in reality, a requirement for sustaining life, especially that of the infant and young child (Fig. 7.8). Relationships vary from intimate, affectional relationships with family and friends to indifferent, coincidental relationships that have no lasting effect upon a person's life. The maternity nurse is most concerned with two categories of relationships: parent–child relationships (particularly mother–infant relationships) and male–female relationships. These types of relationships seem to influence most directly the manner in which a couple, particularly the woman, approaches and copes with pregnancy, childbirth, and parenthood. Parent–child relationships are discussed briefly here and in more detail in Chapter 18; male–female relationships are discussed later in this chapter, as well as in Chapters 8 and 14. Some of the developmental aspects of relationship were discussed in the previous section in association with specific developmental theories and are not repeated here.

Life, for most people, is an interactional experience during which they enter into personal exchanges with many other people. The infant learns quickly that survival is dependent upon another human being to provide it with the essentials like food and love. These early interactions are believed to influence the ways in which the infant, child, and, later, adult relate to and trust other people (Fig. 7.9).

Early relationships are important for another reason as well; from them the young child learns his or her sexual identity. Two early relationships are of particular importance in people's lives for from them they acquire their sexual identity, as well as their sense of trust and belonging: the relationship with their mother or their surrogate care giver and the relationship with their father or the dominant man in their growing-up years. Both parents serve as the first teachers and role models for the child and, as such, profoundly influence the person their child will become. For example, the female child will learn how to be a girl, woman, and mother from her parents, principally her mother; her relationship with and expectations of men throughout her life will be influenced to a great extent by her relationship with her father. The child will also learn to trust (or not to trust) others, to give freely (or to withhold) love and affection, depending on the nature of this early relationship.

As the child grows, other important people will

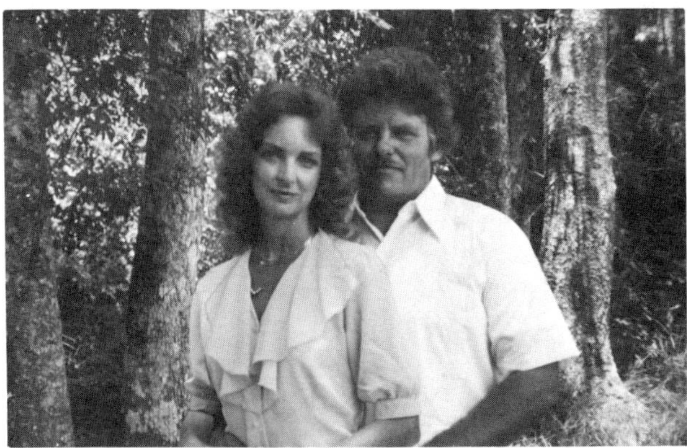

Figure 7.8
The human being relies greatly upon relationships with other people, especially those with whom affectional ties have been established.

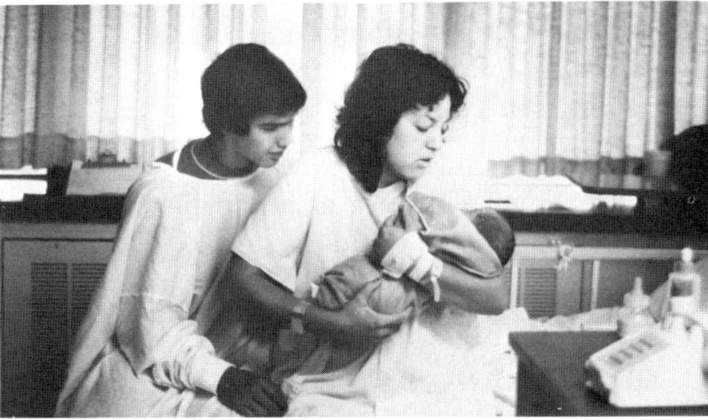

Figure 7.9
Parent–child relationships are of special importance to the child. The mother is most often the first person with whom the infant establishes an affectional relationship.

enter his or her social environment, and the child will learn to establish relationships with relatives, friends, peers of the same sex, and, later, peers of the opposite sex (Fig. 7.10). It is this capacity for entering into and sustaining relationships with other people that prepares the developing child to become adult and take on the demands, first, of the intimate man–woman relationship and, then, of the parent–child relationship. The child who has not learned, through such relationships, to trust others and to give affection and love will often grow into the parent who is unprepared to love and nurture his or her own child.

Relationships with family, friends, and acquaintances also help to lay the foundation for a trusting relationship between the person or couple and the people providing health care to them during events related to human reproduction, such as pregnancy and childbirth. Pregnancy brings the woman into very intimate contact with strangers—the physician, the nurse, and other members of the health care system. The relationships established with these people are personal, almost intimate, experiences that occasionally become an adjunct to or a substitution for some relationships with family members and friends whom the woman may perceive as being less understanding and supportive about her pregnancy.

Affectional relationships serve a number of purposes that help to prepare the person to experience pregnancy, childbirth, and parenthood. Such relationships:

- ▲ Provide the foundations for the child to develop trust or distrust of other people, which are the basis for sustaining old and forming new relationships
- ▲ Are the training grounds for the child to learn sexual identity, role, and function and for guiding self-confidence and self-esteem
- ▲ Enable the child to acquire basic beliefs and values from which he or she will build a personal ideology and value system
- ▲ Are a mechanism for providing love, affection, and support and for teaching the child how to give to and receive or take from another person

The ways in which and the extent to which these purposes are accomplished often determine whether the reproductive experience will be healthy or unhealthy.

Sexual Identification

Sexual identification takes two forms: the recognition by others of a person's gender (role) and the personal identification of self as either male or fe-

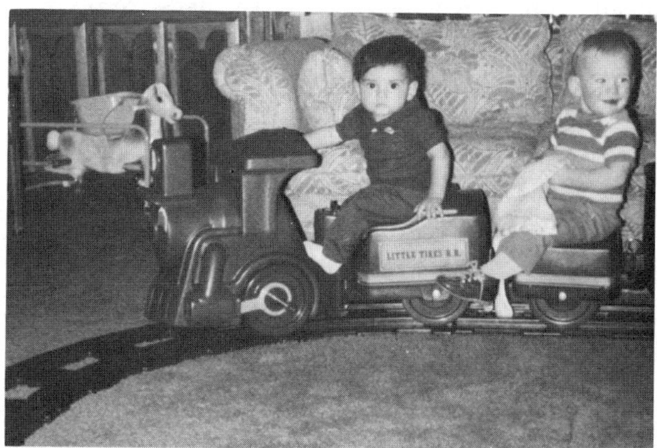

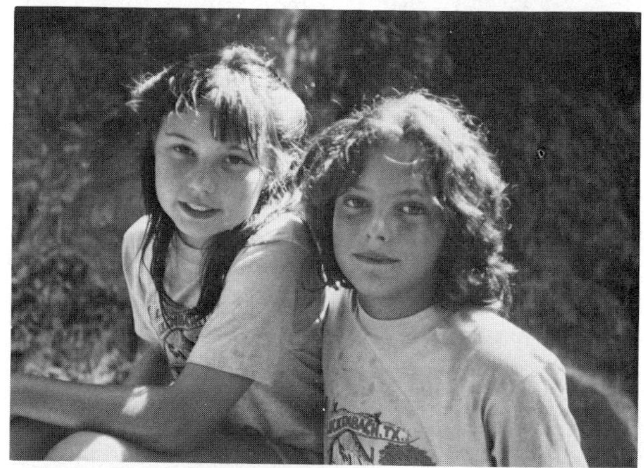

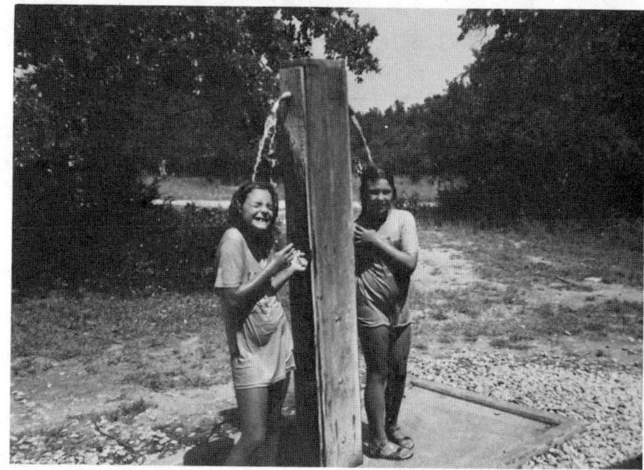

Figure 7.10
Relationships with playmates are a large part of a child's early social experience.

male in regard to our own concept of "ideal" (sexual self-identity). Both of these have a major impact on how a man and woman see themselves as reproductive beings. Perception by others of our sexual self is often colored not only by physical appearance and behavior but also by society's expectations of the role prescribed for that sex. A person's own sexual identity is based on the interrelationship of biologic endowment, socialization to a sex role, total life experiences, and relationships with other people of both sexes, beginning with the primary relationship with the care provider in early infancy, usually the mother (Figs. 7.11 and 7.12).

Genetically, the sex of a person is determined at the moment of conception when the X or Y chromosome from the male parent unites with the X chromosome from the female parent. Sex organ differentiation occurs early in the prenatal life so that the fetal sex is observable in aborted fetuses as early as 12 weeks gestation. Under the influence of testosterone, the male urogenital system develops during fetal life; in the absence of this androgenic hormone, the female develops during fetal life. Studies seem increasingly to support the belief that there is another critical point during fetal life, just preceding birth or in the early months of infancy, during which the fetal or infant brain undergoes a specific process of sex typing, probably as a result of the action of testosterone (Money & Ehrhardt, 1972). This neural sex typing may be the biologic director of some sex-related behavior such as male aggressiveness and female passivity, as well as be the cause for the endocrine development of the male in an acyclic sexual pattern and the female in a cyclic sexual pattern that begins with puberty.

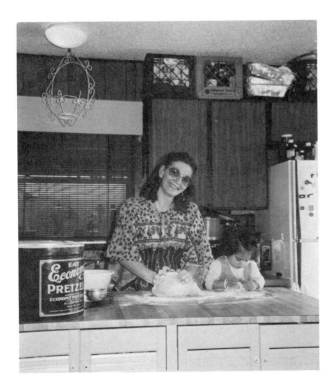

Figure 7.11
The child begins to learn sex role and sexual identification from early relationships with parents. The mother is often a role model for her daughter.

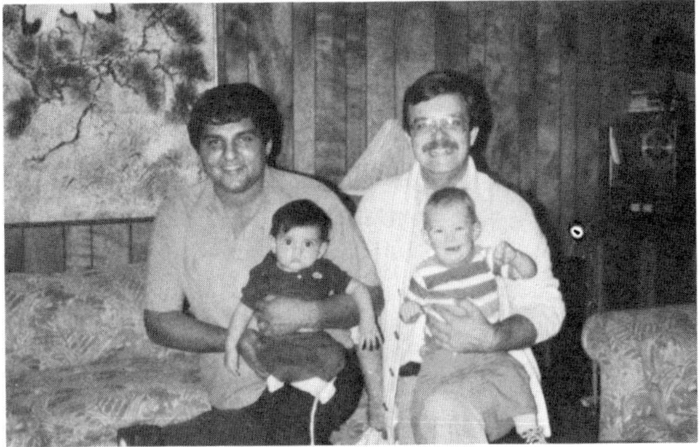

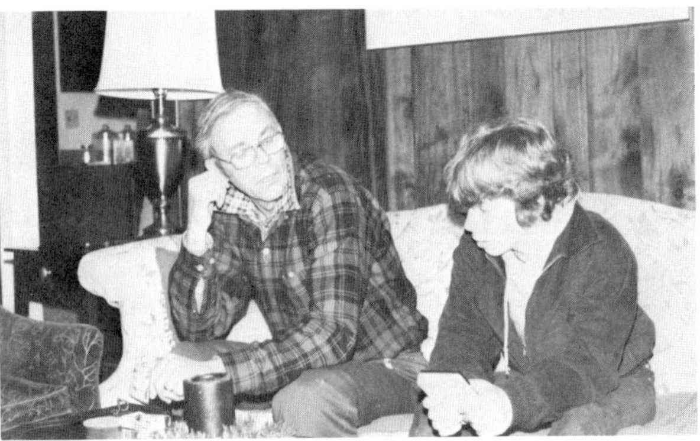

Figure 7.12
The father influences the type of man his son will become.

DIFFERENCES IN BOYS AND GIRLS

Biologic and behavioral differences in boys and girls at birth have been observed and reported (Bardwick, 1971). Most boys are born with greater muscle mass and of a slightly larger size. Boys show more motor activity; girls display less motor activity but greater response to tactile stimulation and pain.

As the infant develops, further differences are noted. By 6 months, girls respond to visual stimulation with longer attention spans; they are generally more socially responsive; they can respond better to complex stimuli such as music; and they attend to the human face better, forming an earlier attachment (fixation) to the mother figure. Boys fixate better on light and attend to intermittent sound tones.

Throughout the first year of life, girl's preference for high-complexity stimuli continues, whereas boys appear to prefer less-complex stimuli. Language development occurs earlier in girls than in the boys, which may be associated with the mother–infant interaction during infancy. Women have been shown to talk more to their girl than to their boy infants. Boys attend to contextual relationships earlier and better.

Boys continue to exhibit greater aggressive behavior than girls. Girls tend to conform better than boys to parental and social demands, even at a very early age. Study has shown that at about 13 months of age, girls respond more actively to the mother figure. When placed in a controlled play situation, they will seek the mother out more readily than will boys and will demonstrate frustration more often when the mother is removed. Girls tend to socialize more with their mothers through touch and vocalization (Goldberg & Lewis, 1972). Boys demonstrate greater early efforts toward independence; they are less likely to conform to parental or societal norms and are more likely to be explorative and adventuresome.

Boys tend to thwart authority more often than do girls and are disciplined more frequently by both parents and school authorities. Harsh methods of discipline are more often used on boys than on girls. Characteristics such as assertiveness and aggressiveness are seen in the adolescent and adult men, particularly in regard to sexual behavior. Girls usually carry their passivity and compliance into their adolescent and adult years, especially when observed and compared with boys.

Behavioral differences between boys and girls from birth through early adulthood are readily documented. Which of these differences are biologically derived and which are influenced by psychosocial factors are not definite. The changing role of men and women in contemporary society may well change some of the findings currently reported, particularly if sex-related behavior is more the result of socialization and social environment.

What is clearly apparent in reported findings is that a prescribed sex role identity exists in most primitive as well as developed societies and that sex role and gender identity, either learned or instinctual, are demonstrated early in life. Children and adults who differ either biologically or behaviorally from expected societal norms are often perceived as different and may be ostracized from normal affectional relationships within their families and peer groups. The sex of the infant is often one of the major concerns of expectant parents and may well influence parental relationships with and expectations of that child.

THEORIES

A number of psychologists have addressed sexual development in their writings. Freud was the first person to describe periods of psychosexual development from infancy through adolescence: Erikson, particularly, has related these periods to his Eight Ages of Man. Newman and Newman (1975) described four stages through which sex role identification is learned and acquired: learning the gender label (I am male or female, boy or girl, man or woman); acquisition of sex role standards (I do as others of my sex do); establishing sex role preference (I want to be a boy; I want to be a girl); and identification with the parent of the same sex (girl: I am like mom; boy: I am like dad).

ROLE MODELS

Because of changing social mores concerning sexuality combined with realignment of roles within the family, parents are often not the principle sexual role models for their developing children. Teachers, acquaintances, relatives, and peers may exert equal or greater influence upon a person's sexual identification. Although it is widely believed that much of a child's sexual identification is determined by age 6, few would argue that influences beyond this age are also great.

The roles and functions of today's parents may differ considerably from the traditional models for mothers and fathers (see Chapter 18). Many mothers who assume roles and responsibilities that take them outside of the home, have given up the role as the child's primary care giver. Some fathers are seeking greater involvement as care givers rather than just as disciplinarians with their children. Reversal of roles is being seen, where the mother takes on the principle provider role and the father assumes the homemaker role. Sex roles are modeled in many different ways in contemporary society, and sex role confusion is always a risk for the young child, and particularly the adolescent.

> *Secure identity allows us to take real risks in intimacy; it allows us to take liberties with our masculinity and feminity. Without that base, however, sex role liberation gets mangled with slipperiness and evasion of responsibility and becomes part of the general slime that laps against the piers of committed relationships.*
>
> *Kilpatrick, 1975, p. 169*

Sexual Response

Theory explaining sexual response in the human is incomplete. What is reported tends to support the viewpoint that sexual response and function in human beings is a result of a combination of emotional and physical factors. This point of view differs from what is known about the sexual response of lower animals, which is essentially under neuroendocrine control.

Sexual response in humans is believed to be tied to motives for sexual behavior. Sexual motivation, like sexual response, is also incompletely understood. What causes the human being to engage in sexual activity? Instinct? Need? Self-gratification? Love? There are no clear, correct responses to such a question. The answer can probably be found in some combination of reasons. Social and biologic scientists have tried for years to provide some answers to sexual motives and responses.

A *motive* is an internal energy force that arises from a physical or psychologic need and that compels a person to behave in such a way that the need is satisfied (Hyde, 1979, p. 9). Motives may be drives such as hunger and thirst.

Sexual motivation is the desire or urge to engage in sexual activity (Goldstein, 1976, p. 95). It precedes puberty and may be present throughout a person's lifetime. It is an individual characteristic and follows no definite pattern. Freud viewed the sex drive as one of two primary forces that governed all behavior.

Most contemporary psychologists accept sex as a basic drive, but few believe that it has an exact correlation to hunger and thirst. Food and water are necessary for survival; individual life can exist when there is sexual abstinence. However, sexual activity is obviously needed in order to maintain the species. Lack of food and water results in a decrease in body stores, eventual depletion of resources, and ultimately death; no such physical trauma is associated with sexual deprivation. One view of sexual motivation is as a learned appetite rather than a basic drive (Hardy, 1964). Another view is that sex is a basic drive but behavior associated with that physiologic need is learned. Although sexual activity is not necessary to sustain life, sexual need is recognized as a part of life from childhood through senescence. Sexual motivation is highly individualized; there is no single pattern that applies to all people.

Much of what is presently known about human sexual response comes from the research by Alfred Kinsey, who studied the psychosocial characteristics of sexual behavior of men and women (Kinsey, 1948, 1953), and from the studies of William Masters and Virginia Johnson (1966, 1970), who focused on the physiology of sexual response.

Kinsey's studies have revealed much about sexual activity that is pertinent today (even though his research is more than 30 years old). Kinsey described sexual practices regarding a number of variables, two of which were petting and nonmarital (premarital) sexual intercourse. A significant number of people reported that they engaged in activities described as petting; many of them also reported feelings of guilt associated with their behavior. Kinsey believed that petting behaviors, particularly among people belonging to Anglo cultures, were restrained as a result of the cultural values that taught children that touching people of the opposite sex was not "nice." This restraint between the sexes was found to carry over into adult sexual relationships. Kinsey also found that lack of skill in love making, particularly poor techniques or approaches by men and restraint of women, accounted for the failure of a significant number of upperclass marriages. Both sexes, but especially women, were found to have had little instruction about sexual matters as they were growing up and had obtained most of their information from peers or courtship experiences such as petting.

Kinsey's data concerning nonmarital or premarital sexual activity showed that the age of the woman was related to the incidence of nonmarital sex, particularly sexual intercourse, with the incidence of intercourse increasing as the age of the women increased. He found no significant differences among women of different social classes and explained this as the result of early marriages among women of the lower social strata. Educational level was a significant factor for men engaging in nonmarital intercourse. College men tended to have nonmarital sexual intercourse less frequently than did their noncollege counterparts.

The maternity nurse must not undermine the importance of Kinsey's work because of changing societal values about sexuality since the time of his studies. Much of what is learned by young people comes from information given to them by their parents, teachers, religious counselors, and others, many of whom still endorse the sexual values that existed at the time of Kinsey's work. Because of the rapidly changing social–sexual climate in the United States, however, the maternity nurse must also be informed about the sexual practices that reflect the values of today's young people.

Masters and Johnson focused on the physiology of sexual activity, particularly sexual intercourse. Much of what is known about sexual intercourse comes from their work. In spite of their contributions, there is still much about physical sexual response that is speculative and often incomplete. Masters and Johnson described four phases associated with the sexual act: excitement, plateau, orgasm, and resolution. The physiology of these phases is similar for both sexes and relies upon two major events: vasoconstriction of tissues and structures and myotonia, reflected by both specific and generalized increased muscle tone.

Excitement may occur from other than physical stimulation. Whether the stimulus is sight, sound, odor, thought, or touch, the same series of activities seem to ensue. Massage of either the male or female genitals, particularly the male glans penis or the female clitoris, leads to sexual sensations. These sensations serve as signals that are mediated through the pudendal nerve and sacral plexus to the sacral segments of the spinal cord and on to the cerebrum. Local areas adjacent to the genitals may also serve as stimuli for the transfer of sexual sensations to the spinal cord. These messages result in the stimulation by the parasympathetic nerves to cause the arteries in the genital area, especially the male penis and the female vulva, to dilate, increasing blood supply to the vessels located in these structures; concurrently, the veins constrict, interfering with venous return of the blood in the vessels and resulting in engorgement of the sexual organs. Similar changes may occur in the vessels in other parts of the body. The penis becomes turgid and may enlarge as much as 50% over its nonerectile state as the blood fills and remains in the cavernous erectile tissue. The clitoris becomes erect, and the vaginal introitus tightens. There is a proportional relationship between the extent and intensity of the stimulus and the degree of excitement.

Plateau is a period during which sexual stimulation is sustained. The engorgement of the penis continues and increases in some cases, as does engorgement of the woman's genital areas. The vulva and especially the labia minora may even change from their bright pink/red color to a deep red hue. The parasympathetic impulses also stimulate some glandular secretions from the Bartholin's glands located bilaterally on each side of the vagina. These secretions lubricate the inside of the vaginal introitus and aide in penile entry, as well as help protect the penis and the vaginal tissues from irritation. The bulbourethral and Littre's glands in the man also secrete a lubricating mucous that is discharged through the man's urethra and aids in lubrication.

Other physiologic changes may appear elsewhere in the body as sexual excitement is maintained. There is an increase in heart rate and blood pressure. Cardiovascular changes seem to be more pronounced in men than in women. Respiratory effort is accelerated, and in the late plateau stage hyperventilation may occur. There is an increase in muscle tone, particularly in the pelvic region, but a generalized myotonia may also occur. The woman's breasts show signs of engorgement, and the nipples become erect. Breast changes in the man are not as pronounced; some men, however, do have nipple erection. Changes in skin color have been described with deepening of skin tone around the darker pigmented areas of the body such as the scrotum and the breast areola and nipple.

Orgasm is the culmination of the sexual act; however, female orgasm is not essential for fertilization to occur as it is in some of the lower animals. Female orgasm is characterized by rhythmic contractions of the perineal muscles possibly as a result of spinal reflex impulses. The fallopian tubes and uterus may also undergo some contraction leading to increased uterine and tubal motility. It has been suggested that oxytocin plays a role in uterine and tubal contractility during orgasm. This theory is not definitive but is based on animal studies. This contractility may in some way aid in transport of sperm to the site of the ovum.

Resolution is the reversion of the man and woman to the physiologic state that existed prior to stimulation and excitement. It is characterized by decongestion of the genital and breast tissue and general body relaxation. Women can usually be reexcited during this period, but men tend to require a longer time before they can respond once more to stimulation. This non-responsive period for the man is simultaneous with resolution.

Sexual identification and response do not occur in isolation from the total man and woman. The relationship between the person and his or her family, as well as the culture of which the person and family are a part, play an influential role in molding sexual identity and affecting sexual function. Sexual relationships between a man and a woman may be transitory or permanent, but they have a profound effect upon the ways in which both will relate to other men and women.

SUMMARY

Psychosocial readiness was defined as the capability of a man and woman to participate rationally in the events related to human reproduction and to establish and maintain affectional relationships and sexual identity and function. Psychosocial readiness was discussed within the context of selected theories of individual development, including the psychoanalytic school of thought, social psychology, humanistic psychology, the cognitive point of view, and organismic psychology. The overview of developmental theory will enable you to compare the different schools of developmental theory.

Affectional relationships were presented briefly in view of the purposes they served: the establishment of trust, sexual identity, and function; mechanisms for giving and receiving love and affection; and personal support. Affectional relationships were also viewed as providing the early and continuing learning fields for the developing person.

Sexual identity was discussed from the perspectives of sex gender, or role, physical sexual response, and sexual self-identification as a man or woman. This discussion relied on selected research, mainly that of Kinsey and Masters and Johnson.

REFERENCES AND READINGS

Baldwin, A. E. *Theories of Child Development.* New York: John Wiley & Sons, 1968.

Bardwick, J. M. *Psychology of Women: A Study of Bio-cultural Conflicts.* New York: Harper & Row, 1971.

Benedek, T. The Psychosomatic Implications of the Primary Unit: Mother–Child Relatedness. *Am J Orthopsychiatry* 19:642, 1949.

Berelson, B., Steiner, G. A. *Human Behavior: An Inventory of Scientific Findings.* New York: Harcourt Brace and World, 1964.

Branfenbrenner, U. *The Ecology of Human Development—Experiments by Nature and Design.* Cambridge,: Harvard University Press, 1979.

Caplan, G. *Concepts of Mental Health and Consultation: Their Application in Public Health Social Work.* Washington, D.C.: Children's Bureau Publication, No. 373, US Department of Health, Education and Welfare, 1959.

Caplan, G. *An Approach to Community Mental Health.* New York: Grune & Stratton, 1961.

Caplan, G. Psychological Aspects of Pregnancy, in Lief, H. L. et al. (Eds.), *The Psychological Basis of Medical Practice.* New York: Harper & Row, 1973.

Clark, A. L., Affonso, D. D. *Childbearing: A Nursing Perspective.* (2nd ed.) Philadelphia: F. A. Davis, 1979.

Deutsch, H. *Psychology of Women: Vol. I, Girlhood; Vol. II, Motherhood.* New York: Grune & Stratton, 1945.

Duvall, E. M., Hill, R. *Report of the Committee on the Dynamics of Family Interaction.* Washington, D.C.: National Conference on Family Life, 1968.

Duvall, E. M. *Marriage and Family Development* (5th ed.). Philadelphia: J. B. Lippincott, 1977. (1st ed.: *Family Development.* 1957.)

Erikson, E. *Childhood and Society.* New York: W. W. Norton, 1950.

Freud, S. *Complete Psychological Works of Sigmund Freud,* Strachey, J. (Trans.). London: Hogarth Press, 1955, Vol. 18.

Goldberg, S., Lewis, M. Play Behavior in the Year-old Infant: Early Sex Differences, in Bardwick, J. M. (ed.) *Readings on the Psychology of Women.* New York: Harper & Row, 1972.

Goldstein, B. *Human Sexuality.* New York: McGraw-Hill, 1976.

Hardy, K. H. An Appetitional Theory of Sexual Motivation. *Psychol Rev* 71:1, 1964.

Harlow, H. The Nature of Love. *Am Psychol* 13:673, 1958.

Havighurst, R. J. *Human Development and Education.* New York: Longmans, Green, 1953.

Howell, J. G. *Advances in Family Psychiatry.* New York: International Universities Press, 1979.

Hyde, J. S. *Understanding Human Sexuality.* New York: McGraw-Hill, 1979.

Illingsworth, R. S. *The Development of the Infant and Young Child.* New York: Churchill Livingstone, 1975.

Kaluger, G., Kaluger, M. F. *Profiles in Human Development.* St. Louis: C. V. Mosby, 1976.

Kaluger, G., Kaluger, M. F. *Human Development—The Span of Life.* St. Louis: C. V. Mosby, 1979.

Kilpatrick, W. *Identity and Intimacy.* New York: Dell, 1975.

Kinsey, A. C., Pomeroy, W. B., Martin, C. W., Gebhard, P. *Sexual Behavior in the Human Female.* Philadelphia: W. B. Saunders, 1953.

Lidz, T. *The Person: His Development Through the Life Span.* New York: Basic Books, 1968.

Maslow, A. *Motivation and Personality.* New York: Harper & Row, 1970.

Masters, W., Johnson, V. *Human Sexual Response.* Boston: Little, Brown, 1966.

Masters, W., Johnson, V. *Human Sexual Inadequacy.* Boston: Little, Brown, 1970.

Money, J., Ehrhardt, A. *Man and Woman; Boy and Girl.* Baltimore: Johns Hopkins University Press, 1972.

Newman, B., Newman, R. *Development Through Life: A Psychological Approach.* Homewood, Ill.: Dorsey Press, 1975.

Parton, D. A. Learning to Imitate in Infancy. *Child Dev* 47:14, 1976.

Piaget, J. *The Construction of Reality in the Child,* Cook, M. (Trans.). New York: Basic Books, 1954.

Piaget, J. *The Origins of Intelligence in Children,* Cook, M. (Trans.). New York: W. W. Norton, 1963.

Rayner. *Human Development* (2nd ed.). London: George Allen & Unwin, 1978.

Rubin, R. Basic Maternal Behavior. *Nurs Outlook* 9:683, 1961.

Rubin, R. Attainment of the Maternal Role: Part I—Processes. *Nurs Res* 16:237, 1967.

Rubin, R. Binding-In the Postpartum Period. *Matern Child Nurs J* 6:67, 1977.

Stein, D. *Motivation and Emotion.* New York: MacMillan, 1974.

Sullivan, H. S. The Interpersonal Theory of Psychiatry, in Perryman, H. S., Gowell, M. L. (Eds.), *The Collected Works of H. S. Sullivan.* New York: W. W. Norton, 1953.

Tanner, L. M. Developmental Tasks of Pregnancy, in Bergerson, B. S. et al. (Eds.), *Current Concepts in Clinical Nursing.* St. Louis: C. V. Mosby, 1969, Vol. 2.

Wholen, R. E. Sexual Motivation. *Psychol Rev* 73:151, 1966.

Yorburg, B. *Sexual Identity—Sex Roles and Social Change.* New York: John Wiley & Sons, 1974.

8

ADOLESCENCE: A PERIOD OF INTEGRATION

Adolescence is the developmental bridge between childhood and maturity (Fig. 8.1); it is a period of biologic and psychosocial integration.

> *During adolescence an individual must master a bewildering variety of familial, social and vocational roles before he [or she] is accepted on equal footing by adult citizenry. Today, advances in technology and social systems pre-empt traditional modes of behavior and demand of the adolescent new attitudes and standards for effective citizenry.*
>
> *Grinder, 1963, p. 17*

A significant number of people for whom the maternity nurse provides care will come from the adolescent age group 12–19 years old. These young people will enter the reproductive health care system, in various stages of readiness, to undertake the responsibilities associated with mature sexual function such as pregnancy and parenthood. Some will seek information about sex-related matters such as contraception and abortion. Others will have health needs that require diagnosis or treatment such as menstrual disorders or venereal disease. Many will already be pregnant and be entering the system for health care for the first time since childhood. The maternity nurse is in a unique position to teach these young people, as well as to minister to their physical/emotional needs.

There is no more important professional relationship into which the maternity nurse will enter than the one that is established with the adolescent client. The adolescent who seeks health care services is an investment in future reproductive health and, as such, deserves recognition and consideration befitting such status. Because adolescence is a period of personal vulnerability, the experience the adolescent patient has with the nurse and other health professionals can either foster good health practices or it can impede them and send the young person out of the health care delivery system never to return voluntarily. The pregnant adolescent is especially vulnerable and is considered to be at reproductive risk for physical, psychosocial, and often economic reasons. This young woman needs help with the pregnancy at hand, as well as with decision making about her emerging role as mother and her potential for future pregnancies. The adolescent expectant father also needs information and support. Both may need to reconsider and often reorder their priorities concerning school, work, and parenthood.

At times, adolescents will require assistance with making decisions about continuation or termination of a pregnancy. The nurse needs to be sensi-

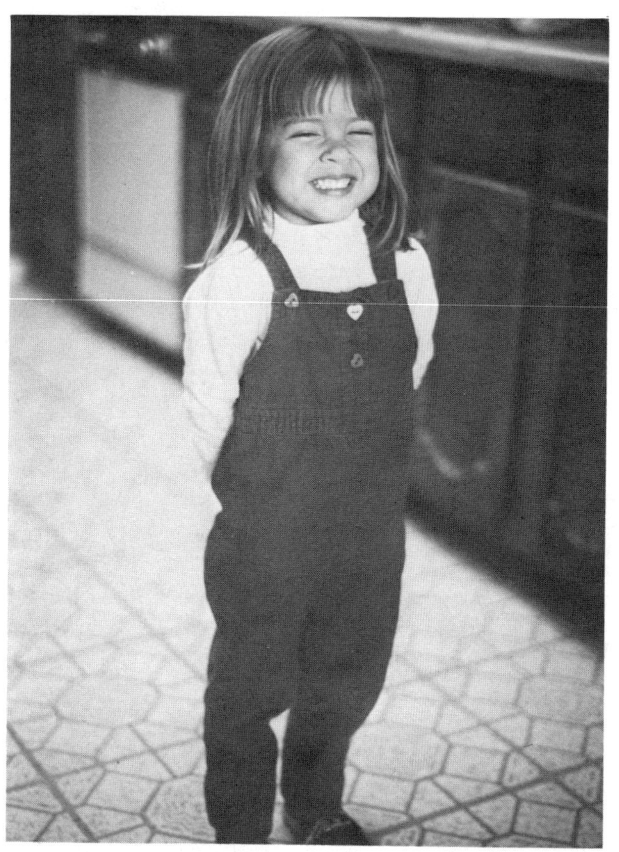

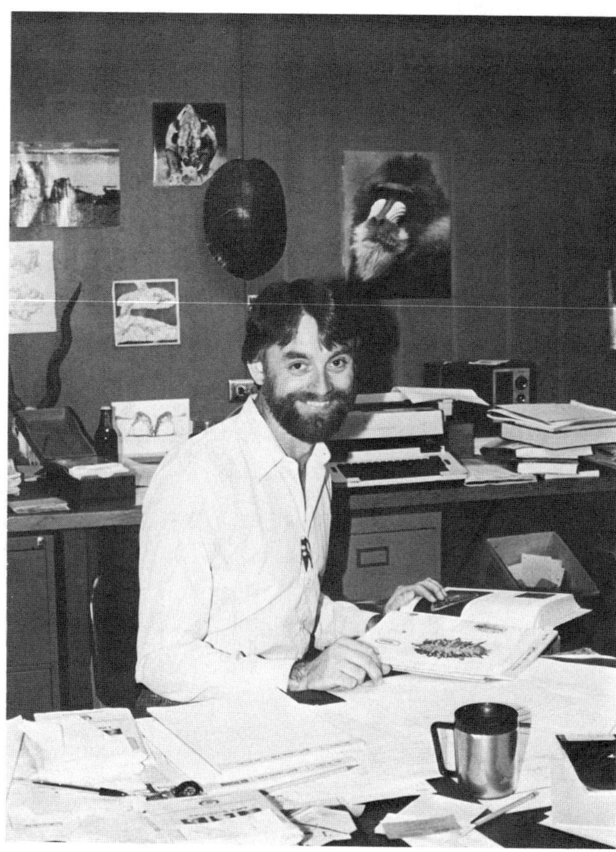

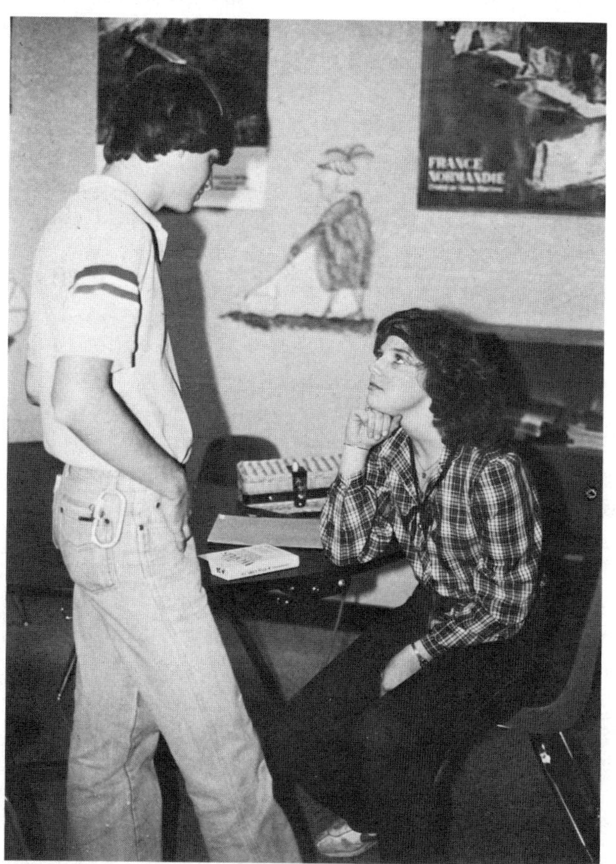

Figure 8.1
Adolescence bridges the gap between childhood and maturity.

tive to the young person, as well as knowledgeable about the options available and the legal constraints associated with any decision.

This chapter will discuss some of the basic information about adolescence that will help the maternity nurse understand, appreciate, and care for the adolescent who needs reproductive health care services. It will center around the physical characteristics of the adolescent and elaborate on adolescence as a developmental period. Adolescent relationships and selected adolescent health needs will be considered.

The goal of this chapter is to help you understand some of the factors that bring about this human metamorphosis and to appreciate the role the maternity nurse can play in easing the transition.

PHYSICAL DEVELOPMENT

Adolescent physical development is noticeable in a number of ways. Changes that occur in connection with development of reproductive and sexual functions are referred to as *puberty* or *pubertal changes.* Puberty in a strict sense, however, consists only of changes that promote functional capability of the male and female sexual and reproductive systems, and the production of the male and female gametes. Changes do occur in most other body systems and are corollary to puberty. There is also a close association among physical changes, psychosocial influences, and adolescent behavior. These somatic changes include alterations in body size and shape, changes in body organs, and alterations in energy levels and nutritional needs.

Puberty

Puberty is an important part of the adolescent period of development. The most apparent pubertal changes are the maturing of the male and female external sex organs and the development of sexual characteristics of an adult man or woman. A more subtle yet important sexual change is the activation of the mechanisms that provide for the production and maturation of the male and female germ cells. Gametogenesis constitutes the "true" puberty.

Maturation of the reproductive organs of both the male and female is known as *primary sexual development.* These are the structures necessary for gametogenesis, copulation, and fertilization. In the female, primary sexual development refers also to the maturity of organs, such as the uterus, which nurtures the developing fetus and facilitates its birth. The reproductive organs exist before puberty but are in an immature nonfunctional state because of the absence of stimulation from the anterior pituitary and gonadal hormones.

Secondary sexual development is a way of classifying other physical changes that support sexual and reproductive function or are associated with the characteristics ascribed to "maleness" and "femaleness." These characteristics include appearance and distribution of body hair, particularly on the pubis, axilla, and the young man's face; increased body height and pelvic bone growth; changes in body shape resulting from the distribution of fat and muscle; increased muscle strength in the man; and breast development in the young woman. See Figures 8.2 and 8.3.

Both primary and secondary sexual development is under the direction and control of the endocrine system, specifically the network comprising the hypothalamus and anterior pituitary gland hormones and their target organs, foremost of which are the male and female gonads. Reproductive endocrine function does not begin until about age 7 or 8. The reasons for its quiescence during childhood are not clearly known. It is believed that hypothalamic function may be restrained during childhood because of central nervous system (CNS) immaturity or the presence of a structure or factor that inhibits hypothalamic hormones. This restraint decreases or disappears as the child matures, allowing for the production of the hypothalamic hormones (releasing factors) that stimulate anterior pituitary gonadotropic hormones that act on the ovaries and the testes. Female sexual maturity is almost always associated with menarche, and male maturity with nocturnal emissions. Menarche, however, is not a true indicator of reproductive maturity for the female. The first menstrual cycles are likely to be irregular and anovulatory. Exceptions to this have been reported, and ovulation has been known to precede the first menstruation. Neither are nocturnal emissions always representative of male sexual maturity. These early emissions may not contain spermatozoa. On the average, male or female gametogenesis is not clearly established until 12–24 months after external indicators of puberty.

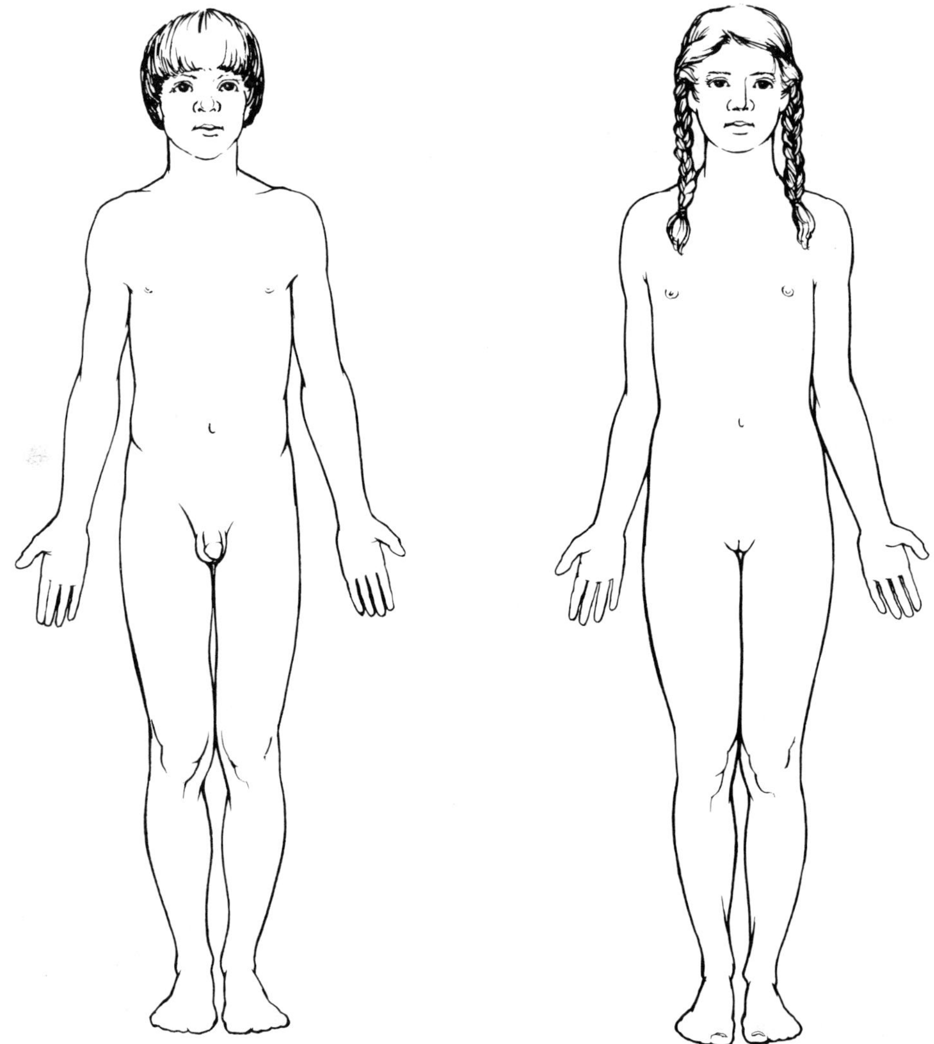

Figure 8.2
Physical characteristics of the prepubertal boy and girl. Note the absence of body hair, lack of breast development, and similarities in general body size and shape.

Puberty has no clearly established timetable but, like adolescence, differs for each person and is influenced by factors of physical, psychosocial, and environmental origin. Male and female puberty are not usually concurrent; the average female puberty precedes the male by about 2 years. Physical reproductive maturity is completed, in most cases, in about 3–5 years after the onset of puberty. Table 8.1 is a comparison of primary and secondary sexual changes in young men and women.

Puberty is the physical "coming together" of the body systems necessary for reproductive function; it represents a clinical summary of reproductive physical development and signifies physical developmental readiness for procreation. Psychosocial development may lag behind physical development in some cases although, most of the time, chronologic, physical, and psychosocial development have been found to correspond. The sex drive becomes more pronounced in both sexes, with sexual exploration and experimentation a usual occurrence. Pregnancy may occur before either partner is psychologically or socially ready to cope with pregnancy, parenthood, and associated demands.

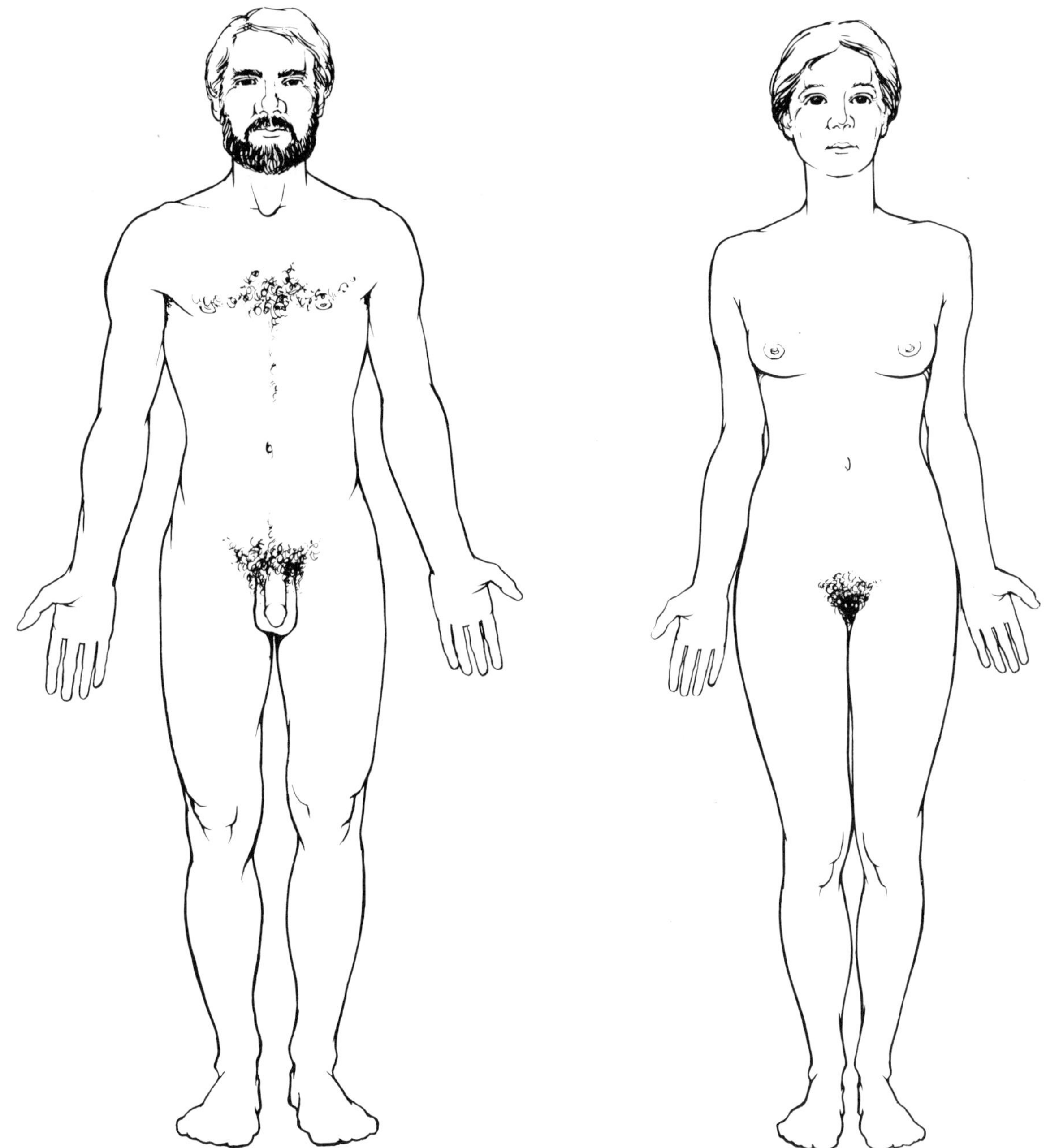

Figure 8.3
The adult, postpubertal, man and woman. Note the normal distribution of body hair, breast development in the woman, and differences in general body size and shape.

Changes in Other Body Systems

Growth is an important aspect of physical change during adolescence. Growth is rapid during the period preceding puberty and has arbitrarily been divided into two stages: the first is the *accelerated growth rate,* or *prepubertal growth spurt,* that is associated with increased production of hormones in late childhood; the second is just before true puberty, during which changes in height are most pronounced (Schuster, 1980).

TABLE 8.1
A COMPARISON OF PRIMARY AND SECONDARY SEXUAL CHANGES IN YOUNG MEN AND WOMEN

General Change	*Young Women*	*Age*[a]	Young Men	Age[a]
Glandular development of breasts	Present but not clinically apparent	8–14	Not apparent in young men	
Skeletal growth	Increase in diameter of internal pelvic planes	9.5–14.5	Increase in height. Pelvic bones increase in weight, thickness, and strength. Shoulder width expands.	10.5–17
Gonadal growth	Growth of ovaries and uterus	12–15	Beginning growth of testes and scrotum; darkened pigmentation of scrotum.	10–12
			Growth of ductile system and continued growth of testes.	12–18
Hyperplasia and hypertrophy of breast	Progressive development from:	8–17	Some boys have brief initial breast enlargement.	12–14
			Recedes after a few months.	14–17
	1. Preadolescent	9		
	2. Breast bud with slightly enlarged nipple and areola; small breast mound	9–11		
	3. Increased size of nipple, areola, and breast mound; pigmentation of areola visible	12–13		
	4. Glandular tissue apparent on palpation, nipple projects; appearance and histology of mature breast	14–17		
Increased hair distribution	Straight, fine, pigmented hair on pubis	10–12	Straight fine pigmented hair on pubis	12–13
	Kinky coarse hair with adult distribution	12.5–14	Kinky, coarse hair with adult distribution	14–15
Axilla	Axillary hair present	14	Axillary hair present	14–16
Face	Not usually present in the young woman; varies with levels of androgens in woman's body		Beard is last hair to appear	17–19

General Change	*Young Women*	*Age*[a]	**Young Men**	**Age**[a]
Growth of external genitalia	Growth of labia and vagina; thin vaginal secretions present, usually preceding menarche	11–12	Penile growth apparent; increase in growth begins; rapid growth	11–17 10–12 12–15
Gametogenesis (usually occurs 12–14 months after external indicators)	Menarche—early periods are often irregular and anovulatory	10.5–15.5 12–18 14–16 17–19	Nocturnal emissions—Early emissions may not contain sperm. Emissions often continue into adult life	13–16
Fatty tissue deposits	Widening of the hips; deposition of fatty tissue to breasts, hips, and upper thighs	12–18		
Voice change	Not a significant change in young women		Deepening of the voice	14–16
Increased muscle mass and size	Not a significant change in young women		Muscle hyperplasia and hypertrophy continues into late adolescence and early maturity. Increased strength apparent	16–21

[a]Average ages and age ranges differ according to source. The ages included here are approximate ranges derived from a variety of sources.

Skeletal growth in the young woman usually precedes that in the young man. Increase in muscle mass, another growth indicator, accounts for much of the change in physical appearance, particularly of the young man. Increased muscle mass ultimately provides the man with significantly more strength than that of the woman. The changes in muscle size in young men seem to be stimulated by the presence of the androgenic hormones. Young women also experience an increase in muscle mass, but rarely of the magnitude seen in the young man.

High energy expenditures are usually associated with the adolescent periods. Parents often see this as a problem. "My child is either in a state of perpetual motion—all over the place—or collapsed somewhere, just worn out." Energy is required for growth to occur. Rapid growth during adolescence, particularly of young men, necessitates an increase in the basal metabolism rate and in turn the consumption of a greater number of calories. It is not uncommon for adolescents to present high energy spurts, on the one hand, and lassitude and fatigue, on the other. Young men and, increasingly, young women channel much of their energy into healthy activities such as sports or community or school events.

Energy concerns are of great importance in the face of an early adolescent pregnancy. The energy requirements of pregnancy necessary to support growth of the fetus and the body system changes in the pregnant young woman, when superimposed on the already high energy requirements associated with adolescent growth place the pregnant adolescent in a vulnerable position.

Nutritional need is a corollary to energy demands at any stage in life, but they are especially important during adolescence. When there is a high energy expenditure, there is likely to be a calorie deficiency unless nutritional intake is adequate to offset the burning up of calories. Young men tend always to be hungry (Fig. 8.4). One parent described her adolescent son in these words, "He goes through the re-

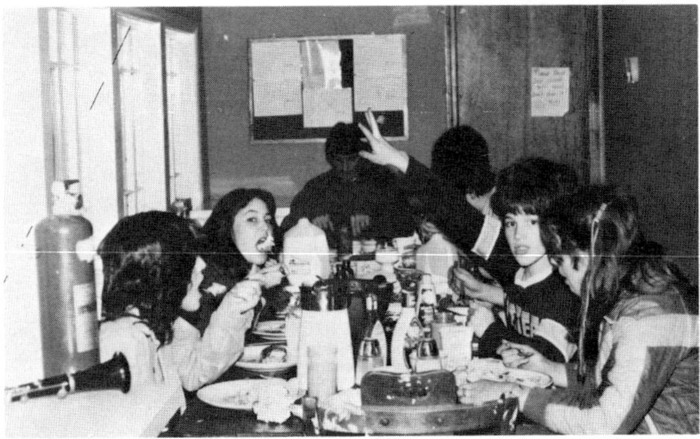

Figure 8.4
Adolescents, particularly young men, often require an enormous amount of food to sustain them.

frigerator like a vacuum cleaner." Young women also have increased appetites, but because of concern with physical appearance they often experiment with fad diets or, as with their male counterparts, ape the food habits of their peer groups (Fig. 8.5). Studies have repeatedly shown that significant numbers of adolescent women are inadequately nourished, presenting as underweight, overweight, and/or anemic. This is a problem of serious concern should the young woman become pregnant. During pregnancy, nutritional deficiency may not be completely corrected, even with a good diet. Nutritional practices, whether good or bad, tend to carry over into pregnancy and later life. Poor maternal nutrition is recognized as a significant factor in regard to the size and health of the growing fetus and the weight of the newborn infant.

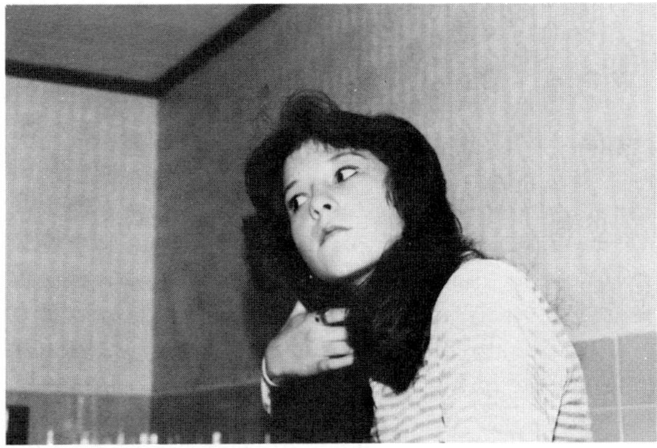

Figure 8.5
The adolescent young woman is often preoccupied with personal appearance and mimics the dress styles of her peers.

All basic food categories are necessary during adolescence, but needs for protein and calcium are significantly increased because of the growth of muscle and bone. Adequate caloric intake should be maintained but not exceeded. With irregular eating habits and "junk" food intake, adolescents are prone to develop poor eating habits early in life.

Other body system changes occur during adolescence, but they are of lesser magnitude than those just discussed. There is general growth of body organs such as the heart, lungs, and stomach. Cardiovascular function is increased to keep pace with the growth of the body systems and the need for vascular perfusion of the new tissues. Lung vital capacity increases in association with the size of the person, and the stomach increases to accommodate the ingestion of adequate food. Central nervous system growth usually precedes adolescence—a logical arrangement since the central nervous system largely directs the other events that occur during adolescence.

PSYCHOSOCIAL AND COGNITIVE DEVELOPMENT

Adolescence places many psychosocial demands on the young man or woman, whose status in society is equivocal to say the least. They are viewed as no longer being children but not yet as adults. Much of adolescent development during this period centers around sexuality: the need to know clearly who they are—boy/man or girl/woman—and to know that they are able to perform according to society's expectations of men and women. Adolescents must attend to more than the acquisition of sexual identity; they must also establish an identity as a person with unique needs and goals in life and function at a more sophisticated cognitive level. Adolescents must accomplish all of these tasks in the face of considerable physical upheaval in which there are significant changes in body image, new energy levels, as well as requirements and demands by society to conform to the values and mores that society prescribes as appropriate. That adolescence is a difficult period for children and parents alike is not surprising; that both groups often survive with body and mind intact is remarkable.

Cognitive Changes

Austin (1980) has described four psychosocial demands placed on the developing adolescent: demonstration of grown-up behavior, management of interpersonal trust in relationships with other people, mastery of sexual impulses in a socially acceptable way, and incorporation of cultural values. To achieve these tasks and demands, the adolescent must have the necessary physical and cognitive capabilities.

Much of what is known about cognitive functioning in children derives from the work of Piaget (1962), who described a cognitive operation as being a guideline or rule that helps a person understand his or her world. Cognitive operations enable a person to process information and give meaning to that information. They are concrete in childhood and move toward the more sophisticated, differentiated formal operations needed for abstract thinking as the child matures. The ability of the person to make this progress is in part the result of physical capability, but it is also influenced by the social dimensions of a person's life, particularly the child's experience with his or her environment. The pace at which a child makes this transition in cognitive function is highly personal; it is difficult to define age-specific times by which this change is accomplished. For example, some 14 year olds may demonstrate a high degree of formal operations, while a 17 year old may still function in a more concrete sense. This necessitates that people—such as nurses—who work with adolescents adjust their expectations of cognitive functioning to each person's ability. Unfortunately, this is not always the case. Nurses may find it easier to use the same style of teaching with each person rather than to assess and adapt to the appropriate level of cognitive functioning for each person.

One way in which a person demonstrates cognitive functioning is in his or her ability to handle an abstract idea or a hypothetical situation. A younger adolescent may not be able to deal with the concept of birth control as well as an older adolescent—the younger person may not be able to comprehend the possibility of a pregnancy occurring if the birth control pill is not taken or may not clearly make the association between sexual promiscuity and venereal disease. Cognitive capability must be associated logically with the way in which health care consumers follow or fail to follow instructions or comply with therapeutic regimens. Readiness for learning new things is closely tied to cognitive capability at any given developmental period. The adolescent is moving not only toward more abstract thinking but also toward thinking in a more comprehensive way, taking into account many more variables or combination of variables. Formal cognitive operations enable the adolescent to analyze situations and problems in a much more complete way.

Adolescent cognitive functioning is paradoxical in a practical sense. Cognitive operations are less concrete and more differentiated, enabling the young person to see the differences between what is and what can be. This capability, however, does not always contribute to the flexibility of adolescents when they must decide between the ideal and the real. Adolescents quite frequently opt for the ideal and refuse to compromise. A classic example is when the maternity nurse encounters an unmarried, pregnant teenager who insists that she keep and care for her infant. Good mothers take care of their babies, and she wants to be a good mother. She may know that an infant needs food and physical care as well as love, but she may be unable to accept the reality of what keeping her baby involves. The ideal goal or standard becomes the important factor in the adolescent's mind, not the reality. The teenagers who wish to marry may be difficult to dissuade because they truly believe that they can manage on their own. The adolescent expectant father will assure the nurse that he can support his wife and child. Realistic decision making is often difficult for the teenager.

Adolescents tend to become more introspective as a part of formal cognitive operations and are able to adapt to the demands of society in relationships with others. Introspection allows adolescents to tolerate the demands of society and to handle the frustrations associated with value conflicts. It increases their levels of tolerance for others and their acceptance of others.

As adolescents move toward maturity, their thoughts begin to include the future and what it can be for them. Goal setting becomes a possibility; thought moves away from "me in the present" to "me and my future." The future is seen as including larger groups of people rather than being focused only on self. Events such as pregnancy will interrupt or interfere with newly set goals and require the adolescents to reorder their priorities and perhaps reset their goals. Goal change is difficult for the teenager. Sarrel (1970) has described the impact of adolescent pregnancy as initiating a cycle of failure, beginning with failure to complete school and including, in sequence, failure to establish a stable family, to be self-supporting, and to prevent future, unwanted pregnancies.

Not only may goals be thwarted by an unplanned pregnancy, but the adolescent who drops out of school to take a job may be cheated out of complete identity consolidation if the decision is in conflict with what the person views as an ideal occupational goal. Such a decision may ultimately affect relationships with a spouse and family who, they perceive, has robbed them of occupational choices such as those requiring a college or high school education.

Another goal for the adolescent is building self-esteem. The teenager will develop positive self-esteem essentially through interpersonal relationships with other people—first, the early relationships with parents or care givers and, then, during adolescence, relationships with peers and with persons of the opposite sex. Adolescents are essentially egocentric. The cognitive ability to be aware of other's thoughts is present. However, personal thoughts tend to dominate thinking and concern is with self and one's own world. Adolescents are obsessed with themselves and believe that others share this preoccupation (Elkind, 1967). With progress toward maturity, the adolescent expands this personal view of self to incorporate the views of other people. Teenagers thrive as a part of a social network comprised of peers, parents, and other adults such as teachers, relatives, and friends.

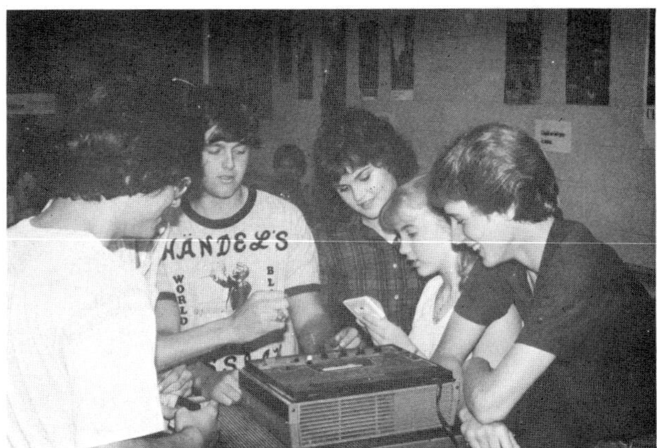

Figure 8.6
Peer groups are important to teenagers.

Relationships with Others

PEER GROUPS

Erikson (1963, 1970) views adolescence as a period in which the basic task is finding one's self—identity vs. role confusion. One way in which adolescents attempt to resolve role confusion and establish identity is through relationships with others, most notably, peer groups, or what Sullivan termed chums, or best friends. Adolescents receive positive or negative feedback through such relationships that helps to confirm that they are what they claim to be or should be. Friend and peer relationships are often the most influential relationships the adolescent experiences; the friend or peer group often sets the standards that direct the adolescent's behavior (Fig. 8.6). These friends and groups may be acquired in association with school experiences, but they more often take the form of private groups or clubs that are disassociated from more formal community organizations. Adolescents tend to have one close friend to whom they relate intimately in a reciprocal giving-and-taking association.

Adults tend to be relegated to a secondary status in the adolescent's social world. This is not to say that the parent's role is obliterated in the mind of their child; however, it is repatterned and diminished in proximate importance. This is especially true during the midadolescent period. Adolescents do see some adults as role models whom they wish to imitate—teachers, coaches, local and national heroes—but the extent of influence by these people is often determined by what the peer group will tolerate. As adolescents near maturity, the adult becomes increasingly important once more.

PARENTS AND OTHER ADULTS

Adolescents are sometimes caught in conflicts between their parents' values and those of their peer groups and friends, particularly concerning sexual matters (Bell, 1970). Much of adolescent behavior can be correctly described as rebellious. Some young people are honestly confused about who they are and what they should be or do. Adults who are part of the adolescent's family, such as parents, are often too close to the person to help him or her chart the most appropriate course. Parents sometimes find it difficult to see their child as an individual rather than an extension of themselves. This separateness is not such a problem in childhood, but in adolescence parents are forced to reexamine their own attitudes toward their child as an individual person. Feelings or conflicts that cannot be shared with a buddy or peer group can sometimes be shared with an objective adult outside of the intimate family circle such as a nurse, physician, teacher, or clergyman.

Freud (1958) believed that adolescence brought a revival of the child's dormant sexual interest in the parent of the opposite sex. In light of the increasing force of the adolescent's sexual drives, separation from the parent may be viewed by the adolescent as an unconscious, necessary move. This sexual conflict was thought to be at the heart of the parent–child antagonism during the adolescent period.

The rebellious nature of adolescents leads to the testing of limits set by adults. The irony of such rebellion is that the person may need and even want such limits established in order to reinforce feelings of security, love, and belonging. Nurses who provide health care for adolescents often experience this same testing of limits within the health care delivery system.

ADOLESCENT SEXUAL RELATIONSHIPS

Relationships with members of the opposite sex are very important to the teenager and take on quite a different meaning than they had in earlier childhood. Sexual relationships are tied to needs associated with the adolescent's budding sexuality. Sexual identity is dependent upon the success of relationships with both members of the opposite and same sexes (Fig. 8.7). Adolescents fall in love frequently and with a variety of different people. Some adolescent sexual relationships develop into lifelong attachments such as the girl and boy who marry their high school sweethearts. Most adolescent sexual relationships are of brief duration. They are, however, potentially explosive because of the intensity of the sex drives and the inexperience of adolescents in understanding and controlling them. Nonmarital sexual intercourse is an increasing occurrence among the adolescent population and often results in an unplanned and unwanted pregnancy. In 1978 more than 10 million adolescents over 15 years old and an increasing number of young people under 15 years old were reported as being sexually active (*McCall's,* 1978). Statistical incidence of adolescent pregnancy in the United States is incomplete, in part because of the failure to report many of the pregnancies. The number of babies born to adolescent mothers each year exceeds half a million. Some of these young mothers have been forced into early marriages; others have married and planned their pregnancies; still others are classified as unmarried mothers with all of the social, economic, legal, and health problems that accompany this state. All relationships between adolescent men and women do not culminate in sexual intercourse. That significant numbers do is verified, not only by the numbers of adolescent pregnancies, but also by the incidence of venereal disease among teenagers.

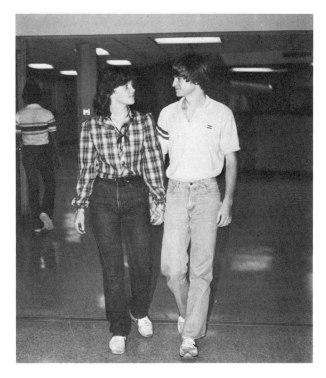

Figure 8.7
Relationships with the opposite sex are a healthy part of growing up.

Woods (1979) sees the psychological aspects of adolescent sexuality as divided into two phases. The early phase is characterized by the strength of the sexual instinct and likely conflicts regarding one's own sexuality. The later phase occurs in the mid-teens and is somewhat more stable. This stability is most likely because of better regulation of biologic and endocrine functions and the ability of adolescents to control sexual impulses.

The nature of adolescent sexual relationships is, in many ways, a response to changes that are taking place within the adolescents and environment. Sexual instincts are strong during adolescence, and the ability of the young man or woman to control these instincts is closely tied to the person's cognitive development. The more differentiated the thinking of adolescents, the better able they are to place sexual drive into an appropriate perspective in their total world. The expectations and values of the peer groups play an important part in sexual as in other behavior. Sexual laxity or promiscuity, when accepted as a group norm, is often the standard the teenager will follow. Personal conflicts with the peer group that cannot be resolved by remaining in the group may cause the adolescent to withdraw from the group. Withdrawal from a valued group of friends is a difficult decision for anyone to make, particularly a teenager. It immediately places the person in the position of outsider and does little to reinforce feelings of self-esteem and belonging. Conflicts concerning appropriate sexual behavior are common among teenagers and are associated with the problem of changing social–sexual standards and a morality that communicates, on the one hand, that liberal sexual behavior is proscribed by society and, on the other hand, that sexual freedom is in. The maternity nurse is likely to encounter adolescent needs that arise from sexual relationships in a number of settings, including school, community, and the more formal health service agencies and institutions.

The adolescent period of development provides a time for the body to undergo the biophysical changes that are needed to move the person from child to adult. It is a time in which most people clearly establish their identity and lay the psychosocial and cognitive foundations for their future identity and life. Realistically, it is a period of physical and emotional highs and lows with emotions often labile and with physical needs vying with cognition for control of decisions and behaviors. Even though adolescence spans a period of 8 to 10 years, it is, in many ways, a period of rapid change, not so much because the changes occur quickly but because so many changes and tasks occur in this period.

REPRODUCTIVE HEALTH NEEDS

Like other periods in life, adolescence generates unique, period-specific health care needs and problems. Four such areas of concern are discussed briefly here, and in more detail in other chapters of this book: birth control, venereal disease, adolescent pregnancy, and drug use and abuse. Other adolescent health concerns, such as depression, suicide, homosexuality, masturbation, developmental aberrations of genetic, teratogenic, or iatrogenic origins, and adolescent diseases or disorder, are important. They are not discussed here since they are more appropriately dealt with in other books.

Birth Control

There are conflicting opinions about the use of birth control for unmarried teenagers (See Chapter 26). One position argues that it is no secret that teenagers engage in sexual intercourse and that pregnancy resulting from such sexual unions should be prevented for a number of reasons. There is a higher incidence of reproductive-related health problems associated with an adolescent pregnancy that lead to damage or even death of the pregnant young woman or possibly her child. Many adolescents are not ready, nor financially able, to take on the adult responsibilities arising from pregnancy and parenthood. Many are also at risk for parenting problems such as child abuse and neglect.

The opposing argument contends that prescribing birth control devices or drugs for adolescents is ignoring the real problem, that of inadequate information about sexual function and too little parental supervision of adolescent behavior. Advocates of this position see parent and sex education programs as the primary need and the appropriate starting point. Some question the use of contraceptive technology such as the birth control pill and the intrauterine device for adolescents because of the limited research showing the long-range effects of such methods. They also oppose starting either of these methods in the teen years because of the likelihood of long-term usage of 30–35 years.

The use of elective abortion to rid the adolescent of an unwanted pregnancy is a highly controversial issue, as is elective abortion per se. Increasing numbers of teenagers resort to this way of managing their needs for contraception. Figures are incomplete concerning the incidence of elective abortions performed in the United States for the general, as well as adolescent, population.

Venereal Disease

Venereal diseases are those infections that are transmitted through sexual contact and include syphillis, gonorrhea, and other less well-known diseases (see Chapter 27). Veneral disease is a reportable health problem of widespread concern in the United States. The incidence of venereal disease has been steadily increasing in all segments of the population. Many of these cases are found among adolescents. Venereal disease has, for many years, been considered to be a social disease that bears a stigma and as such was not openly discussed. This has set the climate for failure to report personal symptomatology, as well as to name others with whom the person has had sexual contact. Diseases such as syphillis may not cause observable symptoms until they are in a well-advanced stage. Treatment given in the late stage of syphillis may not prevent progression of or sequelae to the disease. Transmission of venereal disease is often associated with sexual promiscuity and lack of knowledge about transmission and prevention.

Venereal disease is of particular significance if the girl or woman is pregnant. It can adversely affect the developing fetus in utero, as in the case of syphillis, or at the time of birth, as in the case of gonorrhea. Attitudes toward venereal disease are becoming less jugmental and negative. There is increasing acceptance of sexual matters generally. The maternity nurse is in an excellent position from which to provide health teaching to prevent venereal disease and to support and counsel those who have already contracted the disease or to refer them to the appropriate person for care.

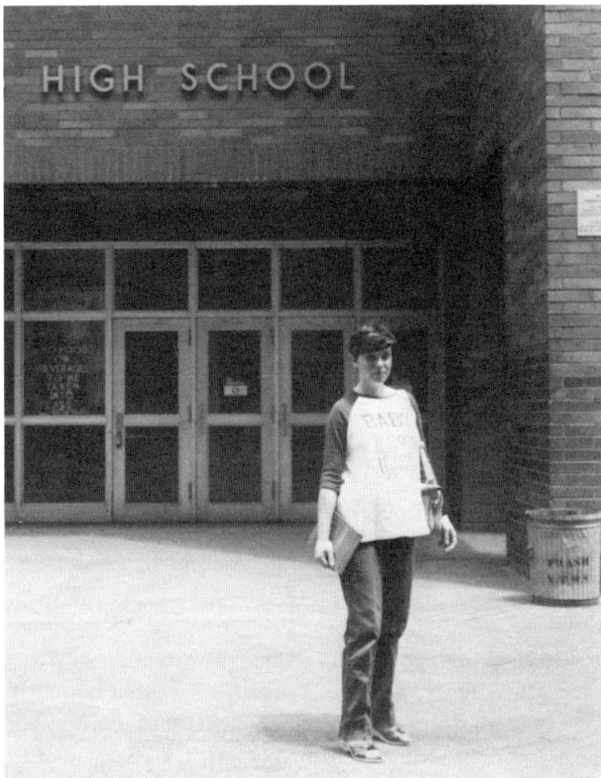

Figure 8.8
Adolescent pregnancy often imposes adult tasks upon a young person who has not yet let go of childhood.

Adolescent Pregnancy

Almost 1 million teenagers, 15–19 years old, become pregnant each year, making adolescent pregnancy one of the major adolescent health problems in the United States. (See Fig. 8.8 and Chapter 12.) Adolescent pregnancy is classified as a reproductive risk for mother and child alike. Pregnant teenagers do not readily report their pregnancies and may not receive prenatal care until the pregnancy is well advanced. Several reasons for the avoidance of health care have been suggested. First, the young woman may not realize that she is pregnant. Lack of information about conception, pregnancy, and childbirth is a frequent occurrence among teenagers, as well as some adults. A young woman may suspect that she is pregnant but irrationally ignore it, protesting that this "can't be happening to me." Adolescent pregnancies are frequently unplanned and often unwanted. Pregnancy is the physical confirmation that the young woman has had sexual intercourse. She may be embarrassed or even frightened to have her pregnancy diagnosed. Diagnosis of pregnancy forces confrontation with reality and often requires that her parents become involved in what has to this point been a personal experience. A significant number of teenage marriages occur because of pregnancy.

Drug Use and Abuse

Drug use is defined as the habitual use of substances such as prescription and nonprescription drugs, alcohol, and tobacco (see Chapter 25). Drug use is widespread in the United States among all age groups (Fig. 8.9). In the 1960s drug use emerged as a problem of some dimensions among adolescents and young adults, particularly young people of college age. It represented a general social revolt against traditional values held by society. The practice of drug use and abuse persisted into the 1970s and

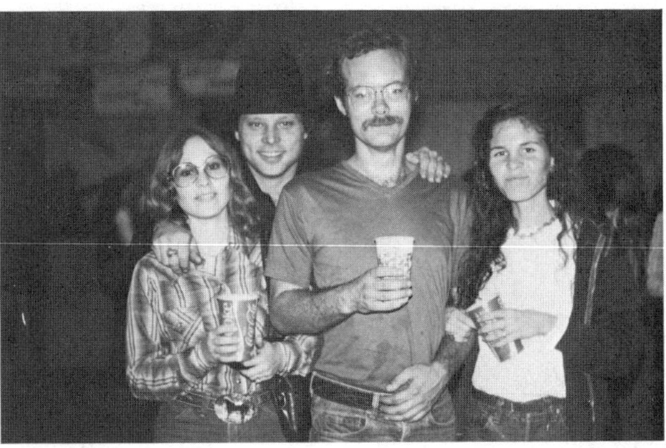

Figure 8.9
Use of alcohol by teenagers is increasing and lays the foundation for multiple social and health problems. It is not uncommon for adolescent drinkers to disguise their drinking in some way, such as the use of soft drink cups.

penetrated the ranks of high school adolescents. Adolescent drug use today is a problem of great concern for society generally. A wide variety of drugs are used by teenagers, including marijuana (pot), amphetamines (speed), and hard drugs such as heroin. Alcohol consumption by teenagers is increasing, and teenage alcoholics are not uncommon today. Drug habituation, repeated use of drugs, is probably the more usual approach to drug use, although drug addiction, a physiologic dependence on drugs, is also on the rise.

Drug use is important to reproductive health because it can severely damage the emotional and physical well-being of the pregnant woman and have a detrimental effect on her unborn and newborn child. Some drugs are believed to affect the male and female gametes thereby influencing reproductive outcome even before the fact of pregnancy.

The sociologic dimensions of the problem of drug use are great, affecting not only the drug user but those closest to him or her. Drug use is a costly habit, and for teenagers into hard drugs, costs are often beyond their incomes. Ways must be found to support the habit. These ways include petty to serious drug-related crimes such as theft or teenage male and female prostitution.

The psychologic effects of drug use vary from giving the person a sense of well-being to severe depression and ultimately suicide. Drug addiction can permanently damage or destroy the quality of life of a person. National and local drug rehabilitation programs have had laudable success in many cases.

Drug use is a legal and moral issue throughout the world. Drug laws vary from country to country and may be more or less severe than those in the United States. Social use of drugs raises questions of morality with heated arguments mounted on both sides of the issue. Some factions believe that social use of drugs such as marijuana and alcohol in moderation should be acceptable and that the use of marijuana should be legalized. Others insist that drug use in any form or for any reason other than medical purposes should be outlawed. These views represent extreme positions. Most authorities dealing with the problem of drug use see it as a symptom of a more complex social problem.

The maternity nurse who comes into contact with pregnant teenagers who are on drugs is faced with the care of two clients, both of whom have guarded prognoses. The nurse can be an objective resource who will provide support, information, and care to these young people.

SUMMARY

This chapter discussed the period of adolescence as a time of integration—a merger of all facets of the person in order to make the transition from childhood to adulthood. Puberty and adolescence are often difficult times for parents as well, many of whom are not prepared to cope with adolescent behavior or to support adolescent needs. Parents and teachers may have a limited or inaccurate understanding of their own sexual and reproductive function and be unprepared to help their child or pupil through this erratic period.

Maternity nurses, in particular, are in a unique position to help adolescents through this period. They have the knowledge and skill related to human development and reproduction. They can serve as teachers of adolescents and their parents and significant others. The nurse may be one of the first members of the health care team with whom the adolescent comes into contact in the health care delivery system. The maternity nurse can be the consistent professional support during adolescent pregnancy and childbirth.

Physical development was viewed as including changes associated with puberty, the time the human being becomes capable of reproducing itself, and general alterations of the body systems. Psychosocial and cognitive development were analyzed with special attention to the change from concrete cognitive operations to more abstract differentiated formal operations. Relationships between the adolescent and other people were included with attention to interpersonal interactions with peers, friends, adults, and members of the opposite sex. The chapter closed with a brief statement about four adolescent health problems that affect human reproduction: birth control, venereal disease, adolescent pregnancy, and drug use and abuse.

REFERENCES AND READINGS

Austin, S. H. Cognitive and Psychosocial Development of Adolescence, in Schuster, C. S. Ashburn, S. S. (Eds.), *The Process of Human Development: A Holistic Approach.* Boston: Little, Brown, 1980, pp. 481–498.

Bell, R. R. Parent–Child Conflicts in Sexual Values, in Mussen, P. H., Conger, J. J., Kagen, J. (Eds.), *Readings in Child Development and Personality.* New York: Harper & Row, 1970. pp. 521–531.

Elkind, D. Egocentricism in Adolescence. *Child Dev* 38:1025, 1967.

Erikson, E. H. *Childhood and Society.* (2nd ed) New York: W. W. Norton, 1963.

Erikson, E. H. Identity vs. Identity Diffusion, in Mussen, P. H., Conger, J. J., Kagen, J. (Eds.), *Readings in Child Development and Personality.* New York: Harper & Row, 1970, pp. 532–537.

Freud, A. Adolescence, in *Psychoanalytic Study of the Child,* vol. 13. New York: International Universities Press, 1958.

Grinder, R. E. (Ed.). *Studies in Adolescence: A Book of Readings in Adolescent Psychology.* New York: MacMillan, 1963.

Hyde, J. S. *Understanding Human Sexuality.* (2nd ed.) New York: McGraw-Hill, 1982.

Inhelder, B., Piaget, J. *The Growth of Logical Thinking from Childhood to Adolescence.* New York: Basic Books, 1958.

Teenager Pregnancy Epidemic. *McCall's* 105(10): 45, 1978.

National Research Council. Food and Nutrition Board. *Recommended Dietary Allowances* (8th ed.). Washington, D.C.: National Acadmy of Sciences, 1974.

Piaget, J. The Stages of the Intellectual Development of the Child. *Bull Menninger Clin* 26(3):120, 1962.

Sarrel, P. Caring for the Pregnant Teenager. *Fam Plann* 3(4), 1970.

Schuster, C. S. Biophysical Development of the Adolescent, in Schuster, C. S. Ashburn, S. S. (Eds.), *The Process of Human Development.* Boston: Little, Brown, 1980, pp. 463–479.

Sullivan, H. S. *The Interpersonal Theory of Psychiatry.* New York: W. W. Norton, 1953.

Tanner, J. M. *Foetus Into Man: Physical Growth From Conception to Maturity.* London: Open Books, 1978.

Valadian, I., Porter, D. *Physical Growth and Development: From Conception to Maturity.* Boston: Little, Brown, 1977.

Woods, N. F. *Human Sexuality in Health and Illness.* St. Louis: C. V. Mosby, 1979.

9

ASSESSMENT OF REPRODUCTIVE READINESS

Assessment of reproductive readiness is defined as the collection and interpretation of information about physical, psychosocial, and cognitive development to determine a person's capability for completing the tasks associated with the reproductive process. It provides the data base from which the nurse and other health care providers make judgments about client needs and appropriate responses to such needs. The purpose of a reproductive health assessment is to evaluate the characteristics of developmental readiness mentioned on pages 135–140. Ideally, this physical assessment should be done before pregnancy and incorporated into the health record as a part of a cumulative data base that begins with birth and continues through maturity. However, the ideal often exists only in the mind, and more times than not, the first real assessment of reproductive capability is made when the woman seeks health care because of suspicion of pregnancy.

Assessment of reproductive readiness is discussed from physical, psychosocial, and cognitive perspectives and includes personal and family health history, physical examination of the male or female reproductive systems, and selected laboratory studies. Genetic screening is also an important part of such an assessment; however, this is not done for everyone. Genetic screening becomes important when there are reasons to suspect that a genetic disorder is present or that there is the potential for transmission of an inherited disorder to the person's children. Chapter 24 discusses methods for genetic screening and some of the transmissable disorders.

TOOLS FOR REPRODUCTIVE HEALTH ASSESSMENT

The tools the nurse uses to assess a person's reproductive health status are principally the health history, physical examination, and laboratory studies. The taking of a personal and a family health history will be familiar to most of you. The extent of knowledge about and skill in performing a physical examination will vary from nurse to nurse. A complete physical examination should not be done by a nurse unless advanced skills have been acquired, such as those of the nurse-midwife or nurse-practitioner. Maternity nurses, however, are likely to participate in various aspects of physical examinations that may include doing parts of the examination, supporting the client, and assisting the physician or other qualified health care providers in the examination. The nurse frequently collects the specimens used for laboratory studies and may do the test. The nurse is often the first person—besides the laboratory technician—to view and interpret the findings. Whether the nurse is responsible for all or part of the health history, physical examination, and laboratory studies or only uses the findings obtained from them to plan and provide nursing care, knowledge about the content, techniques, and procedures of such assessment is needed.

Health History

History is literally a personal account of recollections about what has happened in the past. In this case, it is the client's recall of what has happened to her and her relatives. Rarely are histories completely accurate accounts of past events for time may erode memory or distort recall of events. The client's history is a primary data source from which accurate diagnosis and planning of personalized, safe, health care can be made. Its importance should not be diminished or taken casually. Every effort must be made to obtain the most accurate personal and family history possible. Efforts such as providing privacy for the client during the interview, allowing adequate time for obtaining information, and skilled use of interviewing techniques by the nurse are likely to improve the accuracy of information gathered. Knowledge of the theory underlying human reproduction and about human development and function will direct the course of the interview and enable the nurse to determine the information needed. Inquisitive probing into unrelated and unnecessary areas is both an invasion of the client's privacy and a waste of the client's and nurse's time. The nurse's theory base and the nature of the client's response during the interview will direct the nurse to the areas that require further exploration.

Organized formats for taking a client's history are recommended in most textbooks addressing health assessment. These formats provide assistance with organizing the interview and are particularly helpful to the inexperienced nurse. A general outline will include the following topics: general information about the client and family, biographic data about the client, personal history, and family history.

General information about the client and family includes practical data such as correct name, age, address, and telephone number. People will occasionally use more than one name, so it is important that the name provided to the nurse is correctly spelled and that any aliases are noted. Correct age is also important, not only as a basis from which to assess developmental characteristics but also for legal purposes such as the granting of permission to perform necessary diagnostic or therapeutic procedures or operations. It is not unusual for a person to be lost from the health care delivery system when there remains a need for nursing or other health care follow-up. Reconfirmation of the correct address and telephone number should be done at each contact with the person or family.

Observations about a person's appearance can provide the nurse with an impression of health status. Careful attention to body size, posture, facial characteristics, attire, personal hygiene, and attitude toward self, family, nurse, and others provides a basis for further exploration or confirmation of impressions.

Description of the organization and composition of the family, such as the number of family members, their names, sex, and ages, helps the nurse to understand the position of the person within the family and to identify support resources available to the person or couple. Content categories to guide the nurse in collection of more specific data are suggested in Tables 9.1 and 9.2.

Physical Examination

The human being reaches physical maturity sometime during the period from onset of puberty to the beginning of the young adult years, between the ages of 10–20 years. During this period, the developing adult takes on characteristics and capabilities expected of a mature person. Physical assessment for reproductive readiness focuses on assessment of those characteristics that are indicative of full physical growth.

Complete physical assessment consists of careful, comprehensive scrutiny of body characteristics and functions; it requires the use of clinical, biochemical, electronic, radiographic, and other assessment modalities. Few people—in the absence of apparent physical dysfunction—undergo such a detailed examination; instead most people are likely to experi-

TABLE 9.1
FAMILY ASSESSMENT AREAS

Diseases/Disorders	*Family Organization*	*Family Style*	*Economic Aspects*
▲ Genetic ▲ Viral ▲ Bacterial ▲ Frequency, chronic, or acute characteristics	▲ Roles ▲ Relationships ▲ Responsibilities of family members ▲ Size ▲ Cultural characteristics ▾ Ethnic background ▾ Religion ▾ Childbearing and child rearing practices	▲ Autocratic ▲ Democratic ▲ Activities ▾ Individual ▾ Shared ▾ Goals ▾ Sources of support and affection	▲ Income (in terms of adequacy for support of family needs) ▲ Living accommodations ▾ Provision for privacy (number of rooms) ▾ Safety hazards ▾ Sanitation ▾ Heat and refrigeration

ence selective examinations at different times in their lives, often related to school or work demands as much as to physical problems.

We have made no attempt to discuss health history and physical examination in detail. You will, no doubt, integrate previously acquired knowledge and skill into your personal nursing practice. Our discussion of physical assessment briefly addresses those aspects of physical development and function that are most directly pertinent to human reproduction. Content that is most likely to be used by the maternity nurse is emphasized. Information concerning comprehensive physical assessment can be obtained from the references listed at the end of this chapter.

There are many ways a nurse can approach physical assessment for reproductive readiness. Four categories of data are suggested as one way of organizing information obtained: (1) general physical characteristics, (2) systemic maturity, (3) nutritional status, and (4) activity and rest patterns. It is often difficult to make precise developmental and functional estimations because of a person's individual characteristics. There are available established standards (norms) for normal development and healthy body functioning. These standards represent group rather than individual characteristics. It is common practice, however, to measure a person's characteristics and functions against these standards for they do provide the upper and lower limits for "normal." You are already familiar with many of these norms. Caution is advised that all data collected must be analyzed and evaluated in consideration of the client's genetic endowments, sex, socioeconomic strata, and other personal characteristics and that every effort be made to personalize the assessment rather than fit the client into an already prepared normative box.

General Physical Characteristics

The preceding discussion in this unit has provided you with specific characteristics of sexual maturity. It is the degree of presence or absence of these characteristics that the nurse needs to assess. Body growth and structural changes measured by height, weight, shoulder breadth in the young man, width of the pelvis in the young woman, and fat distribution provide some information about physical maturity. Indicators of pubertal changes such as the growth of the genital organs, secondary sex characteristics, skin texture changes, and glandular activity, particularly the sebaceous, sweat, and mammary glands, should be assessed. Body posture may provide information about muscle tone and skeletal development.

TABLE 9.2
INDIVIDUAL ASSESSMENT AREAS

Physical	*Psychosocial*	*Cognitive*
▲ General. Blood type, serology, hematocrit or hemoglobin, weight, height, race, and general physical development ▲ **Nutrition.** Eating patterns (problems); food habits (preferences, unusual practices); elimination patterns (problems) ▲ **Sexual Practices (if relevant).** Intercourse (frequency, one or more partners); contraception (if used, type, way in which it is used) ▲ **Onset of Puberty.** *Male:* Presence of nocturnal emissions (frequency, characteristics); age at onset; *Female:* Menarche (age of onset); menstrual periods (interval, duration, amount, color, consistency, pain or discomfort) ▲ **Obstetric History.** Number of pregnancies and intervals between pregnancies; course and outcome of pregnancy; age and condition of child	▲ Person's life goals ▲ Interest in childbearing and child rearing ▲ Relationship with others ▲ Expectations of others within or outside of family ▲ Support sources ▲ Role and position within family ▲ Attitudes toward health ▲ Response to stress (coping patterns) ▲ Ways in which person communicates with others	▲ Educational level ▲ Own perception of needs for information and learning ▲ Learning style (way in which person learns best) ▲ Resources used for learning (books, newspapers, magazines, teachers, media, parents, peers) ▲ Language level ▾ congruent with physical and social development ▾ first, second languages spoken

Systemic Development and Function

Ascertainment of the normal or abnormal function of all systems is important for the sensible and safe management of pregnancy and concerns or problems related to reproduction; however, two systems are of particular importance—cardiovascular and genitourinary. The nurse should make a habit of assessing the client's vital signs and be aware of normal ranges of these signs according to age and weight. Hypertension is a major national health problem and is indicative of serious complications should it occur before or during pregnancy (see Chapter 21). There is some evidence that hypertension among adolescents is increasing. Since about one of every five births in the country is from pregnant teenage girls, this increased incidence of hypertension is of serious concern to maternity nurses. Hypertension pre-existing pregnancy places both mother and fetus at risk for various degrees of damage or even death. Adolescent blood pressure norms are 100/50 to 120/70 with 130/90 considered to be the safe upper limit for late adolescence (Batterman et al., 1976). If pregnancy is present, blood pressure increments of +30 systolic and +15 diastolic above the normotensive blood pressure are significant. Pulse rates should also be assessed. Adolescence brings about a slight increase in total cardiovascular activity and an increase in red blood cell mass and hemoglobin. Should pregnancy occur in the adolescent before the cardiovascular system is mature enough to take care of the additional demands, the potential for poor pregnancy outcome exists.

Renal functional maturity is seen through changes in fluid and electrolyte balance. There is increased muscle mass, particularly in the young man, as well as increased bone growth and fatty deposits. Potassium levels rise while exchangeable sodium and chloride levels decline. Total body fluid percentages decrease while intracellular fluid increases. If systemic development is immature or abnormal, pregnancy causes further changes in the renal system that often stress the essentially healthy young woman. The physical capability of coping with all of these changes is strained. Bladder capacity increases with puberty; however, many adolescent and mature women may have inadequate fluid intake on a daily basis, particularly of water ingestion. Although the cause of repeated urinary tract infections is not definitive, there is an association between decreased fluid intake and urinary tract infection. Increased sexual activity has also been associated with bladder infection. Incidence of bladder infections often results in infection of the kidney and ureters. History of urinary tract infections is of importance in the event of pregnancy. Assessment of the male and female reproductive systems is discussed more fully on pages 154–155.

Other systemic changes that are indicative of approaching physical maturity include an increase in the basal metabolic rate, enlargement of the stomach capacity, and increased muscle and skeletal strength, especially in the young man.

Nutritional Status

Adequate and well-balanced nutrition supports human development. Maternal nutritional status influences the end products of pregnancy. The nurse should assess the client for gross evidence of nutritional deficiency, as well as for nutritional aberrations such as being overweight. It is important to remember that the fetus develops from the legacy of its parents. There is ample evidence that correlates poor maternal nutrition with poor pregnancy outcome. A history of diet habits and patterns provides the information to determine client needs. Protein and calcium are especially important for physical development as well as for the support of a pregnancy. Nutritional deficiencies should be corrected before the onset of pregnancy. Pregnancy places increased demands on a body that is normal and much more so on one that is nutritionally deficient. The behaviors associated with malnutrition such as lethargy, fatigue, and irritability do not provide the expectant mother with a sound physical basis for coping with the demands of pregnancy. Poor muscle tone decreases abdominal and uterine efficiency during labor. Poor posture often related to weak muscles is more likely to contribute to backache and respiratory problems during pregnancy. Nutritional anemias ill prepare the woman to cope with hematologic changes during pregnancy, birth, and recovery.

Activity and Rest Patterns

The healthy person is likely to achieve some kind of balance between rest and activity that is right for him or her. Traditionally, the man, particularly the adolescent man, has tended to be more physically active than the adolescent woman. This may be related more to sex role socialization than to physical capabilities or instinct. Physical activity and adequate rest support human development in a number of ways since improved circulation, increased muscle tone, and rest logically allow the body to recuperate successfully from activity. The amount and type of physical activity people engage in are often directly related to the quality of their general health. Pregnancy requires an increased expenditure of physical and emotional energy. Knowledge about activity and rest patterns enables the nurse to help the client adapt to new demands during pregnancy within the framework of existing patterns. Should client rest and activity practices be unhealthy, the nurse can use such information to assist her with health education of the client.

Physical Examination

A complete physical examination is necessary to assess a person's readiness for reproduction accurately. The maternity nurse will usually be involved with the woman's physical examination, which most often will be to diagnose pregnancy and provide prenatal care. Because human reproduction involves both the man and woman, the nurse should be aware of what is involved in the man's examination as well and be capable of participating in either examination. Information about the components of a man's and woman's physical examination is also useful in health teaching. An overview of the examination of the male genitalia and the gynecologic examination of the female are discussed later in this section.

Physical examination necessitates the use of techniques that rely upon sensory as well as psychomotor skill; these include *palpation,* examination of an organ or body area through the use of touch; *percussion,* exploration of the body organs or areas by tapping and then listening with the ear or an instrument in order to determine their size and condition; *inspection,* careful observation of the client's body characteristics and attention to sounds and odors emanating from the body; *auscultation,* listening to sounds produced by the body with the unassisted ear or with the use of instruments that amplify the sound; and *measurement,* collection of data or information that requires the assignment of a numerical value in terms of dimension, quantity, or capacity. The actual procedures for examination of the breasts, the abdomen, and the genitalia varies with examiner and client and is often influenced by the skill and experience of the examiner and the age, size, and physical condition of the client. Recommended procedures for breast, abdominal, and pelvic examinations are covered in texts dealing with physical assessment.

Physical examination of the male and female reproductive systems can be divided into three parts: *gross observation* of body size, shape, and posture, as well as the characteristics of skin and hair; *regional examination* of the reproductive system to include the male and female genitalia, abdomen, and the female breasts; *laboratory analysis,* especially of the blood, urine, and semen.

Physical examination of any part of the body is an intrusion into the client's personal world. The regional examination of the reproductive systems of either the man or woman is often perceived to be even more personal and intrusive than other parts of the examination. With the exception of the mind, the genitals are considered by most people to be their most private parts. It is important for the nurse to remember this and to help others remember it as well.

THE MALE EXAMINATION

Examination of the male genitalia first occurs at birth when the penis is inspected to determine whether or not *circumcision* (surgical removal of the foreskin of the penis) is necessary and the scrotum is palpated to confirm testicular descent (see Chapter 17). Unlike the woman, however, who most likely will use health care services when she becomes pregnant, the man may not undergo genital examination again unless he chooses to participate in periodic physical examination, develops a symptom that requires diagnosis and treatment, develops a problem with infertility, or requires the need for a sterilization procedure such as a vasectomy. The following is an overview of the regional examination of the male reproductive system.

Gross examination of the male includes assessment of body size, shape, and posture. Height is usually the measurement used to determine physical growth in both sexes. Relationships among the sizes of the head, torso, and lower extremities should also be assessed. The ratio of head size to the rest of the body decreases proportionally as maturity is reached; both the torso and limbs lengthen. An ongoing health record reflecting the person's growth and development throughout infancy, childhood, and adolescence is helpful; however, not everyone has had periodic examinations and not all physicians keep developmental records.

The body should be inspected for the amount, distribution, pattern, and characteristics of pubic, axillary, and facial hair. This is important for several reasons: For adolescent young men, this inspection will give some indication of androgenic endocrine function and will help to assess developmental progress during puberty. Sparse or absent hair may be indicative of delayed puberty or endocrine abnormality. In the adult man, with proven fertility, hair may have no reproductive relevance unless there has been a change in the previously existing distribution patterns and characteristics.

The skin should be inspected for color, lesions, and nodes. Skin covering the male genitals, particularly the scrotum, deepens in color during puberty and remains a darker pigmentation during adult life.

Regional examination of the male focuses essentially on the genitals (penis and scrotal sac). Unlike the female, the male breast has no reproductive significance.

The *penis* is examined for the following:

- ▲ Size in relationship to the client's age and general development. In a flaccid as compared with a turgid state, the penis will appear small. Penile size is not a factor in reproduction unless it is conspicuously small when it is in an erect state.
- ▲ Any signs of inflammation or pathology such as swelling, redness, tenderness to touch, lesions, nodules, or abnormal growth or discharge. A common concern with the sexually active man is the presence of syphilitic lesions and discharge from gonorrhea.
- ▲ Presence or absence of circumcision (see Chapter 17). This is more important in regard to personal hygiene than in regard to reproduction.
- ▲ Abnormal position of the male urethra. It is not uncommon to find the urinary meatus displaced to the anterior surface of the penis (epispadias) or to the posterior surface (hypospadias) (see Chapter 23). A thorough examination of the newborn infant at or shortly following birth will often reveal such penile abnormalities.

The *scrotal sac* is examined to determine size, general appearance, and characteristics of its contents.

- ▲ Both testes should be descended at birth or shortly thereafter. If the testes remain undescended, spermatogenesis cannot take place because of the adverse effect of internal body heat.
- ▲ Scrotal contractility and relaxation should be noted. When exposed to cold, the scrotal sac will draw close to the body, with its skin assuming a wrinkled appearance. In the presence of heat, the scrotal sac will be relaxed and will move away from the warmth of the body, with skin appearing smooth.
- ▲ The contents of the scrotum should reveal two testes that feel smooth and regular to touch, are approximately equal in size, and are movable and sensitive to slight pressure. The epididymides are also palpated for size, location, shape, and consistency. The spermatic cords can be assessed by palpation. A light may be placed beneath the scrotal sac to illuminate its contents and provide some visual evaluation.

The examination of the male genitals is done mostly through external palpation and inspection; however, examination of the prostate gland and seminal vesicles occurs transrectally. The prostate can be palpated for size, shape, consistency, sensitivity, and movability. Although the prostate gland serves no major reproductive function, it is a common site for cancer. The normal seminal vesicles appear as soft, amorphic structures and cannot easily be palpated in the absence of abnormality.

THE FEMALE EXAMINATION

Like the male examination, the first assessment of the female genitalia occurs at birth when the newborn infant is examined in order to confirm sex. Because of the nature of the female reproductive function, the woman is more likely to have periodic health examination of the reproductive system than is the man. For many women, examination of the reproductive organs does not occur again until they are approaching marriage, desiring contraception, or suspecting pregnancy. There are still large numbers of women in the reproductive years, however, who do not seek health care services that would diagnose early and likely prevent many of the problems categorized as gynecologic disorders.

Gross examination of the woman is similar to that of the man and includes assessment of body size, shape, and posture. Height is the major indicator of growth used for women as well as for men; average height of the woman is less than that of the man. Access to a cumulative health care record is helpful for this information provides a good baseline from which evaluation can be made.

If the woman is of normal body weight, the presence of fatty deposits in the areas of the breasts, hips, and thighs will provide some information concerning developmental stage. Should the woman be obese or underweight, these observations have less developmental significance, although they may be indicative of a number of other disorders. The body should be inspected for the presence and development of the mammary glands (see following discussion on breasts) and the characteristics of pubic, axillary, and facial hair. In most women, facial hair will be sparce or not apparent. Heavy growth of general body hair and facial hair is unusual in the woman and should lead to further exploration of the endocrine function. Absence of pubic or axillary hair in the woman may be indicative of delayed puberty or endocrine malfunction.

The woman's skin should also be inspected for color, lesions, or abnormal growths. Generally, the abdominal skin reveals the true skin color more often than does the rest of the body and can be used for comparison.

Regional examination of the woman consists of assessment of the breasts, the abdomen, the internal and external genitalia, and the rectum.

Breast examination should begin with puberty and be done at periodic intervals thereafter for the rest of the woman's lifetime. Puberty is the time when the mammary glands begin to develop and become ready for their functional role in childbearing. Both self-examination and periodic examination by the nurse or physician of the breast should become a part of ongoing health assessment practices. The purposes of breast examination are:

- ▲ To assess breast development
- ▲ To diagnose breast pathophysiology such as inflammation or abnormal tumor growth, particularly, carcinoma
- ▲ To evaluate the breast during and following pregnancy to determine its readiness for supplying food for the newborn infant.

The breasts are examined using the techniques of inspection and palpation while the client assumes five different positions during the examination:

- ▲ Sitting with arms at the sides
- ▲ Sitting with arms lifted over the head
- ▲ Sitting and bending forward with the breasts hanging loosely
- ▲ Sitting with hands placed on and pushing into the hips while contracting the pectoral muscles
- ▲ Lying flat on the back with arms abducted

The specific procedure for breast examination is discussed in Chapter 26.

Assessment of the breasts during pregnancy and lactation is adapted to accommodate the changes that occur during these periods, as well as to increase awareness of the problems and conditions that are closely associated with these changes (see Chapters 12 and 17).

Abdominal examination alone, in the absence of pregnancy, provides little information about reproductive readiness. Abdominal examination during pregnancy and labor is of major importance (see Chapter 12). When abdominal assessment is concurrent with the vaginal examination (bimanual vaginal examination) information about the size, position, and condition of the internal female genitalia can be obtained. In a comprehensive abdominal examination, the techniques of inspection, palpation, percussion, and auscultation are all used. Here inspection and palpation of the abdomen are discussed.

The purposes of abdominal examination in regard to reproductive function are to rule out any abdominal pathology that might interfere with reproduction such as tumor growth; to determine the condition of the abdominal muscles; to assess uterine size and fetal age; to diagnose or rule out any abnormal position of the fetus; to assess the abdomen for any lesions or scars from previous surgery such as cesarean section or for unusual skin characteristics; to inspect body hair distribution; and to observe the contour of the abdomen, which is particularly important if pregnancy is suspected.

Abdominal examination is done with the woman lying in supine position and the torso uncovered from the pubis to just below the breasts. The nurse will also observe the abdomen with the woman standing, viewing it from both the frontal and lateral perspectives. Observations of the appearance and characteristics of the skin should be made. Depending upon personal habits, abdominal skin is frequently more protected from the sun than are other parts of the skin. Thus, it may well provide a baseline for comparison of other skin areas. If the skin appears taut and shiny, edema or ascites should be suspected and considered in regard to abdominal contour. Pigment changes such as striae may indicate that the abdominal muscles have undergone stretching such as from pregnancy or obesity. Occasionally, a darkened line *linea nigra,* running vertically along the midabdomen appears in women during pregnancy. This marking usually disappears with the termination of pregnancy; however, its presence should be noted.

Abdominal muscle tone should be noted and further assessment for gastrointestinal (GI) tract symptomatology made since the two are often closely related. Scars that confirm a history of surgery are of particular concern to the maternity nurse. The nurse should note size, location, and shape of the scar and question the patient about it.

The presence of marked abdominal hair in a woman should be reported, for the abdomen, like the breast, is usually covered with sparse amounts of fine, light-colored hair. As mentioned earlier, large amounts of hair generally distributed on the female body is often related to abnormal endocrine function.

In the healthy, nonobese woman, the abdomen should appear essentially flat. There should be no discernible vertical midline separation of the recti muscles *(diastasis)* as is seen in some women following pregnancy. If diastasis is present, the nurse will observe a gathering of loose skin above the separation when the woman contracts her abdominal muscles. If the woman is pregnant, the convex appearance of the abdomen will begin about the fourth month as the gravid uterus begins to displace the abdominal contents and will increase in size as the pregnancy progresses. Abdominal contour may be influenced by a number of factors other than pregnancy. The abdomen may be distended because of flatulence, solid or cystic tumor growth, obesity, feces, and abdominal fluid. The following aid will help you remember the causes of abdominal distention: fluid, flatulence, fat, feces, fibroid tumors, and fetus. Bladder distention will also cause a change in the contour of the lower abdomen.

Good abdominal muscle tone is very important during pregnancy and birth. Poor abdominal muscles will not provide adequate support of the growing uterine contents during pregnancy. This may lead to increased strain on the back and poor alignment of the fetal and maternal long body axes. The abdominal muscles serve as a secondary force for expulsion of the fetus during birth. If they are weak, the efficiency of the forces of the second stage of labor is decreased (see Chapter 16). Some determination of abdominal muscle tone can be made through observation of the abdominal contours and palpation when the woman is lying down. Information about how well the muscles support the abdominal viscera can be obtained through observation of the contour of the abdomen when the client is standing. The contour of the abdomen and spine, including the degree of curvature and the position of the shoulders, can be assessed through viewing the woman from the side (Fig. 9.1). This provides information about proper or improper posture. Poor posture is often the source of several minor discomforts during pregnancy, such as backache and dyspnea.

Abdominal movement will be reflected through the presence of peristaltic activity and sometimes respiratory effort. Markedly visible abdominal movement is usually indicative of a problem such as bowel obstruction or the presence of an active fetus. If the former is suspected, first, auscultation for bowel sounds should be made and, then, the client questioned concerning the presence of pain, tenderness, or other discomfort. If the latter is suspected, pregnancy can be confirmed through the auscultation of the fetal heart beat.

Assessment of the female genitalia is done to confirm developmental maturity; evaluate the tonal quality of the pelvic musculature; diagnose pelvic pathology; and determine the appropriateness of the transvaginal route for performing selected diagnostic, therapeutic, and surgical procedures such as the Papanicolaou (Pap) test for cervical cancer, therapeutic or elective abortion before 12-weeks gestation, or sterilization procedures such as tubal ligation (see Chapters 26 and 27). It is also possible to estimate the dimensions of the bony pelvic planes and cervical changes prior to and during labor. Many of these uses of the vaginal examination are discussed in regard to related content throughout this book.

Examination of the female genitalia consists of inspection of the external genitals, speculum examination of the vagina and cervix, bimanual vagino-abdominal palpation, and inspection and palpation of the rectum. The procedure for pelvic examination is discussed briefly here and in more detail in Chapter 26.

The external genitalia is inspected for appearance and characteristics of the skin. It is important to note the distribution pattern and characteristics of the

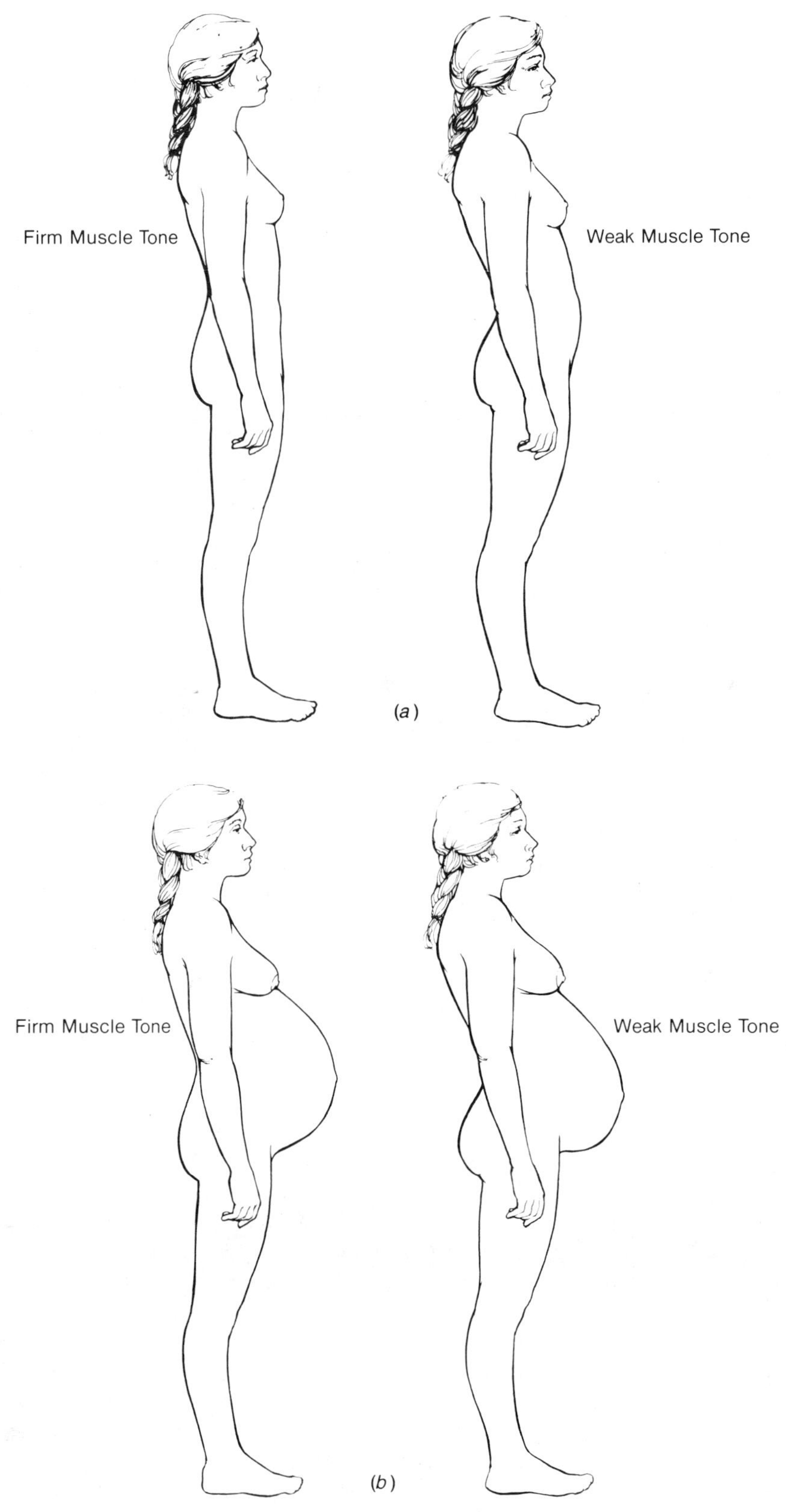

Figure 9.1
Lateral view while standing. Compare position of shoulders, curvature of spine, and abdominal contour in *(a)* nonpregnant woman and *(b)* woman in advanced pregnancy.

pubic hair, looking for adult versus early adolescent patterns; soft/fine hair versus kinky/coarse hair. The skin in the genital area of the female, like that of the male, is normally of a slightly darker pigmentation than elsewhere on the body. Any redness or indication of irritation should be noted, particularly of the inner thigh and vulva. It is not uncommon for irritated areas to be found. The genital area is often moist, receiving less exposure to circulating air. Poor personal hygiene habits and nonporous-fabric lingerie, such as most synthetic materials, contribute to irritations and vaginal infections. Any lesion or abnormal growth should be observed. Infection of hair follicles and other infectious disorders may be found in the pubic area.

The amount of fatty deposit on the mons veneris and the labia may be indicative of developmental progress. You will recall that estrogen is the hormone that supports the deposition of fatty tissue along female lines. The mons veneris tends to be flat and less rounded in the prepubescent girl. The amount of fatty tissue deposits is influenced by obesity and lack of generalized fatty tissue from malnutrition, as well as heredity. Parasites such as lice are sometimes found in the pubic hair.

In some women, varicosities of the entire vulvar and rectal areas will be present. These may be uncomfortable and a problem during pregnancy because of increased cardiovascular activity and often impaired venus return from the pelvis and lower extremities (see Chapter 12).

In the nulligravida, the edges of the labia, particularly the labia majora, are likely to touch or almost touch, whereas the multigravida is more likely to have labia that gape somewhat. The examiner can examine the labia and the rest of the vulva by separating the labia majora with gloved fingers and inspect it for color: the inner aspects of the labia majora and the labia minora should appear as dark pink, moist membranes.

Lesions of the skin such as syphilitic chancre or vesicles are indicative of pathology such as syphilis or herpes. These and other lesions are of particular importance should pregnancy be suspected or apparent since these diseases are transmitted to the developing fetus. Any lesion of the vulva should be noted and reported.

The clitoris should be observed for size and position. The urinary meatus appears as a dimple or slit in the soft tissue inferior to the clitoris. It should be observed for any evidence of abnormal growth or discharge.

The vaginal introitus should be apparent and patent. Occasionally, the hymen will partially to completely occlude this opening. The extent of coverage by the hymen and the consistency of the hymenal tissue will affect the ease and comfort with which first sexual intercourse occurs. An occluded vaginal os will require simple surgical removal of the hymen, *hymenectomy,* before normal sexual relations can occur. The perineum should be observed for the presence of scars such as an old episiotomy or lacerations. The distance between the inferior margin of the vaginal os and the rectum provides some information about the size of the perineum and whether or not tears into the rectum are likely to occur during childbirth.

The rectum should be observed for scars associated with extension of the perineum from laceration or incision and for hemorrhoids.

The external genitalia are palpated to determine the presence of nodules; inflamed Bartholin's or Skene's glands; and cystocele, rectocele, enterocele, or vaginal prolapse. The tone of the pelvic musculature is also assessed through palpation. (See Chapter 26 for further discussion of examination of the external and internal genitalia.)

Speculum examination is performed by inserting a metal instrument, the *speculum,* into the vagina in order to check the vaginal walls and the cervix for any signs of abnormality such as inflammation, abnormal discharge from the uterus and cervix, cervical or vaginal lesions, as well as position, color, size, and surface characteristics of the cervix and shape of the cervical os. Speculum examination also permits the examiner to obtain specimens from the cervix, uterus, and vagina for diagnostic purposes. (see Chapter 26).

Bimanual examination is done to palpate the pelvic contents, particularly the internal genitalia—uterus and adenexae (tubes and ovaries)—between the two hands of the examiner. One hand remains in the vagina while the other hand palpates the lower abdomen. By gently grasping the organs between the two hands, the organs can be assessed for size, position in the pelvis, normal and abnormal surface characteristics, sensitivity to touch (tenderness), movability, consistency, and the presence of any abnormal growths such as solid or cystic tumors. The oviducts are not usually palpable and are sometimes confused with the round ligaments, which are of similar size and shape. Examination of the internal genitalia can provide information about the developmental status of the internal reproductive organs and make possible diagnosis of problems that might interfere with the reproductive process or endanger the client's life.

Rectovaginal examination is done to confirm uterine position, palpate the uterosacral ligaments, and assess the rectovaginal septum and the cul-de-sac located in the posterior part of the vagina. This space enables the examiner to have access to the pelvic organs through the thin walls that separate the vagina from the pelvic and abdominal cavities. Occasionally, it may contain abnormal masses. The rectum is also assessed for the presence of pathology such as polyps, fissures, fistulas, and hemorrhoids. The muscle tone of the rectal sphincter is determined. Any abscesses or masses should be noted and reported.

Laboratory Assessment

There are many laboratory studies available and in use to assess physical health status. Those most often used in regard to reproductive health are blood and urine studies. The most commonly performed blood and urine studies are in Table 9.3; others are discussed throughout the book in relation to the period of pregnancy with which they are closely associated or in conjunction with reproductive risk assessment or gynecologic disorder.

Analysis of semen for sperm activity is not a routinely performed examination. However, when reproductive capability of the man is in question, particularly in cases where infertility is a problem, or in a rare legal case, analysis of the seminal fluid may be done (see Chapter 27).

NURSING RESPONSIBILITIES

Reproductive health assessment, usually done with consent from the client or his or her family, requires the person and family to respond to personal, even intimate, questions and may necessitate exposure of the body to strangers with whom the person may or may not have developed trusting relationships. General physical examination is usually well accepted by the public. Examination of the male or female genitalia is viewed quite differently, however, for this examination truly involves access to the privacy of one's personal self. There appears to be greater acceptance of examination of a woman by a man gynecologist than the examination of a man by a woman physician or nurse practitioner. Since most of the time the maternity nurse practices with the woman as the primary client the following discussion will be from that vantage point.

For many women, the pelvic or gynecologic examination is the first such intimate examination and fear of what the doctor or nurse may reveal through the examination is not unusual. As one young woman expressed it, "I just knew that all of my innermost secrets would be exposed with the examination." It is easy for the nurse and other health providers to fall into the "trap" of viewing the client as an inanimate object to be scrutinized, examined, and discussed. Awareness of and sensitivity to the client as a person, whether male or female, with or without family support, is not only good manners, it is likely to provide an atmosphere to which the client is willing to return for subsequent health care. Cultivating the client's interest in participating in health care supervision is crucial, especially if a diagnosis of pregnancy or a problem or disorder should be uncovered. In any case, it is a good investment toward promoting continuing health care practices.

In addition to performing all or parts of the assessment for reproductive readiness described in the preceding sections of this chapter, or assisting another to do so, the maternity nurse has three other significant responsibilities: the preparation of the client and family for the assessment, particularly the physical examination; support of the client during the examination; and reassurance of the client and family following the assessment.

Preparation of the Client and Family

The goal of the nurse in preparation of the client for the interview and examination is to create a climate that will decrease the client's fear and embarrassment and promote relaxation and cooperation. The maternity nurse may accomplish these goals by following some simple guidelines.

▲ Providing privacy, ideally by using a single examining room or by carefully screening off sections of a room that must accommodate more than one person. Avoidance of probing and unnecessary questions and attention to draping the woman carefully so that only the area being

TABLE 9.3
SELECTED BLOOD AND URINE LABORATORY TESTS

Study	*Purpose*	*Significance*
BLOOD STUDIES		
Type Rh	Determination of maternal and parental blood group and Rh factor to identify blood type and Rh combinations that may affect reproductive outcome.	Occasionally during pregnancy blood incompabilities will occur and result in problems for the woman and particularly the fetus/neonate. (See Chapters 12 and 23.) Hemorrhage of the pregnant woman is always a possibility for consideration. Knowledge of female blood type expedites transfusion therapy if and when needed. Intrauterine fetal or neonatal blood transfusion is sometimes necessary. Knowledge of maternal blood type and Rh is essential.
Serology	Detection of syphilis in the pregnant woman. Provide diagnostic basis for early treatment of syphilis.	Syphilis if detected and treated before 6–18 weeks fetal age will usually result in a nonaffected neonate because of the failure of the spirochete to cross the placental barrier during the first trimester of pregnancy. Failure to diagnose and treat syphilis during the first 20 weeks of pregnancy will likely result in a diseased and possibly damaged neonate.
Hematocrit Hemoglobin	Determination of presence of anemia in the pregnant female. Provide baseline information for direction to do other anemia studies such as ▲ Blood indices ▲ Serum iron content and binding capacity ▲ Folate levels ▲ Sickle cell studies	A number of women in the reproductive years have an iron deficient or nutritional anemia. This may be either aggravated or first noted during pregnancy. Chronic anemia places both mother and fetus/neonate at risk and has been associated with prematurity and infants of low birth weight. Hematocrit of 30 mg% or less or a hemoglobin of 10–11 gm/100 ml or less should alert examiner to potential for anemia. Hemoglobin of 10 gm/100 ml is true anemia.
White blood count (WBC) Differential	Diagnosis of ▲ Infection ▲ Blood abnormalities, e.g., leukemia	Normal increase in WBC during pregnancy and a further increase during labor. Increase or decrease in specific WBC provide assistance with specific diagnosis.
Blood sugar	Diagnosis of CHO metabolic disorders, e.g., diabetes mellitus.	Diabetes mellitus may have an adverse effect on woman or fetus during pregnancy. Diabetes is an inherited disorder so it is important that early diagnosis in men and women be done before pregnancy so that treatment can be instituted and counseling regarding reproduction can be provided.

TABLE 9.3 (continued)

Study	*Purpose*	*Significance*
BLOOD STUDIES		
Rubella	Determination of patient's immune status regarding rubella (German measles).	Rubella, clinical or subclinical during early pregnancy, can cause significant damage to the developing fetus. Live-born neonates may have severe congenital malformations, for example, eye disorders such as cataracts, heart defects, auditory defects, CNS defects, and others. Immunization should be given to women in the childbearing years only if pregnancy can be prevented or a minimal period of 2 months. All women who have received rubella vaccine or who report having had German measles should have a rubella screening prior to pregnancy (1:8—1:10 = + titre).
URINE STUDIES		
Bacteria	Diagnosis of urinary tract infections, particularly pyelonephritis.	Chronic urinary tract infections in the woman are likely to lead to ▲ Renal damage ▲ Infections during pregnancy that will affect the well-being of both woman and unborn child
Protein (Albuminuria)	Determination of renal pathology usually associated with hypertension.	Presence of albumin in the urine is abnormal and is associated with hypertension and other problems. Hypertension pre-existing or during pregnancy may lead to poor reproductive outcome. Measurement of urinary protein is a simple procedure if done by a dipstick (1+ or more on a clean catch urine specimen is significant). Presence of proteinuria should alert the nurse to necessity for carefully assessing patient blood pressure levels and evidence of generalized edema. Generalized edema in the absence of proteinuria and hypertension is likely physiologic rather than pathologic.
Glucose	Determination of CHO metabolic disorders such as diabetes.	Most glucose is reabsorbed in the renal tubules. Glycosuria is usually an abnormal finding in the urine of nonpregnant women. Glycosuria is present in about 30% of pregnant women.

examined is exposed are of particular importance during examination of the genitals. The patient is in a vulnerable, dependent position (Fig. 9.2).

▲ Determining the woman's expectations about the interview and examination. Misconceptions about health care practices abound as do myths concerning sexuality, conception, pregnancy, and childbirth. Often, the nurse can obtain this information by a simple question such as: "Have you had a health history taken before?" or "Have you ever had a vaginal examination before?" If the answer is yes, follow with "What was it like?" If the answer is no, "What do you expect it to be like?"

▲ Carefully explaining the activities to be carried out. The purpose, technical language, and equipment familiar to the nurse are often unfamiliar to other people, particularly those receiving health care. The woman should be encouraged to share her concerns and ask questions before, during, and following the interview and procedures. The best encouragement a nurse can provide is sensitive, clear, willing responses to questions. Vague responses such as follow to questions about a vaginal exam or palpation of the male genitalia are useless to the client.

CLIENT: *"Will it hurt?"*

NURSE: *"Of course not if you relax and do as I tell you."*

Not only does this not answer the client's question, it imposes the threat to the client that if he or she does not do as the nurse says it will hurt. It is much more helpful to the client and ultimately to the nurse to respond honestly and accurate.

CLIENT: *"Will it hurt?"*

NURSE: *"You may feel some discomfort for a moment or two, but I will be there to help you relax."*

▲ Instructing the client in ways in which he or she can participate during the examination. Often the client is not aware of the importance of

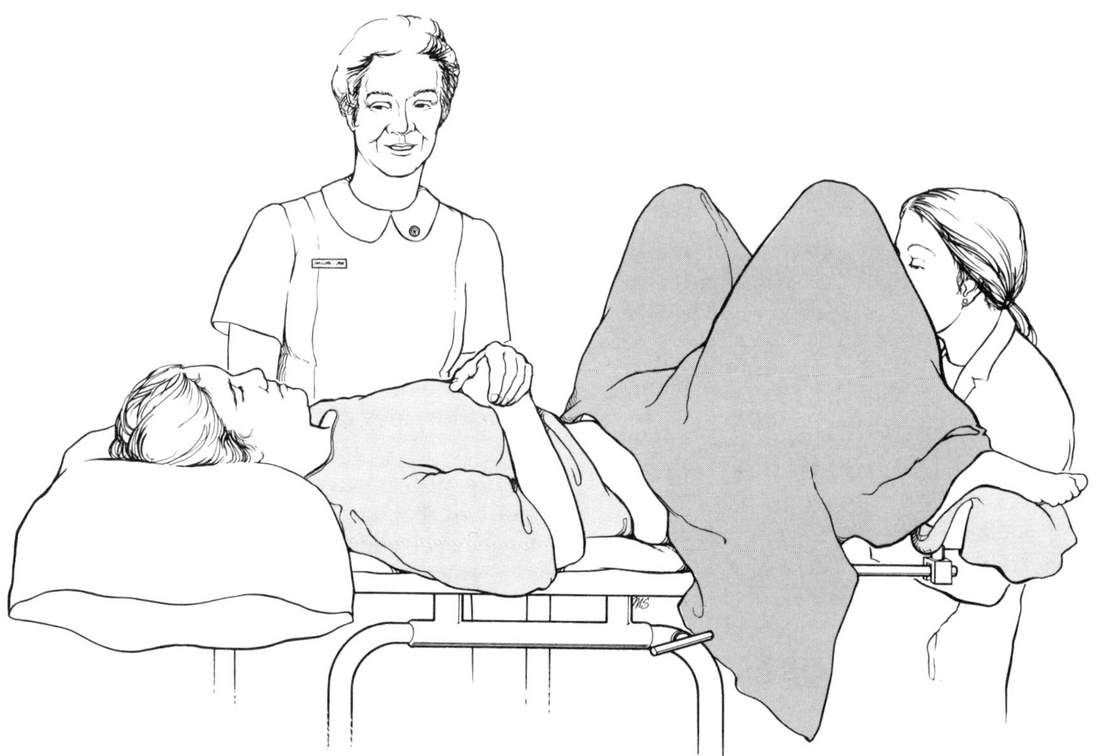

Figure 9.2
Pelvic examination with woman in dorsal recumbent position.

clear accurate responses to questions or of the effect that relaxation has on both the comfort and ease with which the physical examination can progress. Tight pelvic muscles make it difficult for the examiner to assess the female reproductive organs. Taut abdominal muscles make it almost impossible to palpate the abdomen to obtain accurate information. A body that is tense is a resistive force to examination and not only impairs the efficiency of the examiner but is likely to increase the discomfort to the man or woman. Tenseness is often a message from the patient that he or she is frightened or apprehensive. The nurse might give reassurance by providing information or instruction to use breathing techniques in the following way:

"If you can relax and make your body very limp, it will decrease some of the discomfort that you might feel and help the doctor (or nurse) do the examination more quickly and thoroughly. One of the best ways to relax the muscles is to breathe regularly, deeply, and slowly. This increases the oxygen to the muscle and helps it relax."

There are many other techniques for promoting relaxation with which you are familiar. Try them all and repeat the ones that seem to be most effective with the largest number of people. There are times during the examination when the patient is asked to participate in the examination in other ways, such as to contract muscles voluntarily in the abdominal, rectal, and vaginal examinations, or to respond verbally to questions such as "Tell me when you feel pressure."

Support of the Client During the Interview and Examination

Even though a person has been prepared for an interview, physical examination, or the taking of blood and urine for analysis, preparation alone does not obviate all fears and anxieties. The client needs support during the actual experiences, which can be provided in a number of ways.

- ▲ Recognition of the client as an individual is important. In a private health care setting, the client will know the physician or nurse and introductions are unnecessary. Such is not always the case in a public clinical facility. The client may not have met the nurse or physician before this intimate contact. During busy clinical activities, common courtesy is often lost and the nurse may approach the client without clear identification of self or role. The nurse and physician have the advantage over the client, for they have access to the client's health record. Physical examination places a person in a dependent position with little or no personal control. When people are asked to assume various positions during physical examination, such as dorsal recumbent or knee–chest positions, it quite easy to communicate the message unintentionally that only the examination, not the person, is important. This can be avoided if it is clear that the center of initial concern is the person and not the procedures that are to be carried out. Many people submit to physical examination with little or no comment at the time of the examination but are nevertheless influenced by the attitudes of the nurse and physician. If their attitude is friendly, caring, and protective, the man or woman may be more likely to remain in contact with the health care delivery system, otherwise they may not return to any health care facility for further care.
- ▲ Not only is attention to privacy important in preparation of the client for the interview or examination, it is crucial during the actual events. It is of utmost importance to remember that every effort must be made to provide privacy: doors, screens, and drapes should be used.
- ▲ Reinforcement and support of the client's efforts to participate in and cooperate during the examination are also necessary. This may take the form of a smile or nod of encouragement, of squeezing the hand or touching the shoulder, or of verbal encouragement such as "You seem very relaxed. How do you feel?" Repetition of instructions is also useful.
- ▲ Communication of directions needs to be clear and in a voice that can be heard and understood. If the client is frightened or anxious, attention to verbal instructions is likely to be incomplete. Often it is not possible for the nurse to remain beside the client throughout the entire examina-

tion. Reasons for leaving the room and when return can be expected are helpful. Repetition or interpretation of the examiner's instructions may be necessary.

Reassurance of the Client and Family Following Examination

When the examination and the total health assessment are completed, the nurse should see that the client is not left with instructions only for the cashier's office. There are likely to be unanswered or new questions generated by the assessment. Support or an explanation to the family, if present, may be necessary. The nurse may not be able to provide complete information about the outcome of the examination or the assessment; however, reassurance about or instruction for future visits can be given. There are two ways the nurse may do this.

- ▲ If findings from the assessment are clear and definitive, they should be shared with the woman and her family, if this is her wish. Some information such as the result of laboratory tests may not be immediately available, and instruction about when and how to obtain this information should be provided. Often information provided by the physician may not be clearly understood by the client. The nurse is an appropriate person to confirm what was said, clarify it, and reinforce the client's understanding of what was meant or what took place during the reproductive health assessment.
- ▲ Recognition of the client's participation should be given. This may be done through a simple statement of praise, which must be genuine and not given in a condescending manner. Comments like, "You were a very good girl or boy during the examination," to an adult is inappropriate. It is better to say, "Your being relaxed certainly helped the examination go smoothly. I hope that you weren't too uncomfortable."

Assessment for reproductive readiness provides much useful information that can be used in planning a person's health care regimen. It does involve entering into the very private personal world of people and their families. The way in which this assessment is approached may make the difference between people who are interested in the health of themselves and their family and those who are turned off by the health delivery system. Often the nurse is the key to the decision.

SUMMARY

Developmental readiness for reproduction was discussed. Selected content from the biologic and social sciences was used to compare the similarities and differences in reproductive capability of the male and female. This content is used by the maternity nurse in cooperation with other health care providers to assess physical and psychosocial readiness of men and women for their reproductive functions. It also provides the foundation for much of the health care appropriate during pregnancy, childbirth, and recovery.

Reproductive health assessment of developmental readiness involves the collection of information about the person and family through the use of data collection methods such as interview and observation to obtain a health history and physical examination techniques to obtain data through regional physical examination of the male and female genitalia and the female abdomen and breasts and through the laboratory analysis of urine and blood.

The nurse participates in physical assessment of reproductive readiness by using knowledge and skill about physical, psychosocial, and cognitive development. The nurse also participates in reproductive health assessment by preparing the client and family for such an assessment, supporting the client during history taking and physical examination, and judiciously interpreting findings to the client and family independently of and in consultation with other health care providers.

REFERENCES AND READINGS

Bates, B. *A Guide to Physical Examination.* Philadelphia: J. B. Lippincott, 1980.

Batterman, B. M., Seligman, M., Fitz, A. Hypertension: Detection, Evaluation and Treatment. *Nurs Digest* 4(5):55, 1976.

Carlson, C. E., Blackwell, B. *Behavioral Concepts and Nursing Intervention* (2nd ed.). Philadelphia: J. B. Lippincott, 1978

Longo, D. C., Williams, R. A. (Eds.). *Clinical Practice in Psychosocial Nursing Assessment and Intervention.* New York: Appleton-Century-Crofts, 1978.

Malasanos, L., Barkauskas, V., Moss, M., Stoltenber-Allen, K. *Health Assessment.* St. Louis: C. V. Mosby, 1977.

Murray, R. B., Zentner, J. P. *Nursing Assessment and Health Promotion Throughout the Life Span* (2nd ed.). Englewood Cliffs, N.J.: Prentice-Hall, 1979.

Novak, E. R., Jones, G. S., Jones, Jr., H. W. *Textbook of Gynecology.* Baltimore: Williams & Wilkins, 1975.

Stewart, F. H., Stewart, G. K., Guest, F. J., Hatcher, R. A. *My Body, My Health.* New York: John Wiley & Sons, 1979.

UNIT THREE

PREGNANCY

INTRODUCTION

Pregnancy spans a period of 9 calendar months, almost 1 year of a woman's life. During these months the woman experiences events that will change her body and her life. She will learn to be a pregnant woman as well as to be an expectant mother. She will never be the same girl or young woman she was, for as adolescence bridges the gap between childhood and adulthood, pregnancy connects the developmental periods of girlhood and motherhood.

Pregnancy requires much from the woman and her family. There are biophysical demands that affect all of her body systems. Unfamiliar stresses will test the coping skills of the woman and those closest to her. She will experience unfamiliar moods: joys, fears, dreams, frustrations, and hope; she will have emotional highs and lows with periods of introspection and times of uninhibited extroversion.

Pregnancy involves people other than the woman. Her partner experiences a change and even upheaval in his life. He is part of the pregnancy although he is not involved in the same way as is the woman. The family is also a part of the reproductive experience for pregnancy unites generations and has impacts on any other children.

This unit addresses content needed by the maternity nurse to provide comprehensive, sensitive, family-centered nursing care during pregnancy. Unit Three contains six chapters.

Chapter 10, "Development of the Maternal–Fetal Unit," describes fertilization and implantation. The preimplantation period and the development of the placenta and the accessory structures—the umbilical cord and the fetal membranes—are explained. Amniotic fluid is discussed in terms of its purpose and composition. Some implications for the use of this information by nurses is included in the chapter; much more is integrated throughout the book.

Chapter 11, "Pregnancy: Fetal Perspective," continues the discussion begun in Chapter 10 but with a different focus, that of the periods of fetal development from fertilization to birth. The fetal growth of a single conceptus receives considerable attention; however, the subject of twins is also addressed.

Chapter 12, "Pregnancy: Maternal Perspective," is a comprehensive description and analysis of pregnancy as experienced by the woman. Biophysical and psychosocial adjustments are included along with related nursing care. Much attention is given to the manner in which nurses use basic content to provide care to the pregnant woman.

Chapter 13, "Pregnancy: Family Perspective," addresses an event that involves the family in a variety of ways. Contemporary family life-styles and social and ethnic idiosyncrasies are described. Role change within the family, which is important to the maternity nurse, is viewed here predominantly within the context of the nuclear family.

In Chapter 14, "Sexuality and Pregnancy," sexuality and sexual adjustment, important and intimate concerns of couples experiencing pregnancy, are discussed. Practical suggestions for ways in which nurses can help couples make adjustments in a healthy, mutually satisfying way for each partner are emphasized.

Chapter 15, "Preparation for Childbirth," discusses the development of parent education in the United States and contemporary methods for helping expectant parents prepare for childbirth and early parenthood. Considerable attention is given to psychoprophylactic method of childbirth and education.

BEHAVIORAL OUTCOMES

Upon completion of the study of this unit, you should be able to:

- ▲ Describe gamete transport in the man and woman and its goal, fertilization
- ▲ Explain placental development using a contemporary theory base
- ▲ Describe the placenta, accessory structures, the fetal membranes, the umbilical cord, and the amniotic fluid

- ▲ Describe three stages of fetal development
- ▲ Identify two clinical indicators of fetal growth and development
- ▲ Describe physical changes in the pregnant woman by body system
- ▲ Explain the relationship between placental–fetal development and physiologic changes occurring in the mother
- ▲ Describe a woman's psychologic response to pregnancy
- ▲ Explain five major nursing responsibilities for the prenatal care of a pregnant woman
- ▲ Identify three contemporary family life-styles
- ▲ Describe two ways in which pregnancy affects the family
- ▲ Identify two ways in which pregnancy alters usual sexual relationships between a man and a woman
- ▲ Describe three ways in which a nurse can help the couple make a healthy sexual adjustment during pregnancy
- ▲ Identify two methods of preparation for pregnancy and parenthood
- ▲ Explain psychoprophylactic method of childbirth education

10

DEVELOPMENT OF THE MATERNAL-FETAL UNIT

The gamut of human reproduction from fertilization through recovery from childbirth is possible because of a sophisticated physiologic timetable in which each event is, in some way, related to or dependent upon another event. It is no accident that placental development corresponds closely to fetal growth and well-being or that both are associated with changes in maternal biosystems. Knowledge of fertilization, implantation, and placental development and function enables the maternity nurse to understand more completely and appreciate more fully the subsequent processes and events that ensure healthy reproduction. It also enables the nurse to recognize disruptions that may place the mother, fetus, or both in jeopardy of damage or death.

This chapter presents content about fertilization (conception) and some of the conditions that enable fertilization to occur. The preimplantation period between fertilization and implantation is discussed briefly here and in more detail in Chapter 11. The development and function of the placenta and accessory structures such as the fetal membranes and the umbilical cord are included, and the composition and function of the amniotic fluid are explained.

FERTILIZATION

Fertilization is the union of the male and female gametes. Certain conditions are prerequisite to fertilization: (1) maturity of both male and female gametes, (2) timing of sperm deposition, and (3) a climate in the female genital tract that is supportive of sperm survival and transport.

Maturity of the Male and Female Gametes

The process of *gametogenesis* enables the woman's ovum to approach maturity and the man to produce adequate spermatozoa (sperm) to undergo the rigors of travel from his body to the outer portion of the fallopian tube in the woman's generative tract (see Chapters 5 and 6). During the process of gametogenesis, a high number of ova and spermatozoa degenerate and are lost to reproduction. However, millions of spermatozoa do reach maturity and are available for fertilization of a single ovum by one spermatozoon. The female egg completes its maturation after ovulation and fertilization. The completion of sperm maturity is not definitive. In some lower animals such as the rabbit, spermatozoa complete their maturity after being deposited in the female genital tract *(capacitation)*. This incubation of the human spermatozoa has not been clearly demonstrated; however, it is suspected that such a final step may be necessary in the human being as well.

The fertilization capability of the spermatozoon (sperm) and the ovum is dependent upon both their health status and their maturity. Health is used here to mean genetic, morphologic, and physiologic adequacy. The first meiotic division in the ovum *(oocyte)* occurs while the egg is still in the ovary. The second meiotic division proceeds after ovulation as the ovum migrates to the fallopian tube and continues after fertilization. During this period, the ovum is vulnerable to environmental influences that may affect the adequacy of the egg to proceed to maturity or to develop appropriately following fertilization.

The adequacy of the spermatozoa to fertilize the ovum is determined by the number of spermatozoa present in the ejaculate or specimen, by their morphology, and by their motility (Table 10.1). Inadequacy of any of these categories may result in a fertilization failure.

Timing of Sperm Deposit

Appropriate timing in relation to ovulation of the deposit of spermatozoa in the woman's vagina is necessary for fertilization to occur. The lifetime of the ovum awaiting fertilization is approximately 24 hours (or less) and that of the sperm inside the female genital tract rarely exceeds 48 hours. The absence of clinical indicators of ovulation to the woman usually leaves the exact time of ovulation unknown to her and her partner and makes precise control of fertilization difficult for the couple who desires to conceive or who wishes to avoid conception. This omission of clear-cut indicators for ovulation, along with the disassociation between the act of sexual intercourse and conception in the minds of many sexually active couples, causes fertilization—more times than not—to be a random occurrence. Couples who use birth control measures have far more control over the timing of fertilization (see Chapter 26). In most cases, fertilization is possible only within a 72-hour time span surrounding ovulation, that is, deposit of sperm can occur as early as 48 hours preceding ovulation or within the 24-hour period following ovulation (Fig. 10.1).

Climate of the Female Genital Tract

Except for the period surrounding ovulation, the environment of the female genital tract is hostile to spermatozoa, decreasing their life span and impeding their migration to the fallopian tube. Vaginal and cervical secretions, along with decreased contractility of the uterus and fallopian tubes, work in concert to defeat the most ambitious sperm. Around the

TABLE 10.1
SPERM ADEQUACY FOR FERTILIZATION

Category	*Characteristic*
Number	20 million sperm per milliliters of semen or 50 million in total ejaculate or specimen
Morphology	70% are normal in appearance
Motility	50% of total number of sperm are motile and 50% can make a forward motion

Source: Adapted from Page, E. W., Villee, C. A., Villee, D. D. *Human Reproduction—The Core Content of Obstetrics, Gynecology and Perinatal Medicine* (2nd ed.). Philadelphia: W. B. Saunders, 1976, p. 161.

time of ovulation, however, the opposite is true, and these same secretions and structures work to facilitate transport of the sperm to the site of the ovum.

Ordinarily, vaginal and cervical secretions are acidic. The sperm cannot live in an environment that has a low pH. Although the seminal fluid provides agents that work to neutralize the acidity of the vagina, these are often inadequate if the pH of the vagina is low as in the absence of estrogen priming; the presence of progesterone; or, before intercourse, the use of a spermicidal jelly, cream, or foam that is of acid pH.

The consistency of cervical secretions also plays a role in antagonizing or supporting the spermatozoa's effort to fertilize the ovum. At the time of ovulation, these secretions are more copious, a much thinner consistency, and easily penetrable by the sperm. During the luteal phase of the menstrual cycle, they are less abundant, thick, and viscous because of the presence of progesterone; thus they are an impediment to sperm survival and transport, preventing the sperm from migrating beyond the vagina or cervical os.

During much of the menstrual cycle, the musculature of the fallopian tubes and the uterus is in a quiet, noncontractile state. This is particularly true in the second half of the menstrual cycle when the levels of progesterone are high. These structures are much more active during the period of ovulation and are believed to play a role in gamete transport.

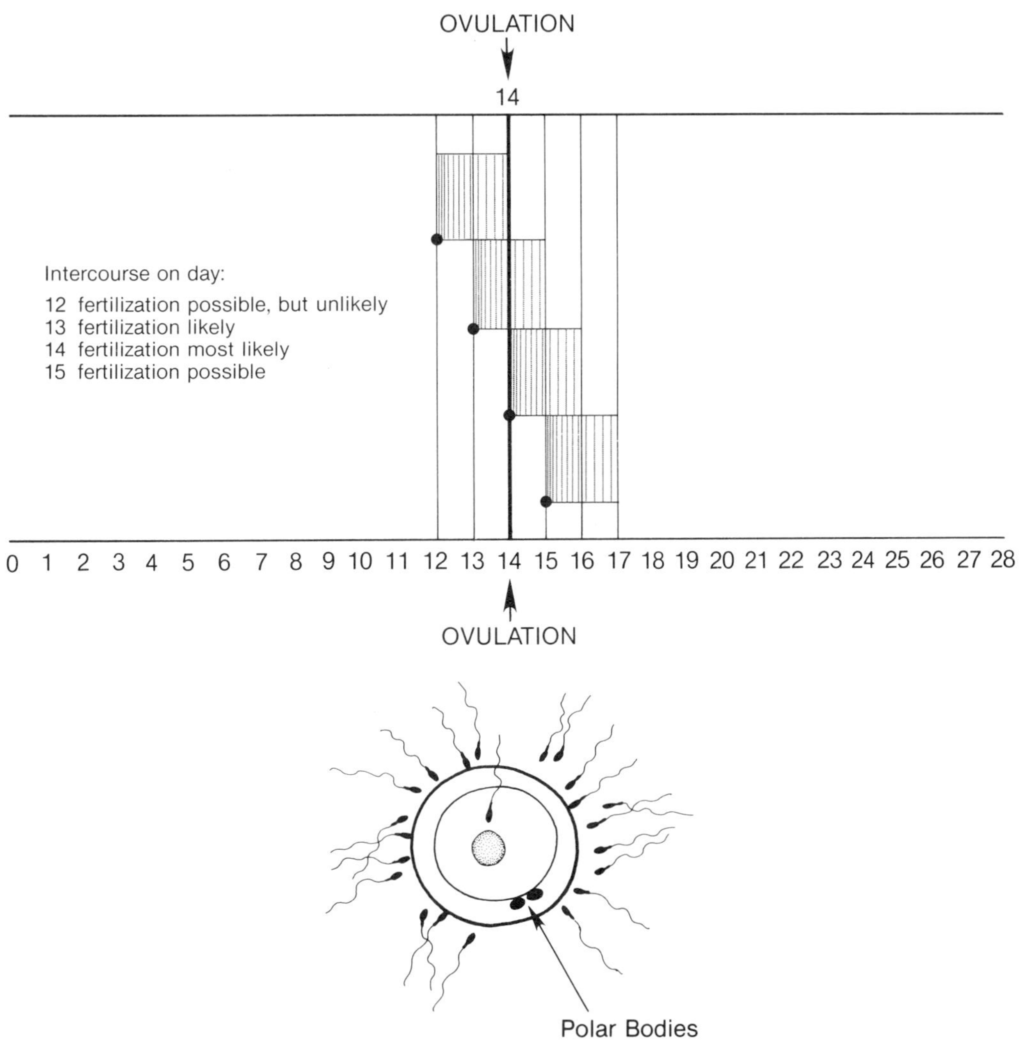

Figure 10.1
Top: Time of fertilization; *bottom:* fertilization.

The distance to be traveled by the ovum is obviously much shorter than that required by the spermatozoa. The mechanism for ovum transport to the ampullary–isthmic junction of the fallopian tube is not completely known. Ciliary action of the tubal epithelium, peristaltic movements of the tube that have been observed to peak at the time of ovulation, and contraction of the ovarian ligament, drawing the ovary and fimbria closer together, enhanced by the creation of a suction, are all believed to play a role in promoting ovum migration into the fallopian tube.

Transport of the spermatozoa is more complex and requires transfer of the sperm from the man to the woman usually through sexual intercourse resulting in ejaculation of semen into the vagina. Artificial insemination by donor sperm may also result in fertilization (see Chapter 27). Once the sperm are deposited in the vagina, they must negotiate the cervical os, the uterine cavity, and the inner two-thirds of the fallopian tube before they reach the ovum. Ejaculation of semen is under the control of the sympathetic nervous system that provides for initiation of a series of rapid contractions that force about 2–5 ml of semen, containing 60–100 million spermatozoa per milliliter out of the man's urethra in response to sexual stimulation (see Chapter 7). Once the spermatozoa enter the female genital tract, they are vulnerable to the environmental factors discussed earlier. Their brief lifetime necessitates rapid movement. Prior to entry into the uterine cavity, they are essentially self-propelled forward by the lashing, whipping motion of their tails. Only a small number of sperm travel beyond the vagina. Once the sperm enter the uterus, it is believed that they receive some assistance by the uterus through a pumping action that gently pushes them forward. Although the most vigorous spermatozoa will reach the ovum within 65–75 minutes, sperm have been reported to reach the outer portion of the fallopian tube as quickly as 5 minutes following deposit. Proximity of deposit of the semen to the cervical os and characteristics of the cervical secretions likely affect this transport time.

The general health of both parents can directly or indirectly affect the act of fertilization and the mechanisms that support it. The health status of the woman is of particular importance. Pathologic or pathophysiologic conditions, congenital anomalies of the reproductive tract, and teratogens can influence both the fact of fertilization and its outcome. Table 10.2 summarizes some of the factors that support or antagonize fertilization.

Fertilization

Fertilization has occurred when one sperm penetrates the vitelline membrane of the ovum and the male and female pronuclei unite. At this time the usual chromosome count of 46 is restored. With the restoration of the chromosome count, the sex chromosomes contributed by each parent combine, and the sex of the new life is determined (Fig. 10.2). All of the inherited traits from both parents are also established at this time. The membranes of the parent pronuclei disintegrate, and the new life is begun. It is now called a zygote.

What happens when the sperm and ovum unite is known; exactly how the sperm manages to enter the ovum is less clear. It is believed that contact between the sperm head and the ovum surface initiates the release of hydrolytic enzymes contained in the acrosome of the sperm. These enzymes in turn have an eroding or disintegrating action on the zona pellucida and the vitelline membrane that enables the sperm to enter the ovum and unite with the pronucleus of the ovum to begin life. Whatever the exact mechanism, only one sperm is believed to enter the ovum, most likely the first sperm to make contact with the ovum surface. Once fertilization has occurred, mitotic cellular division begins, and the single-celled being is on its way to becoming the many-celled unit that will develop into a recognizable human life.

The mechanism surrounding fertilization can be summarized as a series of sequential steps that begins with gametogenesis and ends in the union of the sperm and ovum.

- ▲ Ovulation occurs and the ovum migrates to the outer one-third of the fallopian tube.
- ▲ Millions of spermatozoa are deposited in the vagina at or near the cervical os. (This may precede ovulation by as many as 48 hours. However, the closer to the time of ovulation that the sperm are deposited, the better the chance for fertilization to occur.)
- ▲ Healthy vigorous sperm travel from the site of deposition through the cervix and uterus to the distal one-third of the fallopian tube.
- ▲ Hundreds of spermatozoa reach and surround the ovum.
- ▲ One sperm makes first contact with the surface of the ovum, and the acrosomic reaction is initiated releasing lytic enzymes that act upon the membranes surrounding the ovum.

TABLE 10.2
CONDITIONS AFFECTING FERTILIZATION

Supportive of Fertilization	*Antagonistic to Fertilization*
Intercourse within a 72-hour period surrounding ovulation	Intercourse outside of 72 hours surrounding ovulation
Presence of a mature ovum in the outer one-third of the fallopian tube	Absence of a mature ovum (an anovulatory menstrual cycle)
Adequate numbers of healthy, vigorous sperm	Inadequate numbers of sperm; immature or abnormal sperm; decreased or absent sperm motility
Increased pH of the usual acidic vaginal and cervical secretions	Decreased pH of vaginal and cervical secretions
Increased contractility of uterus and fallopian tubes	Decreased contractility of uterus and fallopian tubes
Absence of pathology, pathophysiology, anomaly in both partners	Presence of pathology, pathophysiology, anomaly in either or both partners

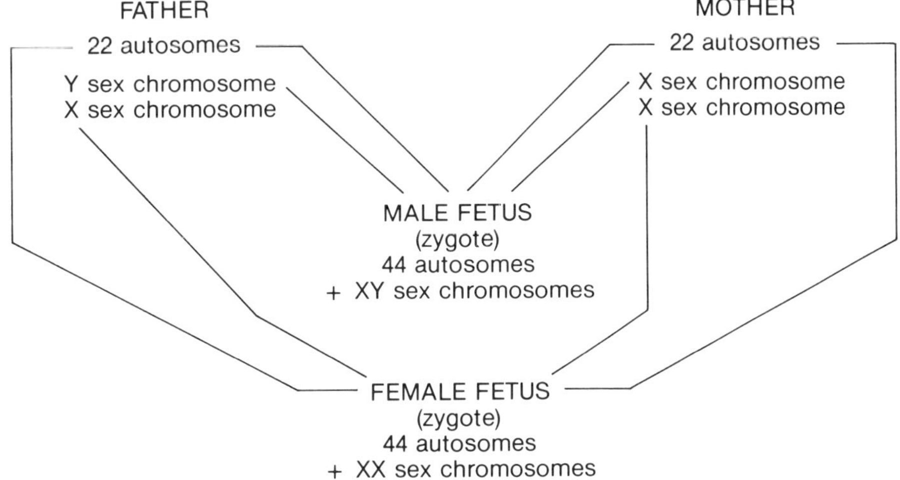

Figure 10.2
Sex determination at the time of conception.

- ▲ The sperm penetrates the vitelline membrane; its head is detached and enlarges; the body and tail are probably absorbed by the cytoplasm of the ovum.
- ▲ The sperm head, now resembling a nucleus (male pronucleus), migrates to the center of the ovum where it merges with the female pronucleus that has been formed as the ovum matures after penetration by the sperm.
- ▲ The two pronuclei interlock restoring the chromosome count to 46 (22 paired homologues and two sex chromosomes). The sex and genetic inheritance is established at this time.

PREIMPLANTATION PERIOD

Following fertilization, several changes occur in the zygote that are necessary to provide the foundations for its survival and later growth and development. The single-celled unit must increase in number and undergo beginning cellular differentiation. It must also travel from the site of fertilization to the uterine cavity where it will attach to the endometrial lining establishing the physiologic communication link with the maternal body systems that will sustain it until separation occurs at the time of birth.

Cell Division and Differentiation

Mitosis is the mechanism whereby the cells divide and replicate themselves in the new life. When fertilization is complete, the ovum becomes known as the *zygote* and must increase from the one cell established by the union of the two parent gametes to 2–4–8–16, and so on, becoming a multicelled unit. It is called a *morula* at this stage because of its resemblance to a mulberry. This process is called *cleavage,* or segmentation, of the zygote into more but smaller cells called *blastomeres.* Cleavage begins at some point during the first 36 hours after fertilization. As the cells increase in number, the structure that was the mature ovum remains encapsulated within the zona pellucida. The corona radiata formed by adherent granulosa cells during gametogenesis disappears before entry of the zygote into the uterine cavity. The zona pellucida remains intact until after the conceptus has entered the uterine cavity and disappears before attachment to the endometrium.

A fluid fills the center of the structure. It forces the cells to reposition themselves. Some cells migrate to the periphery of the sac while others cluster as a cell mass reaching more inward. The structure is now called the *blastodermic vesicle,* or *blastocyst.* The cells that now line the sac comprise a wall of primitive *cytotrophoblasts* that secrete a fluid to aid in the nourishment of the growing life before implantation. These cells will later come into contact with the basal layer of the endometrium and attach there. They will further differentiate and become the precursor to the placenta. The inner cell mass contains cells that are somewhat larger than the cytotrophoblasts. These cells are the basophilic embryonic cells, or *embryoblasts,* that develop into the embryo. At 72 hours of life, there are about 58 cells found within the blastocyst (Hertig et al., 1954). Most of these cells are trophoectodermal cells. Both the embryonic and the trophoectodermal cells continue to increase in number, however, the size of the blastocyst remains unchanged until after implantation. (See also Chapter 11.)

Migration of the Zygote to the Uterus

As cellular division and differentiation are occurring, the fertilized ovum begins its journey from the fallopian tube to the uterine cavity. It is propelled principally by the peristaltic movements of the tubal musculature, not by the cilia lining the tube. The journey of the zygote takes about 3 to 4 days. Once the uterus is reached, another 3 to 4 days pass before the zygote is ready to attach to the uterine lining.

This early preimplantation period is crucial to healthy embryonic and fetal development, for the young life is vulnerable to threats and stresses that can disrupt the rhythm of its processes. This early period of development occurs in secret, for the mother may not yet experience any clinical indicators of pregnancy.

IMPLANTATION

The process whereby the blastocyst attaches to the endometrium of the maternal uterus is known as *nidation,* more commonly referred to as *implantation.* It is believed to occur between the sixth to eighth day after fertilization. The mechanisms that allow implantation to take place are far from clear, although this phenomenon is widely studied. It is an invasive process in which a "foreign" substance attaches to the parent organ without an immunologic rejection and remains attached for a period of months. It is speculated that a fusion of maternal and fetal cells occurs temporarily, which results in a change in the immunologic characteristics in the maternal tissues that prohibits maternal sensitization to fetal antigens (Berhman & Koren, 1968).

Implantation is believed to occur as the result of three factors or episodes. (1) changes in the endometrium (now called the *decidua*) that are preparatory for implantation. The ovarian hormones, particularly progesterone, stimulate the endometrium during the luteal (secretory) phase of the menstrual cycle so that the cells enlarge, with considerable increase in cytoplasm; the glands become thickened and tortuous or twisted; there is generally increased vascularity and glycogen content is increased greatly (see Chapter 5). The endometrium is ready to receive the conceptus and to provide for its nourishment. (2) The blastocyst is readied to become attached to the endometrium through the action of trophoblastic cells that secrete proteolytic and cytolytic enzymes necessary to erode part of the endometrial vessels, glands, and even the stroma (basal layer) so that attachment is possible. (3) Penetration of the endometrium by the trophoblasts is now possible. At this point of invasion, there is a decidual reaction in which the stromal cells become enlarged and pale; some destruction of the endometrial cells occurs. It is believed that the trophoblastic cells take in some substances from the maternal blood, as well as cytoplasm, for purposes that remain unclear; it is suspected that nutrition for the embryo may be the principle reason.

Once the blastocyst settles into the endometrial bed, it is covered over by a layer of decidua *(decidua capsularis)* and rests upon the *decidua basalis.* When the blastocyst is attached to the uterus, the trophoblastic cells proliferate rapidly and the structures that will become the placenta have started to form.

Trophoblastic invasion that facilitates implantation is essentially localized in a single portion of the uterus, usually in the midanterior or midposterior aspect of the upper portion of the uterine cavity. Implantation can be summarized as occurring in three stages or steps:

- ▲ The blastocyst that has been floating free in the uterine cavity approaches and makes contact with the surface of the uterine endometrium. This contact is called *apposition* (Fig. 10.3).

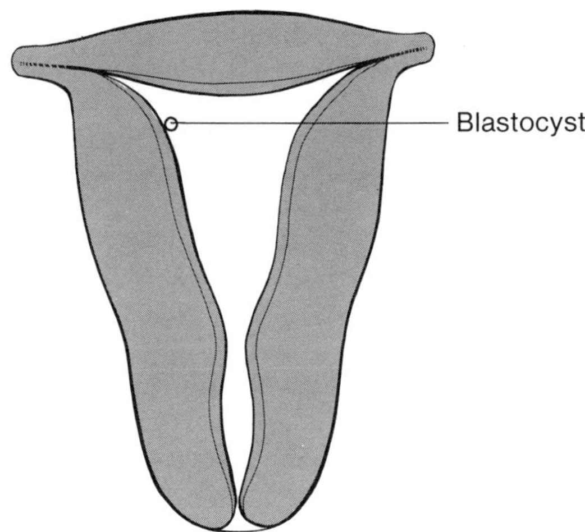

Figure 10.3
Implantation: apposition.

- ▲ Once the blastocyst has made contact with the endometrium, small rudimentary protrusions of trophoblastic cells, called *primary villi,* begin to erode minute areas of the endometrium and insert themselves into the maternal tissues where they adhere. This process of penetration by fetal cells and reception by maternal tissues is known as *adhesion* (Fig. 10.4).
- ▲ Adhesion provides the blastocysts with a base from which the trophoblastic cells proliferate and penetrate wider and deeper into maternal endometrium *(invasion)* (Fig. 10.5). The blastocyst becomes completely covered by endometrial tissue. Numerous microvilli can be found on the chorionic, outer surface of the blastocyst giving it the appearance of a shaggy, tiny ball.

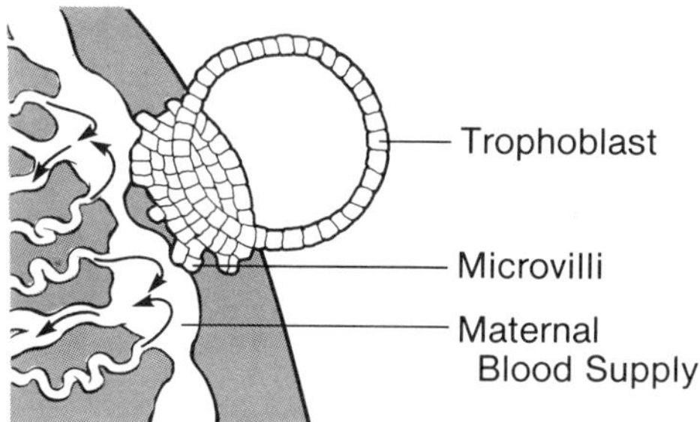

Figure 10.4
Implantation: adhesion.

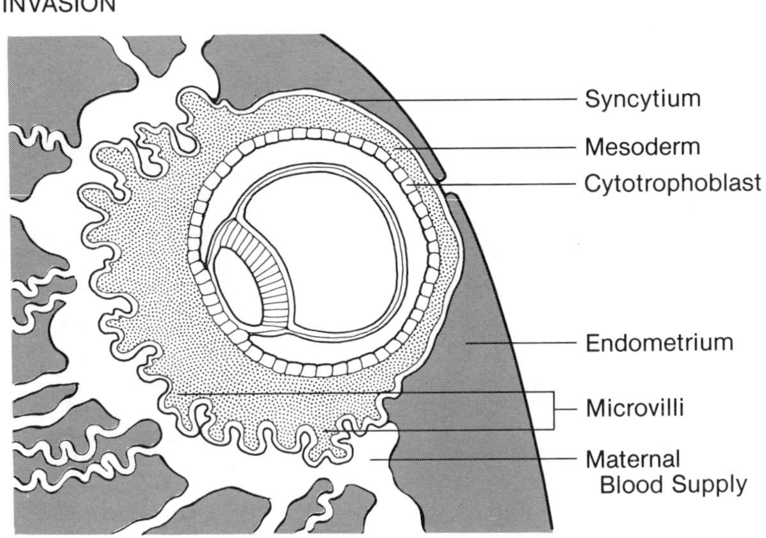

Figure 10.5
Implantation: invasion.

The blastocyst is now positioned so that the *placenta* (afterbirth), the biologic connection between the maternal and fetal systems, can develop. The endometrial lining of the uterus undergoes certain histologic changes associated with its invasion by the trophoblasts. These changes are called decidualization.

THE PLACENTA: DEVELOPMENT AND FUNCTION

The placenta is necessary for survival and subsequent growth and development of the new life. It develops through the union of maternal and embryonic structures and belongs exclusively to neither, but is an important part of both. The placenta serves the fetus; its purpose is physiologic exchange between the mother and fetus, and it has been called the life line of the unborn. The attachment of the blastocyst and the development of the placenta is known as *placentation.* Placentation, in humans, is an incompletely understood process with speculation mixed with fact.

Placental Origin and Development

The mature placenta (Fig. 10.6) is a discoid structure whose diameter is approximately 15–20 cm at term; it weighs 450–600 gm with an approximate average weight of 464 gm (slightly over 1 lb) (Pritchard & MacDonald, 1980). The fetal surface is covered by shiny opaque membranes. The umbilical cord arises from the center of the placenta, and placental vessels are visible beneath the membranous covering of the fetal surface. After separation from the uterine wall, usually following childbirth, the maternal surface, the part of the placenta that was attached to the uterus, resembles a piece of very vascular, red, raw meat. The *cotyledons,* or vascular sections of the placenta, can be readily identified as separate lobes. The flattened rounded appearance of the placenta accounts for its name, which is derived from the Latin and Greek words for flat cake or flat surface.

The placenta is composed of a number of vascular units (Fig. 10.7) with supporting structures that are located between two surfaces, the *basal plate,* the portion next to the uterine wall, and the *chorionic plate,* the upper portion that protrudes into the uterine cavity and is the part of the placenta closest to the fetus. These vascular units are separated by partial partitions, *septa,* that reach upward from the basal plate but do not quite touch the chorionic plate. The

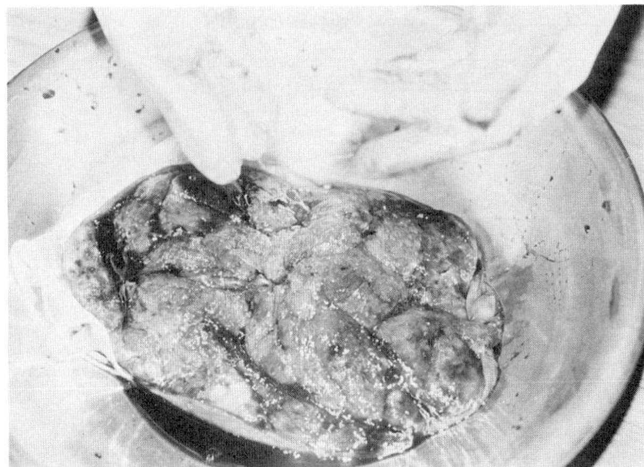

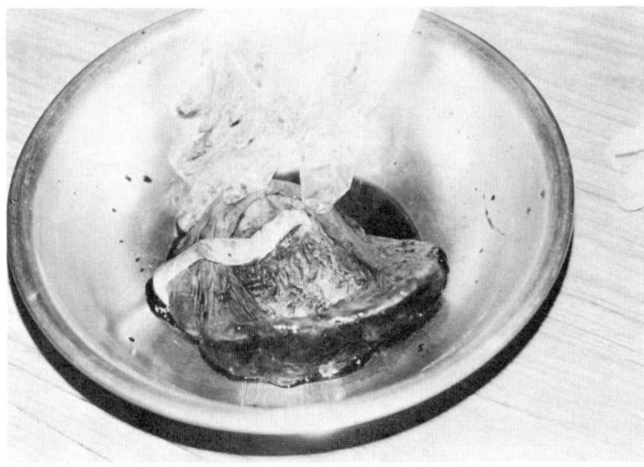

Figure 10.6
Term placenta showing *(top)* maternal side and *(bottom)* fetal side with umbilical cord insertion centrally located.

fetal surface contains a central projection, the *umbilical cord,* that connects the fetus to the placenta; it is covered by opaque membranes.

The placenta derives essentially from the trophoblastic cells that form the outer cell layer of the blastocyst. At the time of implantation, the pole of the blastocyst that contains the embryonic cells penetrates the uterine endometrium. The trophoblasts then undergo a rapid proliferation and are believed to account for three different layers of cells: (1) The *cytotrophoblasts,* or Langhan's cells, are round-shaped cells that are in contact with the *decidua basalis,* the part of the decidua that lies beneath the blastocyst. These cells are the attachment layer and will ultimately anchor the developing placenta to the uterus. (2) Beneath the cytotrophoblasts is a layer of mesynchymal cells called *mesoblasts.* These cells are mostly connective tissue and are probably the basis for the vascular units and the blood-forming elements of the placenta. The mesoblasts seem to remain separate from the trophoblasts above them because of a membrane between the two sets of cells (Hamilton & Boyd, 1970). (3) The third type of cells is the *syncytiotrophoblast* (syncytium), the outer layer of cells. The syncytial cells reflect the merging of a number of cells and appear as a marginless mass of protoplasm peppered with multiple nuclei. The exact function of the syncytiotrophoblasts is not completely known, although they are believed to play a role in embryonic nutrition through protein synthesis, glucose synthesis before the fetal liver functions, and tapping the maternal vessels and beginning the circulation between the mother and embryo. These outer cells appear as soft brush bristles and are called *microvilli.* The primary microvilli may perform a secretory function, as well as a trapping, engulfing function of substances that appear around them.

The microvilli that are in contact with the decidua basalis proliferate quickly, growing from the tips of the villi out and creating columns of trophoblastic cells. These cell columns form a stalk that anchors the developing placenta to the uterine wall. Continued invasion of the microvilli into the uterine muscle is stopped at this time because of the deposit of a band of fibrin caused by erosion of the degenerating maternal and fetal cells. After the anchoring of the microvilli to the decidua basalis, the trophoblastic cells tend to branch laterally with the villi floating freely, giving the structure the appearance of a tree with branches or a leafy fern, *chorion frondosum.* These expanded villi are now called *secondary villi.* The cell columns with their branches develop into one distinct vascular section of the placenta, called a *cotyledon.* The outer microvilli that touch the *decidua capsularis,* the endometrium that lies directly over the blastocyst, become the smooth chorion, *chorion laeve.* The chorion laeve atrophy as the fetal membranes are formed.

As the microvilli invade the decidua, open spaces are left between the fingerlike villus protrusions. Maternal blood and glandular secretions, released because of the eroding action of the trophoblasts, collect in these spaces. Such areas are known as *intervillous spaces.* The syncytial protoplasm also contains open spaces called *vacuoles.* The vacuoles merge to form larger spaces called *lacunae* that are filled with blood that has seeped from the maternal capillaries. The lacunae incorporate the intervillous spaces that are separated by the microvillus stalk and its

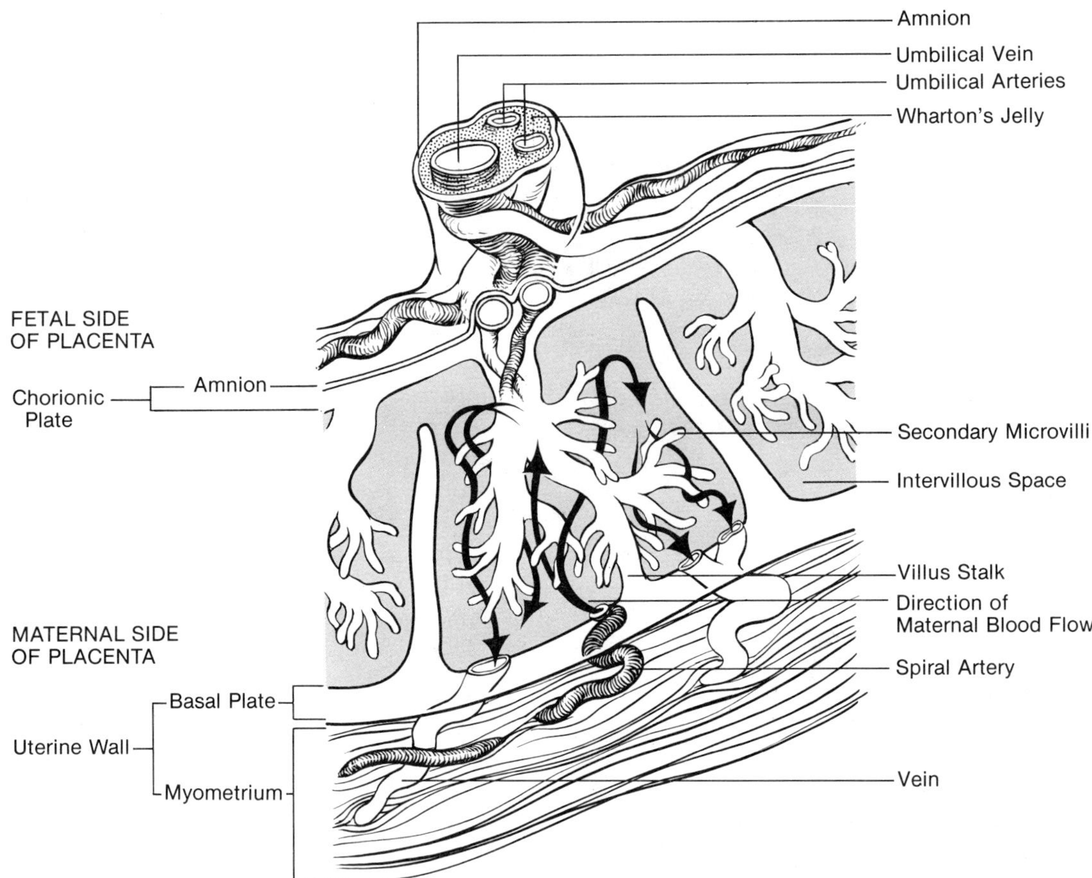

Figure 10.7
Placenta showing vascular unit and direction of circulation and umbilical vessels.

branches, creating areas that are in contact with the maternal spiral arteries and veins. These become the site of maternal–fetal vascular exchange.

Although the placenta is functional with primitive vascular exchange as early as the eighteenth to twenty-first day of embryonic life, it continues to develop and is capable of a low-pressure circulation by the fortieth to fiftieth day (Reynolds, 1966). The placenta continues to develop throughout pregnancy, first by cellular proliferation of the microvilli spreading out from the central core and later by cellular hypertrophy, increasing both the circumference and thickness of the placenta. As the microvilli develop, they contain capillaries and become a functional circulatory channel, now known as *tertiary villi.*

Placental Physiology

The principle function of the placenta is to carry essential substances to and from the fetus. The placenta performs as an endocrine organ as well in that it produces hormones needed for the maintenance of the pregnancy and the support of fetal well-being. The placenta also provides an immunologic service; however, its complete role in this area is not presently understood. To understand the functions of the placenta, it is necessary that the nurse know some basic facts about placental circulatory physiology.

Placental Circulation

Human placental circulatory physiology has puzzled scientists for many years. The characteristics of placental circulation were first confirmed by the research of Dr. Elizabeth Ramsey (Harris & Ramsey, 1966). Since that time, knowledge and research about placental physiology has increased significantly, although there is still much speculation about human placental function. Placental circulation is presently believed to rely upon four factors: maternal arterial blood pressure, uterine contraction patterns, pressure inside of the uterus, and specific action on the walls of the maternal arteries (Pritchard & MacDonald, 1980). Forces that significantly alter any one of these can interfere with placental circulation (see Chapters 16, 21–23).

Placental circulation (see Fig. 10.7) occurs through a series of steps that originates with the mother:

- ▲ Maternal arterial blood pressure forces blood through the spiral arteries into the intervillous spaces. Maternal blood enters these spaces in funnel-shaped spurts.
- ▲ Once the blood has entered the intervillous spaces, the force of the spurt is decreased.
- ▲ When the force of the maternal blood pressure is reduced, the blood is dispersed laterally and around the microvilli where metabolic exchange takes place, providing for the needs of the fetus. Oxygenated blood flows to the fetus through a single umbilical vein and returns to the placenta through two umbilical arteries. (See Chapter 11 for greater discussion on fetal circulation.)
- ▲ Normal maternal blood flow into the placenta is fairly constant, and this continuous influx of maternal blood forces the venous blood into the maternal endometrial veins.

The location and position of the maternal vessels in relation to the vascular units of the placenta are believed to have a significant influence on placental circulation. There is some evidence that maternal arteriolar destruction by the trophoblasts takes place during the early invasion period, which, in turn, decreases the availability of vessels to supply arterial blood to the intervillous spaces. Since this does not occur with the veins, it has been inferred that the trophoblasts may be seeking oxygen-rich blood (Page et al., 1976). Numerous maternal veins are found to open into the basal plate of the cotyledon.

Erratic contractions that occur during the last weeks of pregnancy, *Braxton–Hicks contractions,* are believed to facilitate placental perfusion (Reynolds, 1968). Sustained contractions without periods of rest, however, will significantly reduce placental perfusion (see Chapters 16 and 23).

Transfer of Substances

The placenta provides for circulatory exchange essentially through the maternal arteries and veins and the surface epithelium of the capillaries contained in the microvilli. These structures are in contact with the intervillous spaces of the placental cotyledons making them the principal site for vascular interchange between mother and fetus.

Transfer of substances from the mother to the fetus relies upon the factors mentioned earlier, especially maternal arterial blood pressure and uterine contractions. Maternal blood flow to the placenta is about 50 ml/min at 10-weeks gestation and increases to approximately 500 ml/min in a term gestation. Substances from the maternal blood supply found in the intervillous spaces enter the fetal circulatory system through the surface epithelium of the villi and go on into the capillary endothelium and the capillary canal. From there, the substances are moved to the fetus via the large umbilical artery.

Substances from the fetus going to the placenta depend upon the fetal circulatory system with the fetal heart as the driving force that returns these substances to the placenta through two umbilical arteries. Once the products from fetal metabolic and catabolic processes reach the intervillous spaces, they are picked up by the maternal veins in the basal plate of the placenta and returned to the mother's circulation.

Substances are able to be passed from mother to fetus because of three transfer mechanisms illustrated in Figure 10.8: *diffusion, active transport,* and *pinocytosis.* Occasionally substances will also be transported through breaks in the maternal or fetal tissues that result in leakage of maternal or fetal blood substances. This is an infrequent occurrence. Such leakage is believed to be possible because of the eroding, destructive action of the trophoblasts or defects in maternal or fetal tissues.

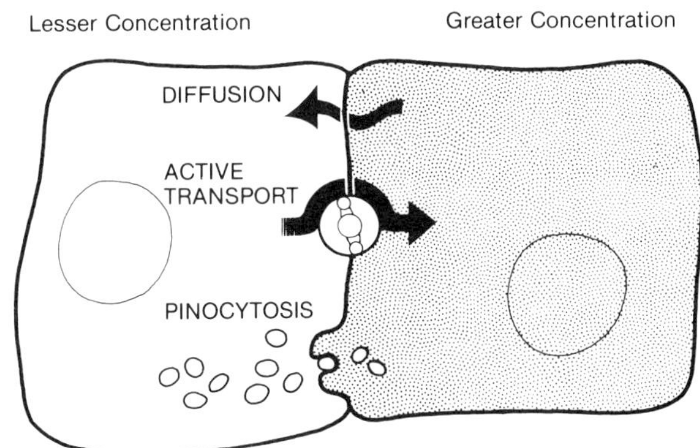

Figure 10.8
Transport mechanisms: diffusion, active transport, and pinocytosis.

DIFFUSION

Substances are transferred by both *simple* (passive) *diffusion,* the movement of a substance from an area of higher molecular concentration to an area of lower molecular concentration, and *facilitated diffusion,* the accelerated transport of substances of greater molecular weight through the assistance of a carrier that aids in transport. The trophoblasts are thought to furnish an aid that is specific to glucose transport. Oxygen, carbon dioxide, and substances of low molecular weight are believed to be transported most often by simple diffusion. Glucose is moved by facilitated diffusion.

ACTIVE TRANSPORT

Active transport is required in situations opposite to those in simple diffusion—the movement of a substance from an area of lower molecular concentration across a membrane to an area of higher molecular concentration. Active transport needs an energy source to expedite movement. It is the mechanism used to transport amino acids, water soluble vitamins, and other substances of high molecular weight such as calcium and iron.

PINOCYTOSIS

Pinocytosis is the mechanism used to transport substances that are quite large such as lipoproteins, phosolipids, and some drugs. These large substances are swallowed up, or engulfed, by the cellular spaces within the cytoplasm. They are then passed across the cell membrane and deposited in the fetal capillaries. Usually only small amounts of these substances are transported to the fetus by pinocytosis. Pinocytosis is not completely understood; it is believed to play a role in placental immunology rather than in fetal nutrition.

The mechanism needed to transfer substances from mother to fetus is frequently determined by the size, molecular weight, and biochemistry of the substance to be transported. However, the size and weight of a substance do not always correspond perfectly to the complexity of the mechanism used for transport. For example, all small substances do not pass through the cell membranes by simple diffusion, and all large substances do not require active transport. Enzymes are known to play a role in breaking large molecules into smaller parts, thereby facilitating their transport.

Placental Hormones

The placenta produces two types of hormones during pregnancy: the *steroid hormones,* estrogen and progesterone, and the *nonsteroid hormones,* human chorionic gonadotropin (HCG) and human chorionic somatomammotropin (HCS), also called human placental lactogen (HPL). They aid in maintaining the pregnancy and in supporting other events associated with pregnancy or fetal development and well-being.

HUMAN CHORIONIC GONADOTROPIN

HCG is produced by the trophoblasts. It has been found in maternal blood and urine early in pregnancy and in maternal plasma within 9–12 days after fertilization. The action of HCG during pregnancy is not definite, but it is believed to play a role in the following:

- ▲ Maintaining the corpus luteum, which in turn secretes estrogen and progesterone needed to sustain the pregnancy during the early period
- ▲ Stimulating the biogenesis of placental steroid hormones, estrogen and progesterone
- ▲ Promoting growth of the fetal adrenals
- ▲ Participating in suppression of maternal lymphocytes that may be antagonistic to fetal invasion

HCG is the hormone found in the blood and urine of pregnant women that makes early diagnosis of pregnancy possible (see Chapter 12). It is also clinically useful in diagnosing conditions such as hydatidiform mole (see Chapter 21) and choriocarcinoma (see Chapter 27).

HUMAN CHORIONIC SOMATOMAMMOTROPIN

HCS (referred to as HPL in earlier literature) appears in the mother's serum about the sixth week of fetal life. It is also secreted by the trophoblasts. HCS acts as an insulinogenic agent and causes maternal insulin levels to rise. It may also divert maternal glucose to the fetus (see Chapters 21 and 22).

ESTROGEN

Estrogen production during pregnancy is principally estriol. During pregnancy estriol increases about 1,000-fold over nonpregnant levels particularly during the latter half of pregnancy. Estradiol also increases, but in significantly smaller amounts. Estrogen production during pregnancy relies upon both maternal and fetal input. The role played by each is not clear at this time, but animal studies have suggested a relationship between maternal and fetal enzyme systems and estrogen biosynthesis. Estriol is one clinical index of normal placental function (see Chapters 20 and 21).

PROGESTERONE

Progesterone, like estrogen, is believed to be the result of maternal–fetal contributions. Progesterone appears significantly elevated in maternal plasma by about the fourth week of fetal life. Except for a brief drop in progesterone levels at about weeks 6 to 7, this hormone rises steadily throughout the pregnancy. Progesterone plays some role in controlling the length of gestation. That role and its function in association with the onset and clinical course of labor are not clearly explained by current research. *Pregnanediol* is the principal metabolite of progesterone.

Both estrogen and progesterone production during normal pregnancy are addressed in Chapter 12.

Placental Immunology

The function of the placenta as an immunologic barrier between mother and fetus has been the subject of much speculation and research. The placenta is an interesting organ for immunologic study since it raises at least two important questions. First, why does the body fail to reject the placenta, which is of fetal origins, as it does other homografts? One possible explanation is that the trophoblastic cells of the placenta create an anatomic and immunologic buffer zone that in some way neutralizes or offsets negative or destructive immunologic responses (Willson & Carrington, 1979). Second, why is the transport of certain substances past the placental barrier possible in spite of their large molecular weight? This question has been partly explained by research of transport mechanisms for moving substances to and from the fetus.

The placenta allows certain antibodies from the mother to pass to the fetus and thereby serves another immunologic function, selective fetal immunity during fetal and early neonatal life. It is known that the newborn acquires IgG antibodies from the mother across the placenta. However, other antibodies that convey immunity to the fetus, such as IgA and IgM, do not pass the placental barrier.

Fetal Membranes

The fetal membranes develop early in fetal life and consist of two loosely adherent but not fused layers —the *amnion* and the *chorion.* The amnion is the innermost layer that forms the sac around the growing fetus. It measures 0.02–0.5 mm in thickness. The outer layer, the chorion, initially is the shell of the blastocyst and the site from which the trophoblasts protrude at the time of implantation. The fetal membranes cover the surface of the fetal side of the placenta, and the amniotic sac distends with the growing fetus until it touches and adheres to the chorion. The chorion eventually lies in contact with the uterine wall. The membranes together resemble thin, but tough, whitish opaque tissues (Fig. 10.9). They can be easily separated. The fetal membranes contain no blood vessels.

The function of the membranes is not definite. They encase the developing fetus and the amniotic fluids that surround the fetus; they indirectly help protect the fetus from external trauma; along with the mucous plug in the cervix (see Chapter 12), they

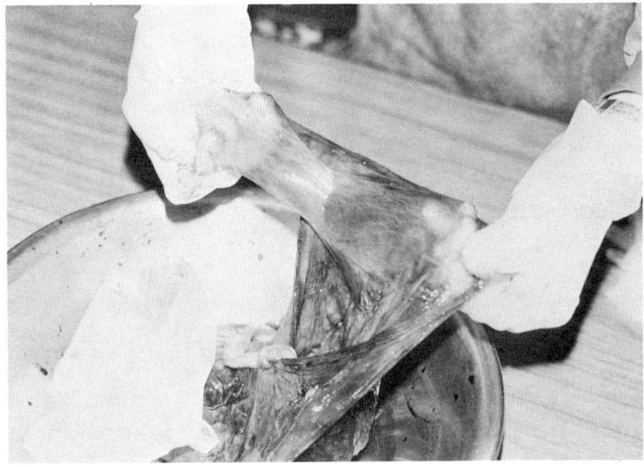

Figure 10.9
Term placenta with membranes showing amnion and chorion.

seal off the vaginal entrance to the uterus and do not allow organisms to go through the vagina or cervix into the uterus. The amnion is believed to play a role in the production of amniotic fluid, although this role is unclear. Phospholipids, containing arachidonic acid, necessary for the synthesis of prostaglandins, are found in the fetal membranes. Prostaglandins are believed to play a role in the initiation of labor (see Chapter 16).

The Umbilical Cord

The umbilical cord is a ropelike structure that connects the fetus and placenta. It contains one vein and two arteries that are encased in a gelatinous mucopolysaccharide substance, called *Wharton's jelly*, and is covered with amnion. The vessels are tortuous in appearance and can be visualized through the glistening, moist membrane that covers them. The umbilical cord is approximately 55 cm long (about 20 in) and about 1.0–2.5 cm wide. Its length can vary greatly, with reported lengths ranging from 30 to 100 cm (Pritchard & MacDonald, 1980). The umbilical cord is the fetal physiologic connection to the mother and, as such, is the only route for transport of oxygen, nutrients, and other substances to the fetus and for elimination of fetal waste products.

The umbilical cord usually comes from the center of the placental fetal surface and is derived from a merger of the body stalk, the *allantois,* a tubular structure off the hind gut of the embryo, the umbilical vessels, and the yolk sac.

The length of the cord permits the fetus to move freely in the fluid medium of the amniotic sac, and consequently fetal position will change frequently during the first 6 months of pregnancy. Occasionally, the umbilical cord will have knots tied in it, most likely from fetal movement. These knots do not pose a problem for the fetus unless they are pulled tight and fetal circulation is interrupted.

Amniotic Fluid

Amniotic fluid is normally a clear fluid with particles of solid matter dispersed throughout. It surrounds the fetus from about the second week of fetal life until birth. The volume of amniotic fluid increases progressively from about 50 ml at 10 weeks, to 200 ml at 16 weeks, to 350 ml at 20 weeks, to as much as 1,000 ml at 38 weeks. It tends to decrease slightly just before term gestation (40 weeks) and to decrease significantly after 42-weeks gestation.

Amniotic fluid is composed of about 98% water and 2% solids and contains a variety of substances, including squamous and fat cells from the fetus; byproducts of fetal metabolism, particularly fetal urine, uric acid, urea, and creatinine; electrolytes, protein, enzymes, respiratory secretions; fetal hair, with particles of *lanugo,* the fine hair that covers the fetal body during the months of pregnancy; and bits of *vernix caseosa,* a creamy white substance that covers the fetus in utero.

The origin of amniotic fluid is unclear, although it has been theorized that the fluid either is secreted by the cells of the amnion or is a transudate from the maternal blood. Its presence and composition during very early fetal life gives some credence to both of these ideas. Fetal urine and the fetal respiratory gastrointestinal tracts have also been cited as sources of amniotic fluid. Since the composition of amniotic fluid changes as the pregnancy progresses, amniotic fluid most likely arises from several sources with different sites having greater importance at various stages of fetal life. Amniotic fluid is produced continuously throughout pregnancy; the water component of the fluid can be completely exchanged in 3 hours and the sodium component can be exchanged in about 15 hours (Vosburgh, 1948).

Amniotic fluid cushions the fetus from any external force by equalizing the intrauterine and extrauterine pressures. It maintains a stable thermal environment for the fetus that corresponds with maternal body temperature, and may play a role in helping cervical change during labor (see Chapter 16).

NURSING IMPLICATIONS

Much of health care supervision during pregnancy relies on as accurate a determination of the date of fertilization as is possible. The time of fertilization is inferred from data about the woman's last menstrual period and time of sexual intercourse.

It is important that the nurse solicit the following information on the woman's menstrual cycle:

- ▲ Age that menstruation began
- ▲ Characteristics of a usual menstrual cycle such as length of bleeding, interval between periods,

amount, color, and consistency of the menstrual flow, and type of discomfort, if any, during or preceding the period

Once the nurse has gathered this information, the patient should be questioned about her *last* menstrual period, particularly regarding the length of that period, the amount, color, and consistency of the menstrual blood, and any unusual happenings. Comparison of this menstrual period with the woman's usual ones enables the nurse to judge whether or not the last bleeding was a normal period or a physiologic response to pregnancy. Once the date of the *first day* of the last normal menstrual period is reasonably confirmed, the approximate date for the onset of labor can be determined through the use of a simple formula (see Chapter 11). Failure to establish accurate dates for the last menstrual period can result in miscalculation of a patient's expected date of confinement (EDC), sometimes referred to as estimated date of labor (EDL) or estimated date of delivery (EDD) with an error of 1 month earlier or later than the baby will be due to arrive. Such an error provides an inaccurate baseline from which prenatal supervision can be planned and fetal growth and development assessed (see Chapters 11 and 12). Women usually have accurate recall concerning their menstrual cycle. However, occasionally a woman will need help from the nurse to recall details about her period. One way in which the nurse may help her is through the use of association such as having her remember other events that occurred concurrently with her period—special activities, guests, unusual circumstances.

Comprehension of gamete transport enables the nurse to respond to patient questions about the relationship between sexual intercourse and fertilization. It also provides the nurse with a basis for understanding problems associated with infertility.

The preimplantation period and the period of nidation are both times of increased vulnerability for the developing conceptus. The nurse must be aware of the need to obtain an accurate history from the woman concerning illnesses occurring during this period, particularly viral infections that can have a teratogenic effect on the development of the fetus. Information about use of drugs, including alcohol, is important as well.

Knowledge about placental development can help the nurse understand the basis for some of the changes that occur in the woman during pregnancy, as well as to help the nurse comprehend the nature of fetal development and survival during interuterine life.

The placenta functions efficiently during a normal pregnancy and is more or less taken for granted. Variations in fetal growth as determined by measuring externally the changes in the size of the maternal abdomen and changes in fetal heart rate (FHR) and maternal blood pressure can alert the care giver to attend to placental function. Factors such as maternal hypertension that decrease the transport of nutrients and oxygen from the mother to fetus can affect fetal growth and well-being. Disruptions in fetal well-being may be clinically evident through changes in placental function, which can be measured through biochemical studies of the placental hormones and enzymes.

The amniotic fluid can provide much information about fetal well-being and maturity through genetic studies, fetal lung maturity studies, fetal metabolism, and other tests. (Studies of the placenta and amniotic fluid are discussed in Chapter 20.) The nurse must understand placental development and function in order to interpret the information obtained through such laboratory analyses to the patient and to other nursing or associated personnel. The nurse also uses such information to make judgments about patient care.

The umbilical cord is a soft structure and, therefore, can be compressed. Pressure that is sufficient to compress the umbilical cord will interfere with fetal circulation. Position of the fetus inside the uterus can cause cord compression. For example, the umbilical cord can become looped around the fetus, especially the neck (nuchal cord) or can become pinned between the fetus and the maternal pelvis, especially in conjunction with premature rupture of the fetal membranes (PROM). The nurse will be aware of cord compression through variations in the normal FHR. Often cord compression can be relieved by having the mother change her position. Abnormalities in the umbilical cord may first be apparent through the characteristics of the FHR. The nurse is often the first person to auscultate the fetal heart. Knowledge about the significance of changes in the FHR is crucial.

The amniotic sac will occasionally rupture before the onset of labor, and there will be leakage of amniotic fluid. Rupture of the sac can open the pathway for infection to the fetus or promote premature labor. If the nurse recognizes the characteristics of the amniotic fluid and knows the significance of early rupture of the fetal membranes, then appropriate action can be taken (see Chapters 12 and 22).

SUMMARY

Knowledge about fertilization, implantation, and development and function of the placenta, accessory structures, and amniotic fluid is important to the maternity nurse for a number of reasons. Accurate reporting and recording of data about the last menstrual period and its characteristics can help to establish a sound basis for understanding and predicting events that occur during pregnancy. The placenta serves not only as a necessary mechanism for fetal survival, but it furnishes the ingredients for diagnostic tests and laboratory evaluation of fetal well-being. The amniotic fluid is the medium from which crucial information concerning fetal maturity and fetal well-being can be obtained.

This chapter provided an overview of the most basic information about fertilization, implantation, and development of the placenta and accessory structures and amniotic fluid to enable the nurse to understand their significance and make proper use of the information. Special attention was given to the development of the placenta as the organ that unites the maternal and fetal units and as the link to the mother that provides for fetal survival, growth, and well-being.

REFERENCES AND READINGS

Berhman, S. J., Koren, Z. Immunology of the Conceptus, in Greenhill, J. P. (Ed.), *Yearbook of Obstetrics and Gynecology. 1967–68.* Chicago: Yearbook Publishers, 1968.

Boyd, J. D., Hamilton, W. J. *The Human Placenta.* Cambridge, England: W. Heffer and Sons, 1970.

DeWolf, F. et al. The Human Placental Bed: Electron Microscopic Study of Trophoblastic Invasion of Spiral Arteries. *Am J Obstet Gynecol* 137(1):58, 1980.

Hamilton, W. J., Boyd, J. D. Development of the Human Placenta, in Philipp, E. E. et al. (Eds.). *Scientific Foundations of Obstetrics and Gynecology.* Philadelphia: F. A. Davis, 1970, Chap. 8, p. 185.

Harris, J. W. S., Ramsey, E. M. The Morphology of Human Uteroplacental Vasculature. *Contrib Embryol* 38:43, 1966.

Henderson-Smart, D. J., Read, D. J. C. Fetal Cardio-Respiratory Physiology, in Shearman, R. P. (Ed.), *Human Reproductive Physiology.* London: Blackwell Scientific Publications, 1979.

Hertig, A. T., Rock, J., Adams, E. C., Mulligan, W. J. On the Preimplantation Stages of the Human Ovum. *Contrib Embryo* 35:199, 1954.

Marrs, R. P., Mishell, D. R. Placental Trophic Hormones. *Clin Obstet Gynecol* 23(3):721, 1980.

Martin, C. B., Jr., Gingervich, B. Utero-Placental Physiology. *J Obstet Gynecol Neonatal Nurs* 5(5):1655 (Sept/Oct suppl), 1976.

Ockleford, C. D., Wakely, J., Badley, R. A. Morphogenesis of Human Placental Chorionic Villi: Cytoskeletal, Syncytioskeletal and Extracellular Matrix Proteins. *Proc Roy Soc Lond* b212(1186):305, 1981.

Page, E. W. Villee, C. A., Villee, D. D. *Human Reproduction: The Core Content of Obstetric, Gynecologic and Perinatal Medicine* (2nd ed.). Philadelphia: W. B. Saunders, 1976.

Pritchard, J. A., MacDonald, P. C. *William's Obstetrics* (16th ed.). New York: Appleton-Century-Crofts, 1980.

Ramsey, E. M. The Story of the Spiral Arteries. *J. Reprod Med* 26(8):393, 1981.

Reynolds, S. R. M. Formation of Fetal Cotyledons in the Hemochorial Placenta. A Theoretical Construct of the Functional Implications of Such an Arrangement. *Am J Obstet Gynecol* 94:425, 1966.

Reynolds, S. R. M. et al. Multiple Simultaneous Intervillous Space Pressures Recorded in Several Regions of the Hemochorial Placenta in Relation to Functional Anatomy of the Fetal Cotyledon. *Am J Obstet Gynecol* 102:1128, 1968.

Rhodes, P. *Reproductive Physiology for Medical Students.* London: J. A. Churchill, 1969.

Simpson, E. R., MacDonald P. C. Endocrine Physiology of the Placenta. *Ann Rev Physiol* 43:163, 1981.

Vosburgh, G. J. et al. The Rate of Renewal in Women of the Water and Sodium of the Amniotic Fluid as Determined by Tracer Techniques. *Am J Obstet Gynecol* 56:1156, 1948.

Willson, R., and Carrington, E. *Obstetrics and Gynecology* (6th ed.). St. Louis: C. V. Mosby, 1979.

Wynn, R. M. Principles of Placentation and Early Human Placental Development, in Gruenwald, P. (Ed.), *The Placenta and its Maternal Supply Line—Effects of Insufficiency on the Fetus.* Baltimore: University Park Press, 1975.

11

PREGNANCY: FETAL PERSPECTIVE

Judith A. Harris

Since World War II, and particularly in the last two decades, knowledge of the fetus and its environment has increased markedly. It has been proven that while in its mother's womb, the baby is not passive, immobile, or unresponsive. The fetus maintains a relatively consistent pattern of waking, sleeping, listening, exercising muscles, and discovering and perfecting functional abilities much as it will do as a newborn. As an important consequence, whether being confined by the uterine environment or adapting to the demands of the birth process, the unborn baby is as much the nurse's patient as is the mother. Therefore, a knowledge of the development and physiology of the embryo and fetus is essential to nursing practice.

Human development during uterine life is viewed as taking place in three successive phases, the pre-embryonic, embryonic, and fetal stages. This chapter will address these three phases in the development of the normal fetus. Anomalies and diseases that affect the fetus and neonate are discussed in Chapters 23 and 24.

ESTIMATION OF GESTATIONAL AGE

The gestational period is commonly measured as 10 lunar months of 4 weeks each, 40 weeks, or 9 calendar months, 3 trimesters of 3 months each. In this chapter, age in weeks refers to the time since fertilization. In clinical practice, however, the term *gestational age* refers to the time since the first day of the last menstrual period. The nurse needs to know the reference point used in order to collect and record accurate data and to help the parents understand their baby's development.

Reasonable estimates of the age of embryos can be determined by the following:

- ▲ Day of onset of the last normal menstrual period
- ▲ Estimated time of fertilization
- ▲ Measurements of the length of the embryo
- ▲ Embryonic external characteristics

Establishing the date at which pregnancy began may be difficult because it depends in part on the mother's memory. Two reference points commonly used for estimating embryonic age are the date of the onset of the mother's last menstrual period (LMP) and the time of fertilization. The probability of error in establishing the last regular menstrual period is highest in women who have become pregnant after discontinuing use of oral contraceptives. This is because the interval between stopping the hormones and ovulation is highly variable. Light vaginal bleeding or "spotting" sometimes occurs after implantation of the blastocyst and may be mistaken for menstruation. Despite the probability of error, LMP is still the most commonly used index for estimating the age of embryos. Because the zygote does not form for approximately 2 weeks after the onset of the last regular menstrual period, 12–14 days must be deducted from the menstrual age to obtain the actual or *fertilization age* of the embryo. The precise time of fertilization is speculative at best.

The ages of embryos recovered after abortion have been determined by examination of external characteristics and measurements of length. The shape of 3- to 4-week-old embryos is nearly straight, which allows for measurements to indicate the *greatest length* (GL) (Fig. 11.1). The sitting height or *crown–rump* length (CR) is most frequently used to measure 5- to 6-week old embryos, while standing height or *crown–heel length* (CH) is used for 7-week and older embryos.

Several formulas have been developed to calculate the estimated date of confinement (EDC). None of them are totally accurate, but used in combination, a fairly close estimation of the anticipated delivery date can be obtained.

- ▲ ***Naegele's Rule.*** Add 7 days to the first day of the LMP, subtract 3 months, and add 1 year.
  - EDC = LMP + 7 days − 3 months + 1 year.
  - An example of this would be if the first day of the LMP were April 2, 1982, the EDC would be January 9, 1983. Naegele's rule assumes a 28-day menstrual cycle with fertilization occurring on the fourteenth day. Therefore, adjustments must be made for cycles longer or shorter than 28 days.
- ▲ ***Fundal Height.*** A gross estimate of the length of pregnancy can be determined during the first 2 trimesters by the measurement of fundal height on the anterior abdominal wall. At 8–10 weeks, the fundus can be palpated slightly above the symphysis pubis. By 16 weeks, the fundus should be halfway between the symphysis and the umbilicus and by 20–22 weeks it should be at the umbilicus.
- ▲ ***McDonald's Maneuvers.*** During the second and third trimesters, use of McDonald's maneuvers adds greater accuracy to the measurement of fundal height in determining gestational age (Fig. 11.2). Using a flexible (nonstretch) tape, measure the height of the fundus from the notch of the symphysis pubis over the top of the fun-

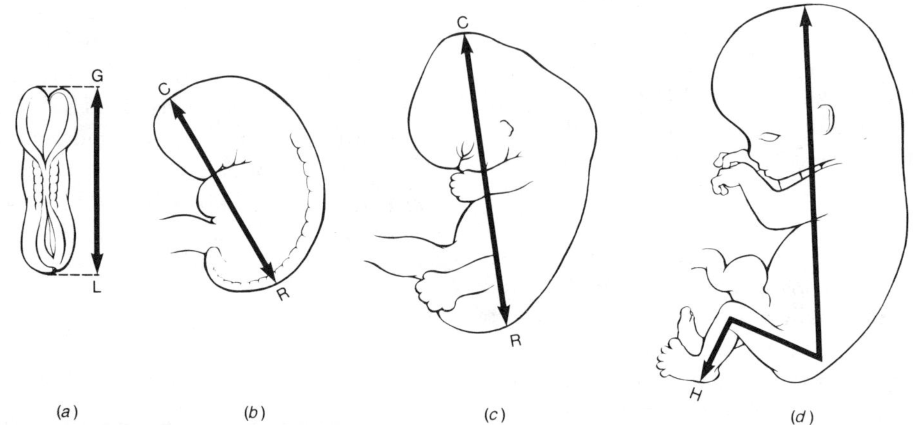

Figure 11.1
Methods of measuring the length of embryos: *(a)* greatest length (GL); *(b* and *c)* crown-rump length (CR); *(d)* crown-heel length (CH).

dus without tipping the corpus back. Calculate as follows:

- Height of fundus (in centimeters) × 2/7 (or ÷ 3.5) = duration of pregnancy in lunar months.
- Height of fundus (in centimeters) × 8/7 = duration of pregnancy in weeks.

The use of this method may help in the identification of high-risk factors such as intrauterine growth retardation, multiple fetuses, and polyhydramnios.

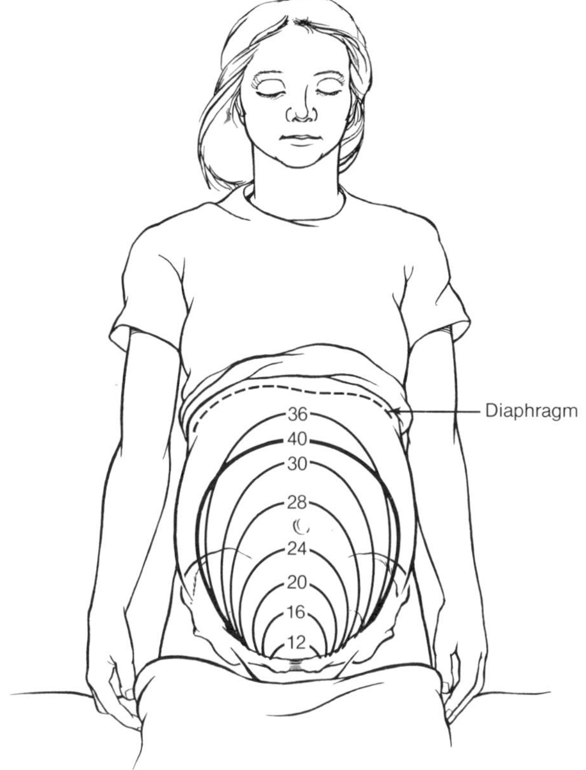

Figure 11.2
Measurement of fundal height using McDonald's maneuvers.

PRE-EMBRYONIC STAGE

The first 14 days of human development are referred to as the *stage of the ovum* or the *pre-embryonic stage.* This period is characterized by extremely rapid growth, differentiation of tissue into essential organs, and development of main external features.

First Week

Fertilization initiates human development by stimulating the *zygote*—the cell that results from fertilization of an ovum by a sperm and is the beginning of a human being—to undergo a series of rapid mitotic cell divisions known as *cleavage.* As the zygote passes down the fallopian tube, it divides into two daughter cells called *blastomeres.* Subsequent divisions follow rapidly, forming progressively smaller blastomeres, until at about 3 days after fertilization a solid ball of 16 or more blastomeres called a *morula* enters the uterus. By the fourth day fluid from the uterine cavity passes into the morula and occupies the intercellular spaces. As the fluid increases, it separates the cells into two parts: (1) an outer cell mass, the *trophoblast,* and (2) a group of centrally located cells known as the inner cell mass, or *embryoblast.* The morula then becomes the *blastocyst*—a hollow sphere of cells enclosing a cavity that is formed when fluid from the uterus enters the morula—and the trophoblastic cells begin to invade the endometrial epithelium. As invasion continues, the trophoblast differentiates into three layers, two of which are of particular importance to embryonic development: (1) the *cytotrophoblast,* an inner germinative cell layer, and (2) the *syncytiotrophoblast,* an outer syncytial layer. The outer cell layer of the invading trophoblast is the beginning of the primitive placenta (see Chapter 10).

While the blastocyst is implanting, early differentiation of the embryoblast occurs. A flattened layer of cells, the *embryonic endoderm,* begins to form on the ventral surface of the inner cell mass. This endodermal layer is the first of three primary germ layers of the embryo that form during the first 3 weeks. All body organs and tissues will come from these three primary germ layers (see Table 11.1). Figure 11.3 illustrates human development during the first week.

Second Week

After about 8 or 9 days, the yolk sac forms as a cavity in the blastocyst. Although the yolk sac has only limited function as a source of nourishment in the human embryo and has virtually disappeared by

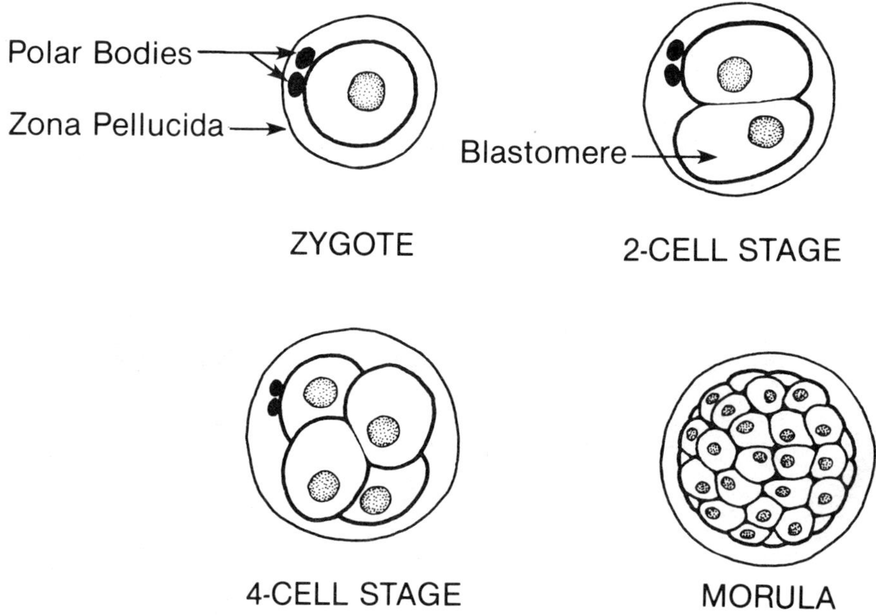

Figure 11.3
First week. Drawings illustrating human development from zygote to morula.

the ninth week after fertilization, its development is essential for the following reasons.

▲ Transfer of nutrients to the embryo occurs during second and third weeks while the uteroplacental circulation is being developed.

▲ Primitive red blood cells begin to form on the walls of the yolk sac during the third week and continue to form until hematopoiesis begins in the liver during the sixth week.

▲ The primitive gut is formed during the fourth week as the dorsal part of the yolk sac is incorporated into the embryo as an endodermal tube. This gives rise to the epithelium of the trachea, bronchi, lungs, and digestive tract.

▲ Primitive reproductive cells appear in the wall of the yolk sac during the third week. In the sixth week, these primitive reproductive cells migrate to the developing gonads where they will differentiate into either spermatogonia or oogonia.

As implantation continues, morphological changes occur in the inner cell mass that result in the formation of the flattened, nearly circular bilaminar *embryonic disk,* composed of embryonic endoderm and *embryonic ectoderm.* The *prochordal plate* develops as a localized thickening of embryonic endoderm and establishes the future cranial region of the embryo and the site of the mouth. Figure 11.4 illustrates human development during the second week.

EMBRYONIC STAGE

The *stage of the embryo* begins with the third week and continues until the end of the seventh week.

Third Week

By the sixteenth day, the third primary germ layer, the *embryonic mesoderm,* begins to appear between the endoderm and ectoderm, converting the bilaminar embryonic disk into a trilaminar embryo.

Early in the third week, the ectodermal cells become taller and thicker, forming the *neural plate* from which the infant's nervous system will develop. The *neural tube* and *neural crest* evolve from the neural plate: the broad cephalic (head) end of the neural tube will become the brain; the narrower caudal (tail) end will become the spinal cord. The neural

TABLE 11.1
DERIVATION OF ORGANS AND TISSUES FROM PRIMARY GERM LAYERS

Endoderm	*Mesoderm*	*Ectoderm*
Epithelium of tympanic membrane and auditory canal	Dermis	Epidermis, including sweat and sebaceous glands, hair, and nails
Alimentary glands, including liver and pancreas	Vascular system—blood, bone marrow, and lymphatic vessels	Central and peripheral nervous systems
Epithelium of respiratory tract	Urogenital system—kidneys, ureters, gonads, and genital ducts	Neuroepithelium of sense organs, including optic lens
Urinary bladder, urethra, prostate and vagina	Body muscles	Epithelium of nasopharynx and mouth
Epithelium of pharynx (excluding nasal), tongue, tonsils, thyroid, thymus, and parathyroid	Connective tissue	Tooth enamel and oral glands
Epithelium of digestive tract	Skeletal tissue	Epithelium of anal canal
	Peritoneum, pleura, and pericardium	
	Teeth (except enamel)	

crest becomes the peripheral nervous system, consisting of cranial, spinal, and autonomic ganglia and nerves. The brain consists of forebrain, midbrain, and hindbrain. The cerebrum develops from the forebrain; the pons, the cerebellum, and the medulla oblongata develop from the hindbrain.

During the third week, another tubelike structure that communicates with the yolk sac arises from the endoderm. This tube will later become the gastrointestinal tract. Concurrently, the *allantois* (Greek, "sausage"), a small fingerlike outpouching of the caudal wall of the yolk sac appears. Although the allantois in the human embryo is very small, it is involved in early blood and blood vessel formation and is associated with development of the urinary bladder.

The cardiovascular system is the first to function in the developing embryo. *Angiogenesis,* or blood vessel formation, begins in the mesoderm of the yolk sac at about 17 or 18 days. Paired endothelial channels, called heart tubes, develop before the end of the third week and begin to fuse into a single primitive heart tube. By the twenty-first day, the primitive heart tube has linked up with blood vessels in the embryo to form the early cardiovascular system, and the circulation of blood has begun. Figure 11.5 illustrates growth of the embryo during the third week.

Fourth Week

The significant event in the fourth week is the folding of the trilaminar embryonic disk into the cylindrical embryo, thus establishing general body form. Rapid growth of the embryo, especially of the neural tube, causes folding in both longitudinal and transverse planes. Surface elevations called *somites* form on either side of the midline of the embryo in a cephalocaudal direction. Somites are the mesodermal precursors of muscles and vertebrae. A slight curve in the embryo is produced by the head and tail folds, and the heart appears as a large ventral prominence. Continued longitudinal and transverse folding throughout the fourth week gives the embryo its characteristic C-shaped curve. By the twenty-eighth day, arm and leg buds become recognizable as small swellings on the lateral body. The primordia of the ear and eye are also present and visible. The special sense organs, especially the eyes, are now very susceptible to teratogenic agents such as viral infections. The most serious sensory organ defects result from developmental disturbances during the fourth to sixth weeks, but sight and hearing defects may also be caused by certain microorganisms during the fetal period.

The *primitive gut* (foregut, midgut, and hindgut) forms during the fourth week. The endoderm of the

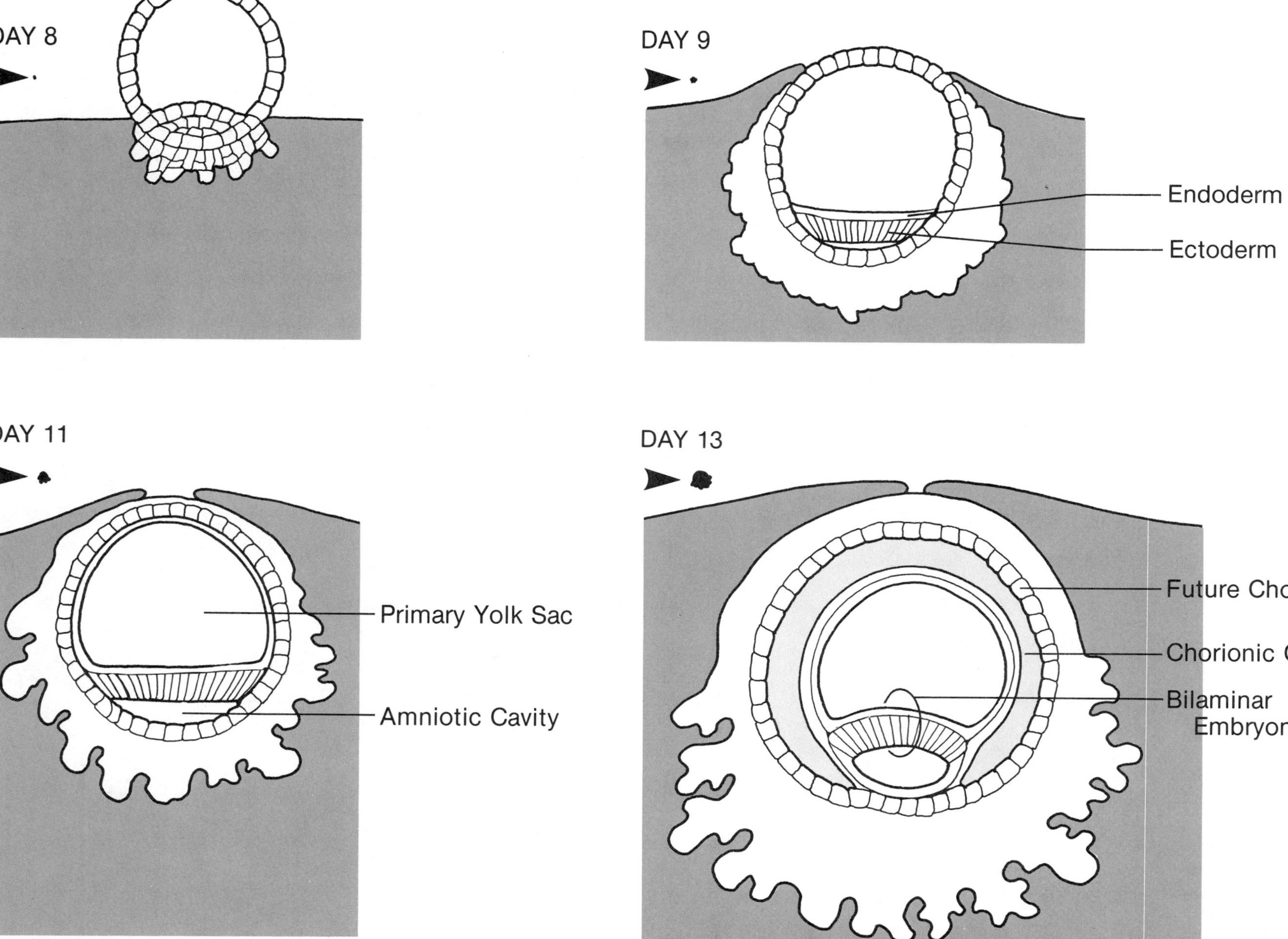

Figure 11.4
Second week. Drawings of sections of human blastocysts during the second week of development; the arrows point to sketches showing the actual sizes of the blastocysts.

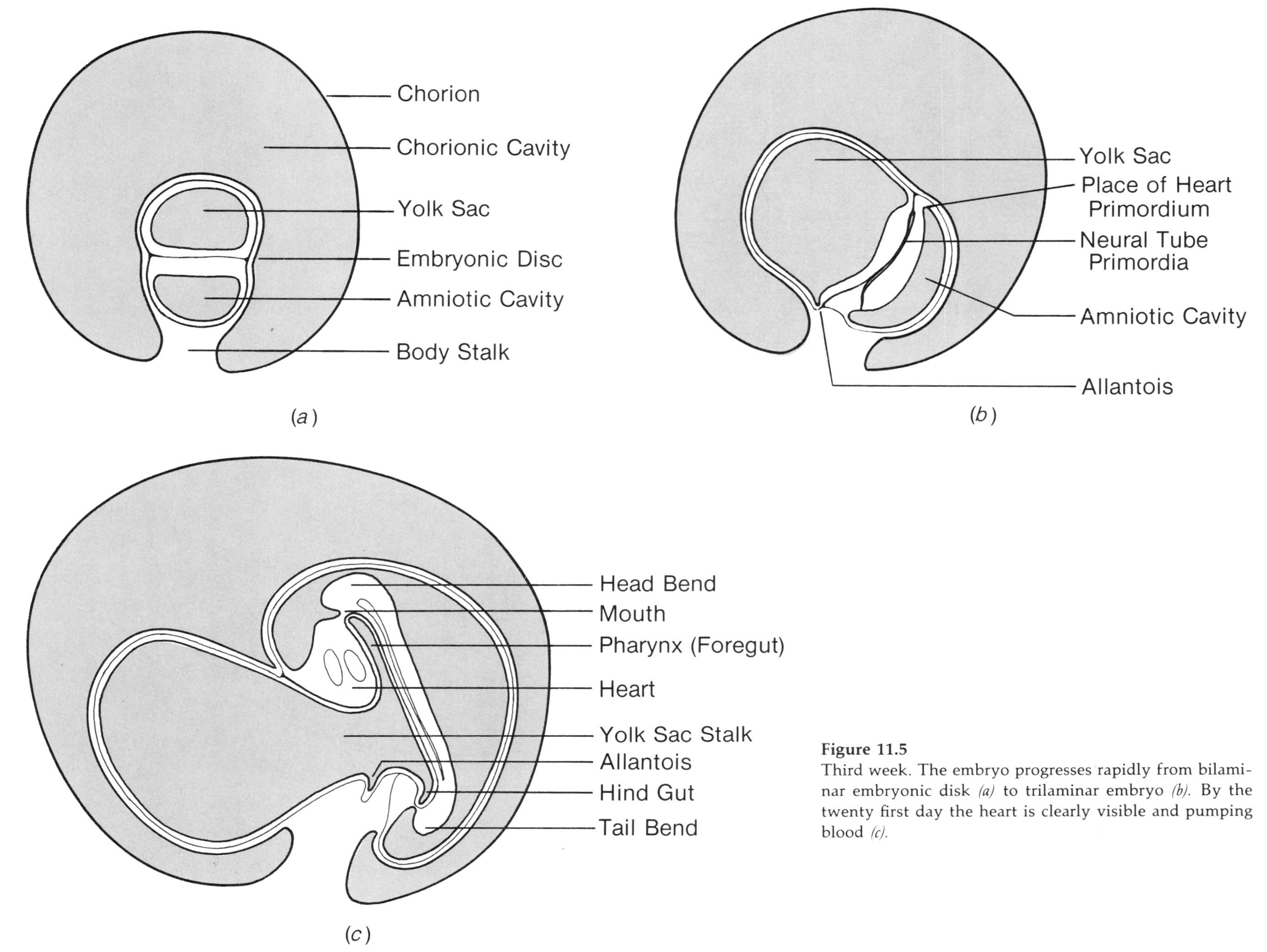

Figure 11.5
Third week. The embryo progresses rapidly from bilaminar embryonic disk *(a)* to trilaminar embryo *(b)*. By the twenty first day the heart is clearly visible and pumping blood *(c)*.

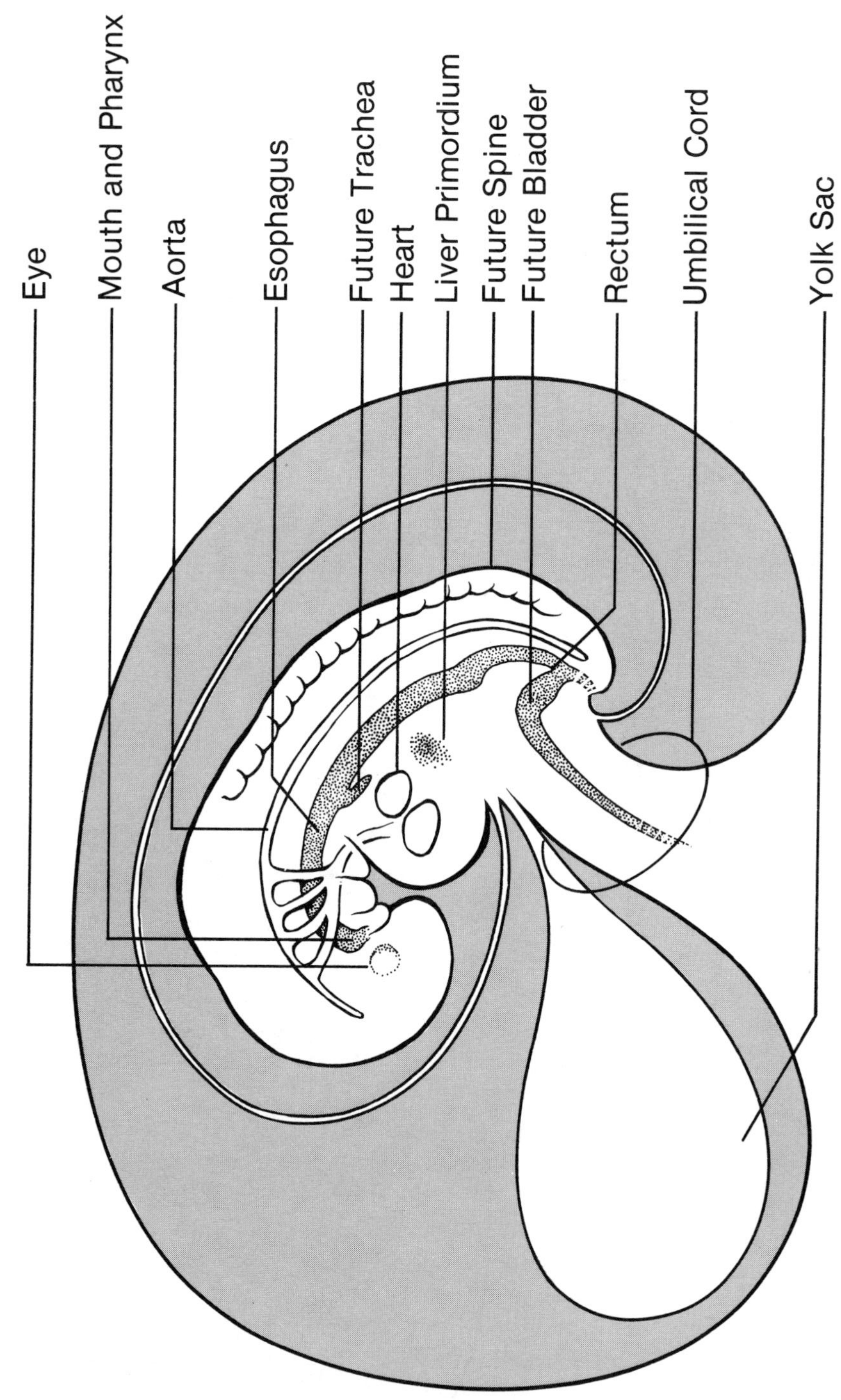

Figure 11.6
Fourth week. Drawing of a lateral view of a 4-week-old embryo.

primitive gut gives rise to the epithelial cells that line the greater part of the digestive tract and biliary tree, as well as the parenchyma of the liver and pancreas.

The *foregut* gives rise to the pharynx and lower respiratory tract, the stomach, the duodenum as far as the common bile duct, the liver, the pancreas, and the biliary tree. The esophagus and trachea have a common origin in the foregut; therefore, incomplete partitioning of the septum between them may result in a tracheoesophageal fistula.

The duodenum, distal to the common bile duct, the jejunum, ileum, cecum, ascending colon, and right half of the transverse colon arise from the *midgut.*

The *hindgut* gives rise to the left half of the transverse colon, the descending and sigmoid colon, and the rectum and upper part of the anal canal. Crown–rump length is 4.0 mm; weight is 400 mg. Figure 11.6 shows a 4-week-old embryo.

Fifth Week

Changes in body form during the fifth week are minor compared to those of the fourth week, but growth of the head exceeds that of other regions. This extensive head growth is the result of rapid growth of the brain, which has now differentiated into five areas in which 10 pairs of cranial nerves are recognizable. Partitioning of the heart begins with the dividing of the atria. The elbow and wrist regions become identifiable and the paddle-shaped hand plates develop digital ridges, which will later become fingers. Nasal pits develop; optic cups and lens vesicles of the eye form and retinal pigment begins to appear, causing the eyes to become more obvious. At this time, the embryo has a marked C-shaped body, accentuated by a rudimentary tail and large head folded over the prominent heart. CR length 8.0 mm; weight 800 mg. Figure 11.7 shows a 5-week-old embryo.

Sixth Week

During the sixth week the head is much larger relative to the trunk; it is bent further over the heart prominence while the trunk is straighter than in earlier stages. The upper and lower jaws are recognizable, and the external nares are well formed. The limbs undergo considerable change during this period. The arms have lengthened and flexed so that

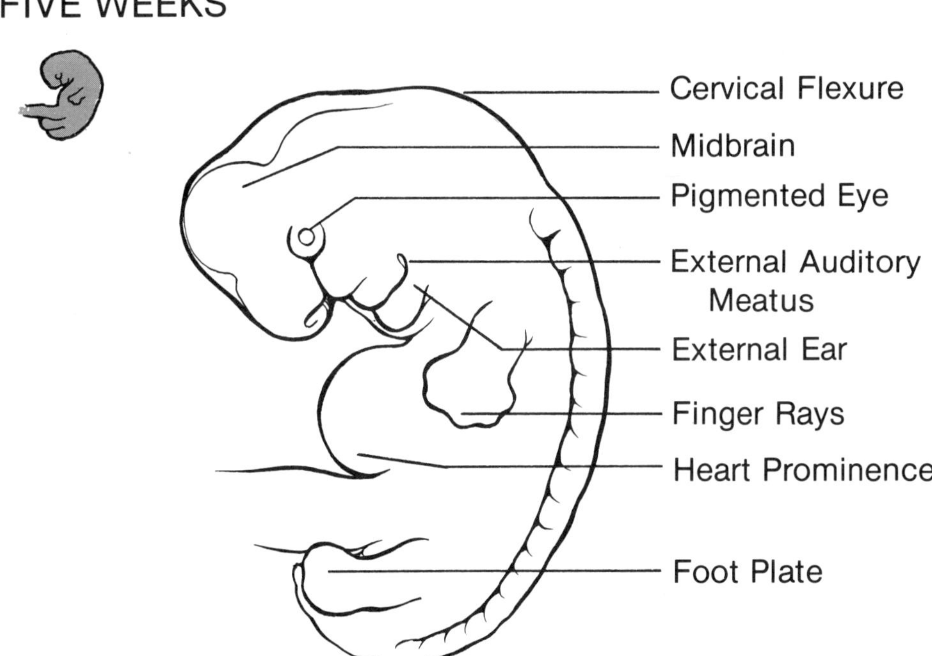

Figure 11.7
Fifth week. Drawing of a lateral view of 5-week-old embryo. Small figure shows actual size.

the fingers reach the nose. Arms and legs have recognizable digits, although they are still webbed. The liver begins to produce blood cells and by 42 days, the somites are no longer visible. The intestines enter the *extraembryonic coelom* (cavity) in the proximal portion of the umbilical cord. The communication between the primitive gut and the yolk sac has been reduced to a relatively small yolk stalk, and the yolk sac begins to degenerate. CR length 12 mm; weight 1200 mg. Figure 11.8 shows a 6-week-old embryo.

Seventh Week

The embryo now has unquestionable human characteristics. The head is more rounded and erect, although it is still disproportionately large. The ears are not fully elevated from the neck area to the sides of the head. The neck region has become established, and the eyelids are beginning to form. The forearms gradually rise above shoulder level, and the hands often cover the mouth and nose region. The palate is almost completed, and the tongue is developing in the mouth. The gastrointestinal and genitourinary tracts have undergone significant changes; before this time the rectal and urogenital passages were one tube that ended in a blind pouch; they now separate into two distinct tubular structures. The abdomen is less protuberant, but the intestine is still in the umbilical cord.

The genetic sex of an embryo is determined at fertilization by the sex chromosome carried in the sperm (see Chapter 10); however, there is no morphologic indication of sex until the seventh week when the gonads begin to acquire sexual characteristics. The reproductive organs in both sexes develop from primordia that appear identical at first. During this indifferent stage an embryo has the potential to develop into a male or female. Figure 11.9 shows a 7-week-old embryo.

Because all major external and internal structures are formed during the embryonic stage, these 5 weeks constitute the most critical period of development. Environmental assaults (viruses, drugs, radiation, etc.) at this time may give rise to major congenital malformations.

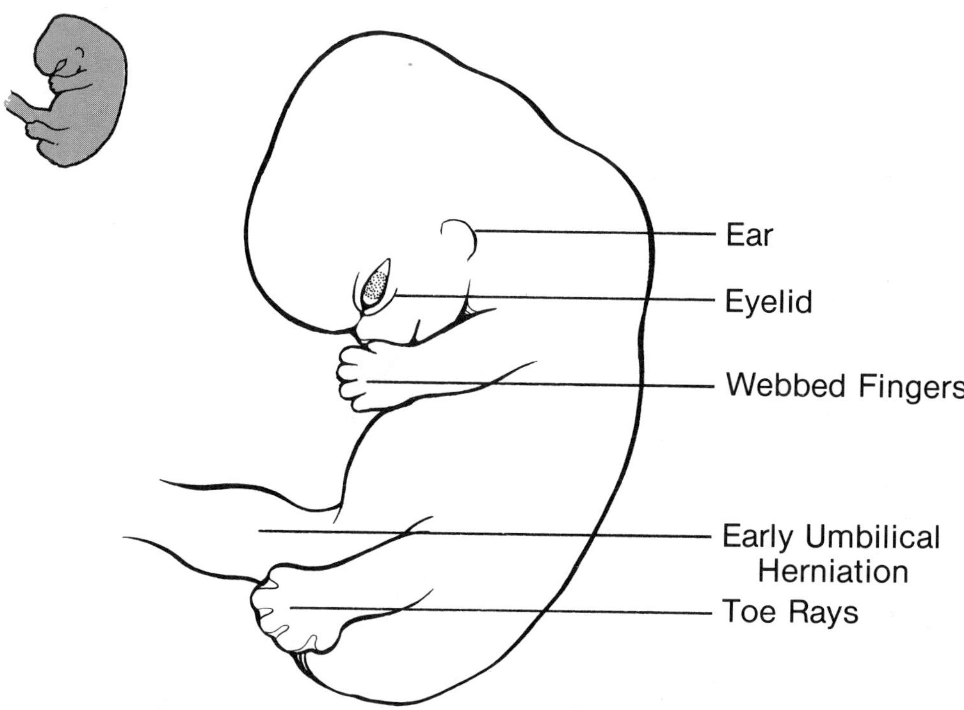

Figure 11.8
Sixth week. Drawing of lateral view of 6-week-old embryo. Small figure shows actual size.

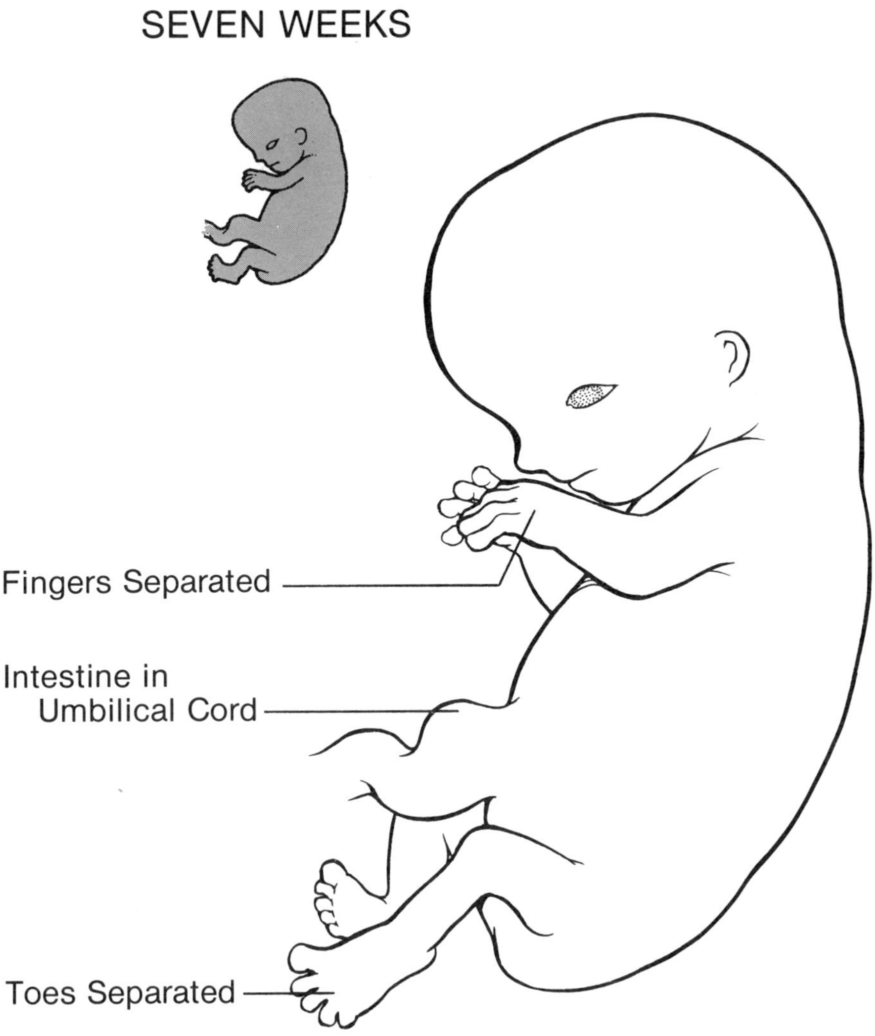

Figure 11.9
Seventh week. Drawing of lateral view of 7-week-old embryo. Small figure shows actual size.

FETAL STAGE

The developmental transition from embryo to *fetus*—the name given to the child in utero from the beginning of the eighth week until birth—is gradual, but the name change is meaningful because it heralds the fact that the growing infant has developed from an undifferentiated mass of cells into a recognizable human being. Also in the fetal stage, the growing child is far less vulnerable to teratogenic effects of drugs, viruses, and radiation than was the embryo. Development during the fetal period is evidenced by growth and maturation of tissues and organs that differentiated during the embryonic stage. Only a few new structures appear during this period. One of the most remarkable aspects of the fetal stage is the incredible rate of body growth, especially between 12 and 16 weeks, and phenomenal weight gain during the last 8 weeks.

Eight to Twelve Weeks (Third Lunar Month)

By the eighth week following fertilization, the fetus clearly resembles a human being, is approximately 2.5 cm long and weighs about 4 gm. By the end of

12 weeks, the CR length will have more than doubled. When the eighth week begins, the head is very large and constitutes almost half of the fetus; from then on growth of the head slows considerably while the body growth accelerates. During this period, the face is broad, eyes are widely separated, and the ears, while still low-set, are acquiring a more adult shape. The eyelids, which have developed from two ectodermal folds, will meet and fuse by about the tenth week and will remain fused until about the twenty-sixth week. During this time, the eyes pass through their most critical stage of development to become functioning visual organs. Long bones are beginning to form, and by the twelfth week the upper limbs have almost reached their final proportional length while the lower limbs are still relatively shorter. The external genitalia of males and females appear similar until the end of the ninth week when changes begin; the sex difference is not evident until the twelfth week. During the middle of the tenth week, the intestine returns to the abdomen and is no longer visible in the umbilical cord. As early as 12 weeks, some sucking movements of the lips have been observed. Tooth buds for all 20 deciduous (baby) teeth are discernible. Although the fetus is now capable of spontaneous movement and responds to external stimuli, its movements are too slight to be felt by the mother. CH length 7–9 cm; weight 5–20 gm. Figures 11.10 and 11.11 shows 9- and 11-week-old fetuses, respectively.

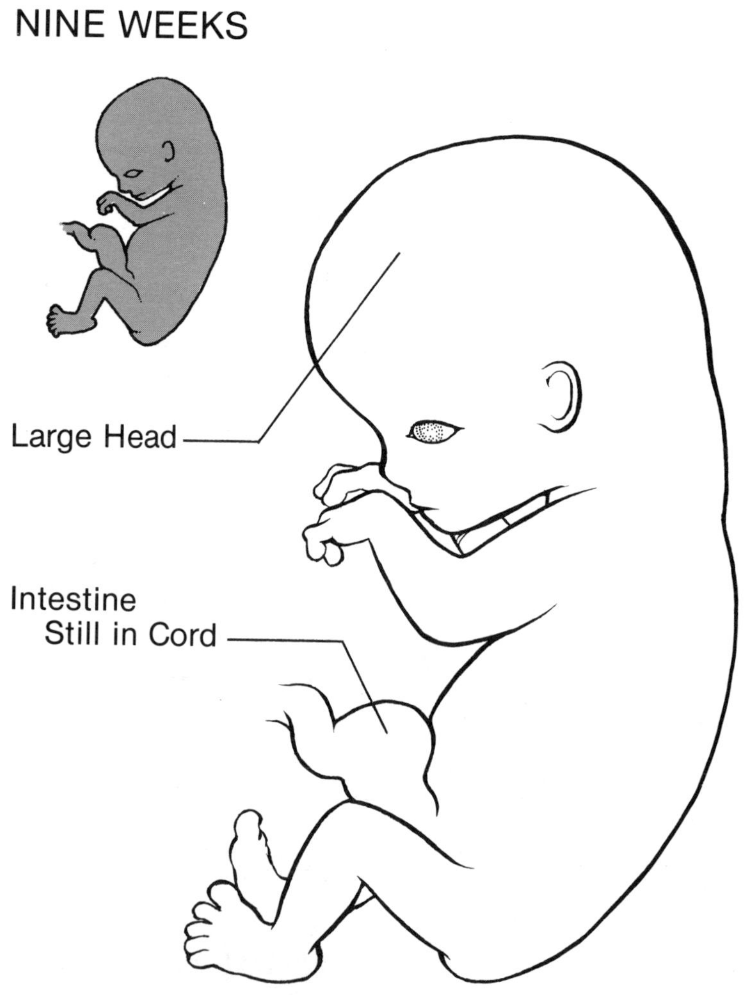

Figure 11.10
Ninth week. Drawing of lateral view of 9-week-old fetus. Small figure shows actual size.

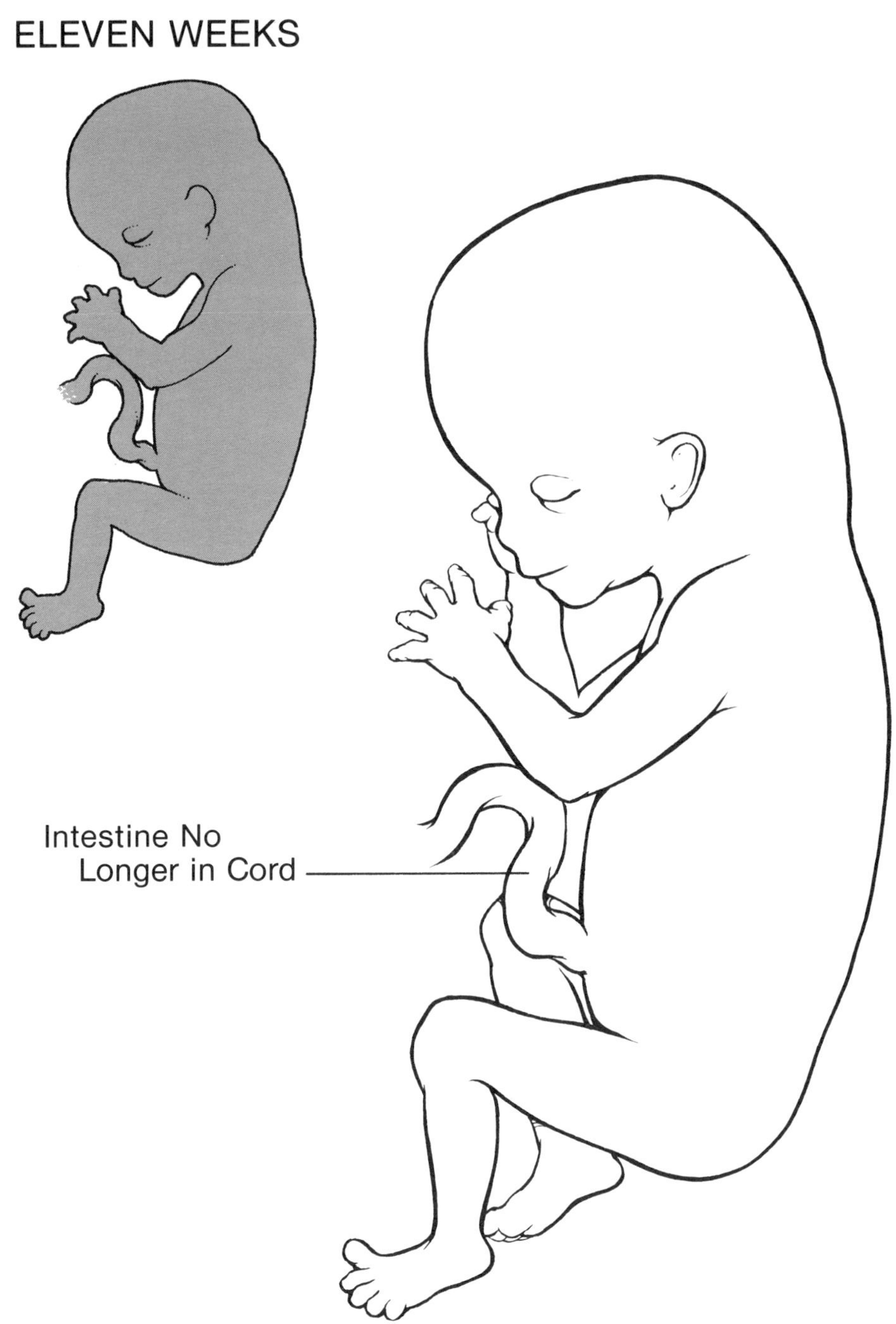

Figure 11.11
Eleventh week. Drawing of lateral view of 11-week-old fetus. Small figure shows actual size.

Thirteen to Sixteen Weeks (Fourth Lunar Month)

Growth of the body is very rapid during the fourth lunar month. By the end of 16 weeks the head is proportionately small when compared to the 12-week-old fetus. Ossification of the fetal skeleton has progressed rapidly and shows clearly on X-ray film by the beginning of the sixteenth week. Blood vessels are clearly visible beneath the nearly transparent skin. The liver and pancreas are producing their appropriate secretions, sweat glands are developing, and bronchial tubes are branching out in the primitive lungs. Even though the fetus now moves about actively in the uterus, stretching and exercising its arms and legs, these movements are usually still too faint to be felt by the mother. The fetal heart beat is discernible using the Doppler method of auscultation or sonography. CH length 10–17 cm; weight 55–120 gm. Figure 11.12 shows the 13-week-old fetus.

THIRTEEN WEEKS (actual size)

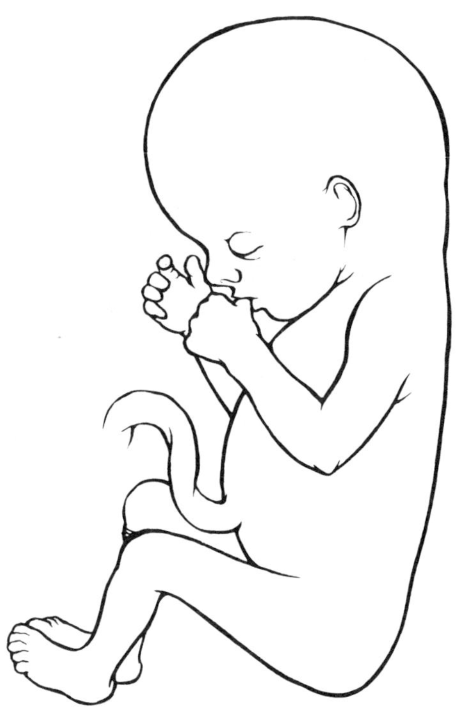

Figure 11.12
Thirteenth week. Actual size of fetus.

Seventeen to Twenty Weeks (Fifth Lunar Month)

Growth slows somewhat during the fifth lunar month, but the fetal CH length will still increase by about 8 cm. The lower limbs have reached their final relative length. The skin is covered with a greasy cheeselike material called *vernix caseosa,* which is a mixture of fatty secretions from the sebaceous glands and dead epidermal cells. Vernix protects the delicate skin of the fetus from hardening, chapping, and abrasions that could result from constant bathing in amniotic fluid. In addition to the vernix, a 20-week old fetus is covered with fine downy hair called *lanugo.* Lanugo is thought to help hold the vernix on the skin. Eyebrows and eyelashes are beginning to form, and head hair is visible. The fetus has now begun to swallow and will excrete the swallowed amniotic fluid by way of the kidneys. Increasing amounts of a substance called *meconium* are found in the fetal intestinal tract. Meconium will be the first stool of the newborn; it is a sterile, dark greenish-black, semisolid residue of bile and embryonic secretions plus squamous epithelial cells, vernix caseosa, and hair swallowed by the fetus in utero. *Brown fat,* which decreases the skin's transparent appearance, forms during this period. Brown fat is a specialized adipose tissue that produces heat by oxidizing fatty acids, particularly in the newborn infant. Brown fat is found primarily on the posterior triangle of the neck surrounding the subclavian and carotid vessels, behind the sternum, and in the perirenal areas. Nails are now visible on fingers and toes. Muscles are well developed, the fetus is active, and fetal movements (known as *quickening*) are now felt by the mother. The fetal heart beat can be heard through a stethoscope. CH length 25 cm; weight 280–300 gm. Figure 11.13 shows the 17-week-old fetus.

Twenty-One to Twenty-Four Weeks (Sixth Lunar Month)

There is a substantial weight gain during the sixth lunar month, and although the body is still lean, it is better proportioned. The eyes are structurally complete and will reopen soon. The skin is wrinkled and red, with very little subcutaneous fat. Distinct footprints and fingerprints have formed on the thickened skin pads of the hands and feet. By 24 weeks, the alveolar cells of the fetal lungs begin to produce *surfactant,* a complex phospholipid substance that lowers the surface tension of alveolar walls. (See page 209.) Although all organs are rather well developed, the 24-week old fetus will rarely survive if born prematurely,, primarily because of the immature respiratory system. CH length 28–34 cm; weight 650–820 gm.

Twenty-Five to Twenty-Eight Weeks (Seventh Lunar Month)

Although the skin is still red, considerable subcutaneous fat has formed under the skin, smoothing out many of the wrinkles (Fig. 11.14). The eyelids reopen during this period, and their motion is under neural control. If the infant is male, the testes begin to descend into the scrotum (Fig. 11.15). Respiratory, circulatory, and central nervous systems have devel-

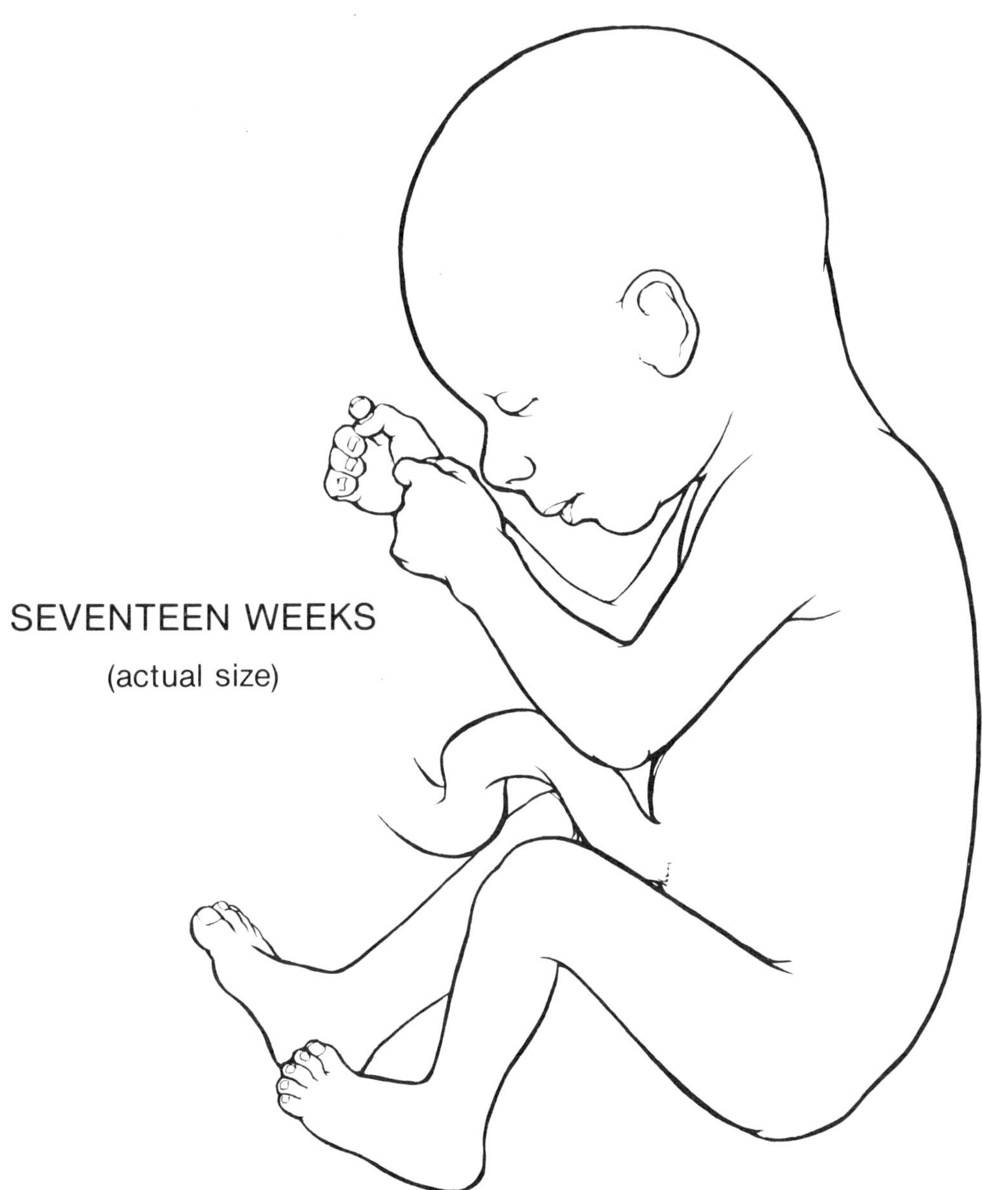

Figure 11.13
Seventeenth week. Actual size of fetus.

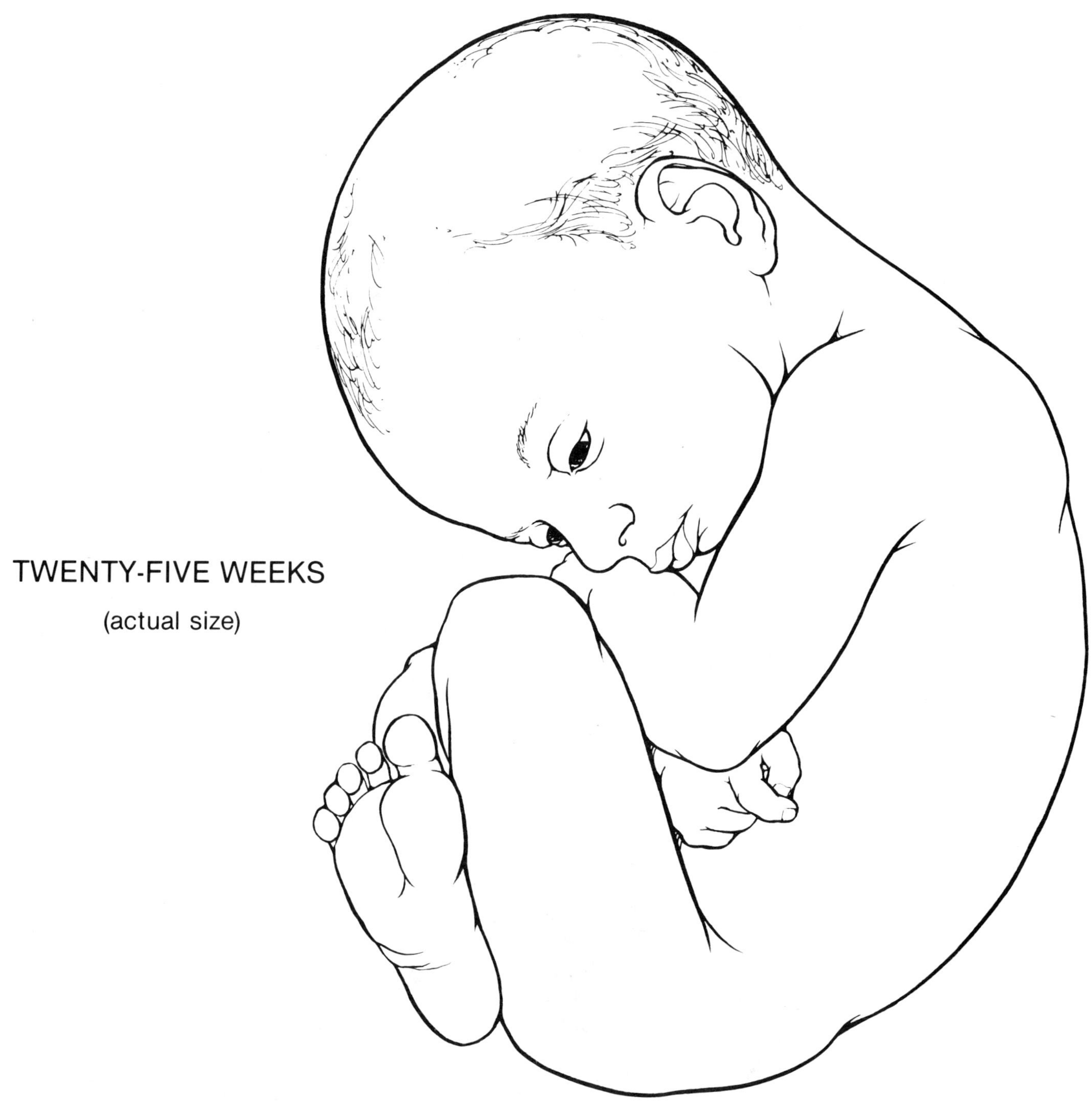

Figure 11.14
Twenty-fifth week. Actual size of fetus.

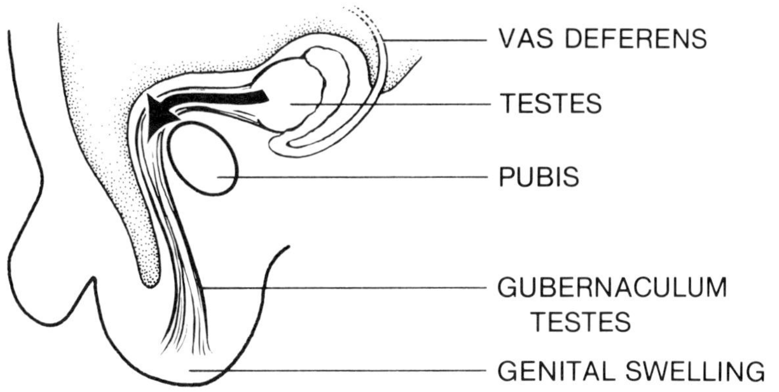

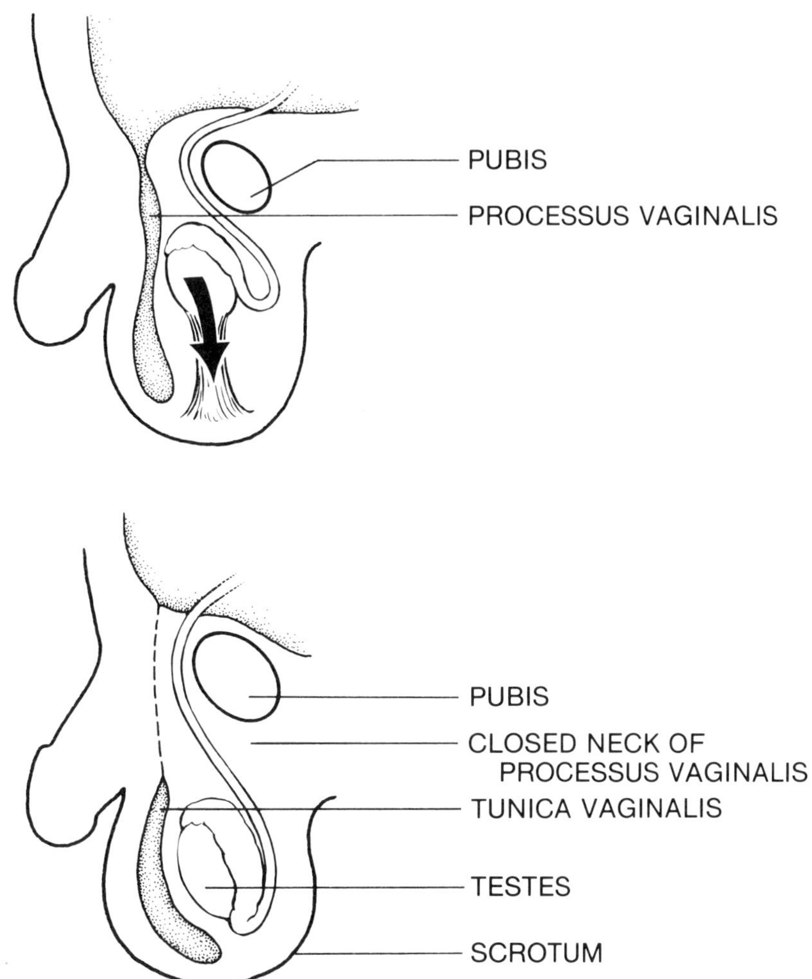

Figure 11.15
Testicular descent.

oped sufficiently to permit the fetus to survive if born at this gestational age. However, the survival rate is only 40–50%, and specialized care is required because the lungs are still relatively immature. CH length 35–38 cm; weight 1,200–1,300 gm.

Twenty-Nine to Thirty-Two Weeks (Eighth Lunar Month)

The fetus continues to gain weight and increase in length as body muscle and fat increases. The skin is usually pink and smooth; it is also pink in fetuses of dark-skinned races because melanin production begins only after exposure of the skin to light. The arms and legs may have a chubby appearance. Bones, although fully developed, are soft and flexible. Mineral storage (iron, calcium, and phosphorus) begins during the eighth lunar month. If born at this time, the fetus has a 60–70% chance of survival with specialized care. CH length 38–43 cm; weight 2,000–2,100 gm.

Thirty-Three to Thirty-Six Weeks (Ninth Lunar Month)

Because of the distribution of subcutaneous fat, the body by this time has become quite plump. Lanugo hair is disappearing, and the skin is usually white or bluish-pink in color. Nails have grown so that they reach the tips of fingers and toes. Infants born at this time have an excellent chance of survival but still require special care. Figure 11.16 shows a 36-week-old fetus.

Thirty-Seven to Forty Weeks (Tenth Lunar Month)

By 38 weeks, the fetus is considered full term. Vernix caseosa is still present in varying amounts, with the thicker deposits found in the folds and creases of the skin. Lanugo hair has disappeared except for what remains on the upper arms and shoulders. The chest, although smaller than the head, is prominent, and mammary glands protrude in both sexes. As the fetal body mass enlarges and fills the uterine cavity, the amniotic fluid diminishes until approximately 500 cc remain at birth. As the time of birth approaches, the fetus assumes a position that is referred to as its *lie;* this is usually a vertical posture with the head down and the fetal spine on the same plane as the mother's spine. The fetus assumes this posture because of the shape of the uterus and because the head is heavier than the feet (see Chapter 16). After the fifth lunar month, the fetus has developed its own feeding, sleeping, and activity patterns, so that at birth the infant has its own body rhythms and unique style of response. CH length 48–52 cm; weight 3,000–3,600 gm.

FETAL CARDIOPULMONARY SYSTEMS

The cardiovascular and respiratory systems provide two of the most crucial developmental capabilities necessary for extrauterine survival of the fetus.

Cardiovascular System

The cardiovascular system is the first system to function in the embryo; blood begins to circulate by the end of the third week. This early activity is necessary to provide the rapidly growing embryo with an efficient methods of acquiring nutrients and disposing wastes. The lungs of the fetus do not function in utero, and a special circulatory system is necessary to bypass the blood supply to the lungs. The placenta assumes this special function by taking away the carbon dioxide excreted by the fetus and returning oxygen and nutrients necessary for fetal development (Chapter 10).

Well-oxygenated blood returns from the placenta in the single umbilical vein. About half of this blood circulates through the liver, entering the inferior vena cava through the hepatic vein. The remainder of the oxygen-rich blood passes directly into the inferior vena cava through the *ductus venosus* where it mixes with deoxygenated blood from the lower limbs, abdomen, and pelvis before entering the right atrium. The blood then flows through the *foramen ovale* into the left atrium and pours into the left ventricle, which pumps it into the ascending aorta. Thus, the vessels of the heart, head, neck, and upper limbs receive well-oxygenated blood. A small amount of oxygenated blood from the inferior vena cava remains in the right atrium where it mixes with deoxygenated blood from the superior vena cava and coronary sinus and then passes into the right ventricle. The blood leaves the right ventricle in the pulmonary artery and passes through the *ductus arteriosus* into the aorta. Most of the mixed blood in the descending aorta passes into the two umbilical arteries to return to the placenta for reoxygenation with only a small amount going to the nonfunctional lungs for nourishment purposes. The remainder of the mixed blood circulates throughout the lower part of the body (Fig. 11.17).

Important cardiovascular changes occur at birth when circulation of fetal blood through the placenta ceases and the fetal lungs begin to function. The foramen ovale, ductus arteriosus, ductus venosus,

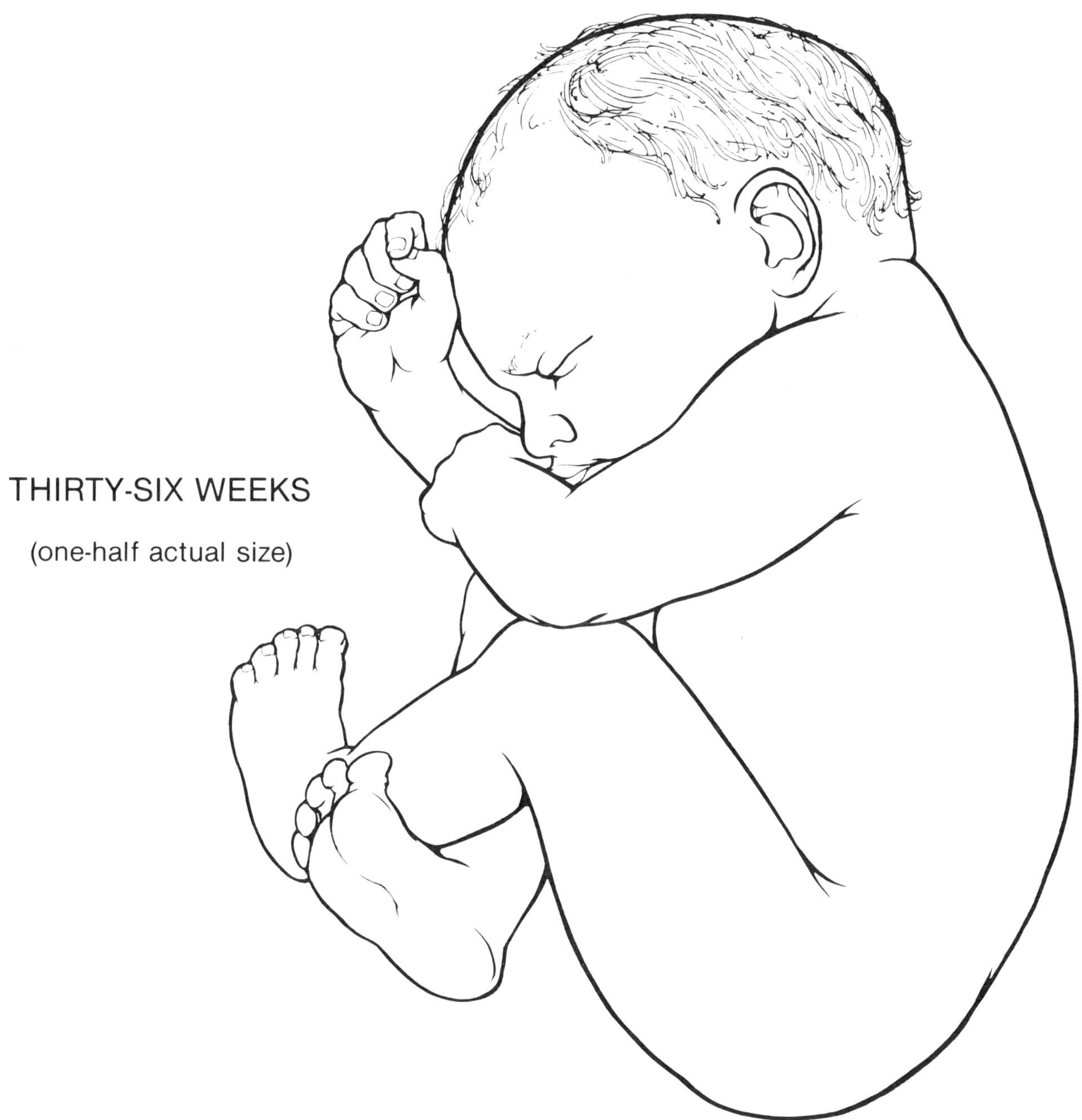

Figure 11.16
Thirty-sixth week. One-half the actual size of fetus.

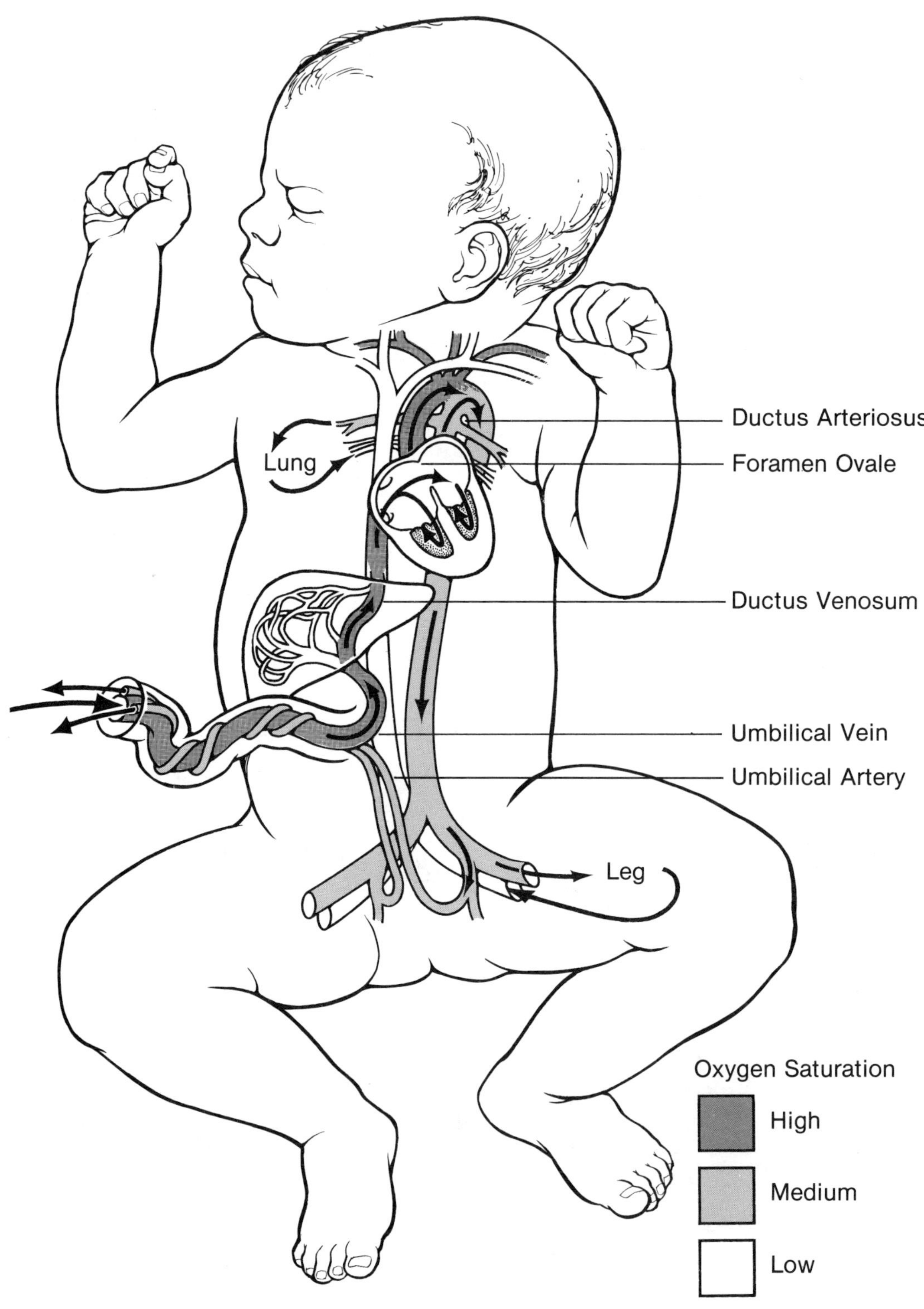

Figure 11.17
Fetal circulation. Schematic drawing of the fetal circulation. Shading indicates the oxygen saturation of the blood, and the arrows show the route of the fetal circulation.

and umbilical vessels are no longer needed. Occlusion of the placental circulation causes an immediate fall of blood pressure in the right atrium and pulmonary artery. Aeration of the lungs is associated with a dramatic fall in pulmonary vascular resistance, a marked rise in pulmonary blood flow, and a progressive thinning of the walls of the pulmonary arteries. As a result of increased pulmonary blood flow, the pressure in the left atrium rises above that in the right. This increased left atrial pressure closes the foramen ovale. The ductus arteriosus constricts at birth, although a small shunt of blood from the aorta to the left pulmonary artery may continue for a few days. The umbilical arteries also constrict at birth to prevent loss of the infant's blood (Fig. 11.18). Table 11.2 gives the fetal cardiovascular system before and after birth.

Respiratory System

Beginning about 24-weeks gestation, pulmonary surfactants are produced in increasing amounts by the aveolar cells. Surfactant lowers the surface tension of alveolar walls, which is essential for initial opening of the alveoli during the first breath and for maintaining alveolar patency, thus preventing *atelectasis* (alveolar collapse).

Absence or deficiency of surfactant is a major factor in respiratory distress syndrome (RDS), the primary cause of death in premature infants. Because fetal lung cells containing surfactant are excreted into the amniotic fluid, it is possible to predict prenatally (through amniocentesis) the maturity of the fetal lung. The principal constituent of surfactant is the phospholipid *lecithin.* Its presence in relation to another phospholipid found in surfactant, *sphingomyelin,* is the indicator by which fetal lung maturity is assessed. At 24 weeks surface-active lecithin concentrations are very slightly above those of sphingomyelin. As the pregnancy progresses, however, lecithin concentration increases while sphingomyelin concentration remains unchanged. Between 30 and 32 weeks, lecithin (L) concentration is 1.2 times greater than sphingomyelin(S) (L/S ratio = 1.2:1). By 35 weeks the L/S ratio = 2:1, signifying pulmonary maturity; this

TABLE 11.2
FETAL CARDIOVASCULAR SYSTEM BEFORE AND AFTER BIRTH

Fetal Structure	*Intrauterine Function*	*Neonatal Function*
Umbilical vein	Transports arterial blood to liver and heart	None; becomes ligamentum teres (round ligament of the liver)
Umbilical arteries	Transport arteriovenous blood to the placenta	None; become hypogastric ligaments on anterior abdominal wall
Ductus venosus	Diverts arterial blood into inferior vena cava	None; becomes ligamentum venosum
Ductus arteriosus	Diverts arterial and some venous blood from pulmonary artery to aorta	None; becomes ligamentum arteriosum
Foramen ovale	Connects right and left atria	None; becomes obliterated at birth
Lungs	Contain very little blood and no air	Oxygen and carbon dioxide exchange necessary for life
Pulmonary arteries	Transport little blood to the lungs	Transport large quantity of blood to the lungs
Aorta	Receives blood from both ventricles	Receives blood from left ventricle only
Inferior vena cava	Transports venous blood from body and arterial blood from placenta	Transports venous blood to right atrium only

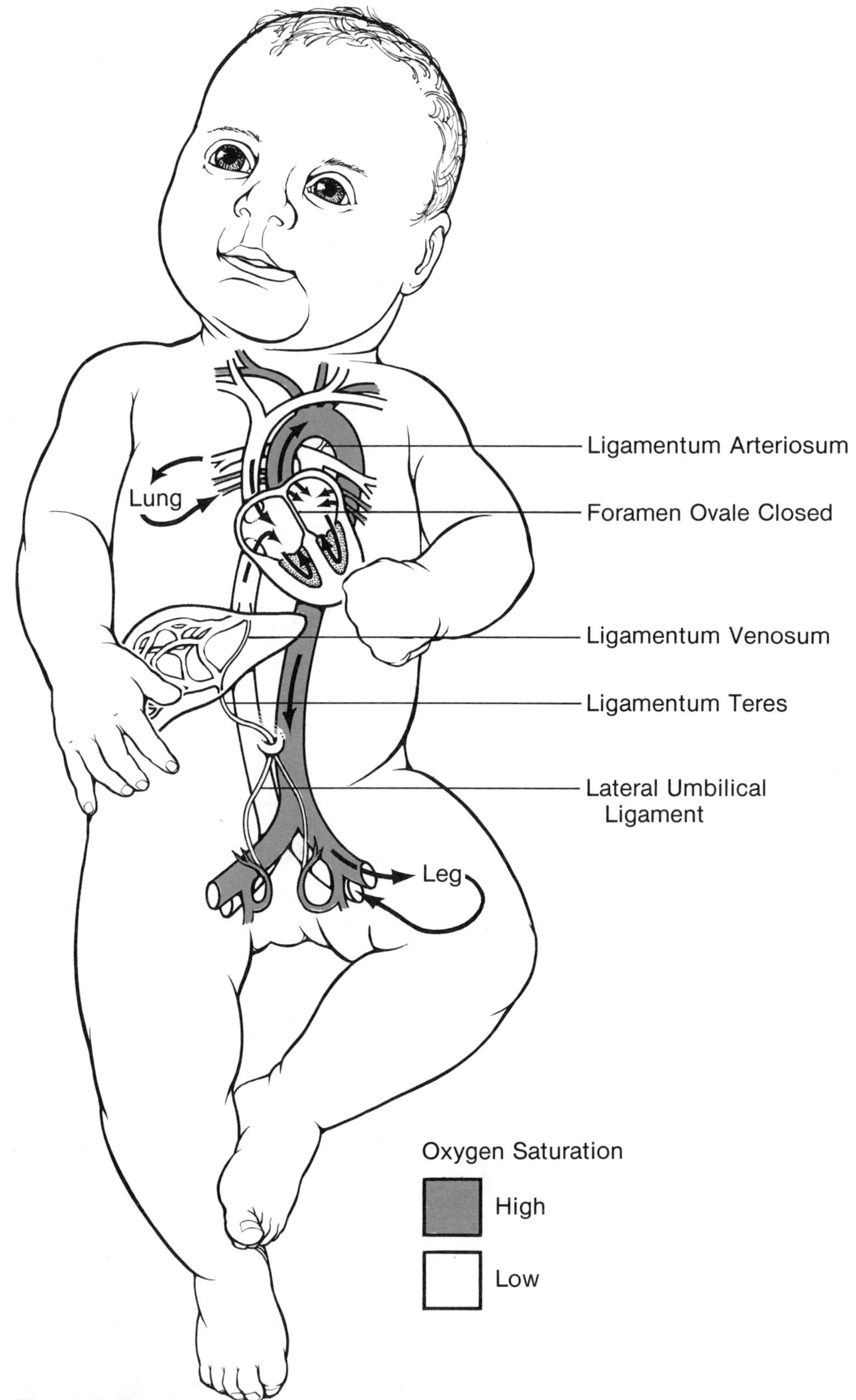

Figure 11.18
Neonatal circulation. Schematic drawing of circulation after birth. The fetal structures and vessels that become nonfunctional at birth are also shown. Arrows show the route of neonatal circulation.

virtually assures that respiratory distress syndrome will not occur after birth.

Fetal hiccough can be seen and palpated, while rhythmic respiratory movements can be demonstrated by ultrasonography late in pregnancy. Fetal squamous cells and lanugo are often found in fetal respiratory passages, indicating that respirations at birth may be an extension of some intrauterine respiratory activity.

MULTIPLE PREGNANCY

Multiple pregnancy is the gestation of two (twins), three (triplets), four (quadruplets), or any other number of infants (except one). These infants may develop from one or more ova. Infants produced from a single ovum are *monozygotic,* or identical, and are always of the same sex. Those produced from two ova are termed *dizygotic,* or fraternal, and may be of the same or opposite sex.

Twinning is the most common multiple gestation, occurring among white North Americans about once in 87 births. The frequency of twin births varies with ethnicity. Twins occur more often among blacks than whites, and more often among caucasians than Orientals. Over 2% of the population are born as twins, but since twins have a higher infant mortality rate than singletons, the incidence of twins found in the general population is less than 2%.

Because dizygotic twins result from fertilization of two separate ova by different sperm, they are no more genetically similar to each other than they would be to siblings born singly. Dizygotic twins always have two amnions and two chorions, but the chorions and placentas may have fused and appear as one (Fig. 11.19).

Since monozygotic twins are produced from the fertilization of a single ovum, they are of the same sex, genetically identical, and very similar in physical appearance. Monozygotic twinning usually begins around the end of the first week and results from division of the embryoblast into two embryonic primordia. Subsequently, two embryos, each with its own amniotic sac, develop within one chorionic sac. These twins have a common placenta and often some of the placental vessels join together, but these anastamoses (joinings) are usually so well balanced that neither twin suffers. Occasionally, however, a large artery-to-artery, vein-to-vein, or artery-to-vein anastamosis exists that causes a circulatory disturbance called *fetal transfusion* or *twin-to-twin transfusion* syndrome. Blood is shunted from one twin to the other, and the twins, although genetically identical, differ greatly in size and appearance.

The donor twin is small, pale, dehydrated, malnourished, and hypovolemic. Severe anemia as a result of chronic blood loss to the other twin is present. The recipient twin is edematous, hypertensive, and ruddy complexioned. Ascites, jaundice, and hypertrophy of heart, liver, and kidneys are associated with this syndrome, and although the recipient may have a healthy appearance, it may die within the first 24 hours after birth from congenital heart failure.

Diagnosis

To ensure proper management of the pregnancy, the diagnosis of multiple pregnancy should be made as early as possible. However, clinical diagnosis is accurate in only about three-fourths of the cases. Correct diagnosis of twins based on the following may be possible by the twenty-fourth to twenty-sixth week.

- ▲ History of dizygous twins on the maternal side of the family
- ▲ Polyhydramnios
- ▲ Excessive weight gain not associated with diet or edema
- ▲ Asynchronous fetal heart beats
- ▲ Palpation of too many small or large parts for a singleton
- ▲ Evidence of more than one fetus by radiography or ultrasonography

Prognosis

Maternal mortality is only slightly increased with multiple pregnancy. However, maternal morbidity is higher, with the primary complications being sepsis, hemorrhage, and trauma.

Perinatal mortality for multiple fetuses is nearly 5 times that of term singletons. Also, neonatal morbidity of multiples is 9–10 times higher than for term

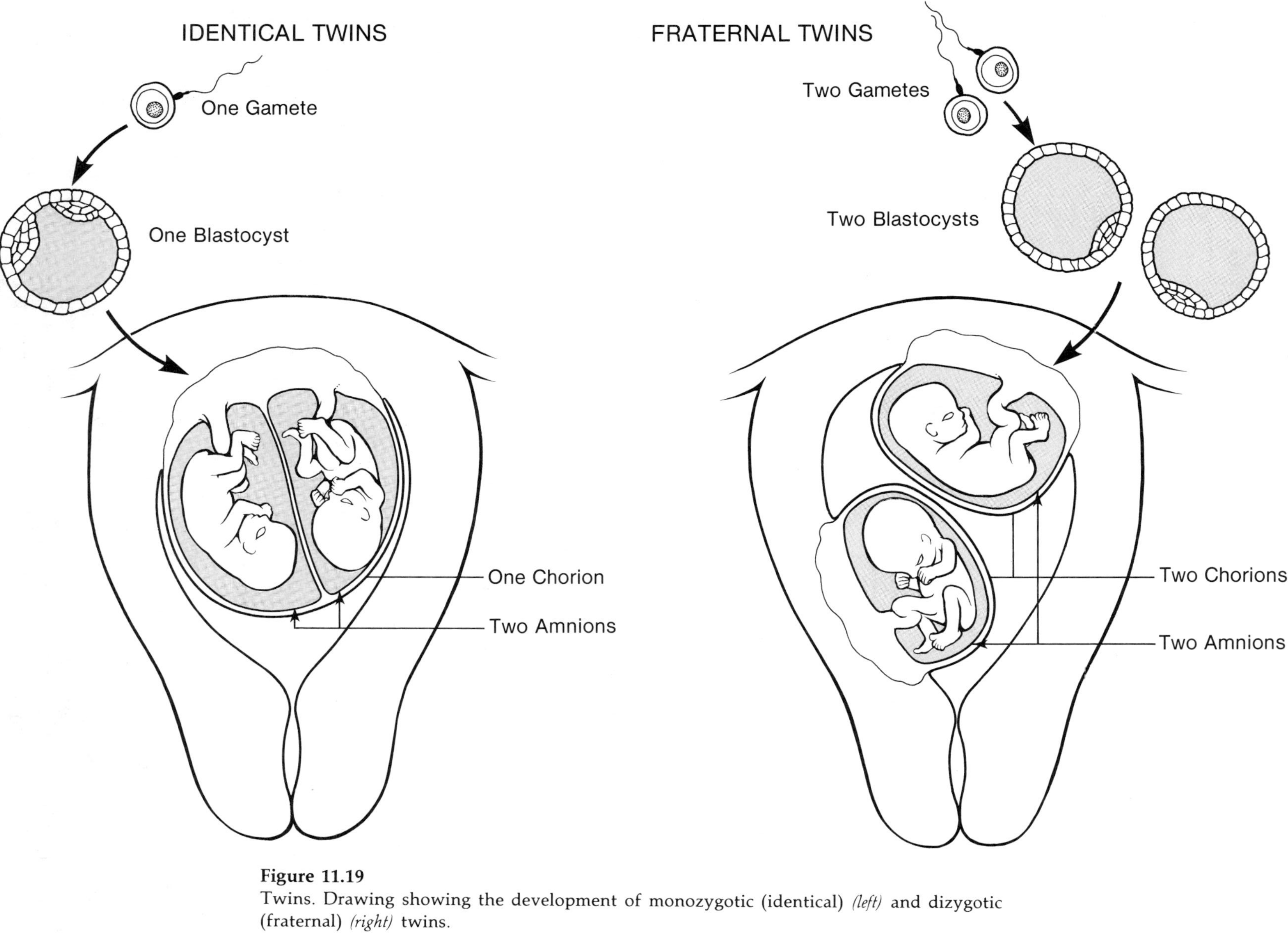

Figure 11.19
Twins. Drawing showing the development of monozygotic (identical) *(left)* and dizygotic (fraternal) *(right)* twins.

singletons, with the primary complication being sepsis.

FACTORS INFLUENCING FETAL GROWTH

Glucose is the primary source of energy for fetal growth and development, but amino acids are also required. All of these substances are transferred from mother to fetus via the placenta. The insulin required for glucose metabolism is secreted by the fetal pancreas, and no significant amount of maternal insulin reaches the fetus. Infants of diabetic mothers tend to be larger than normal, probably because of recurring episodes of hyperglycemia with subsequent hypersecretion of fetal insulin. Therefore, insulin is considered the primary growth-regulating hormone in the fetus.

Other factors that may affect fetal growth are maternal malnutrition, smoking, and alcohol consumption. The fetal alcohol syndrome may occur not only in the offspring of alcohol abusers, but also in those women whose alcohol consumption is less than 60 ml/day. The syndrome is associated with pre- and postnatal growth deficiency, mental and motor retardation, and characteristic facial anomalies (short palpebral fissures, mild microcephaly, maxillary hypoplasia). Because the severity of this syndrome is so variable and because it is virtually impossible to predict which mothers will have affected infants, it is advisable that all women who are either pregnant or planning a pregnancy avoid alcohol consumption altogether. Nicotine is another substance that can cause intrauterine growth retardation, particularly if associated with poor nutrition.

Deficiencies in maternal diet—either total reduction of food intake or lack of specific nutrients—can influence all stages of fetal growth and development. In general, the nutrients required by the fetus come from the mother's diet and not from her bodily reserves, so that temporary deficiencies in diet may cause no symptoms in her but may affect the developing fetus. Monozygotic twins have more of a chance to be growth retarded as the nutritional requirements of more than one infant exceed the nutritional supply available from the one placenta, especially during the third trimester.

Impaired uteroplacental blood flow, which can result from severe chronic maternal hypotension or from maternal hypertension that is caused by vasoconstriction of maternal vessels, for example, can inhibit growth because of fetal starvation. Placental defects, such as infarction or intervillous coagulation, can also produce a growth retarded infant. In effect, these placental changes reduce the total surface area available for exchange of nutrients from mother to fetus (see Chapter 23).

SIGNIFICANCE OF FETAL DEVELOPMENT TO MATERNITY NURSING

The tremendous increase in knowledge about the fetus and its environment has brought a greater awareness that the nurse is caring for the fetus, as well as the pregnant woman. The unborn infant has become a patient in its own right. Although maternal and fetal physiology can be examined independently of each other, mother and fetus can no longer be treated separately by health care providers (see Chapter 12).

To ensure proper care for mother and fetus and to make appropriate assessments of fetal well-being at any time throughout the pregnancy, it is necessary for the nurse to have a thorough knowledge of the growth and development process from zygote to birth. Such knowledge will also allow the nurse to assist the prospective parents toward a greater understanding of the changes that are occurring in their unborn child.

Some of the factors, either favorable or adverse, that affect the fetus in utero are already known. Some are merely speculative. Since the fetal environment can never be made totally free of potential damaging effects, the objective is to reduce the incidence of unnecessary risks to the unborn baby.

Because the maternity nurse cares for the fetus through its mother, special attention should be given to the assessment of maternal nutritional status and preventive or remedial education about proper nutrition. Maternal diet during pregnancy is likely to be supplemented with vitamins, minerals, and iron (see Chapter 12). Finding out about maternal drug use, including alcohol, is of particular importance. The nurse should obtain an accurate and complete history of over-the-counter and prescription drugs taken by the mother. This is a sensitive area for some women, requiring the nurse to use the most tender interviewing techniques. The nurse must be careful not to make the mother feel guilty about drugs that she has used. It is not uncommon for a pregnant woman to worry throughout pregnancy about a single drug taken when she did not know she was pregnant. Health education concerning the use of drugs and alcohol is very important. The nurse can use supportive skills to help the mother who is, or has been, a drug user (see Chapter 25).

The mother should be advised to report any illness such as colds or flu, especially if they occur during the first trimester of pregnancy.

Although the fetus is cushioned by the amniotic fluid, accidents or trauma to the mother, particularly the maternal abdomen, should be reported and described. Fetal status should also be assessed following such trauma.

The fetus is encased in the amniotic sac with the uterus sealed off by a mucous plug in the cervical os, however, any leakage from the maternal vagina should be reported by the mother since it could herald ruptured membranes. Once the amniotic sac has ruptured, there is the possibility for infection of the uterus, the fetal membranes, and even the fetus. Intrauterine infections are often lethal to the fetus.

Fetal activity during the second and third trimesters should be apparent to the mother. Any increase or decrease from the usual fetal activity pattern should be told to the nurse or physician (see Chapter 21).

The fetus is in a dependent position; it must rely for safety on its mother's knowledge about what affects her unborn child and on her perceptual sensitivity to its characteristics and behavior. The maternity nurse needs this same acuity combined with knowledge about fetal development and ability to make sound judgments to ensure optimal fetal growth and well-being.

SUMMARY

Fetal growth and development were discussed with special attention to the pre-embryonic, embryonic, and fetal stages of development. Progressive fetal growth and development by weeks of gestational age and fetal size were shown. Ways of estimating gestational age were included and three rules, or yardsticks, were given for measuring or inferring fetal age: Naegele's rule, fundal height, and McDonald's maneuvers. Each of the fetal cardiopulmonary systems were explained. Fetal circulation and changes in fetal circulation that occur as a result of birth were discussed. The respiratory function of the fetus was addressed, and the role of surfactant in regard to lung maturity was described. This chapter also included information about multiple pregnancy, and factors that influence fetal growth and development such as nutrients, drugs, alcohol, and changes in maternal circulation. The chapter closed with a brief discussion of the significance of fetal development to the practice of maternity nursing. Assessment of maternal diet and drug habits were included along with the importance of consumer education about nutrition, drugs, illnesses, and fetal activity.

REFERENCES AND READINGS

Butnarescu, G. F. *Perinatal Nursing, Vol. I—Reproductive Health.* New York: John Wiley & Sons, 1978.

Dwyer, J. M. *Human Reproduction.* Philadelphia: F. A. Davis, 1976.

Korones, S. *High Risk Newborn Infants* (3rd ed.) St. Louis: C. V. Mosby, 1981.

Moore, K. *The Developing Human.* Philadelphia: W. B. Saunders, 1973.

Moore, K. *Before We Are Born.* Philadelphia: W. B. Saunders, 1974.

Nilsson, L. et al. *A Child is Born.* New York: Dell, 1965.

Patten, B. M., Carlson, B. M. *Foundations of Embryology* (3rd ed.). New York: McGraw-Hill, 1974.

Pritchard, J. A., MacDonald, P. C. *William's Obstetrics,* (16th ed.). New York: Appleton-Century-Crofts, 1981.

Reid, D. E., Ryan, K. J., Benirschke, K. *Principles and Management of Human Reproduction.* Philadelphia: W. B. Saunders, 1972.

Roberts, D. F., Thompson, A. M. (Eds.). *The Biology of Human Fetal Growth.* London: Taylor and Frances, 1976.

Thompson, J. S., Thompson, M. W. *Genetics in Medicine.* Philadelphia: W. B. Saunders, 1980.

Whaley, L. F. *Understanding Inherited Disorders.* St. Louis: C. V. Mosby, 1974.

Winik, M. (Ed). *Nutrition and Fetal Development.* New York: John Wiley & Sons, 1974.

12

PREGNANCY: MATERNAL PERSPECTIVE

According the the report of the *Surgeon General's Workshop on Maternal and Infant Health,* approximately one-fourth of all pregnant women in the United States receive less than adequate care (Surgeon General's Workshop, 1981). Despite this rather gloomy statistic, most pregnancies are normal and terminate with the delivery of a healthy infant by a healthy mother. This chapter focuses on normal pregnancy and discusses physiologic and psychosocial changes during pregnancy. Foundations for healthy reproduction, discussed thoroughly in Unit Two, are built upon when discussing maternal adaptation to pregnancy. After a discussion of pregnancy, duraton of pregnancy, and clinical determinations of gestational age, physiologic and psychosocial characteristics are introduced. A discussion of the minor discomforts of pregnancy is followed by a description of what is involved in data collection for prenatal care. The next section of the chapter focuses on nursing management of pregnancy and includes a discussion of maternal nutritional needs during pregnancy. Pregnancy at either end of the childbearing continuum is highlighted in the last section. You are asked to relate the fetal changes described in Chapter 11 to the physiologic and psychosocial changes occurring in the mother. The purpose is to remind you that although this chapter is "maternal perspective," you cannot exclude the concurrent changes occurring in the human growing in utero.

SIGNS OF PREGNANCY

Traditionally, the student of maternity nursing has had to memorize the signs of pregnancy that are most often described under three headings: presumptive, probable, and positive signs. Since this chapter discusses in detail maternal physiologic adaptation in pregnancy, you can with a little guidance relate these signs of pregnancy to the physiologic changes. Since the positive signs are definitive and fewer in number, we present them in what may be thought of—in relation to tradition—reverse order, that is, positive, probable, and presumptive. Experience has shown us that this is helpful for you in recalling this information.

Positive Signs of Pregnancy

The three positive signs of pregnancy, which emanate from the fetus, are apparent around the eighteenth to twentieth week of pregnancy. They are hearing and counting the fetal heart beat, perceiving fetal movement, and visualizing the skeletal outline on X-ray film or ultrasound by an experienced examiner.

Hearing the fetal heart beat, which should be counted and recorded (normal range 120–160 beats/min), is confirmation of pregnancy. With a head stethoscope *(fetoscope)* the heart is heard at 18–20 weeks; it can be heard by the Doppler method around 12 weeks.

Active movement seen by an objective observer (not the mother) or felt by placing a hand on the abdomen is a positive sign of pregnancy.

Viewing the fetal outline by ultrasonography appears to be a safe and accurate method of diagnosis (see Chapter 20). Although embryos have been identified as early as 4 weeks by this method, it is most clear after the third month. X-ray examination is contraindicated because of the considerable potential of damage to the fetus.

Probable Signs of Pregnancy

Probable signs of pregnancy include uterine enlargement and changes in the size, shape, and consistency of the uterus, Braxton Hicks' contractions, ballottement, and the biochemical pregnancy tests. The abdomen begins to show the effects of the enlarging uterus at about 3 months. Changes in the uterus found by vaginal examination are described under physiologic adaptation and include Hegar's sign and Goodell's sign (see next section). Painless uterine contractions called Braxton Hicks' contractions are sometimes mistaken for early labor by the mother. These occur throughout the antepartum period and are often described as a tightening of the abdomen. *Ballottement* is the rebounding of the fetus when pushed by the examiner's fingers; it can be elicited in the fourth and fifth months when the fetus moves freely in the amniotic fluid. Endocrine pregnancy tests are of two types: immunologic and biologic.

The most accurate pregnancy test is the immunologic radioimmunoassay (RIA) test for the beta subunit of HCG. This test is done on blood plasma, is so sensitive it can be used before the first missed period, and in some references, is listed as a positive sign of pregnancy. It requires about 24 hours to complete and is more expensive than other tests. RIA for HCG (not just for the beta subunit), if done correctly, is accurate but can cross react with the luteinizing hormone making the test inaccurate.

Another immunologic pregnancy test is for the presence of HCG in the urine and relies on antigen antiserum reaction. The two most commonly used tests of this type are hemagglutination-inhibition test (Pregnosticon R) and the latex agglutination tests (Gravindex and Pregnosticon slide test). Hemagglutination is more accurate; it is positive if there is no clumping of cells when the pregnant woman's urine is added to the HCG-sensitized red blood cells of sheep. In the latex agglutination test, latex agglutination is inhibited in the presence of urine containing HCG. The tests are approximately 98% accurate, and there are more false-negative tests than false-positive ones, the most frequent reason being that either there is insufficient hormone production (too early for HCG) or the urine is very dilute. A positive test indicates only that HCG is being produced, which may or may not be caused by a normal pregnancy. Depending on the type of immunologic test, it can be read in 2 minutes or 2 hours.

Presumptive Signs of Pregnancy

The presumptive signs of pregnancy are largely subjective, are observed by the woman herself, and include many of the symptoms demonstrated by the early maternal physiologic adaptations. These include cessation of menstruation, breast changes, nausea and vomiting, frequency of urination, and all of the skin changes associated with pregnancy—Chadwick's sign, striae, increased pigmentation (see next section). Fatigue is often included as a presumptive sign. Because these signs are numerous and not always dependable, a diagnosis of pregnancy may be more accurate if two or more signs are apparent.

DIAGNOSIS OF PREGNANCY AND DETERMINATION OF GESTATIONAL AGE

Determining that the woman is pregnant is done by collecting and interpreting data acquired both directly and indirectly. The exact duration of pregnancy cannot be determined since it can never be known precisely when the ovum was fertilized. Labor usually begins 10 lunar months, 38–42 weeks, or approximately 280 days after the beginning of the last menstrual period. There are numerous ways of estimating the gestation of a pregnancy; clinical diagnosis of pregnancy is dependent on the assessor's ability to interpret presumptive, probable, and positive physical signs and symptoms.

Estimated Date of Delivery*

Indirect or noninvasive methods of determining the estimated date of delivery (EDD) include Naegele's rule, fundal height, McDonald's procedure, and assessment of fetal heart tones and quickening. Naegele's rule, McDonald's procedure, and fundal height are discussed in Chapter 11.

Fundal height affords a gross assessment of gestational age (see Chapter 11). Probably the single most useful thing for the nurse to remember is that after the twentieth week (when the top of the fundus is at the umbilicus), weeks of gestation equals the measurement in centimeters of the height of the fundus (Fig. 12.1). For example, if the height measures 26 cm, you can assume the gestation is 26 weeks. Factors such as intrauterine growth retardation or hydramnios, multiple pregnancies, and maternal obesity can all of course skew this assessment.

Fetal heart tones (FHTs) and *quickening* can help corroborate or refute data obtained by fundal height measurement. FHTs are heard by Doppler method from 11 to 12 weeks and by fetoscope at 20 weeks (Fig. 12.2). Pregnant women describe quickening (the movement of the fetus) from 16 to 20 weeks; the *multigravida* (woman pregnant for her second or subsequent time) describes quickening earlier than the woman who has not been pregnant before.

Direct or invasive methods of determining EDD are ultrasonography, radiography, and amniocentesis. *Ultrasonography* can be used to determine fetal age accurately by measuring the biparietal diameter of the fetal head and correlating it with weeks of gestation. A normal 36-week-old fetus usually has a diameter of 8.7 cm. *Radiography* assessment measures distal femoral ossification centers, which when present indicate a gestational age of 36 weeks. *Amniocentesis,* with subsequent analysis of the amniotic fluid, provides considerable accuracy in assessing fetal age. Ultrasound, radiography, and amniocentesis are discussed in Chapter 20.

*Estimated date of delivery (EDD) is sometimes called expected date of confinement (EDC) or estimated date of labor (EDL).

PHYSIOLOGIC CHARACTERISTICS

Reproductive Adaptation

Physiologic changes in the mother's reproductive system are evident early in pregnancy. Vaginal mucosa becomes edematous, hypertrophied (increased in size because of cell enlargement), and hyperemic (increased blood, distention of vessels). The vagina becomes a deep pink or violet color, known as *Chadwick's sign,* as a result of increased vascularity, which may aid in diagnosis of pregnancy. Both vaginal and cervical secretions increase and combine to form a white discharge. The pH of the vagina becomes acidic as a result of the growth of *Lactobacillus acidophilus,* which thrives on the increased glycogen content of the epithelial cells of the vagina. The lowered pH (5–6) is thought to be bacteriostatic for many of the pathogenic bacteria in the vaginal tract (Huff & Pauerstein, 1979). The cervix changes in consistency and color as early as 4 weeks, becoming softer and cyanotic. The softening of the cervix is called *Goodell's sign.* The cervix also shows increased vascularity, edema, hypertrophy, and hyperplasia (increase in cells) of the cervical glands. There is increased proliferation of the cervical mucosa and decreased thickness of septa between glandular spaces, which become filled with thick, tenacious mucous. A mucous plug seals off the cervical os until the onset of labor (Fig. 12.3). These changes in the cervix decrease compactness and provide for cervical dilation and effacement that occurs during labor and allows for passage of the fetus (see Chapter 16).

The uterine physiologic changes are remarkable. Uterine blood flow (UBF) increases greatly from the time of implantation through the first trimester. At the end of the first trimester, UBF per unit of weight of tissue remains constant. At term, UBF is 500–750 cc/min, 80% of which is going to the placenta. UBF is responsive to cardiac output (perfusion pressure), whereas the uterine vascular bed responds to vasoconstriction stimuli either endoge-

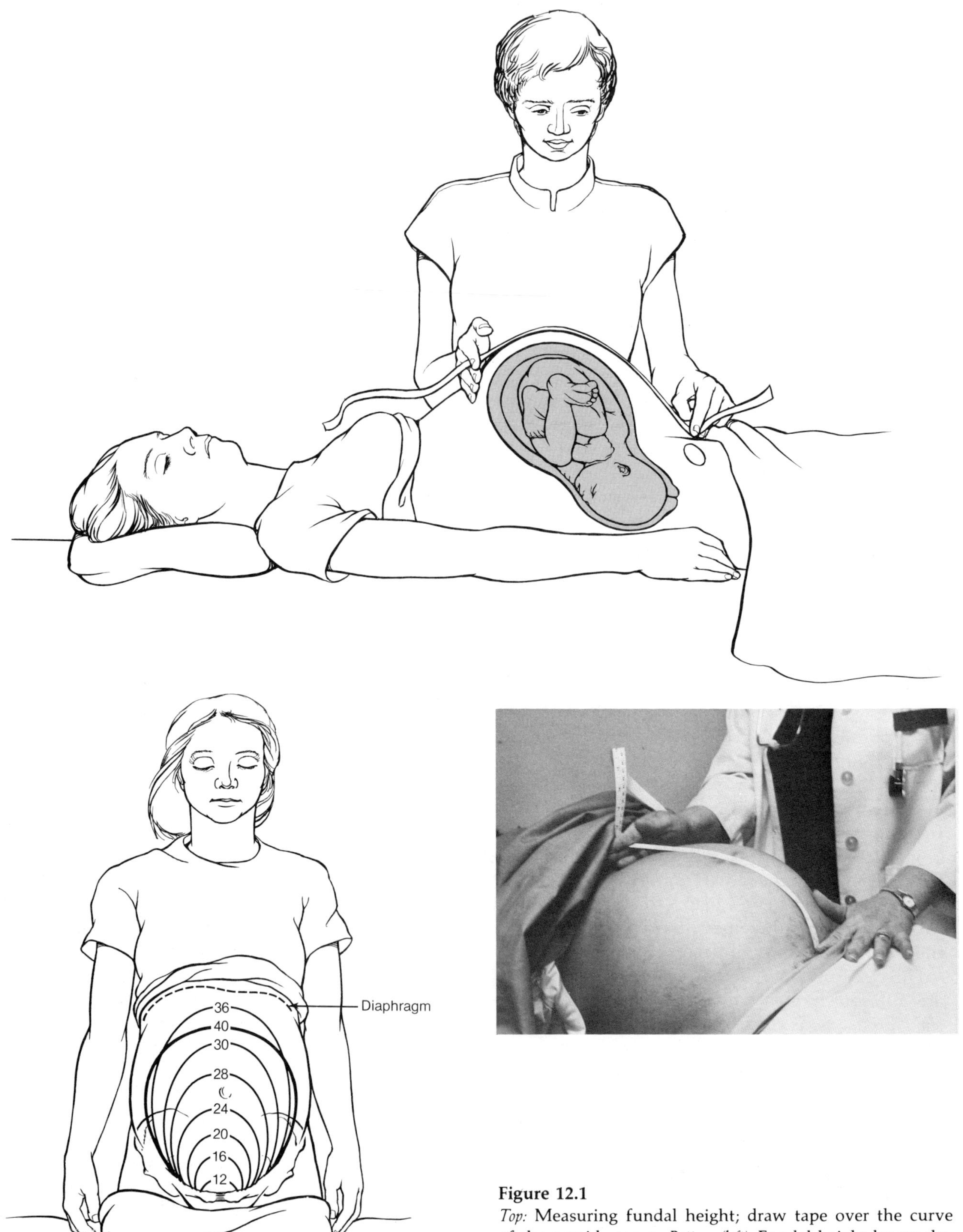

Figure 12.1
Top: Measuring fundal height; draw tape over the curve of the gravid uterus. *Bottom (left):* Fundal height by weeks; *(right)* measuring fundal height; place tape on symphysis pubis.

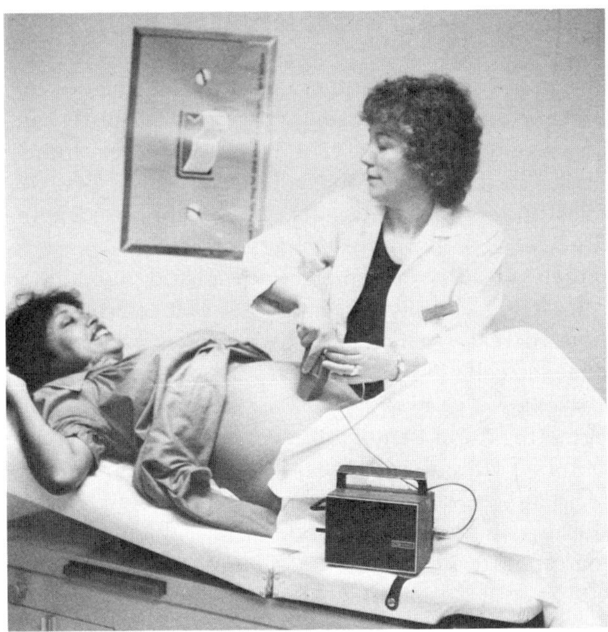

Figure 12.2
Auscultation of the fetal heart using a doptone.

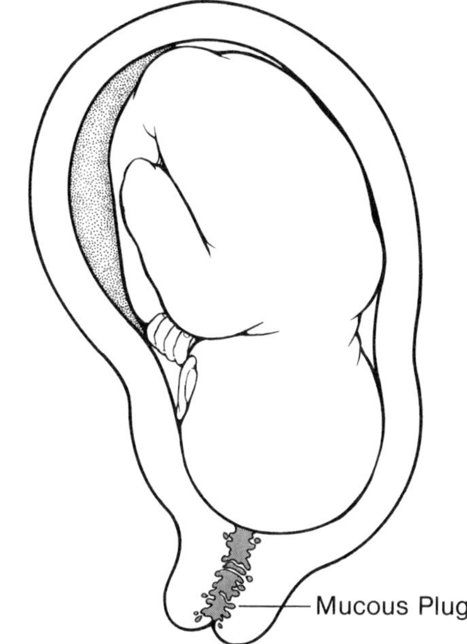

Figure 12.3
Uterine cervix showing mucous plug.

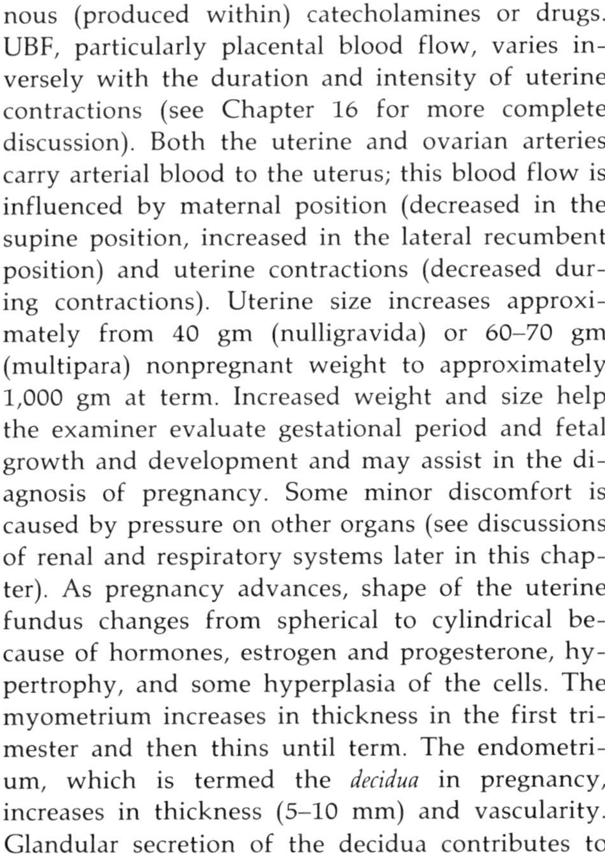

nous (produced within) catecholamines or drugs. UBF, particularly placental blood flow, varies inversely with the duration and intensity of uterine contractions (see Chapter 16 for more complete discussion). Both the uterine and ovarian arteries carry arterial blood to the uterus; this blood flow is influenced by maternal position (decreased in the supine position, increased in the lateral recumbent position) and uterine contractions (decreased during contractions). Uterine size increases approximately from 40 gm (nulligravida) or 60–70 gm (multipara) nonpregnant weight to approximately 1,000 gm at term. Increased weight and size help the examiner evaluate gestational period and fetal growth and development and may assist in the diagnosis of pregnancy. Some minor discomfort is caused by pressure on other organs (see discussions of renal and respiratory systems later in this chapter). As pregnancy advances, shape of the uterine fundus changes from spherical to cylindrical because of hormones, estrogen and progesterone, hypertrophy, and some hyperplasia of the cells. The myometrium increases in thickness in the first trimester and then thins until term. The endometrium, which is termed the *decidua* in pregnancy, increases in thickness (5–10 mm) and vascularity. Glandular secretion of the decidua contributes to the nourishment of the fertilized ovum before the development of fetal–placental circulation. Part of this endometrial lining is eventually shed as *lochia* (vaginal discharge) after delivery (see Chapter 19).

Ovarian follicle maturation ceases during pregnancy. Human chorionic gonadotropin (HCG) secreted by the trophoblasts supports continued functioning of the corpus luteum, and can be detected within 3 days of nidation. Just exactly when the corpus luteum function wanes and the placenta takes over the endocrine support of pregnancy is debated, but it is thought to occur sometimes between the seventh and ninth week after the start of the last menstrual period. Approximately 20% of normal healthy women may notice slight vaginal bleeding at the time of this hormonal shift (Huff & Pauerstein, 1979).

The breasts increase in size during pregnancy as a result of increased vascularity and hypertrophy of the aveoli. The nipples and areola increase in size and show darker pigmentation than in the nonpregnant woman. Montgomery's tubercles, elevations around the areolar, appear more prominent during pregnancy; these tubercles are hypertrophied sebaceous glands. There is development of ductal and glandular systems, and *colostrum* (first milk) is produced. These physiologic changes are preparatory to lactation. The pregnant woman describes breast tenderness and tingling in the early weeks of pregnancy that are the result of the physiologic changes taking place.

Endocrine Adaptation

The hypothalamus releasing factors are intially suppressed by estradiol and progesterone produced by the corpus luteum; continued suppression is a result of the luteotrophic effect of HCG and continued estrogen and progesterone synthesis by the placenta. The anterior lobe of the pituitary enlarges 20–40% in the cells containing prolactin. Although prolactin levels increase, lactation is not initiated during pregnancy probably because of a local blocking effect of estrogen on the breast tissue. The thyroid gland increases in size in about 50% of pregnant women (hyperplasia of glands and increased vacularity). The basal metabolic rate (BMR) increases a little, usually by the end of the sixteenth week of gestation, and increases 10–30% above prepregnancy rate in the third trimester. Goiter formation as a result of iodine deficiency can occur because of increased urinary excretion of iodine and, therefore, iodine nutritional intake is important. There is some increase in circulating thyroid hormones.

Anterior pituitary enlargement has been mentioned, and the posterior lobe also shows increased production of oxytocin and possibly vasopressin (antidiuretic hormone). In the adrenal glands there is an increase in size as a result of hyperplasia of the cortex. Adrenal changes in pregnancy are similar to thyroid changes in that there is no increase in cortisol synthesis (just as there is no increase in thyroid synthesis) but rather an alteration in binding and degradation. Placental estrogens cause an increase in cortisol binding globulins so that cortisol levels are increased in first trimester and again around the seventh month. Aldosterone secretion is markedly increased in pregnancy. Aldosterone increases sodium reabsorption from the renal tubules, which facilitates the needs of pregnancy. Pancreatic function and the usual relationship to carbohydrate metabolism is markedly changed in pregnancy. Pregnancy is noted to be a diabetogenic (diabetes like) state (see Chapter 21). Human chorionic somatomammotropin, HCS (which is the same as HPL, human placental lactogen) has anti insulin properties that are thought to be the cause of the changes in carbohydrate metabolism.

Cardiovascular Adaptation

Pregnancy causes a hypervolemic state; blood volume begins to increase in the first trimester, increases rapidly in the second, and decreases slightly in the third. Total blood volume increases 30–50% over the nonpregnant state, and this increase is influenced by hormonal changes. The increase is largely a result of plasma volume although red blood cell (RBC) volume also increases. The plasma volume increases earlier and to a greater degree than does red cell volume, which results in what is termed *pseudoanemia* or *physiologic anemia* of pregnancy. Both hematocrit and hemoglobin concentrations decrease as blood volume increases. The cellular components of blood differ from the nonpregnant state in that there is increased red blood cells, which increases maternal iron by about 400–500 mg, fetal iron 300–400 mg, and placental iron 100 mg. RBC volume increase however, is less than plasma increase. There is a moderate increase in platelets. Leucocytes elevate slightly in pregnancy and more during labor. Coagulation time decreases during pregnancy; fibrinolytic activity of plasma is prolonged during pregnancy. There is appreciable increase in some clotting factors, notably factors VII, VIII, IX, and X. This increase suggests a hypercoagulable state, but clotting time is relatively unchanged. Mean arterial pressure (mean arterial pressure = diastolic pressure + ⅓ pulse pressure*) is essentially unchanged in the first trimester, reaches its lowest point in the second trimester, and rises slowly in the third trimester. A mean arterial blood pressure (BP) of 90 mm Hg or more in the second trimester and 105 mm Hg or more in the third trimester is indicative of a problem. Peripheral resistance (total) decreases by about 25% after 5-months gestation. Femoral venous pressure tends to increase as the uterus enlarges, but anticubital venous pressure remains unchanged.

The cardiac output (CO), volume of blood circulated by the heart per minute, increases 25–50% (average 35%) by the end of the first trimester, which persists until term. Baseline heart rate usually increases about 10 beats per minute (12%). Increased stroke volume is thought to play a major role in increasing CO. CO increase during labor is thought to be related to both uterine contractile activity and pain.

---

*Pulse pressure = systolic blood pressure − diastolic blood pressure.

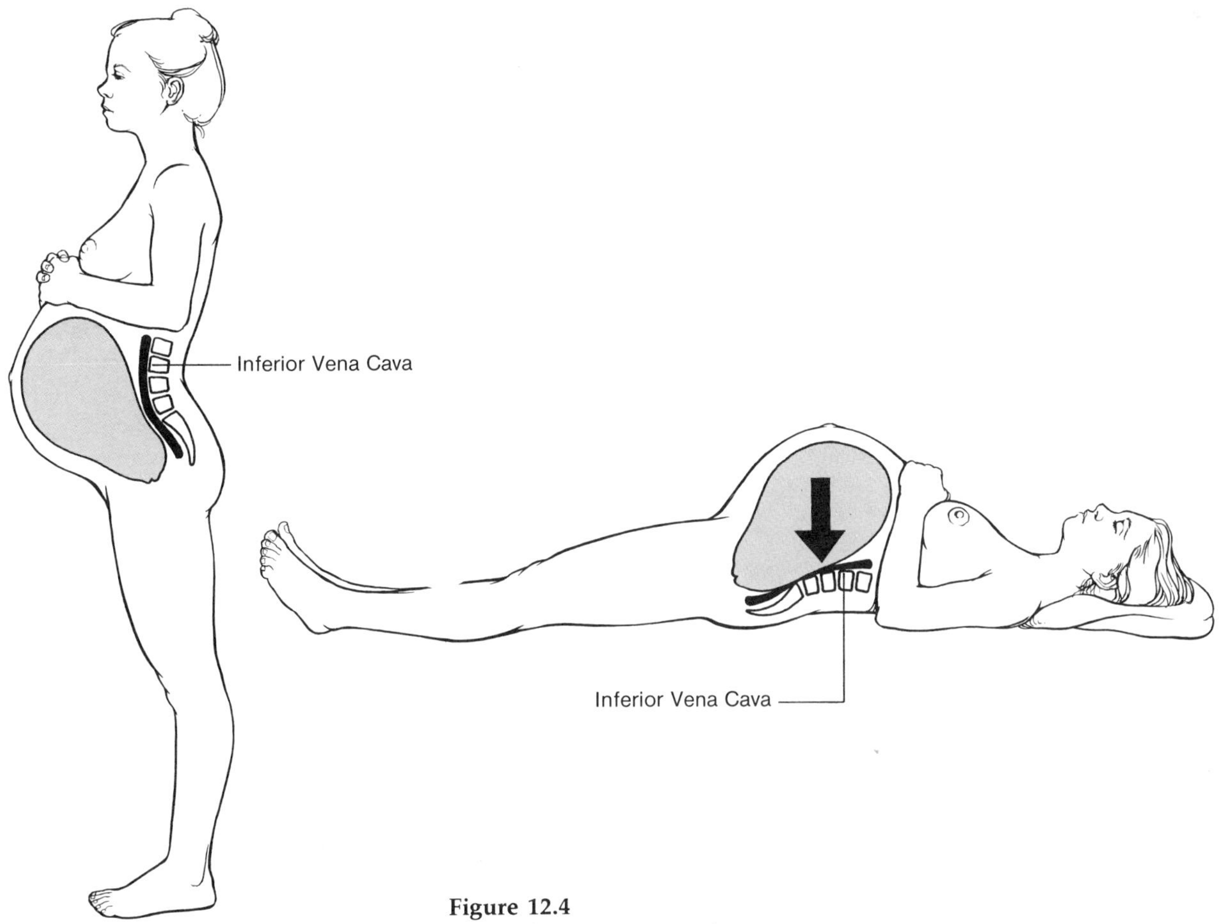

Figure 12.4
Supine hypotensive syndrome.

In summary, the physiologic bases for the changes in CO are thought to be a result of hormonal activity, a low-resistance shunt by uteroplacental circulation during the second half of pregnancy, and decreased peripheral resistance during the second trimester.

BP and CO together are significantly influenced by position of the patient. The gravid uterus of a pregnant woman in a supine position compresses the inferior vena cava against the vertebral column, which can result in a significant decrease in venous return and decreased CO. This sequence of events is termed *supine hypotensive syndrome* (Fig. 12.4). The symptoms that can accompany this syndrome are faintness, anxiety, and hypotension. The condition is corrected by placing the woman on her side or manually displacing the uterus off the vena cava. The bodies of the majority of women compensate for this decrease in venous return by enlarging collateral circulatory channels. It is unknown what is unique about the 11% of pregnant women who experience supine hypotensive syndrome (Huff & Pauerstein, 1979).

Renal blood flow increases approximately 50% in the first trimester, remains relatively unchanged in the second, and decreases in the last trimester, particularly during the last month of pregnancy. Blood flow to the liver and brain is unchanged.

Renal Adaptation

Total body water, discounting edema, increases approximately 7.5 L above normal; most of it is extracellular. This body water increases the need for sodium retention (hence sodium reabsorption is greater) to maintain osmolarity. Capillary filtration increases, particularly in the upright position. The generalized edema of the upper torso and extremities is not significant unless accompanied by elevated BP and proteinuria (see Chapter 21). There is an increase in the glomerular filtration rate (GFR) of about 60–80%, and filtered glucose is reabsorbed into the tubule. The maximal tubular reabsorption of glucose (not altered in pregnancy) is exceeded as the filtered load of glucose is increased. Therefore, about 20% of normal pregnant women demonstrate glycosuria. This glycosuria may contribute to increased size of the infant. It is discussed more fully in the section on diabetes in Chapter 21. The increase in GFR is probably a result of plasma protein concentration, and creatine clearance increases similarly to GFR. Endogenous creatinine clearance can be used as a reliable index of renal function in pregnancy. Determination is made on a 24-hour urine collection; both blood and urine determinations are done. The formula for creatinine clearance is presented below.

$$\frac{\text{Total mg urinary creatinine in 24 hours}}{\text{Plasma creatinine mg/ml} \times 1{,}440 \text{ (minutes in 24 hours)}} = \text{ml/min}$$

Normal pregnancy value is 90–180 ml/min. Renal function tests become of great significance in high-risk pregnancies.

The dilation of the ureters above the pelvic brim up to and including the renal pelves has been demonstrated by pyelogram and postmortem examination. The dilation occurs as early as 10 weeks and does not return to normal until 12-weeks postpartum. There is more dilation on the right side (relates to pyelonephritis, Chapter 21), and again the physiologic change is thought to relate to high progesterone levels that cause generalized atony. Bladder tone is unaffected during pregnancy although the enlarging uterus may result in more frequent urination, particularly in the first trimester, when the uterus is still in the pelvic cavity, and the last trimester, from pressure of the term gravid uterus on the bladder.

The renin–angiotensin system activity is increased in pregnancy, which is probably related to hormones (progesterone and estrogen), the expanded blood volume, increased sodium requirements, or a combination of these and other physiologic changes. The end result is a high level of circulating aldosterone, which affects water and electrolyte balance. BP response to angiotensin seems to decrease during pregnancy. In contrast to glucose, the maximum tubular reabsorption for sodium increases to match the elevated filtration of sodium. In pregnancy, therefore, there is an accumulation of salt and water without significant changes in maternal tissues or serum. The physiology of sodium and water balance in pregnancy is the basis for the fact that sodium intake should not be restricted even in high-risk pregnancies. Tubular sodium reabsorption is influenced by aldosterone and progesterone; aldosterone enhances sodium absorption and potassium loss whereas progesterone counteracts aldosterone and has an overall potassium-sparing action. Maternal position again is a significant factor in water and sodium balance in pregnancy. When a woman turns from side to back (supine) water excretion falls by 50%. Early in pregnancy, increased water intake (1 L) will result in increased output and decreased serum osmolarity. Later in pregnancy, output is unaffected, which suggests that water leaves the blood without stimulating a diuretic response.

Respiratory Adaptation

Residual and total lung volume in pregnancy at term decrease by 20%. Tidal volume increases nearly 40% at term. However, there is an increased inspiratory capacity (tidal volume and reserve volume) of about 5% in late pregnancy. Total oxygen consumption in late pregnancy may increase as much as 20%. Expiratory reserve decreases 15% of the normal volume. There is no change in vital capacity so that tidal volume increases at the expense of expiratory reserve volume. The larger tidal volume drawn into a reduced residual volume results in a more efficient gas exchange so that aveolar ventilation is improved by 65%. Minute volume (tidal volume × respiratory rate) may increase as much as 40–55%. Increased minute ventilation is an important and consistent pulmonary adaptation in pregnancy. It is noted as early as the ninth week and probably is initially related to increased respiratory rate. There are changes that occur in gas exchange probably as a result of increased progesterone levels. Significant changes include increased resting O_2 uptake in pregnancy of 20%. Hyperventilation (increased respiratory rate) results in lowering alveolar partial pressure of carbon dioxide ($P\text{CO}_2$), and although there is decreased arterial $P\text{CO}_2$ reflecting decreased alveolar $P\text{CO}_2$, there is no change in arterial pH because of compensatory renal excretion of bicarbonate lowering the total base by 5 mEq/L. Medullary chemoreceptors are reset to discharge at a lower level; the respiratory center has an increased sensitivity to $P\text{CO}_2$, and as a result respiratory rate is increased. Lowering of arterial PCO_2 and bicarbonates permits optimal fetal respiratory exchange. This exchange is important for normal fetal growth since increasing PCO_2 (or acidosis) can be harmful to the fetus. In the first and second trimesters 60–70% of women complain of *breathlessness*. Behavior simulates that which occurs at high altitudes, yet no pathologic changes have been demonstrated.

Gastrointestinal System

The major change in the gastrointestinal (GI) tract is atony, reduced tone, and as a result, reduced motility. The relaxation of the GI tract is thought to be a result of hormonal influence, and although this decrease in motility allows for more efficient nutrient absorption, the diminished peristaltic action and poor bowel tone contribute to the common complaint of constipation. Relaxation of the cardiac sphincter along with uterine pressure may cause heartburn (regurgitation of undigested food into the lower esophagus). There is decreased secretion of gastric acid (HCL) in the first and second trimesters. Saliva pH is altered from an alkaline to a more acid state, which may contribute indirectly to tooth decay. Hypertyalism (increased salivation) is noted although the reason is unclear. Gallbladder emptying time is increased and cholesterol secretion into bile is increased (because of HCS), which are factors that contribute to the increased incidence of gallstones in parous women.

Metabolic Adaptation

Carbohydrate metabolism is affected by the decreased renal threshold for glucose, and as a result, glycosuria is common in normal pregnant women. Although there is also increased insulin production, there is increased resistance to insulin by free fatty acids and increased destruction of insulin in the placenta, probably because of HCS. Protein metabolism is reflected in positive nitrogen balance, which is noted in the first trimester and increases in the third trimester when fetal needs are the greatest. Maternal protein status can be evaluated by spot and 24-hour urinary urea nitrogen to total nitrogen ratios (UN/TN ratios). Postpartally, blood loss, lactation, and involution tend to contribute to a negative nitrogen balance; nitrogen reserve is maintained by the mother through storage of surplus protein in maternal organs and tissues. Blood lipids (fats) are increased; together with glucose they provide sources of energy to the fetus. There is a progressive increase in free cholesterol until the thirtieth week of gestation, which may result in increased ketonuria if the maternal diet is low in carbohydrate or high in fat. Mineral changes that are significant relate to calcium and phosphorous; the requirement for these minerals doubles during the last half of pregnancy. Half of this increase is absorbed by the fetus and half is stored by the mother. Iron requirements increase to 800 mg; most of the iron is needed in the third trimester. Since dietary intake is never sufficient to meet this need, supplemental iron is routinely prescribed. Anemia in the nonpregnant state is defined as a hemoglobin concentration of less than 12 gm%; in pregnancy, anemia is diagnosed when hemoglobin level falls to 11 gm% (as a result of the physiologic hemodilution of pregnancy). Supplemental iron therapy (in addition to the iron in prenatal vitamins) in the form of iron salts (ferrous sulfate) is used when anemia is diagnosed and should be continued for at least 3 months after delivery until adequate iron stores have been refurbished. Folic acid requirements increase about 5 times that of the nonpregnant state; folic acid is necessary for metabolism of some amino acids and synthesis of nucleic acids. Deficiency of folic acid leads to megaloblastic anemia. Folic acid is commonly found in green leafy vegetables.

Musculoskeletal System

The myometrial cell has the potential for great hypertrophy during pregnancy allowing for extensive uterine growth and for contractility of sufficient force during labor to empty the uterus of its contents (Fig. 12.5). Uterine physiology is discussed in Chapter 16. Bones of the pelvis, symphysis pubis, sacroiliac synchondrosis, and sacrococcygeal joints are widened slightly and are capable of some movement as early as 10–12 weeks of gestation. This mobility is probably a result of the hormone relaxin. Alteration in the center of gravity contributes to the woman's attempt to compensate by moving her shoulders and spine back and projecting her abdomen forward (Fig. 12.6). This results in a lordosis (forward curvature of the lumbar spine), which contributes to backache and poor posture and may cause instability or poor balance. Pressure on the abdomi-

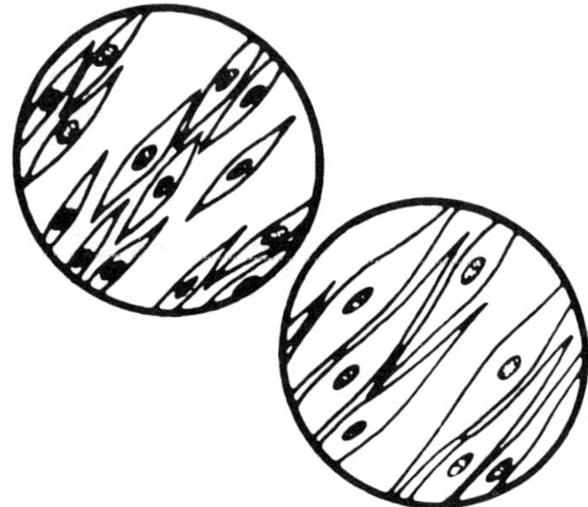

Figure 12.5
Myometrial cells.

nal wall can cause *diastasis recti*—vertical separation of the rectus-abdominis muscles. Wide separation of these muscles can be palpated. Abdominal muscle tone in women with diastasis will result in less efficient voluntary muscular effort during he second stage of labor. The affect that the term pregnancy has on the relationship of organs in the pelvic area and the marked growth of tissue in this region are shown in Figure 12.7.

Skin changes in pregnancy are very common; 50% of all pregnancies result in *striae gravidarum*—reddish brown streaks on abdomen, thighs, and breasts commonly referred to as "stretch marks." Fresh striae are pale pink or bluish in color; after delivery they have a shiny appearance like scar tissue. In a multiparous woman old and new striae may be seen; the striae from former pregnancies, which are silvery and shiny, are called *striae albicantes. Linea nigra,* a brown vertical abdominal line from the sternum to the symphysis pubis, often occurs. *Chloasma,* the mask of pregnancy, is evidenced by dark brown discolorations on the face. Cause is not known but may be related to the presence of melanocyte–stimulating hormone (similar to ACTH), which is present in women from approximately 8 weeks until term. Estrogen and progesterone may also play a role since they may have melanocyte-stimulating effects. Other dermatologic changes induced by pregnancy include herpes gestationis (vesicular or bullous skin eruptions), noninflammatory pruritis of pregnancy, vascular spiders, palmar erythema, and pregnancy granulomas. Skin changes may cause distress in the pregnant woman because of her concern with appearance.

Immunologic Adaptation

It is noted that pregnant women have a higher incidence of bacterial and viral diseases and a higher mortality rate when compared with proper controls (Jensen et al., 1981). Both humoral and cell-mediated changes occur in pregnancy. In general, the major maternal serum immunoglobulin is IgG, which crosses the placenta to the fetus. IgG is reduced in pregnancy, although the reason for this is not clear. Also confusing is the fact that IgM, although it increases in the first trimester, does not change during labor and delivery. IgA, found in plasma and also concentrated in external secretions such as tears, saliva, and mucous, has not been definitively studied in pregnancy. Cell-mediated changes are increases in monocytes, decreases in T-cell activity, and increases in opsonin index. These changes indicate a greater than average need to guard against infection, but the changes in the immunologic system and implications for the pregnant woman need further study.

PSYCHOSOCIAL CHARACTERISTICS

Maternity nursing is concerned not only with the fact of pregnancy or the biopsychosocial capabilities to produce a new life, it is also concerned with values, attitudes, expectations, and motivations of the couple since these have been shown to influence the way in which pregnancy is experienced. The potential for healthy parenting is present in most couples. It is also true, however, that the usual family stresses do not cease when pregnancy occurs and moreover pregnancy itself brings about new stresses. Some of these stresses are increase in family size, circumstances surrounding conception, purpose of the pregnancy, and increased responsibilities. Was fertilization planned or accidental? Is guilt or pleasure the predominant feeling? Is legality or nonlegality of marriage as determined by society a factor? What was the purpose and meaning of *this* pregnancy to *this* couple? Perhaps resolution of marital tension or problems, attention-seeking motivation (by either partner), or demonstration of male–female roles was underlying the desire to become pregnant. Ideally, all pregnancies would be planned and all children

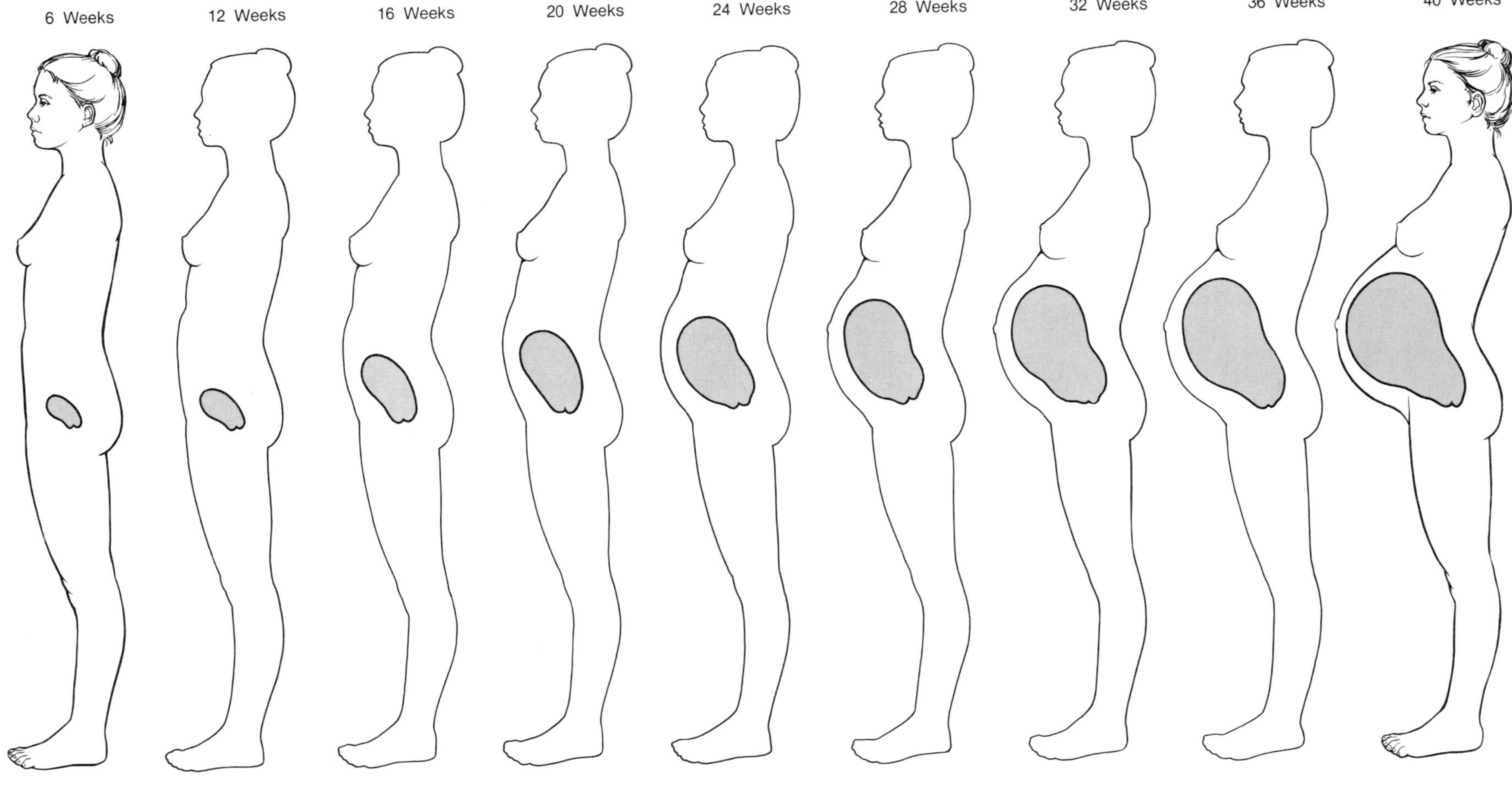

Figure 12.6
Month-by-month enlargement of uterus with related musculoskeletal changes.

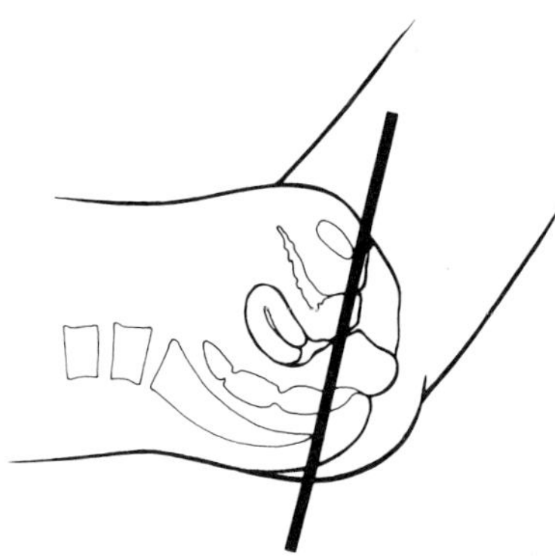

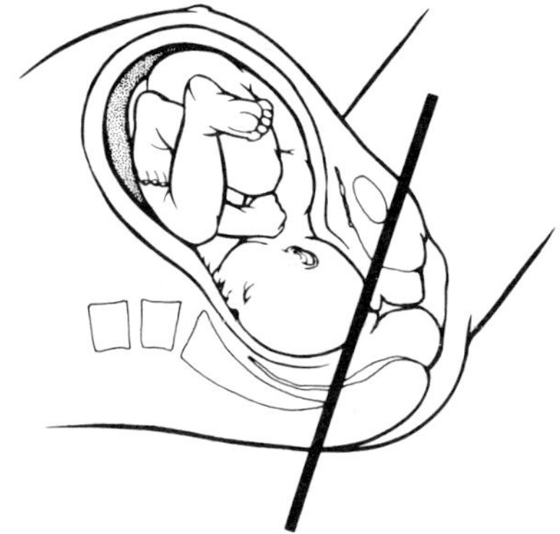

Figure 12.7
Relationship of organs in term vs. nonpregnant pelvis.

would be wanted, and certainly most are, but even in ideal circumstances, stress and ambivalence are present.

Much has been written about the emotional aspects of pregnancy both by nurses and by people in other disciplines (Deutsch, 1945; Caplan, 1961; Benedek, 1970; Rubin, 1970; Clark, 1978). The fact of pregnancy forces a confirmation of the sexual role of the woman. Regardless of the circumstances surrounding the coital act, she is faced either with assuming responsibility for the pregnancy and the child or with terminating the pregnancy. Either way the decision is difficult and sometimes frightening.

Pregnancy is similar to adolescence in that there is always ambivalence, and unresolved fears about feminity may reappear (Deutsch, 1945; Caplan, 1961). There is an increased need for love and attention from partner, family, friends, and others. There is often role conflict. The woman who has unresolved concerns about sexual role identification may have the potential for problems with mother–infant relationships. The woman who is pregnant for the first time often thinks: "This is what it was like when my mother carried me." She wonders about her own beginnings as well as about her child.

As pregnancy is a time for reordering interpersonal relationships for the mother, so too it is for the father. The woman becomes a mother; the man becomes a father; the parents become grandparents. Role identification may lead to feelings of rejection about the pregnancy and, in time, may decrease the quality of care giving following birth. On the other hand, pregnancy may epitomize the most tender and loving feelings and provide opportunities for psychosexual growth resulting in deeper and more meaningful relationships.

Caplan (1961) and LeMasters (1965) refer to pregnancy as a crisis. The term "crisis" carries with it certain characteristics such as social disorganization, decreased coping ability, increased tension, and feelings of helplessness (Rapoport, 1965). These characteristics may include cognitive confusion and even regressive behavior (Benedek, 1970). However, as with any crisis, the potential for a growth-promoting resolution is there, and it is to this end that the maternity nurse intervenes.

Crisis theory differentiates between developmental crisis and situational crisis (Aguilera & Messick, 1978). Examples of developmental crises are parenthood and death; these are expected or inevitable events. Situational crises, on the other hand, are unexpected such as the birth of a premature infant, alcoholism, or divorce. An event is categorized as a crisis when usual patterns of coping are not enough.

Pregnancy is somewhat in the "gray area" in that it certainly qualifies as a developmental crisis but can also border on a situational crisis as it requires shifting of roles and values. The couple who modifies the crisis of pregnancy to the growth-promoting experience will, it is hoped, learn new coping mechanisms, acquire new knowledge, and change and adapt interpersonal relationships. The woman resolving the crisis of pregnancy does it by calling upon her own style of coping as well as support from the culture in which she lives.

Resolving a crisis is work. Several theorists have classified this work into tasks that the woman must complete in order for the developmental crisis of pregnancy to be resolved successfully. Deutsch (1945), Bibring (1961), Caplan (1961), Tanner (1969), and Rubin (1970) have all described tasks or goals. A summary of these tasks gives us three major categories of work to be accomplished that can be related to the three trimesters of pregnancy.

- ▲ Acceptance of the pregnancy (first trimester)
- ▲ Acceptance of the child (second trimester)
- ▲ Assuring safe passage for herself and her child (third trimester)

One final category of work involves adoption of the role of "mother." In order for you to build on previously presented information, it is now useful to recall the work of Erik Erikson presented in Chapter 7. Erikson discusses stages to be mastered at different points in the life cycle and states that failure to master a particular stage may interfere with the ability to meet tasks* at a later stage. The implications for the nurse are tremendous. If the mother-to-be is an adolescent, how well has she mastered the tasks of adolescence? Is she still working on adolescent tasks? If so, anticipatory guidance and goal setting must incorporate the tasks of adolescence with those of pregnancy. The woman who is past 30 and is pregnant for the first time may project very different needs as she continues to master the tasks of young adulthood along with those of pregnancy. Each brings her unique self and her resolution or nonresolution of specific developmental tasks that must be considered by the nurse. Some suggest that the developmental tasks associated with Erikson's theory are not always appropriate. Experientially we know that each period of life has certain predictable challenges, mastery of which is growth promoting. It is with this philosophical understanding that the developmental theorists have provided much important knowledge on which professional nurses can base their practice.

The First Trimester

In a given word the first trimester can be characterized by "ambivalence." Regardless of planned or unplanned pregnancy, ambivalence always is present and has to be resolved. In a planned pregnancy, the couple may ask: "Was this really the right time?" "Why didn't we wait 6 more months?" The fact that she is pregnant requires that the woman doubt herself and her choice of time. In an unplanned pregnancy, ambivalence is somehow easier to comprehend. Feelings of loss of control abound. If she does want the baby, she is destined to experience pregnancy, labor, childbirth, and pain. She will never be just herself again. Adding to the psychologic stresses and role changes is the fact that her physical being is assaulted in many instances. She may be experiencing nausea and vomiting; she undoubtedly is tired; and although she may not be "sick" she may not feel "well." The woman must deal with the acceptance of pregnancy by those around her. What is the reaction of family and friends? Many women can recall years later the "good" friend who said to her at the time of her announcement of pregnancy, "You're kidding, why now or why you?" The support of significant others is crucial for the mother-to-be and allows her to go on to accomplish other tasks. The father realizes that if his partner is going to be a mother, he is going to be a father and also wonders if he is ready. His partner is becoming a mother, which makes him recall his mother. Parents relive their pregnancies, and mortality vs. immortality feelings are aroused.

Generation to generation, roles are shifted and realigned. The family prepares to admit a new member. By the sixteenth week of pregnancy, most women have resolved the ambivalence. If they have not, serious work with the help of professionals may be necessary for the mother, for if the pregnancy is not accepted, the implications for mother–infant attachment are serious.

The Second Trimester

The second trimester normally brings the most advantageous, positive, and outgoing time of pregnancy. Fetal movement is identified, the child becomes "real," and the beginning recognition of another person is initiated. Behaviors demonstrated by the woman accomplishing the second task are the placing of another's hand on her belly so someone else can feel the fetus. The mother dreams of how the infant will look. It is during this period that identification with her own mother is increased, and

*The first use of the concept of "task" in association with Erickson's theory is attributed to Robert Havighurst (1953).

if separated geographically, there is often an increase in letters or phone calls. If the relationship with her mother has not been close, attempts at reconciliation are not unusual. In the second trimester, some introversion begins that continues to increase during the third trimester. Sometimes the preoccupation with self confuses the mother-to-be as well as those around her. A formerly outgoing, giving person who becomes more passive and more interested in receiving may puzzle herself as well as significant others. Increasing dependency needs and introversion may cause fathers to feel shut out. Sexuality and sexual changes in pregnancy can be confusing to the partner, and the couple may need guidance from a professional (see Chapter 14). Fathers state that pregnancy brings about changes in almost every area of their lives, and although the stress may not be overwhelming, it does exist (Marquart, 1976). Nurses need to be careful that the health care setting does not exclude fathers by implication. Are there magazines and signs to welcome him as well as the mother? Is he included in the teaching about pregnancy? Parent education classes have done much to focus on the roles of both parents (see Chapter 15).

The task of the second trimester is accepting the child, and at this time the woman is usually receptive to learning about herself and her baby. However, the emotional lability of pregnancy—mood swings—is evident and the woman can vacillate from being an outgoing, talkative, and interested person to being a withdrawn person quite unexpectedly. Some of this lability is hormonally based, but the fact remains that the woman is sensitive and at times irritable. The openness of the woman in general and her talkativeness, which is evident at this time, provide an opportunity for the nurse to help the mother with her task. The mother's-to-be primary work, that of accepting the child, requires the reordering of relationships, as mentioned before, and for this reason people and interests related to the pregnancy are most important.

The Third Trimester

A sense of vulnerability and concern for herself and her child becomes a focus in the latter part of pregnancy. It is not unusual for the woman to express these safety concerns when flying or riding in an automobile or even when home as evidenced by checking the locks on the doors more carefully. Evidence that she has accepted the child is demonstrated in the care-giving activities she plans, for example, preparing the baby's room and deciding what she will feed the baby. Acceptance of the infant by other family members and siblings is important to her, and she may spend considerable time preparing others for the arrival. By preparing a physical place for the new arrival, she is ultimately preparing an emotional place.

At the end of the pregnancy, in particular, the woman becomes more clumsy and awkward; body boundaries are difficult. For example, in the grocery store, she may bump into the grocery cart or displays or be unable to reach an item because of her size. This awkwardness does not contribute to self-esteem, and by the end of the pregnancy, the woman has come full circle, again displaying ambivalence, anxiety, and eagerness for the pregnancy to end. She is tired of being pregnant in most cases and wants the child but fears birth.

Women have shared how carefully they have planned for other family members "in case something should happen." At this time she is unsure that the father wants the baby; the father wants his wife back whom he feels he has lost to the child. Only open communication between the couple and sharing of feelings will assure them of each other's wishes. Stimulating an open discussion in pregnancy is often the role of the nurse. The nurse can share examples of feelings and promote the environment that says, "It's okay to have these feelings—feelings are legitimate."

The last month brings together the accomplishment of the three tasks—accepting the pregnancy, accepting the child, and providing safe passage for her child and the mother. In most cases, the pregnant woman has sought and received help in preparing herself and her child for this event. If the work has gone well and the tasks have been accomplished, labor will proceed well and the next step, that of mothering, will be carried out. The professional nurse working with the pregnant mother and her supportive others uses two main strategies that are discussed both directly and indirectly throughout this chapter. The nurse must have an understanding of the physiologic and psychosocial changes occurring in order to provide anticipatory guidance to the pregnant woman and her supportive others. Two things—a framework of knowledge (including the physiologic and psychosocial changes occurring) and strategies for providing anticipatory guidance—are keys to successful intervention.

MINOR DISCOMFORTS OF PREGNANCY AND NURSING IMPLICATIONS

In the antepartum period minor discomforts occur that are not serious but do cause physical discomfort with concurrent emotional concern. The overall nursing goal is to teach the patient strategies by which she can manage and combat or ideally prevent discomforts. A discussion of the discomforts, system by system, follows, but it is important for the nurse to remember that any complaint that persists warrants further medical assessment.

Gastrointestinal Discomforts

Nausea and vomiting in early pregnancy is probably the most common complaint, occurring in 50% of pregnancies (Ziegel, 1978). Usually this disappears by the fourteenth week of gestation (Huff, 1979). Symptoms can vary from waves of nausea to persistent and frequent vomiting. Time of day can also vary; some women complain of nausea upon awakening in the morning (morning sickness) while others complain of nausea around suppertime. Undoubtedly, there are both physiologic and psychologic factors; the hormones of pregnancy can contribute to this disturbance, but evidence indicates that tension or emotional factors also play a role. Adequate rest and relaxation, therefore, are an important part of the treatment. Some relief may be obtained by eating small meals more frequently. For early morning nausea, eating dry crackers or toast without liquids first thing upon awakening seems to help. If the woman perceives a pattern to her bouts of nausea, planning to eat 30 minutes earlier seems to help.

Heartburn occurs more often late in pregnancy and is probably related to terminal esophagitis. The reflux, or bubbling back of stomach contents into the lower esophagus, causes a burning sensation in the stomach or in the back of the throat. Usually smaller and more frequent meals are helpful. Sometimes antacids are prescribed. When antacids are used, aluminum hydroxide or magnesium tricilicate may be prescribed; antacids containing sodium (sodium barconbonate, or baking soda) should be avoided as excess sodium intake can affect water balance.

Flatulence, the presence of excessive gas in the stomach or intestine, is fairly common in pregnancy and rather uncomfortable. It is in part a result of bacterial action in the intestines; the decreased peristalsis that occurs in pregnancy contributes to flatulence. Regular bowel habits and avoidance of foods that are gas forming such as cabbage, corn, and fried foods are helpful strategies.

Constipation, another common complaint, can relate to insufficient fluid intake or the deferring of bowel movements. In pregnancy, relaxation of the smooth muscle of the bowel contributes to the problem of constipation; the woman who has a problem before pregnancy is prone to a problem during pregnancy. The intake of fruits, whole grain breads and cereals, and abundant fluids is important. Regular exercise is helpful. Laxatives should be avoided; they may be used in severe instances and then by prescription only.

Genitourinary Complaints

Complaints of urinary frequency are expressed by nearly all pregnant women. Because asymptomatic urinary tract infection is so common, careful questioning and assessment by the nurse is important. Collect data about the frequency of urination, dysuria (painful urination), or hematuria (blood in the urine). Although these symptoms may lead the nurse to suspect urinary tract infection, the diagnosis is based on urinalysis and culture. The loss of urine during coughing, sneezing, or straining is common in multiparous women in the last trimester of pregnancy. This is a good time to remind women of the importance of practicing their Kegel's exercise (Fig. 12.8). When urinating, if the woman can stop her stream and then let it resume, she is contracting the correct muscles. Some childbirth educators compare doing Kegel's exercise of contracting your muscles around the vagina and urethra with holding your breath when going up in an elevator. This mental imagery is sometimes a very useful way to assist the woman in practicing this exercise.

Increased vaginal discharge as a result of the increased amount of cervical mucous at the introitus is another normal part of pregnancy. Usually the white, yellowish discharge is of no significance, and the patient is instructed in good hygiene techniques including regular bathing, rinsing the vulva with warm water after urinating, wearing panties that are all cotton or with a cotton crotch (more absorbent and allows for better air circulation), and sitting in a tub of warm water (sitz bath). If the vaginal dis-

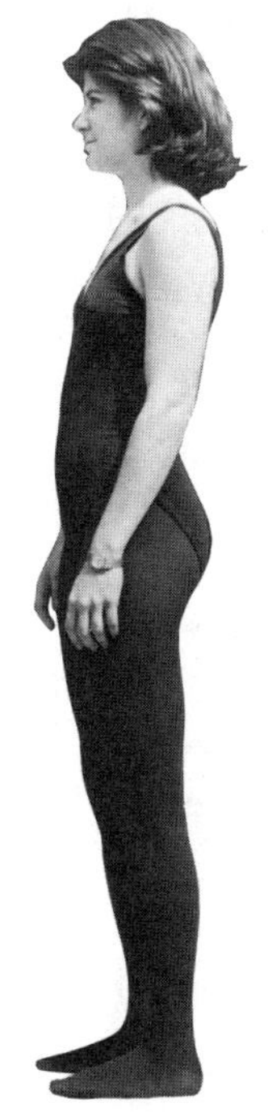

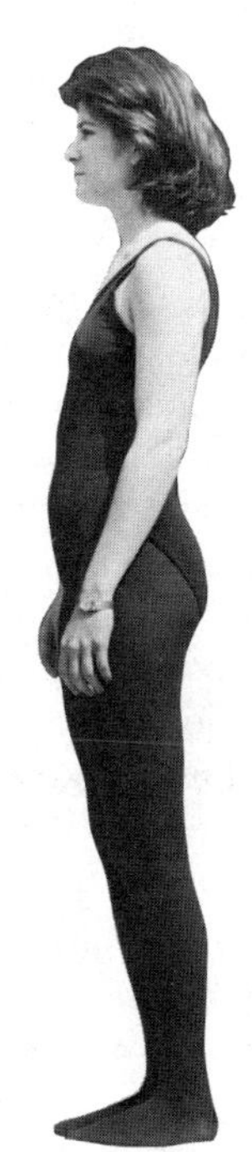

Figure 12.8
Kegel's exercise. *Top:* Tighten vaginal and pelvic muscles and hold for count of 3; *bottom:* relax.

charge becomes profuse and is accompanied by itching or burning, infection is suspected. Commonly encountered vaginal infections and nursing implications are listed in Table 12.1.

Musculoskeletal Discomforts

Backache associated with the increased lumbar lordosis is common among pregnant women. Backache is more severe if abdominal muscle tone is poor as this causes increased strain at the sacroiliac joints. Along with increased lordosis, there is increased kyphosis of the dorsal spine and a thrusting forward of the head and neck. This adds to abdominal muscle strain as well as to long back muscle strain. Instruction in proper body mechanics and good posture is critical. Bending with one knee flexed and keeping the back straight is important. Soaking and relaxing in a warm tub relieves tension and muscle strain. If the lordosis is severe, a maternity girdle to lift the protuberant abdomen may help. If the patient complains of backache in the morning (after sleeping), a firmer mattress may be needed. Wearing shoes with approximately the same heel most of the time is also a good idea since shifting from high heels to low heels can contribute to backache. Exercises to tone muscles, particularly squatting, tailor sitting, and pelvic rock, can help prevent backache. When squatting, the bending should take place at the hips, the back kept straight, and the feet apart and turned slightly outward. Tailor sitting (Fig. 12.9) can be used during some activities such as preparing vegetables or talking on the phone. Pelvic rocking can be done standing, lying down, or on all fours (Fig. 12.10). Since pelvic rocking on all fours can overstrain the muscle of the back, the standing or lying down method is preferred. It is very important to make certain that activities that have to be done (ironing, dishes, desk work) are performed at a convenient level to prevent back strain.

Increase in round ligament pain or lower abdominal or groin pain while walking is common. This is because of the stretching of the ligaments as the uterus enlarges; rest or a change of position usually relieves this pain.

Insomnia, particularly in late pregnancy, is frequently related to musculoskeletal changes. The mother's-to-be large abdomen and active fetus often result in restless sleep. Any tricks or procedures that facilitate sleep can be tried. For example, warm milk, a backrub with a soothing lotion, or a warm bath

TABLE 12.1
VAGINAL INFECTIONS IN PREGNANCY

Condition (Agent)	*Predisposing Factors*	*Symptoms*	*Diagnosis (Dx) Treatment (Rx)*	*Nursing Implications*
Monilia vulvovaginitis *(Candida albicans)*	Pregnancy itself Broad spectrum antibiotics Steroid medications Diabetes	Reddened excoriated vulva "Cottage cheese" discharge from vagina (white, curdy, nonfoul) Vaginal itching	Dx—Microscopic Rx—Nystatin (Mycostatin) Vaginal suppositories No oral mycostatin because of poor GI absorption 1% gentian violet solution (paint the vulva) Other drugs sometimes used are miconazole nitrate (Monistat), candicidin (Vanobid), clotrimazole (Gyne-Lotrimin)	Tell patient not to douche while being treated Gentian violet can stain clothing
Trichomonas vaginitis *(Trichomonas vaginalis)*	Passed between sexual partners	Marked discharge, frothy, yellow-green, malodorous Vaginal and vulvar itching and burning	Dx—Wet smear (microscope) Cervix has "flea-bitten appearance" because of punctate hemorrhage Rx—Metronidazole (Flagyl) contraindicated first trimester; AVC or Sultrin vaginal cream	Note trimester of pregnancy Emphasize good hygiene techniques
Vaginitis (nonspecific) *Hemophilus* Corynebacterium Vaginalis Probably mixed infection	Pregnancy itself (increased glycogen content of vaginal epithelium)	Discharge, itching, burning	Dx—Made when trichimonas and monilia ruled out Rx—douching	Douching lying down in bathtub on doctor's order only—teaching specifics important Ex: No high fluid pressure; bag no higher than 2 ft above hips; nozzle inserted no more than 3 in; no hand bulb syringes
Gonorrheal infection *(Neisseria gonorrhoeae)*	Lower socioeconomic status Sexual transmission Promiscuity	Cervicitis Pelvic inflammatory disease (PID) Purulent cervicovaginal discharge Genital itching Dysuria	Dx—Culture Rx—Penicillin, ampicillin	7–10 days after antibiotic treatment patient should have cultures Sexual partners should also be treated *(Tetracycline contraindicated in pregnancy)*

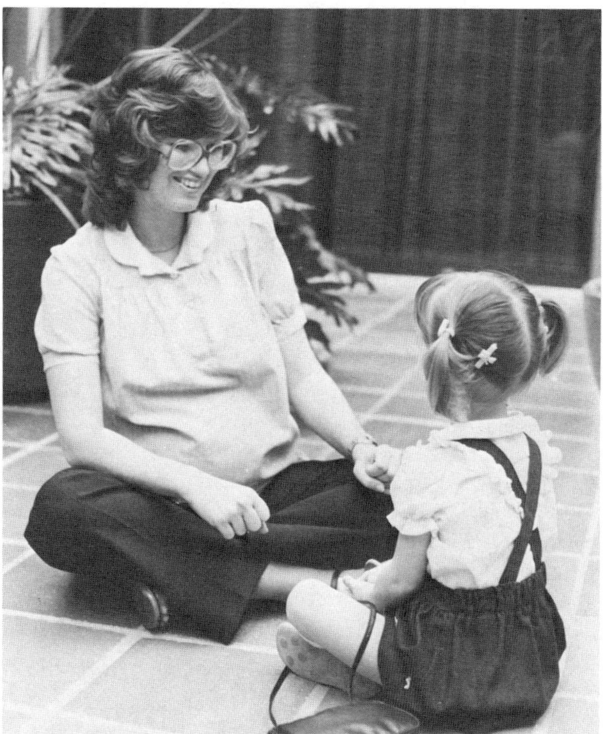

Figure 12.9
Tailor sitting.

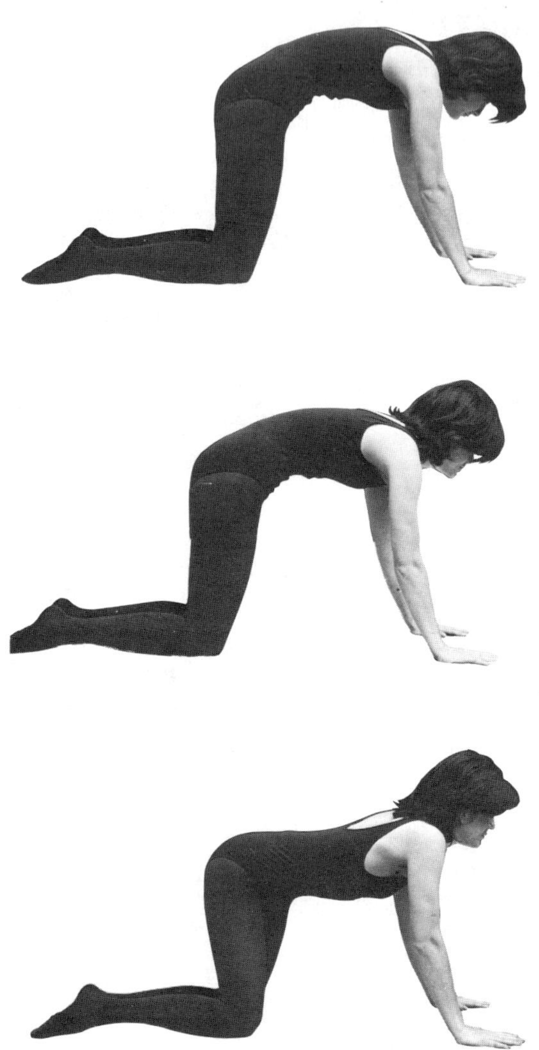

Figure 12.10
Pelvic tilt. *Top:* On hands and knees; *middle:* arching back like a cat; *bottom:* holding pelvic tilt position, wag your behind from side to side, on each side, hold for a count of 5.

may provide relaxation as well as the closeness that the woman needs from her partner (see Chapter 14). Practicing relaxation techniques taught in prenatal class and positioning with pillows may also help (Fig. 12.11). Recall that marked fatigue is a common complaint in early pregnancy because of hormonal change, and this fatigue often recurs in the later pregnancy. Regular periods of exercise and rest throughout the day are helpful in counteracting lost sleep at night.

Cardiovascular Changes

The cardiovascular changes occurring in the antepartum period underlie several of the most common complaints—varicose veins, hemorrhoids, swollen feet, cramps in the legs, and shortness of breath. Varicose veins of the lower extremities, which are permanently dilated portions of the saphenous system along with the veins communicating with the deep (femoral) system, are not unique to pregnancy. They are in part the result of congenital absence of valves in the walls of the veins and are thereby familial (Gibbs & Gibbs, 1979). Dilation of these veins as a result of pregnancy can be seen as early as the tenth week; the patient complains of aching in the calf and thigh, which is worse when standing or sitting. This problem usually worsens as pregnancy advances. The nurse is concerned not only with reducing the symptoms but with preventing further dilation and with detecting thrombophlebitis (inflammation of a vein). For this reason, pain should be assessed at each visit. Further dilation can be decreased by wearing full-length elastic stockings (TED hose) if the veins are in the

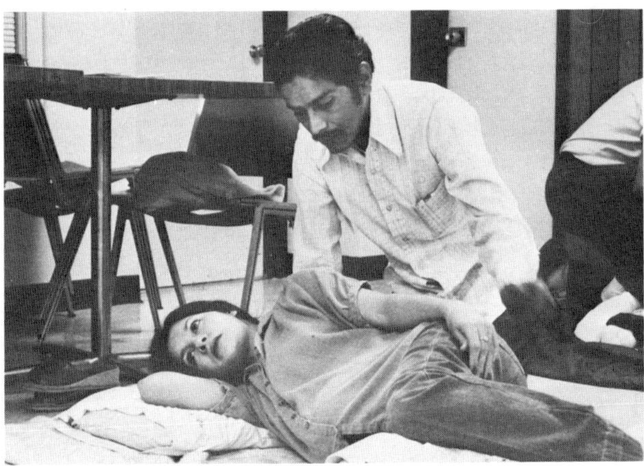

Figure 12.11
Relaxation using position and pillows.

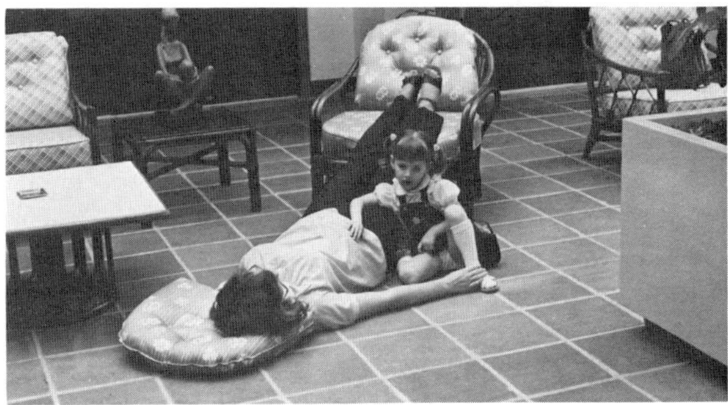

Figure 12.12
Legs elevated at a 45 degree angle.

extremities. Vulvar varicosities are more difficult to compress, and special leotards can be fitted for the patient with severe problems involving the vulva or areas high on the thighs. The best way to relieve the discomfort of varicose veins is for the patient to get off her feet and put her legs up, but this is not always possible. In general, the patient should be advised that walking is better than standing still, that when sitting to put her feet up, and that when she must be on her feet for extended periods of time, to lie down three or four times a day for 5–10 minutes with her legs elevated at a 45 degree angle (Fig. 12.12). This position improves drainage, reduces the varicosities, and lessens aching of the legs. An angle greater than 45 degrees can compress vessels in the groin and interfere with venous return.

Hemorrhoids, or varicosities of the rectum, appear during pregnancy because of vascular engorgement in the pelvis and constipation. Hemorrhoids may cause itching, pain, and bleeding. If the patient notices a lump at the anus, relief can be provided by gently pushing the hemorrhoid back into the rectum. Treatment is aimed at preventing constipation and straining during defecation. Warm sitz baths for 10–15 minutes may relieve the pain and itching. Lying down with the hips elevated on a pillow or cool compresses are other relief measures. When severe hemorrhoids occur, the physician may prescribe topical ointments, creams, or suppositories. Usually hemorrhoids improve markedly after delivery.

Swelling of the feet and lower extremities occurs because of impairment of venous return. The best treatment is for the woman to lie down in a lateral position, which improves venous return and mobilizes fluid from the tissues to the circulatory system. Salt restriction for physiologic edema of pregnancy is not appropriate as it interfers with the normal sodium balance in pregnancy. Depending on the woman's activity, dependent edema in the latter part of the antepartum period can be normal; the nurse, however, needs to be alert to the fact that it can also be a symptom of toxemia of pregnancy and needs to check the woman for other signs of toxemia (see Chapter 21).

Cramps in the legs, which can be strong and painful, occur late in pregnancy. Although the cause is undetermined, it seems to be related to a disturbance in the serum calcium/phosphorous ratio. One treatment is using antacid gels after meals, which decreases phosphorous absorption and restores balance. Other factors that seem to prevent leg cramping are wearing proper shoes and elevating the legs when sitting. Relief of a leg cramp once it occurs is usually found by standing up or extending the leg and dorsiflexing the foot.

Shortness of breath as a result of crowding of the diaphragm can be very bothersome in the later stages of the pregnancy. Lying down compounds the problem so that being propped up on pillows or in a chair is suggested. As mentioned earlier, pregnant women are prone to breathlessness because of increased sensitivity of the respiratory center to the carbon dioxide of the blood. Inspiration, you will recall, is triggered at a lower P_{CO_2} level than when nonpregnant. Often breathlessness will be relieved if the woman lies on her back and raises her arms above her head as this allows for maximum expansion of the thoracic cavity. When lightening occurs (Chapter 16) and the baby descends into the pelvis, pressure on the diaphragm decreases and shortness of breath is lessened.

Supine hypotensive syndrome is mentioned under physiologic changes, but it is also important to remember that this is a cardiovascular-related problem. Again, relief is afforded by turning on the side. The woman who suffers from supine hypotensive syndrome (faintness) needs to be taught that before getting up she should roll quickly to her side for a few minutes, sit up slowly on the side of the bed, and then stand.

It is important for the nurse to realize that many women have few if any of the minor discomforts listed, and when they do experience some they are able to compensate for them. On the other hand, the nurse's knowledge base needs to be complete in order to intervene with each woman appropriately.

PRENATAL CARE

As soon as the woman thinks she is pregnant, an appointment with a physician or certified nurse-midwife should be made. We will define prenatal (or antenatal) care as medical, nursing, and related assistance rendered to mother or unborn child before the onset of labor. According to Huff and Pauerstein (1979), for prenatal care to be judged adequate, it should begin before the twentieth week of pregnancy. The goals of prenatal care are to identify early, prevent, or treat complications, to detect and treat medical–surgical conditions *arising from* the pregnancy or *existing before* the pregnancy, and to prepare the family for birth. Data collection involves three main areas—the health history, the physical examination, and laboratory screening procedures.

The Health History

The purpose of the health history is to determine the physical and mental status of the woman. There are several excellent texts on health history and physical examination; this chapter mainly includes the areas of data collection relevant in maternity nursing.

As with any interview, the surroundings should be pleasant and comfortable and the mother-to-be should know that her partner or other supportive person is welcome if it will make her feel more comfortable. The "set" that is given by the nurse is critical to the validity of the data. For example, the patient must be made aware of the fact that information is being requested in order to provide the best health care possible for her and her baby and that the information is confidential and must be assured that if she wishes to rest at any point or not elaborate on a specific topic, she is free to say so. In other words, the object is for the nurse to be honest and open so that the information the health professional receives is as accurate as possible. Opportunities for teaching often occur during the health history and data collection process.

HEALTH BEFORE CONCEPTION (NONOBSTETRIC)

Information is elicited about previous health events that might affect this pregnancy. Information obtained is in relation to childhood illnesses, surgery, hospitalizations, drug allergies, and medications. The goals at this time are to collect information about medical–surgical conditions that might affect this pregnancy, to be alert to any teratogenic effects that either prescription or nonprescription, legal or illegal drugs might have, and to gain insight into the woman's previous experience with hospitalization and pain. Coping mechanisms of the woman can often be identified in relation to health and illness before conception. It is common during this portion of the history to gain knowledge about the woman's general health habits and practices.

MENSTRUAL HISTORY

Areas of assessment included here are time of onset of *menarche* (onset of first menses); regularity, interval, and flow length; *dysmenorrhea* (painful menstruation) or other complications; date of the last menstrual period (LMP) and, if this was abnormal, date of the previous menstrual period. The first day of the LMP is important for calculating the estimated day of delivery (EDD).

OBSTETRIC HISTORY

Past Pregnancy History. Many clues or insights into potential problems can be learned from past pregnancies. The number of pregnancies or abortions the mother has had, the interval between pregnancies, and birth weights and current health of her children are all relevant and important parts of the health history. A question such as "Did you have any trouble during your pregnancy or during labor?" may prompt information about problems during the pregnancy. Such things as pre-eclampsia, eclampsia, neonatal deaths, hypertension, and bleeding or the need for transfusion are all significant data. If the delivery was forceps or cesarean birth, the type of forceps delivery and the type of cesarean birth (see Chapter 22) should be recorded.

Many times the history of past pregnancies tends to focus on those things that were unpleasant; therefore special attention should be given to obtaining information about positive aspects of past pregnancies. Some review of how the family adapted last time may assist the woman with her developmental tasks at this time.

Some words requires definition before further discussion of the health history.

gravid—pregnancy regardless of duration

para—past pregnancies that continued to viability (capable of living outside the uterus)

primigravida—a woman pregnant for the first time

multigravida—a woman who is in her second or any subsequent pregnancy

nullipara (para 0)—woman who has not borne a viable child

primipara (para 1)—woman who has given birth to one viable child (this term is commonly used incorrectly when the woman is actually a primigravida)

multipara (para II, III, IV, etc.)—woman who has given birth to two or more viable children (again often used incorrectly and applied to the woman who is in her second pregnancy or labor)

parturient—a woman in labor

Several systems are used to record childbearing history. In the two-digit gravida, para system (G_P_), the G stands for gravida and the digit is the total number of pregnancies including the current one. The P stands for para and the digit includes all deliveries following 20 weeks gestation. Sometimes, a third item, Ab, is added to account for abortions. The three-digit system would be G_P_Ab_. There is also a four- and five-digit system. The four-digit system includes P____ and represents a number system that gives the nurse a quick review of past pregnancies. The four digits after the P represent

- ▲ Term deliveries (greater than 37 weeks or greater than 2,500 gm)
- ▲ Premature deliveries (20–36 weeks or 500 to 2,500 gm)
- ▲ Abortions (less than 20 weeks or less than 500 gm)
- ▲ Living children

The five-digit system is the same as the four-digit system except it adds a first number that represents the total number of pregnancies (total of second, third, fourth digits) excluding the present one. Multiple gestations, ectopic pregnancies, and fetal deaths should be noted specifically in the recorded history.

Also included in the past pregnancy history besides the sex, weight and gestational age of the infant, is the neonatal course and present health of the child. Similarly, along with the course of previous pregnancy, one should include data about labor and the postpartum period.

Present Pregnancy History. There are several aspects of the present history that are background information as well as relevant to the current pregnancy. For example, the nurse should ask if there are any twins or disorders, such as, diabetes, cancer, or hypertension, that run in the family. Social history should include demographic data and occupational and mental history. What are the sources of economic and psychologic support? Single-parent as well as nuclear families should have an opportunity to discuss options important to them such as adoption, child care, and available state, federal, or private assistance. The availability of community agencies to meet their needs or to enrich the childbearing experience, for example with childbirth education classes, should be explored. If abortion information is requested early in a pregnancy, the information should be provided.

Nutrition History. A 24-hour diet history elicited by "Tell me what you eat in a typical day," or "Take yesterday for an example and describe what you ate," will give the nurse some clues to nutritional teaching that needs to be introduced, reinforced, or praised. Starting with what the patient generally eats in a 24-hour period and then adapting or correcting for the nutrition needs of pregnancy is much more effective than handing the woman a diet plan (see nutrition history form in appendix). It also demonstrates application of teaching–learning principles in that you are moving from the simple to the complex and building on existing knowledge before introducing new material. During the nutrition history, the nurse is alert to information that might suggest inadequate caloric intake, iron deficiency, vitamin C or protein deficiency, fad foods or pica (see "Nutrition during Pregnancy" in this chapter).

FAMILY PLANNING

Past contraceptive practices as well as future plans for child spacing should be discussed and recorded. Contraceptive failures should be noted. "Planned" vs. "unplanned" pregnancies should be explored, bearing in mind that an unplanned pregnancy is not necessarily an unwanted pregnancy. If sterilization is requested, counseling and discussion of this option can be done in the antepartum period (see Chapter 26).

Needless to say, not all the information required in the health history can be collected on the initial visit, in part because it is time consuming. It is also true that as the nurse begins to collect information in sensitive areas unless trust has been established, which is often difficult to accomplish in one meeting, much of the needed information will not be shared. For this reason, a systematic data collection is begun, which is then supplemented and validated on subsequent visits.

The Physical Examination

Initially baseline data such as, blood pressure, pulse, temperature, respiratory rate, and height are collected and if possible compared with prepregnancy values. Weight should include present and usual nonpregnant weight. The basic guideline for normal nonpregnant weight is 100 lb (45 kg) for a woman 60 in (5 ft or 150 cm) tall. Add 5 pounds (2.5 kg) for each inch over 60 in and subtract 5 pounds for each inch under 60 in (Gibbs & Gibbs, 1979). Variations of less than 10% are insignificant, although this guideline will probably underestimate appropriate weight of a woman who is over 68 in. A further discussion of weight gain in pregnancy is included in the nutritional section later in the chapter.

The physical exam proceeds from head to toe, including extremities, and assessment includes all of the visible physiologic adaptations discussed earlier in the chapter. Head, skin, and scalp should include pregnancy-induced spider nevus, chloasma, and stretch marks. Head, eyes, ears, nose, and throat (HEENT) would pay particular attention to any need for eye or dental referral. Chest examination would include breast exam (see Chapters 9 and 26) and heart and lung auscultation.

Abdominal assessment includes skin assessment (careful to note and record surgical scars) and palpation of the uterus. Fundal height is measured at each visit with a centimeter tape measure and is recorded. Fetal heart tones are assessed; they can be heard at 10–12 weeks gestation with a doptone. Once the uterus is at the umbilicus or above, they can be auscultated with a fetoscope (head stethoscope). Any other palpable masses should be noted. Fetal parts can usually be identified after 27 weeks. Areas of concern would be if the nurse is unable to hear fetal heart tones after 20 weeks or if the uterus seems large or small for estimated gestational age (see Fig. 12.2).

Extremity assessment includes noting any muscle or joint tenderness, edema, and deep tendon reflexes (usually noted by eliciting the knee jerk reflex). The two areas of concern are varicosities (see page 2) and edema. Remember that pretibial edema is usually normal, but pitting edema above the ankle or of the foot (behind the toes) is of concern.

Pelvic exam is discussed fully in Chapters 9 and 26, but the antepartum nurse needs to assess the vulva, vagina, and cervix and note any varicosities, lesions, scars, or congenital anomalies. If signs of inflammation are noted (redness, swelling, tenderness, heat) or if vaginal discharge is profuse, wet smears with saline and 10% potassium hydroxide (KOH) are done to determine causative organism. The cervix is assessed for lesions or dilation and effacement; there should be no effacement noted earlier than 30 weeks. Scars on the cervix from previous pregnancies (commonly noted at the 3 or 9 o'clock positions) should be recorded. Many times a culture for gonorrhea and a Pap smear are also done during the physical examination. The junction of the cervix and the corpus (isthmus) softens during the sixth or seventh week of pregnancy, and this softening is known as Hegar's sign. By 16 weeks the ovaries and fallopian tubes are in the lower abdomen and can be palpated on abdominal exam. Note that clinical pelvimetry, estimation of dimensions of the pelvic outlet by physical examination, is uncomfortable for the patient and not recommended as routine in antepartal care. When the patient is admitted for labor, pelvic examination can be done with greater usefulness and less discomfort; pelvic size and shape are not important in decision making before the beginning of labor. Since we support this view in the management of pregnant women, clinical pelvimetry is not included in this chapter; it can be found in any standard obstetric text. Pelvic dimensions and their significance are given in Chapter 4. The point needs to be made, however, that in some areas where access to technology is difficult or impossible, clinical assessment of the pelvic dimensions may still be done. This assessment should not be performed in early pregnancy, however, and even when done in the later pregnancy, the data are inconclusive.

Laboratory Screening Procedures

Some laboratory tests are necessary for all maternity patients; they are listed here along with significant areas of concern for the nurse.

COMPLETE BLOOD COUNT

Identification of anemia (decrease in red blood cells, hematocrit, or hemoglobin), leukocytosis (increase in white blood cells), leukopenia (decrease in white blood cells), and eosinophilia (excessive, medium-sized leukocytes) is important. Blood count is taken at the initial visit, and hematocrit and hemoglobin are reassessed in the second trimester and again at 36 or 37 weeks, just before delivery. Women whose hematocrit is 34% or above at 28 weeks (hemoglobin above 11 gm/100 ml) rarely become anemic. Hematocrit value can provide information about hidden bleeding or malabsorption of or failure to take iron. Normal values in pregnancy should *not* be lower than hemoglobin 11 mg/100 ml or hematocrit 33%. White blood cell count varies from 5,000 to 15,000/cm. More than five eosinophils per 100 white blood cells is excessive; eosinophilia is seen in allergic states

BLOOD TYPING

Both ABO and Rh blood typing are done to detect rare group and to be alerted to potential antigen–antibody problems. Occasionally, a maternal fetal blood incompatibility will occur. A screening test can be done to determine if maternal antibodies that can be destructive to fetal red blood cells have been formed causing a condition called hemolytic disease of the newborn, also known as erythroblastosis fetalis (see Chapter 23).

RUBELLA SCREEN (HEMAGGLUTINATION INHIBITION, HAI)

A rubella titer is done by serologic exam, and if the titer is greater than 1:8 (or 1:10) the patient can be reasurred that she is immuned. If no antibody is present, the woman is offered rubella vaccine the day after delivery providing she will avoid pregnancy for 90 days. This cannot be given while pregnant as this is a live viral vaccine that is teratogenic.

SEROLOGY

A serology test for syphilis is done at the time of the first visit so that if syphilis is present it can be treated, it is hoped, before the fetus is affected.

URINALYSIS AND URINE CULTURE

A clean catch (cleansing the urethra and labia before voiding) midstream specimen is obtained and examined microscopically. Normal urine examined very soon after being obtained contains no casts, bacteria, sugar, or protein. Up to five WBCs per high-powered microscopic field is considered normal. Urine tests are done in order to assess acute or chronic kidney disease. Since asymptomatic bacteriuria (no symptoms) is common in pregnancy, urine culture is important. Criteria for diagnosing asymptomatic bacteriuria is more than 100,000 col/ml of a pathogen in a patient who is symptomfree. When diagnosed, the patient is usually treated with antibodies to prevent serious urinary tract disease, and a follow-up culture is done.

CERVICAL SMEARS

Cervical smears were mentioned in the section on physical examination. They include smear for gonorrhea and a Papanicolaou (Pap) smear. The former requires treatment with antibiotics; Pap smear is done to detect atypical cells. This is a general part of women's health care and is discussed fully in Chapter 27.

CHEST X-RAY EXAMINATION

Chest x-ray examination is no longer necessary for many Americans but should be done if tuberculosis or other lung disorders are suspected. A chest x-ray study should not be done before the second trimester; abdominal shielding should always be used.

After the data from the health history, physical examination, and laboratory screening are collected and analyzed, a diagnosis is made and plan for care established. Some nurse clinical specialists make the plan independently, confer with a physician colleague, and then discuss management and goals of prenatal care with the woman and her supportive other (Fig. 12.13). At this time, if a risk pregnancy is confirmed, or suspected, other data is collected and appropriate management instituted (see Unit Five, "Reproductive Risk").

NURSING MANAGEMENT—ANTEPARTUM

The general pattern of care for the woman in the antepartum period following the initial visit, is visiting her physician, midwife, or clinical specialist once a month through the first 28 weeks of pregnancy, twice a month from 28 to 36 weeks of gestation, and once a week thereafter. For the woman who is seen in the first trimester, this would mean approximately 12–14 visits.

At each visit, the minimum information to be collected would include a record of any health events since the last visit specifically infections, trauma, or anxieties. If complaints or anxieties are expressed, the nurse should have the woman elaborate on each one. Often this is accomplished by the *who, what, where,* and *when* kind of questions. For example, if the woman is concerned about being unable to sleep, the nurse could ask, When does this happen? Every night? Once a week? What do you do just before you go to sleep? Who is aware of this problem? Who else sleeps in the home with you? Where do you sleep? In general, avoid "why" questions as patients who are anxious cannot usually tell you why. Using who, what, where, and when will allow the patient to see the relationship of events and their significance to her pregnancy and will encourage her to participate in problem solving. For the most part, complaints should be described in the patient's own words. Besides the interval history, a review of problems or concerns noted at the last visit is done and any data, such as laboratory results, that have been added is reviewed with the patient.

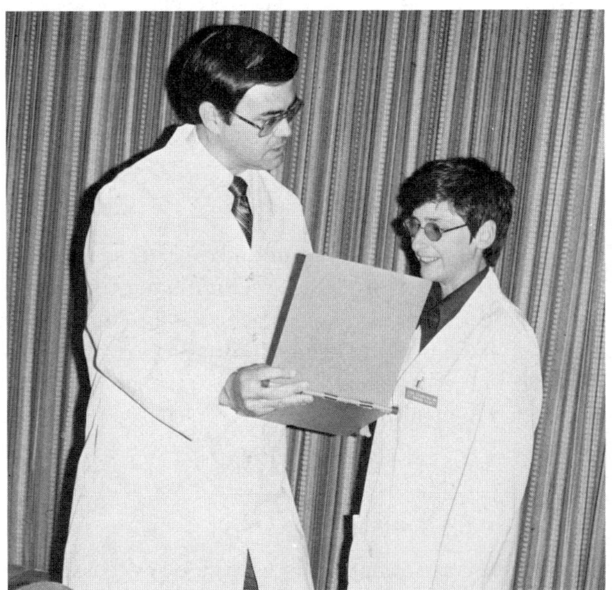

Figure 12.13
Prenatal care is provided by more than one person.

Physical examination on each visit includes blood pressure, weight, and abdominal examination. In general, a weight gain of approximately 4–10 lb trimester-by-trimester is normal. It is important to note that the woman should gain at least 10 lb the first 20 weeks to ensure adequate fetal growth. Blood pressure should be taken in the same position on the same arm each visit, and any significant changes in diastolic (15 mm) or systolic (30 mm) should be noted (see Chapter 21).

The abdominal examination includes measurement of the uterine fundus above the symphysis using a centimeter tape measure and determination of the presence and location of fetal heart tones. The assessment may be made by doptone or fetoscope. After the twenty-eighth week, Leopold's maneuvers should be done. The method and significance of findings are described in Table 12.2 and illustrated in Figure 12.14.

Extremities (legs) are assessed for edema (pretibial, ankle, and foot), and deep tendon reflex (knee jerk) is assessed. Any varicosities or lesions are described. The problem list or plans from the last visit is reviewed and evaluated and new goals established. Any other observations or concerns initiated by the patient are explored.

Laboratory data collected each visit include examination of urine for albumin and sugar; this is usually done using a dipstick. Complete urinalysis or culture should be done if needed.

During the antepartum period, there are significant landmarks that need to be recorded.

- ▲ ***20 Weeks.*** Fetal heart rate should be heard by head stethoscope in 90% of patients weighing under 175 lb at about 20 weeks. If the heart beat is not heard at that visit, the patient should be rescheduled for a visit 1 week later.
- ▲ ***28 Weeks.*** Hemoglobin and hematocrit tests should be done.
- ▲ ***34 Weeks.*** Repeat hematocrit and hemoglobin and test for syphilis (VDRL).

TABLE 12.2
LEOPOLD'S MANEUVERS

Maneuver Number	*Purpose of Maneuver*	*Position of Examiner*	*Description of Procedure*	*Expected Physical Findings*
1	To determine which fetal pole occupies fundus of uterus (head or buttocks)	Facing the patient as she lies in dorsal position	Using entire tactile surface of fingers of both hands to upper abdomen, palpate the outline of the part of the fetus that occupies the fundus of the uterus.	The head is round, firm, smooth, and movable (ballotable) between the two hands. If breech, the examiner feels a softer, more pointed, and not ballottable shaped body.
2	To locate baby's back and small parts (elbows and knees) in relation to mother's right or left side	Facing the patient as she lies in dorsal position	Slide hands down to a lower position on abdomen than in maneuver No. 1, exerting firm, even pressure with palmar surfaces of both hands.	Back is felt as smooth, convex curve that offers resistance. The small parts (hands, feet, elbows, knees) feel like irregular lumps. Motion of extremities may be felt.
3	To confirm findings of maneuver No. 1 To determine if presenting part is floating or not	Facing the patient as she lies in dorsal position	Spread thumb and fingers of one hand as wide as possible just above symphysis pubis. Then bring thumb and fingers together to grasp part of fetus lying between them.	Identify head or breech. Head will be identified as hard round mass. If engaged, presenting part may be difficult to palpate. If lower pole is movable, engagement has not occurred.
4	To locate cephalic prominence, determine flexion, and discover how far presenting part has descended into pelvis	Facing the patient's feet	Place tips of fingers on each side of the midline on lower abdomen. Exert pressure downward in direction of birth canal using gliding motion as hands proceed downward.	The fingers on one side will be stopped by the cephalic prominence, while the fingers of the other hand will continue downward. A cephalic prominence on same side as small parts is the brow, indicating flexed head and that presentation is vertex.

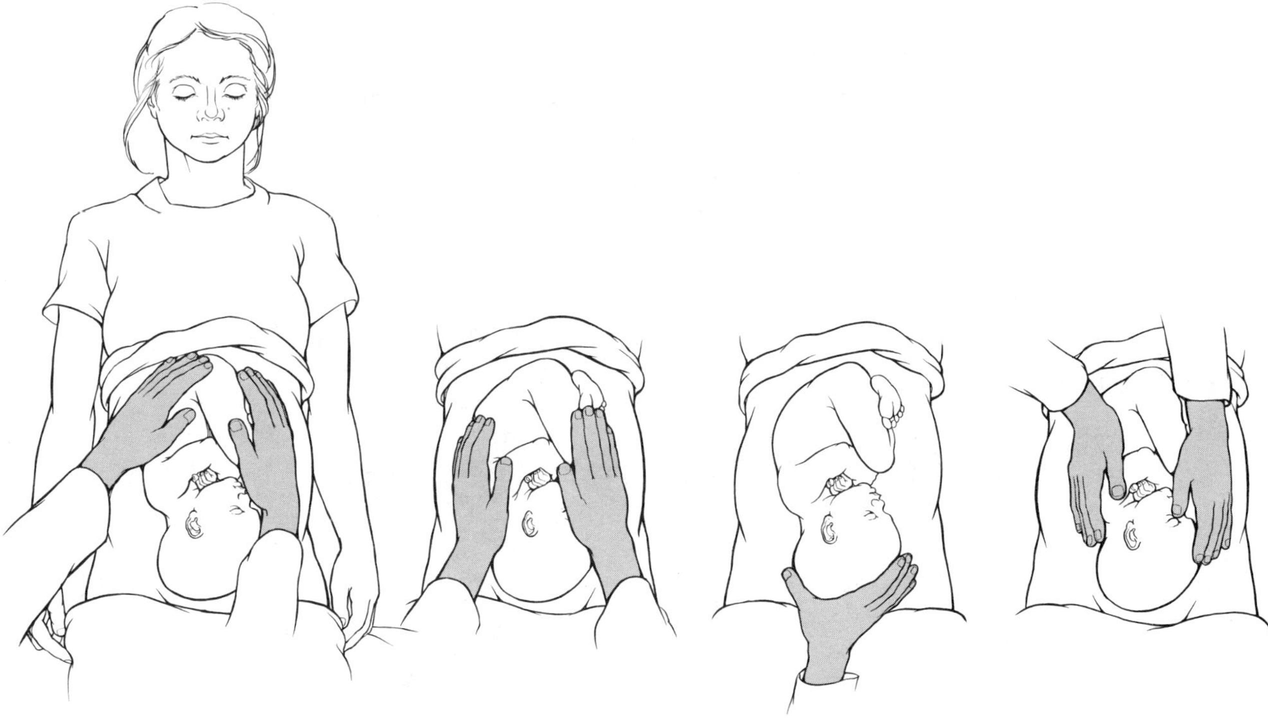

Figure 12.14
Leopold's maneuvers.

The results of the routine physical examination, the laboratory data, and any problems are recorded. An example of an antepartum assessment form for graphic recording is shown in Figure 12.15. Flow sheets and graphs are very helpful in identifying small abnormalities. Blood pressure, weight, and uterine size are plotted against weeks of gestation and provide a readily accessible graphic assessment of the progression of the pregnancy.

The nursing process is the framework for the antepartum management. During each visit after the data are collected, plans or goals are established in relation to identified needs; previous plans are evaluated, deleted if accomplished, or revised according to the new or different needs of the woman or her family (Fig. 12.16). Plans should reflect both physiologic and psychosocial changes and adaptation. The woman should be encouraged to participate in her care, such listening to fetal heart tones and being kept apprised of assessment factors; this involvement reassures her, increases her understanding of pregnancy and fetal development, and promotes self-esteem. Client teaching is a part of each visit, and the maternity nurse should formulate the teaching plan to relate to the tasks of pregnancy while remaining flexible enough to modify or adapt the plan should the woman indicate a need for other kinds of information (Fig. 12.17). There are basic areas of information that need to be shared; each nurse has a personal style for presenting such information and should adapt this presentation to the person's need.

ANTEPARTUM EDUCATION

Clothing

Maternity fashions today allow for comfort and attractiveness, and how the woman looks becomes increasingly important as the pregnancy advances. Fortunately, many women exchange and share maternity wardrobes, which eases the financial strain and provides variety. Girdles are not necessary for most women, but if the abdomen is large and pendu-

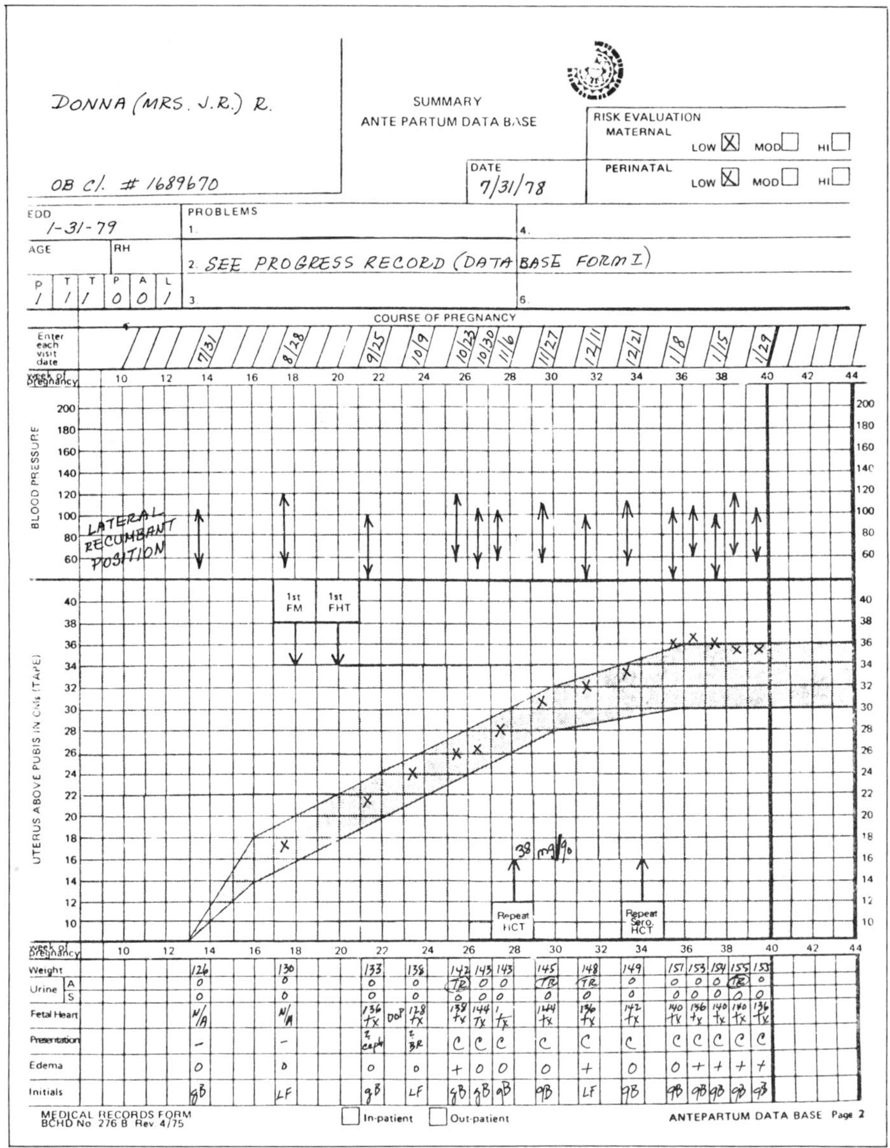

DONNA (MRS. J.R.) R.

OB Cl. # 1689670

SUMMARY
ANTE PARTUM DATA BASE

RISK EVALUATION
MATERNAL LOW [X] MOD [ ] HI [ ]

DATE 7/31/78

PERINATAL LOW [X] MOD [ ] HI [ ]

EDD 1-31-79

AGE | RH

P T T P A L
1 1 1 0 0 1

PROBLEMS
1.
2. SEE PROGRESS RECORD (DATA BASE FORM I)
3.
4.
6.

COURSE OF PREGNANCY

Enter each visit date: 7/31, 8/28, 9/25, 10/9, 10/23, 10/30, 11/6, 11/27, 12/11, 12/21, 1/8, 1/15, 1/29

week of pregnancy: 10 12 14 16 18 20 22 24 26 28 30 32 34 36 38 40 42 44

BLOOD PRESSURE: 200 180 160 140 120 100 80 60

LATERAL RECUMBANT POSITION

1st FM

1st FHT

UTERUS ABOVE PUBIS IN CMS (TAPE): 40 38 36 34 32 30 28 26 24 22 20 18 16 14 12 10

38 mg%

Repeat HCT

Repeat Sero. HCT

Visit	1	2	3	4	5	6	7	8	9	10	11	12	13	14	15
Weight	126	130	133	138	142	143	143	145	148	149	151	153	154	155	153
Urine A	0	0	0	0	TR	0	0	TR	TR	0	0	0	0	TR	0
Urine S	0	0	0	0	0	0	0	0	0	0	0	0	0	0	0
Fetal Heart	N/A	N/A	136 tx DOP	128 tx	138 tx	144 Tx	/ tx	144 tx	136 tx	142 tx	140 tx	136 tx	140 tx	140 tx	136 tx
Presentation	–	–	ē ceph	ē BR	C	C	C	C	C	C	C	C	C	C	C
Edema	0	0	0	0	+	0	0	0	+	0	0	+	+	+	+
Initials	gB	LF	gB	LF	gB	gB	gB	gB	LF	gB	gB	gB	gB	gB	gB

MEDICAL RECORDS FORM
BCHD No. 276 B Rev. 4/75

[ ] In-patient [ ] Out-patient

ANTEPARTUM DATA BASE Page 2

Figure 12.15
Antepartum data base form. Source: Butnarescu, G. F., Tillotson, D. M., Villarreal, P. *Perinatal Nursing: Volume 2—Reproductive Risk.* New York: John Wiley & Sons, 1980. Used with permission. (Norm for growth curve based on patient population from Robert B. Green Hospital, San Antonio, Texas. Patient data simulated.)

lous, a girdle may be comfortable and may aid in preventing backache. Shoes should be comfortable and safe; wearing approximately the same height heel throughout pregnancy will lessen back strain. Clothes should be loose fitting, avoiding any areas of restriction such as elastic sleeves or tight waists. Hose also should be nonrestrictive so as not to predispose the woman to varicosities.

Bathing

There is no contraindication to tub bathing or showers in a normal pregnancy. In fact, because of the increased perspiration and vaginal discharge, daily bathing is important for the woman. The woman may be concerned about slipping in the tub or shower in the last months, so she should take her

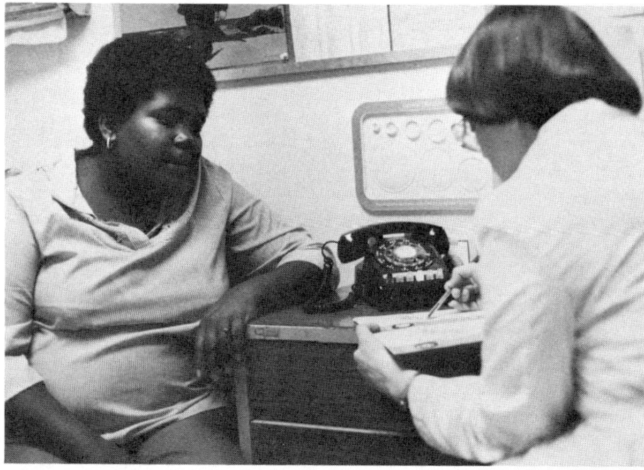

Figure 12.16
Data collection is an important part of prenatal nursing care.

shower or bath when someone is around to assist if needed. Rubber mats and hand holds are helpful aids to prevent slipping and assist when balance is a problem. The only time tub baths are restricted is if the woman has ruptured membranes or vaginal bleeding. This restriction is imposed because of concern about ascending vaginal infection that could be a hazard to the mother and her unborn child.

Breast Care

A good supportive bra is necessary to prevent tissue stretching from the increased size of the breasts. The bra should have wide comfortable straps that will

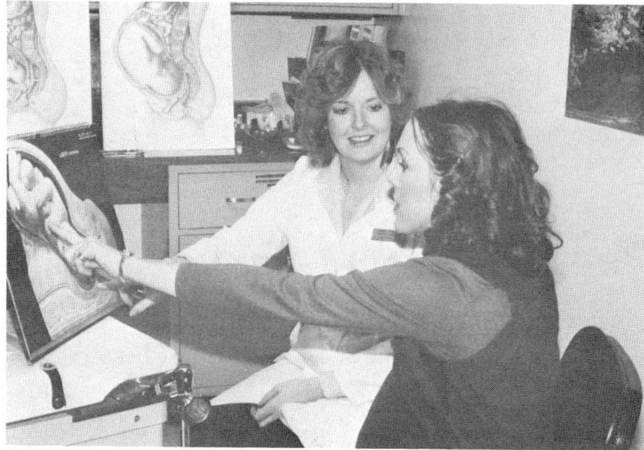

Figure 12.17
Prenatal education is a prominent nursing function.

not stretch with increased weight and a cup into which the entire breast will fit comfortably. There should be at least two and preferably three fasteners in the back. Ideally, the breast is supported so that the nipple line will be halfway between the elbow and shoulder. Many bras today are made from nonporous synthetic fabrics. The expectant and nursing mother may find cotton bras more comfortable.

If the woman is planning to breast-feed, soap should not be used on the nipples since it can cause them to dry and crack. Preparation for breast-feeding includes strategies to toughen the nipples such as exposing them periodically to the air or rubbing them gently with a soft towel after bathing. Oral stimulation by her partner can assist in toughening and preparing the woman's nipples for breast-feeding; if this is pleasurable for the couple, it should be encouraged. Nipple rolling—extending and rolling the nipple between the thumb and forefinger—is also recommended as a method of preparation for breast-feeding.

Employment

Many women work up until the day of delivery, and as long as the environment in which they are employed is not harmful to the fetus, there is no contraindication. Women who have sedentary jobs should be encouraged to put their legs up during breaks or to go for short walks at lunchtime. Continuing to be employed is based both on physical and mental health of the mother, as well as on economic considerations. Avoiding fatigue or excessive physical strain is important, but if a balance between work and rest can be maintained and the mother wishes or needs to be employed, no harm to the fetus should occur.

Travel

As long as the mother is experiencing a normal pregnancy, travel is not contraindicated. Fatigue sometimes becomes a problem on long trips, and an opportunity to get out and stretch her legs every 2–3 hours should be provided. The question of whether or not to wear a seat belt is controversial. The statistics reflect that more severe accidents occur because of ejection from the car, and for this reason seat belts or shoulder harnesses are recommended (Crosby & Costiloe, 1971).

Rest and Exercise

Rest is essential for the pregnant woman and although 8 hours is recommended, people have different needs. Fatigue is a reality early in pregnancy and as the pregnancy advances; it is caused by hormonal shifts. Sleeping becomes difficult, and the need to urinate often interrupts sleep. The nurse can assist the woman in scheduling daily activities to include rest and sleep balanced with exercise. Resting on her side with the upper leg supported by a pillow is not only comfortable but promotes return circulation from the lower extremities. Relaxation techniques used in prenatal class can be practiced and are often helpful in promoting sleep. The practice of contraction and relaxation of muscle groups beginning with the feet and progressing to the head is useful. Walking is an excellent exercise for the pregnant woman; in general, she can continue to do any exercise that she does regularly. Pregnancy is not a good time to take up a new strenuous activity such as tennis or jogging. Exercise and rest in balanced amounts contribute to physical and mental health.

Sexual Activity

See Chapter 14.

Smoking

Many studies have demonstrated the relationship of smoking during pregnancy to low birth weight infants (Fielding, 1978; Deibel, 1980). Carbon monoxide blood levels are higher in mothers who smoke, and carbon monoxide attaches to hemoglobin before oxygen, which affects oxygenation to the fetus. Nicotine's vasoconstrictive action further affects the fetus (Kline et al., 1977). Studies have also indicated that a decrease in smoking can improve fetal outcome (Davies et al., 1976). Therefore, if the mother is a heavy smoker and is unable to stop, the nurse should help her reduce the number of cigarettes she smokes. The relationship of bleeding in pregnancy and smoking is discussed more fully in Chapter 21.

Dental Care

Increased ptyalism during pregnancy may contribute to tooth decay. In addition, hypertrophy and tenderness of the gums associated with the hyperemia of pregnancy may cause the pregnant woman to be careless about dental care. It is important for her to have her teeth checked early in pregnancy. Dental health and hygiene are dependent on good nutrition, particularly calcium and phosphorus intake. X-rays, of course, should be avoided during pregnancy.

Medications

Medications during pregnancy, especially the first 12 weeks when organogenesis is occurring, are contraindicated. No medication or drugs, including alcohol, should be taken during pregnancy. Since a woman is frequently unaware of pregnancy until 8–10 weeks have elapsed, she should stop taking any drugs as soon as she decides to become pregnant. If she happens to have taken a medication that is teratogenic, the effects can be devastating to the fetus. Drug abuse, both legal and illegal, is discussed more fully in Chapter 25. Except for prenatal vitamins with iron, which are generally prescribed by the physician, pregnant women should not take medications unless there is a serious medical problem that must be treated only by drugs such as diabetes.

NUTRITION DURING PREGNANCY

Nutritional needs during pregnancy are directly related to the health of the fetus and mother. The mother's nutritional status before and during pregnancy affects pregnancy growth. The White House Conference on Nutrition in 1969 recognized the need for setting norms for pregnant women and affirmed the right of each woman to have adequate nutrition during pregnancy, both for herself and her infant. Some federal programs such as the WIC Program (special supplemental foods for women, infants, and children) have assisted families in obtaining adequate nutrition. Whether or not federal assistance will continue in the future is a matter of great concern.

Both animal and human studies have demonstrated the interrelationship of nutrition and infant well-being (Committee on Maternal Nutrition, 1970). Research has made it possible to measure the effects of nutritional deficiency on cell and organ growth. As a result of this research, it is theorized that growth occurs in three overlapping stages.

- ▲ Growth by increase in cell size
- ▲ Growth by increase in cell number
- ▲ Growth by increase in cell size and number

This theory has great implications for brain growth. If nutritional status is inadequate when *cell division* is occurring, damage may be permanent; if nutrition is deficient when cells are *enlarging,* the changes can be reversed. Table 12.3 compares recommended dietary allowances for nonpregnant women with those for pregnant and lactating teenage and adult women. You need to be aware of the nutritional requirements of both teenagers and adults since childbearing is occurring in both these groups. We assume that you have a basic understanding of nutrition and food groups, and discussion of nutrition in this chapter only focuses on nutritional adaptation during pregnancy.

Key Nutritional Adaptations Needed During Pregnancy

PROTEIN

Additional protein is needed during pregnancy to support growth and maintenance of the fetus, placenta, and maternal tissues such as the uterus and breasts. An additional 30 gm of protein per day is needed by the pregnant adult. The nonpregnant teenager requires more protein than the nonpregnant adult in order to meet her own growth needs; in pregnancy, an additional 30 gm above that level is recommended. A diet that includes 1 qt of milk, 4 oz of lean meat, 2 slices of bread, and 1 oz of cheddar cheese provides 76 gm of protein, thus meeting daily requirements. It is important that the nurse remember protein equivalents as they are particularly useful if a woman does not like milk but enjoys cheese or yogurt. Protein equivalents equal to 1 cup of milk are

- ▲ 1 cup yogurt
- ▲ 1 1/2 ounces hard or semisoft cheese
- ▲ 1/4 cup (2 oz) cottage cheese
- ▲ 1 1/2 cups ice cream

Animal proteins (meat, fish, eggs, milk) contain all eight essential amino acids and therefore furnish the best building materials.

Planning a diet for the vegetarian that is adequate in protein is very difficult because of the physical bulk inherent in a vegetarian diet coupled with decreased or limited gastric capacity common in pregnancy (Cohn, 1978). At times of physiologic stress (pregnancy is one), "pure" vegetarians often revert to a diet that includes milk and eggs, which certainly makes adequate protein intake more likely.

CARBOHYDRATES AND FATS

Carbohydrates and fats serve as the main sources of food energy for the body. An increase of approximately 300 calories is necessary. Carbohydrates in the form of milk, fruits and vegetables, and whole grain cereals and breads provide bulk as well as energy. Some fat is needed to provide the pregnant woman with essential fatty acids.

CALCIUM AND PHOSPHOROUS

Calcium and phosphorous are important as tissue-building material and in acid–base buffering. Adequate calcium intake provides for fetal needs and allows the mother to store some for lactation. A diet that contains 3–4 cups of milk (or milk substitute) will satisfy the minimum daily requirement of 1,200 mg. Taking large amounts of milk that contains large amounts of phosphorous results in high phosphorous concentration in the blood and a relative hypocalcemia (low calcium). This calcium phosphorous imbalance is thought to contribute to leg cramps. Curtailing milk and meat intake and ensuring that magnesium intake is adequate to allow proper use of calcium will restore this balance.

IRON

Demands for iron are considerably increased in pregnancy, and the Committee on Maternal Nutrition (1970) recommends a simple salt such as ferrous gluconate, ferrous fumorate, or ferrous sulfate be given in amounts of 30–60 mg per day in the second and third trimesters. Supplemental iron is not recommended in the first trimester because of the rapid embryonic development. Foods high in iron such as liver, green leafy vegetables, and cereals high in iron should be encouraged.

ZINC AND MAGNESIUM

Zinc is a nutrient factor affecting growth and is found in milk, liver, shellfish, and wheat bran. Magnesium is essential for cell metabolism and structural growth. Sources include milk, whole grains, peas, beans, and nuts.

TABLE 12.3
RECOMMENDED DIETARY ALLOWANCES FOR WOMEN 15–35 YEARS OF AGE

	Teenage Allowance (15–18 Years)			*Adult Female Allowance (19–35 Years)*		
Nutrient	*Nonpregnant*	*Pregnant*	*Lactating*	*Nonpregnant*	*Pregnant*	*Lactating*
Energy (calories)	2,100	2,400	2,600	2,000	2,300	2,500
Protein (gm)	48	78	68	46	76	66
Vitamin A (IU)	4,000	5,000	6,000	4,000	5,000	6,000
(Re)	800	1,000	1,200	800	1,000	1,200
Vitamin D (IU)	400	400	400	—	400	400
Vitamin E (IU)	12	15	15	21	15	15
Ascorbic acid (mg)	45	60	80	45	60	80
Folacin (mg)[a]	0.4	0.8	0.6	0.4	0.8	0.6
Niacin (mg)	14	16	18	13	15	17
Riboflavin (mg)	1.4	1.7	1.9	1.2	1.5	1.7
Thiamin (mg)	1.1	1.4	1.4	1.0	1.3	1.3
Vitamin B_6 (mg)	2.0	2.5	2.5	2.0	2.5	2.5
Vitamin B_{12} (mg)						
Calcium (mg)	1,200	1,600	1,600	800	1,200	1,200
Phosphorus (mg)	1,200	1,600	1,600	800	1,200	1,200
Iodine (mug)	115	140	165	100	125	150
Iron (mg)[b]	18	18+	18+	18	18+	18
Magnesium (mg)	300	450	450	300	450	450
Zinc (mg)	15	20	25	15	20	25

Source: Food and Nutrition Board. *Recommended Dietary Allowances.* (8th ed.). Washington, D.C.: National Academy of Sciences, National Research Council, 1974.

[a] Folacin allowances refer to dietary sources as determined by lactobacillus casein assay. Pure forms of folacin may be effective in doses less than one-fourth of the recommended dietary allowance.

[b] This iron requirement cannot be met by ordinary diets. Therefore, the use of 30–60 mg supplemental iron is recommended.

IODINE AND SODIUM

As mentioned under physiologic adaptation, iodine is excreted in the urine during pregnancy. Inadequate iodine can cause enlargement of the thyroid gland. Using iodized salt will allow the woman to meet the daily requirement. Sodium ions are critical for proper metabolism, and salt is never curtailed in pregnancy even in pre-eclampsia and eclampsia or hypertensive states. Foods should be seasoned to taste with salt; excessively salty foods such as ham and potato chips can be avoided to eliminate excessive sodium intake.

FAT SOLUBLE VITAMINS

Vitamins A, D, E, and K are all fat soluble and are stored in the liver. The concern with fat soluble vitamins is that excessive intake can be toxic. Symptoms of fat soluble vitamin toxicity are nausea, gastrointestinal upset, dry skin, and loss of hair. It is important, however, that daily minimal requirements of all vitamins be met as each of these has an important role in the body. A balanced diet provides adequate amounts of these vitamins.

WATER SOLUBLE VITAMINS

Only small amounts of water soluble vitamins are stored, so adequate daily intake is important. Vitamin C needs increase in pregnancy from 45 to 60 mg. It functions in the development of connective tissue in the vascular system. The B vitamins function as coenzymes in many activities, including respiration, glucose oxidation, and energy metabolism. Since energy needs increase in pregnancy, so does the need for the B vitamins. Folic acid has been mentioned in relation to cardiovascular changes, and although megaloblastic anemia is not common in the United States, it does occur. Folate deficiency can have serious implications for the embryo and fetus. Folic acid and iron are the only nutritional supplements generally recommended in normal pregnancy.

Factors Affecting Nutrition

There are several factors, such as cultural food patterns, psychosocial factors, economics, life-styles, and food beliefs and habits, that have a significant impact on nutrition. These will all influence the expectant mother's eating patterns.

Myths or beliefs about food often raise the question of pica, which sometimes occurs during pregnancy. *Pica* is a desire for strange foods or substances not usually considered edible or nutritious. The practice of pica is thought to have its roots in myth. Pica occurs more often in low socioeconomic groups, but it is not unique to that group. Substances ingested are starch, dirt, clay, and ice or freezer frost. A common belief is that laundry starch will make the baby lighter in color or make the baby "slide out" more easily in labor (Curda, 1977). Studies have linked pica to anemia since it may cause interference with iron absorption. In some cases, the question has been raised whether pica is a result of anemia or anemia causes pica. It is important that the maternity nurse be aware of the practice and its implications in the nutritional status of her client.

In summary, the nurse needs to remember that nutritional assessment and teaching are integral parts of antepartal care. The patient's weight gain should be monitored, and a diet history should be taken initially and evaluated regularly throughout the pregnancy to be certain that adequate amounts of all key nutrients are included. General physical appearance should be assessed, including skin color, turgor, lesions, and glossy or dull condition of hair.

ADOLESCENT AND ADULT PREGNANCIES

Pregnancy at either end of the continuum of the childbearing years offers unique problems and rewards for the professional nurse and health team. These pregnancies are, therefore, highlighted in this section.

Adolescent Pregnancy: 12–19 Years

Adolescent pregnancy is broadly categorized as a reproductive risk condition. Many teenage pregnancies, however, are as healthy as adult pregnancies, and many of the prenatal nursing care activities for teenagers are the same as those for the mature pregnant woman.

Two themes tend to appear in much of the literature on adolescent pregnancy. First, married and unmarried adolescents with planned and unplanned pregnancies are all treated the same and as if they all require the same nursing care or medical management. Although adolescent needs are similar because of their developmental stage, the expectations and needs arising from a planned pregnancy by two married teenagers do differ from those of an unmarried teenage girl experiencing an unplanned pregnancy or a teenage couple forced into an early marriage because of pregnancy.

The second theme, which is quite similar to the first, is that a teenager is a teenager and as such is only one of a blurred collage of young people who are neither adult nor child. Teenagers are people just like adults, and the nurse must recognize their uniqueness while at the same time rely upon a generalized knowledge base about adolescent growth and development. There is a distinct difference in pregnancy outcome among adolescents 15–19 years old as compared with adolescents under 15 years. The former, particularly those 18–20 years old, tend to follow a clinical course during pregnancy that is quite similar to the more mature young adult 20–24 years old. Pregnant adolescents under 15 years old have a consistently documented higher incidence of complications during pregnancy (Battaglia et al., 1963; Duenhoelter et al, 1975; & Weiner, 1976). Adolescent pregnancy as a reproductive risk condition is addressed in Chapter 21.

Over one-half million births to adolescent mothers 15–19 years old are recorded each year. In 1978 there were 532,635 births to young women in this age group; there were 10,000 births to girls under 15 years of age (Baldwin, 1981). These figures show that adolescent pregnancy has a widespread incidence and that a significant number of these pregnancies are from young adolescent girls. However, a large number of pregnancies are among the older adolescents as well. Nurses tend to manage the young adolescent as a patient at risk and often ignore the adolescent status of the more mature teenager. Both approaches have some merit, but often the needs unique to the adolescent who is having a healthy pregnancy are lost. This section addresses the adolescent couple who is experiencing a healthy pregnancy. There are needs that are peculiar to these young people and that deserve special attention by the nurse, even in the absence of a pregnancy complication.

UNIQUE PHYSICAL NEEDS

Adolescence is a period of growth and energy expenditure. Most adolescent girls reach their full physical maturity by the age of 17. Many of these young women, however, have some form of malnutrition that may not put them in a debilitating condition but that does not provide the best foundation for pregnancy. This is particularly true in regard to deficiencies of iron, calcium, and vitamins A and C. This malnutrition may also appear as adolescent obesity or underweight. The adolescent who is pregnant faces new nutritional demands, which are being placed on a young body that may not be ready to meet them. The nurse must carefully assess nutritional status of the adolescent and provide education, guidance, and support to help her meet her nutritional needs. The nurse does this by taking an accurate history of dietary intake, food habits, and preferences; by interpreting laboratory tests, such as hemoglobin and hematocrit, that provide information concerning nutritional deficiencies such as anemia; by observing general appearance of the young woman with special attention to skin, fingernails, and hair; by determining the adolescent's knowledge about nutrition; by learning about peer group practices; and by involving the young couple, particularly the young woman, in developing a plan that will upgrade or maintain nutrition adequacy during pregnancy. The nurse also needs to know who is responsible for preparing meals. Some adolescent couples live with the parents of the girl or boy and may not need to be concerned with food preparation as such. Others have homes independent of parents and must prepare their own food. Important questions include: Can the young woman plan and prepare meals? Does she need help with meal planning and preparation? The nurse may involve other appropriate health personnel such as a nutritionists or dieticians to help meet any needs. Other resources may be available such as parents, relatives, or teachers.

The adolescent may be susceptible to complications of pregnancy. The nurse, therefore, must augment efforts toward complete prenatal supervision to attend, particularly, to reproductive risk conditions peculiar to the adolescent such as delivering infants of low birth weight (Weiner & Milton, 1976). Careful assessment of gestational age and fetal growth and development is important. This may require reconfirmation of date of last menstrual period and careful measurement of fundal height, taking the fetal heart tones, and questioning the expectant mother about fetal movement.

The adolescent may not be knowledgeable about proper personal hygiene practices. The nurse should assess such knowledge and provide appropriate teaching and counseling. Sexual activity during pregnancy is another area where the adolescent couple may not be as sophisticated as the more mature couple. The nurse should make a special effort to help adolescents regarding sexual adjustment and behavior.

UNIQUE PSYCHOSOCIAL NEEDS

The adolescent couple is caught between two stages of psychosocial development—identity and generativity. Young couples may be holding on to the security of family and home while trying to establish their own homes and families. This often results in frustration and confusion. They may still be struggling with role clarification, both in terms of their sexuality and in regard to roles within the family units they are forming—husband/wife; lover; expectant mother/father.

Pregnant adolescents are frequently suspicious of the nurse as an adult who on the one hand, is not a completely trustworthy peer yet, on the other hand, who may represent the maturity toward which they are striving. The nurse may need to work harder to establish a trust relationship with the young couple than with the mature couple, as well as to be accepted as a person whose judgment upon which the young couple can rely.

Many adolescent couples bring to pregnancy an inadequate basis for taking on the role of parents; others read about child care and plan ahead for their new roles. The nurse must make a particular effort to assess each couple's readiness for parenthood and preparation for undertaking the tasks associated with it.

Unique Learning Needs

Pregnancy, even one that is planned, often interrupts education for both the woman and man. Interruption of education ultimately results in altered career goals that may affect future economic security. The nurse must confirm, rather than assume, that career goals have been interrupted and not impose personal values regarding education and career on the young couple. Some people do not desire a college education, and some couples marry upon completion of high school as a part of their life goals.

The nurse needs to assess capability to perform formal cognitive operations in order to determine the appropriate strategies for teaching the adolescent couple. Decisions such as participation by the adolescent in parent education groups with older couples or exploration and investigation of such services that are designed for the adolescent often can be facilitated by the nurse.

The adolescent couple may be very self-directed concerning their pregnancy and expected child or they may require help with such decision making; the nurse needs to know which and act accordingly.

Nurses who provide care to adolescent couples who are experiencing a healthy pregnancy should be carefully attuned to certain situations.

- ▲ There is a need to establish a climate in which trust and confidence in the nurse and the health care system can be promoted. This requires an openness and honesty that communicates, "I am up front with you, and I care about you." An attitude of condescension can interfere with any relationship but especially one with the adolescent patient.
- ▲ Careful attention to appropriate teaching content and strategy should be given, with particular attention to readiness to learn about pregnancy and parenthood.
- ▲ Since adolescence is a period of challenge of adult authority and even rebellion, careful attention to the type and scope of limits set regarding health care is important. Respect for the influence of adolescent peers on the couple should be evident.
- ▲ Developmental tasks of adolescence, marriage, pregnancy, and parenthood are of special concern. The pregnant adolescent will, out of necessity, be attending to all of these in a healthy or unhealthy way. The nurse must be able to support or redirect their efforts.
- ▲ Assistance is needed in identifying and using appropriate support systems. Parents and peers

are of special importance to the pregnant teenager. The nurse can facilitate healthy use of such groups, particularly in the case of the young couple, by involving parents. Involving peer groups may be an indirect way of providing health education to such groups who may learn about pregnancy and childbirth through the young couple with whom the nurse is working. Because parent–child relationships are sensitive during adolescence, the nurse must approach any suggestions carefully and with support of the couple.

▲ It is important to help the adolescent gain a realistic perspective regarding the demands of pregnancy and parenthood. Adolescents are just learning to accept mature responsibility for self. Pregnancy requires that they now do this for another, far more dependent being—the infant.

▲ Recognition that patterns of health care acceptable to the adolescent are influenced by family attitudes and values is necessary. Adolescents, like all other people, are products of culture as well as heritage.

▲ There are needs for assistance with family planning. Spacing of pregnancies and use of contraceptive techniques may be new to the couple. Careful assessment and guidance regarding acquisition of facts and appropriate use of pharmacologic or technologic methods may be needed.

Nurses can make some general inferences about adolescent pregnancy on the basis of what is known about adolescence, poverty, reproductive risk, and so on, however, the nurse must exercise caution lest the adolescent is not perceived as a person with unique characteristics and needs.

Adult Pregnancy: 30–40 Years

Pregnancy, in what used to be thought of as beyond the childbearing years, the years from 30 to 40, is becoming more evident at this time. In a 1982 issue of *Time* magazine,* it was pointed out that there has been a 15.2% rise in the birth rate of women in the 30–44 age group. Many of the 37 million women in the 25–35 age group have married later than their mothers, have delayed starting their families until education is complete and a career is established, and, as a result, have entered into pregnancy at a different point in time. Couples having a child after 30 may well bring different experiences to the situation, and what implications this has for the health care team in the future is probably not yet fully realized. The fact that pregnancy in the midthirties and later carries a higher biologic risk in some cases is known. However, could it be that the woman who has achieved greater maturity and in some cases greater economic security now realizes that becoming a successful person does not negate the fact that she can also opt to be a successful mother? Does motherhood exclude career and personal success? Or does career and personal success, first, make for better mothering and parenting later?

Certainly, being a parent and a member of the working force have coexisted for a long time, but the option of parenting in the later years after a measure of personal achievement seems to be coming to the fore. It is suspected that some of these women thought a career was what they wanted exclusively and then decided motherhood was something they did not want to miss. One 35-year-old national newscaster after the birth of her child was quoted in *Time* as saying, "I'm now the most boring person to talk to. If you don't want to hear about my baby, you'd better not come around."

Implications for the maternity nurse who works with women in their thirties are unique. If the procedure is based on good data collection and understanding, it will, nevertheless, require the same process as with other pregnant women. If the nurse individualizes her care, adapting to older mothers will be successful. Mothers in their mid- and late-thirties may well experience different biophysical problems. Energy levels during the pregnancy may be affected, and certainly muscle tone and physical activity will have to be evaluated. Economics are important too. It is estimated that the cost of supporting a child to 18 years in 1982 varies from $85,000 to $134,000 in an urban community. Parenting through age 55–60 will become a reality. The underlying motivation in the trend of pregnancy in the later years may be that women see the biologic time clock running out.

**Time,* Cover story, "The Baby Boom," February 22, 1982.

SUMMARY

The positive, probable, and presumptive signs, each of which can often be related to a particular trimester, were discussed. Diagnosis of pregnancy by indirect and direct methods was explained. Clinical methods for determining gestational age were presented, followed by a comprehensive discussion of the physiologic adaptation of the mother to pregnancy. Each maternal system was reviewed, highlighting the physiologic adaptation made in the system to support the pregnancy. Implications for nursing intervention were included.

Psychosocial characteristics were reviewed, including some of the literature that reflects male psychology and paternal roles. The fact that pregnancy is a crisis was explored, and the tasks that the mother must work through in order to prepare herself for her new role—that of a mother with a child—were discussed. The fact that the woman's partner must accomplish certain developmental milestones in order to integrate his role as father was also introduced. Emphasis was placed on the fact that although the nurse could provide guidance about many of the anticipated changes, she must be alert to the uniqueness of the people with whom she interacts. A thorough discussion of the minor discomforts of pregnancy followed.

Prenatal care and management were discussed, and the three major areas of prenatal data collection were described. They are the health history, physical examination, and laboratory tests. Nursing management of the woman throughout the pregnancy followed. Frequency of visits and assessments to be done at each visit were described.

The next section of the chapter discussed antepartal education, including clothing, bathing, breast care, hygiene, exercise, medications, employment, and smoking. The chapter also discussed nutrition in pregnancy. The emphasis was on the nutritional needs that change as a result of pregnancy. The point was made that the nurse needs to be cognizant of individual needs since the pregnant teenager as compared with the adult woman has very specific nutritional needs. Key nutrients and pica were discussed, and a table depicting nonpregnant and pregnant nutritional needs of the teenager and the adult was included.

The last section was devoted to some specific information about needs of mothers-to-be on each end of the childbearing continuum—the pregnant adolescent and the pregnant woman over 30.

REFERENCES AND READINGS

Aguilera, D. G., Messick, J. M. *Crisis Intervention: Theory and Methodology.* St. Louis: C. V. Mosby, 1978.

Baldwin, W. Adolescent Pregnancy and Childbearing—An Overview. *Sem Perinat.* 5:1, 1981.

Bates, B. *A Guide to Physical Examination,* 2nd ed. Philadelphia: J. B. Lippincott Co, 1979.

Battaglia, F. C., Frazier, T. M., Tellegers, A. Obstetric and Pediatric Complications of Juvenile Pregnancy. *Pediatrics* 32:902, 1963.

Benedek, T. The Psychobiology of Pregnancy, in Anthony, E. J., Benedek, T. *Parenthood: Its Psychology and Psychopathology.* Boston: Little Brown, 1970.

Bibring, G. A Study of the Psychological Process in Pregnancy and of the Earliest Mother–Child Relationship. *Psychoanal Study Child* XVI: 1961.

Butnarescu, G. *Perinatal Nursing, Vol. I: Reproductive Health.* New York: John Wiley & Sons, 1978.

Butnarescu, G., Tillotson, D., Villarreal, P. *Perinatal Nursing, Vol. 2: Reproductive Risk.* New York: John Wiley & Sons, 1980.

Caplan, G. *An Approach to Community Mental Health.* New York: Grune & Stratton, 1961.

Card, J. J., Wise, L. L. Teenage Mothers and Teenage Fathers: The Impact of Early Childbearing on the Parent's Personal and Professional Lives. *Fam Plann Perspect* 10:199, 1978.

Carey, J. First Trimester Prenatal Counseling in Private Practice. *Obstet Gynecol Neonatal Nurs* 10(5):336,1981.

Clark, A. L. and Affonso, D. *Childbearing: a Nursing Perspective,* 2nd ed. Philadelphia: F. A. Davis Co. 1979.

Cohn, S. D. *Vegetarian Nutrition: An Overview in Issues in Health Care of Women—Maternal Nutrition.* New York: McGraw-Hill, 1978, Vol. I, No. 1, pp.3–13.

Coleman, A., Coleman, L. Pregnancy as an Altered State of Consciousness. *Birth Fam J* 1:7, Winter 1973–1974.

Crosby, W. M., Costiloe, P. J. Safety of Lapbelt Restraint for Pregnant Victims of Automobile Collisions. *New Engl J Med* 284:632, 1971.

Curda, L. R. What About Pica? *J Nurs Midwifery* 23:8, 1977.

Davies, D. P. et al. Cigarette Smoking in Pregnancy Associated with Weight Gain and Fetal Growth. *Lancet* 1:385, 1976.

Deibel, P. Effects of Cigarette Smoking on Maternal Nutrition and the Fetus. *J Obstet Nurs* 9(6): 333, 1980.

Deutsch, H. *The Psychology of Women: Motherhood.* New York: Bantam Books, 1945.

Duenhoelter, J. H., Jimenez, J., Baumann, G. Pregnancy Performance of Patients Under Fifteen Years of Age. *Obstet Gynecol* 46:49, 1975.

Fielding, J. E. Smoking and Pregnancy. *New Engl J Med* Feb, 9, 1978.

Gibbs, R. S., Gibbs, C. E. *Ambulatory Obstetrics: A Clinical Guide.* New York: John Wiley & Sons, 1979.

Harris, R., Dombro, M. Ryan, C. Therapeutic Uses of Human Figure Drawings by the Pregnant Couple. *Obstet Gynecol Neonatal Nurs* 9 (4): 232, 1980.

Huff, R. W., Pauerstein, C. J. *Human Reproduction, Physiology and Pathophysiology.* New York: John Wiley & Sons, 1979.

Jensen, M. D., Benson, R. C., Bobak, I. M. *Maternity Care: The Nurse and the Family* (2nd ed). St. Louis: C. V. Mosby, 1981.

Kline, J. et al. Smoking: A Risk Factor for Spontaneous Abortion. *New Engl J Med* 297:793, 1977.

Kohn, C., A. Nelson, Weiner, S. Gravidas' Responses to Realtime Ultrasound Fetal Image. *J Obstet Gynecol Neonatal Nurs* 9 (2): 77, 1980.

LeMasters, E. E. Parenthood as Crisis, in Parad, H. J. (Ed.), *Crisis Intervention.* New York: Family Service Association of America, 1965, pp. 312–323.

Luke, B. Guide to Better Evaluation of Antepartum Nutrition. *J Obstet Gynecol Neonatal Nurs* 5(4): 37, 1976.

Marquart, R. K. Expectant Fathers: What Are Their Needs? *Am J Matern Child Nurs* 1(1): 32, 1976.

Marquart, R. K. Nutrition. *Am J Matern Child Nurs* 2(2):85, 1977.

Olds, S. B., London, M. L., Ludewig, P. A., Davidson, S. V. *Obstetric Nursing.* Menlo Park, Calif.: Addison-Wesley, 1980.

Panzarine, S. et al. A Systems Approach to Adolescent Pregnancy. *J Obstet Gynecol Neonatal Nurs* 10(4): 287, 1981.

Phillips, C. R., Anzalone, J. T. *Fathering.* St. Louis: C. V. Mosby, 1975.

Rapoport, L. The State of Crisis: Some Theoretical Considerations, in Parad, H. J. (Ed.), *Crisis Intervention.* New York: Family Service Association of America, 1965, pp. 24–26.

Reed, J. D. The New Baby Boom. Cover story. *Time,* Feb. 22, 1982.

Rubin, R. Cognitive Style in Pregnancy. *Am J Nurs* 70:502, 1970.

Stickler, J. F., Bowden, M. S., Reimer, E. D. Pregnancy: A Shared Emotional Experience. *Am J Matern Child Nurs* 3:153, 1978.

The Surgeon General's Workshop on Maternal and Infant Health Report, U.S. Department of Health and Human Services. Public Health Service DHHS Publication No. (PHS) 81-50161.

Tanner, L. M. Developmental Tasks of Pregnancy, in Bergerson, B. E., Anderson, M., Duffy, M., et al. (eds), *Current Concepts in Clinical Nursing.* St. Louis: C. V. Mosby Co. 1969, pp. 292–297.

Weiner, G., Milton, T. Demographic Correlates of Low Birth Weight. *Am J Epidemiol* 91:148, 1976.

Willson, J. R., Carrington, E. R. *Obstetrics and Gynecology* (6th ed.). St. Louis: C. V. Mosby, 1979.

Ziegel, E., Cranley, M. *Obstetric Nursing* (7th ed.). New York: Macmillan, 1978.

13

PREGNANCY: FAMILY PERSPECTIVE

> *The family is a complete organism, a unity in its own right, as real as an individual. . . . An event in part of this organized system impinges on every part of the rest of the system. . . . Thus childbirth and its attendant pregnancy is an experience that belongs to the family as a whole. . . . Families beget families.*
>
> *Howells, 1972, p. 127*

This generation of families from families is possible since human beings form groups that in turn divide and form new groups. Marriage and pregnancy are two catalysts for this separation of people from their parent groups or families. For many maternity nurses, however, the family is viewed as an appendage to the pregnant woman rather than as an integral part of her life and her reproductive experience. Families are a part of the pregnancy and childbirth experiences. Their influence is seen in the ways in which the expectant parents view themselves, their pregnancy, and their offspring. Each member of the pregnant dyad brings unique contributions to the pregnancy, contributions that have their roots in the families from which each one comes—their families of origin or orientation (Fig. 13.1).

While families contribute to the ways in which the expectant parents view themselves and their pregnancy, families are also affected by the pregnancy, particularly by the birth of the child and all that it symbolizes to them and to the child's parents.

This chapter is concerned with the ways in which an event, such as pregnancy, impacts on the new or developing family, as well as on the families of orientation. The family is viewed by most authorities as being the significant social unit with which a person has sustained contact. There is a reciprocal influence between a person and the family from which that person comes that is unlikely ever to be obliterated completely. The maternity nurse, for these reasons, must view the family as an integral part of the pregnancy and childbirth experiences, understand its influence, and appreciate its needs although contacts with extended family members may be few and often more indirect than direct.

Family is usually defined as two or more persons who are bound together by sociocultural, blood, or affectional ties. This traditional definition will pose problems for those people who view the family as much more than is implied by it. Legal ties do not make a family in a psychosocial sense, nor do blood ties connote a caring, supportive relationship between people; but each of these binds the person to his or her kinship group in some way. Affectional ties may be the strongest bond between two or more people, and caring relationships are believed by many to form the central core that ties the family together. The rules and practices of the society and culture from which the person comes will bind that person to the culture and ethnic group of orientation in both apparent and subtle ways. We see a family as encompassing more than is implied by the scope of legal ties such as marriage and recognize that affectional ties between two or more people may be as strong as legal ties. Blood ties are important to the family, both biophysically and psychosocially; however, adoptive parents, foster parents, and friends replace the biologic family for a significant number of people.

Pregnancy will be discussed here from the perspectives of the married couple expecting its first child, the nuclear family with young and older children, and the extended family. Selected variant family types, such as the unmarried couple, the homosexual family, the commune family, and the migrant family will also be included. The influence of culture on families, generally, will be addressed. Implications for the nursing care of the expectant woman within the context of her family will be the concluding section of the chapter.

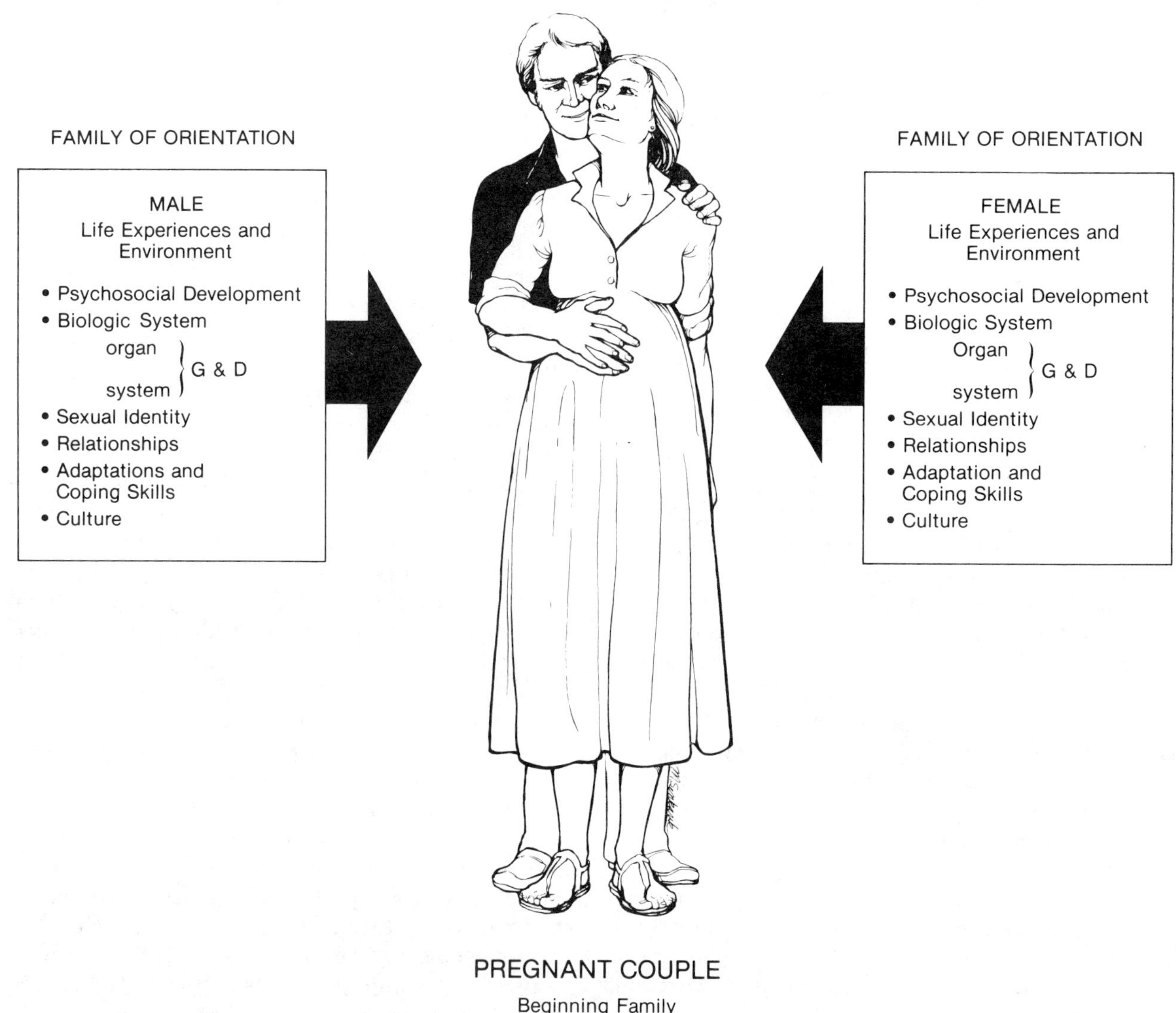

Figure 13.1
Pregnancy brings together biologically, as well as culturally, two separate families of orientation.

THE CONTEMPORARY AMERICAN FAMILY

Families today present a blend of the traditional and contemporary value systems of society. The family can no longer be viewed exclusively as a group of people with legal and blood ties working together toward common goals. Rather, the contemporary American family is an amalgam of unique individuals with diverse interests and goals, interacting with each other through a variety of different, often changing, relational patterns (Fig. 13.2).

Since its inception the United States has received people of diverse national, social, ethnic, and cultural backgrounds. This human collage has merged into the indistinct composit called the American—an industrious individual, motivated by ambition and ingenuity, backed by the love and encouragement of the family who rallies around at the time of crisis and exults at the birth of each new child, the family's investment in the future generation and their assurance of immortality. This characterization of the American has influenced the view of the model American family as being democratic rather than autocratic as is the more traditional European patriarchical family model. The democratic family is characterized as respecting the uniqueness of its members, giving encouragement and support for individual decision making, applauding ambition, and allowing for role flexibility and toleration of differences among its members. Such a representation of the democratic family has been found to be more ideal than real (Koller, 1974). Many of the characteristics of this ideal democratic family are combined with elements of the more traditional family model as it is viewed within the sociocultural heritage of the family. The nurse is most likely to encounter families that are not derived exclusively from one model or concept, but rather, families that are composits of the family organization and values as shaped by preceding generations, contemporary social, political, and economic forces, and unique individual and group needs.

The contemporary family in America is the product of changes that have occurred with each generation in response to the forces that were rampant during that generation. Legacies from past generations have great influence upon the values and attitudes of present generations, particularly in regard to pregnancy, childbirth, and parenthood. There is no prototype of the typical American family around which to develop a model for nursing care that will be appropriate or useful in every situation. Instead, the family is a fluid, ever-changing mixture of the old, the new, and the dreams and aspirations of the future.

Family theory has evolved in an effort to explain the characteristics, functions; structure, and organization of the family. Most of you are familiar with the major theoretical frameworks for viewing families; therefore, this content is not repeated here. Instead the focus will be on characteristics, needs, and goals of the contemporary family.

Characteristics of Contemporary American Families

Characteristics of American families have been influenced by what Tallcott Parsons (1965) refers to as society's "continuing differentiation in its structure, a general process of upgrading of expectations and responsibilities, and the related development of new modes of integration of persons and sub-structures in the increasingly complex society" (p.31). This continuing differentiation is closely correlated with the industrialization of a society and is influenced by events such as wars and nonviolent political or social movements. The greater the industrialization of a society, the more accelerated is the differentiation of its structure. Twentieth-century America has experienced both a significant surge in technologic and industrial growth and the social and political upheaval associated with two world wars and an economic depression (1930s). The women's movement has also influenced the family as it exists today.

Industrialization enabled the family to change its source of income from an agrarian, or farming, income to a salary for employment by an industrial enterprise. The large nuclear family with its closely related kinship network went its separate ways to where jobs were provided by industry. This separation led to dissemination of the family members to different parts of the country where they established smaller nuclear units composed of the husband/wife dyad and their children. Not only did this emigration result in reduction of the total size of the family, it removed the satellite nuclear family from the network of family support, necessitating the establishment of new and different affectional and supportive relationships outside of the kinship group. Today

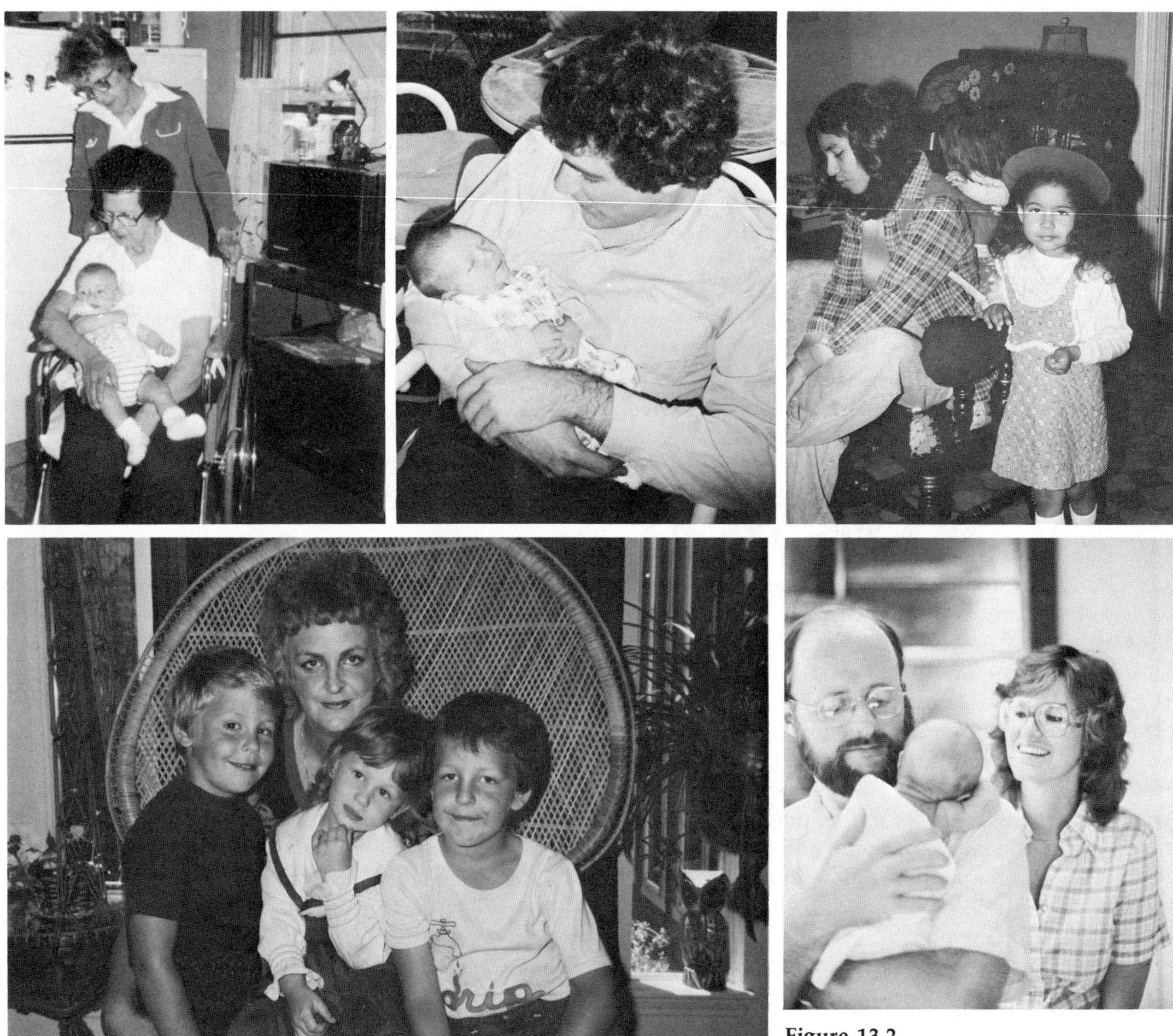

Figure 13.2
Diversity in American families.

the nuclear dyad may be found as married or unmarried couples living in close contact with or in alienation from their families of orientation. Such couples may remain a dyad and may or may not have or adopt children.

Family organization and function are closely related to trends in attitudes toward marriage. The age at which people marry has varied from one historical period to another (Duvall, 1977). Before the widespread use of contraceptives, the age of marriage was closely correlated with the age of first childbirth and the total number of children to which a woman gave birth during her lifetime. Today, young marrieds may delay pregnancy and parenthood because of educational, career, or personal goals. Increasingly, couples are opting out of parenthood or delaying it until their more mature years. (See Chapter 12.) After World War II and on into the 1950s there was a marked reduction in the mean age of marriage. The postwar years saw many teenage marriages. Marriage is more likely now to occur during the early to mid-20s with first pregnancy between 24 and 30 years of age or later.

The birth rate declined significantly between the years 1950 and 1975. This decrease was a result of a number of factors, the most influential one being the availability of contraceptives to poor and affluent alike. The maternity nurse is more likely to care for couples having their first, second, and possibly third child, rather than for families having their fourth, fifth, or beyond child. Many of these expectant parents are better educated and more self-directed, therefore needing a different type of nursing care than what has been traditionally provided.

The geographic dispersal of the family, mentioned earlier, has resulted in decreased access to, control by, and support from kinship groups and the establishment of new and different support sources of which the nurse is one. All nuclear families, however, are not removed from their families of orientation, and the nurse will encounter a significant number of couples with close kinship ties. Dissemination of the family has also resulted in increased population heterogeneity and a blending of cultural values and ethnic practices. The nurse may be providing care to a couple from distinctly different ethnic origins, each of whom brings personal values and beliefs to the union. It is not uncommon for this new family to experience conflicts regarding pregnancy and parenthood because of these differences. The nurse must understand the backgrounds of both members in order to help them successfully establish their new family. The closer the ties to their kinship groups, the greater the influence these groups tend to have on the emerging family. The nurse may find him or herself in the role of buffer for arising conflicts or of a resource person whose judgment is respected by all those involved.

Social change that has affected families has been so accelerated over the past several decades that roles assumed by the man and the woman have become blurred. Men are no longer only breadwinners nor are women only wives, mothers, and homemakers. Today, both men and women are likely to be wage earners; increasingly, household and parenting responsibilities are being shared. (See Chapter 18.) Another aspect of role change is *role reversal* in which the man and woman exchange roles within the family—the woman assumes the role of wage earner while the man takes on the roles of housekeeper and child care giver. This role reorganization can lead to *role confusion,* particularly as roles are perceived by the young children within the family. Role change in families can be expected to influence in some way the growing child's perception of identity and gender role. Much of what is published about parenthood does not take role change, especially role reversal, into account. The working mother may feel that she is shortchanging her family and children and may also try to assume all roles usually associated with wife and mother. She then runs the risk of *role overload* and the frustrations that accompany such a state.

Increasingly women are heading single-parent households with all of the responsibilities associated with such a role. Women sometimes express guilt, which is primarily associated with their role of parent, because their work takes them outside of the home. The long-term effect of role change on the family is not presently known. However, opposing arguments have been mounted ranging from the position that the family is fast becoming an archaic social unit because of change in structure and role to the belief that, even though the organization and function of the family are changing, it is still healthy and viable in today's world.

Contemporary families, on the whole, have increased economic resources and are able to afford a higher standard of living than families a generation ago. This increased purchasing power has enabled many families to afford child-care services outside of the kinship group, once more expanding nonfamily support and decreasing ties to the extended family. Greater purchasing power and its corollary, higher standard of living, are not available to all families. Galanter (1974) has referred to the two groups of Americans as the "haves and have nots," representing a distinct economic dichotomy. Increasingly the gulf is widening between the affluent and poor strata of the population. There is some indication that even the stable middle-class family is gravitating toward one or the other economic poles. National concerns about inflation and recession are widespread. The direction of the national economy in the years ahead is unclear, as is the impact on the family and what it will be able to buy. Health care—except in serious illness or emergency—is increasingly viewed as a luxury, not a necessity, by large numbers of Americans. The effect of the cost of hospitalization for childbirth is already being seen in consumer efforts to shorten hospital stay following birth and in home birth movements and other alternatives to hospital delivery. (See Chapter 28.)

The Influence of Culture on Childbearing Families

Three concepts that are often used interchangeably but that are actually different are culture, ethnic, and ethnicity. *Culture* refers to general characteristics of a society in regard to beliefs, values, attitudes, behaviors, institutions, arts, and other human endeavors that are transmitted from generation to generation. *Ethnic* characteristics are considered to be those definitive characteristics of a social group within the broader culture that gives that group special distinction such as religious beliefs and linguistic and racial characteristics; ethnicity is the association or belonging of a person to that group. The culture of the United States is a variegation of numerous ethnic groups each of which has its own racial heritage and religious and social backgrounds. Many of these groups also have a common language that is different from English. It is not uncommon for the nurse to use the word "culture" to refer to ethnic background or ethnicity of the consumer for whom care is being provided.

Certain cultural characteristics are associated with childbearing practices in the United States. The examples we present here permeate the whole of the American culture. Most women have their children in a hospital. A physician supervises prenatal care and assists with birth or delivers the child through operative procedures such as forceps or cesarean birth; there is widespread use of drugs to control pain during childbirth; and so on. Within the American culture, however, there are numerous ethnic groups who have beliefs perculiar to that group. The maternity nurse is likely to be the liason who helps to reconcile or integrate the American cultural practices with the ethnic behaviors and beliefs of the unique groups. The middle-income, white Anglo-Saxon Protestant (WASP) has frequently been viewed as the prototype for the American culture. In reality, although they are a large segment of the population, they are an ethnic group within the culture. The American Indian, the black, the Mexican–American, the Japanese–American, the Jew, among others, are all ethnic groups within the American culture. Even though their heritages and many of their practices may derive from another culture, they are all Americans. The nurse must be aware of and respect cultural and ethnic beliefs, values and behaviors whether they be different from or similar to those held by the nurse's own ethnic group.

The influences of culture and ethnicity on family structure and function have been clearly established. Historically, a core function of families has been procreation, and the influence of culture on childbearing and child-rearing practices has been profound. Cultural influence from generation to generation has been possible because the family is also the source for teaching a young child the rules of a society—socialization. This is selective education in that the family of orientation determines which rules the child will learn. Each family is a product of its generation and beliefs, and values and attitudes change somewhat from generation to generation. However, some cultural or ethnic traits are perpetuated from one generation to the next through repetition of rituals or behaviors. Many of these rituals and behaviors center around reproduction and related events. Ritual circumcision of Jewish male infants is one example. Food habits during pregnancy are often culturally determined; "eating for two" is a belief in more than one ethnic group. Ethnic groups advocate avoidance of certain activities during pregnancy, such as sexual abstinence for a period during and after the pregnancy or not permitting the woman to hang clothes out to dry because lifting her arms above her head will cause the umbilical cord to twist around the baby's neck and choke the fetus. Attitudes toward labor and behavior during labor are often of cultural or ethnic origin. For example, the pregnant woman of Japanese lineage during labor may appear as a stoic, controlled person, while the woman of Hispanic descent may be very vocal. The mountain woman from Appalachia may place her shoes upside down under the bed after birth in order to decrease the "after-pains." The pregnant woman of German origin may swaddle her infant tightly. The Catholic family may want the infant baptized at the time of birth if there is a concern with the health of the child, whereas the Protestant family may not accept such an action. There are always exceptions to pure ethnic practices for, as mentioned earlier, each generation adds its own cultural dimension to individual and family life. You need only examine the background, beliefs, and practices of your own family and compare them with those of your parents and grandparents to gain an appreciation for the influence of culture on a person.

The following clinical incident is an example of the incorrect assessment of the needs of a certain family concerning education about their newborn twin boys because of the ignorance of a nurse about the family's ethnic background.

Joyce J., a young nurse, had been providing nursing care for Maria G. and her newborn twin boys, Ramon and Riccardo. Maria was 17 years old and her husband Juan was 18. They were bilingual Americans of Mexican descent. Joyce had worked diligently to help prepare Maria and Juan to leave the hospital with their young sons and to be able to take on their parenting responsibilities. The day arrived for Maria to be discharged from the hospital. Joyce was there to see that all was in order for the discharge. As the couple prepared to leave, Maria grapsed the nurse's hand and profusely thanked her for all of her help and instruction. Her words of thanks included: "I'll tell my mother everything you told me since she'll be taking care of my babies for the next three or four weeks while I rest."

Had the nurse been adequately prepared to give nursing care to this young family, she would have understood the ethnic practices and adjusted her plan of care to attend to them. Instead, the nurse imposed her own cultural and ethnic beliefs on the couple, thereby decreasing the immediate usefulness of her teaching to them. Examples of inadequate understanding of culture and its implications for nursing practice are not uncommon.

THE IMPACT OF PREGNANCY ON THE FAMILY

Pregnancy and family are viewed here from two vantage points. First, the impact of pregnancy on selected traditional family types will be discussed with attention to the married couple, the nuclear family, and the extended family. Second, variant family types including the unmarried couple, the unmarried pregnant adult, the homosexual couple, the migrant family, and the commune family, within the context of the pregnancy experience will be addressed briefly. There are many other variations of family life-style seen in the United States today; however, we have chosen to present those mentioned as they represent either emerging family types or family styles of some health or social significance. References and readings included at the end of this chapter will also help you better understand both traditional and variant family styles.

Traditional Family Types

Three family types generally viewed as the most representative in the United States and those with whom the maternity nurse is most likely to come into contact are the married couple, the nuclear family, and the kinship, or extended family.

THE MARRIED COUPLE

The married couple is defined here as a man and woman bound legally by marriage who are expecting their first child—the beginning nuclear family. Pregnancy has a special significance to and impact on this couple. The husband and wife must undergo adjustments that enable them to move from their status as a dyad, concerned principally with their relationship with each other, to a triad that must incorporate and accept their child as part of their life. This change from couple to family is considered by some to be a period of profound change during which the couple must accomplish clearly identifiable developmental tasks (Duvall, 1977). A number of factors influence the ease or discomfort with which the couple makes this transition.

▲ ***Age of the Couple.*** Age at either extreme—early adolescence or middle age—often contributes to the difficulty with which the couple copes with the demands of the first pregnancy. The young teenage couple may still need to work through the tasks associated with adolescence, while the more mature couple may find readjustment of their life-style to incorporate the demands of the infant particularly taxing. The mature young adult who is emotionally and physically ready to receive the child and take on the role of parent is often thought to be better able to cope with the demands of a first pregnancy. Exceptions to either case can be found, for each couple is unique and factors aside from age influence the impact of pregnancy on the couple.

▲ ***Length of the Marriage.*** The longer the period in which the couple has had to adjust to the marriage, the better would seem to be their adjustment to pregnancy. In most cases this is true. If the couple has had the time to work through the demands of the marriage, to learn to know and like—as well as love—each other, and to establish a firm relationship upon which to build their lives as parents, they have a better chance of coping successfully with the birth of their child and with their new roles as parents. The opposite of this is that the couple who has been married for a long time may find the child an intrusion on a life-style that is well established and may resent having to change their relationship with each other and with their peer groups in order to accommodate the demands of the child.

▲ ***Stability of the Marriage.*** A marriage that is stable and in which the partners have mutual respect and love for each other is a sound basis upon which to pursue pregnancy and parenthood. There is clear documentation that couples who use pregnancy and parenthood as a glue to hold an unstable marriage together usually encounter difficulty somewhere along the way and are more likely to fail rather than to succeed.

▲ ***Motivation for Becoming Pregnant.*** Motivation for becoming pregnant has been shown to influence the ways in which the couple cope first with the pregnancy and later with their new roles as parents (Jessner et al., 1970). Rational, positive reasons would seem to be the best basis for becoming pregnant. However, not all pregnancies are planned and not all reasons for becoming pregnant are rational; the real reasons may not even be apparent to the couple or may be irrational. Motives for pregnancy include wanting a child because of the need to complete their family unit or having a child because the couple's friends and relatives are pregnant or have a child or the couple's parents want a grandchild. Pregnancy also occurs without clearly defined reasons. Not all pregnancies are planned; however, most couples adjust to both the planned and unplanned pregnancy. Some pregnancies are accidents. An unplanned pregnancy is not necessarily an unwanted pregnancy nor does it necessarily result in an unwanted child.

▲ ***Circumstances Surrounding the Conception.*** Sometimes pregnancy occurs because one partner imposes a pregnancy on the other, for example the woman who forgets to take her birth control pill or the man who seduces or in some circumstances rapes his partner. Most pregnancies occur because of a strong emotional attachment of the couple to each other. When such an attachment exists, the couple is better able to adjust to the pregnancy and its demands, whether or not the pregnancy was planned or initially wanted at this time.

▲ ***Family Status or Peer Group Pressure.*** It is not unusual for a couple to decide to become pregnant because of the need to maintain the status of the marriage in the eyes of their peers and their relatives. This is especially true if the family has a need to perpetuate the family name or if the child or grandchild is viewed as having a special social or legal significance to the family. Peer group pressure to conform may be overt or subtle, and the married couple whose peers are pregnant may feel that they are excluded from their group of friends if they do not have a child as well.

All of these factors as well as many others have an impact on the way in which the married couple make the adjustment, first to pregnancy and later to parenthood.

Pregnancy requires that the husband and wife not only make many adjustments in their life together, but it also alters their expectations of each other. They have been used to relating only to each other; their focus has been on meeting each other's needs for love, companionship, and sexual gratification; they have not needed other people to make their life complete. Pregnancy requires a significant change in roles within the family. The wife first becomes a pregnant woman, with all of the attendant demands. Then she becomes a mother whose first responsibility is to her dependent child. The husband first becomes an expectant father who may or may not understand the biologic or emotional changes that occur in his wife. Then, he becomes a father, often with little rehearsal for or experience in that role. Pregnancy places his wife in a much more dependent position than she had been in previously. If she had been a wage earner, she may need to leave her job and focus her time and attention on the pregnancy and preparation for the child. The couple may not be certain of what roles each wants the other to assume in regard to the pregnancy or to parenting the child. Because the wife is often emotionally labile during pregnancy, she may not be ready or able to deal with the role change at the same time and in the same way as her husband. Communication patterns will need to be adjusted since the woman may turn to other women—her mother, her friends, the nurse—to help with concerns she otherwise would have discussed with her husband. Biologically, the husband cannot experience the pregnancy, and he may feel left out of activities surrounding his wife and her pregnancy. At the same time, he may find new and different demands placed on him.

Sexual practices will alter because of the pregnancy. (See Chapter 14.) In some cases the sexual relationship will improve for both partners. Other couples may find that their sexual relationship loses something during the pregnancy or deteriorates considerably. The couple may feel either a gain in regard to their love making or a loss of sexual partners who are concerned with satisfying each other's sexual needs.

Pregnancy and childbirth often mark the true entrance of the couple into the world of the mature. If the couple is ready for the responsibility associated with maturity, the adjustment will most likely be assured; if the couple is unprepared, pregnancy will be a stressful period.

Pregnancy is a time of increased stress for the couple, even to the point of being a crisis (Caplan, 1961; LeMasters, 1965). Since pregnancy is only one of many phases in a person's or couple's life, it is not protected from the everyday stresses of life unrelated to the pregnancy, stresses that may be augmented by the pregnancy itself, thereby increasing the number and intensity of stressful events (Howells, 1972). First pregnancy has been clearly documented as a crisis or as a catalyst for crisis (LeMasters, 1965; Dyer, 1965).

Pregnancy may impose a financial burden on some couples, particularly the young pair, who are not yet financially secure. The irony is that the partners are biologically most ready to become parents at a time in their lives when they are economically least secure. Unplanned pregnancy may impose an increased financial burden either because the couple has not saved money to pay for the costs of having a child or because the couple does not have insurance to cover expenses. Many young couples are, however, well prepared to meet the financial demands of an uncomplicated pregnancy.

Once a couple is diagnosed as pregnant and this information is disseminated to friends and relatives, the couple will receive much advice; some of it will result from request, a great deal more will be offered without the couple's solicitation. The attitudes of these family members and friends affects the couple in a number of ways. It assures the future parents of the interest of others in their lives, their well-being, and their expected child; it can reinforce their feelings of security and belonging. Occasionally the values and beliefs of the family will conflict with those of the couple, and frustrations and stresses will arise. The pregnant couple will need to come to agreement upon the roles they want relatives and friends to play in regard to the pregnancy and the extent to which they will allow their influence.

Pregnancy impacts on the married couple in four distinct ways: It precipitates reorganization of the family structure from a two-member unit to a three-member family; it requires the two people to rethink their roles and to reorganize in order to accommodate the demands of the pregnancy and the expected child; it initiates new, and often different, biologic and psychosocial needs in both the man and the woman; and it ushers in a period of decreased marital satisfaction for most couples that is to last for as long as 10 years (Rollins & Cannon, 1974). Pregnancy may be a period of great fulfillment for the couple or it may be a time of upheaval. Evelyn Duvall beautifully described the periods of marriage and parenthood, which are bridged by pregnancy, in the following statement.

> *Marriage involves the risk of failure and the loss of some privacy and autonomy in exchange for the warmth of companionship with a familiar mate over the years. . . . Parenthood has become a courageous leap of faith into the future that only the brave should attempt.*
>
> *Duvall, 1977, p. 481*

THE NUCLEAR FAMILY

The nuclear family is defined here as the parents plus their children. The nuclear family unit in the United States is most likely to consist of a mother, father, and two children ranging in age from infancy through young adulthood. The couple, with one or more children, who becomes pregnant, experiences many of the same adjustments just described in the discussion of the married pregnant couple. However, the nuclear family also experiences pregnancy somewhat differently. Role reorganization is not as great with the second or subsequent child; some role change is needed, however, in order to accommodate another person into the family unit. Motivations for pregnancy are not dissimilar to those discussed earlier. Three areas seem to create the greatest impact on the nuclear family pregnancy: (1) the effect of the pregnancy on the child, or children, within the family and the preparation needed to help them make the adjustment to a sibling; (2) financial considerations in light of the cost of pregnancy and childbearing and child rearing in today's economic environment; and (3) living accommodations as the family increases in size. As more children are added to the family, the parenting responsibilities increase and the marital relationship is likely to become relegated to a position of lessor priority. Increased numbers of children also intensify the stress of the parents in regard to their dual role as marriage partners and parents (Burr, 1970). They have less privacy and less time for each other. Feelings of dissatisfaction by both partners with the marriage, lowered self-esteem, and feelings of unworthiness, especially by the woman, are not uncommon during the parenting years (Rollins & Feldman, 1970). These feelings may be augmented if the second or subsequent pregnancy is unplanned. With the first pregnancy, the couple needed only to attend to the tasks associated with marriage and the addition of a child. Parenthood was a future, but unknown, prospect. With later pregnancies, the couple must continue to deal with the role readjustment that parenthood imposes on any marriage, but they must now experience pregnancy both as parents and as expectant parents, compounding the potential for stressful events.

The response of the child to his or her mother's pregnancy is determined to a great extent by the age and cognitive capability of the child. Children respond to pregnancy in their own unique ways; however, the attitudes of children toward the pregnancy and the ways in which they influence their parents during pregnancy can be divided into two distinct periods that are related to the developmental stage of the child—the preschool period and the adolescent period. Some of the ways in which the child and parents are reciprocally affected during pregnancy are discussed in Chapter 18.

Preschool children whose parents are pregnant may respond with much interest in the pregnancy. They are likely to ask numerous questions about the changes in their mother's body. Most young children look forward to the arrival of a sibling, particularly if they are the only child. Most of the problems associated with pregnancy and the preschool child occur following the birth of the baby when the child must compete with the new brother or sister for the attention of the mother and father. Increasingly, parents are including their young children in discussions about the pregnancy and plans for the new baby. It is not uncommon to see the young child mimic the mother in her preparations for the coming infant. Some families are involving their children, including those of preschool age, in the childbirth experience and are seeking alternative birth methods that provide for this inclusion. (See Chapter 28.)

The school-age child is often interested in the pregnancy but is less concerned with it than the younger child. This is partially explained by the child's interest in other things outside of the family such as school activities and friends. Parents have to guard against expecting too much of their school-age child in terms of understanding and accepting what is going on during the pregnancy. They need to ascertain how their child is responding to the events surrounding the pregnancy and let this guide their response to the child and their inclusion of the child in the experience.

Teenagers and young adults tend to respond to their mother's pregnancy in two ways. On the one hand, they are pleased about the arrival of a new baby in the home and are eager to participate in the pregnancy in helpful ways. On the other hand, they may feel embarrassed about the pregnancy because it confirms that their parents engage in sexual activities, or appear disinterested in what is happening, and even avoid telling their friends about the expected baby. Teenage daughters may appear very interested in what is happening to their mothers. Pregnancies that occur when the other children are adolescents or young adults are often unplanned pregnancies. The parents may have difficulty adjusting to having another child just when their older children are about to leave the home. These parents need the support of their children and their acceptance of the pregnancy.

Children are costly to rear, and the addition of each child imposes increased financial demands on the family. The nuclear family is often better prepared to undertake the costs associated with a second pregnancy than they were with the first. Their readiness to do so may be associated with the intervals between pregnancies. A second pregnancy that closely follows the first may impose additional demands for money when the first pregnancy is not paid for. Health care costs are soaring, and it is not uncommon for a family to go into debt to meet the costs of a first or subsequent pregnancy. The family with a child will have incidental costs the couple did not need to consider, such as baby-sitting fees while the mother goes to the physician or to the hospital. In 1975 *Redbook* magazine reported a categoric analysis of the cost of having a baby. Pregnancy health care costs that include the physician (obstetrician and pediatrician), hospitalization, and drugs, along with the costs for feeding and clothing the infant during the first year of life and incidental costs such as maternity clothing were estimated to be $2,300. Today, with a persistent inflation in double figures, the cost can be adjusted to about $3,000–3,500 depending on the area of the country in which the family resides and whether they live in an urban or rural locale.

Living accommodations may need to be enlarged with a second or third pregnancy. This may require a temporary period of overcrowding until the family can make arrangements for enlarging present living quarters or moving to new ones. A number of families make do with crowded conditions if their children are small, but the family with adolescent children is faced with a different problem since the adolescent is often seeking privacy as he or she searches for personal identity and role. The indigent population who is expecting another child may need assistance with ways in which it can incorporate a new baby into existing family quarters since increasing space or moving to larger quarters is not as likely to be an option.

The nuclear family responds to pregnancy with a different set of needs, sometimes superimposed on needs similar to those experienced with the first pregnancy. They will need to cope with the presence of a child, the increased costs of adding another child, and the crowding of the home to accommodate another member.

THE EXTENDED FAMILY

Large numbers of childbearing families today are likely to maintain close ties with their families of orientation; some of the young families will have parents or other relatives living with them. Pregnancy is not experienced in isolation from these kinship relationships.

The extended family members, especially the parents of the expectant parents, are likely to be intensely interested in the pregnancy of their children whether it be a first or later pregnancy. They are often eager to be involved and are a primary resource for support of the couple or the nuclear family. The extended family's expectations of grandchildren, nieces, or nephews will usually be made known to the pregnant family. If these expectations are complementary to those of the expectant family, there is unlikely to be problems or increased stresses; however, if extended family members have *strong* beliefs about how the pregnancy should be conducted or the child reared that are different from the expectant parents', conflicts are likely to arise. Some of the extended family's areas of interest that could become conflicts are child-rearing practices, food habits, important rituals, education for parenthood, and use of the family for support. In some cultures the grandparents expect to be involved in the care of the child when it is born. They may help the mother's recovery or take charge of the child, if allowed to do so, closing out the new mother and father. The nurse is in a position to help the expectant family determine what roles are preferred for extended family members.

There are some efforts underway to incorporate grandparents into the childbirth experience by providing classes to help them to adjust to grandparenthood, to assist them in understanding the needs of young families, even their own children, and to help them serve as a significant resource to these families. (See Chapter 18.)

It is often healthy for the young child to have contact and relationships with members of a generation twice removed. United States' culture has received criticism by some social anthropologists for its lack of attention to the value of incorporating the older family members into its youth-oriented society.

The key questions the maternity nurse needs to attend to are: "What does the pregnancy mean to the extended family?" "What role does the extended family wish to play in it?" "How does the expectant family feel about the role and involvement of their relatives in the childbearing experience?"

Memories of the relationship of the woman to her mother during her childhood and adolescent periods of development re-emerge during pregnancy. If this relationship was a healthy one, the mother may be a strong necessary support. If the earlier relationship was unhealthy, pregnancy may be the time for old conflicts to resurface to be resolved or further aggravated. Many mothers feel a need to be close to their daughters and to have some role during the pregnancies.

The reciprocal influences of the father/son relationship during pregnancy are not as clear as those of the mother/daughter relationship. This area has not been studied as extensively. It is known that the father has an effect on the way the young boy acquires his gender identity. Some fathers and sons become closer during the daughter's-in-law pregnancy. If the expectant couple's parents look forward to being grandparents, they are likely to involve themselves both in the pregnancy and the parenthood periods. However, the stereotypical grandparent as an elderly, white-haired, retired couple is fading fast. With today's increased life expectancy, many contemporary grandparents are young middle-aged, active people who have both the health and the economic security to lead their own lives. The nurse must be careful not to approach the subject of grandparents with an old-fashioned perspective; instead nurses should try to support the roles agreed upon which are mutually satisfactory to both generations.

Pregnancy is most likely the time that the expectant grandparents are faced with the realization that the expectant parent has been lost to them as their child. They will now have to become a lower priority than their grandchild in their child's life (Howells, 1972). The confirmation of pregnancy may also make them aware that their child's marriage, whether with or without their approval, has been established. The attitudes of the expectant grandparents toward their child's spouse may also influence the way in which the grandparents view and accept or reject the grandchild.

Variant Family Types

A number of variant family types are emerging in the United States. Some of the family styles have been around since the late 1950s; others predated even that period; still others are relatively new. Three of these variant family types are discussed briefly here.

THE UNMARRIED COUPLE

Marriage as a prerequisite for sexual relationships is disappearing as couples establish intimate relationships outside of the legal bonds of matrimony. The increased permissive attitudes toward sex and sexual behavior have enabled young people to live together, engage in sexual intercourse, and establish families without the legal commitment insisted upon by earlier generations.

The unmarried pregnant couple undergoes many of the same experiences with pregnancy that were discussed in the section on the married couple. Some of these couples establish lasting family relationships; others change partners frequently. The social stigma attached to unmarried pregnancy still exists in many parts of the United States. Its influence on health care is seen in hospital policies that deny the unmarried father admission to the labor and delivery rooms regardless of his relationship with the expectant mother. These restrictions, however, are being removed from many institutions throughout the country.

Nursing management of the unmarried couple is basically the same as that of the married couple. There are some unique needs of unmarried pregnant couples, however, about which the nurse should be aware. The name that the baby will assume is one area that should be clarified before birth and certainly shortly thereafter. Unless the expectant father acknowledges paternity and gives authority for the baby to have his name, the newborn will take the name of the mother in most states. Acknowledgment of paternity is usually not as much of a problem with unmarried couples as it may be with single, unmarried mothers. Clarification of the infant's name is necessary, however, before a birth certificate can be issued.

Since the relationship between the members of unmarried pregnant couple is not legally binding until they have lived together openly for a number of years and are recognized as a common-law marriage (requirements for establishing a common-law marriage vary from state to state), a significant number of these relationships terminate after a period of time. Termination of the relationship gives rise to problems concerning child custody and child support. Some such cases have reached the court system; nevertheless, the rights and responsibilities of the unmarried nuclear family to each other in terms of property rights and to the child in terms of custody, support, and inheritance rights have yet to be established clearly.

Since the kinship groups may not approve of the status of the unmarried pregnant couple, reassurance, support, and encouragement may not be forthcoming from the couple's parents or relatives. The nurse and the physician (and sometimes the couple's peer groups) are often the principal support for this couple throughout their pregnancy and early parenting experiences. The nurse needs to call upon other support sources within their peer group and social setting and to treat these people as significant others to this couple.

THE HOMOSEXUAL COUPLE

A variant of the unmarried couple family style is the homosexual couple. This is an arrangement where two men or two women live together in sexual intimacy. Increasingly, homosexual unions are seeking legal recognition and family rights. Since pregnancy is not a concern with such couples, most of the health care needs in relation to reproduction arise in regard to children born to either or both of the partners from an earlier heterosexual union. Homosexual families are also seeking to adopt children. The maternity nurse is less likely to provide nursing care for these families than for some of the others. However, nurses working with families generally or pediatric nurses will find these families among the consumer groups seeking health care. The maternity nurse needs to be aware of some of the unique characteristics of the homosexual family and some of the parenting needs and problems such parents have, for example, roles assumed by each partner and the influence on sex gender identification for the children of the family. Occasionally, the maternity nurse will provide care for a pregnant woman whose heterosexual relationship has terminated and been replaced by a homosexual union. It is important that the nurse understand his or her own values so that sensitive nursing care can be given. The maternity nurse is sometimes sought as a consultant to family life education and parent education courses and should be conversant with emerging family types. However, there are few published resources available to assist the nurse in caring for the homosexual couple regarding pregnancy and parenthood.

THE MIGRANT FAMILY

The migrant family represents a mobile family unit whose residence changes in association with their employment. The migrant family is often poor, large, and geographically removed from their kinship ties beyond the nuclear family. Some migrant family groups, however, do travel as an extended family unit. Although the migrant family may be separated from relatives for various periods of time, they tend to maintain close emotional ties with each other and with their families of orientation.

The migrant family may not readily seek health care supervision during pregnancy and often enters the health care delivery system at the time of childbirth. The pregnant woman may be difficult for the nurse and physician to manage since they usually do not have readily accessible health care records and she is often lost to health care supervision following delivery.

Because the migrant family travels from one part of the country to another, the pregnant woman who does seek prenatal care is likely to encounter inconsistency in health care practices from place to place and may find it difficult to comply with instructions given to her about herself and her unborn child. Migrant families rely on intra-family resources to support them through the childbearing and child-rearing experiences. These families are often large. All members who are able work to support the family, the younger children sometimes becoming the caregivers for those siblings who are younger still.

Migrant worker health care facilities have been established in some states. A large part of the health care services provided are related to childbearing and child-rearing needs. Nurses have been a part of these health care services and have served as health care providers and teachers.

It is important for the nurse to understand the differences between the migrant families who are usually farm workers and the migrant families who move frequently seeking other types of employment because of the economic problems that contribute to high unemployment. Migrant farm families follow the farming industry as a way of work and life. Their life-style is often consistent from year to year. The family who moves because of economic upheaval may be coming from a stable family life-style; they have remained in one location where they have made friends or have relatives. This family may be experiencing more acute stress than the migrant farm family, particularly if the woman is pregnant. The nurse who provides care for either of these groups of mobile families needs to understand their unique characteristics, their life-styles, and their needs.

THE COMMUNE FAMILY

There are two types of communes. One is the commune family in which a group of people have joined together in order to share family responsibilities and functions such as labor and child-care materials, goods, and services. These groups are mostly composed of nuclear family groups in which monogamous marriage is usual and the sharing is limited to social and economic exchange. The second type of commune is the group marriage, or commune marriage. Although this group marriage is not legal in the United States, many contemporary youth groups live together, sharing social, economic, and sexual functions in a de facto group marriage arrangement. The maternity nurse may find consumers from either or both of these communal arrangements seeking reproductive health care.

The commune family presents special family needs to the nurse. Since childbearing in the monogamous marriages closely resembles the events of pregnancy found in any married or nuclear family, the principal problem the nurse may encounter is in regard to education for child-rearing and parenthood. Although there is a clearly defined parent dyad in the commune family, some of childrearing activities are shared, making it difficult for the nurse to assess accurately the needs of the family in regard to its place in the commune. The nurse will work directly with the expectant parents much as with any other expectant parent group and will be aware that the other people in the commune family comprise the essential support system for the pregnant couple.

The commune marriage family presents a different set of needs to the nurse. It is not uncommon for paternity to be unclear in these circumstances. Decisions regarding the role of the expectant father in regard to the pregnancy may be difficult since the nurse may find that she is caring for one pregnant woman and more than one possible expectant father. There may be concerns about the responsibility of the father in terms of legal and health system policy. The rights and responsibilities of the commune members regarding the child are not always clear. Members tend to move in and out of the commune with significant care givers for the child changing frequently.

Both the commune family and the commune marriage have been the target of considerable study by social science disciplines and we suggest that you read further regarding both of these family types.

NURSING CARE FOR FAMILIES WHO ARE EXPERIENCING PREGNANCY

The nursing goals for the care of families, of whatever type, who are experiencing pregnancy are as follows.

- ▲ Facilitate the development of a strong family unit
- ▲ Decrease the intensity of stress the pregnant family is likely to encounter
- ▲ Support family coping through the strategies of teaching, reassurance, and reinforcement of coping efforts
- ▲ Promote family strengths, and moderate family weaknesses
- ▲ Promote the development of self-confidence and self-esteem for family members

The nurse will rely upon a number of nursing approaches to accomplish these and other related goals for the family during pregnancy. One of the most important tools the nurse can rely upon is an accurate and timely *assessment* of the characteristics of the family, including the way in which the family is organized, the roles assumed by its members, the ways in which responsibilities are assigned, and the strengths and weaknesses of the family groups. This assessment of family serves as the basis for planning the nursing care needed for each unique family for whom the nurse provides care.

The nurse will also need to rely upon *anticipatory guidance* to help the family understand and anticipate stresses and events before they happen. Crises associated with pregnancy can be lessened or avoided if the family is aware of pregnancy as a potential for crisis and understands its own strengths in regard to coping with stress and crisis. Families need to learn about pregnancy, childbirth, and parenthood, whatever their family type. The nurse will rely upon appropriate and sound *teaching strategy and methodology* to help families acquire this knowledge.

The nurse may also serve as an objective outsider to whom the family can turn for *support, clarification, reassurance,* and *information.* The pregnant family is the potential investment for the future reproductive health-related events and for the health of the family members generally.

SUMMARY

This chapter examined pregnancy from a family perspective. It began with the contemporary family in the United States and looked at some of the more traditional family types—the married couple, the nuclear family, and the extended family. Characteristics of families were discussed, and a brief description of three variant family types—the unmarried couple (heterosexual and homosexual), the migrant family, and the commune family—were given. The chapter closed with identification of some goals for the maternity nurse and some suggested strategies for assisting pregnant families with health care. It included family health assessment, anticipatory guidance, education, and support. These strategies are elaborated on in other chapters throughout the book and were only mentioned in this chapter to help you associate their use with the care of families, as well as individuals, who are experiencing pregnancy.

REFERENCES AND READINGS

Belsky, J. Early Human Experience: A Family Perspective. *Dev Psych* 17(1):3, 1981.

Bennett, B. Child Rearing Practices of the Communal Family, in Skolnick, A. S. Skolnick, J. H. (Eds.), *Family in Transition.* Boston: Little, Brown, 1971, p. 501.

Burr, W. R. Satisfaction with Various Aspects of Marriage Over the Life Cycle: A Random Middle Class Sample. *J Marriag Fam* 32(1):29, 1970.

Caplan, G. *An Approach to Community Mental Health.* New York: Grune & Stratton, 1961.

Duvall, E. M. *Marriage and Family Development* (5th ed.). Philadelphia: J. B. Lippincott, 1977.

Dyer, E. D. Parenthood as Crisis: A Re-Study, in Parad, H. J. (Ed.), *Crisis Intervention.* New York: Family Service Association of America, 1965, pp. 312–323.

Entwisle, D. R., Doering, D. G. A Longitudinal Study of Family Formation. *Soc Res Child Dev* Newsletter. Fall 1981.

Eshelman, R. *The Family: An Introduction* (2nd ed.). Boston: Allyn & Bacon, 1978.

Galanter, M. Why the Haves Come Out Ahead: Speculation on the Limits of Legal Change. *Law Soc Rev* 9:95, 1974.

Howells, J. G. Childbirth Is A Family Experience, in Howells, J. G. (Ed.), *Modern Perspectives in Psycho-Obstetrics.* New York: Brunner/Mazel, 1972, pp. 127–149.

Jessner, L., Weigert, L., and Foy, J. L. The Development of Parental Attitudes During Pregnancy, in Anthony, E., Benedek, T. (Eds.), *Parenthood: Its Psychology and Psychopathology.* Boston: Little, Brown 1970.

Koller, M. R. *Families: A Multigenerational Approach.* New York: McGraw-Hill, 1974.

LeMasters, E. E. Parenthood as Crisis, in Parad, H. J. (Ed.), *Crisis Intervention.* New York: Family Service Association of America, 1965.

Lewin, E. Lesbianism and Motherhood: Implications for Child Custody. *Hum Organiz* 40(1):6, 1981.

Miller, J. R., Jonosik, E. H. *Family Focused Care.* New York: McGraw-Hill, 1980.

Newton, N., Newton, M. Childbirth in Cross Cultural Perspective, in Howells, J. G. (Ed.), *Modern Perspectives in Psycho-Obstetrics.* New York: Brunner/Mazel, 1972, pp. 150–172.

Parsons, T. The Normal American Family, in Farber, S. M., Mustacchi, P., and Wilson, R. H. L. (Eds.), *Man and Civilization: The Family's Search for Survival.* New York: McGraw-Hill, 1965, pp. 31–50.

Rollins, B. C., Feldman, H. Marital Satisfaction Over the Family Life Cycle. *J Marriag Fam* 32(1):24, 1970.

Rollins, B. C., Cannon, K. L. Marital Satisfaction Over the Life Cycle: A Reevaluation. *J Marriag Fam* 36(2):271, 1974.

Spector, R. E. *Cultural Diversity in Health and Illness.* New York: Appleton-Century-Crofts, 1979.

Spiro, M. Is the Family Universal? *Am Anthropol* 56:840, 1954.

Williams, C. How Much Does a Baby Cost? *Redbook.* April 1976.

14

SEXUALITY AND PREGNANCY

> *Sexual behavior is an important index of a relationship. . . . Men and women undergo profound personal, interpersonal and social changes during pregnancy and the postpartum period. . . . Parenthood makes a shared life more complicated, but it also carries with it the potential to make life together more meaningful as lovemaking goes beyond caring for each other and spreads out to embrace the family unit.*
>
> Bing & Colman, 1977, p. 159

The quote has simple, yet meaningful statements. Sexuality is an integral part of a person's identity and cuts through to the essence of his or her personal self. Pregnancy reveals a woman's sexuality and is confirmation of both male and female sexual capabilities. The maternity nurse may accept pregnancy as a natural and normal event and delight in helping expectant parents cope with the experiences associated with pregnancy and childbirth; this same nurse, however, may lose sight of the fact that pregnancy is, most often, the result of sexual intercourse and, consequently, have difficulty helping pregnant women and their mates with sexual needs during and following pregnancy.

Pregnancy is likely to expose both the man and the woman to new, intensified, or decreased sexual appetites and require changes in their sexual practices if their relationship is to be mutually satisfying. It goes without saying that societal norms, personal values, and cultural practices all affect a person's view of sexuality, which, in turn, has implications for the pregnant woman, her partner, and the nurse.

This chapter will provide the nurse with theory, content, and strategies useful in assisting couples in enhancing sexual adaptation during pregnancy—this period of profound change. Historically, myths, old wives tales, and even instructions about sexuality during pregnancy have been based on hearsay rather than on logic and knowledge. Sexual relationships during the antepartum, intrapartum, and postpartum periods are discussed along with physiologic and psychosocial adaptation during those periods. The role of the nurse in assessing and intervening with sexual needs during and following pregnancy is addressed, with special attention to guidelines for history taking, general assessment, and problem-solving strategies. Anticipatory guidance during pregnancy is also included. The relationship of sexuality, nursing process, and teaching–learning process is presented at the end of the chapter in order to help you interrelate these factors in a way that will make nursing care both effective and sensitive.

DEVELOPMENTAL BACKGROUND

Developmentally, Sigmund Freud has laid the foundation for much of our understanding of human sexuality. He associates the principal source of pleasure during early childhood with the genital organs (Brill, 1935). Freud calls this the phallic stage of development, about 3 or 4 years old. He feels that genital feelings become stronger and more important during this stage and also that it is an important stage in relation to our responses to people later in life. Parental response to the natural sexual curiosities of children in this preschool era also are influential in building the foundation for healthy sexuality in adult life. If the child has a gentle but firm and consistent role model, the child's heterosexual development and good interpersonal relationships in later life will follow.

The 3- or 4-year-old child displays natural curiosity about her or himself and other family members and begins to learn sex roles. The child is curious about where babies come from, explores her or his genital organs, and compares them with friends. *Masturbation,* self-manipulation of one's genitals, is a natural and common learning experience. Discovering the difference between boys and girls is sometimes confusing to the child. Girls may desire a penis; boys may wish for breasts or a baby. Both sexes fear "something may be wrong" because they are "different." Thus, boys enter the phase characterized by the Odeipus complex and girls, the Electra complex. The feelings aroused in boys or girls during this stage are discussed in Chapter 7 and in the works of Freud (Freud, 1933).

At ages 4 and 5, children are highly excitable. The ambivalent feelings about parents and resolution of the complexes are normally followed by internalization of the values of the child's parents and development of the conscience. Thus, as we know from the literature, adequate parenting results in constructive resolution of the complexes. Inadequate parenting may retard full development of conscience and influence later adjustment and life-style. This is why developmental theorists generally agree that the preschool years are crucial for good interpersonal relationships in later life. Erikson talks about this in his stages of development; Sullivan reflects the significance of the early years and development of self-concept in his interpersonal theory (Erikson, 1963, 1968; Sullivan, 1953).

The school years are heavily influenced by schoolmates and are sexually characterized by a somewhat latent period. During adolescence, however, the tasks have clear implications for sexuality (see Chapter 7). Sullivan describes the adolescent period as having three needs: personal security (self-concept depends on how significant others see the person), intimacy, and trust. In other words, a close relationship with another is important, and the adolescent changes from seeking this close relationship from a person of the same sex to that of the opposite sex. Cultural, societal, and personal values are all significant in the accomplishment of the tasks of adolescence. Since pregnancy can occur during either adolescence or adulthood, you need to be aware of the tasks of both periods as you learn and apply information about sexuality and pregnancy.

ANTEPARTUM

Physiologic changes that occur throughout the antepartum period may affect sexual functioning are identified by Masters and Johnson (1966). In the first trimester, breast enlargement occurs as a result of increased vascularity and development of the glands of the breasts. Women experiencing their first pregnancy respond to sexual stimulation with more venous congestion than when nonpregnant. In early pregnancy sometimes breast tenderness during sexual activity reaches severe proportions, noted by turgid nipples and engorged areolae. During the second and third trimesters, breast sensitivity tends to decrease. The pelvic organs, also markedly vascular during pregnancy, are affected by increased sexual activity. In the first trimester, some women report abdominal cramping after orgasm and sometimes low backache. During the second and third trimesters, many women report increased sexual drive and increased interest in coital and manipulative activity. In Masters and Johnson's sample some women described fulminating and multiorgasmic experiences, some for the first time. Almost all women in the Masters and Johnson's sample reported during the second trimester improved sexual performance over their nonpregnant experiences. This included increased awareness, fantasy, and effectiveness of performance. Solberg and associates (1973) reports another viewpoint. In their study women reported a decrease in sexual activity in the antepartum period. It should be noted that this study was a retrospective report of women in the postpartum period.

Some of the changes reported by Masters and Johnson's sample can be related to the phases of the human sexual response cycle (see Chapter 7). The four phases are excitement, plateau, orgasm, and resolution. The human sexual response cycle relies upon two major physiologic events—vasocongestion of tissues and myotonia, increased muscle tone. The physiology of the phases is similar for the man and woman. During the excitement phase, multiparas experience engorgement of the labia majora. The labia minora enlarge 2–3 times their unstimulated size, although this was not evidenced during the third trimester for at this time, the labia minora are chronically engorged with blood. At the end of the first trimester, vaginal lubrication increased both in rapidity and amount. The only visual change noted during the plateau phase was engorgement of the entire vaginal barrel. This intense venous engorgement increases with advanced pregnancy. By the third trimester, the orgasmic platform is so overdistended that objective evidence of contractile efficiency was obscured. During orgasm in the third trimester, spasm of the uterus was observed lasting as long as a minute. Although fetal heart tones slowed, other evidence of fetal distress was not noted (see Chapter 16). In the resolution phase of the pregnant woman the vasocongested pelvis is frequently not relieved. This sustained congestion, along with pelvic pressure from a second or third trimester uterus, may result in a feeling of continued sexual stimulation. The literature suggests that because pelvic vasocongestion is not relieved after orgasm, this may contribute to increased levels of sexual responsiveness as seen and described in the second and third trimesters of pregnancy.

Levels of eroticism and sexual performance reported in the first trimester are varied. Decreased sexual interest in the first trimester seems to be associated with nausea and vomiting, fear of hurting the baby, or fatigue (Woods, 1979). Increased satisfaction in sexual activity during the second trimester seems to be well substantiated in the literature. Sexual awareness and performance were reported significantly improved among both married and unmarried women. In general, during the antepartum period there is decreased coital frequency in the third trimester, which may in part be the result of abstinence prescribed by the physician. Women in the third trimester seem to have more somatic complaints, for example, backache. Some women in the Masters and Johnson's study reported that their husbands withdrew from sex in the third trimester; reasons for this withdrawal were appearance of the woman's large abdomen, concern for personal comfort, and fear of injuring the baby (Bing & Colman, 1977).

The maternity nurse needs to anticipate that coital position will be a necessary sexual behavior change during pregnancy. The man astride position is used less often as pregnancy advances. The woman astride, side by side, and rear entry positions are often used as pregnancy advances (Figs. 14.1, 14.2). It is important that the couple communicate what is pleasant and comfortable in order to adapt and continue to enjoy a sexual experience satisfying to both.

Other studies have supported the fluctuating sexual awareness and activity during the antepartum period (Kenney, 1973; Falicov, 1973; Morris, 1975). The constant seems to be that a woman's sexual behavior during pregnancy varies. One study that looked at sexual attitudes and behaviors of 216 women trimester by trimester seems fairly representative of pregnant women (Tolor & DiGranzia, 1976). It was reported that, in general, women in the first and second trimesters were generally satisfied with the level of sexual activity, whereas women in the third trimester seemed to prefer either an increase or decrease in sexual activity. The women in this study were also administered an Attitude Toward Sex Scale measuring conservatism versus liberalism. Sexual behaviors and attitudes about sex during pregnancy did not relate significantly to either a conservative or liberal attitude about sex.

Two other areas of interest about pregnant women are the need for closeness during pregnancy and the effects of body image changes on the woman and the couple. An increased need for touching behaviors—cuddling and holding—has been noted (Bing & Colman, 1977; Hollender & McGehee, 1974; Ellis, 1980). Women who were surveyed during their pregnancy and retrospectively who described a change in desire for body contact were 2–3 times more likely to report an increase rather than a decrease in desire to be held. Body image changes during pregnancy potentially have much impact on the woman as well as on her partner. The skin changes described in Chapter 12 (linea nigra, striae gravidarum) and breast and abdomen changes can influence

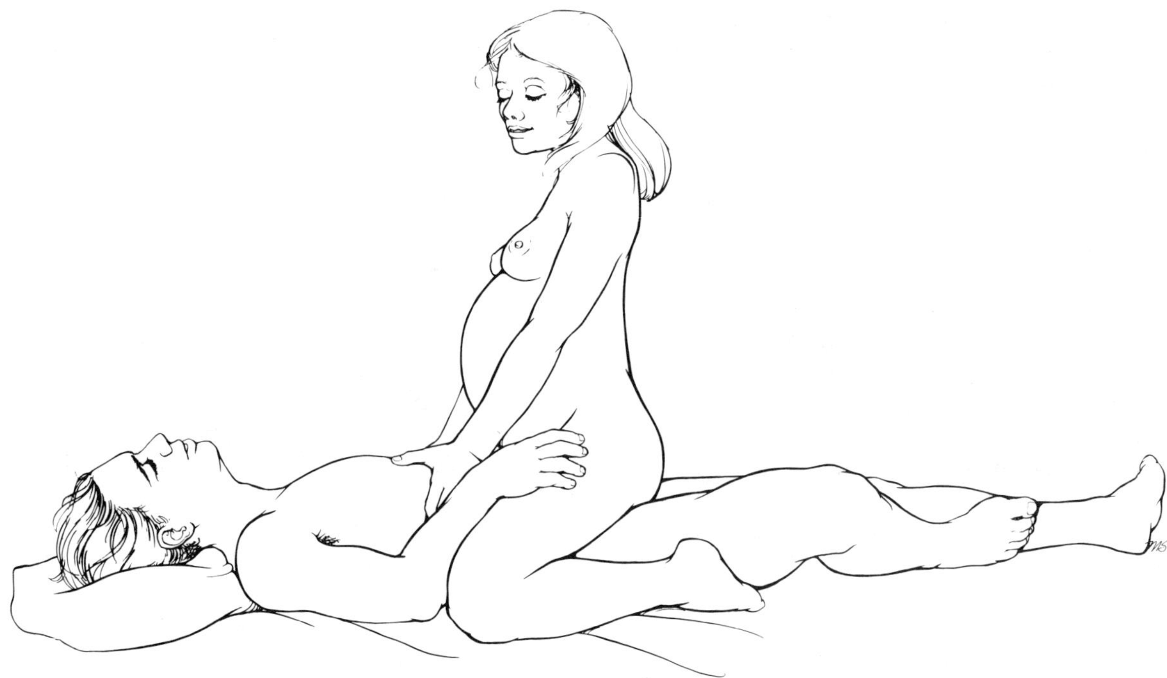

Figure 14.1
Sexual intercourse: woman on top position.

her sexual self-concept and behavior in either direction. She may feel more womanly and find increasing sexual pleasure; or she may question her sexual functioning during and following pregnancy, resulting in decreased self-concept. Some studies have shown that women experiencing nausea, vomiting, and weight gain do continue to enjoy coitus; but women in the weight-gaining group rated themselves lower on attractiveness and were more concerned regarding their husband's fidelity (Semmens, 1971). This finding seems to support other positions in the literature that point out the relationship between body image and sexuality.

Sociologic factors, that is, cultures and values of a given society, significantly shape a couples' response to pregnancy (Mead & Newton, 1967). The response among families and peers varies from culture to culture, and reactions can be as varied as fear and

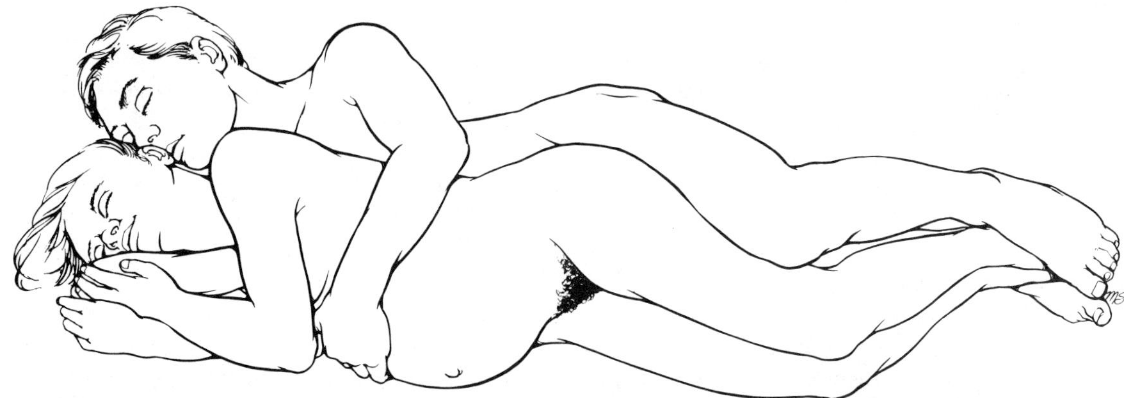

Figure 14.2
Sexual intercourse: side-by-side and rear entry positions.

shame, or ignoring a pregnant woman or viewing pregnancy as proof of sexual adequacy. Nurses who care for pregnant women need to be aware of the cultural patterns of the woman in order to provide effective nursing care. What may seem inappropriate or strange in the nurse's culture may be accepted or necessary in another culture.

Role changes during and following pregnancy, such as woman to mother or wife to mother, are discussed at length in the literature. (See Chapters 12 and 19.) It is interesting to note that humans are the only mammals to mother and enjoy sexual activity at the same time, which, as one author points out, is the basis for the mother/lover conflict (Jessner et al., 1970). The woman's increased dependence on her partner during pregnancy is probably the most well-known role change; and, of course, in many cases this causes protective behavior on the part of the man. Parental influence and childhood concepts of husband and wife will influence sexual behavior patterns. The extended family (see Chapter 13), which in many parts of the United States no longer exists, can no longer provide the cultural support systems that prevailed when the country was largely agrarian. In some cultures, men experience *couvade,* mock labor pains and/or postpartum weakness, which supposedly results in closeness between father and child. The current trend toward fathers' participating more actively in the birth process has been shown to influence their roles as fathers as well as their relationships with their partners positively (Cronenwett & Newmark, 1974).

Concern for the Fetus

Old wive's tales abound about possible dangers to the fetus resulting from coitus during pregnancy. Some research has been done to look at the relationship of intercourse to premature delivery or initiation of labor (Pugh & Fernandez, 1953; Goodlin et al., 1971). You will note that prostaglandins administered intravaginally can stimulate uterine contractions, and some researchers postulate that semen, which contains prostaglandins, may therefore induce labor (Goodlin et al., 1971). (See Chapters 16 and 27.) An increase in peripheral oxytocin levels measured in women experiencing orgasm also supports the possibility that orgasm can cause uterine contractions that are forceful enough to start labor. Some women have reported that postorgasmic uterine contractions were so painful that they discontinued intercourse. Again, no clear relationship between orgasm and labor has been established, but there is enough evidence to require that the nurse be sufficiently informed to provide anticipatory guidance. It does seem prudent, however, to recommend that pregnant women with poor obstetric histories (as far as successful termination of pregnancy is concerned) refrain from having orgasms from cunnilingus, masturbation, as well as coitus. Masters and Johnson reported that orgasms reached by masturbation are of greater intensity than those reached by coitus. Contraindications to sexual intercourse in the antepartum period would be uterine bleeding, a maternal history of abortion, or rupture of the membranes. When sexual intercourse is prohibited, the reasons should be discussed when both husband and wife are present, making sure that the reasons are clearly understood and no unfounded blame or guilt is placed. The wise physician and nurse will be very specific about any allowable alternatives.

INTRAPARTUM

Sexuality during labor has not been studied extensively. Newton (1971) describes a "trebly sensuous" woman and describes delivery of an infant without anesthesia as being similar to the coitus/orgasmic experience. Both are based on neurohormonal reflexes, oxytocin being the hormone involved. Similarities are the woman's breathing becomes deeper, she may hold her breath right before delivery or orgasm, she may make gasping noises, and she may have a tortured or strained expression on her face. Uterine contractions are noted during orgasm and delivery, and abdominal muscle contractions of the bearing-down activity of delivery and coitus are similar. In both experiences, decreased sensory perception (the woman is absorbed in the activity) is followed by feelings of well-being. Newton also notes that the processes of lactation and nursing could be considered analogous to coitus and delivery. The same hormone oxytocin plays a role, uterine contractions are common, and a sense of joy and pleasure with caretaking is usual.

POSTPARTUM

Postpartum sexuality reflects individual differences; many varied responses and descriptions from postpartum women and their partners are quoted by Bing and Colman (1977). Some couples expressed feelings of enhanced sexuality, incorporating both improved physiologic and psychologic experiences (Fig. 14.3).

> *We felt our lives changing for the better after the baby was born. Our sexual adjustment was gradual; it was really months before things were in a good and regular state, and it had more to do with a new openness and security with each other than with babies and birth. Certainly our growing respect and trust of each other as our child's parents helped in this direction—we had grown together.*
>
> *pp. 135–136*

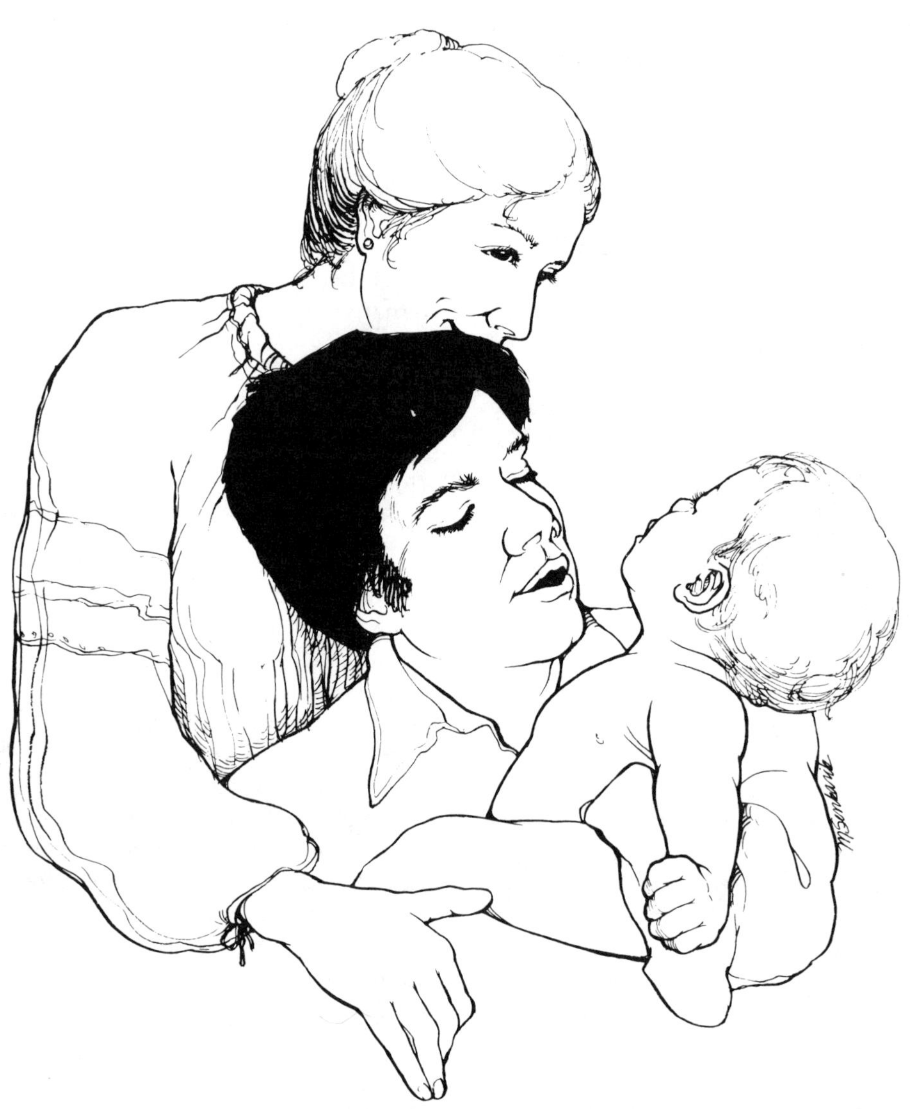

Figure 14.3
Sexuality is a part of family unity.

Other couples described negative feelings, requiring patience and adaptation to resume previous levels of enjoyment.

> *After the birth, there was more of a problem about sex than during pregnancy. At first all of our time and energy went to the baby. But after about two weeks, we both wanted very much to make love, and it was very painful to me. It wasn't completely comfortable until about three months postpartum, and many times I felt depressed—as though I had been ruined by my baby, whom we'd both wanted so much and loved. Things improved steadily when I learned all I had to do was to give my vagina practice in stretching again. I really think more attention ought to be given to this. I've never talked to anyone about it, but I assumed I'd be back to normal within a few weeks.*
>
> *p. 138*

Masters and Johnson report physiologic sexual tension levels by the fourth or fifth postpartum week similar to nonpregnant levels. It is noted that postpartally, female eroticism does not relate to age or parity but can be related to breast-feeding (Fig. 14.4) (Masters & Johnson, 1966). Changes in sexual response are minimal or delayed postpartally. Vasocongestion of the breasts in response to stimulation may not be observed for 6 months. Nursing mothers' breasts may not increase in size during the excitement stage, but there may be involuntary loss of milk particularly during and after orgasm. This may affect the couple by either increasing or decreasing sexual pleasure. During the plateau stage there is delayed vasocongestive reaction; vaginal lubrication develops slowly and quantity is usually less. There are fewer orgasmic platform contractions and less vividness of sex skin reaction in the orgasmic stage. Physiologically, the uterus, vaginal rugae, and labia minora and majora have returned to prepregnancy state. Anatomic dimensions and prepregnancy response to sexual stimulation are complete by 3 months. Most nursing mothers, it was found, resumed intercourse 2–3 weeks after delivery. Falicov (1973) also found that postpartal sexuality including intercourse returned to previous levels of sexual interaction after about 2 months. The usual deterrants to intercourse were perineal pain or discomfort because of the episiotomy or breast discomfort. Sometimes obstetric damage does occur, which can interfere with intercourse. Some postpartal women note a difference in experiencing orgasm that in some cases can be related to fatigue or lack of interest. Other women report concerns about becoming pregnant again, about perceived changes in their sexual organs, and about how their partners perceive them. If there were periods of abstinence before delivery and after delivery, there may be concern about fidelity. In a study of 42 couples postpartally, Hames (1980) asked women what words best described their husbands' behavior following delivery of the baby. Descriptive words used most frequently were understanding, close, sympathetic, and gentle.

It is important to remember that sexual intercourse and breast-feeding or suckling are voluntary behaviors on which the human race depends. In our society, female sexuality is often described in terms of adaptability to males, sometimes neglecting to focus on other aspects of sexuality. Sexuality is a fundamental component of personality, as discussed earlier in this chapter, and includes not only behaviors, fantasies, and feelings about the sexual act and orgasm, but also sensuality and feelings we have about femaleness and maleness. Technology and so-

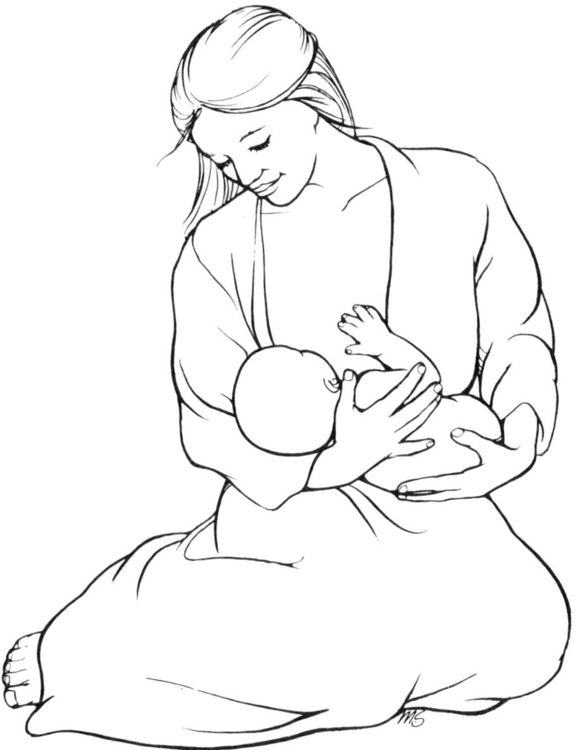

Figure 14.4
Breast-feeding is a part of female sexuality.

cially accepted patterns of childbirth have resulted in practices that inhibit the sexual aspects of labor or lactation. The pregnancy and postpartum periods can provide opportunities for the couple to become more sexually aware of each other and to develop new communication patterns that will enhance childbearing, parenting, and the family relationship. The professional nurse often has the opportunity to play a significant role in fostering mutually satisfying sexual patterns for couples.

NURSING PROCESS AND SEXUALITY

As you recall from Chapter 2, nursing and the teaching–learning processes are closely related, and this relationship is clearly demonstrated in the area of sexuality. When teaching the pregnant woman and her partner about sexual aspects of pregnancy, the postpartum period, and lactation, it is important to collect data about social and personal aspects of pregnancy. As patient data are collected, the nurse needs to know herself and be aware of her own personal biases, values, and interests. General knowledge of the physiologic and psychosocial changes occurring during pregnancy and specific knowledge about sexuality during pregnancy are critical for effective intervention. For example, if nurses are unaware of cunnilingus as an optional method of sexual expression or have personal reservations about it, they need to read about and perhaps view films on the subject to be able to collect the data objectively and handle their own reactions to the interview appropriately (Adams, 1976; Zalar, 1976). Being aware of the language of sexuality is one aspect of personal preparation before collecting information. "With child," "the stork is coming," and "knocked up" can all refer to what is termed clinically as "gestation " (Adams, 1976; Zalar, 1976). Adams points out in her article that "coitus," for example, is a word that is not meaningful to many people. What is important is for the nurse to have and use communication skills to clarify the client's meaning to *her.*

Setting the tone for the interview and the assessment step of the nursing process is important. Sexual history is usually, and should be, part of a general data base. A good rule of thumb is to let the flow of information go in the direction it seems to naturally yet to structure enough to elicit the information needed. For example, sexual history will probably flow from family history and questions about sex education. Some nurses preface initial data collection with overview of what the history taking will include, stating clearly that relevant sexual history is included. At the same time, the client is reminded of the confidentiality of the information and of respect for any limits that the client may set. Often it is suggested that nursing students record a sexual history on a peer to become comfortable with the process. When this process is used, the paper form on which the history is taken may be returned to the "client." After the environmental and psychologic tones are set, the nurse mentally assesses his or her own feelings and values, reminds him or herself to communicate at the appropriate level for the client, and the data collection, the assessment stage begins. History taking by a professional and skilled interviewer usually takes from 1 to 1 ½ hours. Ideally, the interviewer does not need a form for the sexual history; for structure, the interviewer may keep in mind the principles outlined in Chapter 3 and move from the simple complex questioning. An opening question such as "Where did you first learn about sex?" can lead to more specific questions about menstruation, wet dreams, and masturbation. Kinsey (1953) points out that questions framed to include societal norms help prevent pitfalls and avoid denials. For example, "When did you first masturbate?" avoids asking if a person masturbates. Asking people if they do anything can imply that most people do not, and this should be avoided. On the other hand, only in the very sensitive area of sexual experience does the interviewer make assumptions and then only to avoid putting the client on the spot. Also, professional nurses taking sexual histories must be knowledgeable and current in their knowledge of sexual behaviors and the wide range of normal. A general rule of thumb here is if the behaviors are agreeable, pleasant, and satisfying to the partners and do not infringe on others, they are acceptable.

The first areas in the assessment are sex education, developmental history, and family values. The nurse then moves to the areas of current attitudes and practices or, with the pregnant woman, usual prepregnancy practice, and a discussion of attitudes, practices, concerns, and current relationships. This is where the maternity nurse will begin to get a feeling about where the woman is now and how her changing body image and prospective role of parenthood affect her sexuality. Patterns of sexuality begin to emerge as the history evolves, and the nurse can perceive similarities and differences before and during pregnancy, frequently identifying areas of concern. A useful question to find out about expectations is: "What, in your opinion, would be the ideal sexual relationship?" Also useful are: "What is most satisfying?" "What would you change if you could?" From the answers to such questions, the nurse makes the nursing diagnosis (Chapter 2) and goes on to set goals (objectives) with the woman. As mentioned earlier, the interview is free flowing but the interviewer has in mind certain parameters or areas about which to collect information. For example, if the interview is during the antepartum period, the interviewer will gather information about discomfort during intercourse, fatigue, depression, body image changes and the woman's perceptions of those changes, and the woman's and her partner's feelings about sexuality during pregnancy. A postpartum history taking would include all of the physiologic adaptations taking place that affect sexual behaviors. The interviewer can pick up clues by paying careful attention to the words used by the patient and by being alert to those that reflect negativism or ambivalence. The "disgusting leakage of milk from the breasts," for example, should trigger a need for further exploration by the nurse. Teaching is an ongoing part of history taking and nursing process, and the physiologic changes that occur during pregnancy, postpartum, and lactation provide the theoretical basis for the anticipatory guidance that the nurse will do.

Plans, or goal setting, include what the nurse *knows* that the client *needs* to know, as well as what the client says she wants to know. Although some goals are nurse directed, it is hoped, most goals in maternity nursing can be mutually determined by the woman and nurse. Once established, the implementation step of the nursing process begins using all the appropriate human or material resources. Evaluation occurs when the goal is mutually assessed by patient and nurse and when anticipated behavior changes are noted by the nurse to indicate that learning has taken place.

Specific content about sexuality and pregnancy that should be included in the nursing process are as follows.

▲ The individual woman fluctuates in her interest in sexual activities and intercourse throughout pregnancy and for several months after delivery.

▲ Responses to pregnancy and lactation are a result of cultural and societal determinants.

▲ In an uncomplicated pregnancy there is no evidence that intercourse should be prohibited.

▲ Plans for the needs of expectant fathers should be made, including perhaps expectant fathers' groups.

▲ Since anatomic and physiologic changes of the woman during pregnancy may make intercourse uncomfortable, alternate methods of achieving orgasm should be explored. Couples should also be informed that orgasm may result in uterine contraction.

▲ Prohibition of sexual orgasm (intercourse, cunnilingus, or masturbation) is considered if there is uterine bleeding or a history of multiple abortions. When the couple is advised not to have intercourse, the information should be given to them together along with alternatives that can and cannot be used.

▲ Prohibition of sexual intercourse should be considered if it causes vaginal or abdominal pain, if the membranes have ruptured, or if labor has begun.

▲ After childbirth, sexual intercourse can be resumed when bleeding has ceased and it is physically and psychologically comfortable for the woman. Mild obstetric damage or repair should not interfere with sexual functioning. Kegel's exercise (tightening of the pubococcygeus muscle, which improves support to the pelvic organs) should be practiced routinely to restore and improve musculature. (See Chapters 12 and 19.)

▲ The nursing mother should be alerted that there may be spontaneous expression of milk during sexual activity. Sex arousal may also occur when nursing an infant. Lactation is said by some couples to enhance sexuality.

▲ The marriage role and other role relationships are altered by pregnancy. Neither the woman nor the man is ever the same person again, for now they are mother, father, and infant.

When and how the above specific teachings are incorporated into the nursing process depends on the period of gestation and the individual's or couple's readiness for learning (assessed by the nurse). Some facts need to be stressed, repeated, and reinforced; other facts, which are obviously internalized, are seen in behavior changes or are described by the client.

The relationship of the nursing process, teaching–learning, and sexuality is not difficult to understand. Ideally, most of the teaching about sexuality during pregnancy can be done with the couple. Teaching the couple rather than only the woman or the man maximizes time and energy and, more importantly, eliminates information transfer from nurse to patient to partner. Both hear the same information at the same time and, it is hoped, they can share their perceptions and feelings. Moreover, the nurse can then observe the couple's relationships throughout the pregnancy. Findings demonstrate that the sexual counseling provided during pregnancy, based on thorough assessment of the woman and her significant others, can provide real growth for the couple. The nurse has a unique opportunity to contribute positively and significantly to many beginning families.

SUMMARY

This chapter discussed sexuality during pregnancy, the postpartum period, and lactation. A brief description of the developmental aspects of sexuality was included, including the stages of development outlined by Freud. Reference was also made to the contributions of developmental theorists, Erikson and Sullivan.

Antepartum physiologic and psychologic adaptation, trimester by trimester, was discussed. The specific changes in the sexual response cycle were described. The fluctuation of interest in sex demonstrated by pregnant women was discussed; examples of research in this area were included. Body image changes and perceptions on the part of the couple to both the physiologic and psychologic changes of pregnancy were explored. The importance of culture, personal values, and family patterns were pointed out.

The chapter continued by discussing physiologic and psychologic changes and adaptations that occur intrapartum and postpartum. Again, the fact that women can differ greatly, particularly in their adaptation to sexuality postpartally, was discussed. The sexual responses of the nursing mother were also described. Changes in the sexual response cycle after birth were described, including information about when prepregnancy levels of sexual response can be expected. The fact that pregnancy can enhance sexuality by providing an opportunity for sexual growth for the couple was noted.

The last section of the chapter discussed the interrelationships of nursing process, teaching–learning, and sexuality. The steps of the nursing process were reviewed with particular emphasis on assessment as it relates to sexuality. Suggestions for eliciting information about sexuality were given, and specific teaching that we feel should be given to all couples about sexuality during pregnancy, labor, and post-delivery were listed. The fact that the nurse is in a unique position to contribute positively to the emerging family was stressed.

REFERENCES AND READINGS

Adams, G. The Sexual History as an Integral Part of the Patient History. *Am J Matern Child Nurs* 1(3):170, 1976.

Bardwick, J. *Psychology of Women: A Study of Bio-Cultural Conflicts.* New York: Harper & Row, 1971.

Benedek, T. The Psychobiology of Pregnancy, in Anthony, E. J., Benedek, T. *Parenting: Its Psychology and Psychopathology.* Boston: Little, Brown, 1970.

Bing, E., Colman, L. *Making Love During Pregnancy.* New York: Bantam Books, 1977.

Brill, A. (Ed.). *The Basic Writings of Sigmund Freud.* New York: Random House, 1938.

Colman, A., Colman, L. *Pregnancy: The Psychological Experience.* New York: Herder & Herder, 1971.

Cronenwett, L., Newmark, L. Fathers' Responses to Childbirth. *Nurs Res* 23:210, 1974.

Ellis, D. Sexual Needs and Concerns of Expectant Parents. *J Obstet Gynecol Neonatal Nurs* 9(5):306, 1980.

Erikson, E. *Childhood and Society.* New York: W. W. Norton, 1963.

Erikson, E. *Identity, Youth and Crisis.* New York: W. W. Norton, 1968.

Falicov, C. J. Sexual Adjustment During First Pregnancy and Postpartum. *Am J Obstet Gynecol* 117:991, 1973.

Freud, S. *New Introductory Lectures on Psychoanalysis.* New York: W. W. Norton, 1933.

Goodlin, R. C., Keller, D. W. F., Raffin, M. Orgasm During Late Pregnancy: Possible Deleterious Effects. *Obstet Gynecol* 38:916, 1971.

Hames, C. T. Sexual Needs and Interests of Postpartum Couples. *J Obstet Gynecol Neonatal Nurs* 9(5):313, 1980.

Hogan, R. *Human Sexuality: A Nursing Perspective.* New York: Appleton-Century-Crofts, 1980.

Hollender, M. H., McGehee, J. B. The Wish to Be Held During Pregnancy. *J Psychosom Res* 18:193, 1974.

Hott, J. R. The Crisis of Expectant Fatherhood. *Am J Nurs* 1440, 1970.

Iffrig, Sr., M. C. Body Image in Pregnancy: Its Relation to Nursing Functions. *Nurs Clin North Am* 7:631, 1972.

Inglis, T. Postpartum Sexuality. *J Obstet Gynecol Neonatal Nurs* 9(5):298, 1980.

Jessner, L., Weigert, E., Foy, J. L. The Development of Parental Attitides During Pregnancy, in Anthony, E. J., Benedek, T. (Eds.), *Parenthood: Its Psychology and Psychopathology.* Boston: Little, Brown, 1970, pp.209–244.

Kenny, J. A. Sexuality of Pregnant and Breastfeeding Women. *Arch Sex Behav* 2:215, 1973.

Kinsey, A. C. et al. *Sexual Behavior in the Human Female.* Philadelphia: W. B. Saunders, 1953.

Kyndely, H. The Sexuality of Women in Pregnancy: A Review. *J Obstet Gynecol Neonatal Nurs* 7(1):28, 1978.

Lanahan, C. M. C. Eroticism and Orgasm in Pregnancy, in McNall, L. H. Galeener, J. T. (Eds.), *Current Practice in Obstetric and Gynecologic Nursing,* Vol. I. St. Louis: C. V. Mosby, 1976.

Marquart, R. K. Expectant Fathers: What Are Their Needs? *Matern Child Nurs J* 32, 1976.

Masters, W., Johnson, V. *Human Sexual Response.* Boston: Little, Brown, 1966.

Mead, M., Newton, N. Cultural Patterning of Perinatal Behavior, in Richardson, S. A., Guttmacher, A. F. (Eds.), *Childbearing: Its Social and Psychological Aspects.* Baltimore: Williams & Wilkins, 1967, pp.164–169.

Morris, N. M. The Frequency of Sexual Intercourse During Pregnancy. *Arch Sex Behav* 4:501, 1975.

Newton, N. The Trebly Sensuous Woman. *Psychol Today* 5:6, 1971.

Pugh, W. E., Fernandez, F. L. Coitus in Late Pregnancy: A Follow-Up Study of the Effects of Coitus on Late Pregnancy, Delivery and Puerperium. *Obstet Gynecol* 2:636, 1953.

Semmens, J. P. Female Sexuality and Life Situations: An Etiologic Psychosocial–Sexual Profile of Weight Gain and Nausea and Vomiting in Pregnancy. *Obstet Gynecol* 38:555, 1971.

Solberg, D., Butler, J., Wagner, N. Sexual Behavior in Pregnancy. *New Engl J Med* 288:1098, 1973.

Sullivan, H. *Conceptions of Modern Psychiatry.* New York: W. W. Norton, 1953.

Swanson, J. The Marital Sexual Relationship During Pregnancy. *J Obstet Gynecol Neonatal Nurs* 9(5):267, 1980.

Tolor, A., DiGranzia, P. Sexual Attitudes and Behavior Patterns During and Following Pregnancy. *Arch Sex Behav* 5:539, 1976.

Woods, N. F. *Human Sexuality in Health and Illness* (2nd ed.) St. Louis: C. V. Mosby, 1979.

Zalar, M. K. Sexual Counseling For Pregnant Couples. *Am Matern Child Nurs* 1(3):176, 1976.

15

PREPARATION FOR CHILDBIRTH

Dona Pardo

Ideally, no couple should enter the childbirth process without some form of educational preparation, whether it be a one-time hospital prenatal class or extensive instruction in one of the prepared childbirth techniques. There is some evidence that women who are more knowledgeable about the birth process are more relaxed, perceive less pain and, therefore, experience a more positive labor and delivery. Other evidence suggests that men who take a more active part in the birth process—attend classes and participate in labor and delivery—are more apt to become involved in child-rearing activities and experience a better bonding process. Certainly, the more fully prepared the person is, the more able he or she is to deal with the stresses of childbirth and child rearing.

There are many kinds of preparation processes today, and this chapter will discuss those most widely used. Keep in mind that basic class content in most of these processes is the same, and although the focus may be different, the aim is to ensure that the people have enough information to deal effectively with what may prove to be one of the most pleasurable experiences of life—birth.

HISTORY OF PREPARED CHILDBIRTH

As early as the 1920s, an English obstetrician, Grantley Dick-Read, defied tradition by educating his clients for labor and birth, as well as setting up classes for their husbands. Because he was outspoken in many of the unpopular ideas of his times, such as environmental pollution, destruction of the body with drugs, treatment of the client as a "whole person," instruction to teenagers regarding sex, reproduction and family life, and the equality of blacks, he was not viewed favorably by his contemporaries and his theories regarding preparation for childbirth were not readily accepted. In 1933, Dick-Read published *Natural Childbirth,* so titled because of his belief that childbirth is a natural physiologic process not meant to be painful and because he built his teaching around a study of the "laws of nature." Through this widely published book, Dick-Read was misunderstood all over the world and was almost completely rejected by his peers.

In 1944, *Childbirth Without Fear: The Original Approach*

to Natural Childbirth, was published. This book further described Dick-Read's theory regarding the pain of childbirth. In it, he contended that young women, having inquiring minds regarding childbirth, listened to many voices that distorted or destroyed the truth. Their mothers often withheld the true facts of personal unpleasant experiences or shared information of such a negative nature that it was extremely fear producing. Their friends often escalated this fear through discussion of their own martyrdom (recalled in obvious pride). Their husbands often acquired an understandable anxiety over their welfare (formed through similar hearsay) that served to compound this fear. Further, history and religion also supported the idea that suffering was a definite component of the childbirth process. Dick-Read thus contended that women entered pregnancy with the preconceived notion that labor would be extremely painful and something to avoid if at all possible. This fear, he suggested, caused the woman increased tension with a resulting increase in pain. He hypothesized his fear–tension–pain cycle, whereby the increase in pain perception would cause greater fear, which would increase tension, and which would then increase pain (Fig. 15.1). Thus, a viscious cycle would ensue making childbirth a very unpleasant experience. Dick-Read argued that breaking this cycle would allow the woman to relax and, therefore, perceive less pain. Because he felt the initiating fear was caused by negative perceptions about labor and delivery, Dick-Read advocated education to reduce this fear, with exercises in progressive relaxation and breathing directed against the tension part of the cycle. He believed that a completely relaxed woman had no desire for pain medication because she did not have pain.

In 1951, French physician Ferdinand Lamaze, while on a medical visit to the Soviet Union, witnessed the application of the psychoprophylactic method of prepared childbirth (PPM), which he described as painless childbirth and believed it to be the result of physical training and education during pregnancy. Lamaze introduced a modified version of this method to his clients in France, and from the sixth month of pregnancy all women in his care were prepared for "painless childbirth." The *Lamaze method* differs from Dick-Read's in that it is based on the Pavlovian conditioning theory and calls for the standardization of teaching techniques, advocates chest rather than abdominal breathing, and uses relaxation techniques that are based on specific control and distraction rather than on general relaxation.

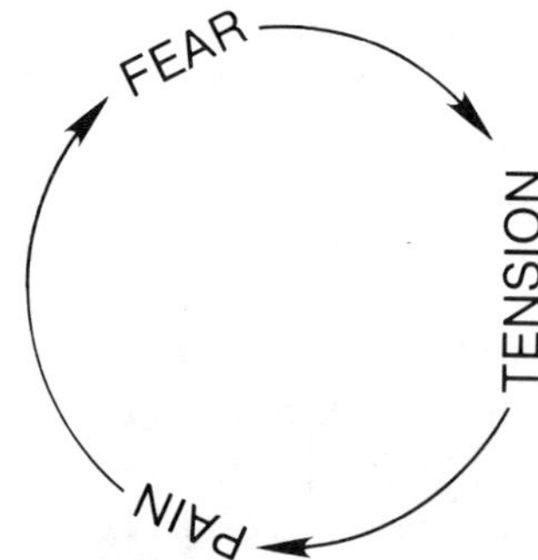

Figure 15.1
Fear–tension–pain cycle.

Lamaze's method spread rapidly in France, was well established in China and the communist countries, and, following sanction by Pope Pius XII in 1956, began to be used in the more Catholic-oriented countries of southern Europe and South America.

In 1958 in the United States Dr. Isador Bernstein published *Psychoprophylactic Preparation for Painless Childbirth,* but the method actually became popular through the efforts of Marjorie Karmel, an American mother and writer. Mrs. Karmel was living in France at the time of the birth of her first child and used the psychoprophylactic method with the help of Dr. Lamaze and a *monitrice* (childbirth educator who also functioned as a coach during labor and delivery). Her second pregnancy occurred when she was living in the United States. She searched all over New York for an obstetrician who would help her deliver her baby the same way she delivered her first child. She finally located a physician who would allow her to try the method, but she had to train herself with her husband as her coach. After a very positive experience, she wrote many magazine articles and the book, *Thank You, Dr. Lamaze,* published in 1959. As a result of public response to her writings, she was instrumental in organizing a group of interested obstetricians and other professionals into the American Society for Psychoprophylaxis in Obstetrics (ASPO) in 1960. This nonprofit organization functions throughout the country to encourage and support the use of PPM by supplying information, sponsoring teacher-training courses, and setting guidelines and recommendations for prepared childbirth. Another supportive organization for prepared childbirth is the International Childbirth Education Association (ICEA). Both organizations seek to standardize the course through specific training of the teachers and require certification. Because PPM is the most prevalent course in this country, the theories and techniques will be discussed in great detail later in this chapter.

Another method of prepared childbirth known as the Bradley Method is used widely in some areas of the United States. This technique is also known as "Husband Coached" prepared childbirth for the wife is required to have a husband as her coach. The founder of this method, Dr. Robert Bradley, an American physician, compares natural childbirth to the peaceful, joyful, birth process of animals and advocates that it is a painless process. During pregnancy, the woman must maintain a special diet in order to protect the fetus and must do extensive body-conditioning exercises to prepare herself for labor. Medication is not allowed during labor (because it is not needed) and abdominal relaxed breathing similar to that established by Dick-Read is taught. The woman is encouraged to walk during labor and to internalize the contractions by closing her eyes, breathing slowly, and focusing on an internal focal point. Her partner walks with her, supports her during contractions, and whispers encouraging words. After delivery, the couple toasts the birth (with orange juice) in the delivery room and walks together to the nursery carrying the newborn.

THE PSYCHOPROPHYLACTIC METHOD OF PREPARED CHILDBIRTH (PPM)

Although the courses for PPM vary depending on the individual instructor, client population, and geographic area, the basic content is standardized as a result of ASPO control. Couples interested in attending prepared childbirth classes should be encouraged to look for those taught by certified instructors so they will be sure to attain the necessary knowledge and learn the appropriate techniques as discussed in the next part of this chapter.

Most of the courses consist of a series of classes begun in the last trimester of pregnancy. The trend today is toward including a prenatal class in the second trimester, but this is often a problem because many of the couples do not register for classes until the latter part of pregnancy. There are usually six classes, completed 1–2 weeks before the anticipated delivery date. This chapter will discuss an example of one series of classes. You should keep in mind, however, that there are many different ways to teach a series. Content is not always taught as suggested here, but it is covered at some point in the course.

Class One

The purpose of having an early pregnancy class is to ensure a healthier more comfortable pregnancy and to introduce the participants to some of the techniques that they will be using throughout labor and delivery. The pregnant woman must be accompanied by another person who will serve as her coach during labor. This person may be her husband, boyfriend, relative or friend.

A popular way of beginning the class is to discuss the characteristics of pregnancy. If the partners can achieve a basic understanding of this content, they may be able to deal more effectively with the ensuing months of the pregnancy. The mother's as well as the father's adjustment to pregnancy are discussed (see Chapters 12 and 13). The information given includes a description of the *couvade syndrome,* which is always of great interest to couples. It is becoming increasingly apparent that fathers experience a wide variety of physical symptoms of pregnancy that disappear once the child is born. Nausea, vomiting (morning sickness), indigestion, backache, toothaches, and weight gain (often as much as 20 lbs—the recommended gain for pregnancy) are a few symptoms that as many as 65% of the "pregnant male" population experiences. The causes of this syndrome are speculative; some suggested possibilities follow.

- The lack of a clearly defined male pregnancy role
- Repressed guilt for the responsibility of causing the pregnancy, particularly if it is an uncomfortable one
- Unconscious suppression of feminine traits (fear of homosexual tendencies)
- Conception envy (jealousy of the woman's ability to bear a child)
- Identification with the pregnancy, which indicates a close relationship with the partner

Some authors suggest that those men experiencing couvade are more likely to take an active part in child-rearing activities because of this closeness to the pregnancy.

Because nutrition is such an important aspect of growth and development, it is discussed in this class with the hope that mother and coach will at least begin to assess their dietary habits and make any necessary modifications. General guidelines for following the basic four food groups are discussed, as well as fluid intake and the avoidance of harmful substances specifically smoking, alcohol, and medications. Recommended weight gain is mentioned, but emphasis is placed on eating appropriately and healthfully rather than strict adherence to specific weight gain. Since nutrition is usually mentioned and reinforced in all the subsequent classes, a short discussion or review of the consumer's knowledge about nutrition is all that is required at this time.

Nutrition leads into another area—the anatomy and physiology of pregnancy. The instructor reviews the female reproductive organs, including a comparison of nonpregnant to pregnant anatomy. This review provides a good basis for a future discussion of the labor and delivery processes, as well as for an immediate discussion of the minor discomforts of pregnancy. Through comparison of the pregnant and nonpregnant anatomy, the expectant parents can understand why the discomforts occur and what measures they can used to rectify them. At this time, fetal development is also discussed along with what should be reported to the physician. This discussion very nicely lends itself to encouraging the partners to verbalize any fears regarding the development of the fetus. The couples will often voice their concerns regarding deformity, something that causes them some anxiety but often is not discussed. It is reassuring to most couples to know that others have these fears as well. Such discussions also give couples information that can be used during future pregnancies so that next time they can actively work to protect the fetus and thus gain a sense of control regarding their child's development.

Discussions of anatomy and physiology also allow for demonstration of good body mechanics. Making the coach responsible for observation of the woman's posture and correction, if improper, also helps to reinforce the coach's role. One very appropriate way of dealing with good posture is by teaching the pelvic tilt (Fig. 15.2*a*). Demonstration of the pelvic tilt and discussion of the stresses pregnancy places on the back emphasize the importance of proper body mechanics. This discussion leads to a demonstration of the other body conditioning techniques and the great variety of exercises encouraged and taught in childbirth classes such as tailor sitting. Shearer feels that even the most well-motivated mothers will do only three exercises no matter how many are taught, so these exercises should be tailored to the needs of each mother. The pelvic tilt and Kegel exercises are the easiest to perform and the ones most beneficial for maintaining the integrity of the back and perineum throughout life.

The instructor begins teaching body conditioning by promoting the use of the focal point and cleansing breaths in order to encourage their use throughout all of the techniques. The *focal point* is simply having the mother stare at an object in the room and concentrate on it, which is the *gate theory of pain control* (a conditioned response will close the gate in the nerve pathways thus dulling pain). The *cleansing breath* is a very deep breath taken in through the nose and expelled through the mouth. It is used at the beginning and end of each series of exercises, and will also be used at the beginning and end of each contraction during labor. The cleansing breath is an excellent signal for the coach that a contraction is beginning; it helps to establish a relaxed state and to oxygenate the mother and fetus.

Relaxation–concentration is essential; if introduced in this class, there will be time for it to become a mind set, thereby facilitating the ease with which the actual breathing method used during delivery can become a conditioned response. Classical conditioning is best remembered through Pavlov's experiment with salivating dogs. The sight of food produces a reflex action of salivation. Ring a bell coincidentally with food presentation, and salivation will become associated with the ringing. Eventually, the bell will produce salivation even without food. The bell has thus become the conditioned stimulus and the salivation the conditioned response. Food must be presented with the bell periodically to reinforce the response or it will undergo progressive extinction.

Operant conditioning is best explained as a reward response. If a behavior elicits a reward, it is more likely to be repeated than if it elicits a punishment. Both theories are used extensively for PPM in that the mother is conditioned to respond to a certain stimulus presented by the coach, and this response is reinforced by reward (Fig. 5.3). For example, a conditioned stimulus may be the coach stroking the expectant mother's forearm in an effort to have her relax her muscles. If relaxation is practiced over and over with the coach using the stroking, eventually the woman will automatically relax

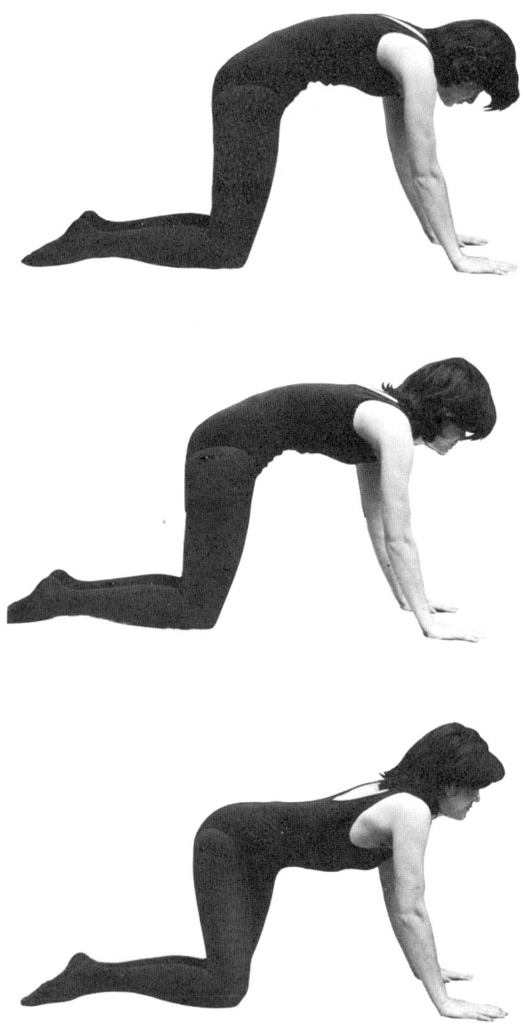

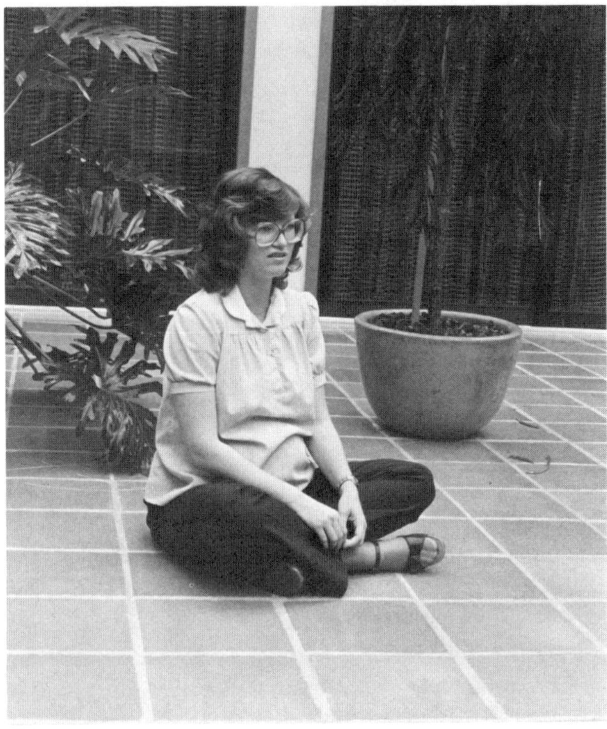

Figure 15.2
Left: Pelvic tilt to develop abdominal muscles and decrease back discomfort. As pregnancy progresses, the woman is often advised to do this exercise standing with back aligned with a wall, or lying flat on her back with knees bent. *Above:* Tailor sitting strengthens the inner thigh muscles and prepares for position during delivery.

once stroked (conditioned response). The coach then gives positive reinforcement to the relaxation by saying "very good," "you're doing great," or some similar response. The woman is then more apt to maintain her state of relaxation (operant conditioning). The expectant mother is also encouraged to continue to use the focal point for relaxation. This helps make the relaxation active rather than passive for she must *concentrate* on that point. The coach then helps her relax every part of her body, progressing from toe to head, by using verbal commands or stroking, whichever the partners choose. Of prime importance is that the same techniques are used over and over thus reinforcing each practice session. Coaches are then asked to assess relaxation by checking the areas of the body in an effort to be able to immediately recognize any tenseness in the woman (Fig. 15.4). This is a great aid in labor for if the coach can recognize the expectant mother's unrelaxed state early, he can work immediately to relax her, thereby increasing her comfort.

It is strongly suggested, that the couples begin practicing at home and continue to do so throughout the rest of the pregnancy (Fig. 15.5). It is hoped that by starting early the conditioned response will be well established by labor. The conditioned response, once established, can be useful during other painful experiences where relaxation is helpful. Couples are encouraged to use relaxation methods.

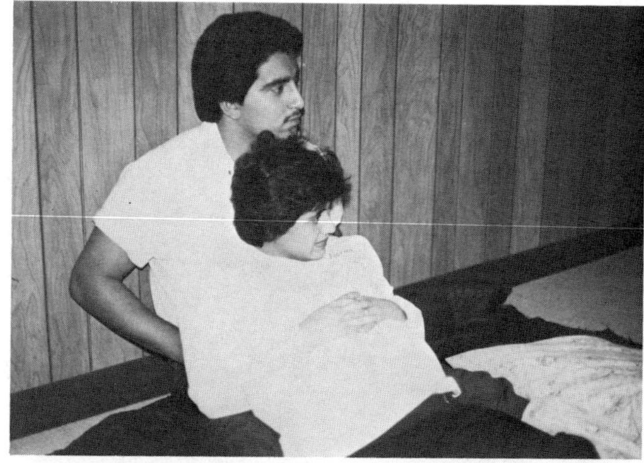

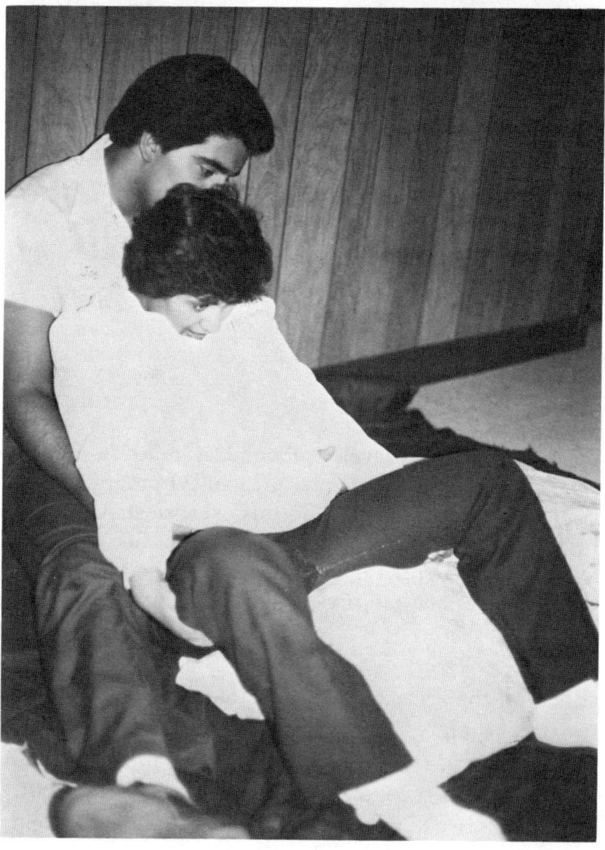

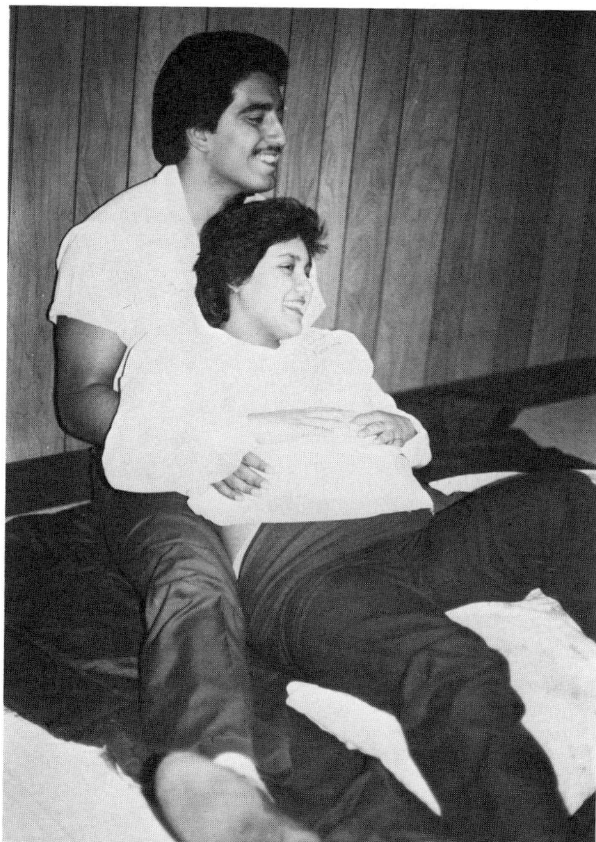

Figure 15.3
Role of the coach is to comprehend process and strategy used and to guide, instruct, encourage, and support before, during, and after childbirth.

Class Two

Class two is generally scheduled 2 months before the expected date of delivery, with one class each successive week for the next 5 weeks, in order to teach the couple all other techniques needed for a prepared labor. A brief history of prepared childbirth along with an overview of the next five classes and a short discussion of the techniques that will be learned is a good beginning for the second class.

In most PPM series, the instructor will now spend some time having the members of the class get acquainted since they will be the same group in each of the following classes. Some couples will have met

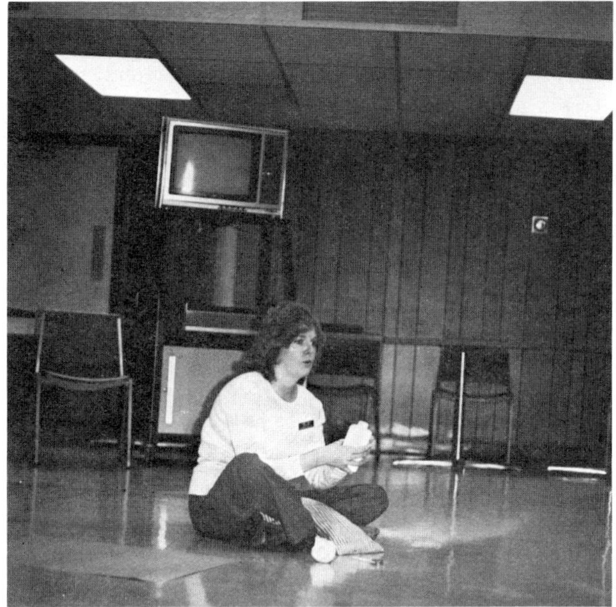

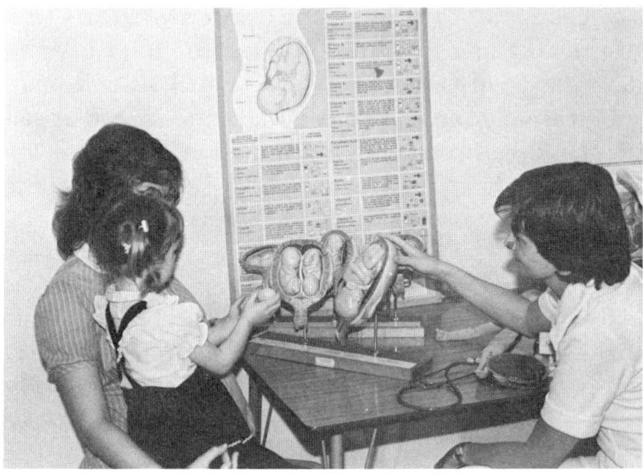

Figure 15.4
Top: Teacher responding to questions. *Bottom:* Teacher with mother and child.

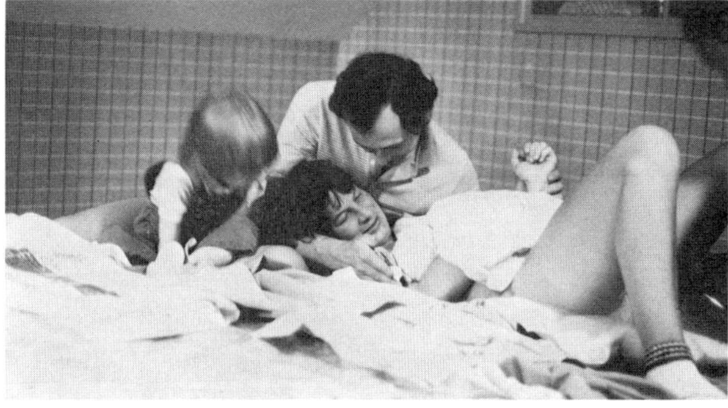

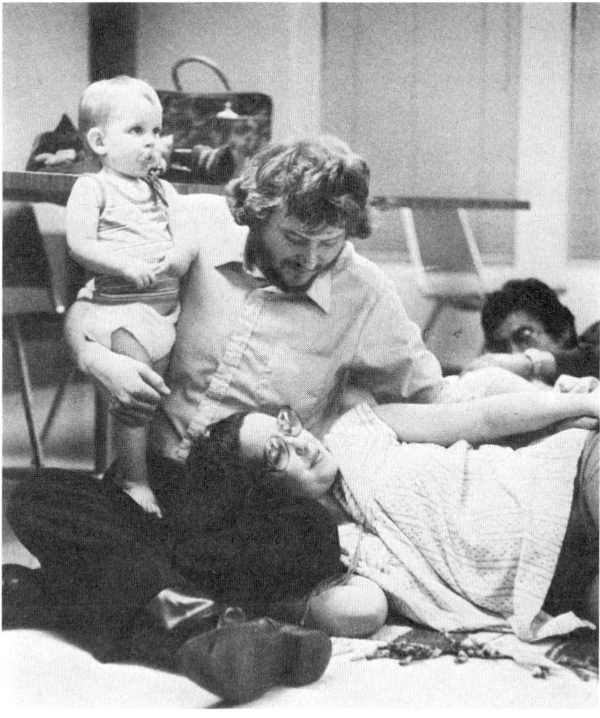

Figure 15.5
Participation by coach and others in childbirth experience is important to the woman during pregnancy, childbirth, and recovery.

in the prenatal class, but many will be new. A sharing of concerns regarding labor and delivery, as well as reasons for attending the classes are good ways of encouraging interaction. The earlier in the series the couples interact, the more relaxed and closer they will become. Anticipatory socialization is an important aspect of prepared childbirth; and the sooner the couples become involved with each other, the more successful their course will be.

Another aim of this class is to begin a deconditioning process regarding labor and delivery because most women today have been raised with the misconception that childbirth is a very painful and negative experience. Through discussion and positive conditioning (by using positive words such as contraction rather than pain), the childbirth educator can move the couples toward viewing childbirth as a pleasant experience. Certain characteristics of labor such as contractions only last a short time (35–90 seconds) and contractions are good because each one brings them that much closer to the birth of their child are reinforced. The woman is encouraged to work *with* the contraction rather than against it; to let her body labor. Sheila Kitzinger (1979) states

> *Uterine contractions are felt by women to sweep towards them, rise in crescendo and then fade away like waves of the sea. . . . A woman must "swim" over the wave and not allow it to envelope her, and to do this she needs to go forward to meet it with her breathing instead of waiting until it is already on her. If she retreats from it, it will almost certainly sweep over her. . . . With each wave of the sea the tide gradually flows farther in bringing nearer the time when her baby will be in her arms.*

The deconditioning phase is begun in this second class and is continued throughout the entire series so that by the time labor begins, it will be viewed as a positive experience.

Because a significant number of the couples attending prepared childbirth classes have not experienced birth before, it is necessary to define the roles they will be expected to assume. Specific role expectations will influence the woman's behavior by inducing conformity and will enable her to know that these behaviors are appropriate and thereby reduce stress. Therefore, procedures are discussed and guides are given to the couples so that they may refer to activities to be accomplished during labor. The guides may be referred to throughout the succeeding classes; the coach is encouraged to refer to it often and to take the guide to the hospital to use as reference.

Couples are encouraged to attend all the classes in the series, as well as to do outside reading so they can get a broad perspective. Many educators have their own lending library or traveling book store to encourage reading. Projects such as viewing a movie or homework are assigned in order to encourage active involvement. The attitude taken is that this course is as important as any other course in which the couple might enroll and they should be serious about it and committed to it.

Since labor and childbirth are the main reasons for enrolling in the series and most couples are eager to get started (readiness for learning), specific content regarding labor is useful in this class. Anatomy and physiology of the female reproductive system and fetal growth and development are briefly reviewed to reinforce as well as review past learning. There can be some discussion of the importance of good nutrition at this time in pregnancy. Reinforcement of women avoiding medication, smoking, alcohol intake, and other harmful chemicals (cleaners, paints, etc.) is also appropriate at this time. (Not allowing the couples to smoke in class will support this.)

The instructor may then introduce the concept of labor, building on past learning about the female anatomy and physiology. The instructor may begin by defining each of the four stages of labor and then provide specific information. Discussion of true versus false labor and the three signs of labor—appearance of show, rupture of membranes, and contractions—will enable the coach to feel more confident about getting the woman to the hospital on time. (A universal fear of most partners is that they will have to deliver their child on the side of the road on the way to the hospital!) The characteristics of a contraction are taught, including how to time and assess each and what to report to the physician or nurse when they are ready to do so. This leads right into a discussion of early labor and demonstration of gear I breathing and effleurage. *Gear* is the term used to describe levels of breathing in which the woman progressively increases her concentration and speed of the breaths taken, in association with the intensity of her contractions (See Table 15.1.) The couples will practice these techniques, and the instructor will check each couple in order to assess the mastery of these skills.

Relaxation is practiced again; at this time it is made more difficult by having the expectant mother contract one limb while keeping the rest of her body relaxed. The coach is encouraged to check the rest of her body and to encourage relaxation through the use of previously initiated techniques (Fig. 15.6). The coach's responsibility for this is emphasized again in an effort to reinforce and assist the role of coach so it will be well integrated by the time labor begins. The cleansing breath and focal point techniques are reviewed, and the coach is taught to *call a contraction* once the woman is relaxed. Here it is emphasized that the woman must always be relaxed before practicing breathing. The coach can use a watch to time contractions and tell the expectant mother that a contraction is beginning and to start her breathing technique. The coach then acknowledges each 15-second interval, which helps the woman to realize which part of the contraction she is breathing for and gives her some guidelines as to how long a contraction lasts. Sixty seconds is the usual allocated practice time, although contractions are not always of that length (see Chapter 16).

TABLE 15.1
BREATHING PATTERNS DURING LABOR

	Stage I			*Stage II*	*Stage III*	*Stage IV*
	Early Phase	***Active Phase***	***Transition***			
CONTRACTIONS						
Intensity Frequency Duration	Mild 15–20 min 30–45 sec	Moderate 3–5 min 45–60 sec	Powerful 2–3 min 60–90 sec	Strong 2–5 min 35–60 sec	Moderate with fundal massage, medication, placental separation, or breast-feeding	Moderate with fundal massage, breast-feeding, or medication
SHOW	Scant → Pink	Moderate → Reddish	Heavy → Bloody	Heavy Bloody		
CERVIX Effacement Dilation	 50–100% 1–4 cm	 100% 5–7 cm	 Complete 8–10 cm	 Complete Complete		
MEMBRANES	May rupture →	→	→	→		
MOTHER'S RESPONSE Physical	 Backache Slowed digestion	 Perspiration Bladder pressure Cold feet Fatigue Thirst	 Profuse perspiration Chills Trembling N/V Leg cramps Sleepiness Urge to push	 Perineal bulge, burning Rectal pressure Urge to push Relief with pushing	 Fatigue Urge to push with placental separation	 Hunger Fatigue
Emotional	Excited Apprehensive Eager to try new skills Secure	Inwardly-directed Questioning Discouraged with plateaus	Irritable "Touchitis" Restless Vague consciousness Discouraged Consumed with urge to push	Rejuvenated Happy Relieved	Excited Joyful Interested in newborn	Satisfied

TABLE 15.1 (continued)

	Stage I			Stage II	Stage III	Stage IV
	Early Phase	*Active Phase*	*Transition*			
Contractions						
ROLES						
Mother's	Relax Walk Conserve energy Drink only clear liquids Focal point Effleurage	Relax Walk or sit upright Rest between contractions Urinate frequently Focal point Effleurage	Relax Walk or sit upright Listen to coach Take ice chips Focal point Effleurage	Relax Assume pushing position with contraction Rest between contractions Listen to coach Push with contraction	Relax Listen to physician Breathe with fundal massage Push when instructed Bond with infant Integrate family Praise coach	Rest Breast-feed if chosen Breathe with fundal massage Enjoy birth Integrate family Praise coach Drink plenty of fluids
	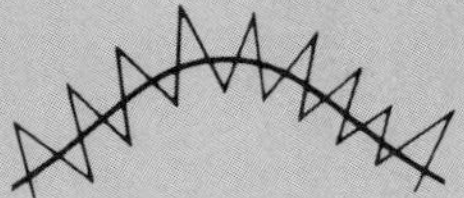 Breathing prn, 6–9 breaths/min nose/mouth	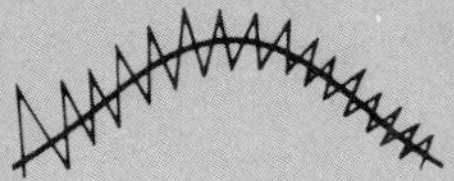 Breathing prn, up to 1/sec nose/mouth	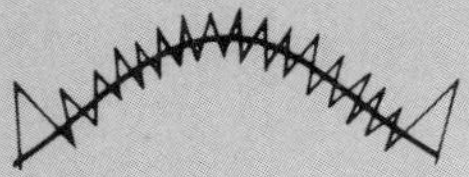 Breathing prn, up to 1/sec 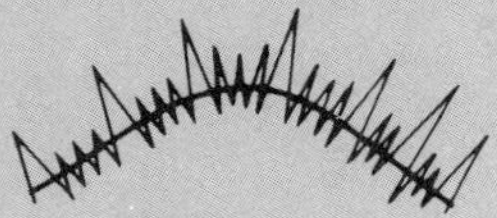 Pant (4 pant 1 blow) 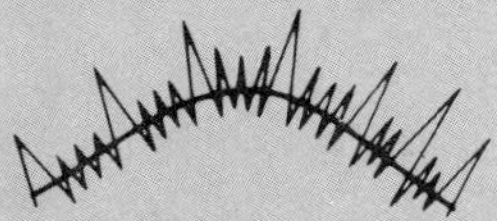 Varied count Pant blow 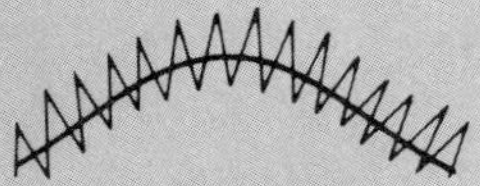 Blowing	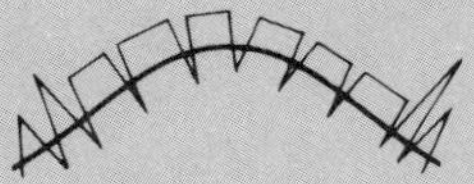 2 cleansing breaths Inhale, bear down 7 sec while exhaling slowly; repeat until urge to push ends 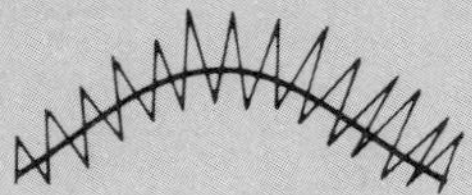 Blowing		

Coach's *	Keep calm Calm mother Time contractions Call 15-sec intervals Notify physician when necessary Assess for relaxation and proper breathing Positive reinforcement	Assess for relaxation and proper breathing Comfort measures Position change Check urination Mouth care Ice chips Lip balm Mouthspray Wash cloth Back rub Medication Give positive reinforcement Time contractions Call 15-sec intervals	Keep her relaxed Breathe with her Positive reinforcement Take command Assess for hperventilation Comfort measures Sponge brow Back rub Encourage to blow when needed Notify nurse when urge to push	Praise for job well done Watch perineum Assist in pushing Give encouragement Remind to relax between contractions Relay physician's instructions	Praise mother Relay physician's instructions Share in joy of birth Bond with infant	Share joy with mother and child Praise mother for job well done
Nurse's	Orient to area Check FHT, BP Explain hospital procedures Answer any questions Inform physician of progress	Acquire needed equipment for coach Ice chips Pillows Check FHT, BP Encourage couple Give positive reinforcement Help coach assess need for medication	Encourage coach Check FHT, BP Give positive reinforcement to couple Assist coach as needed	Assist with pushing Assess for perineal push Check FHT, BP Encourage couple Transfer to delivery room Time birth Care for newborn Share in birth Promote bonding with mother and father	Assess infant Praise couple Encourage bonding Encourage family integration Assist physician Watch for placental separation Assess mother	Assess Fundus Lochia Voiding BP, TPR Praise couple Encourage fluids Supply nourishment Encourage bonding Encourage family integration Allow for breastfeeding

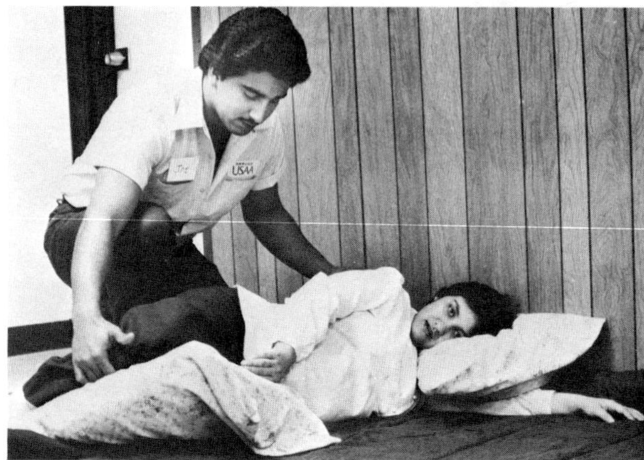

Figure 15.6
Coach checking for relaxation.

All of the breathing techniques are taught as a light chest breathing, which helps raise the diaphragm away from the uterus thereby reducing uterine irritability. This requires greater concentration since most people are abdominal breathers. The *first gear* is a slow nose–mouth breathing.

Effleurage (Fig. 15.7) is simply a light fingertip circular massage of the abdomen. It is done in rhythm with the breathing and is another distractive technique to close the gate. The circular motion may be done on an area of the body other than the abdomen, if preferred.

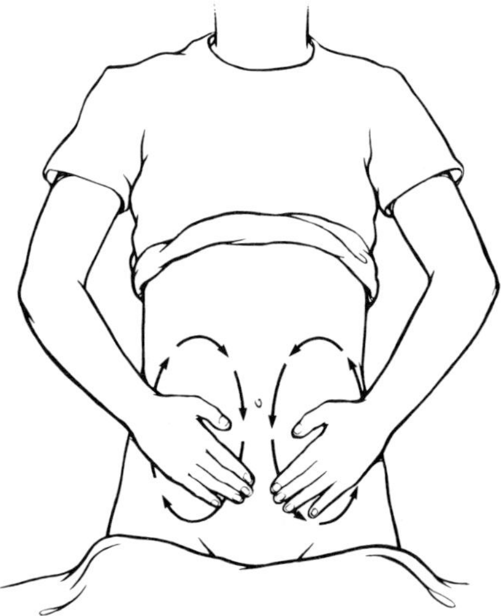

Figure 15.7
Effleurage. Note position of hands.

Emphasis is placed on the coach's role as initiator of practice and the coach's responsibility to set practice times. If the coach can be made to see practice as necessary and beneficial, the coach will be more likely to "call contractions" whenever possible. If there are couples in the class who have used prepared childbirth techniques in a previous pregnancy, they can be encouraged to verbalize and support the need for practice. Equating labor to an athletic event that needs a great deal of training (running a marathon, playing football, hiking) will make practice more meaningful for most coaches because the majority of them are men who at one time engaged in some athletic endeavor requiring such training. There is a fine line separating sufficient emphasis to achieve optimal training and overemphasis that encourages guilt feelings when practice is not done. Each instructor deals with this in an individual manner. In each class, there will be couples who practice very little and later may feel guilty if the labor does not go as well as anticipated. However, the importance of practice does need to be stressed, as training for any physical event must be, and as responsible adults, it is the couple's option to practice or not. One suggestion for making practice less of an ordeal is to practice spontaneously rather than set a definite time each day since labor may initiate at any time. Contractions practiced while driving to a movie or during a commercial break in a television program are better than no practice at all.

In all of the classes, when the couples are practicing their techniques, the instructor will move around the room and check each for mastery. If the coach is asked for an assessment of the mother's mastery, is given suggestions for improvement, and is given positive reinforcement, the role as coach will be reinforced and the coach may go away from this class with the desire to be more assertive toward the practice sessions.

Class Three

The couples have had 1 week to practice the skills they learned in class two and are usually eager to learn more. Part of the content of class two is a continuation of the discussion of the first stage of labor with the focus on the active phase. Since the active phase is usually the time during labor when couples go to the hospital, admission procedures are discussed in order to enable them to be better prepared for some of the very intrusive processes that occur. Routine preps, enemas, intravenous (I.V.) and NPO orders (still used by some of the physicians who support PPM), frequent vaginal exams, and fetal monitoring are generally discussed. This is an excellent time for the childbirth educator to assume a role as consumer advocate by suggesting that the couple negotiate the possibility of avoiding some of these procedures. Although it is often too late to change physicians, if the one they have chosen is nonsupportive, couples can sometimes re-educate their obstetricians to understand and agree to some of their desires. Ideally, such efforts need to begin early.

The third class is a good time to encourage a trip to the hospital so the couples become familiar with the route, any possible detours, and the time it takes to get there (without speeding). They can also tour the maternity unit, which enables them to visualize where they will be while in labor. The visit may also dispel some of the negative misconceptions about labor and delivery rooms (some are actually very cheery!), thereby encouraging a positive attitude and relaxation once admitted. This can also be an opportunity to ask the nurses questions and to begin to place them in a supportive (or nonsupportive) role.

While in the role of consumer advocate, the childbirth educator can suggest the couples start "doctor shopping" for a pediatrician. Since this is one of the few times that couples can take their time and interview and seek an appropriate physician, they should be encouraged to do so. Some suggestions for this include finding a physician located near the home since frequent visits need to be made and making a prenatal appointment to interview the physician in order to assess personality congruence, philosophy of child care, and support or nonsupport of breast-feeding if this is the woman's choice. A mother who needs to be told exactly how to care for a child should not have a pediatrician who is extremely flexible.

At this time the instructor may discuss feeding techniques. Those who will breast-feed are encouraged to seek appropriate information and are informed of community help such as a local La Leche League (there are chapters in most areas). Reference to community agencies, such as Red Cross, offering help with other child-care activities is also beneficial.

Expectant mothers are encouraged to find baby-sitters or house-sitters as needed, to make arrangements for someone to help after the birth, and to pack their suitcases so they are prepared for that unexpected moment. Generally, couples are given a list of things to pack for themselves as well as for the newborn, and they are encouraged to pack a "goody bag" for the labor room. Often, nurses recognize prepared couples by these little bags of comfort measures that they carry with them to the hospital (see Table 15.2).

The goody bag is an excellent lead into a discussion of the active stage of labor since this is when the coach will really begin applying what he or she has learned about making the expectant mother comfortable. All comfort measures are mentioned, including the use of medication. Since PPM does not advocate "no medication" and, in fact, encourages the proper amounts at the appropriate times, it is of

TABLE 15.2
GOODY BAG

Small paperbag (to breathe into to correct hyperventilation)
Talcum powder or lotion (to reduce friction during effleurage or back massage)
Washcloth (for mopping brow, sponging, or sucking on to relieve mouth dryness)
Chapstick, lip balm, or Vaseline (alleviates lip dryness)
Mouth spray or mouthwash (relieves mouth dryness; reduces mouth odor in mother and coach)
Sour lollipops (relieves mouth dryness for mother, supplies energy for coach)
Warm socks (keeps feet warm)
Food for coach (to avoid coach's leaving during needed time)
Small ball, frozen blue ice, tupperware rolling pin (to use in back massage for posterior labor)
Watch (for timing contractions)
Busy work (magazines, books, games, if admitted in early labor)
Focal point
Labor guide

extreme importance that couples leave this class believing that the correct amount of medication can be beneficial. Types of drugs, dosages, side effects, and desired effects are discussed, and couples are encouraged to ask their physicians their particular routine regarding the use of medication. With this information, couples will be able to have active parts in deciding type and amount of medication to be used.

Although the use of medication is supported, the instructor should suggest that all other comfort measures are tried first, including a new type of breathing. After practicing relaxation, couples are taught *gear 1+,* which is just a faster version of *gear 1,* and are encouraged to practice this. The instructor once again visits each couple in the room and assesses its mastery of the technique. Because hyperventilation may be a problem from the faster rate of breathing during gear 1+, the couples are told the symptoms and shown how to rectify it (covering nose and mouth with both hands while continuing to breathe).

During this practice session, relaxation is again assessed and gear 1 and effleurage will again be practiced and assessed. The instructor can generally discern which couples need additional help and/or practice. By now, expectant mothers should be able to relax on command and coaches should have their roles well established, both of which are reinforced by the teacher.

Class Four

During this class in the series, it is usually helpful to discuss some of the variations of labor that may occur. Since induction and augmentation of labor are still widely used today, some knowledge about how this will affect labor might assist the couple. Again, the consumer advocate role may be called into play by having the couples discuss the use of medication, as well as amniotomy, for induction and augmentation and that they may be able to have some input into the physician's decision. Posterior presentations are also mentioned and measures to alleviate discomfort caused by this (position change, application of heat or cold, and back massage) are demonstrated.

Class four will finish the content on the first stage of labor by discussing the transitional phase. Reviewing the latent and active phase helps tie the entire stage together. Because transition is so difficult for most laboring women, the coach needs a great amount of support to help her through this. By emphasizing the positive aspects (it is short and almost the end), the coach may acquire confidence needed during this last part of stage one.

Gears 3, 4, 4+, and blowing to overcome the urge to push are demonstrated and practiced. These are mouth-breathing techniques that are different from the two previous gears and that require greater concentration. Since there are many techniques taught during this class, much time will be spent practicing. The childbirth educator will again assess the individual couples, reinforcing what they are doing and suggesting changes as needed.

Class Five

Content area for class five is concerned mainly with stage two of labor. The mechanism of labor is discussed and demonstrated through use of a pelvis and doll. Appropriate types of anesthesia are discussed since this is the time it is most often used, if at all. Advantages, disadvantages, effects, and side effects of anesthesia are mentioned. Again, the instructor can encourage the couples to question their physicians regarding their preferences.

The coach's and expectant mother's roles in the delivery room are discussed. Procedures such as the possibility of a forceps delivery are also mentioned. Information about the newborn will better prepare the couple for the unexpected look of the child so it will not be as much of a surprise at the time of delivery. Apgar scoring is additional information that couples find most helpful. They are often impressed with knowing terminology that others are not aware of and will very often question the physician in the delivery room as to the rating of their infant. Many fathers score their own children and compare their score with that of the nurse or physician.

Proper pushing technique during labor is demonstrated and practiced (Fig. 15.8). It is advantageous at this time to have the couple practice all the other techniques they have learned to reinforce learning. A demonstration of the success of the techniques usually helps to make the skeptical believers true believers. The coach is asked to apply pressure to some point on the expectant mother (the inner and outer aspects of the knee) in order to cause pain and simulate a contraction. The woman then uses whichever breathing technique she needs to be comfortable, along with relaxation and effleurage, during 1 minute of applied pressure. Once the simulated contraction is completed and the techniques terminated, the coach applies the same amount of pressure to see if the expectant mother notices any difference. The reactions from the mothers are always interesting because generally, up to now, they are apprehensive that their techniques will not work. Noticing the difference in their perception of pain is very encouraging for them to continue practicing. Comments such as, "Were you really pressing that hard?" and "That hurts a lot more!" are very common.

Class Six

All of the techniques have been learned by now and this class can be best used for review and reinforcement. New content is limited to a discussion of the third and fourth stages of labor and the possibility of a cesarean delivery. There has been an increase in the incidence of abdominal deliveries in this century, and most courses have at least one couple who will experience this procedure. In an effort to reduce guilt feelings and encourage a better adjustment to the change in delivery technique, a thorough discussion and verbalization of feelings about cesarean delivery is warranted. There is emphasis on the word *delivery* (rather than section) and a discussion of the positive result of a perhaps healthier baby. One of the main objectives of this discussion is that the couple comes away with the idea that they are not a "Lamaze failure" because their child made an abdominal rather than vaginal entrance into the world. The teacher again encourages the couples to question their physicians regarding type of anesthesia, incision, and projected recovery period. Referral to community support groups such as C/SEC may be beneficial for some couples to allow them to verbalize their feelings of inadequacy after the delivery.

Time is then spent practicing all the techniques learned and reviewing content regarding labor. It is often helpful to describe various situations and ask the coach what to do during them. A good ending for this class is to accentuate the positive by showing a film of prepared labor.

Class Seven

The seventh class is part educational and part social. The content is related to the postpartal period, and although it would be more appropriate after delivery, it is almost impossible to time a class after delivery. Thus, the information is given now hoping that some will be retained and used after delivery.

The physiologic and psychologic changes of involution are included, as well as some suggested coping mechanisms. Postpartum exercises are taught; fam-

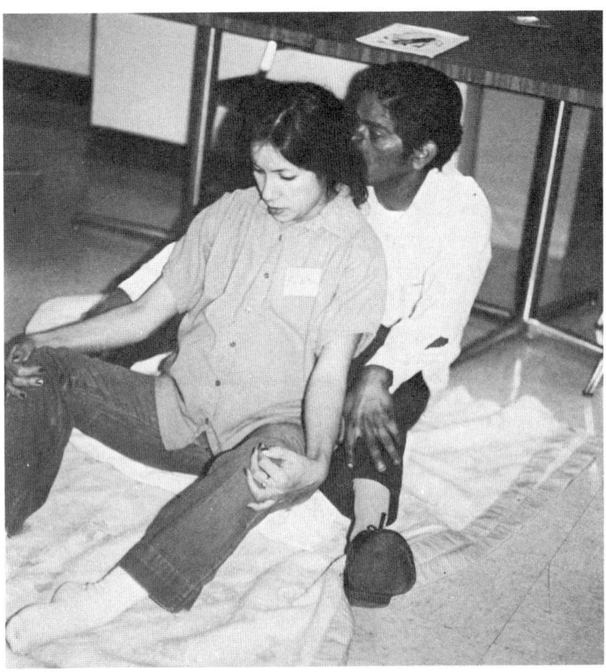

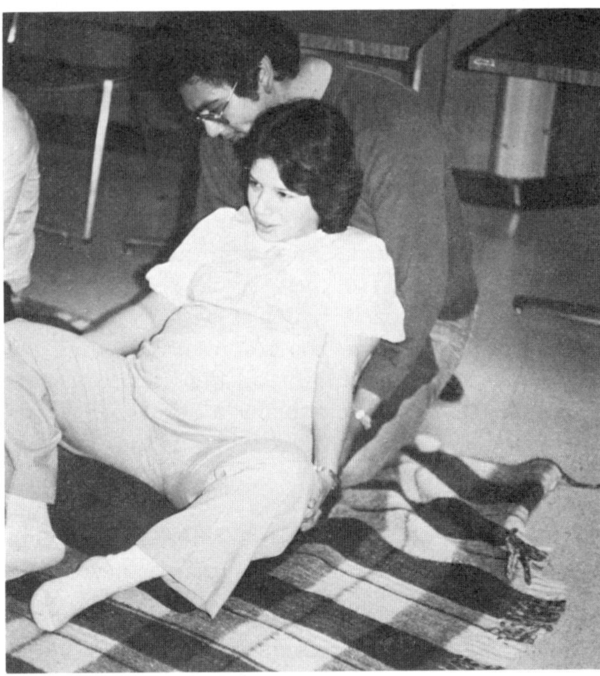

Figure 15.8
Pushing position.

ily planning, bonding, and some parenting techniques are mentioned. This is again a good time to use the experiences of couples who have prior births for they can lend more reality to the discussion. If time allows, additional practice of all the techniques is beneficial.

The social aspect of this class is a visit from a newly delivered couple. If one of the class couples has delivered before this class, they are asked to return; if not, a couple from a past class is usually invited. The couple is encouraged to relate their labor experience and to answer any questions. It is beneficial for the nondelivered couples to see that someone has lived through it and that it was a very positive experience. Having two couples, one vaginal and one cesarean delivery, may more fully prepare the pregnant couple for all possibilities. This lends itself to verbalization of feelings regarding labor.

NURSING INTERVENTION FOR THE PREPARED COUPLE

Regardless of the method used, nursing care is considerably different for couples experiencing a prepared as compared to an unprepared birth. Assessment activities of a prepared birth are the same as with any other labor; the main difference is that the nurse's role is one of supporting the coach. Many coaches experience feelings of helplessness and apprehension if they have not previously experienced a prepared childbirth. At times, nurses assess this inexperience as ineffectiveness and will take over the coaching activities, thus interfering in the couple's relationship. The nurse's role should be one of coaching the coach, which is best accomplished by understanding the coach's role, knowing the techniques, keeping current on the literature concerning new trends, and being a consumer advocate whenever possible. Specific guidelines for care during labor are:

- ▲ Orient the couple to the facility, encouraging the coach to seek supplies or help as needed
- ▲ Introduce the couple to the other personnel who are now members of the team
- ▲ Provide any needed supplies (washcloth, extra pillows, ice chips, mouth swabs, scrubs)
- ▲ Assess labor and inform physician of progress
- ▲ Explain all techniques
- ▲ Inform couple of the progress of labor and answer any questions
- ▲ Allow coach to function and offer suggestions as assessed
- ▲ Be supportive of what the couple is doing and of their decisions
- ▲ Offer positive reinforcement and praise whenever possible (coach needs to know he or she is functioning correctly)
- ▲ Limit distractions in the labor room
- ▲ Encourage the coach to rest and to get nourishment whenever possible
- ▲ Share in the experience of the birth
- ▲ Promote bonding
- ▲ Give positive reinforcement for a job well done

Even though the coach is providing most of the support during labor, the nurse retains the professional and legal responsibilities for safe and appropriate supervision of the couple during their labor and delivery experience. The skilled nurse will find a way to ensure a balance between couple–participant childbirth and assuming nursing responsibilities for care.

SUGGESTIONS FOR THE FUTURE

Preparation for childbirth needs to be started before the woman even becomes pregnant. It should be an integral part of health education, beginning in childhood and early adolescence. Ideally every woman contemplating conception of a child should be able to know what to expect of pregnancy, childbirth, and recovery. A preparation for childbirth and parenting course should be accessible to every woman or couple who wish to participate in such learning activities.

A more realistic goal would be to have couples begin courses in preparation for childbirth as soon as their pregnancy is confirmed. The early classes can contain information regarding nutrition, drugs, and physical and emotional changes during pregnancy. Body conditioning can be started in an effort to help the woman to acquire better physical stamina that will serve her well during the course of labor and childbirth. Beginning classes earlier will also allow for more interaction throughout the pregnancy between the partner and the pregnant woman and provide more time to discuss feelings about starting a family. Parenting techniques can be included in such classes. Involvement of the partner (coach) earlier can encourage a more active role, both during pregnancy and following delivery. Sibling classes can be incorporated into the series so that the rivalry and resentment among siblings can be avoided or reduced. This would also encourage the attitude that childbirth is a family affair.

Postpartal classes can be incorporated into the series to meet the definite need of couples to discuss recovery and readjustment. Often the couple returns home from the hospital with little or no idea of what to do or what to expect. Although some of this content is usually covered in a class before delivery, it has little meaning to couples until the infant arrives and they are faced with the responsibilities of parenthood. Just being able to sit down and talk about problems may help relieve some of the frustrations of child rearing. Special groups of parents with particular problems can come out of such courses. The discussions could continue for as long as necessary or desired by the people involved. Just having an available support system for whatever purpose is reassuring to most couples.

Much information can be acquired during childbirth classes that can be applied to everyday living. The earlier this educational process is started, the more prepared will the woman and family be to deal with reproductive events and the greater the potential for coping successfully with life generally.

Including grandparents in some way in parent and childbirth education seems appropriate as well. These people are often the primary support sources outside of the nuclear family. They could gain greater understanding of prepared childbirth and learn more about their roles as grandparents.

SUMMARY

Preparation for childbirth was discussed from an historical perspective. Some of the popular methods of childbirth education in use today were identified. Special attention was given to describing and explaining the psychoprophylactic method (PPM) of childbirth preparation. A series of classes and ways in which the nurse (or teacher) could be helpful to expectant parents participating in such classes were described. Useful aids to parents during labor were included. The chapter closed with a view of possible changes in approaches to childbirth education, including expansion of existing focus and content to the areas of parenthood and recovery; the participation of siblings in the process; and the involvement of grandparents as a part of the childbirth experience.

REFERENCES AND READINGS

Auerbach, A. B. *Parents Learn Through Discussion.* New York: John Wiley & Sons, 1968.

Bean, C. A. *Methods of Childbirth.* New York: Dolphin Books, 1974.

Bing, E. *Six Practical Lessons for an Easier Childbirth.* New York: Grosset & Dunlap, 1967.

Conklin, M. Discussion Groups as Preparation for Cesarean Section. *J Obstet Gynecol Neonatal Nurs* 6:52, 1977.

Dick-Read, G. *Childbirth Without Fear: The Original Approach to Natural Childbirth.* New York: Harper & Row, 1944.

Ebner, M. *Physiotherapy in Obstetrics.* London: F. and S. Livingstone, 1967.

Edwards, M. *Communications: Dimensions in Childbirth Education.* Seattle: Catalyst Publishing, 1976.

Fawcett, J. Needs of Cesarean Birth Parents. *J Obstet Gynecol Neonatal Nurs* 10:372, 1981.

Felton, G. S., Segelman, F. B. Lamaze Childbirth Training and Changes in Belief About Personal Control. *Birth Fam J* 5:141, 1978.

Hazell, L. *Commonsense Childbirth.* Berkely, Calif.: Berkely Publishing, 1976.

Jimenez, S. M., Jones, L. C., and Jungman, R. G. Prenatal Classes for Repeat Parents: A Distinct Need. *Matern Child Nurs* 4:305, 1979.

Karmel, M. *Thank You, Dr. Lamaze.* Philadelphia: J. B. Lippincott, 1959.

Kitzinger, S. *Education and Counseling for Childbirth.* New York: Schocken, 1979.

Lamaze, F. *Painless Childbirth.* Chicago: Henry Regnery, 1970.

Marquart, R. Expectant Fathers: What Are Their Needs? *Am J Matern Child Nurs* 1:32, 1976.

Shearer, M. Teaching Prenatal Exercise: Part I, Posture. *Birth and Fam Journal* 8:105, 1981.

Shrock, P., Simpkin, P., Shearer, M. Teaching Prenatal Exercises: Part II, Exercises to Think Twice About. *Birth and Fam Journal* 8:167, 1981.

Simkin, P., Reinke, C. *Kaleidoscope of Childbearing: Preparation, Birth, and Nurturing. Highlights of the Tenth Bienneal Convention of the International Childbirth Education Association Inc.* Seattle: The Penny Press, 1978.

Sumner, G. Giving Expectant Parents the Help They Need: The ABCs of Prenatal Education. *Am J Matern Child Nurs* 1:220, 1976.

Sumner, G., Fritsch, J. Postnatal Parental Concerns: The First Six Weeks of Life. *J Obstet Gynecol Neonatal Nurs* 6:27, 1977.

Sweet, P. T. Prenatal Classes Especially for Children. *Am J Matern Child Nurs* 4:82 1979.

Whitley, N. A Comparison of Prepared Childbirth Couples and Conventional Prenatal Class Couples. *J Obstet Gynecol Neonatal Nurs* 8:109, 1979.

UNIT FOUR

CHILDBIRTH, RECOVERY, AND EARLY PARENTHOOD

INTRODUCTION

The onset of labor that culminates in the birth of a child brings the period of pregnancy to an end and ushers in a new reproductive period for the expectant parents. Whereas pregnancy was a more leisurely period during which the expectant parents could work through and adjust to the changes associated with pregnancy, the events of labor are concentrated in an approximately 24-hour period. Recovery takes place in about a 6-week period with major physiologic changes occurring within a 2-week interval after birth. Parenthood, on the other hand, spans the rest of the couple's lives.

Unit Four contains four chapters that will help you comprehend the changes occurring or anticipated during these periods.

Chapter 16, "Labor," discusses the physiology and clinical course of labor, maternal and fetal response to labor, use of analgesia, and the needs of the mother and infant immediately after birth. The role and responsibilities of the maternity nurse are explained within the context of the happenings during labor and their effect on the expectant family.

Chapter 17, "The Neonate," is a detailed discussion of the adjustment of the infant to extrauterine life from both a physiologic and psychosocial view. Both physical and behavioral assessment modalities of the neonate are included. Nursing role and responsibilities regarding the care of the infant are emphasized.

Chapter 18, "Parenthood," discusses parenthood in both traditional and variant family life-styles, such as the single parent. Adoptive parenthood and foster parents and grandparents are also discussed. The nursing focus is on healthy parenthood through the acquisition of adequate and appropriate parenting skills.

Chapter 19, "Maternal Recovery from Pregnancy and Childbirth," addresses the biophysical and psychosocial content needed to understand this rapid period of change. Breast-feeding and early maternal–infant relationships are included. Nursing care focuses on the needs of the woman within the context of her family.

BEHAVIORAL OUTCOMES

Upon completion of this unit, you should be able to:

- ▲ Describe the physiology of normal labor
- ▲ Explain maternal–fetal biophysical and psychosocial responses to labor
- ▲ Describe the impact of labor on the family
- ▲ Comprehend skills essential for the safe care of a mother and her fetus–neonate
- ▲ Explain the biophysical, emotional, and role adjustments of the mother after childbirth
- ▲ Identify learning needs usual for all mothers and families after childbirth
- ▲ Describe the extrauterine biophysical and psychosocial adaptations of the neonate
- ▲ Explain neonatal needs deriving from biophysical, social, and nutritional demands
- ▲ Explain models for gestational age and behavioral assessment of the neonate

- ▲ Identify the tasks of parenthood
- ▲ Describe parenthood in terms of various life-styles
- ▲ Describe mother–infant–father socialization process
- ▲ Explain nursing interventions needed to promote healthy parenthood

16

LABOR

The period of labor that climaxes with the birth of a new life is the culmination of a gestation that has spanned months, and, to many nurses, it is the epitome of maternity nursing. It is indeed a profound time for the pregnant woman and her family, as well as for the maternity nurse. Labor, which is often exciting, frightening, fulfilling, and rewarding, demands the woman's physical and emotional expenditure of energy, while it requires the nurse's intelligent use of knowledge and skills.

Labor is an intensely personal experience, yet the nature of labor is such that most pregnant women do not labor in isolation from other people. One of the primary needs during labor has been identified as the support of a sustaining human presence (Lesser & Keane, 1956). This human presence may be the professional support of the maternity nurse and other health care providers; increasingly, this "supportive other" is being found outside of the professional health care personnel and is more likely to be husband, partner, relative, friend, or childbirth education coach working along side of the maternity nurse (see Chapter 15). The inclusion of a significant other is a reflection of the rapidly changing patterns of family organization and individual life-styles, the trend toward preparation for childbirth through formal and informal methods, and a revolt against the depersonalization of much of the health care services today. Throughout this chapter, this supportive other will not be identified by legal or cultural role, such as husband or boyfriend.

Nurses who work in the labor and delivery area do not practice their art and skill in isolation from the periods that precede labor or follow birth. The truly skillful, effective nurse draws upon concept, theory, and skill from nursing generally, as well as from understandings about the antepartal and postpartal periods; sees the complete picture of pregnancy and understands the various ways in which the pregnant woman and her family may experience the reproductive periods; relies upon the arts and sciences used with the concepts and theories of maternity nursing; and avoids the trap of highly circumscribed practice that is narrow in perspective and scope. In other words, a successful maternity nurse works in the *area* of labor and delivery and is not a labor and delivery nurse. This chapter will focus on normal labor and will include the theory and physiology of labor; maternal biophysical, and psychosocial changes during labor; fetal adaptation throughout labor, and nursing skills necessary for the safe care of mother and fetus/neonate.

THEORIES FOR THE ONSET OF LABOR

Labor is the mechanism by which the products of conception are expelled from the mother's uterus and vagina. It is accomplished mainly by contraction of the uterine muscle, the *myometrium,* which causes the cervix to efface (thin out), dilate (open up), and retract (draw back) helping the fetus, placenta, and membranes to leave the uterus and descend through the birth canal. In most cases, these contractions occur in a regular, rhythmic fashion over a period of about 8–14 hours, depending on whether the woman is having a first or subsequent pregnancy. Occasionally, contractions will be apparent to the pregnant woman or to the examiner through palpation or electronic monitoring but will not cause the changes in the uterus to occur. This is referred to as *false labor.* It is a normal occurrence and is one way in which the body prepares for the event of true labor when uterine changes do occur.

There are several theories for the onset of labor, but what causes its exact onset is not known. Current theories seem to support the belief that there is an interaction between fetal and maternal systems that promotes the event of labor. There seems to be an association between fetal maturity and the onset of labor. Labor rarely occurs if the fetus is immature, unless there is an underlying pathophysiologic cause. For years, it has been believed that the posterior pituitary hormone, oxytocin, played a role in initiating labor; that the uterus stretched to a point at which it could stretch no more and had to evacuate the fetus; that prostaglandins had something to do with labor. It has also been believed that the withdrawal of progesterone, which keeps the myometrium in a quiet state during pregnancy, was the primary precipitator of labor. More recently, the presence of fetal cortisol has been associated with the onset of labor. None of these theories completely explains the phenomenon of the onset of labor. Some of them may be found to be parts of the total picture when all is understood. The characteristics and validity of these theories are presented in Table 16.1 to acquaint you with some of the more current thinking about the onset of labor.

Readiness for Labor

Labor is possible because of factors that have occurred before and during pregnancy. The adequacy of the female bony pelvis to accommodate passage of the term size infant is one such factor. Pelvic size is established before conception and depends on the woman's body build and development (see Chapter 4). The joints between the pelvic bones contain a cartilagelike tissue that is softened somewhat by hormones during pregnancy. This tissue provides for minimal give if not true expansion during labor, increasing pelvic dimensions slightly. For the most part, pelvic size is determined by genetic and other factors predating pregnancy.

Preparation of the uterine myometrium for forceful contractions during labor is an essential prerequisite for labor since the uterine muscle is the primary force for dilation, effacement, and fetal

TABLE 16.1
THEORIES FOR THE ONSET OF HUMAN LABOR

Theory	*Characteristics of Theory*	*Validity*
Oxytocin stimulation	Oxytocin is a peptide released by the posterior pituitary, which acts directly on myometrial fibers causing contraction. In late pregnancy, the uterus is responsive to exogenous oxytocin. Endogenous oxytocin from maternal and/or fetal origins stimulates onset of labor.	No convincing evidence. Oxytocin-calcium-releasing effect.
Uterine distention—Stretch theory	Speculation is that any hollow organ when stretched tends to contract and empty itself.	Provides some basis for the earlier onset of labor in multiple pregnancies and with polyhydramnios.
Fetal-membrane phospholipid—Arachidonic acid-prostaglandin	Prostaglandins are formed biosynthetically from nonesterified polyunsaturated essential fatty acid, arachidonic acid. Uterine decidua has been shown to form prostaglandins.	Speculative only at this time; however, it seems to be biochemically rational.

Theory	*Characteristics of Theory*	*Validity*
	Prostaglandin F_{2a} or prostaglandin E_2 will stimulate uterine contractions at any stage of gestation regardless of route of administration. Levels of prostaglandin have been shown to be increased in amniotic fluid of laboring women. Arachidonic acid increases eightfold in laboring women as opposed to nonlaboring women. Arachidonic acid released by fetal membranes diffuses into the decidua and is speculated to be a precursor for prostaglandin synthesis. High levels of prostaglandins have been found in pregnant women near term and during labor. Prostaglandin, when synthesized by enzymatic activity, enhances labor by ▲ stimulating smooth muscle of the uterus to contract ▲ mediating contractile effects of oxytocin ▲ acting as vasoconstrictor agent creating uterine ischemia and thus initiating contractions ▲ causing progesterone withdrawal thereby transforming myometrium to highly sensitive organ Contractile elements are greater in pregnancy than in nonpregnant states. Progesterone blocks myometrial contractility. Proper estrogen/progesterone balance allows gestation to continue.	
Progesterone withdrawal (estrogen-progesterone concentration)	Withdrawal of progesterone in pregnant rabbits causes labor. Administration of progesterone will prolong pregnancy. Exact mechanism for the estrogen/progesterone balance in humans is not known.	No identifiable decrease in progesterone shown in term human pregnancies.
Fetal cortisol	Has been shown that hypophysectomized or adrenalectomized sheep fetuses resulted in prolonged pregnancy. Administration of cortisol or ACTH to fetal sheep with intact adrenals results in premature labor. There is an association between anencephalic human fetuses and prolonged pregnancy. Blood levels of fetal ACTH do not seem to increase before or during labor.	Cortisol has been shown to play a role in fetal lung maturity; no valid documentation of initiation of labor in humans after the administration of ACTH or cortisol. The fetal role in initiating labor is not clear but implications are that the fetus is an active contributor to the initiation of labor by being a neural trigger for adrenocortical secretions that alter the placenta's endocrine activity to activate myometrial stimulating agents.

descent during labor. The contractile ability of the uterine muscle fibers is dependent on actomyosin, the contractile protein; adenosine triphosphate, which supplies the energy necessary for a contraction; and adenosine triphosphatase, the enzyme that splits adenosine triphosphate to release energy. Estrogen plays a role in contractility, which is supported by the fact that concentrations of contractile elements are greater in the pregnant than the nonpregnant uterus. Lowest concentrations of these elements are in castrates and postmenopausal women, and normal amounts of contractile elements can be restored by administration of estrogen.

The result and desired outcome of uterine contractions are dilatation and effacement of the cervix. *Dilatation* (dilation) is the opening of the cervix by a combination of two factors: (1) Retraction of the upper segment of the uterus, which has become shorter and thicker (see the section on physiology of labor later in this chapter), pulls the lower segment and the dilating cervix upward around the infant's head. (2) The pressure of the contracting uterus forces the infant against the cervix. *Retraction* is the more significant force. *Effacement* is the process by which the cervical canal is progressively shortened to a point of complete obliteration (see Fig. 16.1). The uterine muscles contract some during pregnancy, but these contractions are not usually discernible by the pregnant woman until the latter months of pregnancy. The earlier contraction of the myometrium has been confirmed through electronic monitoring techniques. Contractions during pregnancy are believed to help prepare the uterus for labor by causing some cervical changes before the clinical onset of labor. Contractions occurring during pregnancy are called *Braxton Hicks'* contractions. Changes that take place during these contractions are cervical softening and effacement and some dilatation (Caldeyro-Barcia & Poseiro, 1960; Cibils, 1965). The contractions are much more forceful during labor. The uterine myometrium, being a smooth muscle, is capable of great contractility.

All maternal systems have been prepared to cope with the events of labor. Even though more demands are placed on certain maternal systems than others during labor, all systems are affected in some manner and to some extent. For example, it is known that labor necessitates an increased cardiac workload for the mother and certainly a great expenditure of physical energy. In fact, labor is likened to a 20-mile hike. The muscles have become more elastic and ready for work; the soft tissues, particularly of the pelvis and perineum, are also more elastic and ready to give with the birth of the baby; the respiratory system has compensated for its displacement by the gravid uterus with alterations that enable the mother to tolerate the period of labor without becoming oxygen deficient; blood clotting factors have been altered in a way that will help prevent hemorrhage during and after labor; there seems to be an increase in maternal energy level just before the onset of labor, as if to prepare the mother for work.

There is a psychologic readiness for labor as well. Women appear to become quieter and more in control of themselves as labor nears. They seem to be more task oriented, as evidenced by arranging their homes so that all is ready for the infant. Although many women are anxious and even frightened to some extent, there is a prevailing attitude of "let's get on with this." There is an element of truth in the comic portrayal in films and books of the pregnant woman in early labor getting everything together and then waking her blustering husband.

If the expectant parents (or mother) have attended preparation for childbirth classes in which they have learned about labor and how to help themselves during labor, they are often eager to try out the new techniques learned. The classes often decrease their fears, and they view labor as a challenge with a delightful outcome rather than an ordeal to be endured. Other expectant parents may have read extensively or discussed labor with their nurse or physician rather than attending formal classes. There is no question that preparation for labor is desired for expectant couples and helps them cope more ably with the demands of the childbirth experience.

The fetus gives evidence of readiness for labor. There is a fetal alignment with the maternal pelvis in preparation for descent through this passage. In some cases, particularly with first pregnancies, descent is usually apparent about 4 weeks before the onset of labor. *Lightening,* as this descent is called, is the settling of the fetal head into the upper pelvis. This occurs in the primigravida 2–4 weeks before delivery and coincides with the period of elongation of the lower segment and the effacement of the cervix. In multigravidas, elongation and effacement are less complete at the time of onset of labor; therefore, the fetal head usually remains higher. The fetus often becomes quieter and less active, almost as if there is recognition of what is ahead. The fetus is not an active participant in the process of labor in the

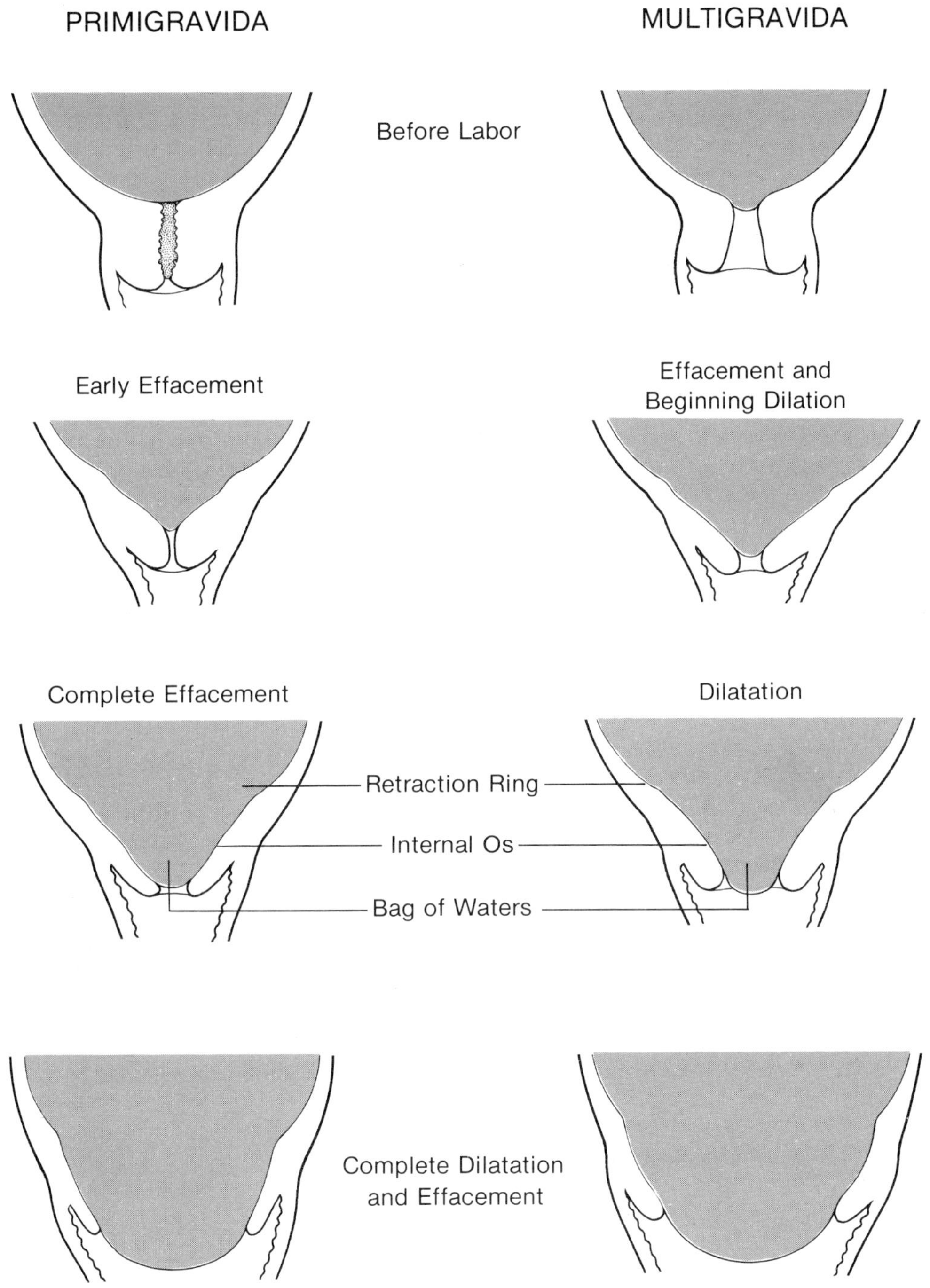

PRIMIGRAVIDA

MULTIGRAVIDA

Before Labor

Early Effacement

Effacement and Beginning Dilation

Complete Effacement

Dilatation

Retraction Ring

Internal Os

Bag of Waters

Complete Dilatation and Effacement

Figure 16.1
Dilation and effacement.

same way the mother is; however, it acts as the recipient of what is ahead and energy will be needed for that. Whatever the reason, decreased fetal activity has been noted before and during normal labor and birth.

Labor—Physiologic Concepts

Physiologically, the uterus contracts throughout pregnancy, and cervical changes including dilatation often take place before labor. After the twentieth week of gestation, the wall of the uterus becomes progressively thinner and the increase in size of the uterus is largely a result of the elongation of muscle fibers. The uterus has two separate divisions: the upper uterine segment, made up of active contracting muscle tissue supplying the force for expulsion; and a thin lower uterine segment, through which the presenting part passes into the pelvic cavity. Uterine muscle fibers have certain characteristics that make them unique and effective for their role in the birth process; namely, they *elongate* (length of a muscle cell increases), they are *elastic* (return to their normal length after uterine distention), and they are able to *contract* (force the products of conception from the uterus). Muscular activity has been studied by measuring the effect of contractions on amniotic fluid pressure. Caldeyro-Barcia and Poseiro (1960) measured intrauterine pressures by means of a polyethylene tube that is inserted into the amniotic fluid. The unit of measure, called a Montevideo unit, is the sum in millimeters of mercury (mm Hg) of all the contractions in a 10-minute period. Caldeyro-Barcia and Poseira's research shows that in early pregnancy, until approximately 30-weeks gestation, uterine activity is less than 20 Montevideo units. Irregular painless contractions (Braxton Hicks) increase from 30 to 80 Montevideo units as the cervix ripens. At the onset of labor, uterine activity is between 80–120 Montevideo units. At the end of labor, when intensity of the contractions are about 50 mm Hg and the frequency is 5 g per 10-minute period, Montevideo units are 250. (Intrauterine pressure and its significance is discussed further under electronic fetal monitoring.) As mentioned earlier, it is the increased muscle activity in the prelabor period that accounts for the changes in the uterine body and cervix (Fig. 16.2). As the muscle fibers of the upper active segment shorten with successive contractions during labor, the fibers in the more passive thin lower segment elongate because the cervix is closed. When the upper segment relaxes as the contraction ends, the lower segment shortens and its wall thickens. This pattern repeats itself until eventually the upper segment becomes shorter and its wall thicker and the lower segment becomes longer and thinner. Eventually, the cervix effaces or is taken up around the membranes and the presenting part and is incorporated into the lower segment. The primary force in labor is the involuntary contraction of the uterine muscles. The contractions have certain characteristics, namely,

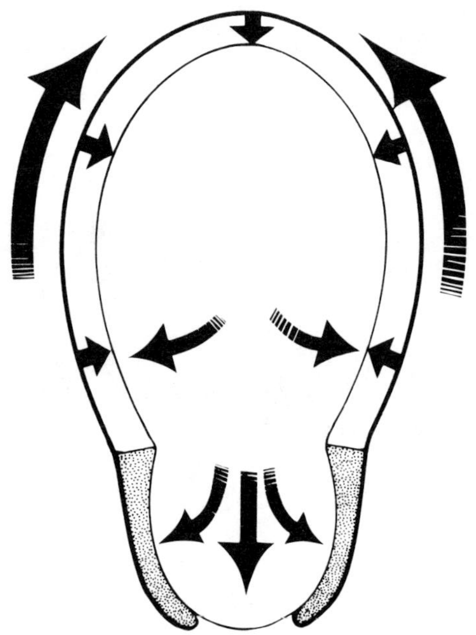

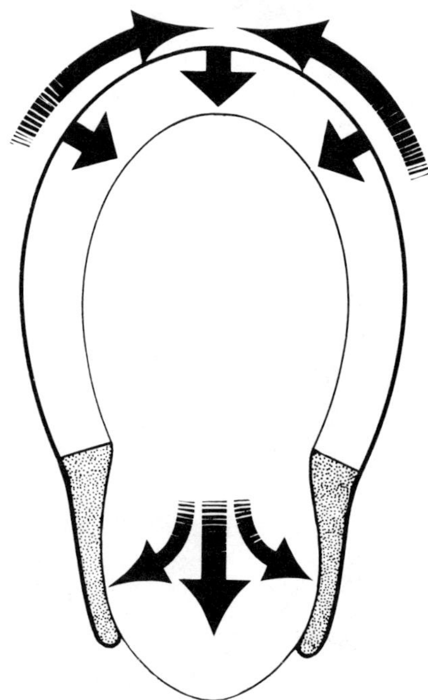

Figure 16.2
Retraction of upper uterine segment. *Left:* partially dilated cervix; *right:* cervical dilatation complete—cervix pulled upward.

they are involuntary, they recur intermittently and rhythmically, and they produce pain. Uterine contractions are presumed to be initiated by one of two pacemakers situated in the cornual areas of the fundus; one pacemaker predominates, and during normal labor each contraction is begun by a single pacemaker. The contraction mechanism is well coordinated so that the peak is reached in all areas of the uterus simultaneously. Hence, the systolic phase is longest in the region of the pacemaker in the fundus, and it progressively shortens in areas more distant. The term *fundal dominance* is used to describe the characteristics of a normal labor contraction. The process is a gradient of force directed from the fundus to the least active and weakest area of the uterus, the cervix. Fundal dominance is reflected on the pattern of the intensity of a contraction. More specifically, each contraction has three phases—increment, acme, and decrement. The *increment phase* is the period in which the intensity increases, the *acme phase* is the peak of the intensity, and the *decrement phase* is the period of decreasing intensity. For the relationship of fundal dominance to phases of a contraction see Figure 16.3. The most important factor in dilating the cervix is retraction of the upper segment of the uterus which is the result of labor contractions.

Labor is traditionally divided in four stages. The *first stage of labor* is the stage of dilatation and is defined as the beginning of labor until complete dilatation of the cervix, or 10 cm, is reached. The primary force during this stage is that of involuntary contraction of the uterine muscles just described. This *first stage* of labor is subdivided into *two phases*—latent and active. The *latent phase* extends from the onset of labor to the beginning of the active phase, identified as that point in time when dilatation takes place more rapidly. The *active phase* is subdivided into three phases—the *acceleration phase,* the *phase of maximum slope,* and the *deceleration phase* (sometimes called transitional phase) (see Fig. 16.4). Almost all cervical dilatation takes place in the active phase. In the latent phase, the curve is almost flat, while it rises sharply in the active phase. The deceleration period during the active phase coincides with the descent of the fetal presenting part (see Fig. 16.5). The deceleration phase is not associated with any true deceleration of myometrial function. Studies show a relatively steady progression of uterine work throughout labor. During the deceleration phase, the cervix is being retracted around the fetal head, and the beginning of the descent pattern (see p. 317) is taking place.

The *second stage of labor,* sometimes called the *expulsive stage,* begins with complete cervical dilatation and ends with the birth of the baby. It is during this stage that the secondary force of labor is used. This force is voluntary, forceful contractions of the abdominal muscles with the diaphragm fixed after forced inspiration. This secondary force is used during the second stage of labor after the cervix is completely dilated. The employment of voluntary abdominal muscles by the mother after forced inspiration (taking a deep breath) increases intra-abdominal pressure and intrauterine pressure. This activity and use of abdominal muscle do not dilate the cervix but aid expulsion of the infant. In summary, labor occurs as a result of the force of muscular contractions. The *primary force* is the involuntary uterine contractions and the *secondary force* is that produced by voluntary intra-abdominal pressure.

The *third stage of labor* is normally a brief period defined as the time from the delivery of the baby to the delivery of the placenta and membranes (the afterbirth). The *fourth stage of labor* is the first hour after delivery, a most important time for the mother and nurse; this stage is discussed more fully later in this chapter.

Friedman (1978) introduced another way of looking at labor, with stages seen as functional divisions rather than sequential events. He points out that only a very small part of the first stage is occupied with cervical dilatation and that the descent is not limited to second stage but begins in the first stage. Friedman divides labor, functionally, into three parts based on their "physiologic objectives," namely, *preparatory, dilatational,* and *pelvic divisions* (Fig. 16.6). This division provides the basis for a logical understanding of the biophysical changes during the first three stages of labor (compare Figs. 16.4 and 16.5 with 16.6).

- ▲ ***Preparatory Division.*** Time during which the contractions become coordinated and the cervix is prepared for intense activity.
- ▲ ***Dilatational Division.*** Period during which the cervix is more actively dilated in a linear manner.
- ▲ ***Pelvic Division.*** Essentially the period of fetal descent during which the pelvis is negotiated and the fetus is able to descend through it and be born.

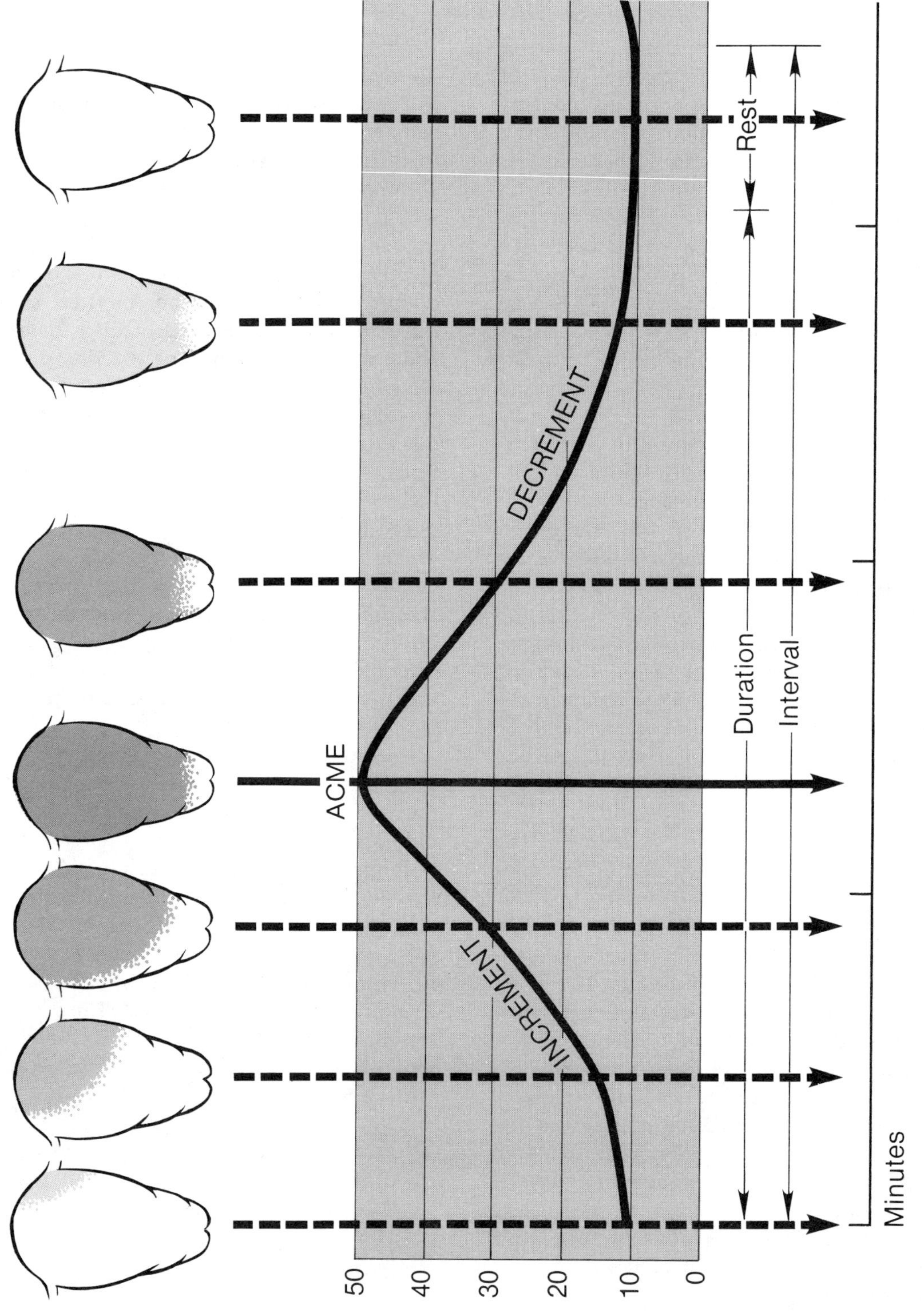

Figure 16.3
Fundal dominance during labor contractions.

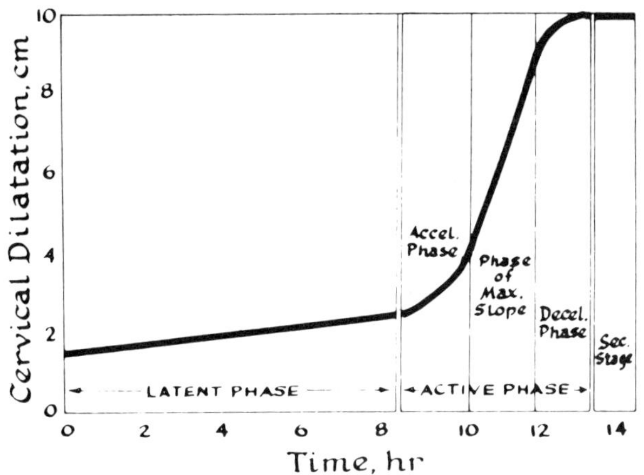

Figure 16.4
Average dilatational curve during labor. Source: Friedman, E. A. *Labor: Clinical Evaluation and Management* (2nd ed.). New York: Appleton-Century-Crofts. Copyright © 1978. Used with permission.

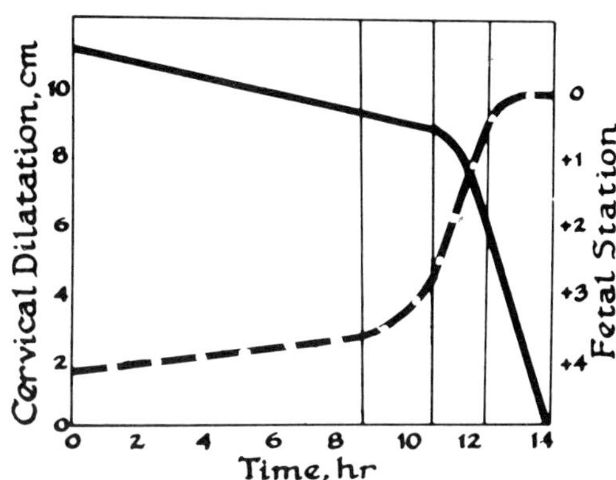

Figure 16.5
Dilatational curve and descent. Source: Friedman, E. A. *Labor: Clinical Evaluation and Management* (2nd ed.). New York: Appleton-Century-Crofts. Copyright © 1978. Used with permission.

Since the divisions are named for their functions, there is little question about what is happening when the woman is said to be in one of these stages of labor. Some analogies between Friedman's work and traditional stages can be made. The preparatory division, like the latent or early part of the first stage of labor, is longer than the other stages. Contractions are felt but are not usually perceived as very painful. There is a longer period of time between contractions, during which the mother can relax and recover. The dilatational division compares with the last part of the first stage, or the active phase of labor, during which contractions are stronger, more frequent, and often felt as more painful. The pelvic division overlaps to some extent both the traditional first and second stages of labor since there is some

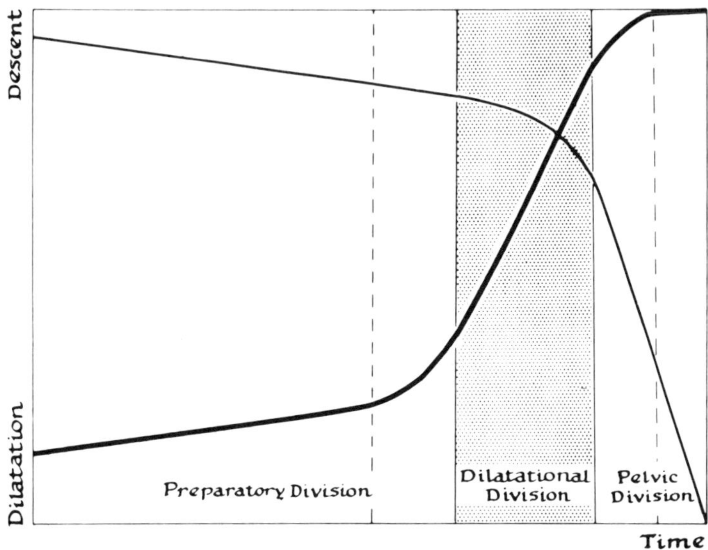

Figure 16.6
Functional divisions of labor and dilatational and descent curves. Source: Friedman, E. A. *Labor: Clinical Evaluation and Management* (2nd ed.). New York: Appleton-Century-Crofts. Copyright © 1978. Used with permission.

descent during these stages and, with the first pregnancy, even more descent before the onset of labor.

Figure 16.6 shows the relationship between the functional divisions of labor and the dilatational and descent curves. Grasping these concepts allows the nurse to assess the client's labor progress. Understanding the physiology of labor is necessary for the comprehension of the normal labor curve that provides part of the theoretical basis for nursing care.

Mechanism of Labor

Mechanism of labor is a term applied to a series of changes in the attitude and position of the fetus during its trip down the birth canal. Although it is necessary to discuss mother and fetus separately, it is very important to remember that labor and the mechanisms of labor are simultaneous events. Fetal descent through the birth canal is possible because of a definite set of maneuvers or adaptations by the fetus to the birth canal. These adaptations need to be understood by maternity nurses in order for them to relate the biophysical and psychosocial changes occurring in the mother during labor.

The *presentation* or *presenting part* of the fetus is the part that comes through the birth canal first. These terms are frequently used interchangeably. *Lie* is the term used to identify the relationships between the long axis of the mother and the long axis of the fetus. For example, *longitudinal lie* occurs when the maternal and fetal spines are parallel; *transverse lie* occurs when the fetal spine is at right angles to the mother's spine; and *oblique lie* occurs when the fetal spine crosses the maternal spine at an acute angle.

Although the terms presenting part and presentation are used interchangeably, presentation indicates the intrauterine situation more specifically and incorporates the lie of the fetus. For example, *occiput presentation* indicates a longitudinal lie where the occiput (back of the skull) is coming first, and *breech presentation* indicates a longitudinal lie with the buttocks coming first. Two other terms are important to understanding the mechanism of labor—attitude and position. *Attitude* refers to the relationship of the fetal parts to each other and is discussed in degrees of flexion. For example, *complete flexion* refers to the fetus with the chin resting on the chest, spine flexed in a smooth curve, arms folded across the chest, and hips and knees flexed. A *deflexed attitude* refers to the position in which the head is extended and the spine curved in less than complete flexion. *Position* is determined by the relationship of an exact fetal part to a fixed area of the maternal pelvis. This relationship is signified in obstetrics by three capital letters, such as LOA (Fig. 16.7). The clue is to remember that the outside letters (e.g., L and A) *always* refer to the fixed maternal landmarks, and the middle letter (e.g., O) *always* refers to the presenting part of the fetus. This determination of position is made most often by direct palpation of the presenting part through a dilated cervix during vaginal examination; for example, LOA indicates that the presenting part of the fetus is the occiput and is located in the left anterior aspect of the mother's pelvis. This chapter deals with the occiput positions only. If the fetus has a

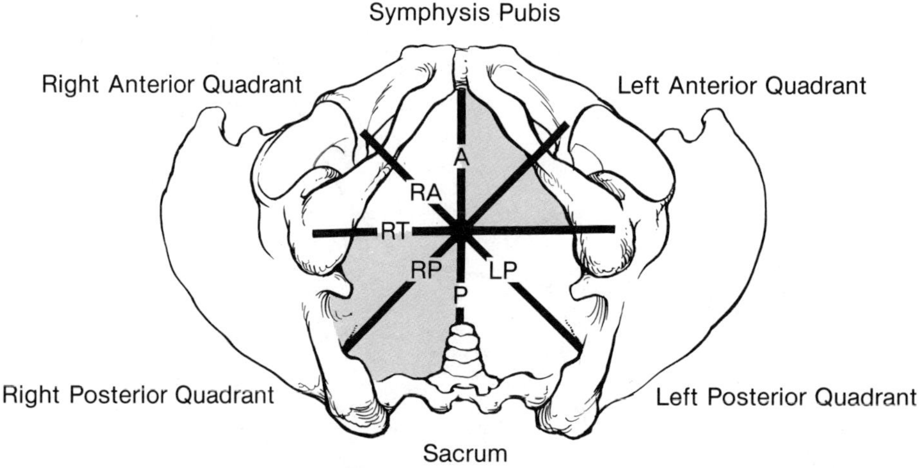

Figure 16.7
Quadrants of the maternal pelvis.

different part of the anatomy presenting, the fetal landmark and middle letter would change. For example, if the sacrum was presenting in the left anterior quadrant of the mother, the position determination would be LSA.

All possible occiput (vertex) positions include the following; see also Figures 16.8–16.13.

Occiput anterior	OA
Occiput posterior	OP
Right occiput posterior	ROP
Right occiput transverse	ROT
Right occiput anterior	ROA
Left occiput posterior	LOP
Left occiput transverse	LOT
Left occiput anterior	LOA

Other fetal indicators are M = mentum or chin; S = sacrum.

RIGHT OCCIPUT POSTERIOR (ROP)

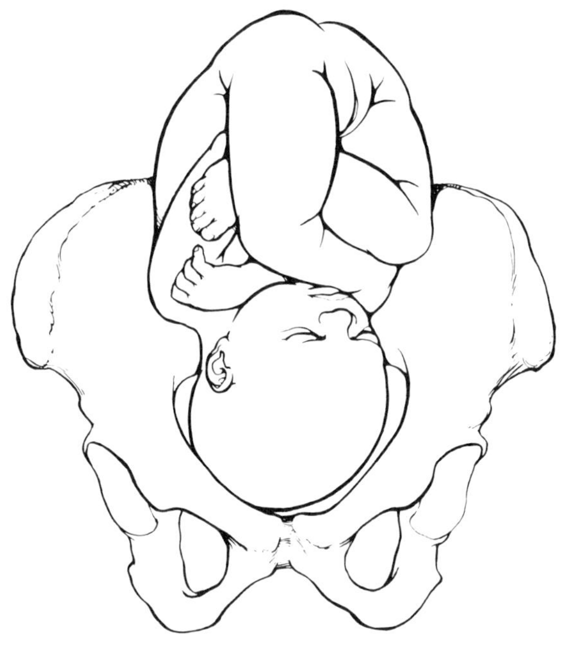

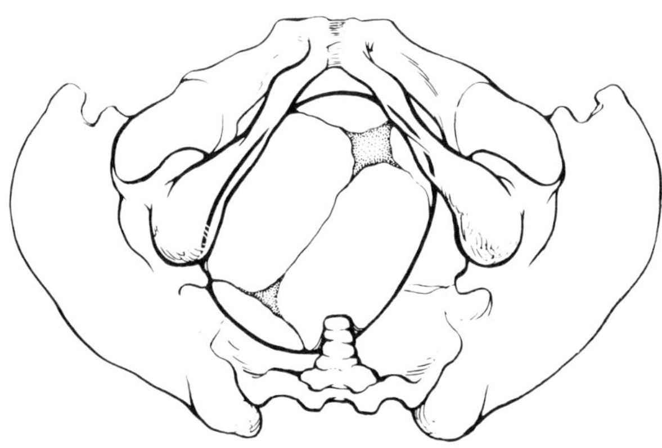

Figure 16.8
Mechanism of labor: ROP.

RIGHT OCCIPUT TRANSVERSE (ROT)

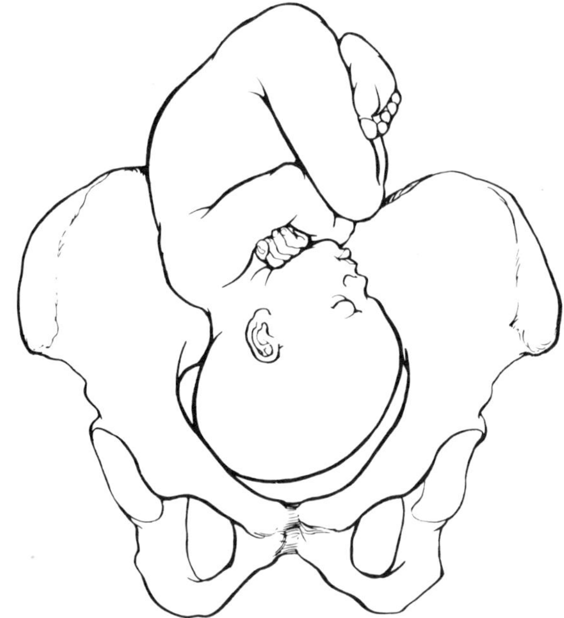

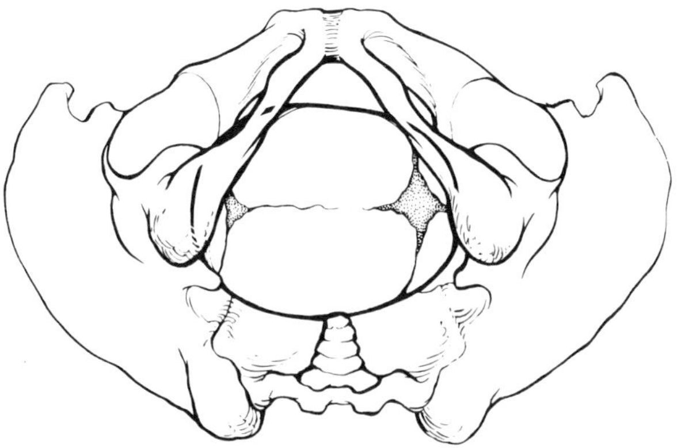

Figure 16.9
Mechanism of labor: ROT.

RIGHT OCCIPUT ANTERIOR (ROA)

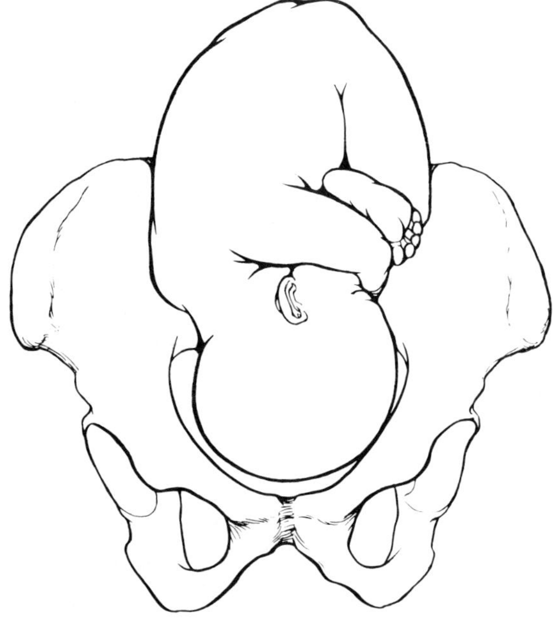

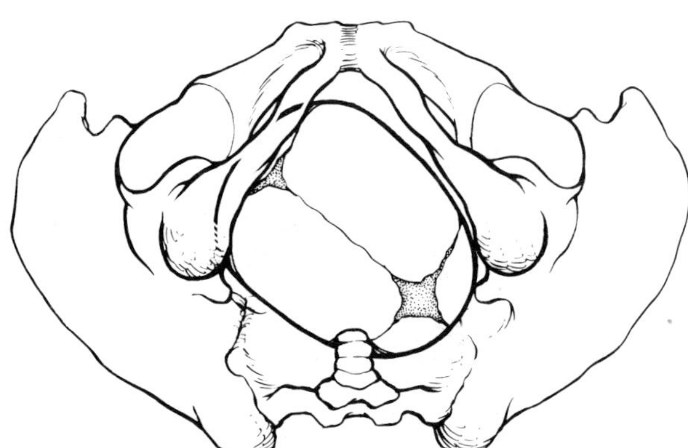

Figure 16.10
Mechanism of labor: ROA.

LEFT OCCIPUT POSTERIOR (LOP)

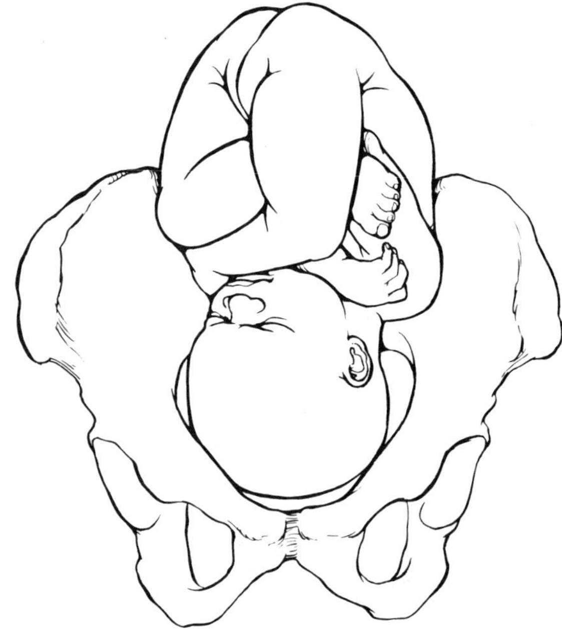

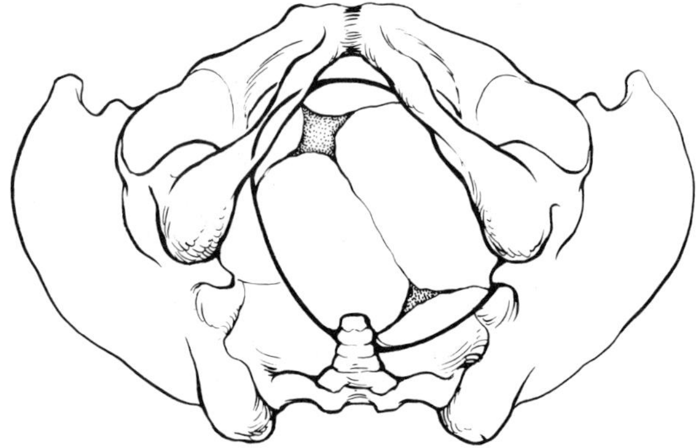

Figure 16.11
Mechanism of labor: LOP.

Presentation position and lie can be determined by three methods—abdominal palpation, auscultation of the fetal heart, and vaginal examination. *Vaginal examination* is the most accurate and will be discussed more specifically under nursing skills. (See Fig. 16.17.) *Abdominal palpation,* including Leopold's maneuvers (Chapter 12), provides a reasonably accurate diagnosis and position of lie and engagement in the last 8 weeks of pregnancy. *Auscultation* of the fetal heart is not an accurate method of determining position, but it may give clues to breech or cephalic presentation.

The passive movements that constitute the mechanism of labor are sequential steps. These positional changes involve twisting and turning motions of the fetal head in its accommodation to the maternal passage. The steps in the mechanism of labor are engagement, descent, flexion, internal rotation, extension, external rotation, and expulsion.

Engagement, descent, and flexion frequently oc-

LEFT OCCIPUT TRANSVERSE (LOT)

LEFT OCCIPUT ANTERIOR (LOA)

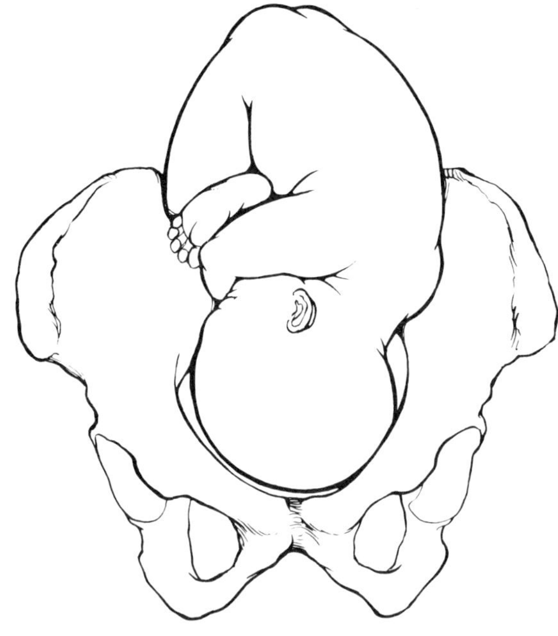

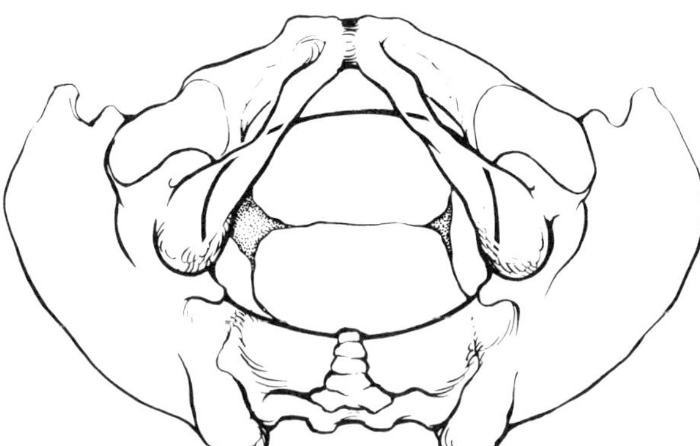

Figure 16.12
Mechanism of labor: LOT.

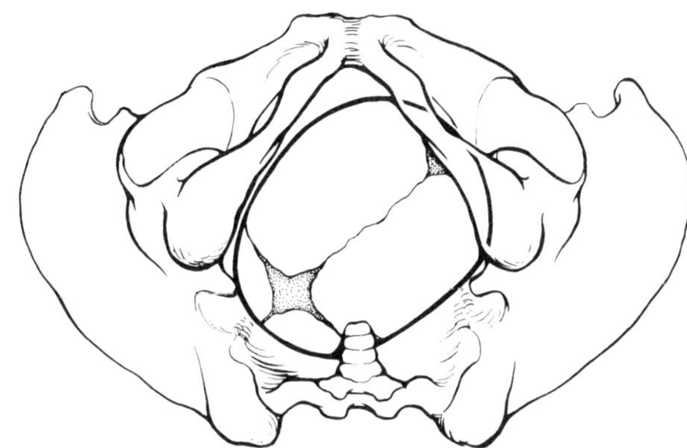

Figure 16.13
Mechanism of labor: LOA.

cur at the same time. *Engagement* means that the widest diameter of the fetal presenting part has passed the maternal pelvic inlet. This often occurs before labor and is the beginning of descent. *Descent* begins with engagement and continues until the delivery of the infant. The degree of descent is designated by the term station. *Station* is expressed in centimeters above (minus) and below (plus) the level of the ischial spines (Fig. 16.14). The fetal head is usually engaged when it is at the level of the ischial spines, or station O. *Flexion* increases during descent, the purpose being to substitute the suboccipitobregmatic diameter (9.5 cm) for the occipitofrontal diameter (10.5–11.0 cm). Because the latter is the widest diameter of the fetal head, it cannot be accommodated by the birth canal as easily. Flexion, the position in which the chin comes closer to the chest (Fig. 16.15), allows the smaller diameter (suboccipitobregmatic) to present first and passage is easier. The point at which

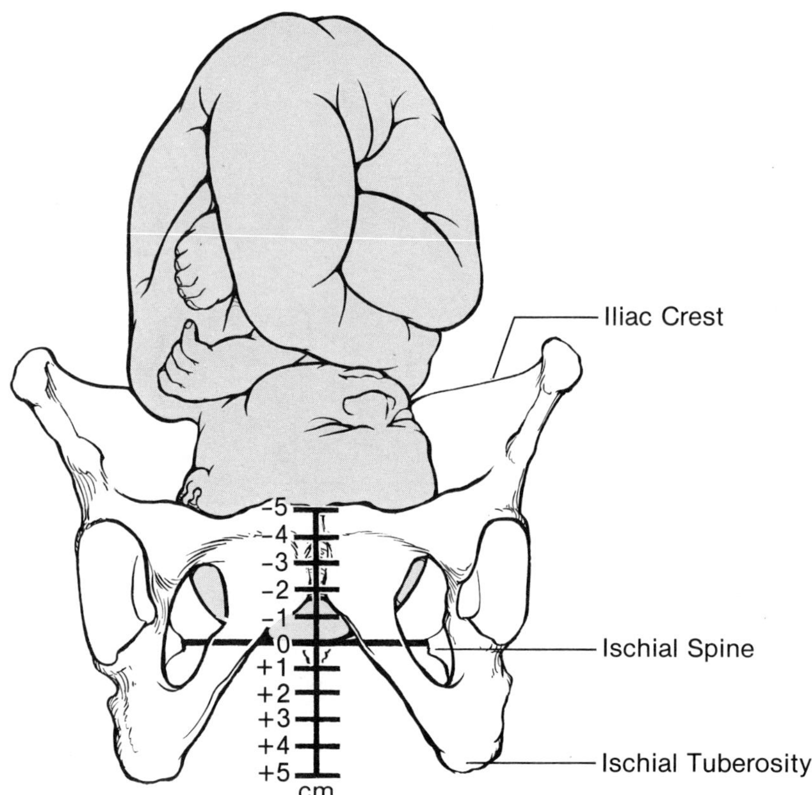

Figure 16.14
Station of the presenting part.

complete flexion takes place varies depending on the pattern of labor and the mother's pelvic structure. If the pelvic inlet is small, the head will meet with resistance and flexion will take place. If only moderate flexion occurs in the pelvic inlet, complete flexion will take place as the head meets the pelvic floor.

Internal rotation is the rotation of the long axis of the fetal skull from the transverse diameter, in which it enters the pelvic inlet, to the anterior–posterior diameter of the pelvic outlet (see Chapter 4 for diameters of pelvic inlet and outlet). Internal rotation takes place sometime during descent and after engagement. The fetal head usually rotates to bring the occiput under the symphysis pubis. This rotation can vary from 45 to 135 degrees depending on whether the head enters the pelvis with its anterior–posterior diameter conforming to the transverse or at an oblique angle to the pelvic inlet and whether the occiput is anterior or posterior. In summary, the sagittal suture of the fetal skull will conform to the widest part of the pelvic inlet and then rotate so that the sagittal suture will conform to the widest part of the pelvic outlet, the anterior–posterior diameter. This turning is the mechanism called internal rotation.

Extension of the head occurs when the suboccipital area of the fetal skull impinges beneath the pubic arch and the forehead slides up the inclined plane formed by the perineum as the head extends. Forehead, face, and chin progressively emerge at the vaginal introitus, and the newborn's face falls posteriorly, freeing the occiput. It is the pressure from the labor contractions that accomplishes this mechanism.

External rotation or *restitution* is the movement of the head, after it is free, 45 degrees to the right or left of the midline to assume normal alignment with its back and shoulders. If the fetal back is on the left, the occiput rotates to the left; if it is on the right, the rotation is to the right. *Expulsion,* or delivery of the shoulders and the rest of the baby, takes place quickly. The mechanism of labor is depicted in Figure 16.16.

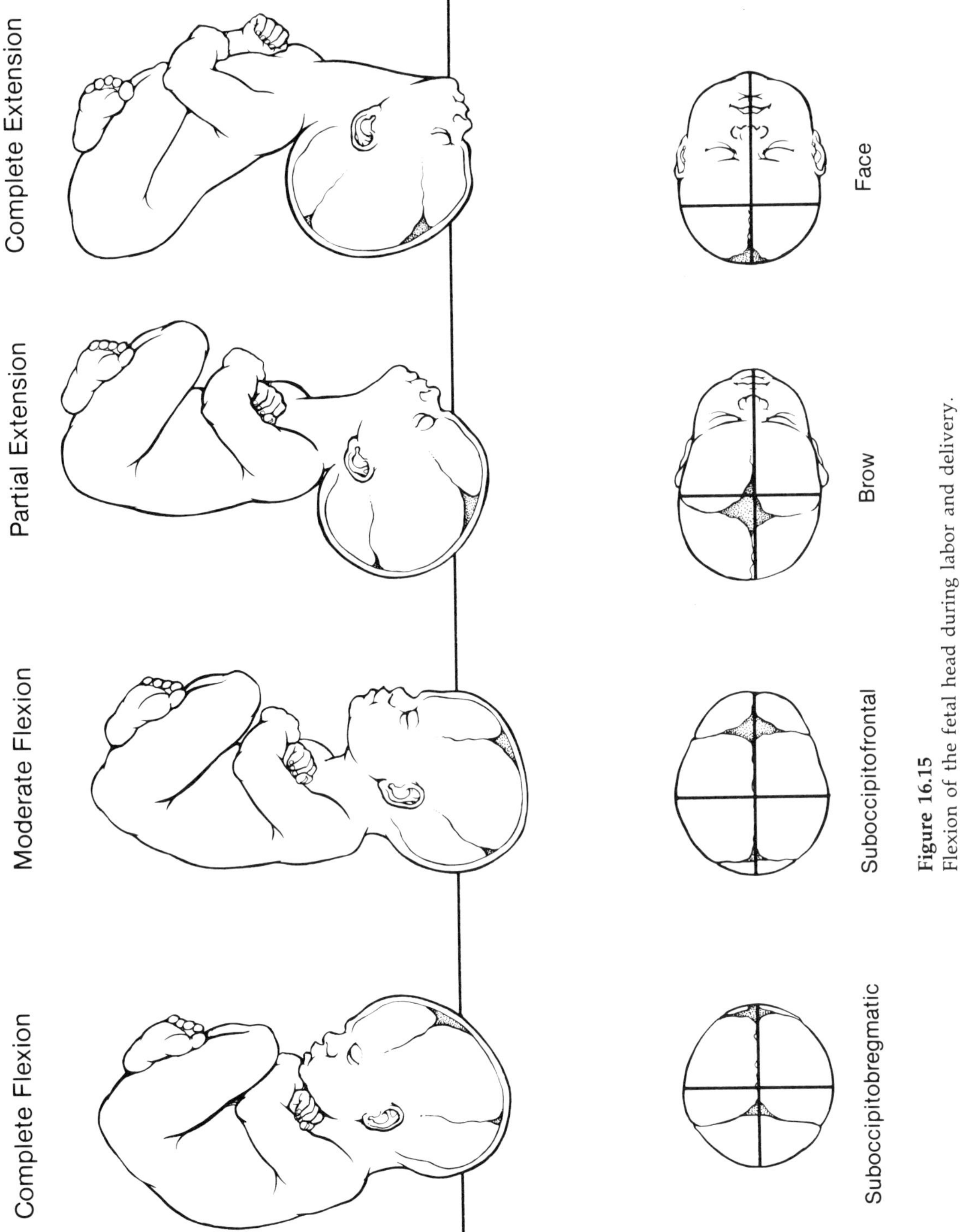

Figure 16.15
Flexion of the fetal head during labor and delivery.

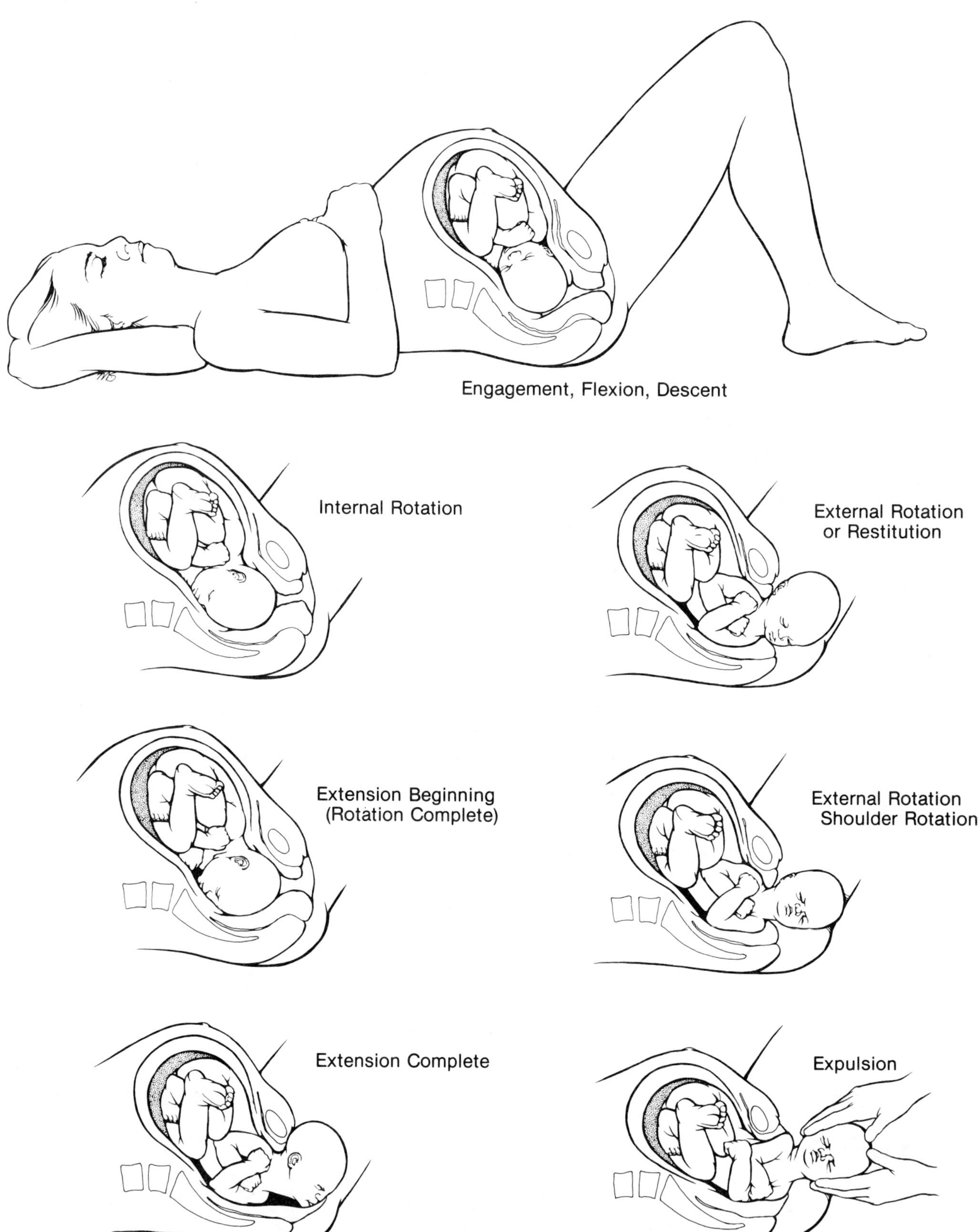

Figure 16.16
Mechanism of labor.

COLOR PLATES

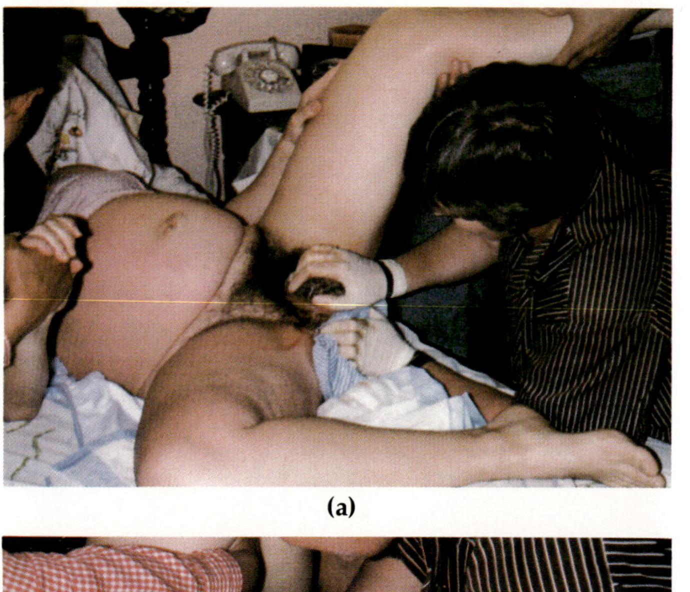

(a)

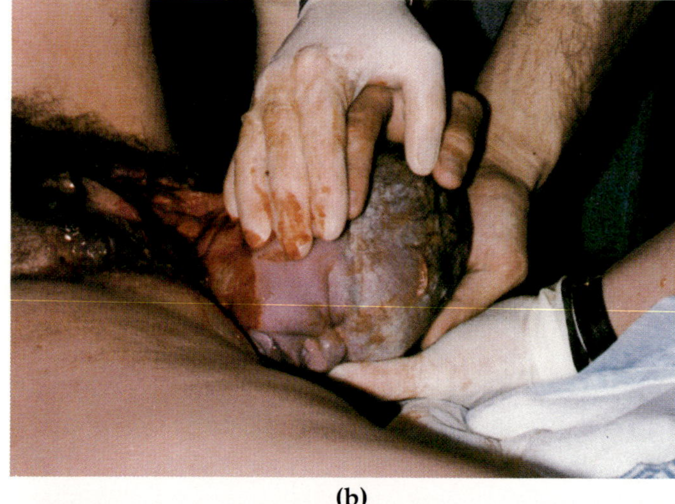

(b)

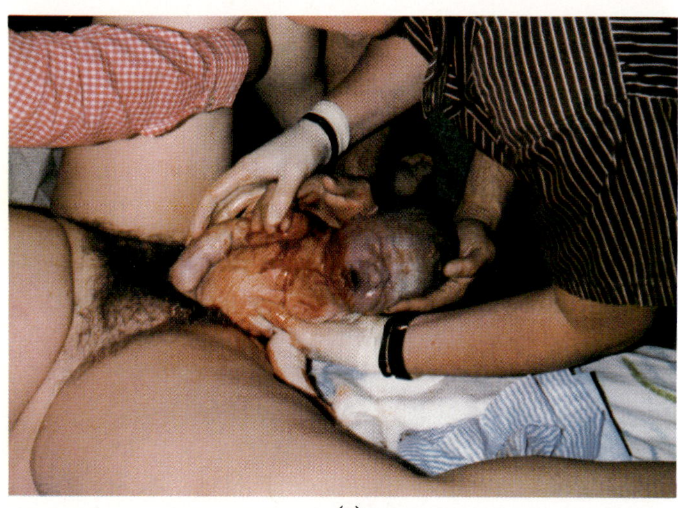

(c)

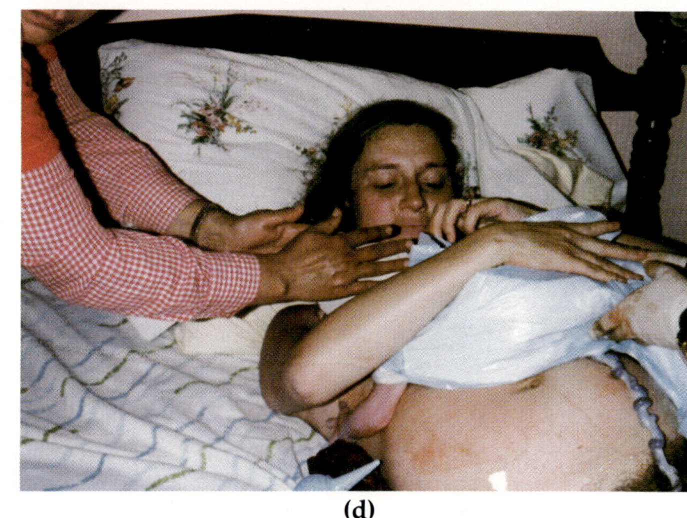

(d)

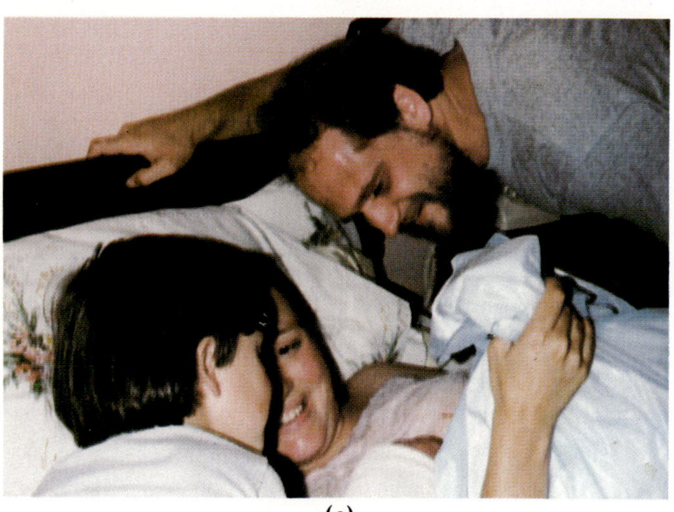

(e)

Plate 1 Home birth.

(a) Home delivery by a nurse–midwife. Note the following: use of the hand to support and control the delivery of the head; the relaxed atmosphere; the support given by a significant other.

(b) Delivery of head. Note support of the head by the nurse-midwife's hands (gloved) and the hands of the father (ungloved). Also note vernix caseosa and the bluish color of the baby's face.

(c) Delivery of shoulder. Note support of father's hands on the baby's head and the color of the baby's skin.

(d) Mother receives infant after delivery. Note mother's eye contact with her infant; umbilical cord (length, color, prominence of umbilical vessels).

(e) Birth is a family affair. Note father and older child.

Photographs courtesy of the Nurse–Midwifery Birthing Service, Eugene, Oregon.

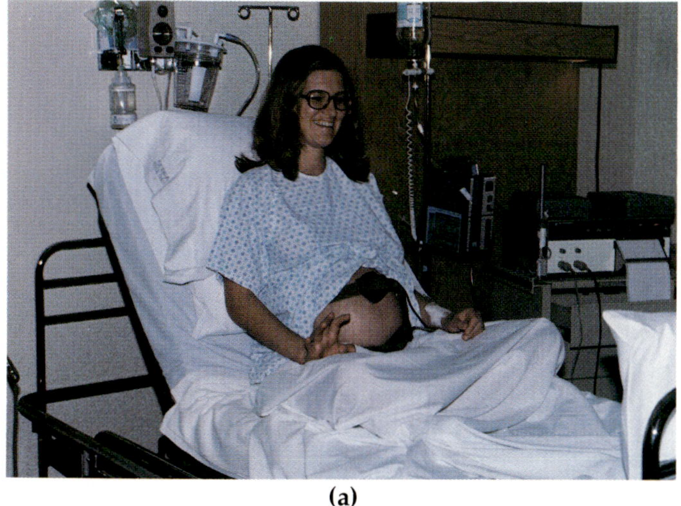
(a)

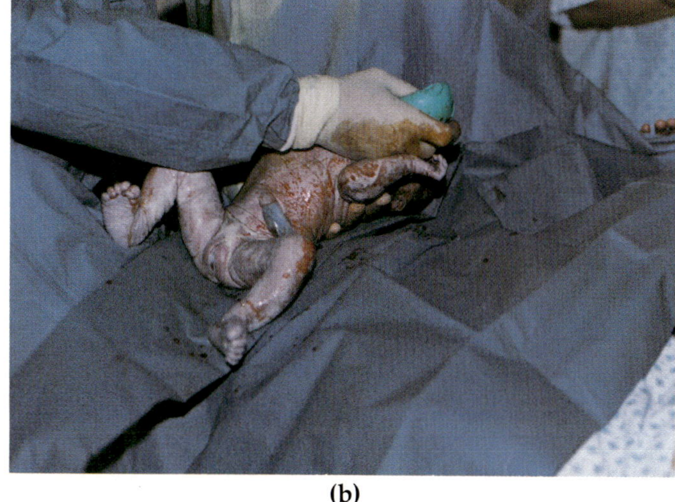
(b)

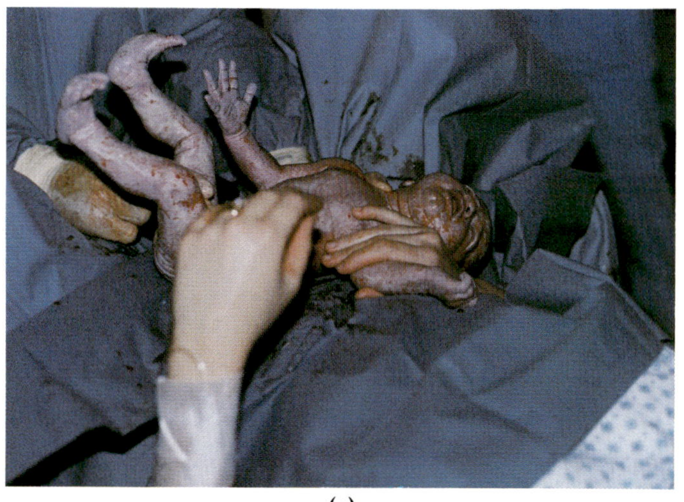
(c)

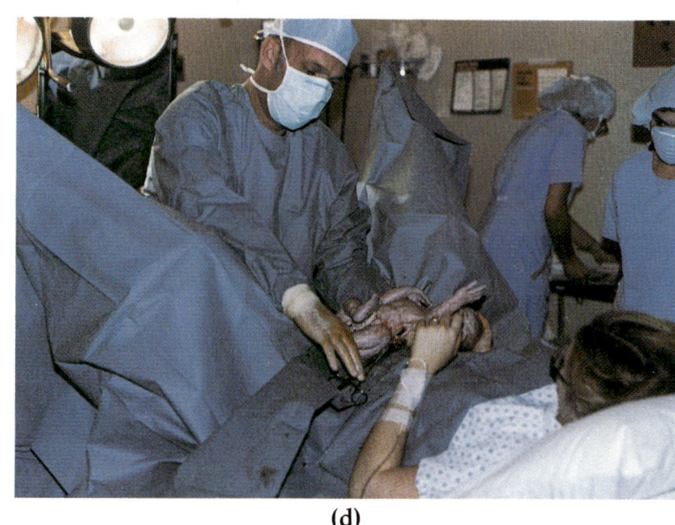
(d)

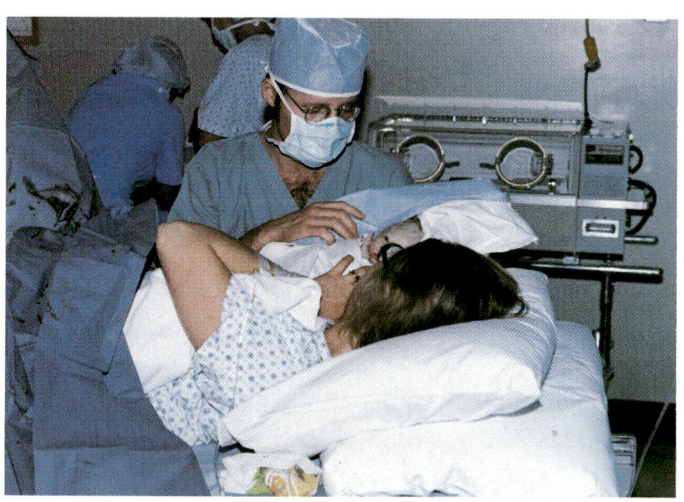
(e)

Plate 2 Hospital birth.

(a) Woman during labor. Technology can be used in concert with woman's participation in labor and childbirth. Mother is awake and alert. Note woman's position and relaxed concentration.

(b) First few moments of extrauterine life. Physician uses bulb syringe to suction baby immediately after birth. Note skin color, presence of vernix caseosa in creases and folds of infant's skin. Also note umbilical cord and color and presence of cord vessels.

(c) First extrauterine contact between mother and infant. Physician places infant on mother's abdomen as mother touches her baby. Contrast color of mother's and baby's skin.

(d) Mother reaches to receive infant. Note again contrast in mother's and infant's skin color and presence of vernix caseosa. Baby's head is lowered slightly to help drainage of secretion from chest.

(e) Childbirth is a family affair. Note mother–infant eye contact and proximity of father to mother and child.

Photographs courtesy of Judy and John Rennick, Las Cruces, N.M.

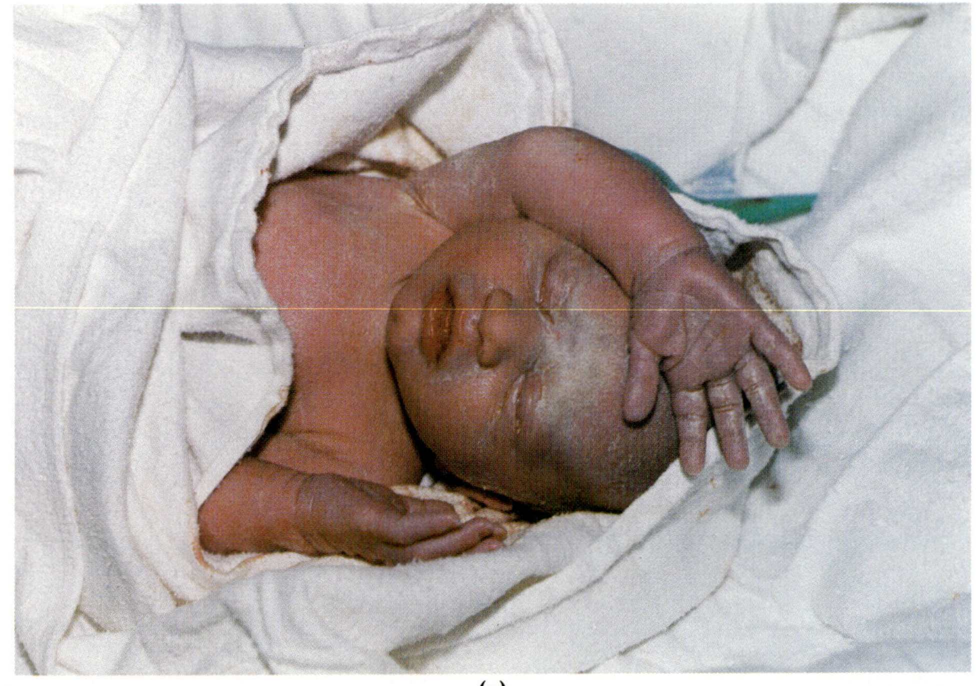

(a)

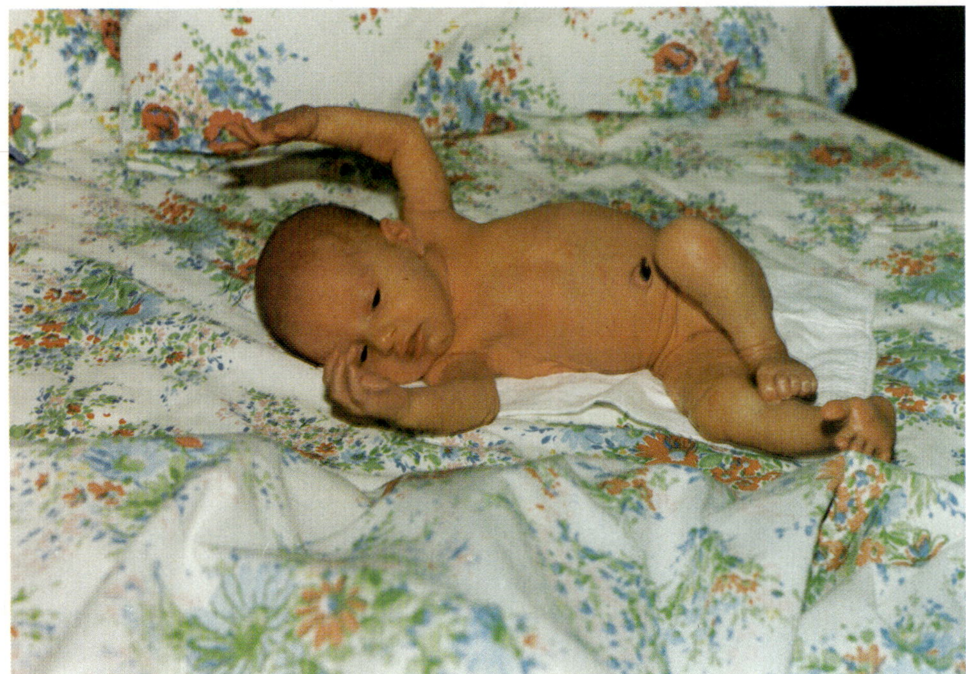

(b)

Plate 3 The newborn infant.

(a) First day of life. Note the following: baby's skin color with slight acrocyanosis of hands; skin creases and body covered with vernix caseosa; edema of eyelids caused by drug used to prevent ophthalmia neonatorum.

(b) Third day of life. Note drying of umbilical cord, skin color showing physiologic jaundice, and partial startle reflex of the baby.

Photographs courtesy of Judy and John Rennick, Las Cruces, N.M.

Maternal–Placental–Fetal Physiologic Concepts

The anatomy and physiology of the placental–fetal unit is discussed in detail in Chapter 10, and it is important to review that material before continuing this discussion. It is useful to recall that the placenta has three major functions; these are transport of essential substances to and from the uterus, provision of an anatomic and immunologic barrier between the mother and fetus, and production of hormones. Blood flow from the uterus to the placenta is approximately 50 ml/min at 10-weeks gestation and about 500 ml/min at term. Blood spurts into the intervillous space of the placenta from the uterine spiral arteries and drains back into the uterine (endometrial) veins. (Fetal blood flows to the placenta via the two umbilical arteries, which branch, divide, and terminate in the chorionic villi dipping into the intervillous space. Blood then returns to the fetus through a single umbilical vein.) It is helpful to recall that uterine veins have thin walls whereas uterine arteries are muscular, fairly thick, and elastic. During a uterine contraction, therefore, uterine venous pressure rises considerably, whereas uterine arterial pressure changes only minimally. More specifically, this means that uterine contractions compress the veins more than the arteries. This increase in venous pressure has the following effects on the maternal fetal unit:

- ↑ venous blood from myometrium
- ↑ venous return to the mother's heart
- ↑ maternal cardiac output during contraction
- ↓ uterine perfusion pressure

The perfusion pressure within the uterus is the uterine arterial blood pressure minus the uterine venous pressure. The formula is expressed as follows:

$$UPP = UABP - UVBP$$

Because venous pressure is raised but arterial pressure is not during a contraction, the difference between the two pressures (UABP − UVBP) is reduced. The significance of this is that uterine perfusion pressure and, subsequently, nourishment and oxygenation of the fetus are reduced. If uterine contractions come too close together so that adequate reoxygenation of the intervillous spaces is not possible or if intrauterine pressure remains high, fetal hypoxia can occur. Normally, a healthy mother and fetus can compensate during contractions, but despite this, "oxygenation saturation of fetal blood steadily declines during the first stage of labor" (Towell, 1976).

Similarities between the fetal and adult hearts can be noted. The intrinsic rate, established by the pacemaker, is influenced by input from the parasympathetic and sympathetic nervous systems. In general, input from the parasympathetic system (via the vagus nerve) slows the heart rate, while stimulation of the sympathetic system increases the heart rate. Baseline fetal heart rate demonstrates a balance between sympathetic and parasympathetic influences. This is measured as a minute-to-minute slowing down or speeding up; it will be discussed more fully in the section on electronic fetal monitoring. The fetal cardiac response to stress, however, differs from the adult's. The adult heart responds to hypercapnia, hypoxia, and acidosis via the sympathetic system with an increase in heart rate. In the fetus, mild hypoxia or initial hypoxia elicits a sympathetic response, but severe changes in Po_2, Pco_2, and pH activates the parasympathetic system causing a decrease in heart rate.

Nursing Care Concepts Relevant to the Stages of Labor

Biophysically and psychosocially, normal labor has a predictable pattern that allows the nurse to use anticipatory guidance and other teaching–learning strategies discussed in Chapter 2. Biophysically, the first stage of labor involves dilatation of the cervix to 10 cm, complete effacement of the cervix (100%), and progressive increase in intensity of uterine contractions to accomplish the preceding two changes. Psychosocially, it is not unusual for the mother to progress from an extroverted, excited, talkative, apprehensive person to an introverted, serious, frustrated, or even depressed and angry person. Obviously, a person's response to labor depends on those same principles discussed in the chapter on teaching–learning; namely past experiences, perception of events, and knowledge. During the second stage of labor, the biophysical process involves the expulsion of the infant and the use of voluntary abdominal muscles to assist during this stage. It is in this stage that most of the mechanism of labor occurs. The mother is psychosocial human being; her reaction at this time may be to be quite introverted, highly suggestible, and sometimes irritable. Perception has narrowed, which, again, has implications for the teaching–learning process. For example, directions need to be stated briefly, and because there is often amnesia between contractions, directions for breathing and pushing must be repeated frequently. Physically and psychologically, there is total involvement with the task of childbirth and, as such, tremendous expenditure of energy.

With the third stage of labor comes physical and psychologic relief; the baby is born and within a short time the placenta is expelled. Contractions, although still occurring, have decreased in intensity so significantly that they are barely perceptible. Basic physiologic needs such as comfort, rest, food, and shelter are great. Psychologically, in the fourth stage a "normal" mother may appear anywhere from elated and laughing to exhausted and in tears. Table 16.2 is a more detailed description of biophysical and psychosocial changes, along with the nursing interventions and supportive other role. It is important to remember that as the mother progresses through labor, her psychologic reaction may be a change from an extrovert personality to an introvert personality, accompanied by a decreased perceptual field; her biophysical reaction moves from experiencing a fetus enclosed in a hollow muscular organ to experiencing its expulsion through the birth canal, requiring a tremendous amount of physical energy. If these psychologic and biophysical concepts can be assimilated, anticipatory guidance in the nursing care of mother and fetus will be possible.

TABLE 16.2
STAGES AND PHASES OF LABOR AND DELIVERY

Stage	*Biophysical Characteristics*	*Psychosocial Characteristics*	*Helpful Activities*	*Supportive Other Role*	*Nurse's Role*
Readiness for labor	Lightening (baby drops). (Primipara 2–4 weeks before delivery.) Increased Braxton Hicks' contractions. Increased vaginal mucous discharge. Weight loss 2–3 lb. Less active baby.	Tired of pregnancy. Feels crowded. Anxious for delivery. Has spurts of energy.	Continue to practice breathing and relaxation exercises. Use Braxton Hicks' for practice. Get ample rest. Pack suitcase. Complete preparations for infant.	Complete any undone items such as hospital preadmission and/or take mother-to-be on hospital tour. Practice coaching. Encourage rest. Provide diversion, such as movies, cards, or walking.	
Onset of labor	Regular progressive contractions. Blood tinged show. Possibly rupture of membranes. Backache or menstrual-like cramps. (Any combination of these symptoms possible.)	Mixture of excitement and apprehension.	No heavy food (eat jello, soup, liquids, if needed). Follow doctor's instruction on when to call. Time contractions. Pack last minute items and include Lamaze "goodie" bag. Rest, relax, do not start "breathing" too soon.	Help with timing and relaxation *if* needed. Put suitcase in car. Take an extra pillow. Provide diversion. Eat.	

Stage	Biophysical Characteristics	Psychosocial Characteristics	Helpful Activities	Supportive Other Role	Nurse's Role
First Stage: Early (latent) phase	Effacement. Dilatation 0–4 cm. Contractions last 20–40 seconds every 15–20 minutes. Head descends to the level of symphysis. Lasts 2–16 hours (50–60% stage 1) Primigravida 8½ hours. Multigravida 5½ hours.	Mixture of excitement and apprehension May enjoy cards, talk, or books. Shows some independent control. Anxiety low—learning can take place.	Slow chest breathing when needed for control. Effleurage added when desired. Report to hospital when doctor advises—but do not be too hurried. Conserve energy.	Take mother-to-be to hospital. Complete admission. Check breathing and relaxation. Continue to time contractions. Adjust bed when necessary. Locate ice chips supply if allowed. Assist with comfort measures, back rub, cool cloth.	Admission Dx and physical assessment. Orient to surroundings. Assess past experience and expectations. Teach about labor. Reinforce breathing techniques. Monitor and record vital signs, BP, P, R, FHR, contractions; intake and output; vaginal secretions; comfort, hygiene. Provide information as needed.
First stage: Active phase	Dilatation 4–8 cm. Membranes often rupture—spontaneously or by doctor (amniotomy). Contractions last 45–60 seconds every 2–5 minutes. 30–40% of stage I. Primigravida 4 hours. Multigravida 2 hours. Period of rapid dilatation. 1.2 cm/hr primigravida. 1.5 cm/hr multigravida.	More serious; short sentences. More need to concentrate on contractions. Dependent; desires companion. Restless or edgy. Contractions may seem endless with little progress or purpose. Regression or increasing dependency. Focus on self.	Switch to accelerated panting when needed. Effleurage as desired. Back pressure if needed for back labor. Medication if desired to increase relaxation and control. Conserve energy during and between contractions. Use the easiest breathing that is effective.	Assess partner's needs and help as needed with her relaxation, timing, and breathing. Keep mother alert enough to catch the beginnings of contractions. Give ice chips at the end of contraction (if doctor orders). Back pressure as needed. Suggest position change occasionally (left side preferably).	Anticipate needs. Comfort measures: cool cloth, clean bed. Praise efforts and inform of progress. Reinforce supportive other's role. Continue to monitor biophysical and psychosocial needs. Check and record FHR every 15 minutes. Administer analgesic if ordered, and monitor for side effects.
First stage: Transition	Dilatation 8–10 cm. Contractions 45–60 seconds long.	Withdrawal. Drowsiness. Depressed. Nausea, trembling.	Switch to pant blow. Continuous blows through urge to push.	Remind partner that she may need to urinate.	Continue physical, psychosocial, and supportive care as above.

TABLE 16.2 (continued)

Stage	*Biophysical Characteristics*	*Psychosocial Characteristics*	*Helpful Activities*	*Supportive Other Role*	*Nurse's Role*
	Contractions every 2–3 minutes. Contractions peak quickly and "breathing" must be started immediately to overcome them. Primigravida 1 hour. Multigravida 15–20 minutes. Total first stage primigravida approximately 12½ hours. Multigravida approximately 7 hours.	Backache, urge to push. Amnesia between contractions. Highly suggestible. Irritable. Increased show. Cannot distinguish beginning or end of contractions.	Keep alert, eyes open with contractions. Do not push until given permission. Maximum concentration required to cope with contractions.	Help mother catch the beginning of a contraction by keeping your hand on her abdomen or anticipating by clock. Pace her breathing if necessary. Back pressure if helpful. Watch for hyperventilation. No distracting conversation except encouragement. Call nurse if patient not recently checked.	Pace breathing or reinforce supportive other doing this. Monitor for hyperventilation. Observe perineum for bulging or caput.
Second stage: delivery of baby	Dilatation is complete. Contractions 50–90 seconds every 1–2 minutes apart. Increasingly expulsive. Bulging of the perineum and gradual presentation of baby. Episiotomy often done. Total second stage *average:* Primigravida—80 minutes. Multigravida—30 minutes.	Totally involved. Relief with pushing. May get second wind. May worry over bowel pressure or "splitting sensation"; panic. Difficulty following directions. Increased amnesia between contractions. Grunts with pushing. May become exhausted.	Push with contractions or as directed by the doctor. *Pant* when told not to push. To push, take two deep breaths, then hold breath and push, while relaxing bottom. Assume pushing position that places abdominal cavity in best position for efficient pushing.	Help partner assume good position—help support head and shoulers if needed. Remind mother to keep elbows out, shoulders down. Remind her to take cleansing breaths. Repeat the doctor's instructions if needed. Call her attention to birth of head if she is too absorbed to notice.	Reinforce supportive other's role and assume if necessary. Continue to monitor vital signs every 3–5 minutes. Observe perineal area. Explain procedures being done. Inform of progress. Praise effort, repeat praise or instructions as often as necessary.
Third stage: Placental delivery	Temporary cessation of contractions. New contraction usually painless.	Exhausted, euphoric, elated. Relieved, cry with joy. Hungry and thirsty.	Push if asked to for delivery of placenta. Will be given an injection to clamp uterus down to slow bleeding.	Share joy and satisfaction of the moment with partner. Be lavish in praise for her effort.	Congratulate. Promote bonding of mother–infant–father. Administer oxytocin.

Stage	Biophysical Characteristics	Psychosocial Characteristics	Helpful Activities	Supportive Other Role	Nurse's Role
	Placenta delivery accompanied by some bleeding. Repair of episiotomy. Total third stage *average:* Primigravida—10 minutes. Multigravida—10 minutes.	Excited over baby. May get chills and shake afterward.	Ask for pain medication if uncomfortable.		Monitor fluids. Coach regarding relaxation. Monitor fundal contraction. Take vital signs every 15 minutes. Meet basic physiologic and psychosocial needs with anticipatory guidance.

Note. The comments listed above are common, but there will be much variation from individual to individual within normal deliveries and even wider variation if unusual factors are influencing this process.

MATERNITY NURSING SKILLS FOR FETAL AND MATERNAL ASSESSMENT

Intrapartum Data Base

Initially, the baseline data including history and physical assessment information should be collected and recorded. This data collection should be as complete as possible, depending on the phase and stage of labor. Ideally, an antepartum record against which the nurse can measure the status of the current vital signs, such as blood pressure (BP) and fetal heart rate (FHR), will be available in the delivery room. (See appendix for sample charting forms.) Information that should be included in an intrapartum data base is listed below.

ASSESSMENT OF PROGRESS DURING LABOR

Uterine Contractions

During labor uterine contractions are monitored for frequency, duration, and strength or intensity. *Frequency* is the time from the beginning of one contraction to the onset of the next one; *duration* is from the beginning of the tightening of the uterus until it relaxes, or how long the contraction lasts; and *intensity* or strength is estimated by firmness of the muscle and is usually expressed as weak or mild and moderate or strong. A weak or mild contraction usually lasts about 30 seconds, a moderate contraction 45 seconds, and a strong contraction 60 seconds. To palpate contractions and determine firmness, the nurse places fingertips or palmar surfaces of the fingers on the abdomen over the fundus of the uterus. A skillful nurse can feel the tightening and relaxation of the uterus often before the mother senses discomfort. The nurse should palpate contractions long enough to collect data about a pattern, that is, frequency, duration, and intensity, which usually requires palpating four to six contractions.

Rupture of Membranes

Whether the membranes rupture spontaneously or are ruptured artificially by the physician, which is called *amniotomy,* specific nursing interventions are important: counting the FHR, observing for prolapse of the umbilical cord, and observing the amniotic fluid. The FHR should remain within the baseline range and should be ausculatated before, during, and after amniotomy. Prolapse of the cord if occult or hidden will be detected by bradycardia in the FHR; if the prolapse is external (vaginal orifice), the assessment can be quickly noted. Nursing actions after prolapse require putting on sterile gloves for palpation of the cord to see if the cord is pulsating, which would indicate oxygenation to the fetus. The mother is assisted into either a Trendelenburg or a knee–chest position, whichever permits the cord to continue to pulsate while the physician and other assistance is sought. Observation of the amniotic fluid for odor, amount, and color is important. A foul odor indicates infection, and a large amount of fluid (which is a subjective evaluation), indicates polyhydramnios, which is sometimes associated with fetal anomalies. A black or blackish-green color in a vertex position indicates hypoxia. Just as is often true with a person who has a seizure, anoxia of the fetus causes relaxation of the anal sphincter and elimination of meconium into the amniotic fluid. If the amniotic fluid in a vertex presentation is meconium (first stool of neonate, which is black) stained, there has been at least one episode of anoxia and perhaps more. The labor then needs to be monitored more frequently and, if not already instituted, electronic fetal monitoring needs to be started.

Abdominal Assessment

Abdominal palpation is an important nursing assessment skill. Abdominal assessment of the labor patient includes palpation of uterine contractions and Leopold's maneuvers (discussed in the section on mechanism of labor and in Chapter 12). Assessment of the abdomen for fundal height in relation to weeks of gestation is also important.

Vaginal Secretions

Show, the pinkish mucous discharge from the cervix, increases as labor progresses and may contain a small amount of bright red blood in the transitional phase as the capillaries in the cervix rupture. Nursing measures involve good hygiene, keeping the perineal area as clean as possible by cleaning from front to back (perineum toward the anus). The use of a clean, disposable paper pad underneath the buttocks, which is changed frequently, is effective. If the membranes have ruptured, there may be leakage of amniotic fluid with each contraction. There are two methods of assessing for rupture of the membranes. In one method, litmus paper impregnated with phenaphthazine (nitrazine test) changes color when placed in contact with amniotic fluid. The nitrazine test is based on the fact that the pH of normal vaginal secretions ranges from 4.5 to 5.5 and the pH of amniotic fluid ranges from 7.0 to 7.5. This test can be misleading if bloody show, which is alkaline, is in contact with the indicator paper. For a more accurate reading, the litmus paper should be inserted into the posterior fornix of the vagina during a vaginal exam.

The other method is called the *fern test.* Vaginal secretions are placed on a glass slide, allowed to dry, and then examined microscopically. A ferning pattern is observed when amniotic fluid is present because of the sodium chloride in the fluid. Blood and other vaginal secretions can obscure both tests.

Vaginal Examination

Vaginal examinations are frequently used as a method of determining the progress of labor. Information assessed is about effacement, dilatation, station, and presenting part. The initial examination is made on admission and repeated when necessary during labor. Since it is inevitable that bacteria is introduced from the introitus and vagina to the interior of the uterus during labor, it is important that vaginal examinations be performed properly and be limited in number. Vaginal examinations can be done in the labor bed with the woman in dorsal recumbent position. The examiner wears sterile gloves and uses an antiseptic solution to cleanse the vulva and act as a lubricant. The labia are separated with the fingers of one hand; two fingers of the other hand are inserted into the vagina, being careful to avoid contact with the rectum (Fig. 16.17). Since the examiner is seeking information about dilatation station, effacement, and the presenting part (if the cervix is dilated enough), the cervix, ischial spines, and presenting part are palpated directly. The cervical opening is felt as a circular rim around a depression. The amount of cervical dilatation is estimated in centimeters. The amount of effacement is estimated by determining the thickness of the cervical rim and is expressed as 50%, 70%, and so on. Consistency of the cervix is also noted; a soft cervix usually thins out or effaces faster. A firm cervix (which effaces more slowly) feels similar to the tip of a nose. When examining the cervix, the status of the

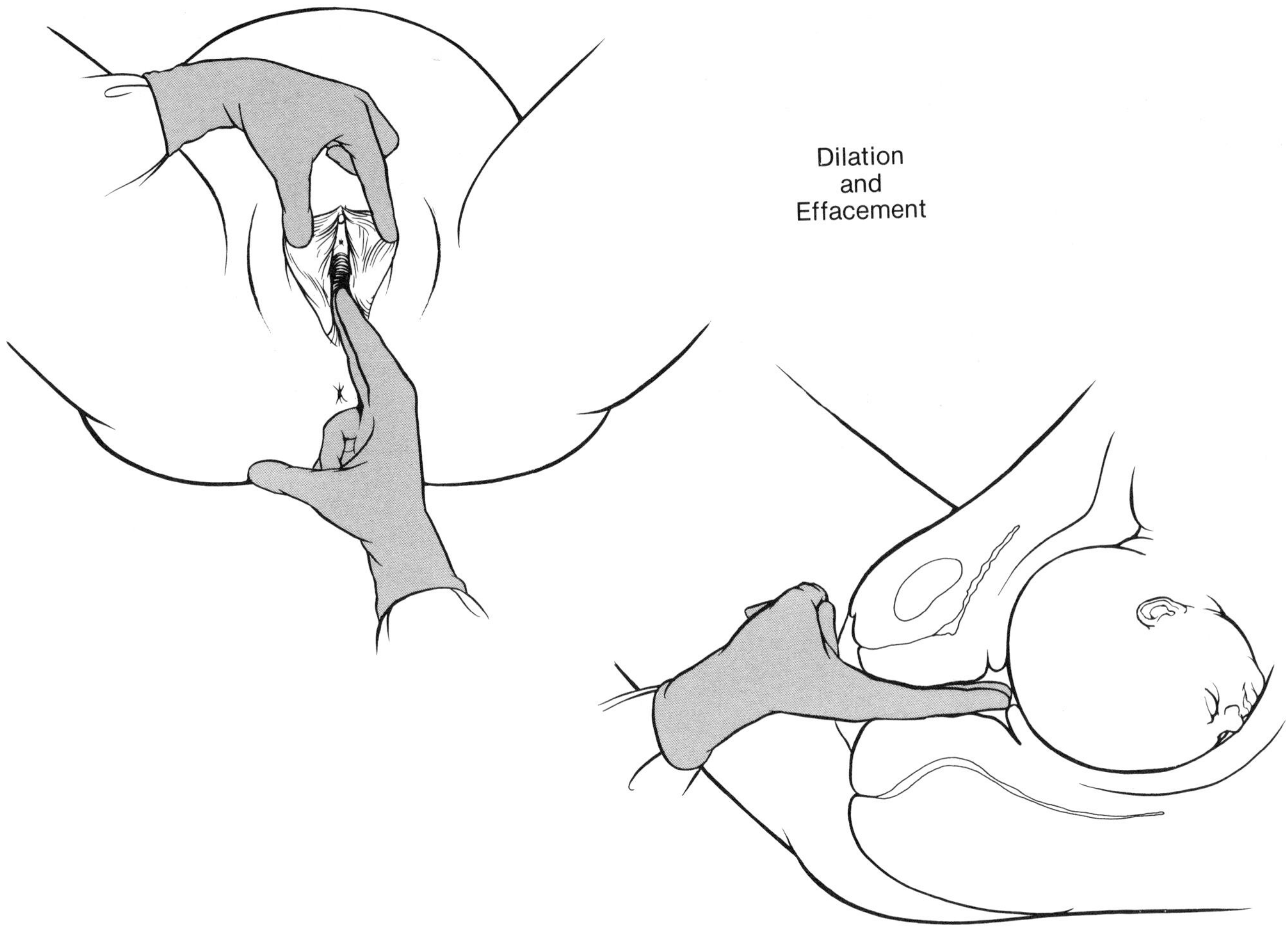

Figure 16.17
Vaginal exam to determine dilation and effacement.

membranes is assessed, that is, intact or ruptured. If intact, the fetal membranes often can be felt bulging through the cervical depression; if ruptured, amniotic fluid may drain out through the vagina. *Station,* degree of descent of the fetal head, is determined by locating the ischial spines and feeling to see if the fetal head is at the level of the spines or above or below them.

It is helpful to know that most often the spines are felt as a notch or projection that can be located by palpating the pelvic outlet at approximately the 4 o'clock and 8 o'clock positions. Because people vary anatomically, some spines are more easily felt. The position of the baby can be determined if the cervix is well dilated. In order to assess position, search for landmarks on the presenting part. In the vertex position, you can usually locate the sagittal suture and follow it to a Y or its juncture with the lamboidal suture, which is the posterior fontanel. Because there is often molding and edema of the fetal skull, sometimes the landmarks are difficult to determine. Recall that in labor the head is normally flexed, therefore, the posterior fontanel of the fetus is palpated during the vaginal exam. Then the examiner determines in which quadrant of the mother's pelvis the occiput is and makes a determination of position, for example, LOA. Vaginal examination can be made either during or between contractions and may provide different data as the force of the contraction will maximize the dilatation (Fig. 16.18). Dilatation, station (descent), and effacement should be plotted on a labor graph to provide recorded data about the progress of labor. Graphs make deviations from normal more easily seen, which can provide a sound basis for decision making. (See appendix for sample form.)

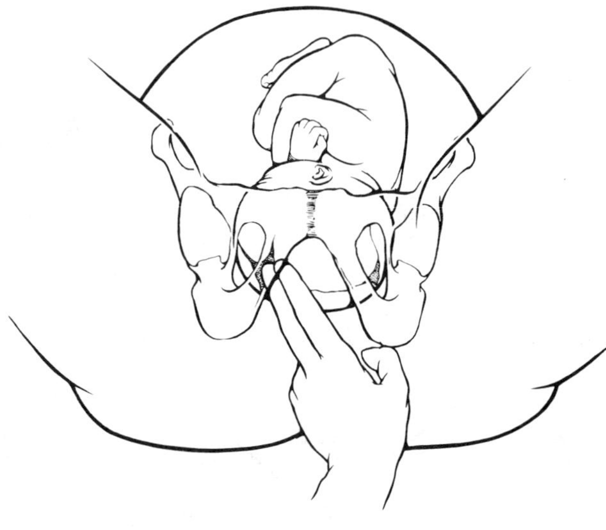

Anterior Fontanel

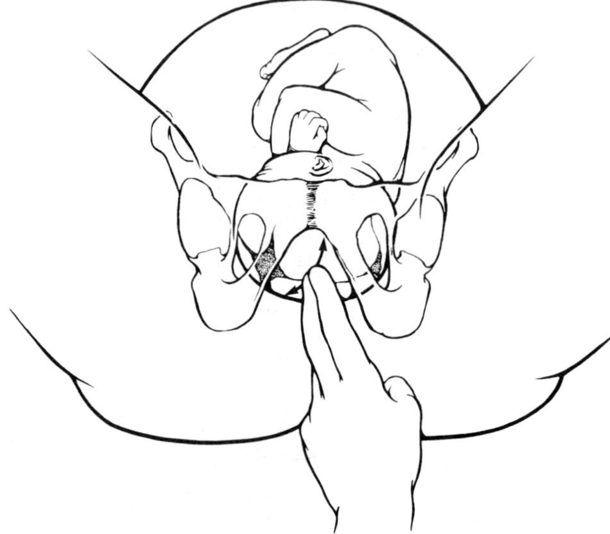

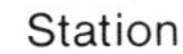

Station

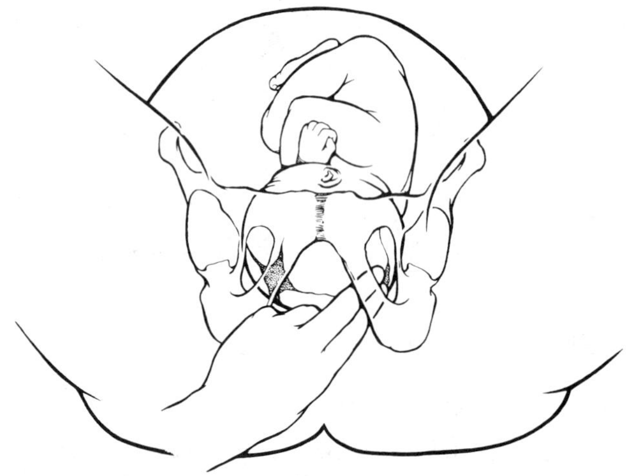

Posterior Fontanel

Figure 16.18
Vaginal exam to determine position and station.

ASSESSMENT OF MATERNAL–FETAL RESPONSE TO LABOR

Blood Pressure, Temperature, Pulse, and Respirations

Blood pressure, pulse, and respirations are checked every hour during labor unless there is indication of elevation or maternal history necessitating more frequent assessment. Pulse and respirations change relatively little during a normal labor. Blood pressure should be taken between contractions (during the relaxation phase of the contraction cycle) since there may be an increase of 5–10 mm Hg during a contraction. Temperature is taken every 4 hours unless it is elevated or membranes are ruptured after which it should be taken every hour.

Hyperventilation

Hyperventilation, an increase in the rate and depth of breathing, is common during stressful periods; as you will recall, hyperventilation is sometimes associated with fright or anxiety. Physiologically, hyperventilation causes loss of carbon dioxide leading to respiratory alkalosis. Besides being related to stress, hyperventilation can also occur in labor when breathing techniques are not being used correctly. Education for childbirth and breathing techniques are discussed more fully in Chapter 15. The mother complains of feeling dizzy or faint or of a tingling in her extremities. The implications for the fetus are compromise of the uteroplacental exchange. Hyperventilation can be corrected easily by having the mother breath into a paper bag or cupping her hands over her nose and mouth thus reabsorbing carbon dioxide.

Hypotension

Hypotension, or low blood perfusion, is a concern in labor because of the obvious implications for the fetus. The significance of having a maternal baseline blood pressure in order to identify hypotension in the woman is obvious. Hypotension is often related to regional anesthesia (see Chapter 22) such as caudal, paracervical, or epidural and is in these instances related to sympathetic nerve block and systemic toxic reaction from excessive and rapid absorption of a drug. As mentioned earlier, during active labor the blood pressure should be taken at least every 30 minutes and the nurse should be particularly alert to signs of hypotension after administration of analgesics or anesthetics, after administration of oxytocin (see Chapter 22), or when contractions are stronger and more frequent (increased stress). Nursing interventions for hypotension are:

- ▲ Position the mother on her side, which relieves pressure on the inferior vena cava and improves venous return.
- ▲ Elevate the legs (or lower the head), which decreases venous pressure and improves peripheral circulation.
- ▲ Increase the intravenous flow rate, which increases fluid volume of the circulatory system.
- ▲ Administer oxygen by nasal catheter (or mask) at 6–8 liters if positional changes do not improve hypotension.

These measures raise the maternal arterial pressure increasing intervillous space blood flow, thereby improving fetal oxygenation, which, because of the maternal hypotension, may be seriously compromised.

Fetal Heart Rate

Auscultation of the fetal heart rate gives evidence of how the fetus is responding to the stress of labor. To count the FHR, the bell of a stethoscope is placed on the mother's abdomen at the spot where the heartbeat can be heard most clearly. A head stethoscope, which allows for the augmentation of bone conduction, is usually used. Auscultation can be done using a fetoscope, bell stethoscope, or doptone (an electronic device) (see Fig. 16.19). Move the stethoscope over the abdomen until the point of maximum intensity is located. Information obtained during Leopold's maneuvers is useful. Namely, in cephalic presentations, heart rate is usually best heard below the

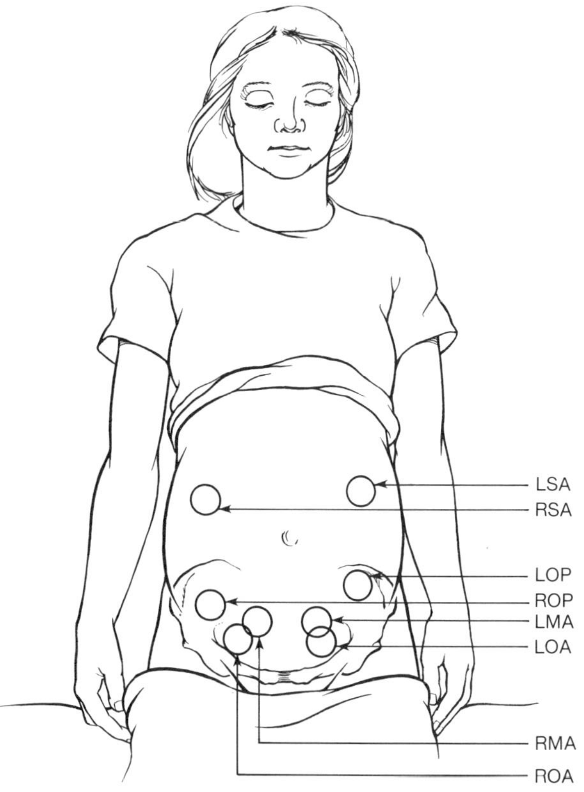

Figure 16.19
Location of fetal heart rate for auscultation in different positions.

umbilicus; in breech, above the umbilicus. The heartbeat is transmitted through the fetal chest wall, and in vertex and breech presentations the beat would be most audible on the side where the fetal back has been located.

The FHR is heard as a double sound. It may sound distant and is sometimes described as a watch ticking under a pillow. Fetal heart rate should be between 120–160 beats per minute. This rate should remain constant (within 4–6 beats per minute) during labor if adequate placental exchange is occurring.

There are four sounds that need to be differentiated in auscultating the pregnant abdomen. The FHR needs to be differentiated from the maternal pulse, which can also be heard abdominally. Checking the mother's radial pulse at the same time as abdominal auscultation and listening for synchronization clarifies this. The two other sounds, uterine (or maternal) souffle and funic (or fetal) souffle are sounds made by blood swishing through a vessel and can be distinguished from the heart rate that is a more clipped, distinct sound. The *uterine souffle* is blood flowing through the uterine vessels and is synchronous with the mother's pulse rate. The *funic souffle* is blood flowing through the umbilical vessels and is synchronous with the FHR. Both of these souffles are bruits, which you may have identified during physical assessment learning.

During the first phase of the first stage of labor, the FHR should be counted and recorded every 30 minutes; after 5 cm of dilatation if FHR is within normal range and characteristics, it should be counted every 15 minutes or more often. Auscultation of FHR should be done before, during, and immediately after a contraction because interference with oxygenation can usually first be detected during uterine activity.

Electronic Fetal Monitoring

For years maternity nurses have monitored the fetus during labor using a stethoscope to determine the FHR and manual palpation to assess frequency, strength, and duration of uterine contractions. Electronic fetal monitors were designed in the late 1960s that monitor both uterine contractility and FHR. As with any technology, fetal monitoring cannot replace good clinical nursing care; it is an adjunct to the safe care of the maternal–fetal unit. Research supports that machines can augment but not replace good clinical care by knowledgable personnel (Haverkamp et al., 1976).

Electronic monitoring may be done directly (internally) or indirectly (externally). The external method of fetal monitoring is noninvasive and can be used before the membranes are ruptured.

External monitor recording is seldom as clear as internal or direct monitoring. Advantages of external fetal monitoring are that the membranes do not have to be ruptured or the cervix dilated and the fetal part does not have to be in the pelvis. The disadvantages of external fetal monitoring are that the FHR and contraction recordings are easily disturbed by fetal or maternal movements. Externally, uterine pressure is monitored with a pressure transducer held against the abdomen at the fundus of the uterus by an adjustable strap that circles the abdo-

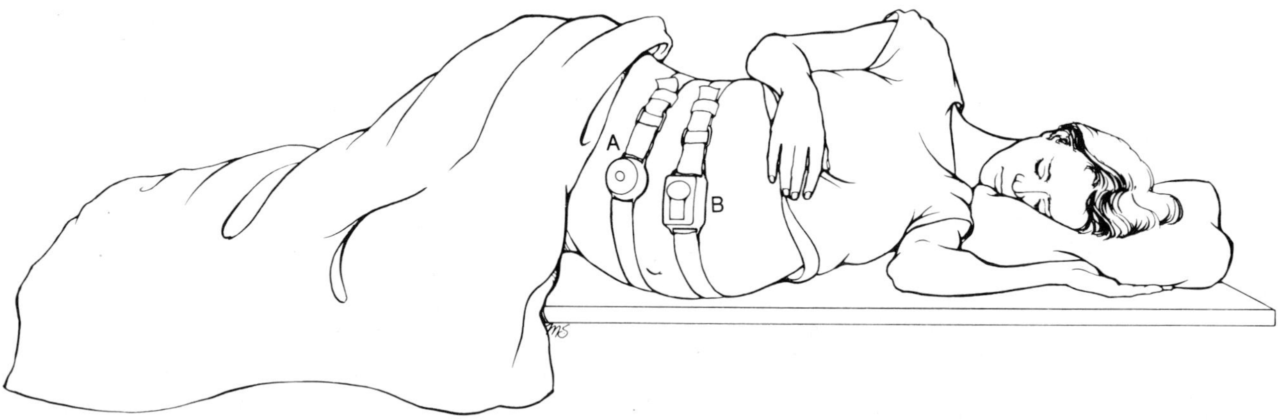

Figure 16.20
External fetal monitor—indirect monitoring. A: Ultrasonic transducer (FHR); B: Taco dynamometer (contraction pressure).

men (Fig. 16.20). The transducer converts the pressure of the uterus into an electric signal that is subsequently recorded on graph paper. For an accurate recording it is important that the transducer be placed on the fundus where contractility is the greatest. The FHR measured externally requires a transducer placed similarly on the abdomen over the spot where the fetal heart sounds are the clearest.

There are three ways of monitoring the fetus indirectly: phonocardiography, ultrasound, and fetal electrocardiography. The phonocardiographic transducer transmits the FHR through a contact microphone. This transducer is easily positioned but picks up noises from the environment resulting in a graphic recording with many artifacts. Ultrasound reflects a lower energy ultrasonic beam that bounces off blood moving from the fetal heart back to the receiver on the maternal abdomen. It is easiest to use but is easily disturbed by movement and requires frequent adjustment. Fetal electrocardiography records the FHR by calculating the interval between each fetal R-wave. Disadvantages are that it sometimes interprets the maternal signal instead of the fetal, and movement by the woman can be recorded that may obliterate the fetal electrocardiogram (ECG) signal. The most commonly used method of monitoring FHR is by ultrasound or Doppler.

Direct or internal monitoring requires that certain physiologic conditions be present in the mother; namely that the membranes be ruptured, that the cervix be dilated at least 2–3 cm, and that the presenting part be at the cervix. Contractions are monitored directly by inserting a fluid-filled catheter into the uterus (Fig. 16.21). The catheter is connected to an external transducer (strain gauge) located on the side of the monitor. Uterine contractions cause a rise in fluid pressure in the catheter. The pressure is converted to an electric signal by the external transducer. This changed signal is recorded on the fetal monitor graph paper as a curved line measured in millimeters of mercury (mm Hg)—the changes from the resting uterine pressure. The FHR is measured by a spiral electrode inserted into the fetal epidermis of the presenting part. This electrode measures the ECG. Signals are converted by a cardiotachometer into an instantaneous heart rate and recorded on the fetal monitor graph paper. Both the uterine catheter insertion and spiral electrode application are inva-

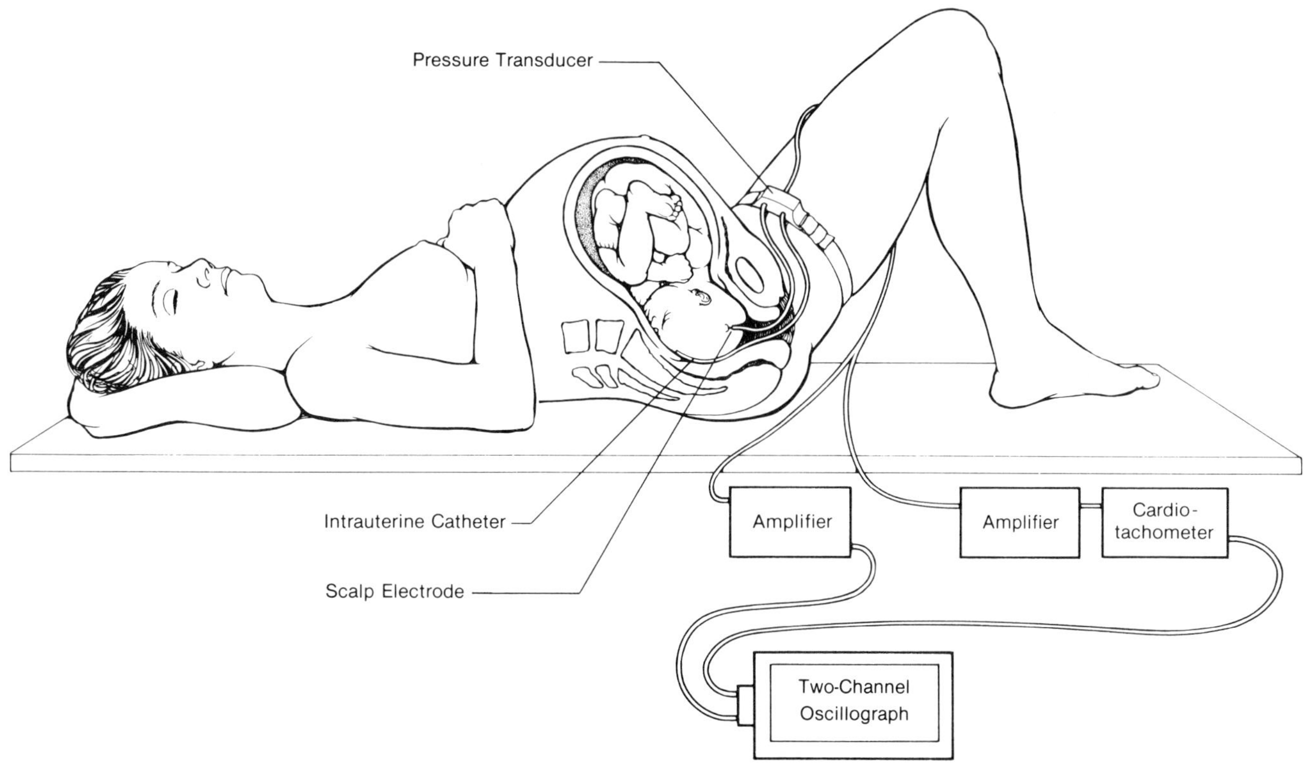

Figure 16.21
Internal fetal monitor—direct monitoring.

sive procedures and must be done under sterile conditions. The nurse clinician or physician applying the electrode must identify the presenting part and take care to avoid applying the scalp electrode over a fontanelle or suture line. The direct (internal) monitor provides an accurate method of monitoring FHR and uterine contractions and allows the mother to move in labor.

While detailed evaluation of fetal monitor patterns are beyond the scope of this text, it is important that you know the three basic patterns and the fact that monitor records should be read systematically. To read systematically, start with reading the contraction pattern and then move to reading the FHR.

CONTRACTION PATTERN

1. Determine the baseline intrauterine pressure by reading the pressure between contractions. Normal resting pressure is 6–15 mm Hg. (This reading is accurate only in direct monitoring.)
2. Determine the duration of the contraction by noting the point where the pressure leaves the baseline and returns to the baseline.
3. Determine the frequency of contractions by noting the time from the beginning of one contraction to the beginning of the next.
4. Determine the relaxation period by noting how long the baseline pressure is maintained between contractions.

FETAL HEART RATE

1. Determine the baseline heart rate by reading the rate between contractions. Normal heart rate is between 120–160 beats per minute.
2. Determine if there is tachycardia or bradycardia of the FHR by noting persistent rates above 160 beats per minute (tachycardia) or below 120 beats per minute (bradycardia). In addition to the criteria of 160 for tachycardia and 120 for bradycardia, the nurse should note a rise or drop of 10% from the previous baseline. This can alert the nurse to impending problems.
3. Determine the reactivity of the baseline heart rate by assessing beat-to-beat variability. Contrary to heart tracings in the adult, a persistent smooth heart tracing in fetal monitoring is an omnious sign. A reactive baseline, one that fluctuates more than 5 beats per minute, indicates a fetal nervous system that is responsive—a favorable sign. A previously reactive baseline can "flatten out" when the fetus sleeps or in response to analgesics given to the mother. Accurate measurement of reactivity, or beat-to-beat variability, is possible only in direct monitoring. However, causes of loss of beat-to-beat variability should be pursued in external monitoring as the actual reactivity is never greater than recorded. See Figure 16.22 for summary of reading a fetal monitor.

After reading the two tracings on the fetal monitor separately, that is, the contraction pattern and the FHR, the two tracings are evaluated in relation to each other. Periodic changes in the FHR in relation to uterine contractions are differentiated by describing the three basic patterns in fetal monitoring first described by Hon (1973).

EARLY DECELERATION

Early deceleration (Fig. 16.23) is associated with head compression. This pattern (early deceleration) is identified by its smooth waveform in which the FHR mirrors the pattern of the contraction. The key factor in identifying an early deceleration pattern is that the FHR deceleration begins with the onset of the contraction and returns to baseline within 30 seconds of the end of that contraction. This is a benign pattern, not requiring treatment and usually indicating that the woman is at least 6–7-cm dilated.

LATE DECELERATION

Late deceleration (Fig. 16.24) is associated with uteroplacental insufficiency and is identified by a deceleration in FHR that persists after the end of the contraction. In other words, the FHR has *not* returned to the baseline rate within 30 seconds of the end of the contraction. The waveform pattern can be subtle with gradual onset and recovery. Late deceleration is differentiated from early deceleration by the fact that late deceleration commences after the onset of contraction and returns to the baseline after the end of the contraction. Any late deceleration is omnious, and treatment focuses on improving uteroplacental blood flow. Turning the mother on her side,

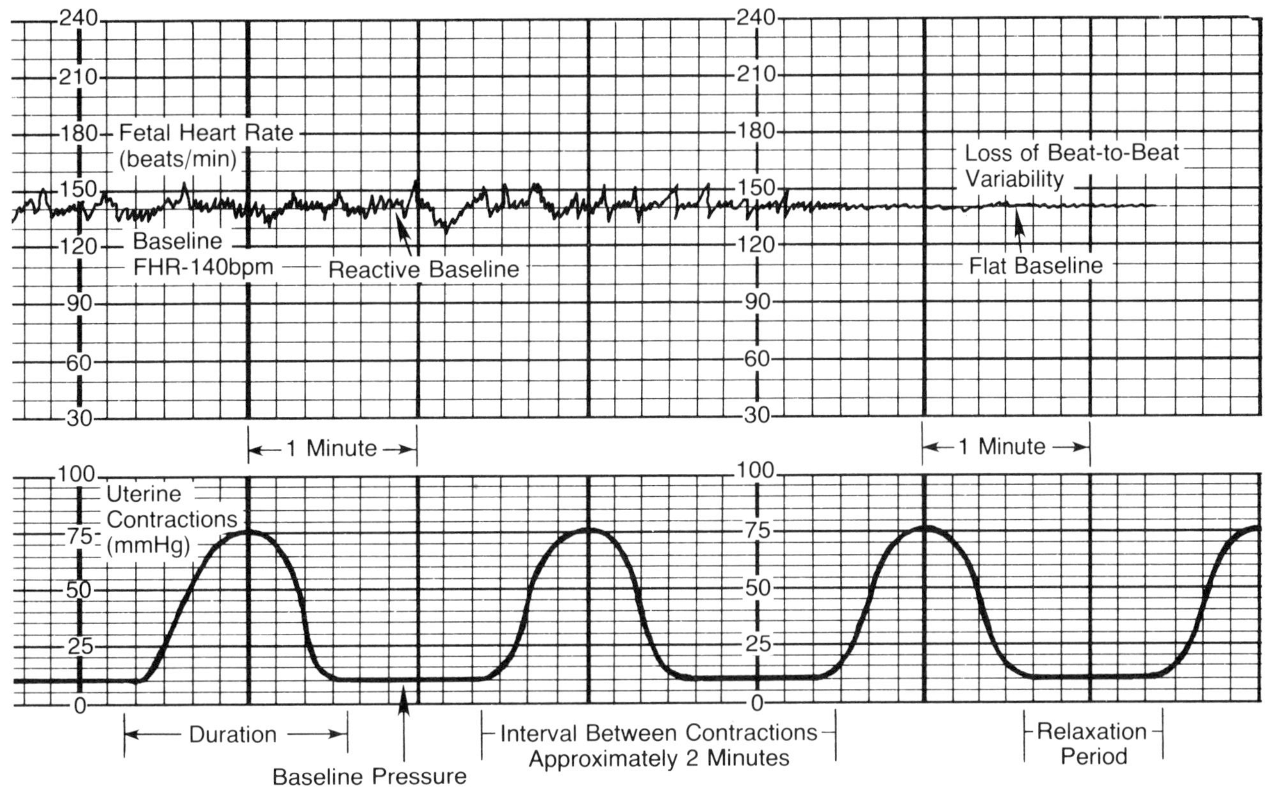

Figure 16.22
Summary reading of electronic fetal monitoring.

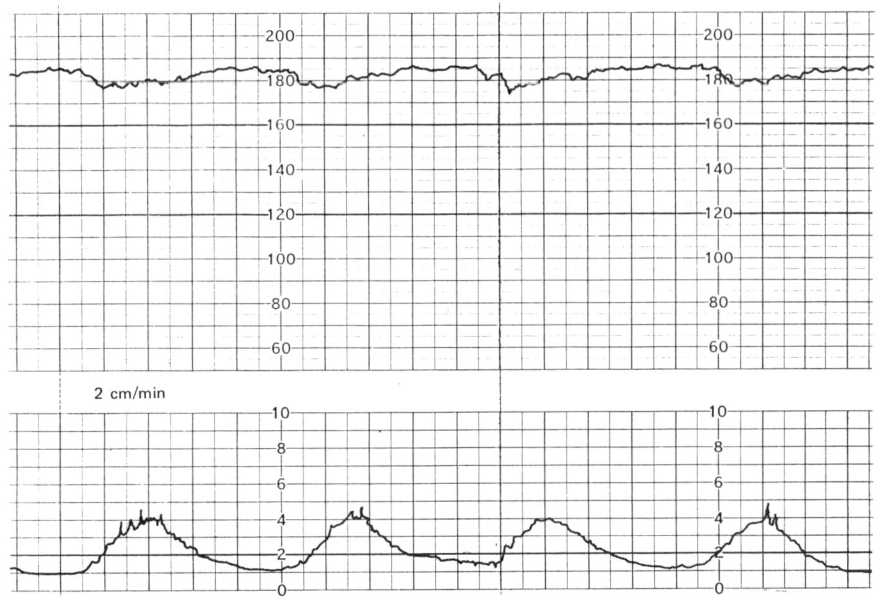

Figure 16.23
Early deceleration of the FHR. Source: Butnarescu, G. F., Tillotson, D. M., Villarreal, P. P. *Perinatal Nursing Volume 2. Reproductive Risk.* New York: John Wiley & Sons, 1980, p. 75. Used with permission.

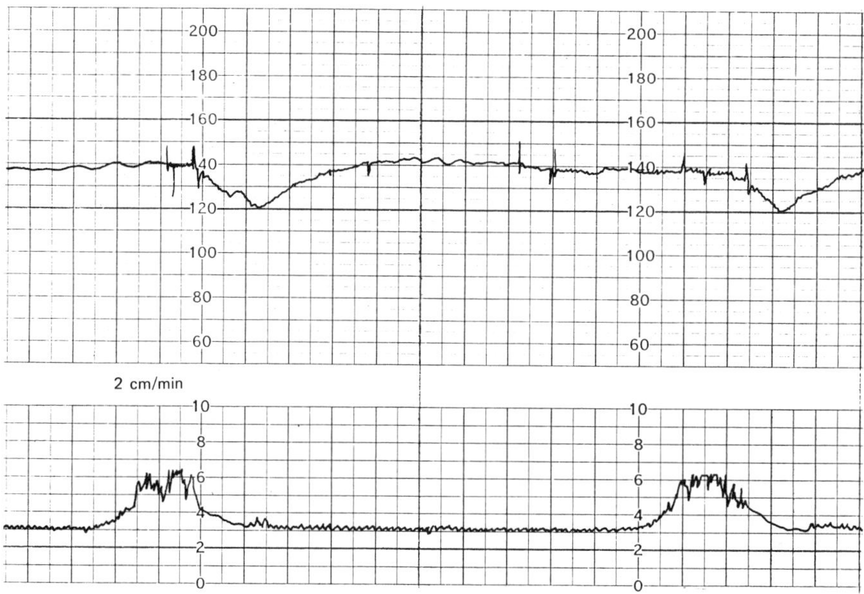

Figure 16.24
Late deceleration of the FHR. Source: Butnarescu, G. F., Tillotson, D. M., Villarreal, P. P. *Perinatal Nursing Volume 2. Reproductive Risk.* New York: John Wiley & Sons, 1980, p. 77. Used with permission.

administering oxygen, correcting maternal hypotension, and reducing uterine activity by discontinuing oxytocin may correct the pattern.

VARIABLE DECELERATION

Variable decelerations (Fig. 16.25) are associated with cord compression, which indicates a disturbance in umbilical vessel circulation. This pattern has a precipitous onset and recovery of heart rate deceleration, occurs anytime during a contraction cycle, and gives a jagged V-shaped waveform. The lower the drop in FHR and the longer the return to baseline FHR, the more serious the problem. The treatment for variable deceleration, which you will remember is caused by cord compression, is to relieve pressure on the cord by changing the maternal position. This may require several position changes. Severe variable decelerations, those lasting more than 1 minute, may necessitate Trendelenburg or knee–chest position before correction. Preparations for immediate delivery must be made if, in the cases of persistent variable and late deceleration, the pattern cannot be corrected.

You have now been introduced to basic reading of fetal monitor tracings and the three basic patterns. Successful interpretation of monitor tracings of the mother and fetus comes with time, experience, and a sophisticated knowledge base, similar to successful interpretation of adult cardiac monitoring strips. Besides the interpretation of the monitor tracings to recognize problems and institute treatment, the physical and psychologic responses of the woman must be monitored. Positioning the abdominal belts to minimize discomfort when external monitoring is being used, being alert to the pressure of the gravid uterus on the major blood vessels, and maintaining the transducer in place when mother or fetus moves are all nursing concerns. During internal monitoring, care must be taken to avoid infection. In addition to sterile techniques during insertion of the uterine catheter and the fetal electrode, the bed should be kept clean and fluid balance maintained, with attention to possible bladder distention. Research indicates that monitoring per se does not increase infection. Psychologic effects of monitoring have not been widely investigated, but studies by Starkman (1977) and Dulock and Herron (1976) have indicated that reactions to monitoring are generally more positive than negative. Some mothers have reported more secure feelings when electronic monitoring was used. It is interesting to note that fetal monitoring is now being discussed during education for childbirth classes more often than in

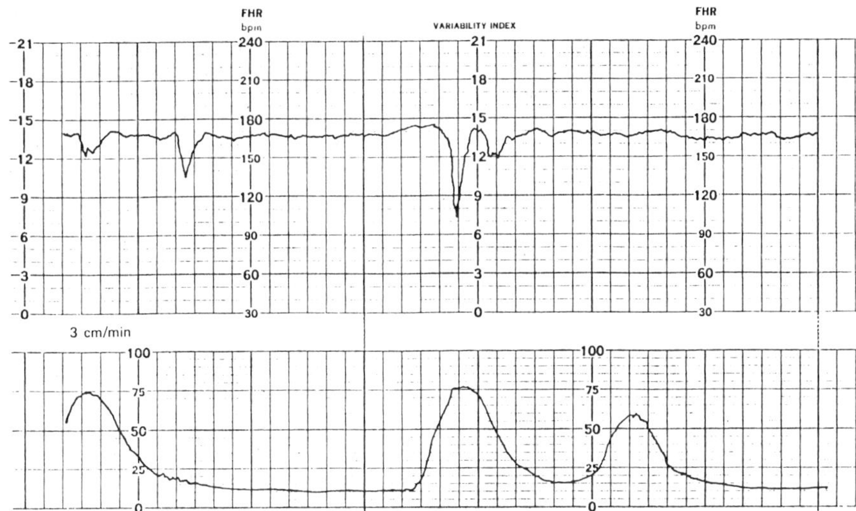

Figure 16.25
Variable deceleration of the FHR. Source: Butnarescu, G. F., Tillotson, D. M., Villarreal, P. P. *Perinatal Nursing Volume 2. Reproductive Risk.* New York: John Wiley & Sons, 1980. p. 78. Used with permission.

previous years. Explanation of procedures being carried out and respecting the woman's privacy, both facets of nursing care discussed extensively throughout this text, must be attended to throughout the labor and delivery process. You only have to project yourself into the place of the woman with the constant reminder of "how would I feel" or "what would I wish" in order to use a common sense professional approach.

Fetal Scalp Blood Sampling

Information about the acid–base status of the fetus is needed when a suspicious or worsening FHR pattern is seen on the monitor record. A sample of fetal blood is obtained by collecting a few drops of capillary blood from the fetal scalp through a small incision made in the scalp. Repeated samples can be obtained if the monitor pattern worsens. Frequently, information from sampling is used to determine the need for emergency cesarean section. After sampling, the pH is immediately determined and anything below 7.2 is evidence of fetal distress (normal fetal pH is 7.25–7.35). The blood sample may be analyzed for P_{CO_2} and base excess or deficit as well as for pH. The sample is, of course, an indication of the status of the fetus only at the moment it was taken. Although bleeding is not usually a problem, a lower pH (acidosis) compromises the clotting mechanism so the acidotic fetus is more likely to have continued oozing of blood. Also, nursery personnel should be notified of invasive procedures done on the infant so they can assess for complications following birth.

PROCEDURES TO FACILITATE LABOR PROGRESSION OR SUPPORT

Mother–Fetus Well-Being

ENEMA

The case for the enema in labor is controversial and, as with the issue of shaving the vulva (see below), more research is needed. The indication from the literature is that in some cases an enema is beneficial in that it empties the colon and permits easier descent of the fetal head; it also prevents contamination at the time of delivery (Whitley & Mack, 1980). The type of enema ordered depends on physician's order or hospital policy.

PREPARATION OF THE VULVA

Cleaning of the vulva for delivery by shaving of the pubic and vulva hair upon admission to the labor and delivery unit is still common practice in many institutions. More often, a partial, sometimes called *moustache prep* or *mini prep* is done, which leaves the hair on the mons veneris and removes the hair from the labia majora, the perineal area, and around the anus. Proponents of shaving believe that it provides a cleaner, more visible area for delivery or is necessary in the event of episiotomy. When shaving, you need to keep the area well lubricated with soap and water and the razor parallel to the skin to prevent nicking. Obviously, a break in skin will increase the chance of infection by opening a portal for organisms. Many nurse-midwives and some physicians no longer shave the perineal area.

POSITIONING OF THE PATIENT

Mothers in early labor can be in or out of bed, but as labor advances they are generally more comfortable in bed. It is preferable for a mother to labor on her side, not on her back. The pressure of the enlarged uterus impedes vena cava blood flow in the dorsal position. In other words, positioning a pregnant woman on her back affects the maternal circulation—venous return is drastically impeded and maternal cardiac output is reduced. Other advantages to having a mother labor on her side are comfort, more effective uterine contractions, better uterine perfusion, and improved fetal gas exchange.

FOOD AND FLUIDS

Gastric emptying time during labor is delayed, and analgesia or sedative drugs delay it even more. If labor is prolonged, intravenous fluids and glucose appropriate to meet energy needs are required.

BLADDER

As the lower segment of the uterus lengthens and the cervix retracts, the bladder is pulled upward. Because of other stimuli during labor, such as pain, the urge to urinate may be decreased and careful assessment for urinary retention needs to be made by the nurse. A distended bladder appears as a fluctuate mass just above the symphysis pubis and is easily observed and palpated. A full bladder may retard the descent of the fetus, as well as predispose the woman to urinary infection because of stasis. If the mother is unable to void spontaneously, catheterization is needed. Care must be taken to prevent infection, that is, strict asepsis as well as a small catheter (14 F) to minimize discomfort is important. The catheter is inserted between contractions; the insertion is somewhat more posterior and downward than in the nonpregnant female because of the stretching of the urethra by the proximity of the fetal head.

Analgesia

Although painless labors do occur, they are the exception rather than the rule. Pain during labor is caused by the uterine contractions that are necessary for labor and childbirth; therefore, the goal is not to relieve the pain source but to decrease the stimulus; to block the pain pathway; or to decrease pain perception, interpretation, or reaction. Since biblical times and undoubtedly before, childbirth has been considered a painful experience. More recently, the view that pain in labor is inherent has been disputed, and social, cultural, and emotional influences have been looked at. Nevertheless, in all cultures and even in primate and animal societies, the pain of childbirth is related to the physiologic process. The pain of the first stage of labor is related to dilatation of the cervix and contractions; this pain travels by way of sensory pathways through several routes to the spinal cord. Pain is felt in the lower abdominal wall, lumbar spine, and upper sacrum. As intensity of the uterine contractions increases, pain may spread to include the thighs, midsacrum, and umbilical area. Pain during the second stage of labor is caused by distention of the lower birth canal and perineum. This pain is transmitted by sensory fibers that are components of the pudendal nerves. (This fact has relevance for pudendal anesthesia; see Chapter 22.) Pain and its relationship to education for childbirth are discussed in Chapter 15. Pain relief for the woman needs to be selected according to her specific pattern, which may vary considerably during the course of labor.

Systemic drugs are administered to most women in labor to reduce the discomfort of uterine contractions. In general, drugs used are cerebral depressants, and since most of them cross the placenta, they also affect the fetal brain. If placental exchange is adequate while the fetus remains in utero, this placental transfer is not generally a problem. The concern for depression of the fetal respiratory center occurs when medication is given late in labor or when the mother delivers more rapidly than anticipated. The most appropriate time for administration of analgesia is in the active phase of the first stage of labor. The need for analgesia depends on the mother's perception of pain, which is influenced by her attitude toward pregnancy, delivery, and motherhood in general. Emotionally secure women who approach childbirth with a good understanding of the process and are only moderately apprehensive usually require little medication. Childbirth education does much to promote this emotional climate (see Chapter 15). Understanding about medication by the mother, father, and/or supportive other, appropriate insight into the mother's wishes, and correct administration by the nurse are all necessary for successful use of analgesia. Pharmacologic support in its proper perspective is an adjunct to successful labor and delivery. There is no one suitable drug or method, and Table 16.3 lists drugs used commonly and some sedatives and amnesic drugs occasionally used in labor. Many of the drugs used in labor you will have used elsewhere in nursing. There are some general rules of thumb to guide you in the administration of analgesic drugs.

- ▲ Remember, there are always *two* patients when giving medication in labor.
- ▲ Give medication to the mother only when labor is well established—in the primigravida after 4 or 5 cm; in the multigravida, sometimes earlier.
- ▲ Try never to give sedation within 2 hours of delivery—easier to gauge in the primigravida than multigravida.
- ▲ Give analgesia only when the mother can be observed constantly.
- ▲ Give only enough medication to provide rest and relief between contractions, not enough to depress the infant's respiratory center or reduce efficiency of uterine contractions.
- ▲ Give intravenously or intramuscularly as gastric motility and emptying time are considerably reduced in labor.
- ▲ Know the medication and the physiologic effects of the preparations administered.

Before leaving the discussion of care during the first stage of labor and proceeding to the discussion of care in the delivery room, we will summarize the signs of transitional phase (8–10 cm) since they are unique and important and, once observed, never forgotten.

- ▲ Increase in bloody show
- ▲ Nausea or dry heaves
- ▲ Increasing discomfort from contractions and an urge to push, often expressed as "I need to move my bowels," which is the pressure of the baby's head on the perineum
- ▲ Anal distention followed by perineal bulging
- ▲ Involuntary pushing and grunting
- ▲ Perhaps most significant and always important, the mother saying: "The baby is coming"

Many nurses unfortunately have ignored this last statement assessing from previous data "this could not be so" only to find it was indeed true. The axiom for the novice: Always believe the mother, particularly the multipara until what she is saying has been disproven. Psychosocial support, important throughout the first stage of labor, becomes critical during the active and transitional periods. As mentioned earlier, the mother has progressed from an extroverted talkative person to an introverted sometimes irritable person. Women frequently say retrospectively: "As contractions became more intense and closer together, I was unable to determine when one contraction began or ended." They also say: "They told me to push only with a contraction" or "Don't push because you're not fully dilated. All I knew was I hurt all the time and I wanted labor to be over." Frequently, the nurse is the recipient of comments such as: "Get out of here." "You're not helping." "Nobody helps me." "Can't you do something?" This is when the experienced nurse knows that the woman should *not* be left and that she really needs the nurse more than ever. Statements such as "You are 9-cm dilated, which means you have only a bit more to dilate," and "I will help you through the next contractions" can be very useful. Or perhaps the nurse encourages the father, supportive other, or coach to assist the mother. Perceptual field is narrowed so although the mother who has had analgesia may be relaxing between contractions, each time a contraction begins she may become

TABLE 16.3
COMMON ANALGESICS, SEDATIVES, AND AMNESICS USED IN LABOR

Drug	*Dose*	*Desired Effect*	*Side Effects on Mother*	*Effects on Fetus/Newborn*	*Comments*
SEDATIVES Barbiturates	100 mg IM[a] 50 mg IV[b]	Sedation Hypnotic sleep	None with RD[c] With severe pain, can cause restlessness	None with RD Oversedation causes depression	Sometimes used in early (latent) phase of first stage if mother is tense
Phenothiazine derivatives (Vistaril, Atarax, Phenergan)	Dose varies depending on drug	Sedation Tranquility Antiemetic	None except occasional hypotension.	Same as above	Useful during early labor Can be used in conjunction with narcotic, which requires a smaller amount of drug Tranquilizers are synergestic when used with narcotics
Diazepam (Valium)	15–20 mg IM	Sedation, muscle relaxant	None with RD[c] Overdose can cause respiratory depression	Same as above	Same as above—can be used with narcotic but with caution because of respiratory side effects
AMNESICS Scopolamine	0.3 mg (1/200 grain)	Amnesia sedation	Excitement, restless with contraction Dry mouth		Contraindicated in obstetrics generally because of side effects Only justification is amnesic effect Mother must have someone with her *constantly*
NARCOTICS Meperidine (Demerol)	25–50 mg IM or IV	Sedation Euphoria Decreased anxiety	Mild respiratory or circulatory depression Delays gastric emptying	Mild depression with RD Severe with overdose	Effective pain relief in 75% of patients; should be given in active labor (4–5 cm) so as not to slow labor; should not be given just before delivery to prevent fetal depression

[a] IM—Intramuscular.
[b] IV—Intravenous.
[c] RD—Reasonable dose.

disoriented. The nurse, knowing that amnesia is common, may need to repeat instructions with each contraction such as, "Mrs. B your contraction is beginning and I want you to start your breathing technique and I'm here to help you." Once the nurse has supported the mother through the contraction, she praises the mother's effort and repeats the stage of progress. This step-by-step verbal support given with a calm voice along with touching make this toughest part of the labor experience productive and positive. The presence and support of another caring human being is critical.

The Second Stage of Labor

The second stage, which ends with delivery of the infant, can be quite brief—a few minutes in the multigravida or as long as an hour in the primigravida. At this point the secondary force of labor, the use of abdominal muscles, is added. Techniques for pushing with correlated breathing techniques are discussed in Chapter 15. In general, multigravidas are taken to the delivery room when they are 8- or 9-cm dilated, primigravidas are taken when there is caput (head) or "50 cents worth" of the baby's hair showing at the vaginal orifice. Because in the primigravida the birth canal has not been traversed before, more resistance from soft tissues is encountered; therefore the trip for the neonate and the work of the mother is usually more difficult.

Delivery Room (Second and Third Stages of Labor)

Nursing care of the mother and infant in the delivery room involves both psychosocial and physical support as does the whole labor and delivery experience (Fig. 16.26). In this room, part of second and all of third stages of labor usually take place. Maintenance of aseptic technique to prevent infection is crucial, and all personnel and family members, if they are included, should wear a cap that covers the hair and a face mask that covers the nose and mouth. Those participating directly in the delivery should wear sterile surgical gowns and gloves. Others in the room, for example, the father, must wear clean surgical clothes. A mother should *never* be left alone in the delivery room. She needs constant attention and support, both physical, such as frequent checking of the FHR, and psychosocial, such as information, encouragement, and praise, as well as monitoring for expulsive efforts that could result in delivery of the infant. When spontaneous delivery is imminent, the mother is positioned appropriately. Dorsal recumbant position (Fig. 16.27) is satisfactory, particularly for multiparas, as is the side lying position, which is often used in other countries and by certified nurse midwives in the United States. Both of these positions result in less tension on the perineum, hence lacerations are less likely to occur. *Episiotomy* (surgical incision of the perineum to provide more room for the infant's head; see Chapter 22) can be performed in this position, but repair is difficult to perform since it is difficult to expose the area to be sutured. The lithotomy position is more uncomfortable for the patient but it provides a better view of the perineum and therefore better inspection of the birth canal during and following delivery. The lithotomy position is essential for operative delivery

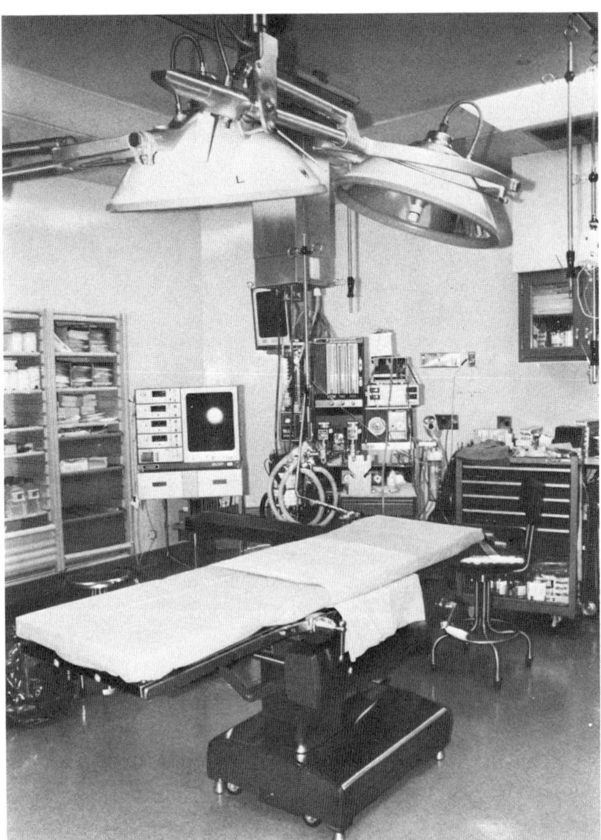

Figure 16.26
Labor and delivery room.

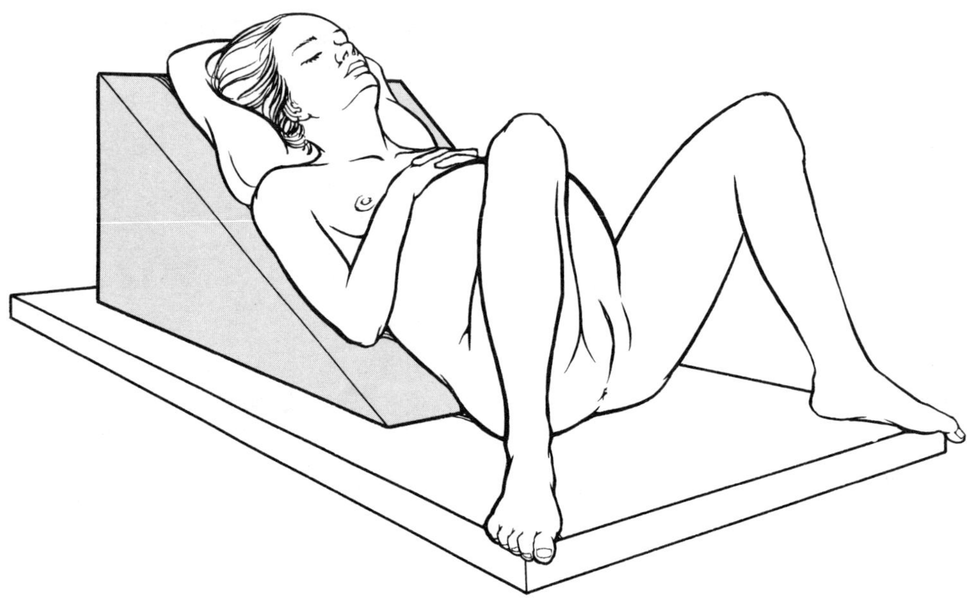

Figure 16.27
Dorsal recumbent position.

(e.g., forceps, see Chapter 22) and for repair of more than a superficial episiotomy or tear. Care must be taken when raising or lowering the mother's legs into stirrups as strain or tension on muscle or ligaments can cause injury. Also, leaving the patient in lithotomy position for extensive periods of time, more than 1 hour, will cause pooling of blood in the pelvic region and impaired venous return. This is a contributing factor to pelvic thrombophlebitis. Movement of the legs should be simultaneous, recalling normal range of motion. Sometimes in lithotomy position, the mother's hands are restrained to prevent contamination of the sterile field. Hand restraints are demeaning and less used today, but are necessary in some instances. When used, explanation and care that the restraints are not too tight are important. Frequently, there are handles adjacent to the restraints, which provide a hold that assists the mother in the expulsive process.

The vulva and anus, the upper postion of thighs, and the skin over the pubis and lower abdomen are cleansed with soap and water and antiseptic solution. Cleansing motions are always from the center outward (most clean to least clean) and from anterior to posterior, discarding the cotton cleansing sponge after each stroke. An acceptable pattern of the cleansing sequence is diagrammed in Figure 16.28. No attempt is made to cleanse the vagina since the constant flow of amniotic fluid with contractions provides a cleansing force. Sterile leggings and sheets are put in place; it is common practice to use paper or disposable sterile gowns and drapes. Some delivery tables have an end section that drops down and slides underneath the section that the mother's back is on, much like a drawer. This lower half of the table is never removed until someone is positioned constantly at the vaginal orifice. Sliding back the lower half of the table permits the physician or nurse-midwife closer access to the mother.

While the mother is being prepared for delivery, other preparations are occurring simultaneously. An area is being prepared to receive the infant, and the physician or nurse-midwife prepares hands and arms as for surgery and dons sterile gown and gloves. If a local anesthetic is to be used, it is administered at this time. If episiotomy is to be performed, it is done after the perineum has been flattened out by crowning of the fetal head. *Crowning* is when the widest diameter of the fetal head is surrounded by the vaginal opening. Delivery of the head is controlled by the physician and rapid expulsion is prevented. During delivery of the head, the mother is encouraged to pant while the nurse reassures her delivery is imminent. After the head is out the next step for the person delivering is to check to see if the cord is around the neonate's neck and, if so, to slip it over the head

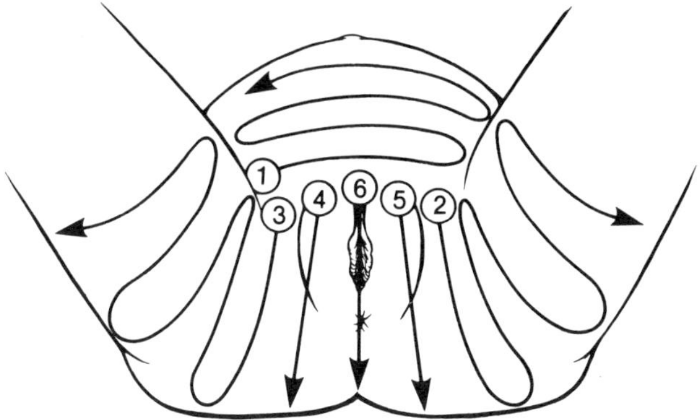

Figure 16.28
Cleansing the perineum.

preventing tension on the cord. After the head is delivered, the anterior shoulder, posterior shoulder, and remainder of the body is delivered, and the newborn is held with head in dependent position (downward) to facilitate postural drainage. Some delay in clamping the cord is probably beneficial in the normal newborn. When held at the level of the vaginal introitus, blood will infuse from the placental vessels to the baby permitting as much as 75–100 cc increase in blood volume. After this brief interval, two clamps are placed on the umbilical cord and it is cut between the clamps. The baby who has cried spontaneously is dried and placed in a heated crib or on the mother's abdomen, preferably skin to skin for warmth.

For the mother, the third stage of delivery can be the most serious time since abnormalities in separation and expulsion of the placenta can result in maternal death. Normally, blood loss during delivery is 250–350 cc; it is common practice to diagnose postpartum hemorrhage when bleeding exceeds 500 cc in the first 24 hours after delivery. The following are signs that the placenta is separating from the uterine wall (see Fig. 16.29).

- ▲ A gush of blood flows from the vagina as the placenta separates.
- ▲ The cord lengthens at the vaginal introitus as the placenta moves to the lower uterus.
- ▲ The fundus rises as the placenta separates.
- ▲ The fundus changes shape from flat to globular as the placenta drops into the lower uterine segment.

The steps of expulsion of the placenta depict how once the placenta separates it slides into the lower segment of the uterus. At this time expulsion is assisted by uterine contraction and by the physician placing a hand on the fundus and applying manual pressure downward. The placenta appears at the introitus with either the fetal or the maternal surface first. If the fetal side is first, it is known as Schultze's mechanism; if the roughened (cotelydons) maternal side is first, it is called Duncan's mechanism. (See Fig. 10.6.) Duncan's mechanism is less common and is usually accompanied by more bleeding. At this point, the mother is physically tired but usually alert and emotionally can be anywhere from laughter to tears. Usually, there is a great need to see her child, which should be allowed. In Chapters 17–19, mother–infant bonding is discussed in detail. Remember that it is important for the delivery room nurse to observe and record the first interaction between mother and infant. This recording should note touching, talking, eye contact, and mother's observations of the infant such as "Your eyes are shut; you're so small." It is important for the nurse to note the time of events in the delivery room. Most labor and delivery room records have a place to note time and to record events such as the length of each stage of labor, the time of delivery of the infant and of the placenta, and any medications administered. An example of a labor and delivery record is included in the appendix.

Care of the Infant in the Delivery Room

The priority for newborn care is the establishment of respirations, which normally is accomplished within 1 minute of birth. The mouth and nose are cleared of secretions as soon as the head is out, and most newborns cry vigorously at birth. Additional secretions are removed from the mouth and nose following birth by postural drainage, that is, holding the infant in a head dependent position with the neck extended. Frequently, a bulb syringe which is the first choice of suction methods, is used by the physician. Suction catheters, either a catheter attached to mechanical suction or a De Lee mucous trap can also be used. When suction is employed, the mouth is suctioned first and then the nose because nasal stimulation may cause the neonate to gasp and aspirate secretions. Any type

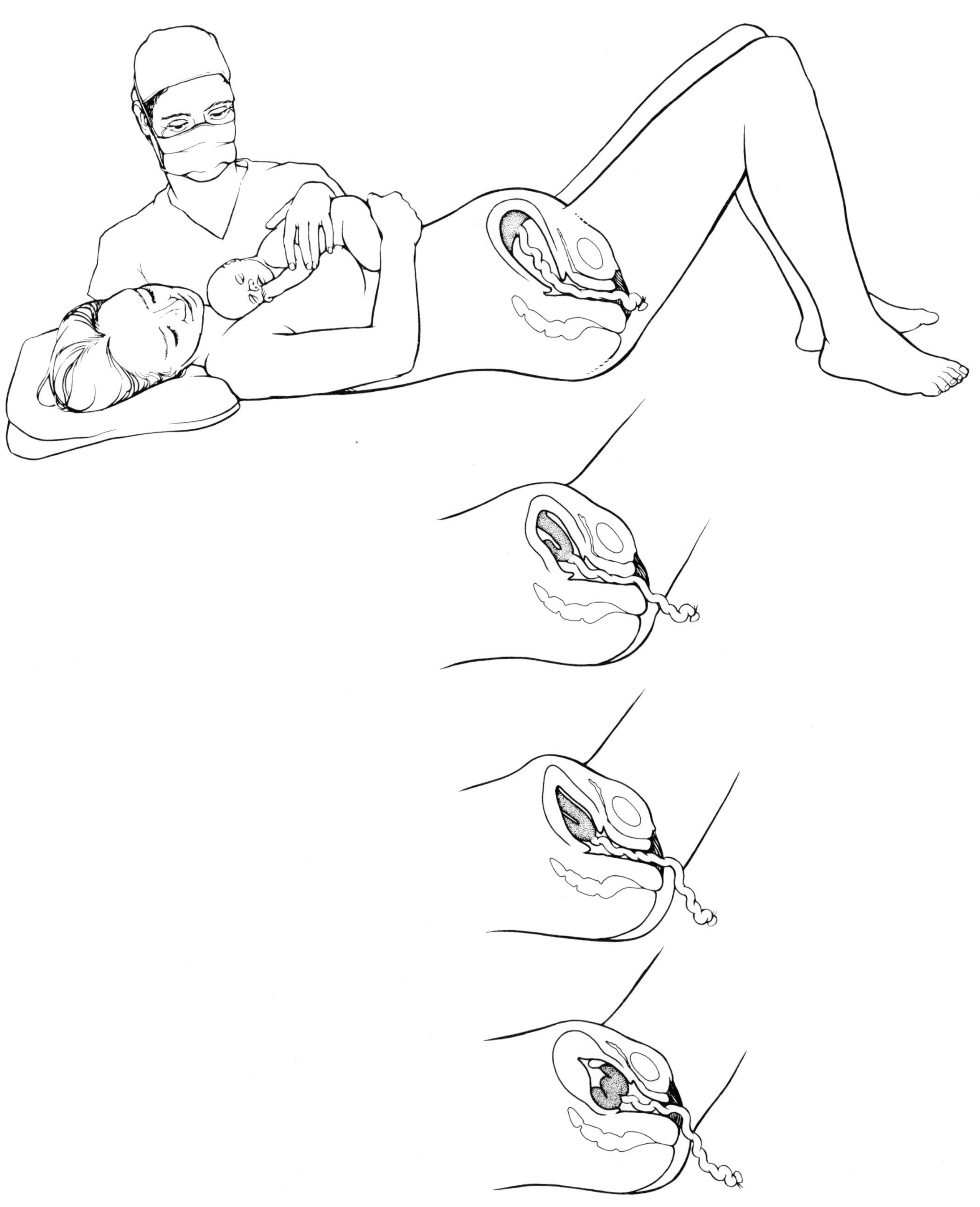

Figure 16.29
Stages of placental separation.

of suctioning should be gentle and brief, less than 1 minute. If prolonged suctioning is employed, the result can be laryngeal spasm, bradycardia, and cardiac arrhythmias, physiologically caused by vagal stimulation and lack of oxygen. Almost simultaneously with the establishment of respirations, attention should be given to temperature control. In order to minimize evaporative heat loss, the infant should be dried and placed under a radiant heat warmer (Fig. 16.30).

Doctor Virginia Apgar (1952) developed a standardized assessment of the newborn that should be done 1 minute after birth and then again 5 minutes after birth. The Apgar Score is used as an initial screening tool to see how well the infant is doing. The 1-minute score indicates what assistance the infant needs, and the 5-minute score indicates how the infant is responding following the stress of labor. The 5-minute score is also an indication of how the infant will do in neonatal life. This is particularly true in the infant who requires resuscitation because a higher score at 5 minutes, after a low score initially, indicates that resuscitative measures have been effective. Conversely, a 5-minute Apgar score that is lower than the 1-minute score is indicative of a problem. The *normal* neonate who has been assessed accurately at 1 minute will not have a lower score at 5 minutes. A more detailed account of the neonate's adaptation to extrauterine life is in Chapter 17. In this chapter, discussion is confined to immediate assessment and care of the normal neonate in the delivery room.

In Apgar Scoring there are five objective signs; each is evaluated and a score of 0, 1, or 2 is given; the highest possible score is 10. Most healthy infants score between 7 and 10. Lower scores indicate an increasing degree of asphyxia and depression. Scores between 4 and 7 indicate that the muscle tone is reduced and the infant cyanotic; scores below 4 indicate that the infant is severely depressed and requires prompt medical intervention to prevent sequellae.

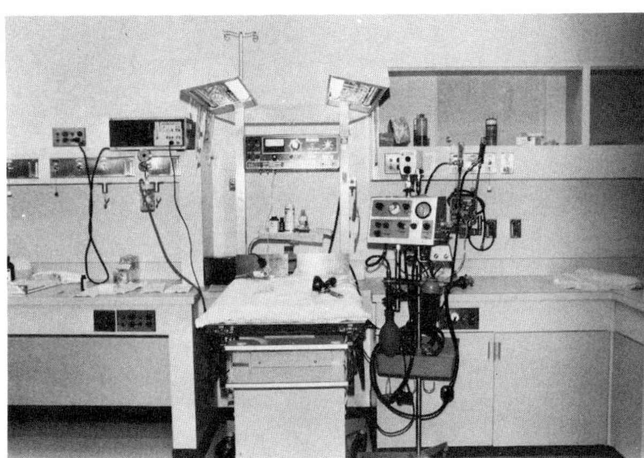

Figure 16.30
Radiant heater warmer.

Criteria Used in Apgar Scoring

HEART RATE

The heart rate sign is the most significant indication of the neonate's oxygenation and is evaluated by palpating the pulse at the juncture of the umbilical cord and abdominal wall or by auscultation with a stethoscope. A heart rate below 100 is serious, and resuscitation measures are instituted. If bradycardia is present, the other criteria are absent or only minimally present. If the heart rate does not improve with artificial ventilation, the prognosis is poor. Resuscitation steps are the establishment of an airway, the delivery of oxygen, and the establishment of ventilation. The most efficient method of ventilation in a newborn is the bag-to-endotracheal tube, but because the intubation process takes skill and time, the bag-to-mask ventilation method is usually used first. (See Chapter 23.)

RESPIRATORY EFFORT

Respiratory effort, the second most important sign, is usually established in the normal newborn by 1 minute. A lusty cry is followed quickly by respiratory efforts in the normal newborn.

MUSCLE TONE

Muscle tone is evaluated by the amount of flexion of the extremities. A healthy newborn has arms and legs flexed and an attempt to extend the legs meets with resistance. Poor muscle tone is evidence of acidosis.

REFLEX IRRITABILITY

Reflex irritability is tested by tapping the sole of the foot or by placing the tip of a catheter in a nostril. The vigorous baby responds with a cry to the slap on the sole and with a cough or sneeze to the catheter in the nostril. A less-active baby will respond with a grimace.

COLOR

Color is the least significant of the criteria and the one that changes the quickest. Rarely is a newborn completely pink at 1 minute and many times not at 5 minutes. For these reasons, many healthy babies may have an Apgar score of 9, having received a 2 in all criteria except color.

NURSING CARE OF THE NEONATE IN DELIVERY ROOM

Blood volume in the term newborn is 250–300 cc and, as a result, blood loss from the cord must be avoided. The cord should be tied or clamped approximately 2 cm from the skin edge. The umbilical cord can be ligated with a metal or plastic clamp or tied in a square knot with a strong, heavy cord. The blood vessels are easily visible at the end of the cut umbilical cord. The nurse should assess to be sure there are *two arteries* and *one vein.* One artery only is usually indicative of congenital anomalies. Even if there are no obvious or gross anomalies when only one artery and one vein are present, the fact should be noted and recorded as it is sometimes indicative of internal urinary tract anomalies. No dressing is applied to the cord, but an application of antiseptic such as alcohol is applied several times a day to keep the cord dry. Other measures to prevent infection such as washing hands before care of the infant are important.

CARE OF THE EYES

In 1884, Crede instituted the use of silver nitrate ($AgNO_3$) in the eyes of the newborn to prevent gonorrheal ophthalmia, also called *ophthalmia neonatorum.* If gonococci are present in the mother's birth canal and the infant becomes infected during birth, blindness can result. Eye treatment is a legal responsibility in most states. Some agencies, where state law permits, treat the newborn prophylactically with antibiotic ointment instead of silver nitrate 1%. Before eye treatment, the outer surface of the eyelid should be cleansed of blood and vernix with a cotton ball and sterile water. Silver nitrate usually is packaged in a wax ampule, which is punctured with a needle to open. The medication is put in each eye by pulling down the lower lid and instilling one or two drops of silver nitrate in the conjunctival sac. The American Academy of Pediatrics recommends no rinse following silver nitrate. If antibiotic ointment is employed, the procedure is the same. Expiration date of the medication should always be noted before using it. In many hospitals, treatment of the eyes is delayed for 1 or 2 hours so as not to interfere with mother–infant bonding.

IDENTIFICATION

Before mother and infant are separated, each must be identified. A method commonly used is identification bands with identical numbers for mother and infant. After mother's surname, date, time of delivery, and sex of the infant are recorded and inserted into three plastic identification bands, each with the same number, two are placed on the infant, one on the arm and one on the leg, and one is placed on the mother's wrist. Some bands include a place for the physician's name. Identibands are checked with a second person to prevent error. The infant's band is checked with the mother's each time they are separated and reunited. Footprinting of the infant is mandatory in some states and may be done in the delivery room or at a later time.

GROSS PHYSICAL ASSESSMENT

Before a more systematic assessment is done (see Chapter 17), a gross assessment for anomalies is carried out in the delivery room. Besides checking the three cord vessels, a head-to-foot assessment for such things as extra digits, hypospadias, imperforate anus, and birthmarks is done. General behavior and color of the infant is observed constantly or frequently during the time in the delivery room.

In summary, care of the newborn in the delivery room includes establishment of an airway and attention to warmth (see thermo-regulation, Chapter 17). Apgar scoring at 1 and 5 minutes is done and recorded. Cord care, eye care, and a brief physical assessment and identification of mother and infant are completed. Once the airway is established and the infant is dried, an opportunity for bonding is provided as quickly as possible.

The Fourth Stage of Labor

The fourth stage of labor, or the first hour after delivery, is a crucial time for the mother, and for all intents and purposes, the mother is treated like an intensive care patient with vital signs, perineal checks, fundal assessment, and intake and output assessed every 15 minutes. The assessment focuses on the mother's reaction to the stress of labor and on the ascertainment that the fundus remains firmly contracted. An oxytocic drug is usually given to all mothers following delivery of the placenta to stimulate contraction of the uterus; this is the specific physiologic action of oxytocic drugs. There are three oxytocic drugs that can be used postpartally: ergonovine maleate (Ergotrate), methylergonovine maleate (Methergine), and oxytocin (Pitocin). Ergotrate is a powerful stimulant to uterine contraction whose action is quick (a few minutes following intramuscular injection and within 5–10 minutes following oral administration) and sustained, lasting for hours. Methergine is a synthetic derivative of ergonovine and can be used in place of Ergotrate. Both Ergotrate and Methergine can be administered parenterally or orally. The usual dosage is 0.2 mg. These drugs (ergot derivatives) are contraindicated in the hypertensive woman, and blood pressure should be checked before administering. Ergot preparations are not used as frequently postpartum as they once were, but they are important obstetric drugs and should be learned. Intravenous administration of these drugs is contraindicated as they can cause hypertension as a result of cerebral vasospasm.

Oxytocin, the oxytocic hormone of the posterior pituitary, is the drug used most often to control postpartum bleeding. Although this drug occurs naturally, oxytocin is produced synthetically (Pitocin or Synctocin), and it is this synthetic preparation that is used. Pitocin comes in an aqueous solution, 10 United States Pharmacopeia (USP) units per 1 cc. It is administered intravenously or intramuscularly. Unlike ergonovine, Pitocin does not have a long sustained effect, and it is most frequently administered by continuous intravenous infusion, 10 units (or 1 cc) in 500 cc of intravenous solution. A large single dose intravenously can cause profound hypotension (oxytocin is the same drug used for induction of labor and is discussed in Chapter 22). It is the physician's decision to administer an oxytocic drug. It is, however, the nurse's responsibility to know the drug being used and its action and side effects. In general, it is much safer to administer oxytocics after the delivery of the placenta.

Besides administering oxytocin, the care during the fourth stage of labor involves cleansing the vulva, thighs, and buttocks and applying a perineal pad. The perineal area is cleansed from front to back with care to avoid contamination and to prevent infection. The mother is moved from the delivery room to a recovery area and is put into a clean bed. Whether or not the infant accompanies her depends on hospital policy. The mother's vital signs—blood pressure, pulse, and respirations—are taken every 15 minutes and recorded. Fundal assessment is done each time also. To palpate the fundus, one hand is placed above the symphysis pubis as a guard and the other hand is placed on the top of the fundus so that the uterus is virtually held between the two hands (See Fig. 16.31). The uterus is palpated as a firm round object in the abdomen not unlike an orange or grapefruit. Immediately after delivery, the top of the fundus is located halfway between the symphysis and the umbilicus. Thereafter, in the immediate postpartum period, the height of the fundus is at or just below the umbilicus. If it is not easily detected, the uterus is massaged with a gentle circular motion until it contracts, but only until it is firm. The uterus is a muscle and overstimulation causes relaxation. Once the uterus is felt, the height above the pubis is recorded in centimeters by the use of a paper measuring tape. This is a more accurate method than measuring by finger breadths as each person's

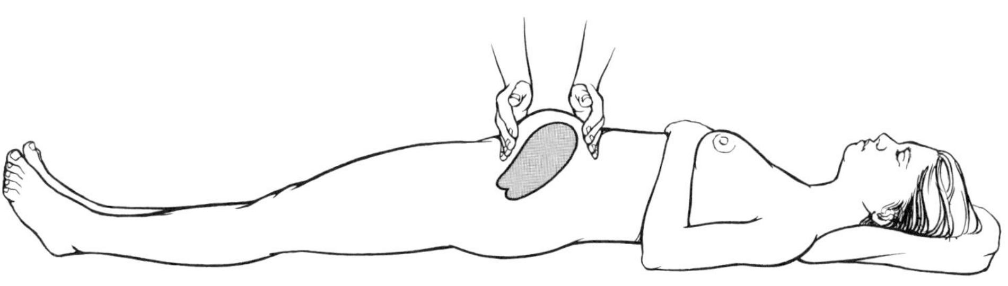

Figure 16.31
Palpation of the fundus.

fingers are different, and involution can be assessed more accurately. The end of the tape is held at the top of the pubic bone and the height is recorded in centimeters. As long as the uterus is contracted, blood vessels will be constricted and blood loss will be minimal. If the uterus becomes relaxed or "boggy," bleeding is more likely to occur. Observation of size, height, and consistency of the fundus is made and recorded every 15 minutes. The mother should be taught how to palpate her uterus and how it feels when contracted. Each time the fundus is checked, the perineal pad should be observed. Turning the patient to assess bleeding that may have occurred and collected under the buttocks is important. Saturation of two perineal pads in 15 minutes or three in 30 minutes is an indication for closer assessment. Intake and output should be monitored, especially if intravenous fluids have been absorbed fairly quickly. Because of the shift in intra-abdominal pressure, the mother frequently is unable to feel a full bladder. A fundus that is rising in the abdomen, noted by fundal height measurement, or a fundus that is displaced to the right or the left frequently is caused by a full bladder. Explanations of all postpartal assessment procedures should be shared with the mother.

Following delivery, mothers are frequently exhausted and sore; generalized discomfort and perineal pain may be reduced by use of an analgesic drug. Basic physiologic needs, including food, warmth, shelter, comfort, and what Maslow calls love and belonging needs must be met. Family relationships should be fostered and re-established. Opportunity for the baby to visit again in the recovery room (if the neonate is not allowed to remain) should be made with the father having an opportunity to touch and hold the infant.

Table 16.2, mentioned before, depicting the stages of labor, the biophysical and psychosocial changes, and interventions, is a summary and guide.

SUMMARY

Chapter 16 on normal labor discussed theories for the onset of human labor, pointing out that current theories suggest that interaction between fetal and maternal systems initiate labor. Characteristics and validity of current theories were presented in Table 16.1. Readiness for labor, both biophysical and psychosocial, was introduced and was followed by a discussion of the physiologic concepts surrounding labor. The muscular activity of the uterus, the primary force in labor, and characteristics and physiology of uterine contractions were explained. The four stages of labor and the mechanisms of labor, that is, the series of passive positional adaptations that the fetus makes on its trip through the birth canal, were discussed in detail. Maternal–placental–fetal physiologic concepts such as blood flow and oxygenation of the fetal unit during labor and more specifically during a contraction were explained.

The latter part of the chapter discussed maternity nursing skills for fetal and maternal assessment, assessment of maternal–fetal response to labor including nursing interventions, and procedures to facilitate labor progression or support maternal–fetal well-being. Electronic fetal monitoring was discussed in detail, along with nursing skills commonly encountered in maternity nursing. Analgesia during labor was discussed briefly. Care of the mother and infant in the third stage, immediately before and after delivery including infant care in the delivery room, was outlined. Apgar scoring and the use of oxytocic drugs was discussed. Psychosocial and biophysical care of the mother in the fourth stage was explained. Table 16.2, a summary of the stages and phases of labor and delivery, incorporates biophysical characteristics, psychosocial characteristics, helpful activities and the role of supportive other.

REFERENCES AND READINGS

Beck, C. T. Patient Acceptance of Fetal Monitoring as a Helpful Tool. *Obstet Gynecol Neonatal Nurs,* 9(6):350, 1980.

Brown, M. S. A Cross-Cultural Look at Pregnancy, Labor and Delivery. *J Obstet Gynecol Neonatal Nurs* 5(5):35, 1976.

Butnarescu, G. F. *Perinatal Nursing—Volume 1—I—Reproductive Health.* New York: John Wiley & Sons, 1978.

Butnarescu, G. F., Tillotson, D. M., Villarreal, P. P. *Perinatal Nursing—Volume 2—Reproductive Risk.* New York: John Wiley & Sons, 1980.

Caldeyro-Barcia, R., Poseiro, J. J. Physiology of the Uterine Contraction. *Clin Obstet Gynecol* 3:386, 1960.

Clark, A. L., Affonso, D. D. *Childbearing: A Nursing Perspective* (2nd ed.). Philadelphia: F. A. Davis, 1979.

Cranston, C. S. Obstetrical Nurses' Attitudes Toward Fetal Monitoring. *J Obstet Gynecol Neonatal Nurs* 9(6):344, 1980.

Dulock, H. L., Herron, M. Women's response to fetal monitoring. JOGN Nursing 5 (suppl): 685–705 (September–October), 1976.

Friedman, E. A. *Labor: Clinical Evaluation and Management* (2nd ed.). New York: Appleton-Century-Crofts, 1978.

Gardner, S. The Mother as an Incubation—After Delivery. *J Obstet Gynecol Neonatal Nurs* 8(3):174, 1979.

Goodin, J. A., Godden, J. O. Chance, G. W. *Perinatal Medicine.* Baltimore: Williams & Wilkins, 1976.

Haire, D. Cultural Warping of Childbirth. *Int Childbirth Assoc* Spring 1972.

Haverkamp, A. D., Thompson, H. E., McFee, J. G., Citrula, C. The Evaluation of Continuous Fetal Heart Rate Monitoring in High-Risk Pregnancy. *Am J Obstet Gynecol* 125:310, 1976.

Hazle, N. Parent's Response to Fetal Monitoring. *Am J Matern Child Nurs* 6(1):32, 1981.

Highley, B. L., Mercer, R. T. Safeguarding the Laboring Woman's Sense of Control. *Am J Matern Child Nurs* 3(1):39, 1978.

Hill, S. T., Shronk, L. K. The Effect of Early Parent–Infant Contact on Newborn Body Temperature. *J Obstet Gynecol Neonatal Nurs* 8(5):287, 1979.

Hon, E. H. *An Introduction to Fetal Heart Rate Monitoring.* Los Angeles: University of Southern California, 1973.

Huff, R. W., Pauerstein, C. J. *Human Reproductive Physiology and Pathophysiology.* New York: John Wiley & Sons, 1979.

Jensen, M. D., Benson, R. C., Bobak, I. M. *Maternity Care.* St. Louis: C. V. Mosby, 1977.

Landry, K. E., Kilpatrick, D. M. Why Shave a Mother Before She Gives Birth? *Am J Matern Child Nurs* 2(3):189, 1977.

Lesser, M. S., Keane, J. R. *Nurse–Patient Relationship in a Hospital Maternity Service.* St. Louis: C. V. Mosby, 1956.

Liu, V. C. Effects of an Upright Position During Labor. *Am J Nurs* 74:2202, 1974.

Pritchard, J., MacDonald, P. C. *Williams Obstetrics* (16th ed.). New York: Appleton–Century–Crofts, 1980.

Roberts, J. E. Maternal Positions for Childbirth. *J Obstet Gynecol Neonatal Nurs* 8(1):24, 1979.

Shannon-Babitz, M. Addressing the Needs of Fathers During Labor and Delivery. *Am J Matern Child Nurs* 4(6):378, 1979.

Starkman, M. Fetal monitoring: Psychologic consequences and management recommendations. *Obstet Gynecol* 50:500–504, 1977.

Whitley, N., Mack, E. Are Enemas Justified for Women in Labor? *Am J Nurs* 80(7): 1339, 1980.

Willson, J. R., Carrington, E. R. *Obstetrics and Gynecology* (6th ed.). St. Louis: C. V. Mosby, 1979.

17

THE NEONATE

The fertilization of a single human cell, an ovum, by a sperm, and the subsequent division of that ovum into trillions of highly specialized cells 9 months later results in the miracle of human birth, the newborn. Although in the 1980s we live in a technologic world full of constantly amazing inventions, no human event or product can rival this synchronized achievement of nature.

During the transition from intrauterine to extrauterine life the neonate must make the adjustment from a warm, dark liquid environment, to one that is often chilly, filled with bright lights, dry and full of new external stimuli. Internal environmental changes are equally dramatic. Conversion from a dependent physiologic state to independent functioning of all human systems calls for massive reorganization in a brief period of time. Probably no other 24-hour period in the life of a normal healthy person is more momentous. Equally important during the first 24 hours is the psychosocial adaptation of the newborn. There seems to be evidence that there is a sensitive period in the first minutes and hours of life during which close contact with mother and father is important for later development to be optimal (Klaus & Kennell, 1976). Although opinions in the literature differ as to when the critical period or periods occur, the fact that *human* interaction very early in life *is* critical is not disputed.

The neonatal period, the first 28 days after birth, represents an extremely critical period for the newborn. In fact, two-thirds of the deaths that occur in the first year of life occur during this 28-day period. This chapter discusses neonatal adjustment to extrauterine life; physiologic adaptation; physical, gestational and behavioral assessment; and infant care giving. In order for maternity nurses to practice effectively, they need to know the predictable patterns of adjustment and the developmental stages of the neonate. This knowledge base allows nurses to provide opportunities for optimum physiologic and psychosocial adjustment, as well as to be alert to deviations from the normal that may call for different actions on the part of the health care team.

ADJUSTMENT TO EXTRAUTERINE LIFE

The First Six Hours

The neonate proceeds through three predictable periods during the first 6 hours of life: *reactivity, inactivity,* and *reactivity* (Arnold, 1965). During the first reactivity period that lasts 15–30 minutes neonates have been observed crying vigorously, sucking their fists, and being alert and interested in the environment. Frequently, the neonate's eyes are open; this provides an optimum opportunity for parental contact. The sucking reflex, which is active, provides a chance to begin breast-feeding. The healthy newborn usually suckles easily during the first 30 minutes, and this is a satisfying experience for both mother and infant. Because this initial 30-minute reactivity period is followed by a relatively inactive period, it is reasonable for the nurse to use this initial active time to enhance mother–infant bonding. The period of inactivity is a state of calm and sleep for the neonate, which is reflected by a decrease in heart rate, respiratory rate, and body temperature. The period of sleep is not a good time to undress or bathe the neonate because of temperature instability. This 30 minute to 2 hour period of inactivity is then followed by a second period of reactivity. The second reactivity period is a time of physiologic stabilization; the infant is awake and alert and heart and respiratory rates increase. This reactivity period lasts from 2 to 6 hours and provides another ideal opportunity for parental contact and interaction. Research in 1971 has shown that mothers who have had an extended period of initial contact with their newborn, have engaged in more eye-to-eye contact and fondling and have showed more reluctance to leave their infants with someone else. This research was reaffirmed by follow-up study a year later (Klaus, 1972). Table 17.1 summarizes the extrauterine adaptations of the healthy neonate in the first 6 hours of life.

TABLE 17.1
EXTRAUTERINE ADAPTATIONS OF HEALTHY NEONATE

Assessment Factor	*Initial Period of Reactivity (First 15–30 Minutes)*	*Period of Inactivity (30 Minutes–2 Hours)*	*Second Period of Reactivity (2–6 Hours)*
Respirations	Irregular, abdominal, shallow Rate rapid (60–90 per minute) Rales, rhonchi, nasal flaring, grunting or thoracic retraction (may be sternal reaction); brief periods of apnea	Rate declines, periods of rapid respirations or dyspnea, clear respiration "barreling" of chest observable	Variable rates related to activity May be rapid respirations and/or irregular with brief periods of apnea
Heart rate	Tachycardia—peak 180, loud and forceful	Heart rate declines to 120–140; increases if crying	Swings from bradycardia to tachycardia, depending on activity and/or stimuli
Color	Brief cyanosis Some acrocyanosis common	Color more pink Flushed when crying	Abrupt color changes, may change from pink to cyanotic quickly
Stool	Present at delivery		Meconium passage
Peristalsis	Absent first 15 minutes	Present May be visible	Variable Sounds increase—bowel cleared of meconium
Temperature	Begins to drop	Continues to fall and reaches low	Begins to rise Variable
Muscle tone and posture	Increase in tone	Upper extremities flexed, lower extended	Relaxed sleep Variable, depending on stimuli
Activity	Alert, eyes open, vigorous	Sleeps—does not respond easily to stimuli	More responsive Variable activity

PHYSIOLOGIC CHARACTERISTICS

Respiratory Adaptation

As mentioned in the introduction, the most profound adjustment of the neonate is from a placental supported, or dependent, system to an independent system, which coincides with initiation of breathing. Respiratory onset is triggered by chemical and thermal factors. In a normal delivery, where the mother has not had a lot of medication or anesthesia, the newborn begins to breathe as the head and chest are delivered. The sudden chilling exposure of the neonate probably stimulates peripheral impulses in the skin that are transmitted to the respiratory center. The fetus leaves an environment of 37°C (98.6°F) in the uterus, and the neonate enters a delivery room with a temperature of 21–23°C (70–75°F). Chemical factors also trigger the neonatal respiratory center. Chemoreceptors in the carotid artery or aorta respond to low oxygen tension (arterial Po_2 decreases from 80 to 15 mm Hg), high carbon dioxide tension (arterial Pco_2 increases from 40 to 70 mm Hg), and low pH (arterial pH below 7.35) by initiating neurologic responses. In most instances, respiratory reaction of the neonate follows within 1 minute of birth.

As the infant takes his or her first breath, negative intrathoracic pressure (up to 50 mm Hg) occurs, and about half of this remains as residual pulmonary volume. The lungs, largely nonfunctional in utero since oxygen and carbon dioxide exchange occurs via the placenta, now respond to the increase in negative pressure and the aveoli are opened. In other words, air is substituted for fluid in the aveoli. Once the aveoli open, further respiration of less force allows them to remain open and respiratory effort stabilizes. Surfactant is a very significant factor in expansion of the aveoli. *Surfactant,* a lipoprotein film produced by the aveolar epithelium, decreases surface tension of the alveoli; it acts like a detergent, reducing the surface tension of fluids. The surface tension effect of surfactant is inversely proportional to the size of the alveoli; that is, the smaller the aveoli the greater the effect of surfactant. This relationship is fortunate since the aveoli decrease in size during expiration. The relationship of surfactant to aveoli must be understood in order to understand respiratory distress syndrome (see Chapter 23). Another factor that affects entry of air into the lungs is the viscosity of fluid in the respiratory tract. As much as 7–24 cc of this fluid is squeezed from the respiratory tract during vaginal delivery (Aladjem et al., 1979). The rest of the fluid is rapidly absorbed by the alveolar capillaries and the lymphatic system. This absorption is accomplished rather easily because of the fact that the lung fluid is less viscous and has a lower protein content than amniotic fluid.

Respirations in the neonate are shallow and irregular and vary from 30 to 60 per minute. Periods of apnea (less than 15 seconds) are normal, but all apneic periods should be evaluated. Neonatal respirations are largely abdominal because of the horizontal position of the ribs. In the adult, the usual lateral and downward position of the ribs is changed to horizontal by contraction of the intercostal muscles, which increases the chest cavity. In the infant, the opposite is true. Since the ribs are already horizontal, contraction of the intercostal muscles (raising the ribs more) decreases chest diameter. The newborn respirations are seen as diaphragmatic—abdominal breathing—since during inspiration the diaphragm is forced downward increasing space for lung expansion (Fig. 17.1). Other differences between the neonate and the adult are that neonates are obligate nose breathers, respiratory secretions are more abundant in neonates, and all openings in the respiratory tract are smaller and therefore more easily collapsed in neonates. The mucous membrane lining of the tract is more delicate in the neonate and more susceptible to trauma. This friability is reflected in the capillary system, which is not fully developed and does not constrict and dilate like an adult's. Because the aveoli are delicate, they are more sensitive to pressure changes. Finally, it is useful to note that the infant's tongue is proportionately large (macroglossia) whereas the trachea and glottis are small. In summary, the contrast between the adult and the neonate is a result of both developmental and neurologic immaturity of the neonate and needs to be understood in order to assess and plan appropriate nursing care.

Circulatory Adaptations

The physiologic cardiovascular changes that occur in the adaptation from fetal to adult circulation have been discussed in detail in Chapter 11. At term the neonate's heart is midway between the crown of the head and the buttocks. By the age of 3, the cardiac

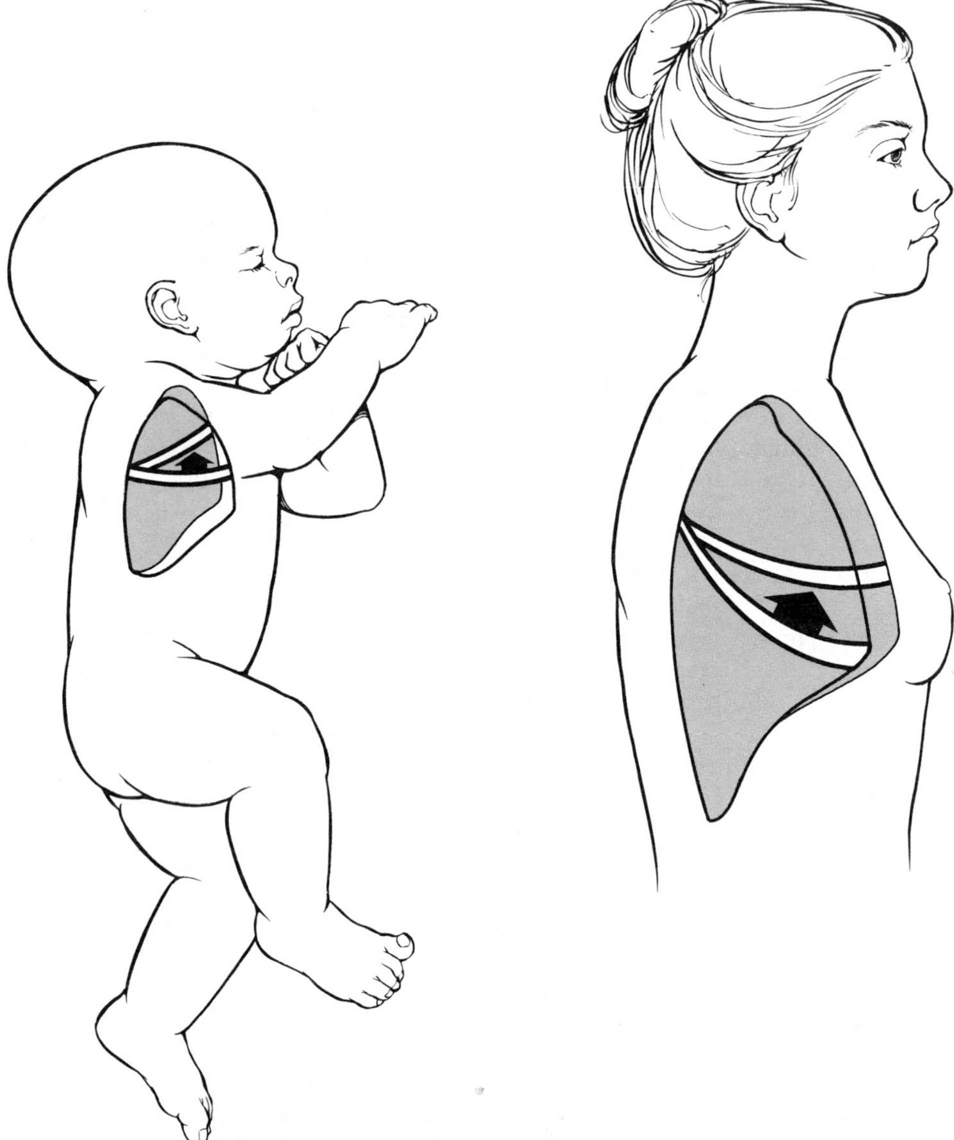

Figure 17.1
Newborn respiratory excursion: neonate versus adult.

shadow on x-ray examination is the same as for the adult. In adulthood the apex of the heart and the point of maximum impulse (PMI) are located in the fifth intercostal space, midclavicular line. Initially, however, the heart is more horizontal, and, as a result, the PMI is located at the third to fourth intercostal space lateral to the midclavicular line.

The heart rate of the newborn is considered normal between 120–160 beats per minute with a peak of 180 being typical during the first 30 minutes of life. By the second day of life, the range is from 90 to 160 beats per minute depending on activity of the neonate. Upon auscultation with a stethoscope, heart sounds in the neonate are higher pitched, stronger, and of shorter duration than those in the adult. It is not unusual to hear a systolic murmur that is caused by incomplete closure of the anatomic shunts and that usually disappears by the end of the first month. Because of the rapid rate and shorter duration of heart beat, accurate counting of neonatal heart rate takes practice. The apical pulse rate should always be counted for at least a full minute.

Hematopoietic Adaptation

Total blood volume of the term neonate ranges from 80 to 110 cc/kg (average after birth 300 cc) and doubles by the end of the first year.

Red blood cell (RBC) count, hemoglobin (Hgb), and hematocrit (Hct) are all significantly higher in the newborn than in the adult. The RBC averages 5 million/mm^3 and depends somewhat on the amount of placental transfusion at birth. If delayed clamping of the cord is practiced, the hemoglobin and hematocrit will be higher. Another factor in the blood count is the source of the sample. Capillary blood, usually obtained from heel or toe, will result in higher values, which are believed to be a result of the sluggish peripheral circulation. Warming the heel before the sample is drawn, as well as discarding the first few drops of blood, improves the accuracy of the sample. The fact remains that capillary samples must not be compared with venous or arterial ones. The high RBC in the fetus assures adequate oxygenation in utero, but few red blood cells are produced for approximately 6–8 weeks after birth so that the RBC falls to 3–4 million/mm^3 by the eighth or tenth week of neonatal life. This state is often referred to as *physiologic anemia.* In the term newborn, fortunately, there are sufficient iron stores to maintain normal red blood cell production for approximately 6 months. There is a decrease in hematocrit and hemoglobin as well as in red blood cells. At birth the average hemoglobin value is 16–18 g/100 cc of blood, the average hematocrit is 45–50% of blood, and the average white blood count is first 20,000/mm^3 and then decreases rapidly. There is a wide range of normal newborn blood values given in the literature. *Bilirubin,* the by-product of red blood cell breakdown, rises in the neonate from a normal level of 1 mg/100 cc of blood to an average of 5 mg/100 cc. This elevation of serum bilirubin occurs on the second to fourth day and results in what is called *physiologic* or *neonatal jaundice.* The buildup of bilirubin in the serum is a result of the fact that the newborn liver is immature and incapable of *conjugating* (changing *insoluble,* or unconjugated bilirubin to conjugated, or *soluble,* bilirubin) large quantities of bilirubin with glucuronic acid for excretion into the bile. Platelet count and aggregation in the neonate are the same as in the adult, and, unless there has been a marked vitamin K deficiency, the blood clots normally. Because vitamin K is synthesized in the gut after production of normal flora (initially the bowel is sterile), the newborn is frequently given a vitamin K preparation intramuscularly after delivery.

Renal, Fluid, and Electrolyte Adaptation

Anatomically, in the neonate all renal system components are present. The bladder is both a pelvic and abdominal organ. The first voiding should occur within the first 24 hours and should be recorded. Although the total urine volume is only 300 cc per 24 hours by the end of the first week, the neonate's bladder involuntarily empties when stretched by 15 cc. For this reason, the neonate may void as many as 20 times a day. The urine of the neonate normally is colorless and odorless and has a specific gravity of about 1.008. Occasionally, the urine of the neonate may cause a brick red stain on the diaper. This is because of limited glomerular function and urate precipitation. Poor phosphate clearance causes excessive uric acid to precipitate as uric acid infarcts, which in turn may block the renal tubules. When this brick red color is noted, fluid intake of the neonate should be increased.

The kidneys of the newborn are not able to concentrate urine and adapt to fluid and electrolyte stress. Nephrons are functionally developed at approximately 1 month. The tubules are short and narrow and do not mature for approximately 5 months, which affects urine concentration. The posterior pituitary production of antidiuretic hormone (ADH), or vasopressin, is also limited. Vasopressin inhibits diuresis, and along with the inability of the immature kidney to concentrate urine, the neonate is susceptible to dehydration.

The term infant is 73% water as compared to the adult who is 58% water. But even more significant is the fact that the neonate has a proportionately higher ratio of extracellular-to-intracellular fluid. Because of this, the neonate has higher levels of total body sodium and chloride and lower levels of potassium, magnesium, and phosphate. There are several other factors that influence fluid and electrolyte balance, namely, the neonatal extracellular fluid rate exchange is seven times greater than the adult. For example, newborns take in and excrete 600–700 cc of water, which is 20% of their body weight and 50% of their extracellular fluid. Adults exchange 2,000 cc of water, which is 5% of their body weight and 14% of their extracellular fluid. As a result, twice as much acid is formed in the neonate, providing a situation where acidosis can occur rapidly. Add to this the infant's rate of metabolism (twice as high as the adult's per body weight) and it is understandable why the neonate has a minimum range of safety. In summary, the renal system of the neonate when compared with that of the adult differs in the following areas: the relationship of extracellular-to-intracellular fluid, rate of exchange of extracellular fluids, composition of body fluids, glomerular filtration rate, and ability to concentrate urine.

Digestive Adaptation

The mucous membrane of the mouth of a term infant is pink and moist. The neonate's ability to eat, digest, and metabolize food at birth is adequate. The gastrointestinal tract is limited functionally in that elasticity, musculature, and control mechanisms continue to develop until age 2–3 when adult level functioning is achieved. The gut of the newborn is proportionately longer than that of the adult and at birth contains no bacteria. This proportionately longer length provides a larger surface area for absorption than in the adult. Within 24 hours, oral and anal orifices permit air and bacteria to enter. Peristalsis and bowel sounds can be auscultated usually an hour after birth. Peristalsis in the esophagus is uncoordinated initially but quickly becomes coordinated in normal infants. The stomach has a capacity of about 90 cc, which increases to 125 cc by 1 month and to 360 cc by 1 year. Since peristalsis is rapid and emptying time is short, food passes quickly through the gastrointestinal tract. It is not unusual for the newborn to have a bowel movement after each feeding. Time and type of feeding, volume, temperature, and psychic stress may all affect feeding and emptying time of the stomach.

Enzymes to digest carbohydrates and proteins are present at birth with the exception of amylaze, which is not produced by the salivary glands until the infant is approximately 3 months. For this reason, polysaccharides are not digested. Deficiency of pancreatic lipase inhibits absorption of fats, especially those fats with a high saturated fatty acid content such as cow's milk. The neonate can digest simple carbohydrates and proteins but has a limited ability to digest fats.

The fact that the liver of the neonate is immature functionally results in several gastrointestinal implications. As mentioned earlier (hematopoietic adaptation), the liver conjugates bilirubin poorly and is deficient in forming plasma proteins, which results in decreased plasma protein concentration. It is thought that this hypoproteinemia contributes to the edema seen in the neonate. A very important consequence of the liver immaturity is deficient gluconeogenesis. Because of this, the blood sugar level in the unfed neonate drops to 30–40 mg/100 cc. Since the brain is dependent on carbohydrates, the importance of early feeding is obvious. Until fed, the neonate is dependent on fat stores for energy. The liver is also deficient in prothrombin and factor VII formation needed for blood coagulation.

Thermoregulation and Adaptation

Heat regulation in the neonate is critical, and although the capacity for heat production is present at birth, it is affected by several important factors. Heat production in the neonate is accomplished by increased metabolic activity, particularly in the heart, brain, and liver, whereas the mechanism for heat production in the adult is shivering. The metabolic rate of the infant is approximately twice that of the adult, and there is a larger body surface to body weight (mass) ratio than in the adult. The significant issue in *thermogenesis* is, therefore, to minimize the difference between heat production and heat loss.

In addition to increased metabolic rate, a source of heat unique to the neonate is *brown fat* (Davis, 1980). Superficial brown fat is located between the scapula, around the neck, and behind the sternum with deeper deposits around the kidneys and adrenals. Brown fat has a rich nerve and blood supply and generates heat that is distributed by the blood as it passes to other body parts. Brown fat reserves, usually present for several weeks after birth, can be rapidly depleted during cold stress.

Heat loss occurs in four ways defined below.

convection—the flow of heat from body surface to cooler environmental air

radiation—the flow of heat from body surface to cooler solid objects not in direct contact

evaporation—the loss of heat when liquid changes to vapor

conduction—the flow of heat from body surface to cooler surfaces in direct contact

Loss of heat, which must be directed toward each of these routes of heat loss, is addressed more specifically in the section on nursing care (p. 382). The infant has only a thin layer of subcutaneous fat and is less able to conserve body heat. Body flexion, the normal neonatal position, reduces body surface area exposed to the environment and is a way of conserving heat.

Cold stress affects all infants and calls upon heat production activity, which, if the cold stress continues, cannot be met. Physiologically, in conditions of continued cold stress, oxygen consumption and energy are diverted from maintaining brain and cardiac functioning to thermogenesis for survival. With decreased oxygenation of tissue, vasoconstriction follows, which jeopardizes pulmonary perfusion. Blood gases become abnormal with decreased PO_2, and increased PCO_2 and decreased pH. The metabolic rate increases to compensate, but if cold stress continues there is anaerobic acidosis and increase in production of acids. The infant can easily go into metabolic acidosis with other complications ensuing; these are discussed more fully in Chapter 23.

Integumentary Adaptation

Immaturity of the integumentary system as well as the other systems discussed poses unique problems. The dermis and epidermis are loosely bound together and very thin. Even slight rubbing can cause separation and blistering. The vernix caseosa is fused with the *stratum corneum* and for this reason should not be removed. The stratum corneum becomes the effective skin barrier.

Caput succedaneum, a localized edematous area of the scalp, is caused by the pressure of the head against the cervix during labor. This pressure compresses blood vessels slowing venous return. The resulting swelling caused by the decrease in venous return, often present at birth, extends across the suture lines of the skull and disappears spontaneously in 2–3 days. (See Chapter 23, Figure 23.9).

Sebaceous (sweat) glands are active in late fetal life and early infancy. Probably because of the hormonal influence of pregnancy, there is some sebaceous gland hyperplasia and, as a result, sebum production. However, as the sebaceous glands are immature, they do not function effectively. Sebaceous glands are located more densely on the scalp, face, and genitalia. Plugging these glands on the face results in *milia* (see discussion of skin in the section on physical examination) and on the scalp causes *cradle cap.* The eccrine glands, which produce sweat in response to heat and emotional stimuli, are initially nonfunctional; they become active in a few days although sweat production is minimal until puberty. This reduction in sweat production prevents fluid loss via evaporation. The skin functions as a barrier to infection, which is fairly effective in the neonate. Since sebum and sweat production is minimal, the skin is dry, decreasing the opportunity for bacterial growth. Only in the genital region, where moisture from urine and feces is present, is the growth of bacteria favored. There are other integumentary manifestations that are unique to the neonate; they are discussed in detail in the physical assessment section of this chapter.

Reproductive Adaptation

In the female neonate there are thousands of primitive germ cells (oocytes) that represent all potential ova that the female will have. The number of ova from birth to maturity decreases by approximately 90%. Mothers' increased estrogen production during pregnancy can cause swelling of breast tissue (breast engorgement) in neonates of either sex. Sometimes a thin discharge from the breast is seen; it is sometimes called *witch's milk.* This engorgement or discharge is of no significance and disappears without treatment as the maternal hormones are eliminated from the newborn's body. Maternal estrogen sometimes causes a mucous vaginal discharge that may contain a small amount of blood called *pseudomenstruation.*

In 90% of male neonates testes are in the scrotum. The incidence of undescended testicle is less than 1% at the end of a year. It is common in the male newborn for the foreskin to adhere to the penis, and it may not be able to be retracted for 1 or 2 weeks. The foreskin (prepuce) is retracted to expose the glans penis during cleansing and is then replaced.

Adaptation Against Infection

Passive immunity in the neonate is dependent on the amount of IgG in the maternal system and the sensitivity to that agent to antibodies. In general, most infants are protected against the major childhood diseases such as diphtheria, measles, and smallpox for approximately 6 months. Pertussis (whooping cough) immunity is rarely sufficient; therefore, protection is given exogeneously to the infant early in the immunization schedule. Breast-fed infants may also receive additional immunity through IgA in early breast secretion colostrum. IgA may promote immunity to such diseases as mumps, polio, influenza, and chickenpox.

Research continues to indicate that the neonate may have a capacity for active immunity (produce antibodies in response to specific antigens), but this response is less vigorous than in the older child or adult. *Opsonins* (complement components and specific antibodies), which facilitate phagocytosis, are present at birth in the term infant. The process of phagocytosis is mature at birth, but the inflammatory response of the tissues to localized infection is immature; the reasons for this are obscure (Whaley & Wong, 1979). The first line of defense, the skin, has been discussed under integument. The reticuloendothelial system, which produces cells capable of attacking pathogens, also plays a role in protection against infection.

Neurologic Adaptation

The nervous system at birth is complete but immature and is incompletely integrated. Initially, most functioning is that of primitive reflexes. Autonomic nervous system functioning is important at birth because it stimulates respiration, assists in acid–base balance, and contributes to temperature control. All cranial nerves are present at birth and all are myelinated except for the olfactory and optic nerves. The brain at birth is 25% of its eventual size and comprises 12% of total body weight. In the adult, the brain is 2.5% of body weight.

Nervous system growth follows a predictable cephalocaudal proximal–distal pattern. In other words, growth and development is from head to toe, from midline to tip of extremity, and is related to observed mastery of gross and fine motor skills. Sensory, cerebellar, and extrapyramidal tracts develop myelin first, which accounts for the acute sense of taste, smell, and hearing in the neonate. Myelin is essential for effective transmission of nerve impulses.

Spontaneous motor activity is noted in transient tremors of mouth, chin, and extremities. Persistent tremors or twitching, especially of the whole body, need to be evaluated for pathologic basis. Some evidence of neurologic control is noted by the fact that when infants are placed on their stomachs, they lift their heads to the side to maintain an airway. Also when in a supine position, raised by their hands and arms off the mattress, they attempt to hold their heads in line with their bodies.

Musculoskeletal Adaptation

The skeletal system of the neonate contains more cartilage than ossified bone. The six skull bones are soft and not yet joined. Between these six bones are areas of bands of connective tissue, called *sutures.* Wider areas of connective tissue, one anteriorly on the skull and one posteriorly at the junction of the sutures, are called *fontanelles.* The sinuses, ethmoidal, maxillary, and sphenoidal are incompletely formed (see p. 361).

In contrast to the skeletal system, the muscular system is almost completely formed. Muscle growth results in hyperplasia, and as muscies increase in size strength increases, providing for the progression of the neonate from lying to rolling to sitting to standing to walking. Integration of musculoskeletal and neurologic systems is necessary for development.

Sensory Functions

Complete differentiation of the fovea centralis does not take place until approximately 4 months of age, at which time the infant's vision is approximately 20/200. Coordination and control of the eyes are immature and the neonate's eyes appear to stray or wonder. Actually, better focus is achieved in the neonate by glancing away, which permits the image to focus more directly on the fovea. The clearest vision appears to be at a distance of 7–8 inches (17–20 cm), which is one reason why the mother's face becomes so significant in the early months. The pupils react to light, and blink and corneal reflexes are present. Lacrimal ducts (tear glands) do not function for 2–4 weeks. Eye color can usually be determined at about 3 months, but pigmentation is not complete for 1 year.

Eye-to-eye contact is extremely significant in mother–infant interaction, and psychosocial aspects are discussed more fully in Chapter 19 (Robson, 1967). It has been determined that at 2 weeks infants can distinguish a pattern with strips one-eighth inch apart, and by 6 months of age an infant's vision is as acute as an adult's (Frantz & Miranda, 1975).

After the amniotic fluid has been drained from the ears, the neonate hears as well as an adult. Some research has shown that high-pitched voices elicit increased motor activity and alertness and low-pitched sounds are soothing (Lang, 1972). At about 2 weeks crying in response to a human voice may cease. More specialized cortical activity related to hearing (or other senses) is dependent on myelination of the neural pathways.

Research regarding smell is limited, but there seems to be evidence that breast-fed infants can detect breast milk and, in some instances, can distinguish their mother's milk from other mothers' milk.

A neonate can distinguish sweet from sour or bitter as determined by facial expression. Taste buds in the early years are located mostly on the tip of the tongue.

There is much evidence indicating that touch is essential for normal growth and development. Behavioral response and development of the neonate received much attention in the 1970s and undoubtedly will continue to be an area of research. There are experts who feel that behavioral assessment is more indicative of cortical control than Apgar scoring and reflex assessment (Brazelton, 1973). In other words, 10 years ago parents were told what to expect of their newborn, whereas today the focus is not only on what to expect but what role their interaction has in their child's development. It is no longer as valid to focus on the sameness of neonates but instead to see each neonate as unique, whose patterns and needs are individual.

ASSESSMENT OF THE NEONATE

In Chapter 16 there is a description of the assessment of the newborn in the delivery room, which includes criteria for Apgar scoring, immediate care of the newborn, and gross physical assessment. Thorough head-to-toe physical, gestational age, and behavioral assessments are important at the earliest possible opportunity. This is usually done in the nursery, ideally under a radiant heater, within the first 2–6 hours after respirations appear stabilized. The activities involved in physical, gestational age, and behavioral assessments may be combined and many neonatal nurses establish a systematic assessment system that incorporates all three areas. We will, however, discuss each assessment separately for clarity.

We include gestational age assessment in this chapter on the normal neonate because of our belief that you need to assess the normal neonate successfully in order to be alert to deviations from the normal. Gestational age assessment is easily performed by the nurse and provides good information for anticipatory guidance, as do all three types of assessment. It is relatively easy for the nurse in the large medical center to validate findings with an intern, resident, clinical specialist, or physician, but in the 50-bed community hospital at three o'clock in the morning when there is often only a nurse, it is important that the assessment skills be performed with skill and confidence. Repeated practice with normal infants improves this skill.

Although there is individuality among nurses in the way they assess infants, there must also be consistency. In any physical examination, the four techniques of observation, percussion, palpation, and auscultation are used. Moreover, the assessment process must include all facets of the examination and, in most instances, the assessment is carried out head to toe. It is suggested for the beginner that a head-to-toe, proximal-to-distal pattern be used as a way of assuring that no step is missed. It is usually wise to listen to heart, lungs, and abdomen first since undressing the neonate may initiate crying. It is useful to do head, chest, and length measurements at the same time since it reinforces the relationship of these measurements. To weigh the infant, place the unclothed infant on the scale after it has been balanced with a cloth or paper barrier as shown in Figure 17.2a. During assessment, the neonate may need to be picked up and cuddled, provided with a pacifier (nipple), or allowed to suck on the examiner's gloved finger to soothe him or her when fussy. These general strategies, which may or may not be adopted, have been found useful by other nurses. The point we wish to reinforce is that you establish a routine that promotes efficiency of time and energy and eliminates omission of specifics that are important in the examination.

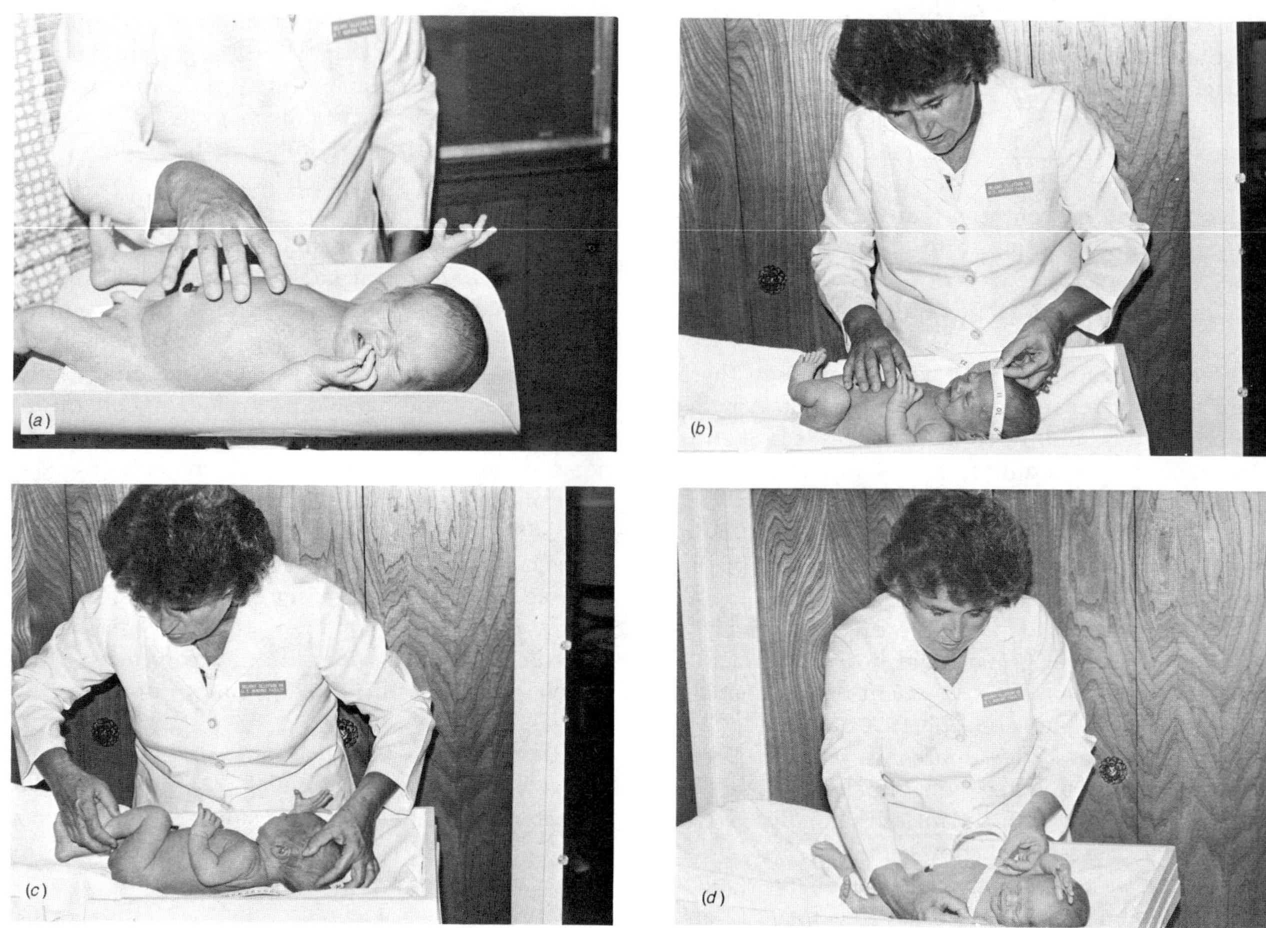

Figure 17.2
(a) Weighing the infant; *(b)* measuring the head; *(c)* measuring the crown–rump length; *(d)* measuring the chest.

PHYSICAL EXAMINATION

A general evaluation of appearance, posture, maturity, activity, and overall well-being is made at the beginning of the physical examination. In other words, how does this neonate look? Are color and respirations all right? Does the neonate seem to be a term infant? Is the cry normal? The skill needed to appraise normalcy quickly comes with experience and reflects back to what was discussed in the teaching–learning chapter in relation to nursing process. The nurse who says, "this is an O.K. newborn" actually has processed a huge amount of data, evaluated the infant, and arrived at this conclusion because of a reliable knowledge base. Nursing practice is not intuitive; it is based on logical and methodical processing of data using theory and knowledge appropriately.

Appearance

Posture, color, and behavior are all part of the neonate's appearance. The position of the normal neonate born from a vertex presentation is flexion, which is a consequence of his position in the uterus. The arms and legs are flexed at the elbows and knees, respectively, and the hands are in a clenched or fisted position. The chin rests on the chest, and the hips are flexed so that the thighs are on the lower abdomen. Infants who do not assume a position of flexion should be evaluated for an abnormal position in utero such as breech, for prematurity, or for hypoxia.

In general, color of the neonate becomes more reddish-pink during crying. An infant that is experiencing a temperature decrease will appear cyanotic because of vasoconstriction. Acrocyanosis is observed when the hands and feet are bluish and the rest of the infant is pink. This occurs quite commonly in the newborn and is thought to be caused by venous stasis and not hypoxia. *Harlequin sign* is when a transient pink color appears on half of the body, the midline being the dividing point. When the infant is placed on the side, the infant demonstrating Harlequin sign is noticeably pinker on the dependent side than on the superior half. Although not common, this is seen sometimes between 48–96 hours after birth. This condition has no known physiologic basis and is not seen when the infant is prone or supine. Color changes have to be evaluated, keeping in mind ethnic background. Neonatal behavior should be carefully noted. Is the infant alert, drowsy, or irritable? Does the infant respond positively to being held or cuddled? Is the infant startled by loud noises? In other words, the nurse needs to determine if behavioral responses are expected and normal.

Measurements

Measurements of the neonate are important individually, in relation to other measurements, and in relation to graphs or tables that represent national norms. Many basic measurements, such as height and weight, are graphed from the neonatal period through the first year and longer. Average head size is 35.5 cm (13–14 in.) and may be smaller initially because of molding. Chest circumference is 30.5–33.0 cm (12–13 in.). In general, the head is 2–3 cm (1 in.) larger than the chest. On initial assessment, the chest and head numbers may be the same, again because of molding. A significant difference, that is, the head much larger or smaller than the chest, may indicate *hydrocephalus* (distention of the cerebral ventricles with cerebrospinal fluid from obstruction within the ventricular system) or *microcephalus* (characterized by a small head whose circumference is less than two standard deviations below mean for age and sex). The premature or malnourished infant often has a much larger head circumference than chest; this is because of a decreased chest size (German et al., 1976). Probably the more reliable comparison is that of the crown-to-rump length to head circumference; they should be approximately equal. *Crown-to-rump length* (or sitting height) is 31–35 cm (12.5–14.0 in.). Head-to-heel measurement of the neonate is also done, and the nurse needs to be sure to extend the leg. The average newborn length is 48–53 cm (19–21 in.). The normal neonate weighs between 2,700–4,000 gm (6–9 lb); term newborns weighing less than 2,500 gm (5.5 lb) are considered low birth weight. The relationship of weight to gestational age is of more significance than weight alone and will be discussed in detail later in this chapter. Newborns lose approximately 10% of their body weight the first 3–4 days; this loss is because of excessive extracellular fluid and meconium loss combined with limited food intake. Neonates are generally back to birth weight by their tenth day.

Vital signs are another important category of measurement. Axillary temperatures should be taken. The only rationale for a rectal temperature is to check anal patency, which can best be assessed by observation. If a rectal temperature is taken, it must be done carefully with only the tip of the thermometer inserted and the nurse supporting and holding the infant's legs during the entire procedure. Not only is the rectum very small, but the mucosa can be perforated if the procedure is not done correctly. Axillary temperatures range from 35.5 to 37.0°C (97.6–98.6°F). Pulse and respirations should be taken for a full minute, and the heart rate should be auscultated apically. Heart rate is usually 120–160 beats/min and respiratory rate 30–60.

Heart and Lungs

Respirations in the neonate, as mentioned earlier, are chiefly abdominal, irregular in depth and rate, and with occasional periods of apnea. The average respiratory rate is 30–60 breaths per minute and can be assessed through observation. Auscultation of breath sounds is difficult because the chest is so small and cardiac and bowel sounds are transmitted to all parts of the pleural cavity. Auscultation should be practiced; the beginner sometimes finds it useful to auscultate by dividing the chest into four quadrants and listening both anteriorly and posteriorly. Bronchial breath sounds should be auscultated bilaterally in the midaxillary line. *Rales* may be heard soon after birth and may indicate areas of atelectasis. *Ronchi* are sometimes caused by fluid in the larger bronchi. These may be important if aspiration of feeding is feared.

The heart rate is normally from 120 to 160 beats/min and may range from 100 to 180 beats/min in the early hours of life. The apex is palpated or auscultated in the third or fourth intercostal space. Differentiation of specific heart sounds is difficult, but the first and second heart sounds should be clearly heard; the second sound is characteristically described as somewhat higher in pitch and sharper than the first sound. Murmurs are not unusual in the neonate; they should always be noted and recorded, however. Murmurs are usually a result of incomplete closure of fetal structures and are usually heard at the base of the heart or at the left sternal border in the third or fourth interspace.

Skin

Skin assessment of the neonate provides normal variations that introduce a descriptive vocabulary largely unique to the newborn. The vocabulary and definitions are listed below for quick reference.*

acrocyanosis—symmetric mottled cyanosis of the hands and feet associated with coldness

cutis marmorata—blue or purple mottling of the skin

ecchymosis—extravasion of blood into the subcutaneous tissues; discoloration of the skin; commonly referred to as a bruise

erythema toxicum neonatorum—pink, papular rash with vesicles, superimposed mottling

Harlequin sign—a sign of transient vasomotor disturbance in young infants; flushing of the body on the dependent side and pallor on the upward side

hemangioma—an angioma made up of blood vessels

***jaundice* (icterus)**—yellowness of the skin, mucous membranes and secretions

lanugo—the downlike hair that covers the fetus from about the fifth month of gestation

milia—a minute epidermal cyst; appear as white papules mostly on the nose, chin, and cheeks

mongolian spot—a focal bluish-gray discoloration of the skin of the lower back, aberrantly on the face, present at birth and fades gradually

nevus—any lesion containing melanocytes, a birthmark

pallor—paleness, especially of the skin and mucous membranes

petechiae—minute, rounded spots of hemorrhage on a surface such as skin or mucous membrane or on cross-sectional surface of an organ

telangiectasis—dilatation of groups of capillaries

vernix caseosa—a cheesy deposit of grayish white substance on the surface of the fetus; may have insulating and protective functions

Head

Assessment of the head is important since molding occurs in almost all vaginal deliveries. In other words, not until 1 or 2 days postdelivery does the head assume its normal round shape. Because the bones of the cranium are not fused, the skull adapts to the birth passage during labor, and on palpation you can often feel overriding or overlapping of the sutures of the skull. Figure 17.3 illustrates skull landmarks on the infant's head.

The nurse palpates all bones and sutures, which feel like cracks between the bones. The anterior fontanel is diamondlike in shape, and the skull sutures do not approximate one another. The posterior fontanel is smaller and triangular and may be closed because of the molding. The tip of the index finger is used to trace the sutures and the fontanels. Two other masses found on the skull are important to note: *caput succedaneum* and *cephalhematoma. Cephalhematoma* is a clearly outlined fluctuant mass caused by extravasation of blood between a scalp bone and the periosteum. Cephalhematoma usually appears on the first or second day of life and are most common over the parietal bone. In contrast to *caput succedaneum,* which is present at birth, does cross suture lines, and disappears quickly, cephalhematoma does not appear immediately, does *not* cross suture lines, and may last several weeks or even months. Differentiation of these is important in order to provide anticipatory guidance to parents. Neither condition requires treatment. (See Figure 23.9.)

Eyes, Ears, Nose

The eyes of the infant should be examined for symmetry and *hypertelorism* (excessive width between two organs or parts). Distance between the inner canthi

*Definitions are from *McGraw-Hill Nursing Dictionary,* 1979.

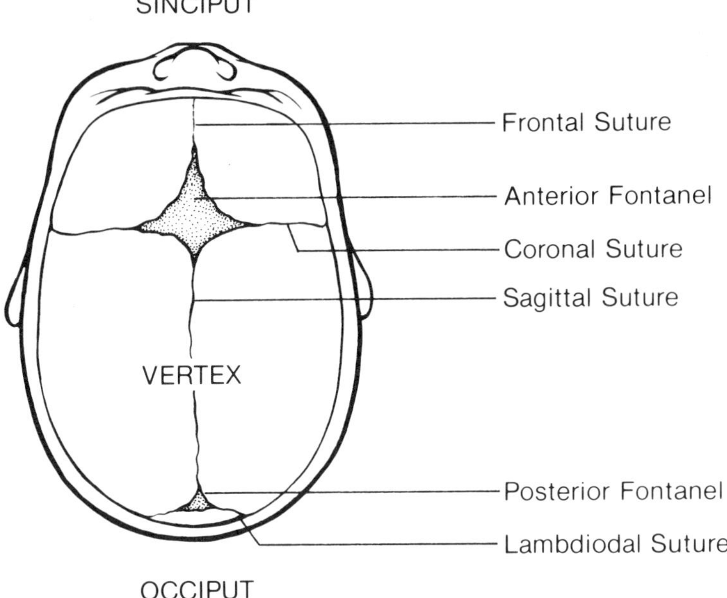

Figure 17.3
Skull landmarks on the infant's head.

greater than 3 cm is considered to be ocular hypertelorism (Laestadius et al. 1969). The mean distance is 2 cm. As newborns usually keep their eyes tightly closed, when checking the eyes it is useful to hold them supine and slowly lower their heads. Usually the eyes will open and the sclera can be observed for conjunctival hemorrhage. This is common and occurs during the stress of labor; it requires no treatment and disappears spontaneously. Although corneal reflex is present, it is not routinely elicited in the normal newborn. The pupils should react to light by constricting, and a red reflex should be elicited to rule out congenital cataracts. Until 6 months of age, occasional strabismus is common. Sometimes discharge is observed and should be noted; purulent discharge related to infection or chemical irritation as a result of silver nitrate instillation needs to be assessed.

The infant's nose, after birth, is quite flat, and patency can be assessed by occluding one naris at a time. Sneezing is common in neonates; it is their way of blowing their noses. Flaring of the nares, the earliest sign of respiratory distress, should always be noted and reported immediately.

The ear should be examined for position, structure, and function. The top of the pinna should be in line with the outer canthus of the eye (or above it). (Low set ears are associated with mental retardation and renal anomalies.) An infant with intact hearing will respond to a loud, sharp noise with a startle reflex. Presence and extent of cartilage formation is discussed under gestational age assessment.

Reflexes often assessed at this time in the assessment process are as follows.

▲ ***Moro Reflex.*** Elicited by sudden jarring or change in equilibrium. The response of the neonate is extension and abduction of the extremities and fanning of the fingers with the index and thumb forming a "c" followed by flexion and abduction of extremities. Persistance of the Moro reflex past 6 months may indicate brain damage. This reflex is strongest in the first 2 months. Asymmetric Moro is associated with injury to clavicle or injury to the brachial plexus (see Chapter 23).

▲ ***Startle Reflex.*** Elicited by a loud noise. The response is abduction of the arms with flexion of elbows and the hands remaining clenched. It disappears by 4 months.

▲ ***Pupillary Reflex.*** Elicited by shining bright light. Response is constriction of pupil. Remains throughout life. Unequal constriction or fixed dilated pupil requires further assessment.

- ▲ ***Blink Reflex.*** Elicited by bright light or object approaching the eye. Persists throughout life.
- ▲ ***Doll's Eye.*** Elicited by moving the head slowly to right or left, eyes normally do not move. Disappears as fixation develops.
- ▲ ***Sneeze Reflex.*** Spontaneously elicited by newborn in response to irritation or obstruction. Persists throughout life.

Mouth and Throat

One of the most significant reasons for inspecting the mouth is to assess for cleft palate. (See Chapter 23.) This is done by observation, using a small flash light, and by palpation. There are also normal variations that are important to know and describe. The following are important areas of assessment.

- ▲ ***Teeth.*** Rarely are present, but may be and if loose need to be removed.
- ▲ ***Epstein's Pearls.*** Small, white epithelial cysts located either side of the midline of the hard palate. They are insignificant.
- ▲ ***Inclusion Cysts.*** Gray, round lesions on the gum margins that are sometimes mistaken for teeth; disappear in a few weeks.
- ▲ ***Monilia.*** Appear as flat, white spots that look like milk but do not rub off (contracted from infected birth canal during delivery). Monilial infection requires medical treatment.
- ▲ ***Frenulum.*** A thin ridge of tissue that goes from the base of the tongue in the midline to the lingual surface of the mouth. If the frenulum is attached near the tip of the tongue, it sometimes is of concern to parents and may restrict protrusion of the tongue but does not hinder sucking, feeding, or speech.
- ▲ ***Frenum.*** Tissue that attaches under the inner surface of the upper lip to the maxillary aveolar ridge. Can be observed during smiling or yawning.
- ▲ ***Uvula.*** The conical appendix hanging from the free edge of the soft palate is best observed when the neonate is crying.

Reflexes assessed during mouth and throat assessment are as follows.

- ▲ ***Extrusion Reflex.*** Elicited by touching or depressing the tongue; the neonatal response is to force the tongue out. Constant protrusion of the tongue may suggest trisomy 21 (see Chapter 24).
- ▲ ***Yawn Reflex.*** Can be spontaneously elicited by the neonate in response to decreased oxygen by increasing amount of inspired air. Persists throughout life.
- ▲ ***Cough Reflex.*** Elicited by irritation to mucous membrane, larynx, or trachea. Present after the first day and persists throughout life.
- ▲ ***Sucking Reflex.*** Can be elicited by placing a nipple or a gloved finger in the mouth. Persists throughout infancy.
- ▲ ***Rooting Reflex.*** Elicited by stroking the cheek; the response of the neonate is to turn head to the side stimulated and to suck. Disappears at about 4 months.
- ▲ ***Gag Reflex.*** Not routinely elicited but present and observed during suctioning or sometimes feeding. Persists throughout life.

Neck

The newborn's neck appears short because it is usually covered by folds of skin. Allowing the head to fall back while supporting the back makes assessment possible. The clavicles should be palpated for a mass that may indicate fracture. Careful palpation along the bone may elicit crepitation. Infants with a fractured clavicle will have an asymmetrical moro reflex; they typically will not raise the arm on the affected side (see Chapter 23). Another finding, which is uncommon, is torticollis, a deformity of the neck most commonly a result of contraction of the sternocleidomastoid muscle unilaterally. This may be observed or palpated during neck assessment as a muscle mass.

Abdomen

The abdomen appears as rounded and prominent since the abdominal musculature is not developed. The umbilical cord should be carefully inspected for two arteries and one vein, as well as for any signs of infection. Appearance of the cord at birth should be bluish-white and glistening. The liver is usually palpable 2–3 cm below the ribs (right costal margin). Kidneys can be palpated by the trained examiner by flexing the legs (to relax the abdomen); they are normally located 1–2 cm above the umbilicus. The bladder can be palpated and percussed if distention is observed or suspected. The newborn should void in the first 24 hours. Femoral pulse palpation is part of the abdominal exam; pulses should be strong and bilaterally equal.

Genitalia

In both sexes, genitalia should be inspected for any anomalies. In the female infant the urethra should be located below the clitoris. In the male infant location of the urethral opening is ascertained to rule out *hypospadias* (opening on the ventral side of the penis) or *epispadias* (opening on the dorsal surface of the penis) (Fig. 17.4). Normally the *prepuce* (foreskin) is tight and cannot be retracted. Smegma, a white cheesy substance, is frequently seen around the glans penis. The scrotum is observed and palpated to ascertain if the testes have descended.

Back and Rectum

The infant should be placed in a prone position and the spine inspected for abnormal openings or masses after the head-to-toe assessment with the infant supine (spina bifida and pilonidal sinus are discussed in Chapter 23). The spine of the neonate is gently rounded (not the S curve of the adult). When stroked along the back on one side of the vertebral column, infants will move their hips to the stimulated side (see trunk incurvation reflex, p. 364). The infant should pass meconium stool in the first 24 hours, which indicates anal patency. If anal fissures (cracks) are present, they can be observed by gently separating the buttocks with the infant in the prone position. Anal fissures can be caused by constipation; asymmetry of the sphinctal mucosa is suspicious of fissures.

Extremities

Symmetry, range of motion, muscle tone, and signs of malformation are all part of the assessment of the extremities. Although *polydactyly* (extra digits) and *syndactyly* (fusion of digits) are usually part of the delivery room assessment, toes and fingers should be assessed again carefully. Range of motion and hyper- or hypoflexibility of joints are noted. Nail beds are observed; their color gives an indication of oxygenation (they should be pink). Yellowing of the nail requires further assessment in relation to intrauterine distress or postmaturity. Creases on the palms of the hands and soles of the feet are important and are discussed under gestational age assessment. The most frequent sources of fracture are the clavicles, humerus, and femur, where visible deformity or limitation of movement may be seen. (See Chapter 23.)

Hip dislocation is carefully assessed by two maneuvers called Ortolani's sign and Allis's sign. *Ortolani's sign* is demonstrated by an audible click

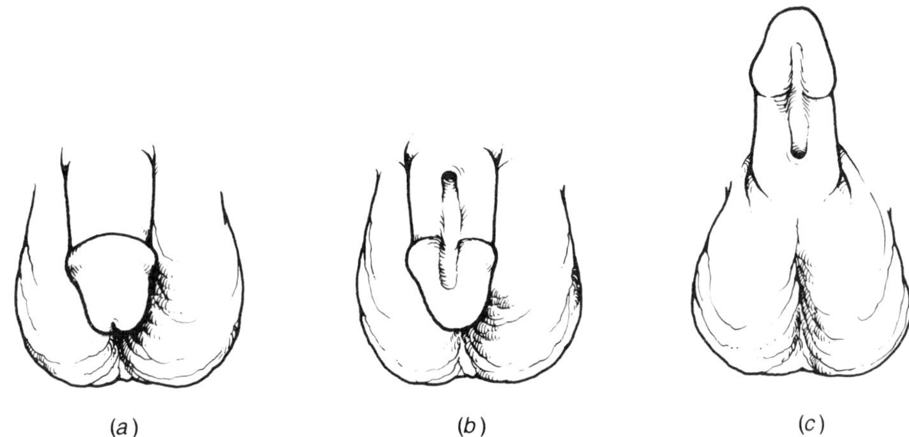

Figure 17.4
(a) Normal urethra; *(b)* epispadias; *(c)* hypospadias.

on abduction. With the infant supine, flex the legs at the hips and knees and abduct at least 175 degrees or almost flat on the mattress. If abduction is limited and/or the click is heard, hip dislocation is suspected. Another way to check or validate hip dislocation is with the infant prone; extend the legs and check gluteal and leg folds for symmetry. The folds are asymmetrical in congenital dislocated hip. *Allis's sign,* shortening of the affected leg, is demonstrated with the neotate supine; flex the hips and knees and place the neonate's feet flat on the table. The knee on the affected side (where the hip is dislocated) is higher.

Reflexes assessed during examination of the extremities are as follows.

- ▲ ***Grasp Reflex.*** Elicited by touching palms of hands or soles of feet near the base of the digits. Response is flexion of toes or fingers. Replaced by voluntary movement by 8 months of age.
- ▲ ***Babinski's Reflex.*** Can be elicited by beginning at the heel and stroking upward along lateral aspect of sole and across the ball of the foot. The response is hyperextension or fanning of toes. Disappears after 1 year of age.

Generalized reflexes assessed during physical examination, in addition to Moro andStartle included earlier, are as follows.

- ▲ ***Tonic Neck Reflex.*** Elicited with neonates on their backs (supine). As the head is turned quickly to one side, the arm and leg on that side extend and the opposite arm and leg remain flexed. Disappears by 4 months.
- ▲ ***Perex Reflex.*** Elicited with infant prone on firm surface by pressing thumb along spine from neck to sacrum. Response is crying, flexing of extremities, and raising head and pelvis. Disappears by 6 months.
- ▲ ***Neck-Righting Reflex.*** Elicited with infant supine; head is turned to one side. The shoulders and trunk will turn followed by pelvis. Disappears by 10 months.
- ▲ ***Trunk Incurvation Flex (Galant Reflex).*** Elicited with infant prone by stroking alongside the spine. Expected response is that the hips will move to stimulated side. Disappears by 4 weeks.
- ▲ ***Otolith-Righting Reflex.*** Elicited by tilting the body of erect infant. Response is infant's head will return to upright, erect position.
- ▲ ***Dance or Step Reflex.*** Elicited by holding infant so that foot touches a hard surface. The response is flexion and extension of the leg as if the infant is walking. Disappears after 4 weeks.
- ▲ ***Crawling Reflex.*** Elicited by placing infant prone. Expected response is a crawling movement with arms and legs. Disappears by 6 weeks.

Table 17.2 summarizes physical assessment of the newborn including implications for the nurse.

Gestational Age Assessment

Gestational age assessment, that is, the determination of gestational age by physical examination, is best determined between 2 and 8 hours of age. The infant needs about 2 hours to recover from the stress of birth, and after 48 hours some responses change significantly. In 1977 Dubowitz and Dubowitz first described the procedure for assessment. They described the results of the assessment done by trained nurses, which showed that when taught correctly, nurses can accurately determine gestational age by examination of the newborn. There are vocabulary terms important to the understanding gestational age assessment.

Preterm (premature)—neonate born before 37-weeks gestation (conception to 37 weeks)

Term—neonate born between 38 and 42-weeks gestation (start of week 38 through week 42)

Postterm—neonate born after 42-weeks gestation (start of week 43)

There is a normal weight range for each gestational week. An infant is classified as large for gestational age (LGA) if at any week his or her weight is above the ninetieth percentile, which indicates two or more standard deviations above the norm. An infant is classified as small for gestational age (SGA) if at any week his or her weight is below the tenth percentile, which indicates two or more standard deviations below the norm. If the newborn's weight falls between the tenth and the ninetieth percentiles at any

TABLE 17.2
NEONATE SUMMARY ASSESSMENT

Assessment	*Usual Findings*	*Common Deviations*	*Abnormalities*	*Nursing Actions*
General appearance	Posture—flexion of head and extremities Readily assumes prenatal position Resists extension Moves all extremities Moro reflex	Frank breech—extended legs, flattened head Quivering or momentary tremors	Limp posture Extension of extremities Paralysis Hypotonia Tremors, twitches, and myoclonic jerks	*Record all assessment; record and report any abnormalities or deviations* Observe resting posture Look for symmetry of movement
Apical pulse	120–160 beats/min Regular rate changes with activity	Murmurs sinus arrhythmia Irregular rhythm following physical or emotional stimulus	Sounds of poor quality Extra sounds Dextrocardia Persistent tachycardia (>170) or bradycardia (<120)	Take heart rate apically and count for full 60 seconds Pulse rate should be related to activity, i.e., sleeping, crying Quality should be sharp, clear First sound—closure of mitral and tricuspid valves Second sound—closure of aortic and pulmonic valves
Breath sounds	Lusty cry, 30–60 breaths/minute; varies with activities Abdominal respirations/nasal breather Bilateral bronchial breath sounds Shallow, effortless, quiet, symmetrical chest and abdominal movement	Increases with crying Rate and depth may be irregular Momentary apneic spells < 15/sec Rales shortly after birth	Apnea > 15 sec Dyspnea rate ↓20 Rate ↑160 when quiet Persistent irregular breathing Repeated apneic spells Grunting respirations Deep sighing respiration Seesaw respirations Persistent fine rales Rhonchi Diminished breath sounds	Respiratory rate should be taken for full 60 seconds Respirations can be noted by observation or ausculation by stethoscope Respiratory rate should be related to activity of infant
Blood pressure	Systolic, 50–80 mm Hg Diastolic, 40–50 mm Hg	Varies with activity level	Low BP Hypovolemic shock	Size and width of cuff affects accuracy of reading; 1-inch cuff and palpation of radial pulse can be done Blood pressure readings relate to activity

TABLE 17.2 (continued)

Assessment	*Usual Findings*	*Common Deviations*	*Abnormalities*	*Nursing Actions*
Axillary temperature	97.5–98.6°F (36.4–37.0°C) Heat loss by evaporation, convection, conduction, and radiation	Elevated temperature—room too hot or overdressed Subnormal temperature may indicate low environmental temperature, inadequate clothing	Elevated temperature—too hot (room or clothes), dehydration, sepsis, brain damage Subnormal temperature with infection, brain damage, cold	Should be taken for at least 3 minutes Parent teaching should include how to take temperature and read thermometer and possible causes of elevated temperatures
Skin	COLOR Cyanotic at birth →↑ Pink 1 minute Later dependent upon ethnicity Vernix caseosa, milia, lanugo Edema—eyes, face, legs, hands, feet, scrotum or labia TURGOR Skin returns to its former position after release of grasp between thumb and index finger	Acrocyanosis, plethora when crying Harlequin color change Mongolian spots (infants of black, Oriental, and American Indian) Petechiae caused by birth trauma—usually on head or presenting part Mottling Erythema toxicum neonatorum (newborn rash) Desquamation Jaundice after first 24 hours (i.e., bilirubin level), nose, face, abdomen, and legs Telangiectasis (stock bites or capillary hemangiomas) Ecchymosis (bruises from trauma) Forcep marks	Generalized cyanosis Grayness Pallor Petechiae that persists and purpura indicates hemorrhagic tendency Tinted vernix caseosa Nevus Cafe au lait Jaundice within first 24 hours is pathologic (i.e., bilirubin level >12 mg/100 ml blood) Hemangiomas (vascular tumors) Nevus flammens (port wine stain) Strawberry mark Cavernous hemangiomas	Inspect skin in well-lighted area Avoid drafts Discuss with parents all normal newborn skin changes and variations To check for jaundice (hyperbilirubinemia) blanch over bony prominences, e.g., forehead, sternum For all birthmarks, inspect and palpate; record location, size, distribution, characteristics, color
	TEXTURE Smooth, soft, may have dry hands and feet	Generalized cracked and peeling skin May be SGA–LGA or postmature	Papules, pustules, ulcers	Assess gestational age Check maternal history
Head (shape and size)	33–35 cm (13–14 in.) circumference (2–3 cm larger than chest) Round, symmetrical, moves easily Fontanel—flat, solt, and	Molding may decrease circumference Head and chest may be equal for 1–2 days after birth Asymmetry	<32 cm—microcephaly >38 cm—macrocephaly or ≥4 cm more than chest	Measure circumference Compare head and chest measurements Record measurements on growth chart Inform parents of any

	firm Anterior fontanel diamond-shaped, 2.5–4.0 cm (1.00–1.75 in.) Posterior fontanel triangular shaped 0.5—1.0 cm. (0.2–0.4 in.) Sutures—felt as flat ridges, may feel open	Fontanel—bulging because of crying Posterior may be closed Sutures—may be overriding because of molding Caput succedaneum Cephalhematoma Petechiae over scalp Scalp probe lesion (from fetal monitor or scalp pH)	SUTURES Fused—craniosynastosis Widened—hydrocephaly	common deviations (caput) as a result of birth process and when they will disappear Discuss with parents closure times of fontanels Dispel myths about soft spot Check hydration status Instruct parents on care of head and scalp
	Head lag while sitting, but momentary ability to hold head erect			Marked head lag Instruct parents about need for head support
	Hair—smooth and fine texture	Hair amounts vary Texture relates to ethnicity		Coarse, brittle, dry Instruct parents on care of hair
Face	Symmetry between left and right side	Asymmetry from uterine molding	Congenital malformation Hemiplegia Movement of only one side when crying—facial nerve palsy	Assess symmetry—record and/or report lack of symmetry Assess for signs of chromosomal aberrations
Ears	Position—top of pinna on horizontal line with outer canthus or eye Well formed Pinna flexible, cartilage present Startle reflex elicited by loud, sudden noise	Preauricular papillomas Pinna flat against head, crumpled Inability to visualize tympanic membrane because of filled canals	Low placement—malformation Nodules Cysts Sinus tracts No response to sound	Assess for trisomy 13 or 18 if ears are low set of renal anomalies
Nose	Midline of face Flattened Nasal patency Discharge—thin white mucous Sneezing	Bruised Milia Telangiectatic nevus on bridge	Deviated to right or left Malformation Nonpatent choanalatresia Thick blood discharge Flaring of nares—respiratory distress	Assess for patency of nares by occluding one and then the other
Eyes	Symmetric size, shape, movement, and placement on face in relation to each other		Centered or deviated to right or left Agenesis—absence of one or both	

TABLE 17.2 (continued)

Assessment	Usual Findings	Common Deviations	Abnormalities	Nursing Actions
	Lids edematous Bluish-white sclera Usually closed	Discoloration and swelling because of silver nitrate Telangiectatic nevus on lids	Drooping eyelids (ptosis) Marked edema Mongoloid slant/Brushfield's spots Jaundiced sclera	Assure parent that strabismus (deviation of the eye from a normal positon of focus) is normal up to 6 months
	Color—slate grey, dark blue, brown Absence of tears No discharge Red reflex present Pupillary reflex Blink reflex Follow objects to midline/momentarily focuses Doll's eyes (when head is turned eye movement lags behind)	Subconjunctival hemorrhages Searching hystagmus or strabismus Moderate discharge because of silver nitrate Pseudostrabismus	Pink color of iris Congenital cataracts Purulent discharge No red reflex No pupillary reflex—constricted or dilated fixed pupil, unequal Inability to follow to midline "Setting-sun" (hydrocephaly) Upward slant, epicanthal folds	Assess for other signs of disease or congenital anomalies (trisomy 21, cri-du-chat) (see Chapter 24)
Mouth	Intact high-arched palate, uvula in midline Frenulum of tongue Gums pink Absent or minimal salivation Sucking pads in cheeks Tongue pink, mobile, does not protrude	Short frenulum Inclusion cysts Epstein's pearls Transient circumoral cyanosis	Cleft palate Frenulum extending to tip of tongue (may interfere with sucking) Precocious teeth Salivation excessive and frothy (tracheoesophageal fistula) Tongue large and thick (macroglossia) Down's syndrome Thrush	Exploration and referral for parents if anomalies assessed Reassure about normal deviation such as Epstein's pearls Differentiate between mild curd and thrush Assess tongue movement and reassure parents it can vary Assess reflexes (sucking, rooting) Assess for abnormalities
	Lips pink, symmetrical movement Reflexes present Sucking, rooting gag, extrusion, range of motion	Lips may have transient circumoral cyanosis Reflexes dependent on hunger, wakefulness	Cleft lip Loss of sucking reflex Micrognathia—Pierre Robin's or other syndrome	
Neck	Short, straight, thick, full range of motion	Transient deformity from position in utero	Torticollis (wry neck) Masses, cysts	Assess for congenital anomalies (Turner's

	Turns head to side when prone Trachea midline Reflexes—tonic neck, neck-righting, otolith-righting, head lag while sitting—momentarily able to hold head erect	Head can be moved passively Marked head lag Abnormally short neck	Distended veins Edema Absence of reflexes Opisthotonus Turner's syndrome, trisomy 18 or 21 (see Chapter 24)	syndrome, trisomy 18 or 21)
	Clavicle symmetrical Thyroid not palpable		Clavicles asymmetrical or fractured	Can be assessed by palpation and suspected by asymmetrical Moro reflex
Thorax	Almost circular and symmetric Xiphoid process evident Circumference 30.5–33.0 cm (12–13 in.) 2–3 cm smaller than head	Circumference—may exceed head circumference in large infants (over 8½ lbs)	Asymmetric, check expansion Depressed sternum Marked retractions of chest and intercostal area Funnel chest Pigeon chest Barrel chest	Assess respiratory and circulatory signs Assess for disease or congenital syndrome
Breasts	Breast enlargement 3–10 mm Nipples symmetrical, prominent, well formed (approximately 6 mm)	Secretion of milky substance (witch's milk) Supernumerary nipples Breast nodule 3–10 mm Engorgement	Redness and firmness around nipples Asymmetrical placement of nipples Lack of breast tissue (prematurity)	Reassure parents that breast engorgement is normal
Abdomen	Cylindrical in shape and prominent No distention Bowel sounds 1 hour after birth Femoral pulse Symmetrical	Diastasis recti (due to poor muscle development) Visible veins Visible peristalsis	Scaphoid or concave Asymmetry Distention Localized bulging—hernia or distended vein Gastroschisis	Teach parents about feeding Auscultate bowel sounds Assess passage of meconium Appraise for hip Dysplasia, color, temperature, or mottling of legs Palpate femoral pulses with hand flexed on infant's hips; palpate along inguinal ligament, halfway between symphysis pubis and iliac crest; palpate bilaterally and concurrently
	Umbilical stump—3 vessels (2 arteries, 1 vein) Dry around base Odorless Whitish gray	Umbilical hernia that is reducible	Redness, bleeding, odor Meconium stained Less than 3 vessels	Assess for bleeding and infection Teach parents care of the cord

TABLE 17.2 (continued)

Assessment	*Usual Findings*	*Common Deviations*	*Abnormalities*	*Nursing Actions*
Liver	1–2 cm below right costal margin		Enlarged liver	Record any enlargement or tenderness
Spleen	Tip felt under left costal margin		Enlarged spleen	Record any enlargement or tenderness
Kidneys	Posterior flank Oval, firm mass		Displaced kidney Wilms' tumor	To palpate kidneys (first 4–6 hours) place one finger behind flank and press gently from front Leg should be flexed to relax abdomen
Bladder	Urine—no odor	Mild—not unpleasant odor	Failure to void in 24 hours	Assess voiding
Genitalia	FEMALE Labia and clitoris edematous Labia minora smaller than labia majora Hymenal tag—mucoid discharge Vernix caseosa between labia Smegma Orifices open (vagina, urethra)	Edema, ecchymosis following breech delivery Pink-stained urine (uricacid crystals) Blood-tinged discharge—pseudomenstruation	Enlarged clitoris with urethral meatus at tip Fused labia Absence of vaginal opening Fecal discharge from vagina Ambiguous genitals	Assess if there is bleeding to be certain from where it is coming Refer to genetic studies if necessary Teach parents to clean genital area from front to back
	MALE Urethral opening at tip of glans penis Testes palpable in scrotum Scrotum large edematous and pendulos Deeply pigmented rugae Smegma under prepuce Phimosis to some degree Erection	Urethral opening covered by prepuce Testes in inguinal canal Scrotum small Hydrocele Size of genitals wide variation Edema and ecchymosis if breech	Hypospadias Epispadias Testes not palpable—enlarged or small Inguinal hernia Ambiguous genitals Cryptorchidism (undescended testicles)	Assess voiding if circumcision, teach parents care
Extremities	Flexed position Full range of motion—muscle tone	Athetoitic posturing and movements Slight tremors—some	Limp extremities Limitation of movement of any joint or hypermobility	Assess and evaluate all extremities and reflexes that are pertinent

	Symmetry of extremities—equal in length Ten fingers and toes Nail beds pink with transient cyanosis immediately after birth Creases on anterior two-thirds of sole Mild degree of bowing or medial rotation of legs Fist clenched with thumbs in C position Feet held in varus or valgus attitude but can be straightened with forceful manual stretching Babinski reflex Grasp reflex—palmar/plantar Stepping reflex	acrocyanosis Partial syndactyly between second and third toe Clinodactyly of second toe with overlapping into third toe Deep crease on plantar surface of foot between first and second toe Dorsiflexion and shortness of hallux May turn in but can be manually turned out Asymmetric length of toes	Asymmetry of extremities Unequal muscle tone or range of motion Polydactyly Syndactyly Persistent cyanosis of nail beds Yellowing of nailbed Dislocated hip Limitation in hip abduction Unequal leg length Audible click on abduction (Ortolani's sign) Fractures Malformations Phocomelia Palmar creases	
WITH INFANT PRONE				
Spine	Straight, easily flexes Intact, no opening, masses or prominent curves Can raise head momentarily	Pilonidal cyst or sinus	Pigmented nevus at base of spine Spina bifida Meningocele Myelomeningocele	Assess and evaluate Instruct parents accordingly
Hip	Symmetry of gluteal folds		Unequal gluteal or leg folds—dislocated hip	
Anus	Patent opening Meconium stool in 24 hours	Anal fissures	Imperforate anus	Instruct parents about cleansing Note passage of meconium
IN APPROPRIATE POSITION				
Weight	2,500–4,000 gm (5 lb 8 oz–8 lb 13 oz) 5–10% weight loss Regains birth weight in 2 weeks		Weight <2500 gm ($5y_2$ lb) = prematurity SGA, fetal alcohol syndrome Weight 4,000 gm (8 lb 13 oz) += LGA, IDM	Balance and adjust scale with paper liner (or cloth) in place Protect neonate from heat loss Use safety measures Weight same time each day
Length	45–55 cm (18–22 in.)			Measure length from top of head to heel

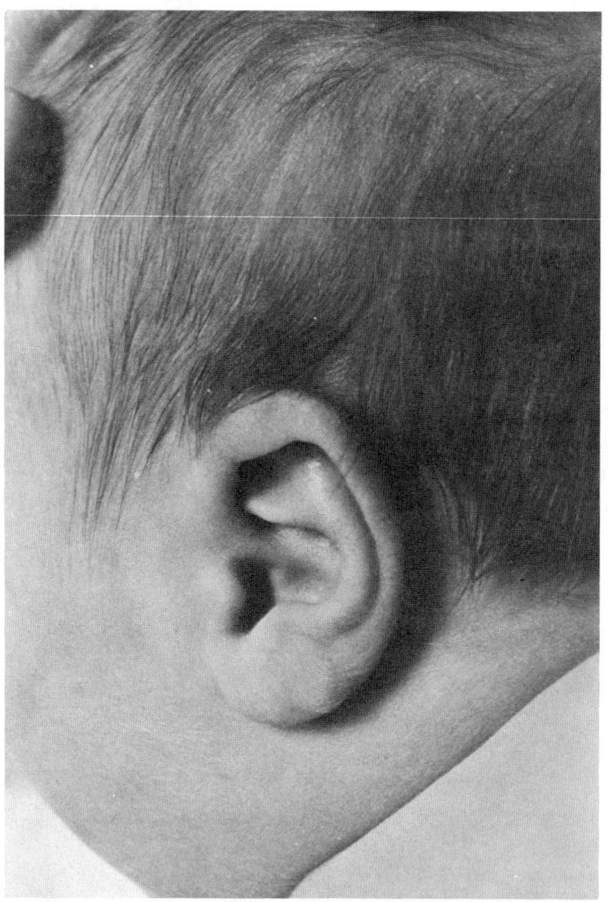

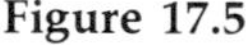

Figure 17.5

Term infant. At less than 34-weeks gestation infants have very flat, relatively shapeless ears. Shape develops over time so that an infant between 34 and 36 weeks has a slight incurving of the superior part of the ear; the term infant is characterized by incurving of two-thirds of the pinna; in an infant older than 39 weeks the incurving continues to the lobe. If the extremely premature infant's ear is folded over, it will stay folded. Cartilage begins to appear at approximately 32 weeks so that the ear returns slowly to its original position. In an infant of more than 40-weeks gestation there is enough ear cartilage so that the ear stands erect away from the head and returns quickly when folded. (When folding the ear over in this portion of the examination be certain that the surrounding area is wiped clear or the ear may adhere to the vernix.) Courtesy of Dr. Richard Schreiner, Indiana University School of Medicine. Indianapolis, Ind. Used with permission.

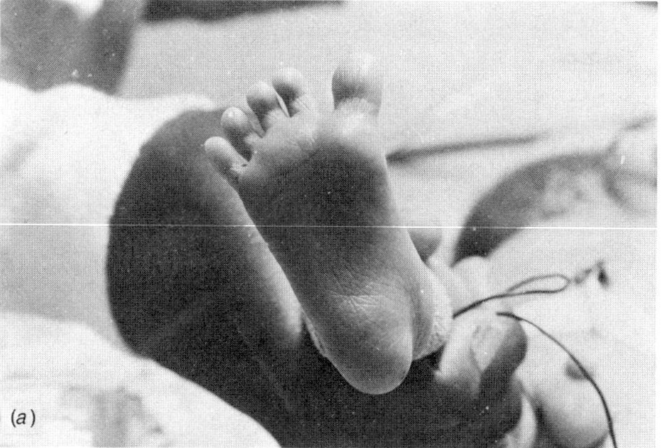

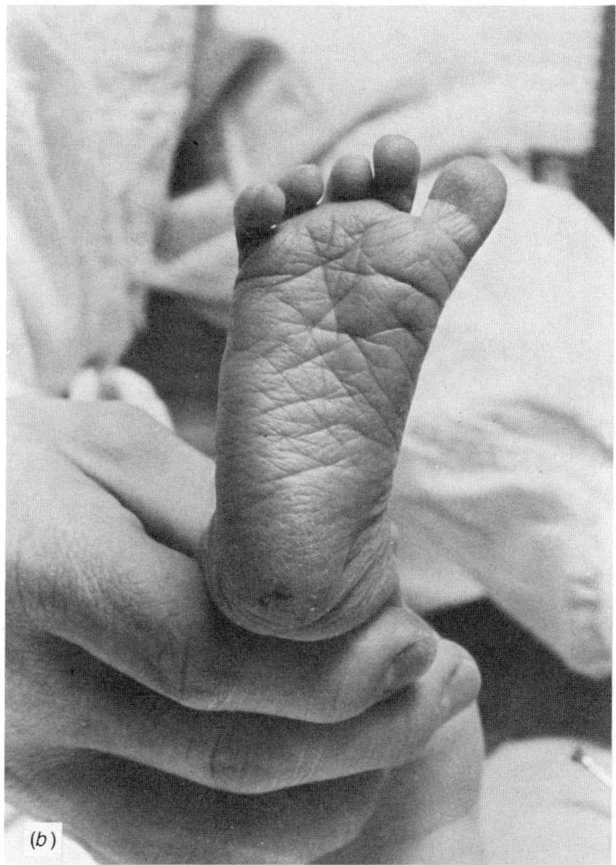

Figure 17.6

(a) Premature infant; *(b)* term infant. Sole creases. The sole of the premature infant has very few or no creases. With increasing gestational age, the number and depth of sole creases multiply so that the term baby has creases involving the heel. (Wrinkles that occur after 24 hours can sometimes be confused with true creases.) Courtesy of Dr. Richard Schreiner, Indiana University School of Medicine. Indianapolis, Ind. Used with permission.

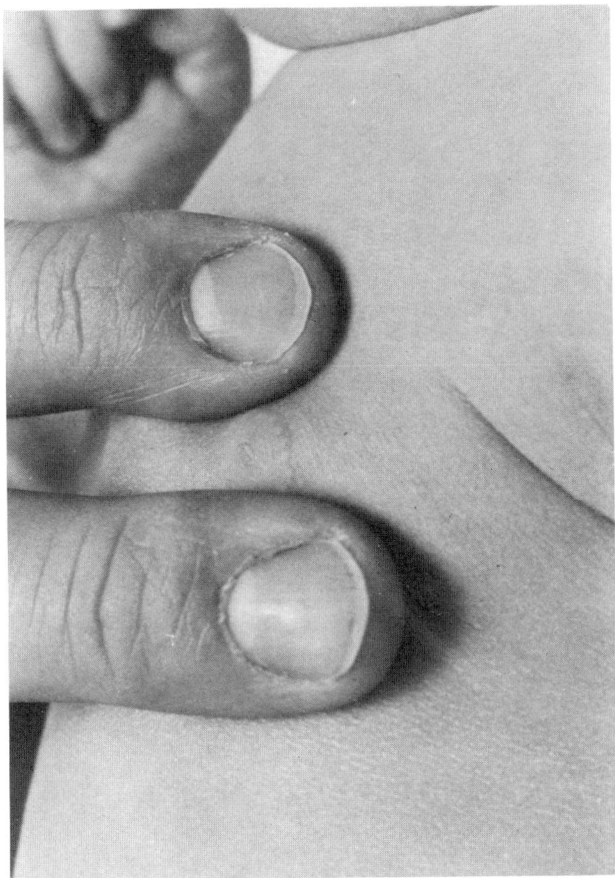

Figure 17.7
Nipples and breast—term infant. In infants younger than 34-weeks gestation the areola and nipple are barely visible. After 34 weeks the areola becomes raised. Also, the infant of less than 36-weeks gestation has no breast tissue. Breast tissue arises with increasing gestational age as a result of maternal hormonal stimulation. Thus, an infant of 39–40 weeks will have 5–6 mm of breast tissue, and this amount will increase with age. Courtesy of Dr. Richard Schreiner, Indiana University School of Medicine. Indianapolis, Ind. Used with permission.

week of gestation, the infant is classified as appropriate for gestational age (AGA). Although fetal growth, gestational age, and fetal maturity are related, they are *not* synonymous. Maturity implies functional capacity; therefore, gestational age is more closely related to fetal maturity than to birth weight. In other words, the LGA infant is presumed to have grown at an accelerated rate and the SGA at a decelerated rate during fetal life. The relationship of gestational age to weight gives additional information regarding potential risk for the newborn. Problems of LGA and SGA infants are discussed more completely in Chapter 23. The gestational age assessment examination requires assessment of physical and neurologic signs and the assignment of a score for each based on the criteria defined in the assessment tool. There are several tools used by nurses for gestational age assessment, but all use combined neurologic and physical assessment criteria to make a determination of LGA, AGA, or SGA. (See Appendix D.) As with psychomotor and cognitive skills, practice makes perfect, and the nurse should be able to determine gestational age of an infant accurately within 2 weeks. Physical characteristics assessed and assessment factors are shown and described in Figures 17.5 through 17.12. Neurologic

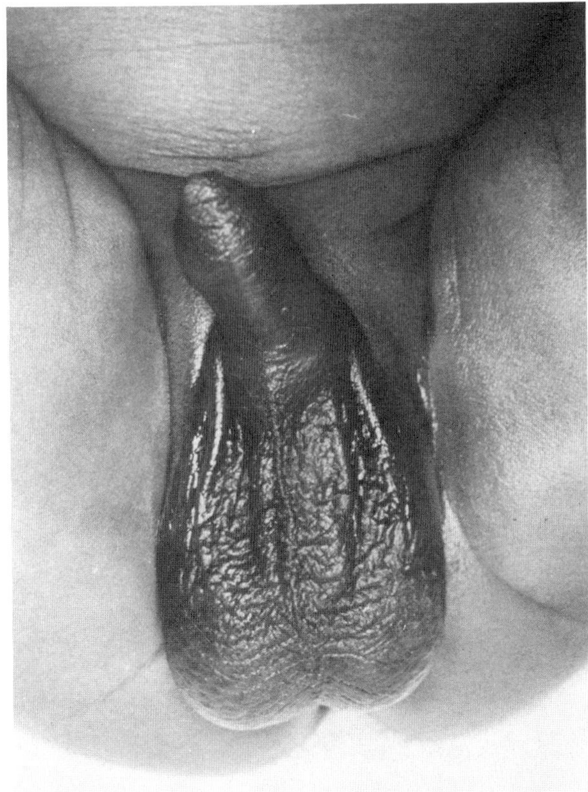

Figure 17.8
Male genitalia—term infant. In the premature male the testes are very high in the inguinal canal and there are very few rugae on the scrotum. The term infant's testes are lower in the scrotum and many rugae have developed. Courtesy of Dr. Richard Schreiner, Indiana University School of Medicine. Indianapolis, Ind. Used with permission.

characteristics assessed and a description of the assessment techniques are pictured and described in Figures 17.13 through 17.22. Infants should be in a quiet, restful state for neurologic examination.

BEHAVIORAL ASSESSMENT

Newborns today are being recognized as the unique human beings they are. To expect every adult to behave like every other adult is ridiculous, but at

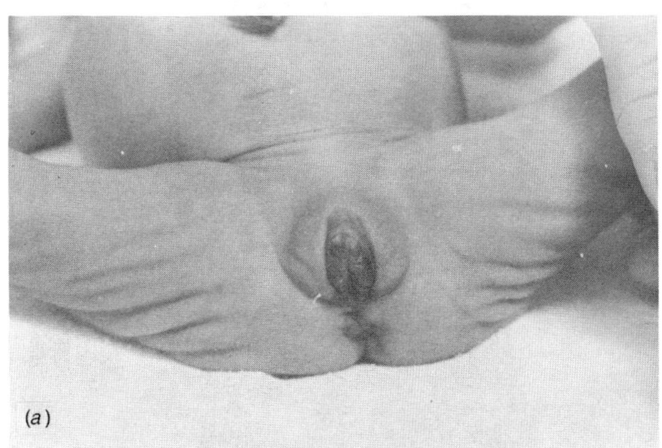

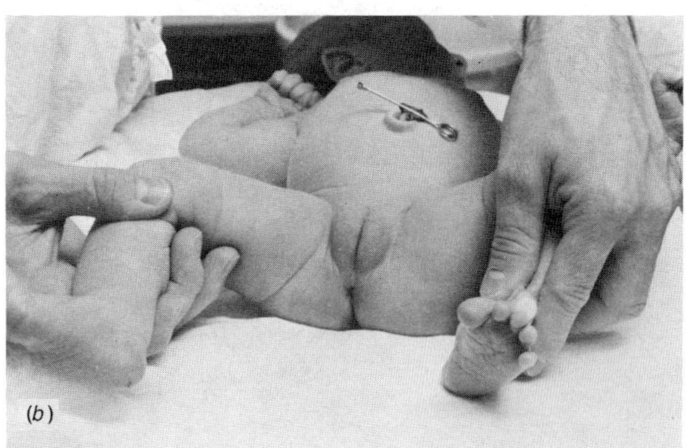

Figure 17.9
Female genitalia: *(a)* premature female; *(b)* term female. When the premature female is positioned on her back with hips adducted, the clitoris is very prominent and the labia majora are very small and widely separated. The labia minora and the clitoris are covered by the labia majora in the term infant. Courtesy of Dr. Richard Schreiner, Indiana University School of Medicine. Indianapolis, Ind. Used with permission.

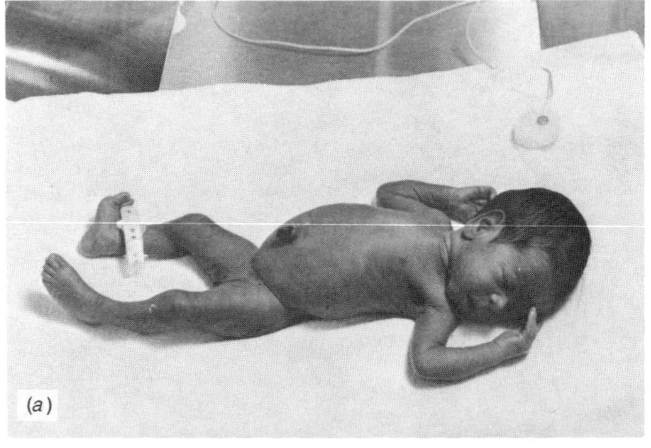

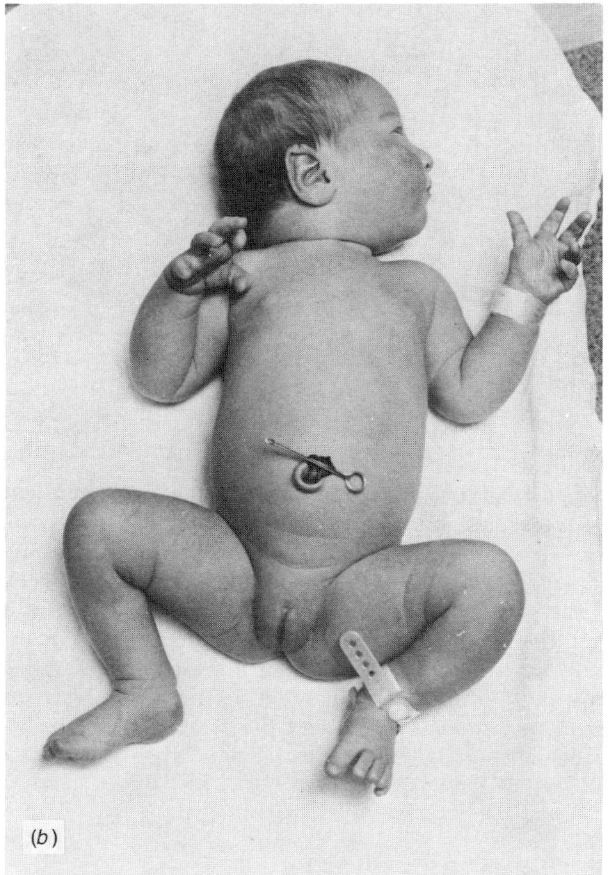

Figure 17.10
Resting posture: *(a)* premature infant; *(b)* term infant. The premature infant is characterized by very little, if any, flexion in the upper extremities and only partial flexion in the lower extremities. The term infant exhibits flexion in all four extremities. Courtesy of Dr. Richard Schreiner, Indiana University School of Medicine. Indianapolis, Ind. Used with permission.

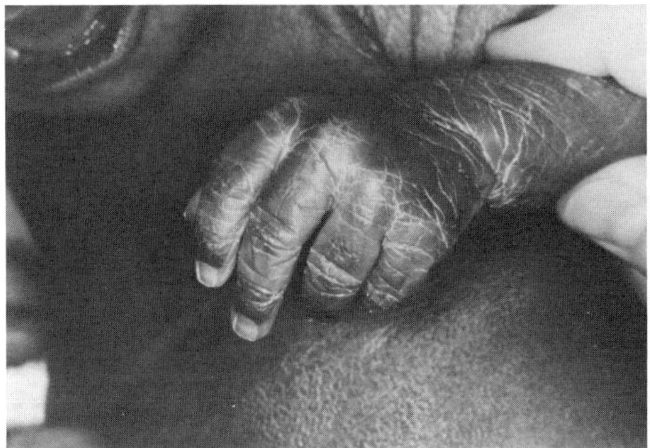

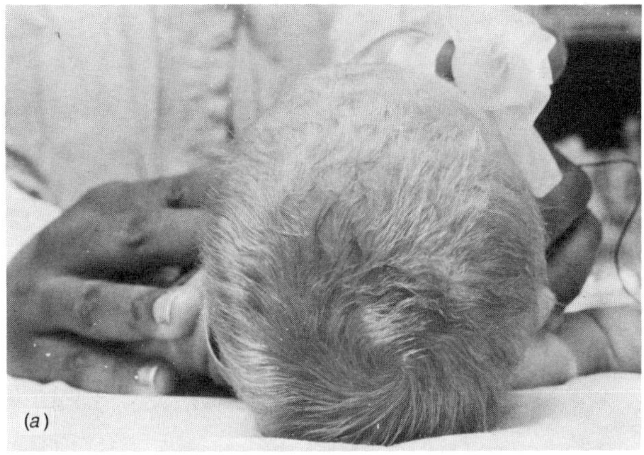

Figure 17.11
Skin and vernix—postmature infant. The skin of the premature infant is smooth, may be edematous, and blood vessels may be visible through it. In the postmature infant the skin is thick and pale and there is marked desquamation over the entire body. It is also meconium stained. Vernix caseosa, a white cheesy material on the infant's skin, appears early in gestation and begins decreasing in quantity later in gestation. After 42 weeks no vernix remains. Courtesy of Dr. Richard Schreiner, Indiana University School of Medicine. Indianapolis, Ind. Used with permission.

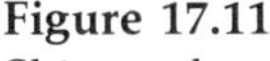

one time that was the expectation with newborns. However, study of the behavior of the newborn and the attachment process has provided us with a greater appreciation of the newborn as a person.

The process of parent–infant attachment has been stated from two aspects, that is, the attachment of infant to parent (or significant other) and the attachment of parent to infant (Bowlby, 1969; Ainsworth, 1973; Klaus & Kennel, 1976; Rubin, 1961). According to Bowlby (1969), there are four major steps in the infant's process of attachment. In the first step infants use their proximity and contact–promoting behaviors to bring their mothers in contact with them. These behaviors occur during the first 2–3 months. The second behaviorial step is the infant's ability to discriminate clearly between familiar people and to respond differentially to each. This occurs 2–6 months of age. In the third step (6 months to 2 years) the infant promotes contact and proximity with the attachment person. During the fourth step infants begin to understand the factors that influence their mothers' behaviors and can initiate activities that change mothers' behaviors.

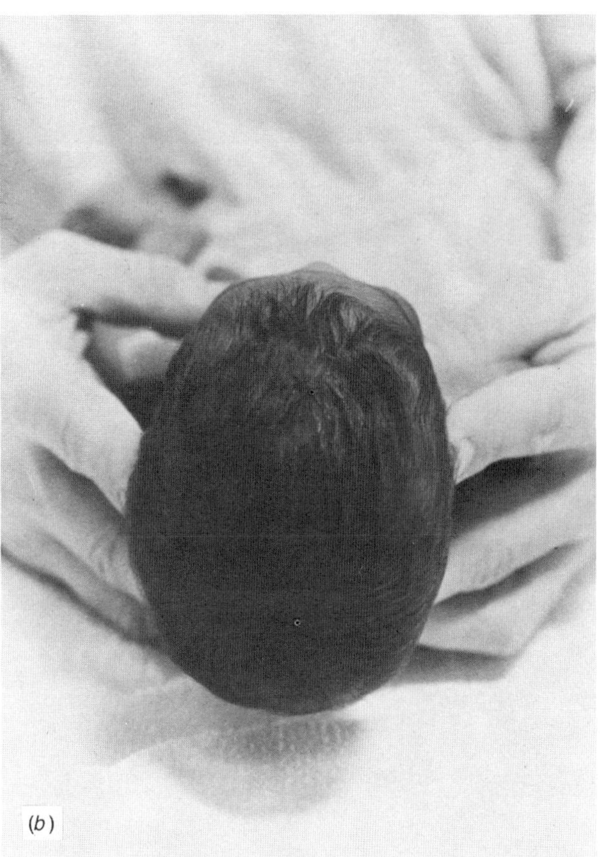

Figure 17.12
Hair: *(a)* premature infant; *(b)* term infant. The premature infant has very fine wooly hair that occurs in bunches. The term infant has very silky hair that occurs in single strands and lays flat. (Hair must be thoroughly cleansed of vernix or appearances may be deceptive in this observation.) Courtesy of Dr. Richard Schreiner, Indiana University School of Medicine. Indianapolis, Ind. Used with permission.

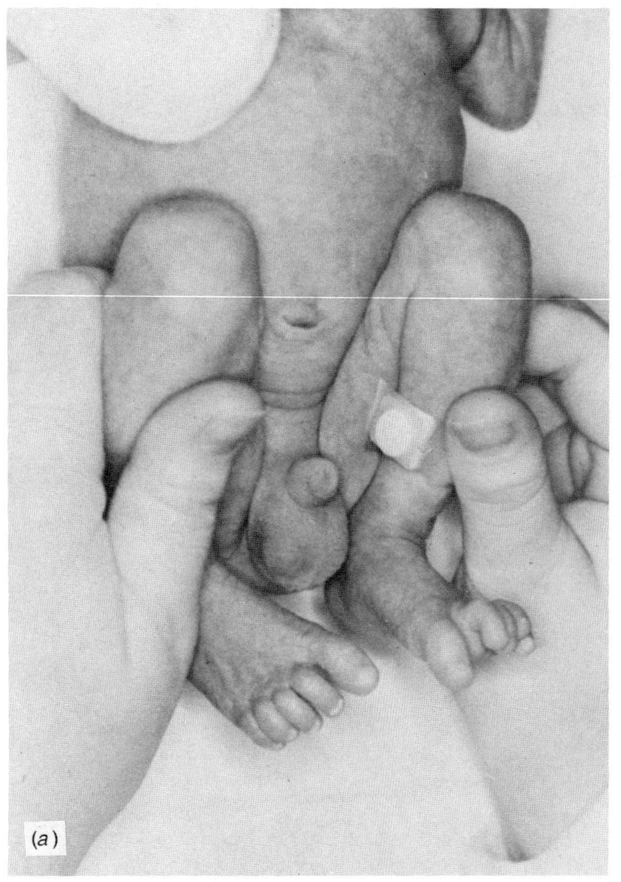

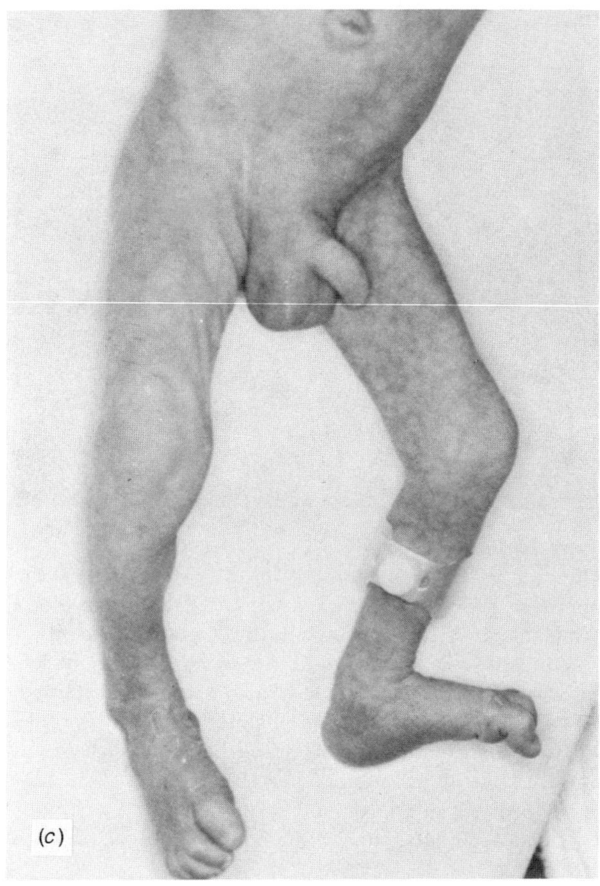

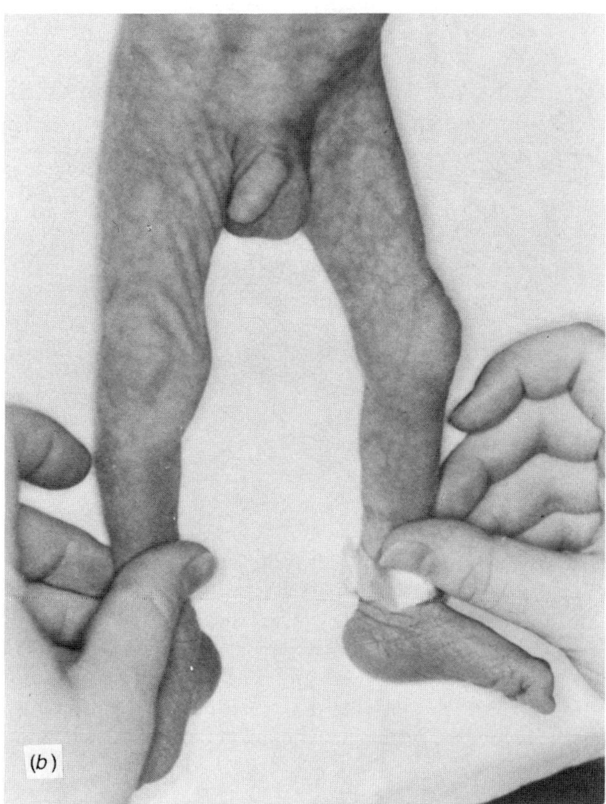

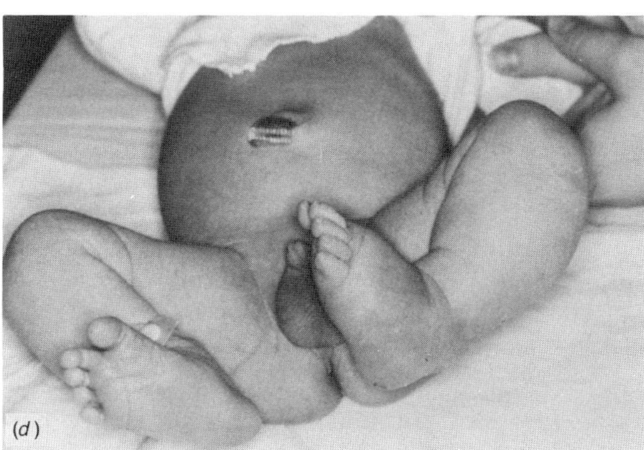

Figure 17.13
Recoil of extremities: *(a)* flex extremities and hold; *(b)* extend; *(c)* response in premature infant; *(d)* response in term infant. Place the infant supine. To test recoil of the legs (1) flex the legs and knees fully and hold for 5 seconds; (2) extend by pulling on the feet; (3) release. To test the arms, flex forearms and follow same procedure. In the premature infant response is minimal or absent; in the term infant extremities return briskly to full flexion. Courtesy of Dr. Richard Schreiner, Indiana University School of Medicine. Indianapolis, Ind. Used with permission.

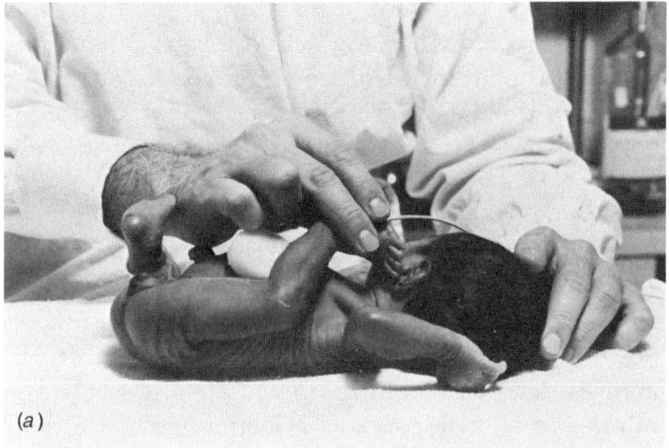

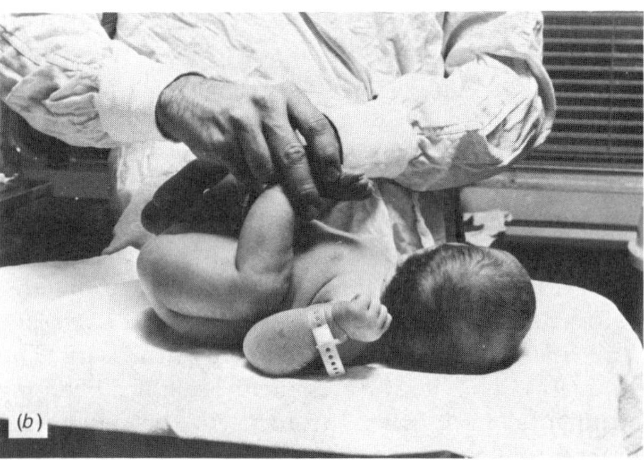

Figure 17.14
Heel to ear: *(a)* premature infant; *(b)* term infant. With the baby supine and hips positioned flat on the bed, draw the baby's foot as near to ear as it will go without forcing it. Observe the distance between the foot and head, as well as the degree of extension at the knee. In the premature infant very little resistance will be met. In the term infant there will be marked resistance; it will be impossible to draw the baby's foot to the ear. Courtesy of Dr. Richard Schreiner, Indiana University School of Medicine. Indianapolis, Ind. Used with permission.

Ainsworth (1973) describes three groups of behaviors initiated by neonates because of their perceptions and ability to process stimuli from people. These behaviors are described as orienting behaviors, active physical contact behaviors, and signaling behaviors. An example of *orienting behaviors* is the establishment of eye-to-eye contact; the newborn can fixate on an object and track it. Rooting and sucking are orienting behaviors that not only promote attachment but are significant in maintaining infant–mother contact. *Active physical contact behaviors* of the infant such as embracing, grasping, and clinging are quite easily identified. It is interesting to note that Ainsworth and her colleagues suggest that the infant's discrimination of people may be more tactile than visual. *Signaling behaviors*—crying, smiling, vocalizing—are the newborn's ways of signaling mother to come. The smile, of course, stimulates positive social behaviors or responses on the part of the mother.

Klaus and Kennell (1976) and Rubin (1961) have focused on the attachment of parent to infant. Klaus and Kennell describe a "sensitive period" in the first

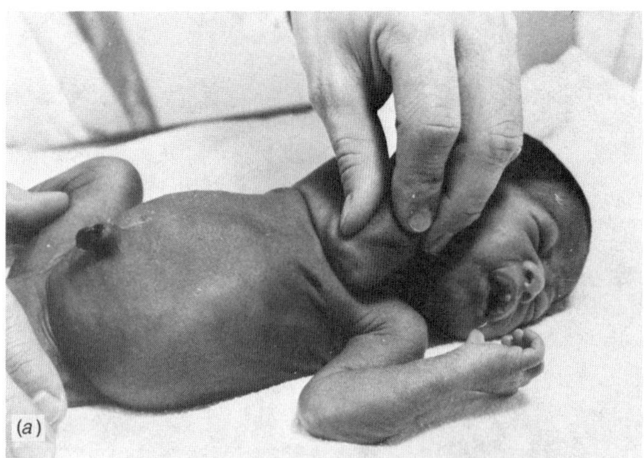

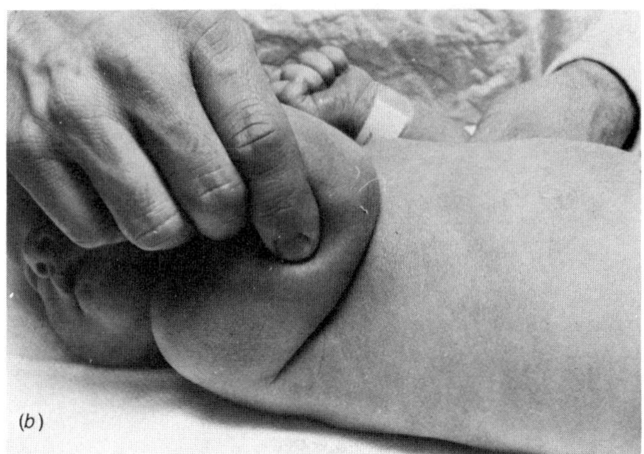

Figure 17.15
Scarf sign: *(a)* premature infant; *(b)* term infant. Hold the baby supine, take the hand and try to place it around the neck and above the opposite shoulder as far posteriorly as possible. Assist this maneuver by lifting the elbow across the body. See how far across the chest the elbow will go. In the premature infant the elbow will reach near or across the midline. In the term infant the elbow will not reach the midline. Courtesy of Dr. Richard Schreiner, Indiana University School of Medicine. Indianapolis, Ind. Used with permission.

minutes and hours after birth during which mothers demonstrate a sequence of attachment behaviors unique to human mothers. They describe the behaviors as touching, massaging and stroking, and palm contact with the newborn's trunk. Maternal behavior as described by Rubin is often used to assess maternal–infant attachment postpartally. The progressions of touching from fingertips to palmar surfaces and from holding with the arms extended to drawing the infant close are observed and evaluated as part of the data concerning attachment. Undoubtedly, the most significant attachment behavior is eye contact; this gives the infant personification and is rewarding for the mother. The quality of mother eye contact in both frequency and degree is significant. The mother's affect can be described as flat, warm, anxious, inquisitive, or fixed. If eye-to-eye contact is not established or the contact is distressful, attachment is delayed and both immediate and long-term human relationships can be jeopardized. Mother's reactions to all of the infant's verbal and nonverbal behaviors are important to observe. Does the mother call the infant by name or is the newborn identified with other family members (positively or negatively)? What does she do when the infant cries, yawns, gags, or grunts? What is the tone of her voice?

There are two tools currently available that are helpful in assessing behavioral characteristics of the newborn—the *Neonatal Behavioral Assessment Scale* developed by Brazelton (1973, 1974) and the *Neonatal Perception Inventory* (NPI) developed by Broussard. The Neonatal Behavioral Assessment Scale has been instrumental in shifting the focus to the newborn's inherent neurologic abilities, as well as responses to stimuli. It is important to realize that correct use of the tool requires training. An examiner is required to practice 10 ratings before the reliability of the ratings can be assumed. The scale measures 27 items in six categories of assessment. Each item is repeated several times, and the infant is scored on his or her *best,* not average, performance. Before discussing the

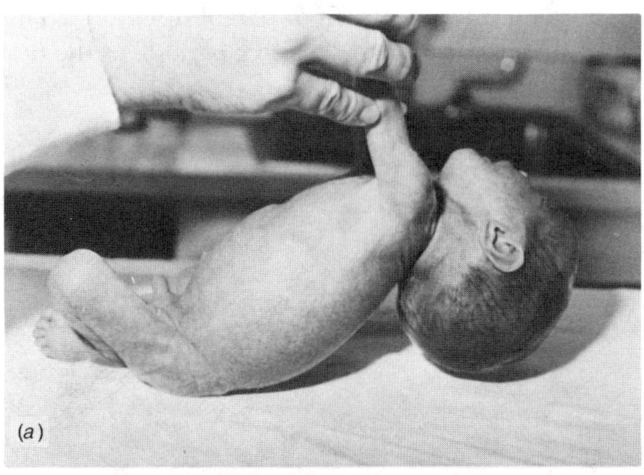

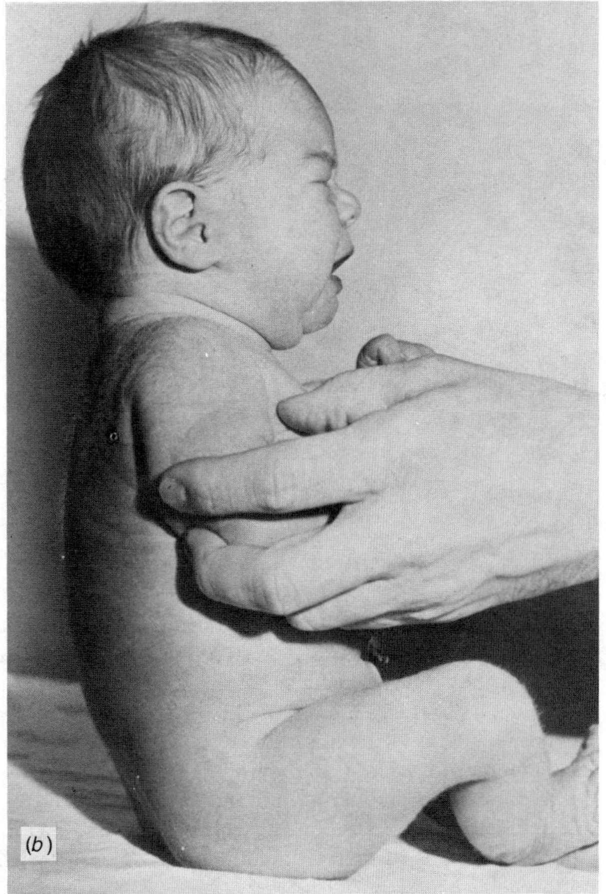

Figure 17.16
Neck flexors and extensors: *(a)* premature infant; *(b)* term infant. Neck flexors. Place the baby supine, grasp hands (or arms if infant is very small) and pull slowly to a sitting position. Observe the position of the head in relation to the trunk. In a premature infant there will be no flexion of the neck. The term infant will hold his head erect. Neck extensors. The infant held in the sitting position is observed for the degree to which he or she maintains head in the upright position. In the premature infant the head will bend forward whereas in the term infant head will be held erect for a few seconds. Courtesy of Dr. Richard Schreiner, Indiana University School of Medicine. Indianapolis, Ind. Used with permission.

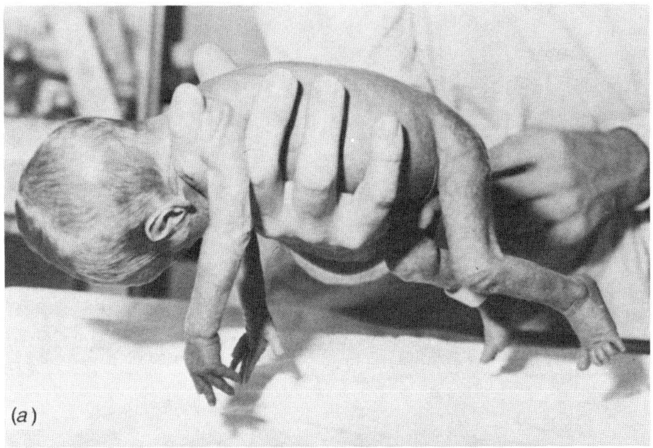

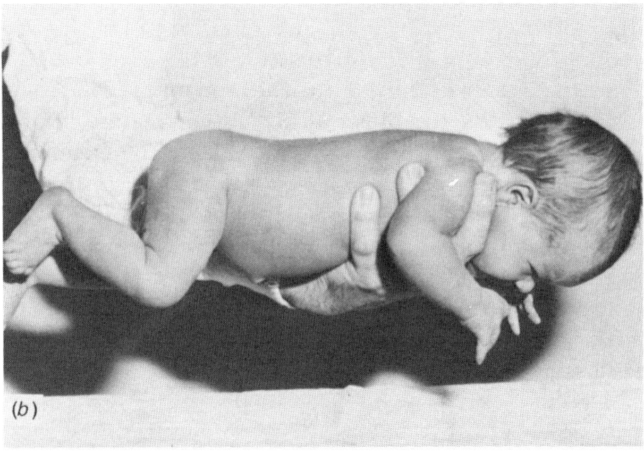

Figure 17.17
Horizontal position: *(a)* premature infant; *(b)* term infant. The infant is suspended in the prone position with the examiner's hand under the chest. One hand is used for a small infant, two for a larger infant. Observe the degree of extension of the back and head and the amount of flexion of the arms and legs. Also note the relation of the posture of the trunk and extremities. The premature infant will be limp with arms and legs almost straight and back rounded, whereas the term infant will exhibit flexion of the extremities, extension of the head, and a straight back. Courtesy of Dr. Richard Schreiner, Indiana University School of Medicine. Indianapolis, Ind. Used with permission.

six categories of assessment, you need to understand the asleep and awake states of the newborn since the Brazelton tool correlates with these.

There are two asleep states and four awake states identified. The *pattern of states,* as well as transition from one state to another, is important as ability to respond during a particular state is predictable. The first asleep state, *regular* or *deep sleep,* is when the eyes are closed and there is no movement except sudden jerky motions. In regular sleep, which comprises 4–5 hours a day, the routine noises of the environment will not rouse the neonate. If a very loud noise does awaken the infant during this part of the sleep cycle, the infant will go back to sleep if left alone. The second asleep state, *irregular* or *light sleep,* is characterized by closed eyes, irregular breathing, and slight muscle twitching. This state lasts 12–15 hours a day. During this state, external stimuli may minimally

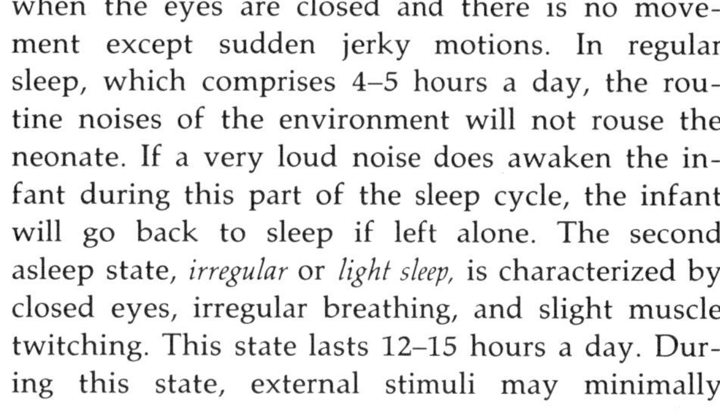

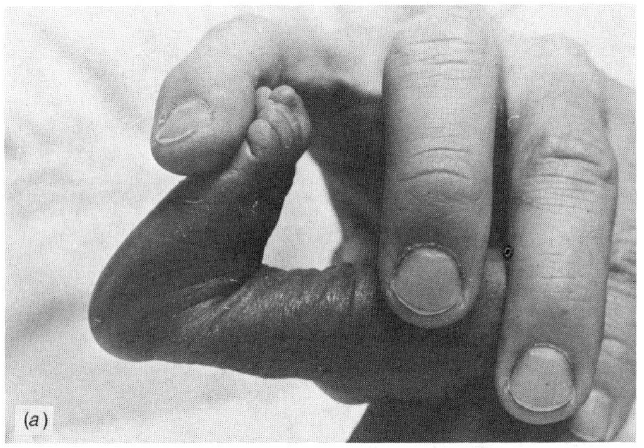

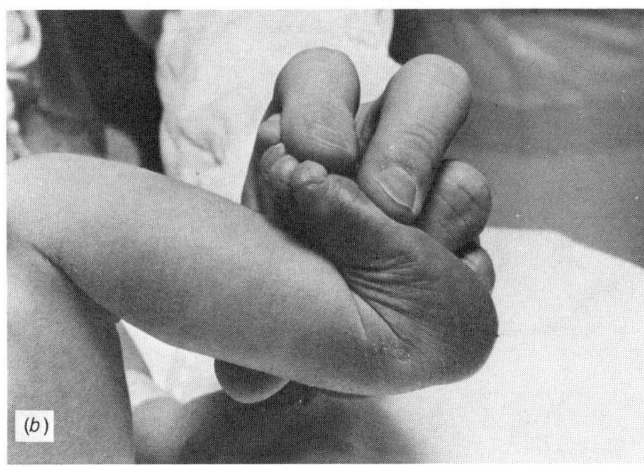

Figure 17.18
Ankle flexion: *(a)* premature infant; *(b)* term infant. The foot is pushed onto the anterior aspect of the leg. Enough pressure is applied to get as full flexion as possible. The angle between the dorsum of the foot and the anterior of the leg is measured. In the premature infant there will be an angle of 45–90 degrees. In the term infant it will be possible to flex the foot until it touches the leg. Courtesy of Dr. Richard Schreiner, Indiana University School of Medicine. Indianapolis, Ind. Used with permission.

arouse the infant so that he or she moans, smiles, or cries out. During the third state, *drowziness,* the eyes may be open and there is active body movement and irregular breathing. Most stimuli will arouse the infant during this time. When aroused, it is an appropriate time to pick the infant up. *Alertness* with a bright look is the fourth state; it lasts 2–3 hours a day and is characterized by active body movements and staring at nearby objects. During this period, the infant should be where the household activity is taking place. Stimuli should be provided; objects for viewing should be placed 7 or 8 in. away. Hunger needs, as well as other physiologic and psychosocial needs, should be met. The fifth state is *eyes open* during which the infant exhibits vigorous movement of arms and legs. The infant will react to external stimuli with increase in motor activity, and it is difficult to distinguish discrete reactions. The last (sixth) state, *crying,* is easily identified by parents. Both internal stimuli (hunger, pain, and cold) and external stimuli (pulling the bottle away while sucking) triggers angry crying and vigorous movement. Until the primary stimulus is satiated or basic needs met, attempts to quiet the infant may be unsuccessful.

In general, 75% of an infant's sleep is the irregular state. Sleep cycles vary from 45 minutes to 2 hours, divided into periods of about 15 minutes of regular sleep and approximately 40 minutes of irregular

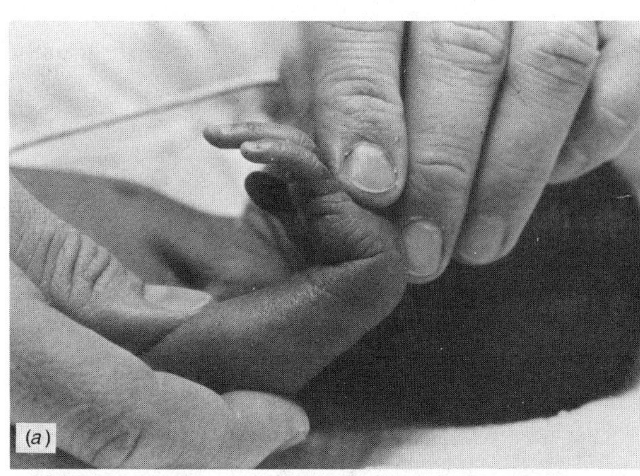

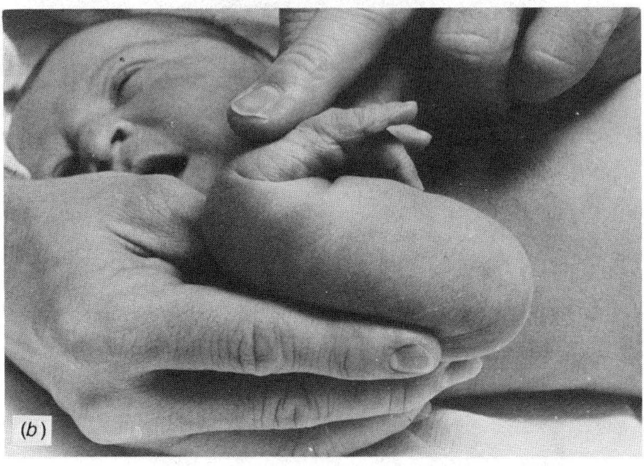

Figure 17.19
Wrist flexion: *(a)* premature infant 28–32 weeks; *(b)* term infant. The wrist is flexed, applying enough pressure to get the hand as close to the forearm as possible. The angle between the hypothenar eminence and the ventral aspect of the forearm is measured. (Care must be taken not to rotate the infant's wrist.) The premature infant at 28–32 weeks gestation will exhibit a 90 degree angle. With the term infant it is possible to flex the hand onto the arm. Courtesy of Dr. Richard Schreiner, Indiana University School of Medicine, Indianapolis, Ind. Used with permission.

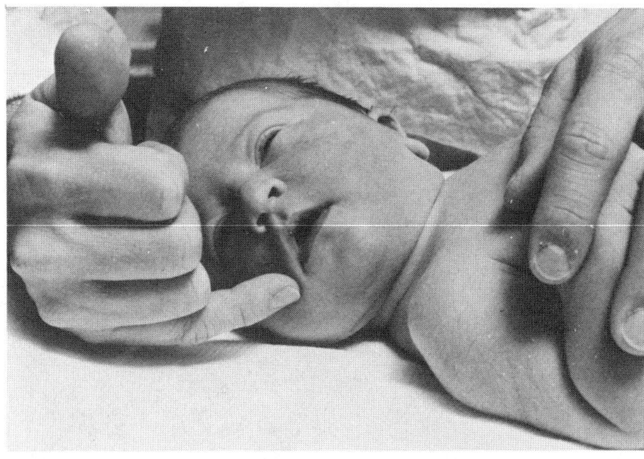

Figure 17.20
Rooting reflex. Testing for this consists of stroking the cheek to one side of the mouth. The term infant will move head toward the stimulus quickly; the premature infant will respond more slowly. Sucking reflex. The examiner inserts a nipple or a finger covered with a finger cloth into the infant's mouth to determine the presence and strength of the sucking reflex. In the premature infant response will be weak if present at all; in the term infant sucking will be strong. Courtesy of Dr. Richard Schreiner, Indiana University School of Medicine. Indianapolis, Ind. Used with permission.

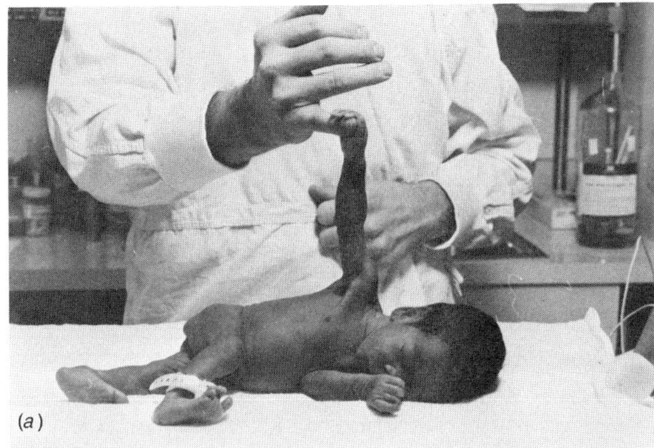

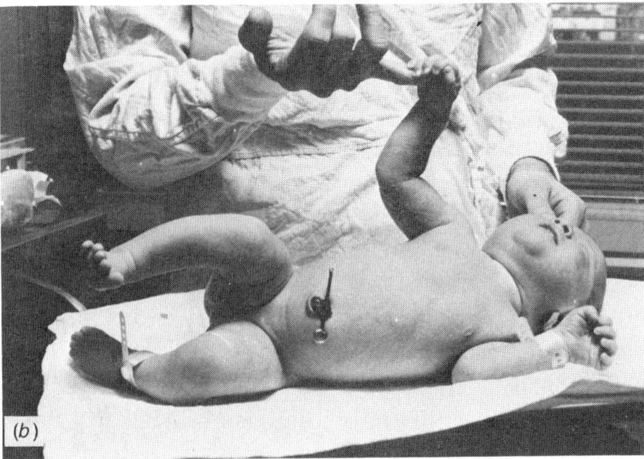

Figure 17.21
Grasp reflex: *(a)* premature infant; *(b)* term infant. The examiner places a finger in the palm of the infant's hand and evaluates the strength of the infant's hold. The term infant's grasp will be so strong that the infant can be lifted off the bed. In the premature infant there will be a grasp reflex but the examiner will not be able to lift the infant off the bed. Courtesy of Dr. Richard Schreiner, Indiana University School of Medicine. Indianapolis, Ind. Used with permission.

sleep. These cycles correlate with rapid eye movement (REM) and non-REM sleep. In general, it is noted that the first 6 weeks of the newborn's life involve a decrease in the amount of active REM sleep to total sleep and an increase in the quiet sleep time. At the same time, there is a 25% increase over the first 4 weeks in wakefulness. Initially, these wakeful periods are dictated by hunger, but as time passes the need for socialization becomes apparent. At the end of 4–6 weeks some infants are awake from one feeding to another. A child reaches the adult sleep pattern around age 4 or 5.

Items to be assessed in the Neonatal Behavioral Assessment Scale are divided into the following six categories. The state in which the behaviors should be assessed is noted.

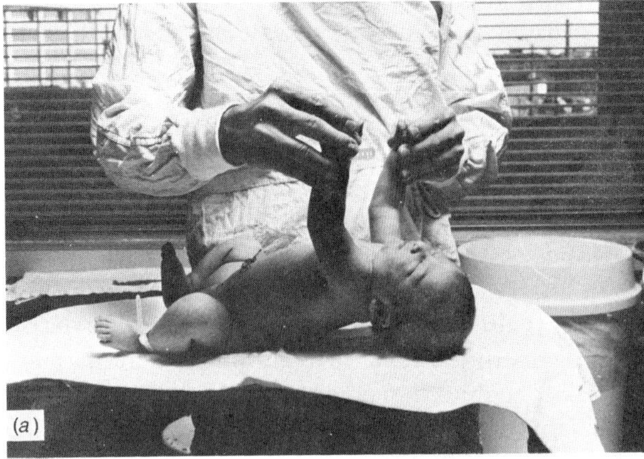

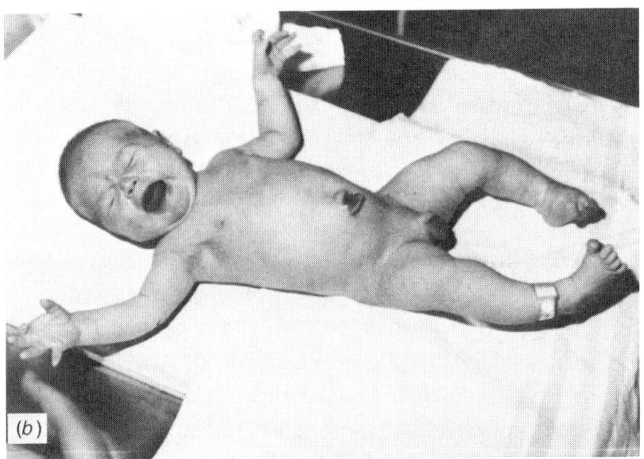

Figure 17.22
Moro reflex: *(a)* lift infant and release; *(b)* response in term infant. This reflex may be elicited by lifting the baby either by the arms until shoulders are 1–2 in. above the bed or by lifting head slightly and then suddenly releasing. The normal response in the term infant is that of an initial extension of the arms and legs and fanning of the fingers and toes followed by a flexion of the knees and embraced posture of the arms. Frequently the infant also cries. Response in the premature infant is weak. (Asymmetry in the response may indicate a nerve palsy or skeletal fracture.) Courtesy of Dr. Richard Schreiner, Indiana University School of Medicine. Indianapolis, Ind. Used with permission.

- ▲ ***Habituation.*** How quickly the infant diminishes or shuts down responses to specific repeated stimuli, for example, rattle, bell, light, pinprick. Normal newborns can stop responding, demonstrating their ability to control the environment. (Assessed in state 1, 2, or 3.)
- ▲ ***Orientation.*** How frequently and when the infant attends to visual or auditory stimuli. Ability to fix and follow objects and respond to visual and auditory stimuli is assessed. This ability and parental appreciation of it is extremely important in promoting the attachment process. (Assessed in state 4 or 5.)
- ▲ ***Motor Maturity.*** How well the infant controls and coordinates motor activities. This involves overall assessment of body tone as the infant reacts to stimuli. Motor maturity seen by range of movement—smooth versus jerky movement. Premature infant demonstrates jerky, coglike movement that is floppy and not balanced. (Assessed in state 4 *not* in state 6.)
- ▲ ***Variation.*** How often the infant demonstrates alertness, color changes, state changes, and peaks of excitement. *Alerting* is defined as brightening and widening of eyes; *orienting* is identified as the response of turning toward the direction of the stimulus (Brazelton, 1973). (Assessed in state 4 only.)
- ▲ ***Self-Quieting Abilities.*** How often, how soon, and how effectively the infants can use their own resources to quiet and comfort themselves. Behaviors demonstrated and assessed include putting hand to mouth and sucking on fist or pacifier. (Assessed in states 6 and 5 to 4, 3, 2.)
- ▲ ***Social Behaviors.*** How often or how much the newborn smiles and cuddles. These behaviors include the infant's need to be held, which in turn enhance the parent's self-esteem and influences the parent–infant feedback system. (Assessed in states 4, 5.)

The *Brazelton assessment* should be carried out in a quiet, dimly lit room after assessing the infant's asleep or awake state. Scoring and introduction of selected items must be correlated with asleep or awake states. The assessment takes about 30 minutes and is frequently not done before the third day as some infant's early movements are uncoordinated. Every attempt is made to obtain the best response and to elicit the highest possible score. The tool is important in that it focuses on the newborn's capabilities and responses and provides an excellent teaching tool for parents. It can promote positive beginnings for parent–child relationships by making parents aware of their critical role and at the same time adding to their confidence as parents.

The other assessment tool, the Neonatal Perception Inventory, aims to promote the mental health of the newborn and to serve as an aid to early care giving. A mother's idea of the "average" baby is compared to her perceptions of her own infant. The assumption is that the mother who does not see her infant as better than average indicates a mother–infant dyad that needs immediate intervention as the infant may be at risk (Clark, 1976). The intervention focuses on drawing the mother's attention to the positive aspects of her particular neonate in a kind and supportive way. Further implications are that the mother who does not see her infant as better than average may not view herself positively. Systematic behavioral assessment of the newborn has promoted objective, individual observations and has done much to unfound the myths about the newborn. Nurses are now more knowledgeable about and more aware of the neonate's abilities and have developed their assessment skills, which in turn have provided more complete information and better anticipatory guidance for parents.

NURSING CARE OF THE NEONATE

The goals of nursing care of the newborn focus on maintaining homeostasis or body equilibrium. Establishment of the airway has been noted in Chapter 16 as the first priority, and subsequent concerns are stabilizing the body temperature, providing safety against both injury and infection, providing adequate nutrition and promoting the parent–neonate attachment process. Figure 17.23 illustrates safe ways to hold a newborn. Immediate care in the delivery room was discussed in Chapter 16. Subsequent stages of care are frequently subdivided into care during the transitional stage (through the first 6 hours) and care until discharge.

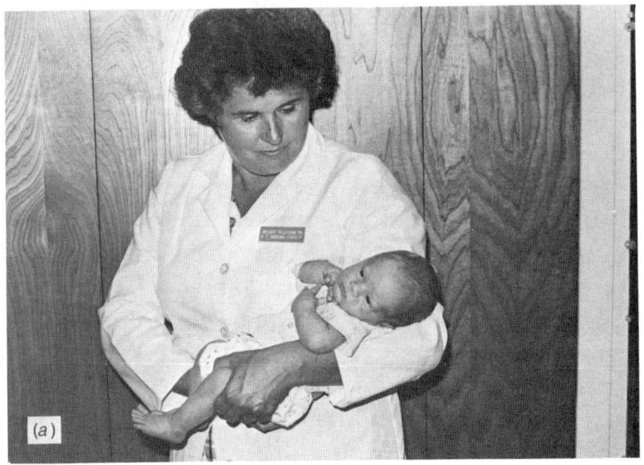

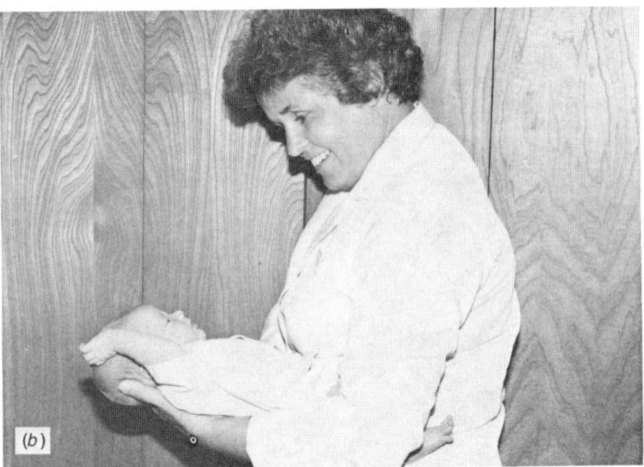

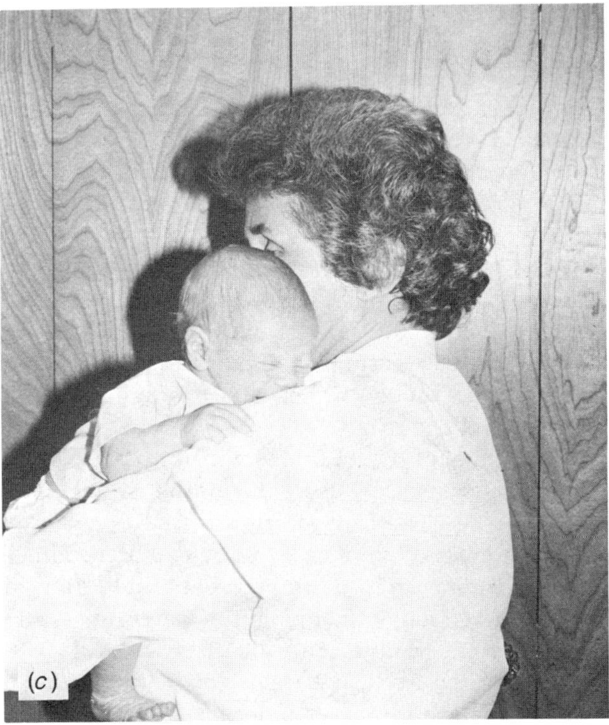

Transitional Care

If the nurse conceptually considers the newborn as an intensive care patient for approximately the first 6 hours, the maternity/neonatal nurse should automatically realize this implies frequent observation and assessment. A minimal safe schedule for vital signs (apical pulse, respirations, temperature) would be every 15 minutes during the first hour of life, every 30 minutes during the second hour, and every hour for the first 6–8 hours. The pattern after the first 8 hours usually changes to every 4 hours through the first 24 hours of life and then 3 times a day until discharge. Any change in color, behavior, or muscle tone is an indication that more frequent assessment is necessary. Axillary temperatures are preferred over rectal to prevent trauma to the rectum. If digital or electronic devices are used, it is important to ascertain that the device is working properly. A good axiom for the maternity nurse in any setting is that *any* electronic device is *only* an adjunct to human assessment; careful human assessment by an educated professional is the best. Respirations, temperature, and heart rate are assessed at the same time, on the schedule described; blood pressure is usually taken once during the first 6 hours; unless there is a cause for concern, is not monitored routinely (refer to Table 17.2 for normal ranges of vital signs).

Medications for the Newborn

The two medications routinely administered to the newborn are vitamin K (see physiologic adaptation) and silver nitrate. Vitamin K is usually administered during the first 2 hours and is given intramuscularly in the muscles of either the upper arm or thigh (preferably the vastus lateralis muscle), using a small (27-gauge) short needle since the infant's muscle mass is not developed. Administration of silver nitrate ($AgNO_3$) consists of one drop of a 1% solution in each eye. This administration should *not* be followed by a rinse as this is ineffective in diminishing con-

Figure 17.23
Three safe methods of holding a newborn infant. Note the two contact points that provide support—the head and the rump. *(a)* The "cradle hold"; *(b)* the "football" hold; *(c)* the upright hold with head resting on the mother's shoulder.

junctivitis (Lum et al., 1980). The procedure may be delayed during the first hours, providing time for the parents and newborn to become acquainted.

Bathing

The first bath is generally done during the transitional period after the vital signs are stabilized. It is particularly important that the infant's temperature be stabilized (Williams & Lancaster, 1976; Iles & McCrary, 1976). Some nurseries use guidelines such as "Once you have two successive temperature readings of 97–98°F axillary at 30 minute intervals, the bath is given." Plain warm water should be used, and cleansing should proceed from head to toe. The eyes are cleaned from the inner canthus to the outer and the washcloth turned so that a clean area is used for each stroke. The scalp should be wiped and, depending on the amount of hair and matter, may be lightly shampooed by positioning the head over a small basin where the soap can then be throughly rinsed by using a cup and slowly pouring water over the scalp. The rest of the body is covered when shampooing the scalp. After the shampoo the head should be thoroughly dried to prevent evaporative heat loss. Ears and nose can be cleaned with the twisted end of the cloth or cotton-tipped swabs, being careful not to insert swabs into orifices. The rest of the body is washed with warm water, being careful to wash gently and pat, not rub, dry as the epidermis is thin. Care must be given to clean in the creases (neck, axillae, joints) where vernix and dried matter may collect. Again, the process is to wipe clean and not attempt to remove all vernix vigorously, as vernix probably has bacteriostatic and insulating functions. Fingernails and toenails when long may be cut with manicure scissors to prevent the neonates from scratching themselves. This is more easily done when the infant is asleep and is usually necessary during the first few days of life.

The genitalia require careful cleansing; on the female the labia are separated and the vernix is removed. Frequently there is a period of several diaper changes before all vernix is removed. If there is considerable accumulation of matter in the genital area, the infant may be placed in a few inches of water, like a sitz bath; care must be taken to keep the umbilical area dry and to prevent chilling. Cleansing of the genital area is always from front to back, as in the adult. Bathing the male genitalia involves washing the penis and the scrotum. Normally the foreskin or prepuce of the newborn is tight and should never be forcibly retracted. When pulled back to cleanse the smegma that sometimes collects, the foreskin should be returned to its original position. Leaving the foreskin retracted in the neonate can restrict blood flow and cause edema.

The buttocks and anal area of the neonate must be kept free of fecal material. Urine and feces on the skin can cause excoriation. If not cleansed frequently, the warm, moist, dark environment fosters the growth of bacteria. *Dermatitis* (diaper rash) caused by inadequate cleansing can lead to secondary bacterial infection. Plastic pants and plastic-lined disposable diapers can foster diaper rash by increasing warmth and preventing air circulation. Allergy to plastic diapers and diaper rash can frequently be differentiated from other allergies by assessing the area affected. Allergy usually involves the whole area covered by the irritant, whereas diaper rash is confined to the anal–genital area. When diapering a neonate, the diaper should overlap from back to front to avoid restricting leg flexion. In males the extra fold should be in the front to provide more absorbency; in females the folds may be in the front or back, depending on whether she is to be placed in prone or supine position.

The bathing and diapering processes provide excellent opportunities for teaching and for encouraging the mother to raise questions about her newborn. Individual characteristics of the newborn can be pointed out to the mother, and the normalcy of such things as erythema toxicum or caput succedaneum can be discussed. Explanations about sensory development and gastrointestinal and urinary tract functioning can be given. Progressive changes in the stool cycle from meconium (sticky and greenish black) to transitional (greenish brown to yellow-brown) to the typical yellow milk stool should be discussed. The difference between milk-fed and breast-fed baby's stool should be described; the former is pale yellow, firmer, and has more odor; the latter is yellow-to-golden color and pasty. Cleansing the genitalia of the infant from front to back and the fact that this is a principle the mother should use in her own hygiene care can be stressed.

Economics of child care can be explored. This includes the fact that perfumed soaps and lotions are not more effective than plain tap water. In addition, although the convenience of disposable diapers is evident, their exclusive use can be many times more expensive than home laundering.

Limitless opportunities for teaching and learning on the part of the nurse and the parents occur, and the nurse should plan for and use these opportunities. Explanations provide information and also demonstrate interest on the part of the nurse. During the intervention the nurse can assess the mother's interests and concerns and, by her interventions, establish a relationship to promote positive mother–infant attachment.

Care of the Umbilicus

As discussed in Chapter 16, the umbilical cord is clamped and cut after delivery. Normally, the cord dries and falls off within 7–10 days, but because the stump is a potential medium for bacterial growth, it should be kept as clean and dry as possible by exposing it to the air. Care should be taken that clothing not irritate the cord. The diaper should always be secured below the umbilicus since a diaper that is wet with urine could increase the opportunity for infection. Any signs of purulent (pus-like) or watery drainage or any odor should be recorded and reported. After the cord falls off, the stump requires a few weeks to heal. During this time, cleaning the area with mild soap and water during the bath will prevent infection.

Clothing and Positioning the Newborn

In the nursery, sufficient clothing consists of a shirt and diaper with the infant either wrapped in or covered by a cotton blanket. Diapers, clothing, and blanket should be loose enough to permit maximum lung expansion and snug enough to prevent heat loss. The infant, particularly after feeding, should be placed on the abdomen or right side (helps passage of food to small intestine) with a blanket roll or other support to the back so the side lying position is maintained. In between feedings, or throughout the day, the neonate's position should be changed to front-to-back and side-to-side positions since the infant cannot do this. It is important to make sure that after feeding the baby is not left on the back which risks spitting up and choking on the milk or formula. Adequate clothing after the infant goes home is a shirt and diaper and a cotton blanket. The mother should use common sense about clothing, basing the need for additional clothing on the temperature and the environment. In colder climates, bonnets or head coverings and extra blankets are important to prevent heat loss. The goal is to maintain balance and not allow the infant to be overheated or chilled.

Care of the Circumcision

Circumcision, or surgical removal of the foreskin, began as a traditional Jewish ceremony that takes place on the eighth day of life and is performed by a *moel,* a man especially trained and skilled in the procedure. Although routine circumcision is done in many hospitals before discharge, the American Academy of Pediatrics in 1975 reaffirmed its position that no valid medical indication for circumcision exists. Grimes (1980) opposes the routine circumcision of newborns and feels the risks outweigh the benefits. The three types of complications he pointed out are hemorrhage, infection, and surgical trauma. There is evidence that infant behavior and psychobiology is affected by circumcision (Emde et al., 1971; Anders and Chalemain, 1974; Talbert, 1976). It is important, however, that the maternity nurse know what is involved in the care of the circumcised as well as the uncircumcised neonate. The decision about whether or not to circumcise the infant is the parent's; selection of infants for circumcision seems to be based primarily on the preference of the mother (Patel, 1966). Nursing care of the neonate and teaching of the parents is the nurse's purview. As mentioned earlier, the foreskin of the uncircumcised male infant will retract on its own 99% of the time (Kaplan, 1977). Forcible retraction of the foreskin can result in scarring with subsequent phimosis making circumcision necessary. The nurse should inform parents of the necessity for cleanliness so

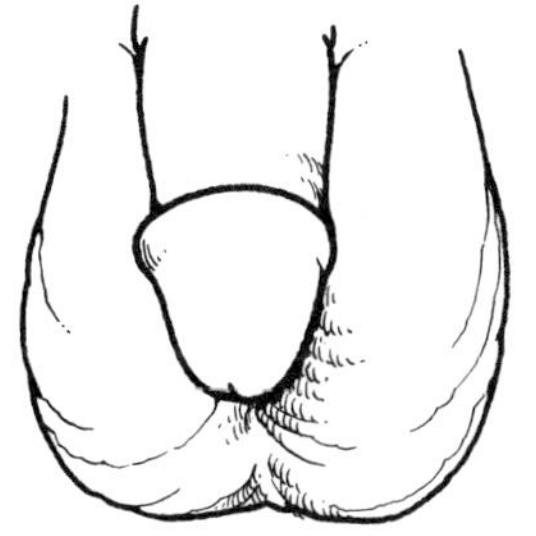

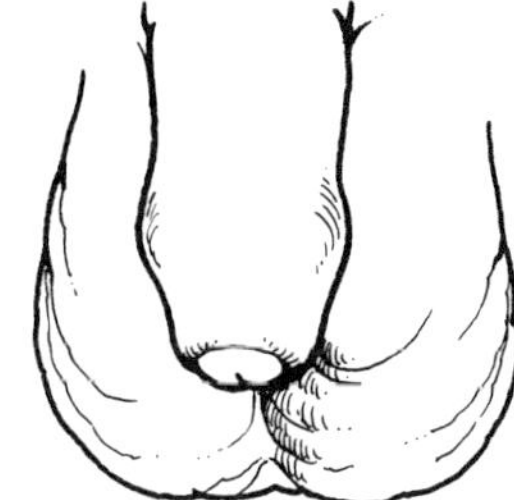

Figure 17.24
Comparison of *(left)* circumcised penis and *(right)* uncircumcised penis.

that its importance will be instilled in the child. General guidelines should include that starting at age 3, the foreskin should be pushed back gently once a week and by age 10 the child should be washing under his foreskin daily (Poole, 1979). No force should be used in retracting the foreskin, and should it retract and not return to its former position, the physician should be notified immediately.

The circumcised neonate must be observed for signs of hemorrhage during the first 12 hours after surgery. During hospitalization, the newborn is also observed for signs of infection and inability to void. On the second day, a yellowish white exudate, which is a normal part of the healing process, may be observed. This exudate may persist for 2–3 days. The penis may be gently washed and patted dry, but no attempt should be made to remove the exudate.

Parent teaching involves telling the parents that special care is required for approximately 10 days. The actual procedure, freeing and removal of the foreskin from the glans penis, can be accomplished by using a scalpel, Yellen or Gomco clamp, or a Hollister plastibell. The infant is placed in a restraining device (usually molded plastic that is padded for comfort) to prevent movement during the procedure and is held and cuddled immediately after the circumcision. The clamp crushes nerve endings and blood vessels, which minimizes trauma and promotes physiologic adaptation. Usually a petrolatum gauze dressing is applied. The dressing is removed after 24 hours; if the dressing is dry it may be moistened with water or hydrogen peroxide before removal. Some physicians prefer that the circumcision dressing be changed with each diaper change; ointment may or may not be ordered. In general, parents should be instructed to keep the area clean and dry and to change the diaper frequently. No plastic pants should be used as they tend to retain heat and moisture, which promotes bacterial growth. Special products to reduce bacteria in the diapers such as commercial antibacterial products or bleach can be used. Care must be taken to be sure the diapers are rinsed thoroughly as bleach can irritate the newborn's skin. Sunlight and high-temperature dryers also assist in reducing bacterial count. The newborn's voidings should be observed for any possible meatal stenosis. The normal voiding by the male infant is in a high arching stream. Parents whose infants have been circumcised are advised to notify the physician if the baby's temperature is greater than 101°F rectally, if he is not urinating, or if there is a continued bright red bleeding.

Feeding the Newborn

Although hereditary factors are responsible for much of the ultimate growth of a person, it goes without saying that nutrition in early infancy is extremely important and that optimal nutrition for all infants is the goal. Much research regarding infant nutrition is being done, and the maternity nurse needs to keep abreast of this information. The mother and father, with guidance, make the decision regarding feeding methods of their infant. Generally, there are three acceptable choices—human milk, cow's milk, and commercially prepared cow's milk formula. The physiologic requirement for growth is protein. Cow's milk contains 3 times more protein than human milk, and commercially prepared formulas have approximately 2 times as much protein as human milk. The quality of protein in human milk, however, is better for the neonate. The higher protein content in cow's milk is illustrated by weight gain; an infant on formula doubles birth weight at 3½–4 months while the breast-fed infant doubles birth weight at 5 months (Slattery, 1977). Overeating is a nutritional hazard of bottle-feeding, and research continues on the relationship of overfeeding in infancy to obesity in later life. The breast-feeding mother does not know how much the baby consumes, whereas the bottle-fed infant is often encouraged to drink "it all up." The *type* of protein in human versus cow's milk is also different. Human milk contains more lactalbumin, which has a higher percentage of amino acids and is therefore a more complete protein. Cow's milk contains casein, which results in the formation of large hard curds requiring longer digestion time. Since the protein in human milk is more easily digested, the stomach emptying time is shorter and the baby usually has more frequent feedings. The amount of fat in human versus cow's milk is similar but different in type. Human milk contains more monounsaturated fatty acids, mainly oleic acid, whereas cow's milk has more polysaturated fatty acids. Unsaturated fatty acids (human milk) enhance absorption of fat and calcium and may also be related to decreasing atherosclerosis in later life (Whaley & Wong, 1979).

Cow's and human milk both provide 20 kcal/oz. Both calcium and phosphorus are critical minerals for optimal growth, and the proportion of these minerals in both types of milk is sufficient. In cow's milk, there is a higher ratio of phosphorus to calcium; in human milk, higher ratio of calcium to phosphorus. Excess phosphorus is difficult for the neonate to eliminate because of physiologic hypoparathyroidism. You will recall that parathyroid hormone is necessary for the excretion of phosphorus. So if phosphorus increases in the blood, calcium is eliminated resulting in low serum calcium or tetany. The term neonate is born with an iron reserve that should last 5–6 months. Both human and cow's milk contain adequate amounts of iron, but it is advised that the infant's diet be evaluated periodically in relation to iron since iron deficiency is common in the United States.

Approximately 75% of the infants in the United States are bottle-fed despite the fact that breast milk is certainly the most perfect form of nutrition for the neonate. Mothers make their decisions based on a combination of factors or variables, and the nursing role is to assist in the decision making by providing the information regarding breast- and bottle-feeding on which the mother can make an informed decision. Nursing care and teaching for the mother who is breast-feeding and bottle-feeding are discussed more fully in Chapter 19. The appropriate amount of formula for the bottle-fed baby is easily calculated. Infants need approximately 117 calories/kg (51 calories/lb) from birth to 5 months (Slattery, 1977). The formula used to calculate the amount of formula needed is

$$\text{Weight (kg)} \times 110 \text{ kcal/kg} = \text{total number oz/day}$$
$$(1 \text{ oz formula} = 20 \text{ kcal})$$

Fluid requirement calculation is also important to ensure proper hydration. The newborn requires 150 ml/kg (70 ml/lb) of fluid per day. The fluid requirement formula is

$$\text{Weight (kg)} \times 150 \text{ ml} = \text{total number ml/day}$$
$$(30 \text{ ml} = 1 \text{ oz})$$

A normal newborn ordinarily will fulfill fluid requirements by taking adequate breast- or bottle-feedings. To use a simple example, if a baby at the time of discharge weighs 8 lb, his or her caloric requirements will be approximately 410 calories per 24 hours. Breast milk and most formulas contain 20 calories per ounce; therefore, the 8-lb baby needs 20½ oz of formula, which can be subdivided into approximately six feedings of approximately 3½ oz each. Formulas that are commercially prepared (for example, Similac, Enfamil, SMA) are milk-based formulas prepared to simulate human milk and come in three basic preparations. The first is a ready-to-use form in cans or bottles, the second is a concentrated preparation that has to be diluted with water, and the third is a powdered preparation. Commercially prepared formulas are about twice as expensive as evaporated milk, and for this reason the latter is often used. Evaporated milk has advantages over whole cow's milk, which is unsuited for infant nutrition. Whole cow's milk would have to be diluted to meet the protein requirement, and when this is done it does not meet caloric requirements. Evaporated milk undiluted is approximately 44 kcal/oz; adding 15½ oz of sterile water will give a formula of about 20 kcal/oz. Sugar or karo syrup is often added to prevent constipation and the resulting formula is

13 oz evaporated milk + 17 oz water + 1–2 tsp sugar = 20 kcal/ounce

Preparation of Formula

The two traditional methods of preparing formula are the aseptic technique and the terminal heat method. These are important where water supply or sanitary conditions are questionable. In the *aseptic technique,* the equipment is sterilized and then the formula is prepared and poured into sterile containers. This necessitates knowledge of asepsis and some skill in being able to differentiate sterile, unsterile, and clean. The *terminal heat method,* which is much more widely used, requires that all utensils and formula are assembled and then sterilized together. The already filled bottles are placed in a sterilizer, or deep kettle, containing 2–3 in. water, covered, and boiled gently for 25 minutes. Because of improved sanitary conditions, in many instances, it is not necessary to use either of the above methods. Many times, the formula is bought ready to serve (or perhaps just diluted) and tap water and clean bottles are all that are required. This one bottle at a time preparation, or single method, is safest when you are using clean method preparation as opposed to sterilization. The method of choice often depends on the physician's advice to the mother.

Distinctive feeding behaviors have been identified (O'Grady, 1971). These are prefeeding behavior, approach behavior, attachment behavior, consummatory behavior, and satiety behavior. *Prefeeding behaviors* as the name implies, identify those behaviors that occur before feeding such as fussiness or crying. In early infancy, *approach behaviors* included the rooting reflex or any sucking noises. In later infancy, an approach behavior would be recognition of the bottle. *Attachment behaviors* include all behaviors from the time the infant receives the nipple until he or she sucks. *Consummatory behaviors* are those identified by coordinated sucking and swallowing. And *satiety behavior* would be identified when the neonate indicates he or she is satisfied, most clearly by falling asleep. These five steps have been identified in successful feeding; assessment of the steps can assist nurses in identifying feeding problems.

Feeding Schedules

Just as sleeping schedules differ from neonate to neonate, so do feeding schedules. Ideally, the newborn should be fed when hungry. Hospitals frequently arbitrarily place newborns on a 4-hour feeding schedule, which usually is fairly satisfactory for bottle-fed babies but not so for breast-fed babies (see Chapter 19). Feeding when the neonate is hungry is called *demand feeding.* In reality, most newborns are fed on a combination of demand and scheduled feedings depending on the life-style of the parents. Good advice to parents may be do not feed more often than every 3 hours and do not let the neonate sleep longer than 5 hours during the day if you are aiming for a reasonable pattern of feeding.

Vitamin Supplements

The question of vitamin supplements has to be answered in relation to the formula to be used. For example, infant's receiving commercially prepared cow's milk or soy formulas receive more than the recommended amounts of vitamins A, D, C, thiamine, riboflavin, niacin, and ascorbic acid. However, human milk is lacking in vitamin D, and 400 IU of vitamin D supplement daily is recommended. Both iron and flouride need to be supplemented for the breast-fed baby. If the intake of the infant is pure cow's milk, ascorbic acid is needed and can be obtained from baby juices. As mentioned earlier, iron deficiency anemia is a common problem in the United States and most experts feel that an iron supplement (7 mg) for those infants receiving human or cow's milk is appropriate from age 4 weeks through 12 months (Slattery, 1977).

Summary of Nursing Care Goals of the Newborn

In reviewing the goals of newborn care discussed at the beginning of this section, you will recall that airway establishment is primary. Suctioning of the oropharynx, positioning the neonate on the side to ease drainage of mucus, and assessing vital signs every 15 minutes are all important. Maintaining a stable body temperature is supported by drying and then clothing the infant in diaper and shirt and covering the infant or placing him or her under a radiant heat warmer, taking care to reduce radiant heat loss. Bathing and other procedures (footprinting, circumcision, etc.) should be postponed until the infant's temperature is stable. Protection from infection and injury focuses on good handwashing before and after handling the infant. Close inspection of the cut surface of the umbilical cord for the presence of one vein and two arteries is necessary. Vitamin K and silver nitrate given to the neonate help protect the infant from trauma and infection. On a daily basis, eye care, cleaning the genital area after voiding or stool, and bathing are all important. If the neonate has been circumcised, the area and the dressing should be kept clean. Injury to the neonate is avoided by being sure that the infant is never left unsupervised, particularly on a surface without sides or during weighing. The identification bracelet should be checked to assure correct identity. Diaper pins need to be kept closed and pointed or sharp objects kept out of reach. Uncoordinated as the neonate may be, the grasp reflex is strong. Adequate nutrition is provided via breast or bottle. Breast-fed infants should be taken from the nursery to the mother every 2–3 hours (unless the mother has rooming-in and the neonate is near). Both parents should participate in the feeding whenever possible. Positioning the infant after feeding is important. The stool pattern should be assessed. The last goal, that of promoting mother–infant attachment is an ongoing activity, occurring each time there is opportunity for mother–infant contact. Specific behaviors to be assessed and nursing interventions that foster the attachment process are discussed fully in the behavioral assessment section.

SUMMARY

This chapter on the neonate initially discussed adjustment to extrauterine life. The periods of reactivity, inactivity, and reactivity that occupy the first 6 hours of life were explained, and the behaviors seen in the neonate during this time were described. This was followed by a discussion of the physiologic characteristics of the newborn. The physiologic and chemical basis of respiratory adaptation, the most profound adaptation, was described. Changes in the pulmonary system, pressure changes, the role of oxygen and carbon dioxide, and the relationship of surfactant to the aveoli and its significance were emphasized. Respiratory effort of the neonate was contrasted with that of the adult. Next, circulatory adaptation was discussed and contrasted with the adult circulatory system. Cardiac location and auscultation were described. Hematopoietic adaptation was discussed along with blood components, including cells, iron stores, and the significance of bilirubin and vitamin K in the newborn. Renal, fluid, and electrolyte adaptation was included in a discussion of the urinary system in the neonate and again this was contrasted with the adult. The composition of body fluids in the neonate versus the adult and rate of fluid exchange were discussed. Digestive adaptation traced the function of the gastrointestinal tract from the mouth to the anus. Enzymes to digest carbohydrates, fats, and proteins were described, and the relationship of the immature liver to gluconeogenesis and its significance were mentioned. Thermoregulation, heat production, stability, and metabolic activity were contrasted with the adult. The uniqueness and significance of brown fat in the neonate was noted. Methods of heat loss and the physiologic effect of cold stress were described. Integumentary adaptation pointing out the immaturity of the integumentary system and the unique problems this poses were described. Reproductive adaptation and the effect of maternal hormones on this system were explained. Adaptation against infection and a brief discussion of the immune properties of the neonate followed. The discussion of neurologic adaptation included the fact that although the nervous system is intact at birth, it is immature. Growth and development of the nervous system were described briefly. Musculoskeletal adaption discussion followed, noting that integration of musculoskeletal and neurologic systems was necessary for development. The last section under physiologic characteristics was sensory function. Functional ability of eyes and ears and sense of smell and taste were described. The significance of touch was stressed.

Following the description of the system-by-system physiologic characteristics, the chapter moved to the area of assessment of the newborn—physical, gestational, and behavioral. Physical assessment carried out by the nurse was described with some guidelines for the nurse regarding the process of assessment. The section then described areas of assessment in the physical exam, including appearance and measurements. Heart and lung assessment and the importance of auscultation were described. Skin assessment followed, and the vocabulary critical to skin assessment in the neonate was listed. Head, eye, ear, and nose were followed by neck and abdomen assessment factors. Assessment of genitalia, back, and rectum were included. Significant factors to be assessed in relation to the extremities were described, and appropriate methods for eliciting the many reflexes of the newborn and the significance of these reflexes were included. The section on physical assessment was summarized in Table 17.2, noting assessment factor or area, usual findings, common deviations, abnormalities, and nursing actions.

The next section on gestational age assessment stressed the importance of the nurse being able to assess gestational age in order to predict any potential problems related to LGA or SGA infants. Definitions of preterm, term, and postterm were given. Neurologic signs and physical characteristics assessed were listed, and many figures with the relevant captions illustrated how to proceed with gestational age assessment.

Behavioral assessment emphasized the reciprocity of the mother–infant and parent–infant attachment process. This section included Bowlby and Ainsworth's review of the infant as well as Klaus and Kennell's and Broussard's work on maternal–infant attachment. A discussion of awake and asleep states of the neonate was included, and the relationship of these states to the Neonatal Behavioral Assessment Scale was explained. Behaviors of infants to be assessed, as well as how and when the Brazelton tool should be used, were described. The Neonatal Perception Inventory and its aim were discussed briefly.

The behavioral assessment section stressed the mutuality of the attachment process and emphasized the role of the nurse in the education of parents regarding their infants.

The last section of the chapter described nursing care of the neonate, pointing out that the goal of nursing care is to maintain homeostasis in the newborn. Subsequent goals were establishing an airway, stabilizing body temperature, providing safety against injury or infection, providing nutrition, and promoting the parent–neonate attachment process. Transitional care and care of the normal neonate followed. Areas discussed were nursing assessment of vital signs, bathing, care of the umbilicus, clothing and positioning, care of the circumcision, feeding and the importance of feeding schedules. Nutritive values of breast versus cow's milk and other milk formulas were explored, and vitamin and mineral adequacy or deficits of milk preparations were discussed. The techniques of breast- and bottle-feeding and nursing interventions regarding this with new mothers are discussed more fully in Chapter 19.

REFERENCES AND READINGS

Ainsworth, M. D. The Development of Infant–Mother Attachment, in Caldwell, B., Ricuid, H. N. (Eds.), *Review of Child Development Research.* Chicago: University of Chicago Press, 1973, pp. 1–94.

Aladjem, S. A., Brown, A. K., Sureau, C. *Clinical Perinatology* (2nd ed.) St. Louis: C. V. Mosby, 1979.

American Academy of Pediatrics. Committee on Fetus and Newborn. Report of the Ad Hoc Task Force on Circumcision. *Pediatr* 56:610, 1975.

Anders, T. F., Chalemain, R. J. The Effects of Circumcision on Sleep Wake States in Human Neonates. *Psychosom Med* 36:174, 1974.

Anderson, G. C. The Mother and Her Newborn: Mutual Caregivers. *J Obstet Gynecol Neonatal Nurs* 6(5):50, 1977.

Arnold, H. W. et al. The Newborn: Transition to Extrauterine Life. *Am J Nurs* 65:77, 1965.

Bowlby, J. *Attachment and Loss, Volume I.* New York: Basic Books, 1969.

Brazelton, T. Mother–Infant Reciprocity, in Klaus, M. et al. (Eds.), *Maternal Attachments and Mothering Disorders.* New Brunswick, N.J.: Johnson and Johnson Baby Products, 1974.

Brazelton, T. *Neonatal Behavioral Assessment Scale.* Philadelphia: International Ideas, 1974, pp. 5–8.

Brazelton, T. *The Neonatal Behavioral Assessment Scale.* Philadelphia: J. B. Lippincott, 1973.

Broussard, E. R., Sturgeon, M.S. Further Considerations Regarding Maternal Perception of the First Born, Exceptional Infant: Studies in Abnormalities, Vol. 2, Hellmuth, J. (Ed.). New York: Brunner/Mazel, 1971.

Clark, A. Recognizing Discord Between Mother and Child and Changing it to Harmony. *Am J Matern Child Nurs* I(2):100, 1976.

Clark, A., Affonso, D. *Childbearing: A Nursing Perspective.* Philadelphia: F. A. Davis, 1976.

Clark, A., Affonso, D. Infant Behavior and Maternal Attachment: Two Sides to the Coin. *Am J Matern Child Nurs* I(2):94, 1976.

Dagher, R. et al. Carcinoma of the Penis and the Anti-Circumcision Crusade. *J Urol* 110:79, 1973.

Davis, V. The Structure and Function of Brown Adipose Tissue in the Neonate. *J Obstet Gynecol Neonatal Nurs* 9(6):368, 1980.

Dubowitz, L. M. S., Dubowitz, V., and Goldberg, C. Clinical assessment of gestational age in the newborn infant. *J Pediatr* 77:1–10, 1970.

Emde, R. et al. Stress and Neonatal Sleep. *Psychosom Med* 33:491, 1971.

Erickson, M. P. Trends in Assessing the Newborn and His Parents. *Matern Child Nurs* 3(2):99, 1978.

Frantz, R., Miranda, S. B. Newborn Infant Attention to Form and Contour. *Child Dev* 46:224, 1975.

German, L. D., Mason, P. A., Rosman, N. P. Reliability of Head Circumference Measurement in the Newborn. *Clin Pediatr* 15:891, 1976.

Greenberg, M. Morris, N. Engrossment: The Newborn's Impact Upon the Father. *Am J Orthopsychiatry* 44(4):520, 1974.

Grimes, D. A. Routine Circumcision Reconsidered. *Am J Nurs* 80(1):108, 1980.

Guyton, A. *Textbook of Medical Physiology.* Philadelphia: W. B. Saunders, 1976.

Hugo, M. J. A Look at Maternal Position During Labor. *J Nurse Midwifery* 22:26, 1977.

Iles, J. P., McCrary, M. Cuddle Bathing Can Be Fun. *Matern Child Nurs* I(6):350, 1976.

Jenkins, R. L., Westhus, N. K. The Nurse's Role in Parent–Infant Bonding: Overview, Assessment, Intervention. *J Obstet Gynecol Neonatal Nurs* 10(2):114, 1981.

Jensen, M. D., Benson, R. C., Bobak, I. M. *Maternity Care, The Nurse and the Family* (2nd ed.). St. Louis: C. V. Mosby, 1981.

Johnson, N. W. Breast Feeding at One Hour of Age. *Matern Child Nurs* I(1):12, 1976.

Johnston, M. Cultural Variations in Professional and Parenting Patterns. *J Obstet Gynecol Neonatal Nurs* 9(1):9, 1980.

Kaplan, G. Circumcision: An Overview. *Curr Probl Pediatr* 7:1, 1977.

Kempe, C. H., Helfer, R. E. *Helping the Battered Child and His Family.* Philadelphia: J. B. Lippincott, 1972.

Klaus, M., Kennell, J. *Maternal–Infant Bonding.* St. Louis: C. V. Mosby, 1976.

Klaus, M., et al. Maternal Attachment: Importance of the First Postpartum Days. *New Engl J Med* 286:460, 1972.

Laestadius, N., Aase, J., Smith, D. Normal Innercostal and Outer Orbital Dimensions. *J Pediatr* 74:465, 1969.

Lang, R. *Birth Book.* Ben Lomond, Calif.: Genesis Press, 1972.

Leonard, S. W. How First-Time Fathers Feel Toward Their Newborns. *Matern Child Nurs* I(6):361, 1976.

Lum, B., Batzel, R. L., Barnett, E. Reappraising Newborn Eye Care. *Am J Nurs* 80(9):-1602, 1980.

O'Grady, R. Feeding Behavior in Infants. *Am J Nurs* 71(4):736, 1971.

Olds, S. B., London, M. L., Ladewig, P. A., Davidson, S. V. *Obstetric Nursing.* Menlo Park, Calif.: Addison-Wesley, 1980.

Ostwald, P., Paltemen, P. The Cry of the Human Infant. *Sci Am* 230(3):84, 1974.

Patel, H. The Problem of Routine Circumcision. *Can Med Assoc J* 95:576, 1966.

Pedersen, D. R., Ter Urugt, D. The Influence of Amplitude and Frequency of Vestibular Stimulation on the Activity of Two-Month Old Infants. *Child Dev* 44:122, 1973.

Poole, C. J. Neonatal Circumcision. *J Obstet Gynecol Neonatal Nurs* 8(4):207, 1979.

Riesch, S. Enhancement of Mother–Infant Social Interaction. *J Obstet Gynecol Neonatal Nurs* 8(4):242, 1979.

Robson, H. S. The Role of Eye-to-Eye Contact in Maternal–Infant Attachment. *J Child Psychol Psychiatry* 8:13, 1967.

Ruber, V. D. Is the Nuturing Role Natural to Fathers? *Matern Child Nurs* I(6):366, 1976.

Rubin, R. Basic Maternal Behavior. *Nurs Outlook* 9:683, 1961.

Slattery, J. S. Nutrition for the Normal Healthy Infant. *Matern Child Nurs* 2(2):105, 1977.

Talbert, L. M. et al. Adrenal Cortical Response to Circumcision in the Neonate. *Obstet Gynecol* 48:208, 1976.

Whaley, L. F., D. L., Wong. *Nursing Care of Infants and Children.* St. Louis: C. V. Mosby, 1979.

Williams, J. K., Lancaster, J. Thermoregulation of the Newborn. *Matern Child Nurs* I(6):355, 1976.

18

PARENTHOOD

Patricia P. Villareal

Parenthood is a normal stage in the family life cycle. This "normal" stage, though, causes major role readjustment, stress, and uncertainty for the mother and father. Nurses have the significant role of assisting new parents in adapting to the demands of parenthood, which is a family developmental stage.

A *parent* is one who begets an offspring or adopts a child as his or her own. *Parenthood* is a position or a state of being, while *parenting* are the activities that a parent carries out in raising a child. This chapter explores various facets of parenthood. A historic overview of the family is given. Motivation and readiness for parenting, as well as the roles of mothering, fathering, grandparenting, and sibling, are examined. Various parenting situations, such as adoptive parenting, parenting in reconstituted families, single parenting, parenting a newborn in the middle years, and parenting twins, are discussed. Emphasis is placed on the role and intervention that nurses assume in each of these parenting situations.

MOTIVATION FOR PARENTING

The establishment phase of parenthood is from the time the couple is married or living together to the awareness of the first pregnancy. Early marriage (or living together) is a stage characterized by happiness, close intimacy, joint activity, and future planning. This future often includes the birth of a child. It is at this time that couples who are living together may formalize the relationship with a legal marriage. Most husbands and wives want to procreate and become parents. Today, many children result from planned pregnancies. The number of children born to a couple is a function of the number desired and the degree to which contraception is practiced. It is important to remember that unplanned pregnancies do occur. A man and woman make the purposeful decision to get married, but often one becomes a parent without intentionally wanting the role.

The deliberate decision to have children is one influenced by societal pressure. Traditional views of the family are for the purpose of procreation. Table 18.1 gives reasons for having children as sited by subjects in a study done by Hoffman and Hoffman (1973).

Society, in general, values children. Nurses, doctors, friends, and relatives believe that a new baby brings nothing but joy into the lives of parents. Little recognition is given to the fact that moving from a dyadic relationship to a triadic one may cause great difficulties for the parents. The process of becoming a parent is a complex experience involving gratification, stress, and potential dysfunction.

PREPARATION FOR PARENTING

For many years, American society has directed all attention to the baby. Classes for new mothers

TABLE 18.1
VALUES INSTRUMENTAL TO THE CHILDBEARING DECISION

1. Children, by their presence, confirm adult status and give people, particularly women, a recognized social identity.
2. Children provide a means for continuation of the self, a kind of immortality.
3. Children tie parents to the community through children's activities in school, public recreation programs, and the neighborhood.
4. Children show, according to religious doctrine, that couples are moral beings. Children are evidence that parents place others' welfare before their own and contribute to the continuity of the group.
5. Children protect parents from loneliness in an impersonal world.
6. Children supply novelty and fun to family life that keeps it interesting.
7. Children, with their attendant socialization requirements, develop competencies in parents and give them a sense of accomplishment.
8. Children provide scope to parents for demonstrating creative child-rearing strategies.
9. Children permit parents to exercise power over others, as well as to gain prestige since parents usually receive more social approval than do childless people.
10. Children give some parents a sense of vicarious achievement through their children's accomplishments.
11. Children can be of economic help, especially to elderly parents who need financial aid or a home.

Source: Hoffman, L. W., Hoffman, M. L. The Value of Children to Parents, in Fawcett, F. T. (Ed.), *Psychological Perspective on Population.* New York: Basic Books, 1973, pp. 46–47.

focused on activities such as bathing, diapering, and feeding the infant. More recently, childbirth preparation classes (see Chapter 15) have become a commonplace activity for expectant parents. Unfortunately, there are no classes that educate parents about what to do in relation to role transition and the impact of parenting on the marriage. It is known that marital satisfaction generally decreases after the birth of a baby. Mothers have less time to devote to their partners. Fathers often feel displaced. Both partners wonder when things will return to normal. The true answer is *never.* Parents are not always prepared to make the adaptation to a triadic relationship.

High schools across the country have attempted to prepare teenagers for their potential role as parents through family life classes. The motivation for learning about parenting at this period in life, however, is usually low. Swendsen et al. (1978) have described an approach to helping first-time parents master the role. The program is called *Preventive Role Supplementation.* Nurses conduct meetings for expectant parents in the third trimester of pregnancy. The goals of the group are to provide didactic information to the parents, opportunity for group discussion, and role modeling situations and role rehearsal. In addition to the group meetings, nurses make at least two home visits after the baby is born to assess family adaptation to parenthood. A couple who is experiencing successful parenting visits a group session of the parents-to-be. This gives the group an opportunity to see a role model. There is discussion on how they would handle various situations that are likely to occur in the early parenting stage. Evaluation of this program to date indicates a favorable response from parents. Couples have stated a decrease in anxiety and increase in self-confidence concerning preparation for parenthood.

TRANSITION TO PARENTHOOD

Marriages may be made and broken, but parenthood is irrevocable in our society. The responsibility for parenting is present from the birth of the infant to the death of both parents. The tasks of parenting vary dramatically over this time span. The major responsibilities of the parents occur early in the child's life.

Evelyn Duvall (1977) has described the developmental tasks of families along the age continuum. Important to the discussion in this chapter is the review of the tasks of the family in the establishment phase (see Table 18.2). While these are tasks primarily for middle-class traditional families, many of them are also true for nontraditional families. Confirmation of a pregnancy leads to the expectant phase, which brings a whole new set of developmental tasks to the family (Table 18.3).

It is important for each nurse to assess the family in relation to the developmental tasks outlined here. If a family is failing to meet one or more of these tasks, there is danger to the integrity of that family. Nursing intervention must be directed at assisting the family in accomplishing the developmental tasks.

Clarke-Stewart (1977) has set forth certain family policy propositions derived from reviewing child developmental research (Table 18.4). This set of propositions shows the importance of the integrity of the family to the welfare of the child. Nurses have an important role in actualizing these propositions. The nurse is directly responsible for including the father, for providing for early mother–father–infant contact, and for offering parenting classes. Indirectly, the nurse can be a parent advocate by supporting public laws that provide needed services to families.

Families today are choosing to have fewer children. Since couples will experience parenthood fewer times, they are demanding and expecting quality experiences. No longer does a mother want to "be delivered," she now wants to "give birth." This implies active participation of the mother in the childbirth experience. Nurses must provide for this consumer demand by helping couples through the metamorphosis that leads to parenthood. Health care providers must remember that couples need more than simple facts to survive the transition to parenthood.

THE HISTORY OF THE AMERICAN FAMILY

During the twentieth century, some interesting changes have occurred in the family. Despite what modern alarmists say, the family is not dying. It is merely undergoing some functional changes that allow it to survive in our society today.

Before the twentieth century, people married later and had more children spread over a longer time. Since they had shorter life spans, child rearing often took place over the parents' entire lives. Children

TABLE 18.2
FAMILY TASKS: ESTABLISHMENT PHASE

Phase of Family Development	*Developmental Tasks*
Beginning family Establishment phase: from marriage to first pregnancy	1. Establishing a home base in a place to call their own 2. Establishing mutually satisfactory systems for getting and spending money 3. Establishing mutually acceptable patterns of who does what and who is accountable to whom 4. Establishing a continuity of a mutually satisfying sex relationship 5. Establishing systems of intellectual and emotional communication 6. Establishing workable relationships with relatives 7. Establishing ways of interacting with friends, associates, and community organizations 8. Facing the possibility of children and planning for their coming 9. Establishing a workable philosophy of life as a couple

TABLE 18.3
FAMILY TASKS: EXPECTANT PHASE

Phase of Family Development	*Developmental Tasks*
Beginning family Expectant phase: from awareness of pregnancy to birth of first child	1. Arranging for the physical care of the expected baby 2. Developing new patterns for getting and spending income 3. Re-evaluating procedures for determining who does what and where authority rests 4. Adapting patterns of sexual relationship to pregnancy 5. Expanding communication systems for present and anticipated emotional needs 6. Reorienting relationships with relatives 7. Adapting relationships with friends, associates, and community activities to the realities of pregnancy 8. Acquiring knowledge about and planning for the specifics of pregnancy, childbirth, and parenthood 9. Maintaining morale and a workable philosophy of life

grew up with a number of siblings. Older siblings often served as surrogate parents. Parents frequently died, particularly the father, before the youngest child reached adulthood. Many mothers died during or immediately after childbirth.

Nineteenth-century families raised children with the expectation that they would start to work as soon as possible. There was no pension system in those days, and it was expected that children would support their parents in their old age. The obligation to the family always came before individual interests. The family relationship was often based on economic needs and tasks. There was little time or energy to worry over emotional satisfaction in relationships among family members.

During the twentieth century there has been a more orderly transition into family roles. Today there is a specific time for entering and exiting from school, for choosing an occupation, for getting a job, for leaving parents' household, for marrying, for starting a family, and for retiring. Before, the major transition in a woman's life was seen as marriage, not parenthood. Today the time between marriage and the birth of the first child has increased so the transition to parenthood has taken on more significance. The decision to get married does not necessarily mean the inevitable parenthood role 9 months after the marriage vows. Since the timing of children can be planned more accurately, marriages are occurring earlier. Modern families have fewer children more closely spaced. Thus, only a small proportion of an adult's life may be spent in the parenting role.

This newer trend has brought with it the empty nest syndrome. The *empty nest syndrome* is when the last child has left the family of origin. The parents must once again focus their energies on a dyadic relationship. For some, this transition can present problems that may end in the dissolution of the marriage, even after 25 years. For others, this period of life may be viewed as a time of freedom to travel and to do what they have always dreamed of doing but never could when their children were smaller. The couple may take on some "daring" activities such as camping their way across the country. The children now have a chance to worry about their parents.

Since the modern American family does not depend on children for economic support, there is a greater focus on the individual rather than on the family as a group. Social systems such as pension plans and social security help provide for retired parents. Social structures such as retirement havens

TABLE 18.4
PROPOSITION FOR CHILD CARE IN THE FAMILY

- ▲ A child should be given help in developing a secure attachment to his or her parents and then, increasingly, be given opportunities to interact with other adults and children.
- ▲ Policy should promote the parents' attachment to the baby from the beginning.
- ▲ Services should be provided to help parents plan their families and raise their children.
- ▲ Support services, work practices, and income maintenance should be provided so that mothers can choose whether they want to work or to stay home.
- ▲ Fathers should be encouraged to spend more time parenting and to adopt a more nurturant role, if they choose to.
- ▲ Parent education programs should be improved and made available to all parents and prospective parents who want them.
- ▲ A wide variety of "quality" day-care arrangements should be provided to accommodate the different needs of parents and children.
- ▲ Policy should encourage adoption rather than foster care, early rather than late adoption, and adoption by adults who are or can be competent caregivers.
- ▲ Policy should make services available but not dictate their use. Provision of adequate family "support" is preferred to direct or involuntary intervention.

Source: Clarke-Stewart, A. *Child Care in the Family.* New York: Academic Press, 1977.

and nursing homes remove from children the burden of caring for their aged parents in their own homes. Since many of the physical needs of people are being met, the family today can focus on the emotional needs of its members. Family members look to each other for emotional support and nurturing. The obligation now is more for personal affection than for material welfare. Members of the modern, somewhat isolated nuclear family must turn to one another for help. Society views today's family as a retreat from the tension-filled outside world. This is an unrealistic expectation to place on the family. This ideal can cause distress to family members that can lead to discord and divorce. Divorce rates have steadily increased. This increase does not necessarily mean that families are weaker than in previous times. It does mean that society now allows for divorce without the social taboos of previous times. Divorces have been steadily climbing, reaching a 4.7 per 1,000 population level in 1975.

What does the future hold for the family? Only time will tell for sure. There does seem to be the continued trend to privateness, to a focus on the needs of the individual, and to a highly technical computerized home life. Knowledge and technology will continue to increase at a rapid rate. We hope that society will not dehumanize its members but will find ways to humanize and personalize services to increase the feelings of worth of every member of the family.

MOTHERHOOD

"Why did you want a baby?" If the nurse asked this question of potential mothers, likely responses would be: "To be fulfilled as a woman." "To have someone to share our love with and to love us back." "So I could experience motherhood." The word *mother* denotes the role taken on by a woman after the birth of a baby. *Motherhood* is the state of being a mother, while *mothering* involves all the tasks and activities in raising a child. Motherhood, like most other things, has undergone tremendous changes. The motivation for motherhood may range from the traditional to a highly modern view. Society, especially the women's movement, has impacted heavily on the role of mother. Mothers range from the woman who stays home and devotes her time to her children to the woman who combines motherhood with a full status career. There are many styles for mothering, all of which can lead to successful parenting. The nurse has the responsibility to help each woman define her style and to support her as she assumes the role.

Taking on the Role

No longer is the belief commonly held that mothering is instinctual. With biologic motherhood, psychologic motherhood is *not* conferred. The role of the mother must be learned.

The process of assuming the maternal role was studied by a nurse in the early 1960s (Rubin, 1963). Rubin identified three phases of adjustment to the maternal role. During the first phase, taking in, the mother focuses on her physiologic and psychologic needs. She wants to discuss her labor and delivery with friends and nurses. The second phase, taking hold, occurs around the third postpartum day. At this time the mother wants to learn the mothering tasks of diapering, feeding, and bathing her infant. The last phase, letting go, occurs about 10 days after birth and continues for a couple of months. In this phase the mother comes to see her infant as a separate person with his or her own personality.

Women have often experienced bouts of depression and crying in the early postpartum period. Some experts attribute this to a physiologic shifting of hormones; others attribute it to the psychologic need to let go of previous roles and assume the new one. There is some grief work that goes on at this time. The mother looses the fantasized ideas of what her baby will be like and now must deal with the reality of how her baby looks and acts.

Rubin (1963) was one of the first to describe the maternal acquaintance process. She states that a mother becomes acquainted with her infant by first exploring the infant with her fingertips; next using her palms, hands, and whole arms; and finally enfolding the child in her arms. It was believed that this process took several days, now it is known often to occur within a few minutes.

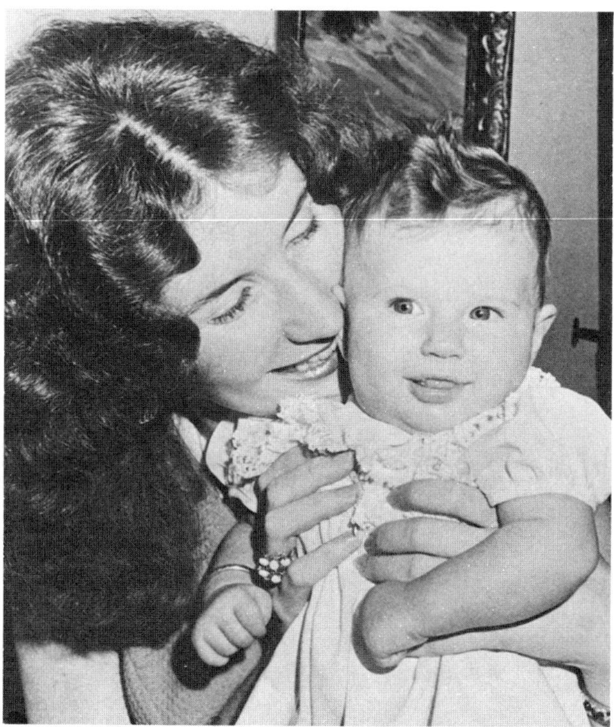

Figure 18.1
The mother–infant relationship is a very special one.

Maternal Attachment

Recently there has been overwhelming attention given to how a mother attaches to her baby (Fig. 18.1). Before discussing the current attachment literature, it would be helpful to look at a historic perspective of this topic.

In the early 1950s, Bowlby (1969) first used the term *attachment* to refer to the patterns of behavior that lead a child to attain or maintain closer proximity to the mother. The purpose of this behavior is to protect the young against predators and thus increase the chances for the offspring to survive. Ainsworth and associates (1978) expanded this concept when they studied in detail the child's development of attachment to the mother figure during the first 2 years of life. They also examined the child's response to separation from the mother. Their comprehensive report is contained in *Patterns of Attachment.* Recently, attention has been given to how the mother attaches to her infant rather than how the infant attaches to her.

Perhaps one of the most significant studies of this century was done by Kennell and colleagues in 1974. Their study served as the basis for changing maternity hospital policies across the country. The researchers took one group of mothers and allowed them extended contact with their infants immediately after birth in the early postpartum period. When this experimental group was compared with the mothers who followed the usual hospital routine (late contact group), several significant findings emerged. One month later at a well-child examination, the early contact mothers were found to stand close to their infants and watch the examination, to soothe the infant more, to engage in more eye-to-eye contact in the *en face position*—eye-to-eye contact that occurs between infant and adult where the adult rotates his or her head to be in the same vertical plane as that of the infant's eye—to fondle more during feeding, and to be more reluctant to leave their infants. At 2 years, mothers in the early contact group were found to use more questions, more words per proposition, more adjectives, and fewer commands when speaking to their children than mothers in the late contact group used (Ringer et al., 1975). Many other studies have looked at the significance of early postpartum contact. It appears that all mothers benefit from early contact with their infants. Early contact helps to form a bond between mother and infant that then helps in the process of attachment.

These findings have caused Kennell et al. (1974) and Klaus to propose that there exists a sensitive period right after birth where the mother is particularly attuned to bond with her infant. The existence of this sensitive period is yet to be proven. The discussion that has taken place concerning this sensitive period has filtered over to the lay literature and has caused a great deal of concern to mothers. Mothers who have failed to have this early contact, have expressed worries that they have failed as a mother and all is lost. They feel they will never be able to establish a close relationship with their children. Of course, this is not true. It is known that mothers have attached well to their infants even after prolonged separations. Adoptive parents have excellent parent–infant relationships.

It is known that infants who have been separated from their parents because of prematurity or other serious illnesses are more likely to be the objects of parental abuse. This fact has caused most hospital nurseries to change their policies. Parents and grandparents are now encouraged to visit, touch, and hold their infants no matter how ill the infant is and no matter what are the chances for recovery.

Another problem that has befallen this area is the professional's and lay person's interchangeable use of the words bonding and attachment. Kennell and Klaus's work focuses primarily on bonding. *Bonding* refers to the relationship established with the infant during the sensitive period (Fig. 18.2). It is measured by a yes/no phenomenon: *maternal–infant* bonding occurred or did not occur. In contrast, *attachment* is a process that occurs over time. The parent–child relationship grows and develops into a close, powerful tie.

What the Mother Brings to the Relationship

A woman's first experience with motherhood is influenced by many factors. Her culture, personality, physical status, and past experiences all have a tremendous impact on the role she plays as a mother. Various cultures contribute values and attitudes that can attract or detract from the maternal role. In cultures where the extended family is common, mothers have been supported in their mothering roles by other people they trust and in whom they have confidence. In the United States, motherhood is fraught with myths such as all mothers should look like Hollywood starlets and mothers have inborn maternal instincts making it possible to raise perfect babies.

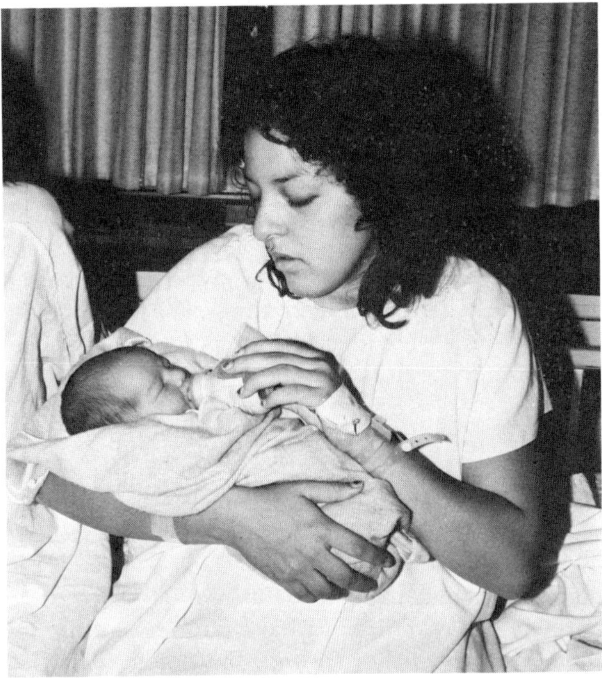

Figure 18.2
Early mother–infant relationships are an important part of maternal–infant bonding.

The demands of motherhood require that a mother have an ample supply of energy. One of the needs of mothers is to recover from the birth process. Nurses need to use postpartum assessment (see Chapter 16) to assure that satisfactory physical recovery is occurring.

Recent past experiences such as the length and ease of her labor help to shape the woman's perspective on motherhood. Early life experiences of the mother also determine the mothering cycle. It has often been said that we learn to parent as we have been parented. Mothers enter the role with a perception of mother formed long ago by how their mothers took care of them.

Motherhood is a radical change in a woman's life. The woman's ability to adapt her life-style to the demands of the role depend, in part, on her basic personality type. Although women with varying personalities find success in motherhood, some personality traits make it easier to adapt to certain aspects of the maternal role. The easy-going, patient woman may find it easier to adapt to some challenges, while the "go get them" type adapts better to other challenges of parenting. The main attribute the nurse should encourage is that the woman have confidence in her mothering skills.

What the Infant Brings to the Relationship

It is well accepted today that the infant can affect the mother's behavior. Infants have far greater abilities than was previously believed. Physiologically, the infant induces oxytocin release in the mother that causes uterine contractions when he or she sucks her breast. Even the infant cry can induce the "let down" reflex necessary for milk flow in the mother's breast.

There is conflicting research concerning early behaviors of male and female infants. It is known that mothers (fathers too) respond differently to female infants than to male infants. It is also believed that infants born first may act differently from those born later.

Infants can see at birth and will engage in eye-to-eye contact with adults. Infants prefer the human face to inanimate objects but will track both when presented with this challenge. Infants focus best when objects are about 8 in. away from them. This is the same distance that an infant is from mother during feeding. The eye-to-eye contact that a mother and infant establish is one of the most powerful agents of interaction and attachment.

It is known that infants will be alert to and turn to a high-pitched female voice in preference to a lower-toned voice. Infants selectively attend to auditory stimuli from as early as 2 days of life. Infants' sense of smell is developed sufficiently by 1 week for them to distinguish the smell of their mothers' breast pads over that of other smells.

Another characteristic of infants that enhances the mother's view of herself and her confidence as a mother is the infant's ability to cuddle. Some infants innately cuddle and mold to the holder's body. This serves as a reinforcer to the mother that she is capable of supporting and comforting her baby.

A great deal of work has been done in the area of infant temperament. Carey (1972) defines *temperament* as "the emotional reactivity or behavioral style displayed in the early months of life" (p. 823). He has developed a questionnaire* that he gives to mothers. He asks mothers to rate their infants' behaviors in specific situations, such as feeding. There are nine categories of temperament in this questionnaire: activity, rhythmicity, adaptability, approach, sensory threshold, intensity, mood, distractability, and presistence. The infant is then classified as (1) difficult, (2) intermediate high, (3) intermediate low, or (4) easy. Although there is nothing that can be done to change an infant's temperament, this information does help the nurse to support, counsel, and give anticipatory guidance to the mother.

The Neonatal Behavioral Assessment Scale (Brazelton, 1973) was developed to assess the infant's response to the environment. Since it readily demonstrates the infant's behavioral characteristics, many nurses use parts of the scale to show parents what their infants are capable of doing. The scale also shows parents how to elicit responses from their infant. In this way, the nurse can increase the mother's knowledge about her baby and help her to form a satisfying relationship with her infant.

Reciprocal Effects of Mother–Infant Interaction

The main responsibility of a mother is to interpret the cues her infant sends correctly and the main responsibilities of an infant are to send clear cues denoting needs and to respond to the care the mother gives (Fig. 18.3). When the two are in harmony, there is a synchronous interaction that Brazelton (1973) has "likened to waltzing." Other terms used to describe this interaction are temporal phasing, cyclic behavior, and being in tune with each other. The mother must develop a sense of her infant's need for attention and need to withdraw. This synchronous behavior can be observed in vocal interactions with the baby as well as tactile and pause/delays during feedings.

* *The Infant Temperament Questionnaire* (4–8-month-old infants); revised 1977 by W. B. Carey and S. C. McDevitt. It can be obtained for $5.00 from William B. Carey, M.D., 319 W. Front Street, Media, Pennsylvania 19063, Telephone: (215) 566-6691.

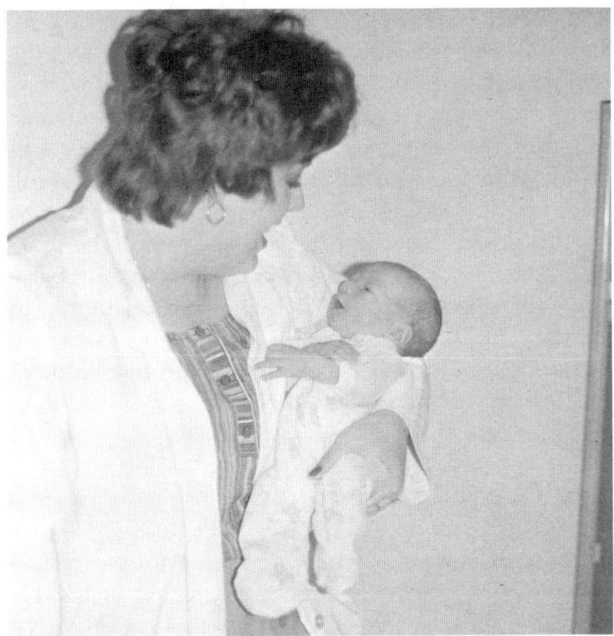

Figure 18.3
Mother–infant relationships are reciprocal.

An important question remains for nursing practitioners: How do we apply these findings to improve the parenting capabilities of families? Many tools have been developed for assessing maternal attachment. Some tools, based on clinical experiences, have not undergone the rigorous research techniques to make them valid and reliable. Other tools that have been proven valid and reliable may be too long and cumbersome for the nurse to use. Regardless of the tool, the essential behaviors of mothers that nurses observe in the early postpartum period are eye-to-eye contact, calling the infant by name, smiling at the infant, and expressing some joy about the infant, such as the sex, physical characteristics, or temperament. The waltzing described earlier may take a few weeks to develop between the infant and mother.

Perhaps one of the most useful and reliable set of scales has come from The Nursing Child Assessment Project conducted by Kathryn Barnard and colleagues (1974, 1979), a nurse at the University of Washington. There are four scales* that assess early parent-infant interaction.

*For information on training in the use of these tools, write to Georgina Sumner, NCAST, T436A, Health Sciences Building, SC-74, University of Washington, Seattle, Washington 98195.

- ▲ Nursing Child Assessment of Sleep Activity Record (NCASAR)
- ▲ Nursing Child Assessment of Teaching Scale (NCATS)
- ▲ Nursing Child Assessment of Feeding Scale (NCAFS)
- ▲ Home Observation for Measurement of the Environment (HOME)†
  Nurses must take a course in order to use these assessment techniques reliably and accurately.

The NCASAR is a way a mother can compare her baby to the average baby's time spent in sleep. This record allows the nurse to help the mother understand her baby's asleep/awake cycles and to plan accordingly.

The NCATS and NCAFS assess the mother's (caregiver's) sensitivity to the infant's cues; response to infant's distress; and social, emotional, and cognitive growth-fostering behavior and the infant's clarity of cues and responsiveness to the parent.

The HOME measures the caregiver's emotional and verbal responsiveness, involvement with the child, organization of the environment, provision of appropriate play material, provision of opportunities for varied daily stimulation, and avoidance of restriction and punishment.

Together these scales provide an excellent data base from which the nurse can make inferences, develop family-centered goals, and apply nursing intervention. Motherhood, without a doubt, is a complex and demanding job, and nurses must intervene effectively so optimal role attainment can be achieved.

FATHERHOOD

"Do I really want to be a father?" Almost all men will ask this question during their partner's pregnancy. The acceptance of the role of *father* initiates a change in the marital relationship. Prospective fathers realize they must give up some of the freedom they enjoyed as part of a couple. The father must "compete" with the child for the mother's attention. Frequently, there is financial worry about the cost of the new baby. Prospective fathers must

†Originally developed by Betty Caldwell (1970).

adapt to a change in the sexual relationship in their marriage (see Chapter 14). At this time most couples experience a decline in sexual intercourse. Men report, however, that their relationship with their partners is closer and more interdependent. Men tend to want to socialize more with other expectant or actual fathers during the time of pregnancy. Most men will have some fear about the emotional responsibility of becoming a parent and a father. The expectant father may doubt his capacity to father and be unclear as to what behaviors are expected of fathers. All fathers, though, have some degree of pride in their masculinity and potency. Table 18.5 summarizes the concerns of men related to fatherhood.

Fatherhood, the state of being a father, depends on a process that must be guided and allowed to blossom. *Fathering* can be defined as the process of providing for physical, emotional, and psychologic needs of the offspring. Nurses can play an important role with prospective fathers in three areas: nurturing, providing, and teaching. The first thing nurses can do is to include the father in all aspects of the pregnancy, labor, and delivery. Nurses must examine the physical environment to determine if it is father centered. Are there appropriate reading materials in the waiting areas for the father? Is the attitude of health care providers couple directed or mother directed?

Fathers need to discuss sexuality during the pregnancy and after the birth. Men may be reluctant to bring this topic up, so nurses should provide the opportunity. A comment such as "pregnancy and a newborn may change the sexual relationship you have with your wife" can provide the opportunity for a discussion.

Parenting centers and childbirth education organizations should recognize a man's need to socialize with other expectant or actual fathers. Setting up activities such as father's night could provide the opportunity for prospective fathers to share concerns and interests about parenting. Fathers engage in many activities, such as observing and talking to other fathers, attending childbirth and/or parenting classes, and reading about parenting in preparation for fathering. Expectant fathers will adjust the family budget in order to make purchases for the baby and will alter the physical living arrangements. In addition, they will anticipate their role as father by thinking about life-style changes, planning child activities, and dreaming about their expected child.

TABLE 18.5
CONCERNS RELATED TO FATHERHOOD

- ▲ Adequacy as a father
- ▲ Baby's effect in the martial dyad
- ▲ Financial responsibilities
- ▲ Infant-care skills

The Couvade Syndrome

The *couvade syndrome* refers to the various physical symptoms a man experiences any time during his partner's pregnancy. The symptoms usually reported are nausea, vomiting, anorexia, headaches, and abdominal pains. There seems to be no real physical basis for these symptoms, and they disappear after the birth of the child. It is believed that subconsciously men are experiencing the same discomforts as their partners. The intervention given is supportive care directed at relieving the symptoms. The interesting aspect of these male pregnancy symptoms is the relationship to ritual couvade. In primitive societies and in ancient times, men went through certain rituals, including going to bed and simulating groans while relatives and friends pampered them while their wives labored and delivered.

Fathers and Their Infants

Many myths exist about fatherhood. One is the belief that fathers are less nurturant and competent in caring for an infant. Another myth is that fathers are not interested in the caretaking role associated with a newborn. Parke and Sawin (1976) have conducted many studies that have dispelled these myths. They found that fathers respond appropriately to the baby's signals. Fathers tend to talk back to the infants rather than take some actions as most mothers do. Fathers slow their speech, use short phrases and repeat themselves as they talk to infants. Fathers tend to talk more to rather than touch their infants after a vocalization episode. Mothers do more touching. During feedings fathers respond to infant cues of distress. Infants take as much food from their fathers as they do from their mothers. During feedings fathers tend to wipe the infant's mouth less often than mothers do.

No matter how modern a couple's views of family roles are before the birth of the child, in most cases they tend to adopt traditional roles after the birth of their child. This means that mothers will spend more time than the fathers in caretaking activities even if she also works outside the home. It has been found, though, that fathers will spend more time in infant caretaking if their partners have had a cesarean section.

Most of the time the father spends with his baby will be in play. Fathers, as compared to mothers, tend to be more tactile and less verbal in play sessions. A play session may be father throwing his baby in the air; in general, fathers have a "jazzing up" approach to their babies.

Fathers respond differently to sons than to daughters. Some of the sex-type differences include talking to, looking at, and stimulating boys more than girls and holding girls closer to their bodies than boys. Mothers do just the opposite. They talk to and stimulate their daughters more than their sons. This does not mean that fathers neglect their daughters nor that mothers neglect their sons. But during a day fathers play approximately one-half hour more with their sons than with their daughters. Fathers are probably responsible for their sons adopting culturally ascribed behavior as they grow up.

Fathers have an important relationship to their offspring during infancy (Fig. 18.4). Fathers who attend childbirth classes and are present at the birth of their children are more involved with their babies. It has been said that these fathers are more engrossed with their newborns. It must also be noted that parental participation is influenced by the marital relationship and sex and temperament of the baby. The early postpartum period has always been recognized by nurses as an important time for intervention with the mother. This concept should be extended to fathers. Fathers need as much support as mothers during this early parenting period. Nurses should see that fathers are provided extended contact with their newborns. Paternity leaves should be a standard in our society. Men should be guided and given the opportunity to practice caretaking skills. Parenting classes should be directed to include content pertinent to fathers.

Parke (1981) showed a group of fathers a videotape of father–infant interaction during the postpartum hospital period. The videotape demonstrated the capabilities of infants and ways you can play and interact with the baby. The fathers who saw the film were compared to fathers who did not. The "film fathers" vocalized more to their infants, did more caretaking activities, and were less disturbed about the disruption the infant caused in their lives.

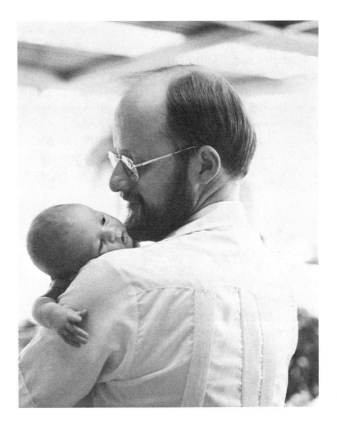

Figure 18.4
Fathers are parents too.

As with all nursing intervention, it must be individualized to meet the needs of the specific family. Opportunities must be provided to increase fathers' involvement. It must also be recognized that not every father will want this close involvement, and nurses must *not* equate this with poor fathering. It is simply a different style of fathering, a style that must be respected. Role conflict and disruption could occur if nurses are not careful to preserve systems that work well within each family.

GRANDPARENTHOOD

Despite an increase of research regarding various aspects of the family, the role of *grandparenting* has received little attention. Most of the information comes from two main sources: informal, popular magazines and scientific literature concerning problem-oriented families.

In our culture, grandparents are viewed as plump, gray-haired, happy-go-lucky people who lavish gifts on their grandchildren. Recently, more grandparents are attaining this role in their late 30s or early 40s. These young grandparents may have difficulty seeing themselves in the traditional role society has assigned to grandparents.

There are several responses to the birth of a grandchild. If the grandparents are generally satisfied with their lives, this event may be viewed as another accomplishment. Another perception of the birth may be that of being given a second chance, that of giving this grandchild the time, education, and money that could not be given to their own child.

Grandparents may become a teacher and role model. Children can then develop a sense of history and ancestry. In addition, it is believed that children who know older people may face the life-maturing processes with less fear (Craig, 1980).

Grandparents can assume the role of mother or father again and help the parents (Fig. 18.5). They often relive their parenting experiences through their grandchildren, but with less stress since they do not have direct responsibility for the child. An instinctual wish to survive is gratified through the grandchild. Often, there is personal pleasure in seeing oneself reincarnated. Remarks about the newborn such as "he has my eyes" reflect these feelings. Grandparents seem to enjoy their grandchildren more than their own children.

One recent study on grandmothers (Robertson, 1977) has shown that grandchildren help curb loneliness and carry on the family heritage. The younger the grandparent, the more the fun seeking and the more the parent-surrogate role is played. Grandparents are also often babysitters. They also fulfill the kinship role of families. It is the grandmother who keeps the various family members informed of what is happening to other family members.

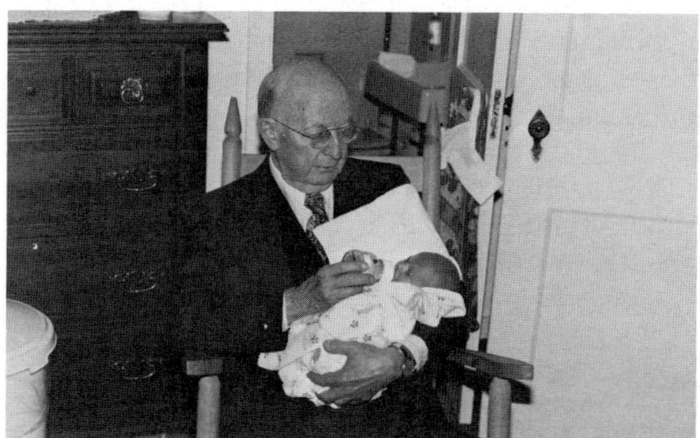

Figure 18.5
Grandparents have a role to play in the infant's world.

Grandparents can sometimes serve as stabilizers in families undergoing the developmental crises of birth. Young mothers will often look to their mothers for help in acquiring the necessary parenting skills. Intergenerational influences on parenting a child are yet to be elucidated in research. It is known that mothers often mother their children in much the same way they were mothered. If health care providers accept this premise, then attention should be given to grandparents in the perinatal stage. Every effort should be made to incorporate grandparents in the childbearing cycle. Parenting centers have offered sessions for grandparents in an effort to help them define their roles. Visiting hours on maternity units should be unrestricted for grandparents. Nurses should help grandparents be support systems for the new parents. In doing this, it may be necessary to update grandmothers, in particular, on the newer trends in child health care. Nurses can assist in strengthening the family if consideration is given to the grandparents of the infant.

PARENTHOOD BY ADOPTION

Adoption is a legal and social means of taking a child from another set of biologic parents into your family. This gives children of couples or single parents who cannot adequately provide for them a chance to be raised in a potentially secure family. Most adoptions today are done through an agency or by an intermediary person (such as a physician or lawyer). An agency screens the adopting family in order to determine their suitability for parenting a child. An agency also helps the natural mother with health care and other problems she may have. The agency acts as an advocate for the child and tries to provide protection to the child and to the natural and adoptive parents.

In the past 10 years there have emerged many new trends concerning the adoption of children. Single parents have adopted children. Couples have adopted children to complete their families. Due to liberalized abortion laws, better contraception techniques, and increased social acceptance of single parenthood, there are fewer newborns available for adoption. Since there are fewer "healthy white infants" available for adoption, many couples have opted to raise an older child, a handicapped infant, or a biracial child. Adoption agencies have more flexible policies today. At one time families had to pass rigorous interviews and home visits to be accepted as potential parents. Now a more sympathetic view is taken of potential adopting parents. No longer must the mother give up her career and stay at home to rear the adopted child. No longer must the family fit the mold of what an idealized American family should be. Adoptive families can have diverse interests and careers. The important characteristic an agency wishes a family to have is the capacity to love the child within a home environment that is conducive to normal growth and development. Nurses must remember that adoptive parents are real parents. They have all the needs, concerns, and fears about parenting that any biologic parent has.

In some ways, adoptive parents may be put at a disadvantage by the current system of adoption agencies. After a couple qualifies for adoption, there may be a long wait, even up to 2 years, for a baby. During this time, the couple carries on its life's activities. One day the phone rings and the couple is asked to pick up a child the next day. The suddenness of this conferred parenthood may leave the couple in crisis. It must be remembered that adoptive parents do not go through the usual rites of parenthood such as preparation for childbirth classes, baby showers, and postpartum classes on baby care. Most couples have not bought baby clothes or other necessities. There are no classes on preparing for parenthood when a couple is adopting a baby. Maternity leaves and insurance coverage may not be readily available to the adopting couple, thus making it even more difficult.

In a recent study, Walker (1981) determined that the needs of adoptive parents for information about childrearing were great, especially if the couple had no previous experience with parenting. Usually, the first contact the adoptive parents have with the health care system is on the first well-child visit. By this time, the parents have already had to struggle through bathing, diapering, feeding, sleeping schedules, finding a suitable pediatrician, and wondering if the infant's behavior is normal. Nurses could meet some very special needs by conducting classes for adoptive parents and providing an on call telephone line for the parents when the baby arrives. The classes could cover the typical skills needed to care for a young child, information about growth and development and how to handle the various situations (i.e., what to do about excessive crying, what are the signs of illness, is the child eating enough) that concern young parents appropriately. Classes would also provide adoptive parents the opportunity to meet with other couples who have adopted a child.

Once parents have made the decision to adopt, two large problems loom in their minds. Parents, especially mothers, are concerned about becoming attached to their adopted baby. Much of the current literature insinuates that a mother goes through a hormonal-sensitive period after biologic motherhood that allows her to bond to her baby. Adoptive mothers must be reminded by the nurse that attachment is a process. It is not "quick glue" where you feel immediately cemented to your newborn. One adoptive mother stated that attachment is having and holding the baby and being responsible for the baby's entire future. Attachment grows and blossoms for both biologic and adoptive parents.

The second problem that concerns adoptive parents is how to tell children they are adopted. Over the past decades, well meaning, but poor, advice, such as never tell your child he or she is adopted or the child will hate you, has been given to adoptive parents. Today it is believed that parents need to be given help and support as to when and how to tell children they are adopted. Many adoptive parents today simply rear their children with the knowledge that they are adopted. The first time children ask about where they were born, the parents simply tell the truth. One excellent short story (Zimmerman, 1977) shows a clear and simple way to explain adoption to a young child. Baby books are available for the adopted child, which treat the adoption as a matter-of-fact occurrence. In addition, adoptive parents should have some knowledge about the child's background. Children will go through a period of wanting to know about their biologic mothers. Parents should be assured that this is normal. Children should be allowed to discuss their feelings about being adopted with other adults.

Society has come a long way in accepting adoptive parents and their children. No longer is the adoptive parent stigmatized as being different and not a *real* parent. Nurses must also make some modern transitions with interventions directed at adopting parents. No longer can nursing, as a profession, ignore the needs of adoptive families. Nurses must work directly with the parents, child, and grandparents to help each make a smooth role transition.

PARENTHOOD THE SECOND TIME AROUND

At first it may appear that a multipara has an easier time with her pregnancy and infant than a primipara. After all, the stages of labor are shorter for a multipara and she knows what to expect. But does she really know what to expect in parenting the second time?

The parents who are having a second (or another) child are increasing the complexity of their total relationship. Suddenly they are going from a mother and father with a child to a family with two children. The number of possible interactions with people suddenly multiplies not only for the parents but also for the first child. If this is a third or fourth baby, the complexity increases even more.

The decision to have another child may be arrived at by relenting to social pressure to have the "ideal" two-child family, from wanting a sibling for the other child, or for some other reason. Every mother, though, will question her ability to love this second child as much as she loves her firstborn. She will have concerns about the demands on her time and energy that a second child necessitates. She will tend to have a very realistic view of motherhood and its demands. The mystical view of motherhood was dispelled the first week home with her first child.

The multipara may have concerns about how this pregnancy is differing from her first pregnancy. If this baby is more active than her first baby, she may believe something is wrong. She may be more fatigued or have more backaches and general discomforts with this pregnancy. The nurse must remember that multiparas need support and education too. Childbirth educators could assist multiparas by having special classes for them. This allows the mothers to focus on their special concerns and interests. It allows them to explore what they want to do differently with this child. They can reminisce about the great things and the not so great things that happened with their first child.

Perhaps the overriding concern of mothers and fathers is how to prepare the first child for the new baby's coming. Fathers often play an important role with the coming of the second or third child. Men can spend that little bit of extra time that is needed with the other children. Mothers often have feelings of being a traitor to their first child. Women need to express these ideas and discover that other second-time mothers feel the same.

One of the greatest let downs for a multipara may be the unenthusiastic response she gets from friends and relatives about her second pregnancy. Even her partner may not display that special spark he had when he learned he was going to be a father for the first time. This matter-of-fact acceptance of her second pregnancy may dampen the mother's emotional mood. It can take away from her special feelings about carrying a child in her body.

Health care providers may be guilty of neglecting the feelings and needs of the multipara. Nurses are quick to stress the importance of attending childbirth classes for the primipara but may forget that multiparas need to be prepared for childbirth too. In general, health care providers seem to give more attention to the primipara than the multipara. Though nurses may say to their patients that each pregnancy and child is different, they may fail to carry this belief out when dealing with multiparas.

Nursing intervention for a multipara should be directed at giving anticipatory guidance about the possible effect of this child on the family roles and relationships (Fig. 18.6). One question the nurse might ask is: What changes do you think this baby is going to make in your family? This will often let the nurse know what concerns the mother is having in this area, as well as what other areas the mother

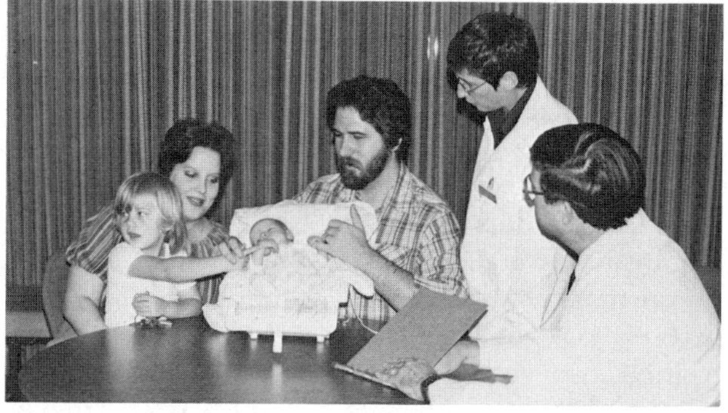

Figure 18.6
The nurse can be a real help to parents the second time around.

should be thinking about. It is extremely important that the nurse take an accurate history of the mother's impression of the labor and delivery of the first pregnancy. Although by medical standards the first pregnancy may have been low risk, the mother's perception of the experience may be quite different. If the mother perceives her first birth experience as an ordeal, she may approach her second birth with fear.

OLDER MULTIPARAS

If a pregnancy occurs after a woman is 40, there will be a whole different set of maternal needs that must be met by the nurse. First, the mother may be caught totally off guard by a pregnancy. She may have already entered the development tasks of another stage of the family life cycle. Suddenly, she is thrown back to the tasks of the expectant mother. Since most pregnancies occur before this age, the mother may feel she has no one her age with whom to share her thoughts, concerns, and feelings. It is an important task of pregnancy to be able to share concerns with other pregnant women. Society dictates that childbearing occurs in youth. The older mother and father may feel embarrassment or even shame about her being pregnant. Parents will have great concern for the welfare of their unborn child. Medically, the pregnancy will be classified as high risk. The occurrence of birth defects, especially Down's syndrome, increases dramatically after age 40.

The initial shock may give way to excitement as all of the memories of the joys of young children flood the mother's mind. Conversely, depression can occur if she does not feel she can meet the challenges an infant presents. She may look far to the future and calculate her age in relation to when this child will graduate from high school or college or get married. She may display a hopelessness that she is just too old to go through this. Her husband and older children can be a huge support to her. Her husband can give her the emotional support and respect she so desperately needs. Adolescent children often meet this announcement with great excitement and pride in their mothers. They will take on many responsibilities joyfully to ease their mothers' burdens. In general, this event can draw the family together and give it a common goal for which to prepare and look forward to.

SIBLING INTERACTION IN A FAMILY

Little attention has been given to the influence sibling relationships have on the family (Fig. 18.7). Factors such as age, sex, birth order, and number of siblings serve to make this area very complex. According to Smart and Smart (1976), siblings play the following roles: companions and playmates, teacher–learner, protector, role model, leader, and adversary. Within these roles some obvious behaviors emerge. The firstborn holds high power with other siblings. Sibling rivalry is the attempt of each child to struggle for the love and attention of one or both parents. If family disorganization exists, siblings will turn to each other for support and protection. Siblings may serve as role models for what they want to be like or for what they reject: "I am not like my brother. I'm different." Safe experimentation can go on within sibling relationships. Children can try on roles and use each other for sounding boards. Often siblings know things about each other that are kept from the parents. It is interesting to watch the bargaining power between children. The threat of tattling can be a powerful behavior modifier.

It is interesting to note that in the average middle-class family siblings spend more time with each other than they do with their parents. Sibling interaction may change dramatically when parents are not present. There are obviously strong bonds formed at this time. It must be remembered that sibling relationships last 60 or more years while parent–child relationships often last a much shorter time. It appears that the larger the family, the more

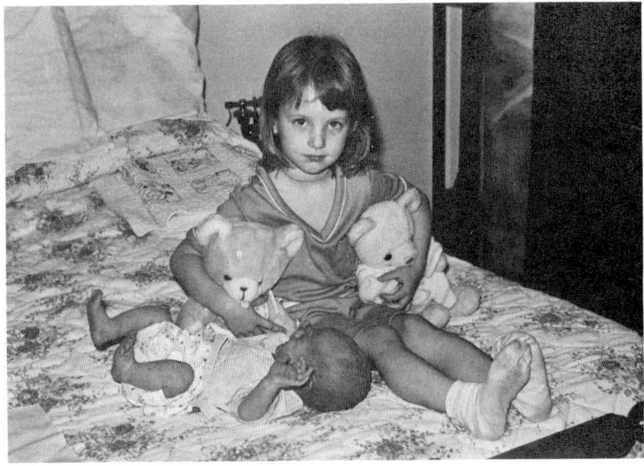

Figure 18.7
Siblings are interested in the newborn infant too.

important the sibling relationship especially for socialization. Nurses need to be aware of new research in this area so that they can help parents better understand the dynamics within the family.

THE IMPACT OF TWINS ON PARENTING

Two does make a difference. If you do not believe parenting twins is twice as difficult, just ask the parents of twins. The arrival of twins makes a dramatic difference on the relationships within the family. Suddenly parents are faced with a double dose of everything. More time and energy are spent in the caretaking of twins. Research shows (Lylton, 1980) that there is less time spent with each twin when compared to time spent with a singleton child. It is also known that parents of one child speak more to that child than parents of twins speak to each twin. Twins score lower on verbal tests than singletons. Researchers believe that this is a result of the environment, not genetic or perinatal factors. There are many stresses placed on parents, thus it is easy to see why the attention given to each child is reduced when dealing with two children of the same age. On the whole, twins become competent adults who make good social adjustments to life.

It has been noted that parents respond to the differences in twins as the infants display differences. Since identical twins look, act, and respond more similarly than fraternal twins, it is not surprising to find that parents treat monozygous twins more alike than they do dizygous twins.

Without a doubt, twinship has a great impact on the infants' socialization. Parents of twins verbalize many concerns about parenting in this special situation. Parents will need support and help from relatives and friends who can relieve them of the caretaking responsibilities from time to time. Parents will have many questions about child-rearing practices, such as: "Should I dress them alike?" "I find myself spending more time with one twin than the other, is this bad?" Nurses can often give support and encouragement to these families just by listening. When twins are term and healthy at birth, there is no need for any special child-rearing techniques. The one thing research has shown and that nurses can incorporate into practice is to encourage parents to spend time talking to each child individually. Many of the other problems encountered will be similar to those problems in families where the children are close together in age. The Mothers of Twins Club, a national organization, has provided invaluable material things (extra cribs, strollers, etc.) and emotional help to new mothers. This organization allows parents a chance to socialize with other parents of twins and to share helpful hints and give moral support and encouragement to one another.

THE ONE-PARENT FAMILY

The one-parent family may exist because of divorce, desertion, death, or an out-of-wedlock birth. Today there is an ever-increasing number of *single-parent families* (Fig. 18.8). Most consist of a mother with one or more children. More than one-fourth of single-parent, mother-headed households are classified as poor. There is a great deal written about single-parent families and the problems they must endure.

Two of the most overwhelming problems faced by the single-parent families are providing for the economic needs of the family and attempting to fulfill the roles of both father and mother. The economic burden of maintaining a household and feeding and clothing one or more children may exceed the capabilities of one parent. Inflation is contributing to this stress. It must also be remembered that a woman is more likely to have a lower paying job than a man. There may be extra costs incurred for a working single parents. They must provide for child care costs, transportation, and suitable work clothes for themselves. Since there is less time to prepare meals, many single parents resort to fast convenience foods

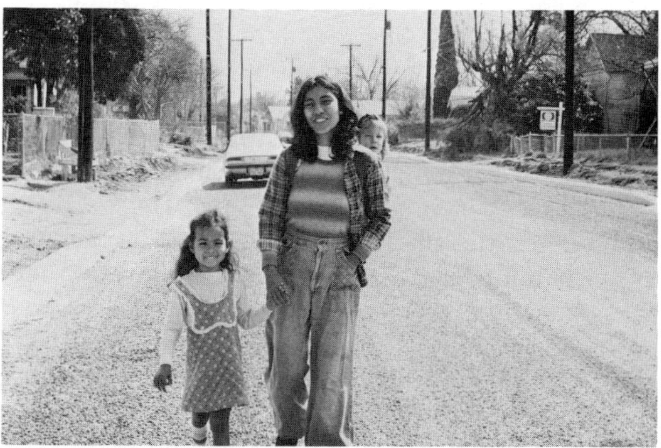

Figure 18.8
One-parent families are seen more frequently today.

that tend to be more expensive. The General Mills Report on The American Family (Yankelovich, Shelly and White, Inc., 1979) found that although all families were cutting back on health-related items to cope with inflation, single-parent families were cutting back more than any other type of families. It is obvious that nurses need to stress the cost effectiveness of prevention and early intervention to this group of families.

A single parent may feel overwhelmed and at a loss to carry out the roles of both mother and father. These families must be helped to realize that this expectation of themselves is unrealistic. The single parents can be directed to such groups as Big Brothers, Big Sisters as a way of helping their children have a role model of the other sex. This organization also helps to relieve some of the responsibility of parenting simply by allowing the parent more "time off." Single parents find little time to be away from their children and often feel trapped.

There are other problem areas that exist for single-parent families. Communication within this family structure is basically one sided. The parent generally does not have another adult in the home to share the concerns and frustrations that exist in the work setting. Social contacts may be limited since little time or energy may be left for such activities. The single parent has no one to discuss parenting or tactics to handle the behavior the children display. The children will generally be exposed to other adults at day care or school. The children, however, do not get the benefit of two adults interacting together in the home setting. It is believed that many cultural values are transmitted by two-way interaction in the home.

Another significant factor in a single-parent family is that the child sees only the one parent as the authority figure. In the case of mother-headed households, discipline is carried out only by the female sex. If the child identified authority too closely with one sex, there is the possibility of adjustment problems later in life.

The affectional needs of children can be well met in a one-parent family. It is often the parent whose emotional needs are unmet. The single parent must continually give love and support and act as an outlet for negative feelings. The child's love may be gratifying, but it is not supportive for the many stresses incurred by the single parent. A single parent must find other ways to vent negative feelings since children are not an appropriate outlet.

Perhaps one of the biggest helps to single-parent families would be prevention. Society needs to make readily available low-cost marriage counseling. Better premarital education would also help people who are considering marriage. It is far better to get to the root of the problem before a marriage is destroyed. It is necessary for people to know themselves so they can better cope with the dilemmas that occur in any marriage.

The nurse can play a strong advocacy role by supporting legislation that addresses the needs of the single-parent family. One community issue is the need for better child care for working mothers, especially those raising children alone. Nurses can also refer single parents to appropriate counseling services. Self-help groups such as Parents Without Partners can be particularly helpful.

RECONSTITUTED FAMILIES: IMPLICATIONS FOR PARENTING

A *reconstituted family* occurs when a woman (or man) with children from a previous marriage marries a man (or woman) who may or may not have been married before or a woman with children of her own marries a man with children of his own. Nurses will often come into contact with these families when the man and woman are having another child of their own. In the popular literature, this is often referred to as "yours, mine, and ours." It is beyond the scope of this chapter to discuss in detail the complexity of the problems that can exist in such families, but we will outline some problems that the nurse should be alert for while taking a nursing history.

Reconstituted families can be as happy and well adjusted as other families. Certain myths of our culture, however, may impose greater stresses on this type of family. Despite the fairytale *Cinderella,* all stepmothers (stepfathers) are not wicked and cruel. But it must be remembered that stepparents are not immediately accepted. Like any relationship, it takes time and effort on the part of the children and the stepparent to develop a sense of trust and friendship. If the natural parent is still seen by the children it may be unrealistic for the stepparent to assume the role of the "missing" parent.

It is always best to prepare and discuss with the children the upcoming marriage. Although children do not have a right to make a decision about the parent's marriage, there should be some open discussion about what this will mean in their lives. A child who has been living with one parent for a period of time will have developed a special closeness to that parent. With a remarriage, some of that closeness must be relinquished. This can lead to a feeling of being displaced and present adjustment problems for the child.

Two of the major problems that reconstituted families must deal with are nurturance and discipline. A stepparent's efforts to give affection and nurturance to the stepchild may be met with rejection. Stepchildren may view such behavior as an effort to make them betray or be disloyal to the first parent. Stepchildren may be wary of establishing close bonds. They may feel the first parent abandoned them and that it may happen again. The stepparent must be aware that these feelings can exist. The "warming up" period may take up to 1 year.

It is difficult for the stepparent to apply discipline to stepchildren. It is often helpful for the husband and wife to have detailed discussions of discipline practices and beliefs. The parents need to make a special effort to share the responsibility for limit setting and to be consistent and supportive of each other.

The reconstituted family is a growing trend in our society. There is a high incidence of remarriage among single parents. These men and women bring certain strengths to the second marriage, including a more realistic view of marriage, an awareness of how the prior marital discord affected the children, and a willingness to work hard to make a second marriage work. The major problem to be overcome is the integration of the various roles in a new family. Health care providers should support these families and direct them to the services they need to fulfill the roles of the various family members.

THE ONLY CHILD

Society has generally disapproved of families with only one child. The only child has been stereotyped with such characteristics as selfishness, attention seeking, overly dependent, unhappy, unlikeable, and generally maladapted. Yet more families today are choosing to have only one child. Economics is one major reason for this. Other reasons may be infertility or unwillingness of parents to change their life-style or career patterns to accommodate more than one child.

Is the only child compromised in the family? There is very little research in this area. Falbo (1972) has conducted some recent research. Her findings on only children compared to children with one or more siblings in the area of interpersonal relationships found that only children reported fewer friends, the same number of close friends, and membership in fewer clubs but leadership in those organizations. Further, only children reported feeling comfortable with others and they received positive peer ratings. In general, only children receive greater affection and attention from parents and others and, therefore, have a lower need for affiliation.

Another finding is that intelligence tends to be higher for only children than for children in large families. The only child has a slightly lower intelligence than those in families with two children. The explanation often given for this is that in a family of two children, there is the opportunity for sibling tutoring. Nowhere is there evidence to support the stereotype society has given to the only child. It is important for the nurse to know these facts and to support parents who have concerns about an only child.

SUMMARY

This chapter presented the many issues facing parents today. A short historic perspective was given so you could understand from where the family came. Parenthood, as a development stage in the family life cycle, was reviewed. The current data on the roles of motherhood, fatherhood, and grandparenthood were discussed with an emphasis on the role of the nurse. Alternate parenting styles (adoption, single parents, reconstituted families, parenting twins, and parenting the only child) were reviewed. Sibling interaction and having a second child were special topics covered. It is hoped that by presenting a synthesis of the current understanding of parenthood the nurse will be better prepared to give effective and enlightened nursing care to families in the maternity setting.

REFERENCES AND READINGS

Ainsworth, M. D. S. et al. *Patterns of Attachment.* Hillsdale, N. J.: Lawrence Erlbaum, 1978.

Barnard, K. E., Douglas, H. B. (Eds.). *Child Health Assessment, Part I: A Literature Review,* U. S. Department of Health, Education and Welfare, Public Health Service, Health Resources Administration. Bureau of Health Resources Development, Division of Nursing. DHEW No. (HRA)75–30. Bethesda, Md., December 1974.

Barnard, K. E., Eyres, S. J. (Eds.). *Child Health Assessment, Part II: The First Year of Life.* U. S. Department of Health, Education and Welfare, Public Health Service, Health Resources Administration. Bureau of Health Resources Development, Division of Nursing. DHEW No. (HRA)79–25, Hyattsville, Md., June 1979.

Bowlby, J. *Attachment and Loss, Volume I: Attachment.* London: Hogarth Press, 1969.

Brazelton, T. B. Neonatal Behavioral Assessment Scale. *Clin Develop Med,* (No. 50). Philadelphia: J. B. Lippincott, 1973.

Caldwell, B. M. *Instruction Manual Inventory for Infants (Home Observation for Measurement of the Environment).* Little Rock, Ark., 1970.

Carey, W. B. Clinical Applications of Infant Temperament Measurement. *J Pediatr* 81(4):823, 1972.

Clarke-Stewart, A. *Child Care in the Family.* New York: Academic Press, 1977.

Craig, J. Birth of a Grandchild Brings Time of Reflection. *Menninger Perspect* 23, 1980.

Duvall, E. *Family Development.* Philadelphia: J. B. Lippincott, 1977.

Eyres, J., Barnard, K. E., Gray, C. A. (Eds.). *Child Health Assessment, Part III: Two–Four Years,* U. S. Department of Health, Education and Welfare, Public Health Service, Health Resources Administration. Bureau of Health Resources Development, Division of Nursing. Bethesda, Md., 1980.

Falbo, T. Only Children and Interpersonal Behavior: An Experimental and Survey Study. *J Appl Soc Psychol* 8(3):244, 1978.

Falbo, T. Sibling Tutoring and Other Explanations for Intelligence Discontinuities of Only the Last Borns. *Popul: Behav Soc Environ Issues,* I(4):349, 1978.

Hoffman, L. W., Hoffman, M. L. The Value of Children to Parents, in Fawcett, J. T. (Ed.), *Psychological Perspectives on Population.* New York: Basic Books, 1973.

Kennell, J. H. et al. Maternal Behavior One Year After Early and Extended Postpartum Contact. *Dev Med Child Neurol* 16:172, 1974.

Lylton, H. *Parent–Child Interaction.* New York: Plenum Press, 1980.

Parke, R. D., Hymel, S., Power, T. A., et al. Fathers and Risk: A Hospital Based Model of Intervention, in Sawin, D., Hawkins, R. C. (Eds.), *Psychosocial Risks During Pregnancy and Early Infancy.* (In press)

Parke, R. D., Sawin, D. The Father's Role in Infancy: A Reevaluation. *Fam Coord* 365, 1976.

Ringer, N. M., Kennell, J. H., Jarvella, Navokosky, B. J., and Klaus, M. H. Mother to Child Speech at Two Years—Effects of Early Postnatal Contact. *Behav Pediatr* 86: 141, 1975.

Robertson, J. F. Grandmotherhood: A Study of Role Conception. *J. Marriag Fam,* 39:165, 1977

Rubin, R. Attainment of Maternal Role: Part I, Processes. *Nurs Res,* 16(3):237, 1967.

Rubin, R. Maternal Touch. *Nurs Outlook* 11(11): 828, 1963.

Smart, M. S., Smart, L. S. *Families Developing Relationships.* New York: MacMillan, 1976.

Swendsen, L. A., Meleis, A. J., Jones, D. Role Supplementation for New Parents: A Role Mastering Plan. *Am J Matern Child Nurs,* 3(2):84, 1978.

Walker, L. Identifying Parents in Need: An Approach to Adoptive Parenting. *Am J Matern Child Nurs* 6(2):118, 1981.

Yankelovich, Shelly and White, Inc. *The General Mills American Family Report, 1978–1979: Family Health In an Era of Stress.* Minneapolis: General Mills, 1979.

Zimmerman, B. M. Billie and His Sad and Happy Mommies. *Am J Matern Child Nurs,* 2(3):193, 1977.

19

MATERNAL RECOVERY FROM PREGNANCY AND CHILDBIRTH

The postpartum period (or puerperium) is seen by some as a less exciting phase of maternity nursing, or perhaps it is somewhat anticlimatic following the 9 months of pregnancy and the excitement of the delivery itself. In the opinion of many nurses, however, the care of the postpartal family has many challenges and rewards, and in recent years the beginning family has been receiving the focus it deserves.

After delivery, the obstetrician is less evident and the mother feels some let down. However, during the first 24 hours and on into the first 6 weeks of this new beginning family, opportunities for nursing are exciting. The joy of watching the new mother and father absorb the realities of this new human being that is a part of both of them is fascinating. Moreover, there is no doubt that nurses are the people who impact most on this new family unit and, by their assessment and intervention, have the potential to influence the people in this family unit significantly. The crucial events occurring in the mother–infant, father–infant attachment process are now well documented in the literature, and nurses can play a significant role in facilitating this attachment process.

The *puerperium* is that period of time from the end of the third stage of labor until the time at which the pelvic organs have returned to normal, about 6 weeks postpartum. This chapter discusses physiologic and psychosocial adaptation postpartum, including nursing care and education of the postpartal woman. Breast- or bottle-feeding the infant and teaching the parents about infant feeding is included. Complications that can occur in the postpartum period, discharge planning, and the anticipated needs of the new family during the first 6 weeks after delivery are discussed.

PHYSIOLOGIC CHARACTERISTICS

Uterus

At term the uterus, which weighs about 1,000 gm returns to its normal prepregnant weight of about 60–80 gm by a process known as *involution.* Changes in weight of the uterus are striking, decreasing to 500 gm at the end of the first week to 350 gm at the end of the second, and to 100 gm by the third week after delivery. During pregnancy, the woman is in a state of positive nitrogen balance, the retained nitrogen being used for growth and development of the fetus, placenta, uterus, and breasts. This excess protein in uterine muscle cells after delivery is broken down by a process called *autolysis.* If the patient is lactating, the metabolized protein may be used, otherwise it is excreted in the urine. The number of muscle cells does not change during involution, but each cell decreases in size approximately 90% (Willson & Carrington, 1979).

At about 12 hours after delivery, the fundus can be palpated at the level of the umbilicus. It then continues to decrease in size (about 1 cm per day), and by the tenth to twelfth day it cannot be palpated above the symphysis pubis (Fig. 19.1). The superficial layer of the decidua becomes necrotic and sloughs; the bases of the glands that dip into the uterine muscle remain intact. New epithelium, which eventually will reline the uterine cavity, generates from the remaining glandular epithelium.

After delivery of the placenta, the placental site becomes progressively smaller, measuring 3–4 cm by the end of the second week. Immediately after delivery of the placenta, bleeding of the choriodecidual sinuses is contained by compression and kinking of the blood vessels that lead to the site. After the stricture of blood vessels, a clot forms, the placental site, including a superficial layer of myometrium beneath the site, is infiltrated by leucocytes, and necrosis begins. This process results in a crust composed of decidua, thrombosed vessels, endometrial glands, and myometrium, which separates from the normal uterine wall beneath. Thus healing of the placental site occurs with no significant scarring, and regeneration of endometrium and glandular tissue begins on the third day and continues rapidly from then on. The uterine cavity, except for the placental site, has a new endometrial lining by 3 weeks, and the placental site is epithelialized in another 3 weeks.

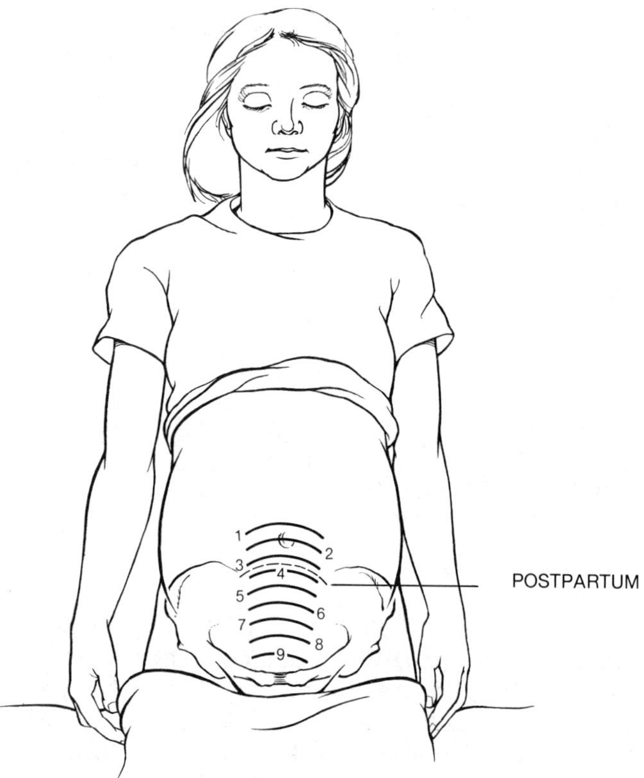

Figure 19.1
Postpartum involution of the uterus day by day.

Uterine discharge postpartally is called *lochia,* which is made up of blood and debris from decidual necrosis. Lochial flow is classified as lochia rubra, lochia serosa, and lochia alba. *Lochia rubra* is bright red, pure blood, and necrotic decidua, which gradually changes to *lochia serosa,* which is less red or pinkish. *Lochia serosa,* which is serosanguinous lochia, contains less blood, eventually becomes tan in color, and finally changes to serous (thin watery secretion) or *lochia alba.* The progression from *lochia rubra* to *lochia alba* takes approximately 10 days in the normal postpartal woman.

Ovarian Function and Menstruation

Recall that during pregnancy the ovaries are inactive and the placenta produces estrogen and progesterone. Following delivery, the inhibiting effects of placental estrogen and progesterone are removed and gonadotropin secretion resumes. Most women who do not nurse their babies will have a period of bleeding within 4–6 weeks; however, the exact time required for return of normal ovarian function is determined by how rapidly the pituitary gland activity and ovarian response are restored. Some lactating mothers may be amenorrheic as long as they nurse. Return of menstruation by 3 months is reported by Sharman (1951) in 91% of nonlactating primiparas. Multiparas are apt to start menstruating earlier, even if nursing their infants. Usually, the first menstrual period is no heavier than usual and may be anovulatory, but by the third or fourth menses, flow and ovulation should have returned to normal. It is important for the nurse to know that ovulation does occur in women who are breast-feeding (Perez et al., 1972). Perez reported that 14.1% of women on a full nursing schedule and 28.8% of women partially nursing ovulated. Ovulation can occur even though menstruation has not resumed. The implications for the nurse regarding contraception information are obvious.

Cervix and Vagina and Perineum

The cervix, which is flabby and relaxed after delivery, regains its tone fairly rapidly. The cervical canal reforms as the internal and external os contract, and at the end of 2 weeks, the canal is narrow. Lacerations of the cervix heal by proliferation of fibroblasts.

The vagina never returns completely to the pregravid stage. Tags of tissue called *carunculae myrtiformes* that represent the hymenal rings now exist. These torn edges of the hymen remain separate and heal and these carunculae myrtiformes are indicative of a previous vaginal birth. The vaginal epithelium is thin and smooth, resembling that of postmenopausal women, and this appearance changes as the ovaries begin to function and estrogen is produced. A mother who is breast-feeding may have delayed estrogen production and, as a result, thin, more friable vaginal mucosa, which has implications for sexual intercourse (see Chapter 14). In the nonlactating mother, ovarian estrogen production may begin in 3–4 weeks. Vaginal rugae return in 3–4 weeks, and tightening of the vaginal orifice is dependent in part on perineal tightening exercises (see Kegel's exercise, Chapter 12).

Perineal changes are related to the fact that the pelvic floor muscles are thinned and stretched by the pressure of the presenting fetal part, which is usually the head. This pressure is greater in primigravidas and in women with big babies. It is common in the United States for the woman to have an episiotomy (incising of perineum, see Chapter 22) to alleviate perineal pressure and stretching and perhaps prevent tearing of the perineum. Midwives are more often apt to deliver the woman in a side lying position, which is physiologically better, decreases stretching of the perineum, and lessens the need for an episiotomy (Fig. 19.2). Edema and bruising of the perineum and vulva are common following delivery.

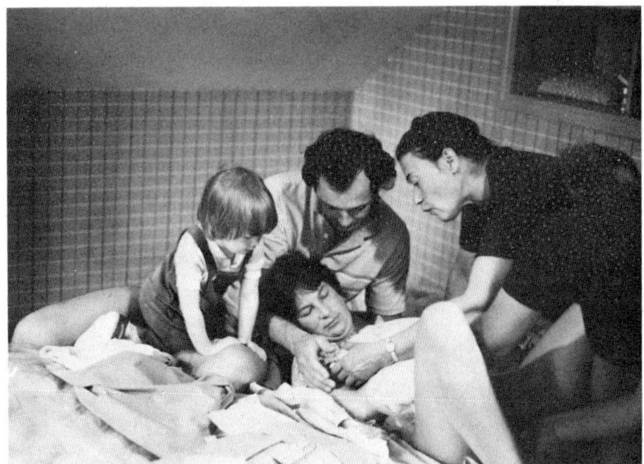

Figure 19.2
Midwife delivery. Note mother's relaxed position.

Urinary Tract

After delivery, the bladder may be edematous and hyperemic, and there may be swelling and bruising of tissue around the urethra. There is increased capacity for fluid but a decreased sensation to fluid pressure and buildup, so that the postpartal woman is prone to overdistention or incomplete emptying of the bladder with subsequent buildup of residual urine. Women with conduction anesthesia (see Chapter 22) are more prone to bladder problems because of the inhibiting neural effects of the anesthesia. The hydronephrosis and hydroureters return to normal within 2–3 weeks if there is no urinary tract anomaly.

The profound diuresis that occurs in the first 12–24 hours postpartum is important for the maternity nurse to understand. The kidneys must eliminate the 2,000–3,000 ml of extracellular fluid that accumulates during normal pregnancy; this amount of fluid retention can be even greater if the woman has been edematous such as in pregnancy-induced hypertension (see Chapter 21). Bladder elimination and assessment of voidings are critical. Recall that if stasis (or residual urine) exists the chance of urinary tract infection is greater because of the physiologic changes of pregnancy that have not had time to return to the non-pregnant state. Specifically, these are bacteriuria, and dilated ureters and renal pelves that persist for 4 weeks postpartum (Pritchard & MacDonald, 1976). Accompanying the profound diuresis is *diaphoresis,* the elimination of excess fluid and waste products via the skin. Diaphoretic episodes characteristically occur at night and the woman may awaken drenched with perspiration. The anxiety caused by the diuresis and diaphoresis can be minimized by anticipatory guidance and the nurse explaining what may happen to the woman.

Gastrointestinal Adaptation

After delivery, the woman is often hungry and thirsty and will eat and drink as soon as food and drink are provided. Muscle tone in the intestinal tract is sluggish because of decreased hormones, less muscle tone, and decreased intra-abdominal pressure. Re-establisning bowel habits is often a concern, as women feel that bearing down efforts may increase perineal or episiotomy discomfort. Attention to diet, ambulation, and fluids in order to prevent constipation is important. Stool softeners may be ordered by the physician in order to increase bulk and moisture and to help evacuation of the bowel.

Breasts

During the antepartum period, glandular and ductal tissues are stimulated by rising concentrations of estrogen, progesterone, HCG, prolactin, cortisol, and insulin. After delivery, the levels of these hormones circulating in the postpartal woman drop dramatically. Lactation begins from the third to fifth postpartum day. The interaction between the various hormones and breast tissue is not clear, but the evidence indicates that prolactin is essential for lactation. Willson and Carrington (1979) point out that women whose anterior pituitary has been destroyed do not produce prolactin and do not lactate. *Colostrum,* the thin yellowish fluid that is the first milk, is secreted late in pregnancy and during the first few days postpartum. On the third or fourth day postpartum, the breasts become engorged (distended, firm, tender), and milk can be expressed from the nipples. Some women experience engorgement so significantly that it involves axillary breast tissue. This engorgement is primarily a result of engorgement of blood and lymph systems rather than of milk.

The mechanism of breast-feeding involves two important components—the let-down reflex and the supply–demand response (Riordan & Countryman, 1980). The *let-down reflex* is initiated by the infant's suckling, which triggers a nervous stimulus from the nipple to the hypothalamus that releases oxytocin from the posterior pituitary (Fig. 19.3). Oxytocin stimulates the myoepithelial cells surrounding the mammary glands to contract, which forces milk into the ducts and from the nipples. The let-down reflex (sometimes referred to as milk ejection) in some instances can be triggered by the baby crying or even the mother thinking of nursing the infant. The psychogenic factors of the let-down reflex should be noted by the nurse; she may observe that the mother who is anxious, insecure, tired, or in pain often has difficulty letting down her milk, while the mother who is confident and relaxed has sufficient milk production for the neonate.

The *supply–demand response* relates to the fact that the baby's sucking primarily controls the amount of milk produced. This fact has implications for nursing interventions, which are discussed later in the chapter. It is important to remember that both quan-

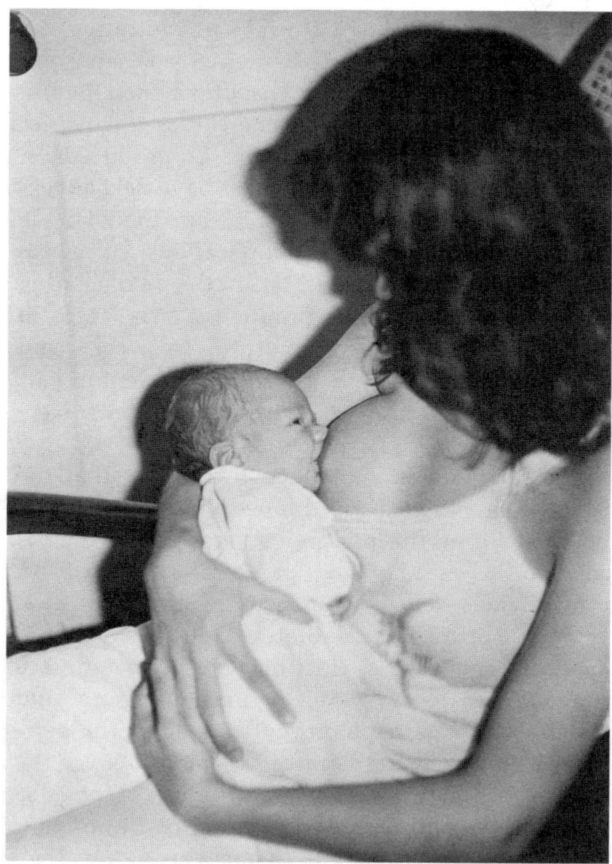

Figure 19.3
Mother sitting and nursing baby.

tity and quality of milk can be altered by diet, activity, and emotional situations.

Vital Signs

Normally, there is no great change in body temperature during the postpartum period. Sometimes a temperature elevation is reported in the first 24 hours postpartum, which is normally related to dehydration or the fatigue of labor (see postpartum complications for discussion of infection). The pulse rate is normally low following delivery (50–70 beats/min), which may be related to increased stroke volume, decreased cardiac stress, or the decreased vascular bed after delivery. A rapid pulse rate may be indicative of excessive blood loss. Blood pressure should change only slightly in normal women. A slight decrease is related to decreased intrapelvic pressure or uterine bleeding.

Blood

White blood cell count may increase to as high as 20,000–30,000 WBC, especially if labor has been prolonged, because of an increase in granulocytes. Normally, blood volume loss with a vaginal delivery is 300–400 cc and with cesarean section is 750–1,000 cc. As the plasma volume, which increases so significantly during pregnancy, decreases, the hemoglobin and red blood cell count will rise. Blood values should return to prepregnant levels by the end of the first week postpartum.

Body Weight

After delivery, there is an immediate weight loss of 10–12 lb (4.8–5.8 kg); by the end of the first week, there is an additional 4–5 lb (1.9–2.4 kg) loss as excess tissue fluid is eliminated. Further weight loss follows as the uterus continues its involution and plasma volume contracts. Many women who have gained the usual 20–25 lb are back to their prepregnant weight between 6–8 weeks postpartum.

Endocrine Status

Hormone production changes significantly after delivery. Hormones produced by the trophoblastic cells are all reduced.

- ↓ ***Chorionic gonadotropin.*** Only a small amount detected in the urine after the first day.
- ↓ ***Estrogen*** Placental production ceases with delivery
  - ▾ ***Estrone.*** Nonpregnant level 1 week
  - ▾ ***Estradiol.*** Nonpregnant level 1 week
  - ▾ ***Estriol.*** Decreases more slowly; present for 2–3 weeks
- ↓ ***Progesterone.*** Nonpregnant level 1 week

Adrenal function returns to normal fairly rapidly after delivery; prepregnancy levels of thyroid functioning resumes more slowly. Anterior pituitary gonadotropic hormones gradually resume prepregnancy functioning; only prolactin and oxytocin (increased by suckling) are changed after delivery.

PSYCHOSOCIAL CHARACTERISTICS

It is difficult to address psychosocial adaptation after delivery separately from the biophysical changes because, as always, they are intertwined. The system-by-system physiologic changes fit neatly into the time frame of the postpartum period, but the psychosocial changes, although evident immediately after childbirth—for example, the role changes—seem to occur over at least the first 3 or 4 months. In fact, some refer to this period as the "fourth trimester." Chapter 18 discussed parenthood in detail; roles of father, mother, siblings, and grandparents were discussed in relation to different family life-style patterns. In this chapter the more immediate psychosocial characteristics are explored. The early maternal tasks involve each of the following areas.

- ▲ Reviewing the events of pregnancy, labor, and delivery
- ▲ Regenerating physiologic and physical energy
- ▲ Learning to care for the infant
- ▲ Re-establishing and defining relationships and roles

Rubin (1961) discusses the phases of taking-in, taking-hold, and letting go, which describe the progression of maternal roles. It is helpful to recall that during labor the woman progresses from extroversion in the early phase of labor to introversion during the second stage—a quite rapid progression, in fact, in most instances, less than a day. The behavior of the woman in the postpartum period is from dependence (or introversion) to independence, although this progression requires more time. Just as in labor, the nurse's understanding of the phases and the maternal tasks to be accomplished makes specific interventions more logical and appropriate. How each woman adjusts and experiences the puerperium depends on several factors, such as her self-concept, her own parenting and childhood, her relationship with the infant's father, and the number of children she has had. Although each postpartum experience is unique, there is a pattern of adjustment that provides an operational framework for the nurse.

Taking-In Phase

During the *taking-in phase* the woman is described as passive and dependent, accepting assistance for both her physical and emotional needs. Her energy level is low, and food, attention, rest, and other basic physiologic needs are great. During this time, the woman has a great need to review the labor experience, as if she has to rate and evaluate her performance. She relates her experience in relation to a previous labor (if she has delivered before) or to other women's—her sister's, her mother's, or her friend's—labors. Affonso (1977) suggests the mother has a need to fill in the missing pieces of her experience. Other authors have described the mother's task of relinquishing expectations of herself and her infant and adapting to the reality of motherhood as *grief work.* Frequently, the fantasy baby and the real baby are not alike in the mother's eye. Also, the mother's expectation of being svelte and slim again may not coincide with her less firm abdomen and distended breasts. If the baby is the sex hoped for and the expected size and appearance, the task of reconciling fantasy baby with real baby takes less time. If the infant is not as expected, or is ill, or has an anomaly, or the nurse hears the mother say, "Oh, she is so tiny," the gap between expectation and reality is predictable. Nursing interventions are based as always on the nurse's assessment of the mother's progression toward the accomplishment of the maternal tasks.

Taking-Hold Phase

As physical recovery occurs, that is, muscle soreness becomes less, bladder and bowel functioning is reestablished, breast tenderness lessens, and fatigue becomes less evident, the mother is able to focus on the acquaintance process with her infant. Nurses may notice behavior changes such as the mother getting out of bed on her own, showering, putting on makeup, and eagerly attending to feeding and caring for her infant. As the mother remasters her own body and its functions, she moves on to the task of mothering her infant. These behaviors indicate that independence is returning, taking-in is over, and *taking-hold* is beginning. (Fig. 19.4). According to Rubin (1961a), the mother now has a strong urge to get on with the caretaking tasks, even though anxiety is also present. "How can I care for this new human being?" she asks herself. Eventually, the mother begins to make plans for the trip home; she is now the initiator, not the receiver.

The maternal behaviors involved in caring for an infant are caused by anxiety. As mentioned earlier, the new mother is anxious, and how to care for a newborn is something you learn, not something that happens spontaneously at the moment of birth. The nurse observing the primipara with her newborn can observe "the sweating palms, flushed or perspiring face, the body held tense and rigid throughout the act, the predominantly silent concentration with which she carries out her task" (Rubin 1961a, p. 684). These behaviors can often be seen with each new task—feeding, changing the diaper, or bathing. It is the wise nurse who allows the mother to con-

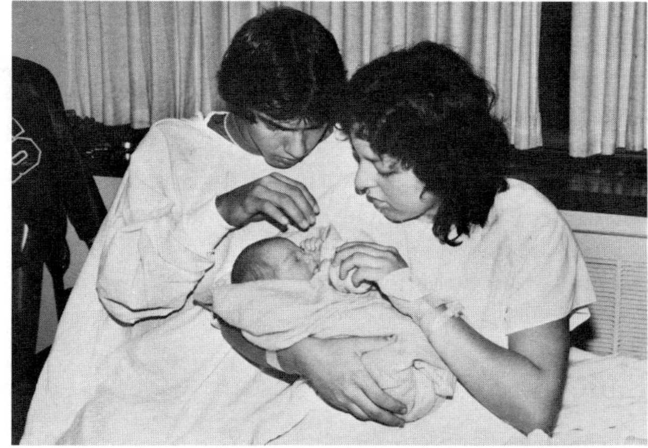

Figure 19.4
Taking-hold phase.

tinue her learning process, even if she is clumsy. The professional nurse needs to resist the urge to take over since the competent, efficient role model may contribute to lowering self-esteem in the mother who is already sensitive.

Mood swings are common in the taking-hold phase and wax and wane with successes and frustrations. As the mother assumes more and more of the infant caretaking, depression, fatigue, and an awesome sense of responsibility can occur. Hormonal shifts, physical discomfort, and some lessening of attention all contribute to mood changes. It is useful to reassure the mother that these feelings are normal and to offer positive feedback on things she is doing well.

Initially, the mother looks for approval for mastery of her tasks from the "experts" around her. As the mother continues in the taking-hold phase, she begins to move from needing the praise of outsiders to receiving her reward from the neonate. This is a turning point; the successful burp, eye contact with the infant, and the satisfied neonate she sees sleeping after being fed are all reinforcements for the new mother.

Many mothers today are discharged from the hospital in 2 or 3 days, some even within the first 24 hours. Those that go home during the first postpartum day are undoubtedly in the taking-in phase. Even mothers who return home 2–4 days postpartum undoubtedly have not achieved stability in the taking-hold phase. Depending on the mother's previous experience with child care, her personality, and her supportive others, the taking-hold phase may extend for several days. It is important for the nurse to assess the behaviors that identify accomplishment of the maternal tasks and provide continuing support, such as printed materials and outreach services, when needed.

Letting-Go Phase

In the *letting-go phase,* the mother lets go of herself as she was before childbirth and deals with who she is and her relationships with those around her now. In a phrase, it is the redefining of roles (Mercer, 1981). The mother's relationship with the baby's father, including sex and role behaviors, has to be re-established. At the same time the mother is caring for her neonate, she is trying to establish a mutually satisfying adult relationship. Again, this is unique in each situation; the unwed mother, the teenager, and the older primipara who has been married for about 10 years each brings her special needs to this task of defining her new role as mother. The more people who are closely involved with the new mother, such as baby's father, father's parents, mother's parents, grandparents, siblings, and friends, the more roles that need to be re-established and the more energy that is required. Probably the most overwhelming realization of all is the fact that she will never be the exact same person again for she will hereafter be a mother.

POSTPARTUM NURSING MANAGEMENT

Postpartum management includes physical assessment, psychosocial assessment, and nursing interventions related to the occurring physical and psychosocial adaptation. In each section of the assessment process discussed here health teaching is included. Care of the mother during the first hour after delivery has been discussed in Chapter 16.

Vital Signs

The mother's temperature may be elevated during the first 24 hours after giving birth; the upper unit of a normal elevation is usually 100.4°F (38°C). (Criteria for morbidity, as an indication of puerperal infection, is discussed in the section on postpartum complications.) Pulse rate is normally slow and is referred to as puerperal bradycardia. Tachycardia, pulse rate over 100, can indicate impending hemorrhage, infection, or pulmonary embolism and warrants immediate attention. All vital signs—temperature, pulse, respirations, and blood pressure—should be taken 3 or 4 times during the first 24 hours and evaluated in relation to other subjective and objective signs of the patient, as well as to predelivery values.

Breasts

A supportive nursing or nonnursing bra should be worn by the mother after delivery both for comfort and to prevent stretching of connective tissue and ligaments. The nurse should palpate the breasts gently for heat, tenderness, engorgement, or caking (swelling of a lobule because of blockage, occurring most commonly in the upper outer quadrant of the breast). The nipple should be inspected for fissures (cracks), soreness, and degree of erectness. When the nipple is gently pulled out from the breast and released, erectility can be assessed. Milk production can be assessed by expressing a small amount of milk; colostrum is ivory or darker in color than milk, which is bluish-white. To express milk, the thumb and forefinger are placed on either side of the areola, the skin and tissue are displaced back, and the areola is gently squeezed. Nursing mothers can keep their nipples supple with lanolin-based creams. Nipples should be cleaned with water since soap can dry them; exposing the nipples to air helps toughen them for nursing. Nonnursing mothers should be checked for discomfort from engorgement. Medications to suppress lactation such as TACE or Diatate may be given. A good supportive bra and the use of ice packs or analgesics may be helpful. Heat and massage will encourage milk flow and should be avoided in nonnursing mothers.

Abdomen and Fundus

After delivery the abdomen is soft and flabby, which may be a major concern to the newly delivered mother who wants to regain her figure as quickly as possible. Sometimes the abdominal wall is stretched so much that *diastasis recti,* separation in the midline of the two rectus abdominis muscles, occurs. This condition is easily noted when palpating the abdomen. Assessment should include length and width of the diastasis, which can be measured with a paper measuring tape, similarly to the fundal height. The length of the diastasis above and below the umbilicus and the width are recorded.

Key fundal assessment factors include location, height above the symphysis pubis, and firmness. The progress of uterine involution is estimated by the size and consistency of the uterus and the character, amount, and odor of the lochia. The height of the uterus is most accurately measured by using a paper tape. Zero point on the tape is placed at the top of the symphysis pubis, and the distance to the top of the uterus is measured in centimeters. Many texts suggest recording the height by finger breadths above or below the umbilicus, and in many instances this is done. However, the width of people's hands and fingers vary, and a more accurate picture of involution is obtained if everyone uses the same measuring device. Recall that immediately after delivery the fundus is often halfway between the symphysis pubis and the umbilicus; within several hours it rises to the level of the umbilicus and it remains at that level for a day or two. Day-by-day descent is illustrated in Figure 19.1. It is important to have the mother void before assessing fundal height since the stretched uterine ligaments allow the uterus to move about easily. A uterus located to the left or the right of the midline is usually displaced because of a full bladder. Consistency is noted and recorded as firm (feels like an orange or grapefruit) or boggy (difficult to determine the boundaries and not firm). Since the uterus responds to tactile stimulation, a boggy uterus should become firm when massaged briefly with circular motion at the fundus. Correct position of hands for palpating the fundus is shown in Figure 19.5. One hand should be placed just above the symphysis pubis and the other on the top, or fundus, of the uterus. Assessment of the lochia provides additional data regarding involution. Lochia decreases in amount and changes from lochia rubra to lochia serosa in a few days. Amount (small or scant, moderate, large) and color are recorded daily. At first lochia is profuse; during the puerperium it gradually disappears. If the lochia remains bright red after the first 3 or 4 days, it may indicate involution is not progressing well. After sitting for a period of time or upon arising in the morning, it is not unusual for a mother to experience a gush of blood. Whether nursing or not, lochia flow varies from person to person. Usually perineal pads (or tampons when insertion is not uncomfortable at approximately 3–4 weeks) are required for approximately 6 weeks. Odor should be nonoffensive; if a bad odor is noted, infection is suspected.

Afterpains, alternating contractions and relaxation of the uterine muscle, are common in multiparas and unusual in primiparas. Because of oxytocin release, afterpains are more severe when a mother is nursing. They usually disappear after 2–3 days. Analgesics are sometimes given to lessen pain; since the amount transmitted in breast milk is minimal, they may be given to nursing mothers as well. Certainly other comfort and pain relief measures should be tried first. Since pain and tenseness can inhibit the letdown mechanism, the nurse needs to collect all the data in order to intervene appropriately.

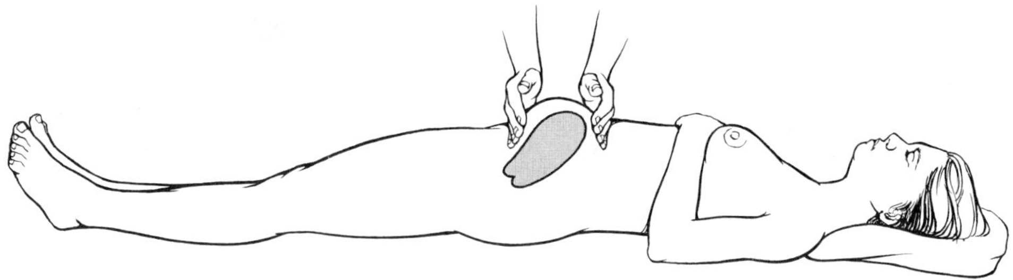

Figure 19.5
Palpation of uterine fundus after birth. Note position of hands.

Perineum

Looking at and assessing the perineum is done most comfortably and efficiently by having the woman turn to either side and lie in the Sims' position with her top leg positioned over her bottom leg. By lifting her buttock, the perineum and anus are exposed without undue loss of privacy. The incision from an episiotomy or any perineal tears are assessed.

Davidson (1974) describes REEDA, redness, edema, ecchymosis, discharge, and approximation, as the five criteria for assessment, each one indicating a stage of healing. Each should be evaluated on a three-point scale and the results recorded. Approximation, for example, refers to the fact that within 24 hours skin edges in an episiotomy should be glued together so that gentle pressure does not cause them to separate.

Applications of heat or cold are sometimes used for perineal discomfort. Sitz baths and showers, where water can flow over the sore and tender areas, are relaxing and healing. Hemorrhoids, which become large and painful in the later months of pregnancy if not present before the pregnancy, usually disappear completely. They should be assessed for size, number, pain, or tenderness. Mothers are frequently not aware that episiotomy sutures as a rule are absorbable, and often wonder silently when their stitches will be removed. When perineal care is taught, cleaning of the perineum from front to back and general hygiene principles can also be reviewed. Most hospitals provide a plastic squeeze bottle that the mother fills with tap water to rinse her perineum each time she voids or defecates. Perineal pads should be applied from front to back and changed at each voiding. Perineal heat lamps are sometimes used to promote healing.

Ambulation

Because of the increase in clotting factors (see complications postpartum), the risk of thrombophlebitis is high in postpartum women. Therefore, assessment of the lower extremities for redness, skin temperature, pain, and edema should be done daily. Early ambulation has reduced the incidence of thrombophlebitis, and a regimen of progressive ambulation is important. Passive leg exercise is important for mothers on bedrest.

Rest and Sleep

It has been said by parent educator groups that labor is like a 12-mile hike; therefore, the need for rest in the postpartum woman is great. Recall that after delivery a mother may be euphoric or reticent and even depressed. Physical fatigue influences many physical and psychosocial adjustments, and the astute nurse needs to assess each woman and to advocate rest. It is important to organize caretaking activities to provide for periods of rest and to minimize interruptions. Basically, mothers should rest when their infants rest, which is a good pattern to continue even after they return home.

Mothers are frequently eager to initiate an exercise plan in order to regain muscle tone, and the nurse should help them plan and pace their exercise programs (Fig. 19.6). Abdominal breathing (contracting the abdominal wall) can progress to head raising (raise head and touch chin), to perineal tightening, and to stretching; all can be initiated early. More strenuous exercises such as leg raising, leg exercises, pelvic rocking, and pelvic tilt should be started later; sit ups may be delayed for at least 2 weeks.

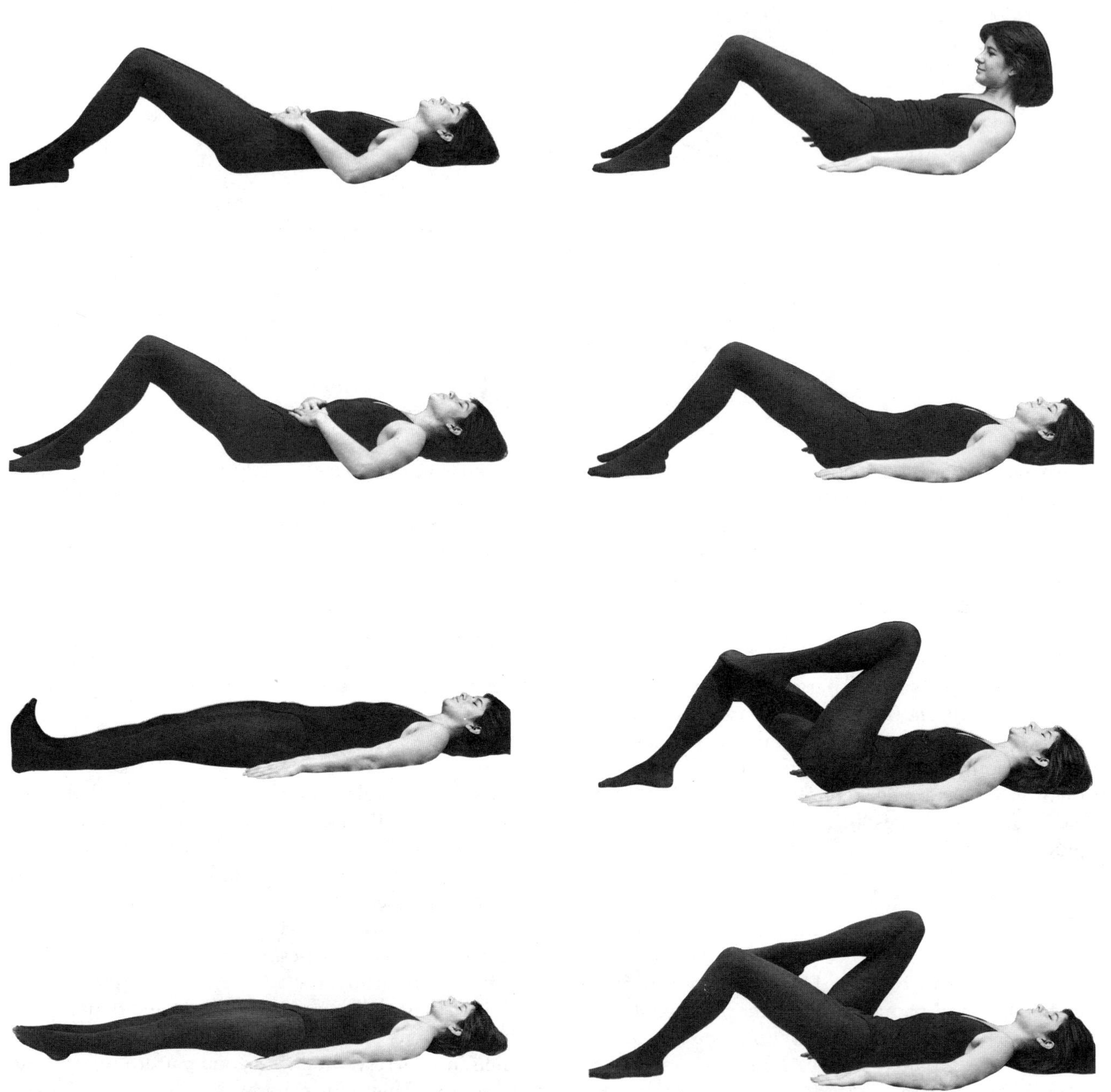

Figure 19.6

Postpartum exercise series. These exercises become progressively more difficult for the woman to do. *Breathing exercises.* Lie on back with legs flexed and hand on stomach. Breathe deeply so hand is pushed up. Exhale. (See *a1* and *a2.*) *Calf pumping.* Lie on back with legs straight. Move feet up and down at ankles. (See *b1* and *b2.*) *Abdominal exercises.* Lie on back, knees bent, arms at sides. *(c1)* Lift head, touch chin to chest, hold for count of 3. *(c2)* Squeeze buttocks together as if trying to stop bowel movement. *(c3)* Pelvic tilt: tighten abdominal and gluteal muscles while pressing lower back down on floor. Hold for count of 3; relax. *(c4)* Do pelvic tilt *(c3)*, hold and bring right knee toward chest. Return foot to starting position; repeat with left knee.

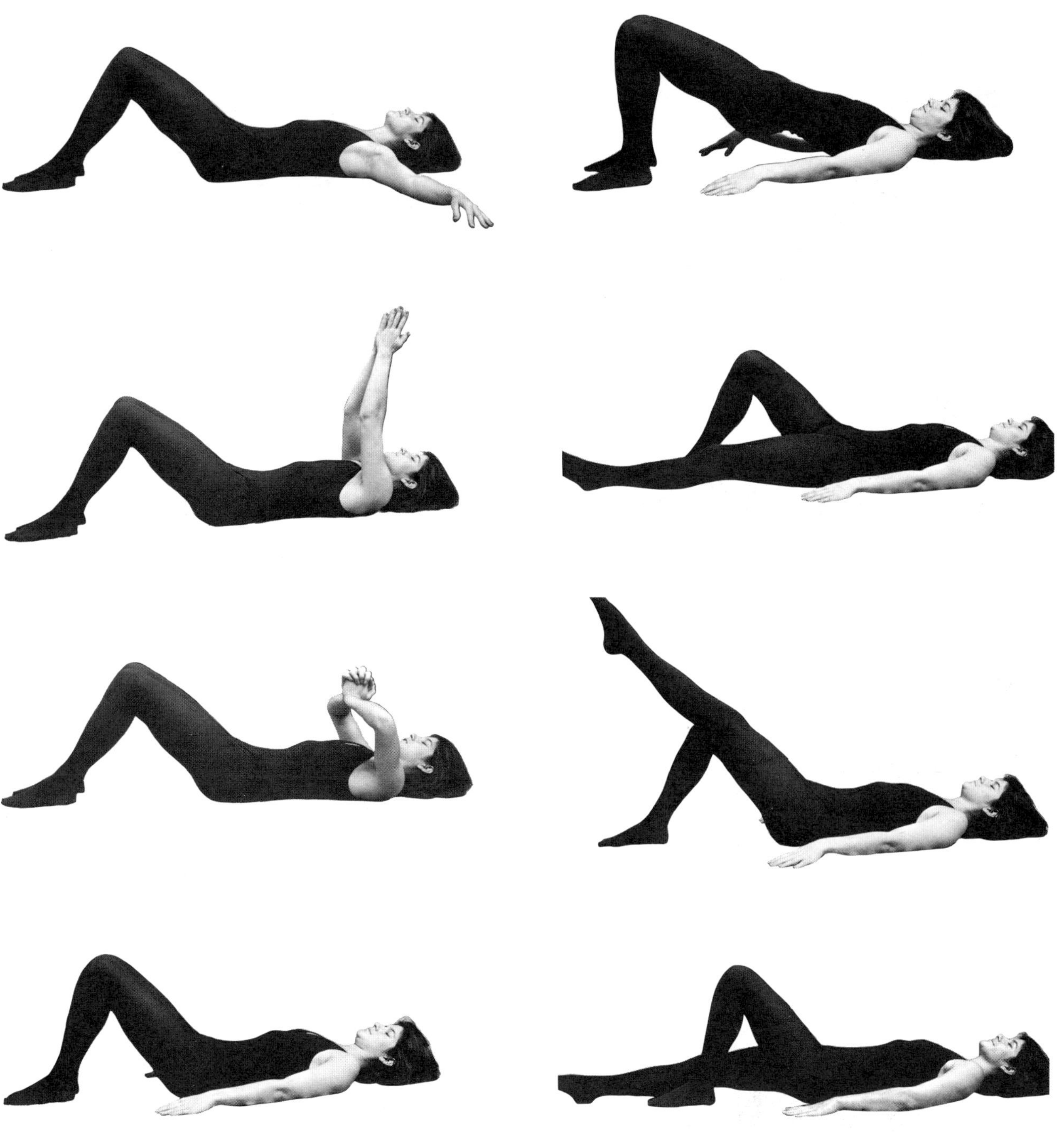

Figure 19.6 (continued)
Chest exercises. (d1) Lie on back, arms straight. *(d2)* Keep elbows straight; bring hands together directly above chest; return to starting position. *(d3)* Clasp hands in front of chest with elbows bent; press hands together; hold for count of 3; relax. *Bridging. (e1)* Lie on back with knees bent, feet on floor, arms at side. *(e2)* Push down with feet; raise hips off floor; hold for count of 5; relax. *Straight leg raise. (f1)* Lie on back, right knee bent; left leg straight. Do pelvic tilt and hold. *(f2)* Raise left leg keeping knee straight; lower leg and relax. *(f3)* Bend left knee and repeat with right leg *(f4)*.

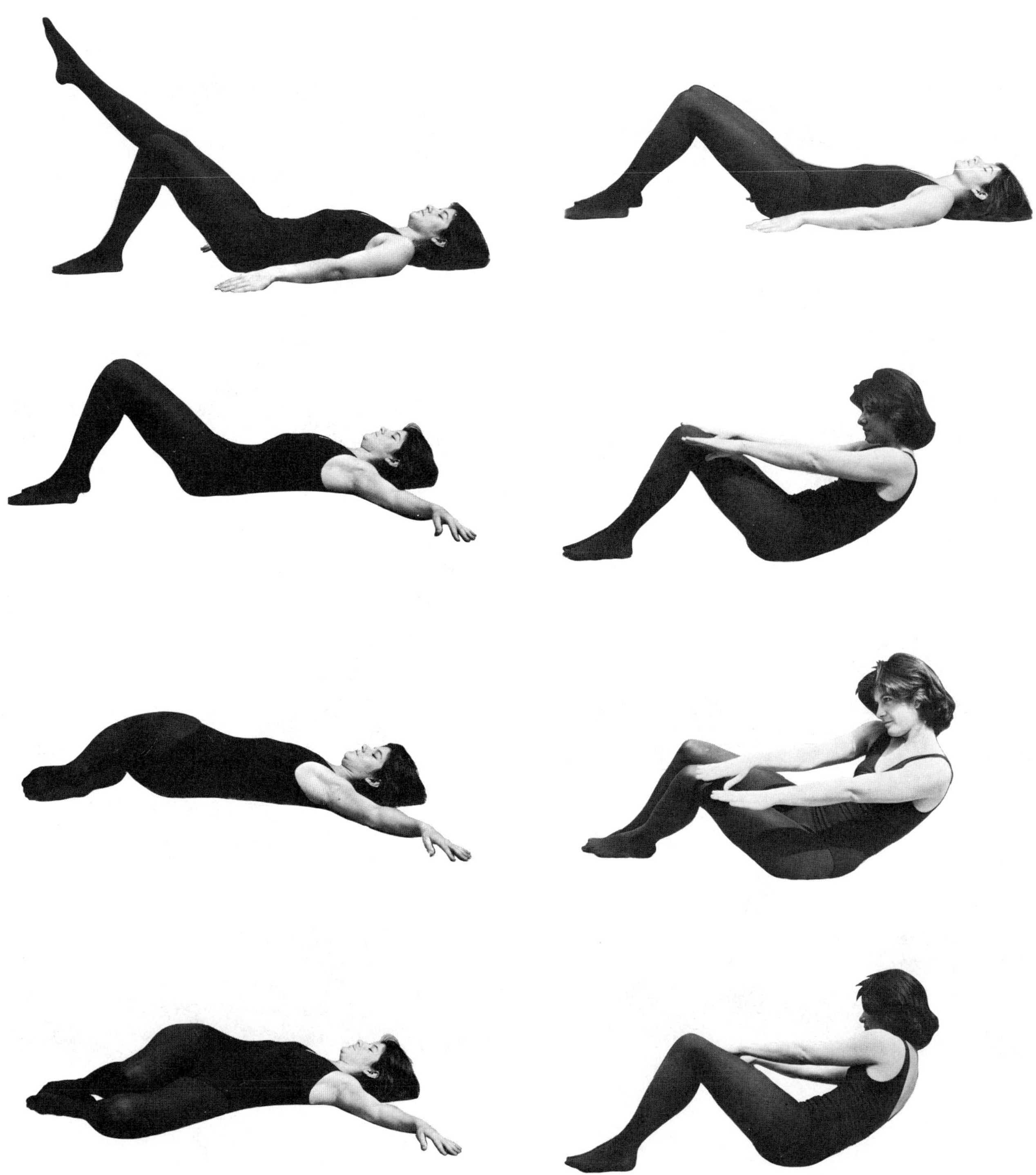

Figure 19.6 (continued)
Straight leg raise (con't). (f4) Raise right leg. *Lower trunk rotation. (g1)* Lie on back with knees bent, feet on floor. *(g2) and (g3)* Keep knees together; roll slowly from side to side trying to touch floor with knees. *Sit-ups. (h1)* Remain on back with knees bent, feet on floor. *(h2)* Reach forward with both arms. *(h3)* Curl up to partial sitting. Keep chin tucked in and uncurl. *(h4)* Repeat, but twist body as you curl reaching hands to knee.

Psychosocial Nursing Management

Again, postpartal physiologic and psychosocial adaptation cannot really be separated except for discussion. Recall that one of the major maternal tasks is integrating the labor and delivery experience, and the nurse can provide an opportunity for the woman to do this. The skilled nurse can give the mother the opportunity to review what happened without embarrassment. The mother who says, "I am so embarrassed, I know I yelled at the doctors and nurses in the labor room," is seeking resolution and evaluating her experience. The nurse who says "Everyone does that" or "I know how you feel" closes the door to further conversation. The nurse who says, "I can understand that" acknowledges that it is really impossible to know how another feels exactly but understands that the mother does feel embarrassed and allows her to discuss her feelings while not being judgmental. The mother will thus be able to resolve her feelings.

Assisting with the grief work of motherhood is helpful. Comments, such as "Oh, but my husband wanted a boy" or "I wanted a girl," do not mean the mother or father will not bond but merely that there is work to be done. Remember that attachment is a process, and pointing out the specialness of their new baby will aid the process. Fantasy baby becomes actual baby!

Recall also that basic physiologic needs must be met in order to deal with love and belongingness or higher needs (Maslow, 1970). Physical care, care of the episiotomy, exercise suggestions for the flabby abdomen, palpation of the fundus are all procedures that need to be shared, described, and appraised. Telling the mother that the episiotomy is not red and that when nursing it is not the time to diet are important and often provide relief for the new mother. Pampering is important; and even though there are things that need to be done, rest is important.

Helping the mother acquire caretaking skills is an important part of the nurse's role. Obtaining a balance between role modeling and taking over can sometimes be difficult. Assessing where the mother is in learning her caretaking role and commenting on that which she is doing well are critical. Making the mother think ahead not only provides an opportunity for anticipatory guidance, but assists in new role conceptualization. "What do *you* think your day will be like when you get home?" "How do you think the baby will change the daily activities of the others in your home?" The nurse can help the mother think about how to divide up chores, and make plans for some time alone, or away from the newborn. Re-energizing is a very large concern for the new mother as sleep deprivation, even with the normal well baby, is a reality. Many new mothers find a friend, not a family member, as the most helpful person. Giving the new mother a phone number that she can call 24 hours a day—nurses work 24 hours a day—often gives her the opportunity to resolve that question at 3:00 A.M., which may not be big or important enough to call the physician. Nurses in many hospitals initiate a follow-up telephone call to their maternity clients after discharge just to ask "How are things going?"

Nurses can also help fathers to think through how life may change with a new baby—diapers, feedings, less sleep. This kind of anticipatory guidance may forestall short tempers that sometimes come with lack of sleep and sensory overload. If the nurse can succeed in assisting the mother to feel good about herself, those around her will benefit, and positive reinforcement will become cyclic.

Education of Parents

All of the teaching–learning principles described in Chapter 2 should be recalled and used when teaching postpartal families. The nurse needs to assess the learner and emphasize principles, not teach step-by-step procedures that are impossible to remember and will increase anxiety. Principles involved with giving the newborn a bath are cleaning the genitals from front to back, preventing exposure that will chill, using a safe tub or sink, and never leaving a newborn alone unless in a crib or restraining device. Recall that during the taking-hold phase the mother is beginning to focus on the neonate, therefore, teaching should take place at this time. In the taking-in phase, the mother is exhausted and in pain and receptivity to new learning will be low; both teacher and learner will be frustrated at this time (Petrowski, 1981).

Bottle-Feeding

Teaching infant feeding is an important part of postpartum education. The importance of assessing readiness to learn has already been mentioned, and identifying what the parents know about feeding a newborn is also important. Recall that building on previous knowledge is an important principle. For example, if this is the fourth child the mother is bottle-feeding, the nurse's approach will be different than for the new mother with no infant caretaking experiences. Making the mother comfortable and having her wash her hands before feeding are prerequisites. If the mother has had a cesarean birth, positioning her so that she can comfortably support the neonate will contribute to her success. It is hoped that most care settings allow for flexible feeding patterns so that the infant is fed when ready, not when the hospital deems it is time. Bottle-feeding is a unique opportunity for father participation. There are several things to consider in helping parents who elect to bottle-feed.

- ▲ Bottles should always be held, not propped. Otitis media can develop if an infant drinks from a propped bottle since milk may block the eustachian tube.
- ▲ The nipple should be placed on the top of the tongue and inserted straight in, not toward the roof of the mouth. This position provides better suction and less air intake. To further reduce air ingestion, the nipple should be kept full of milk at all times.
- ▲ Holes in the nipple should be large enough for the milk to flow freely but not pour out.
- ▲ It is important to burp the infant at intervals. The infant needs to be positioned upright so the air bubble will rise to the top of the stomach. Patting or rubbing the back may help the burping.
- ▲ Force feeding, or finishing all the bottle, should be avoided. A fat baby is not necessarily a healthy baby.

Sterilization and types of formulas are discussed in Chapter 17. The critical aspect of bottle-feeding, besides the milk or nutritional nourishment, is the socialization process. The infant's need for touch and closeness are met, which evokes and meets reciprocal needs in the mother or father. Close physical contact and eye contact facilitate bonding and contribute significantly to the attachment process. For the mother who chooses to bottle-feed, it is important to reassure her that these needs—holding, touching, bonding—can and do occur equally well in breast- and bottle-feeding, providing infants are held during feedings.

Breast-Feeding

Ideally, the baby who will be breast-fed is put to breast as soon as possible after delivery. Although some neonates are not terribly interested in nursing, the psychologic and physiologic benefits are many. The reality of seeing, holding, and touching their newborn is psychologically beneficial for both mothers and fathers. This contact between parent and child is psychologically beneficial for the neonate too. Colostrum has nutrients and immunoglobulins, which are physiologically beneficial for the neonate.

Assisting the breast-feeding mother requires certain skills on the part of the nurse. The goals of the instruction should be that the newborn receives adequate nutrition, that the mother has an adequate milk supply, and that trauma to the nipple is avoided. Helping the mother assume a comfortable position is important. Many women are comfortable nursing lying down on their side with the head of the infant slightly elevated (Fig. 19.7). Whether lying down or sitting comfortably, the nipple should be directed straight into the mouth with as much of

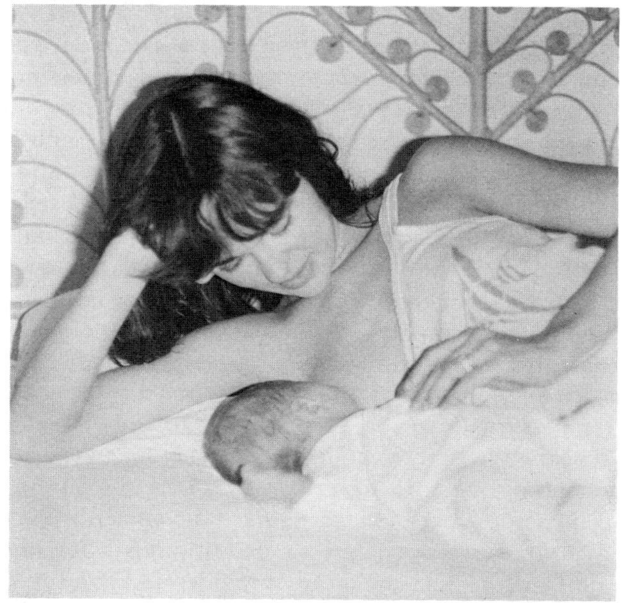

Figure 19.7
Nursing lying down.

the areola inserted as possible. Ideally, the jaws of the neonate compress the ducts that are beneath the areolar. If the mother grasps her breast between her forefinger and third finger, she can direct the breast into the infant's mouth (Fig. 19.8). Expressing some milk may further encourage the neonate to nurse since the sense of smell is well developed in the neonate. If the neonate's nose (newborns are obligate nose breathers) is compressed against breast tissue, the mother should put her finger against the breast pushing it back from the baby's nose.

It is at the beginning of the feeding when the baby latches on and the sucking reflex is strong that the mother may feel uncomfortable. As her nipples become tougher and more resilient, this initial discomfort decreases. Rotating feeding positions lessens stress as the greatest stress occurs in a line from the nipple to the baby's chin. Rotating from cradle hold, to football hold, to maternal side-lying, changes the stress focus and contributes to complete breast emptying (see Chapter 17, Figure 17.23).

Most of the milk is emptied from the breast in the first 5 or 10 minutes of nursing, and the infant can be nursed on the other breast at this time. Nursing time should progress, first, from 3 to 5 minutes to 5 minutes on each side, then from 7 to 10 minutes to 10 minutes on each side. The infant in this way will empty the milk on each side (stimulating milk supply), as well as meet oral satisfaction needs. As the mother becomes more comfortable with breast-feeding, the baby can remain longer on the second breast assuring that oral needs are completely satisfied. Alternating the starting breast at each feeding changes the extended nursing time from one breast to the other. In other words, the baby nurses on both sides at each feeding but spends the extended time on the second breast. Many mothers attach a small safety pin to the bra strap of the breast that they will start with next time since it is sometiems difficult to keep track of the feeding routine.

In addition to teaching the mother about alternating breasts during feedings and the time frame for nursing, the nurse should teach her about breaking the suction by inserting a finger into the baby's mouth before removing the neonate in order to avoid nipple trauma. The nurse should also give instructions about positions for burping (see Fig. 19.9) and the fact that burping between feedings on each breast and at the end of feeding are important. A crying infant should be burped before feeding if possible.

When beginning breast-feeding, supplemental formula feedings should not be given since the infant can become confused with the different stimuli. Parents need to be taught that even though they cannot see how much is taken, satisfaction can be measured in other ways. Weighing the infant and having the mother see the weight gain is helpful. Informing the mother that because breast milk is more easily digested, the neonate becomes hungry sooner, and increasing feedings usually resolves the supply-and-demand balance. There are many types

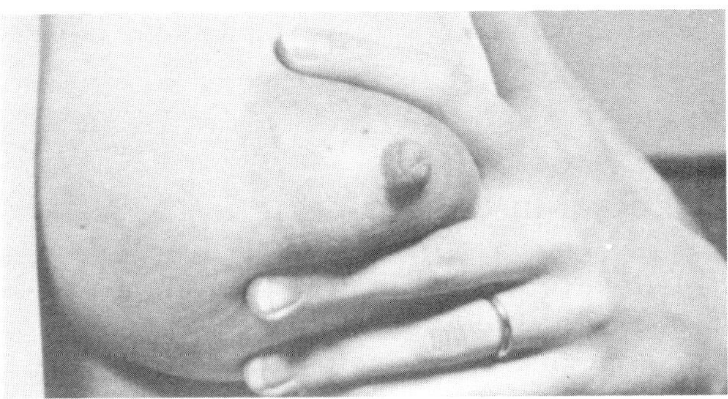

Figure 19.8
Expressing milk between forefinger and third finger. Courtesy of Ross Laboratories. Used by permission.

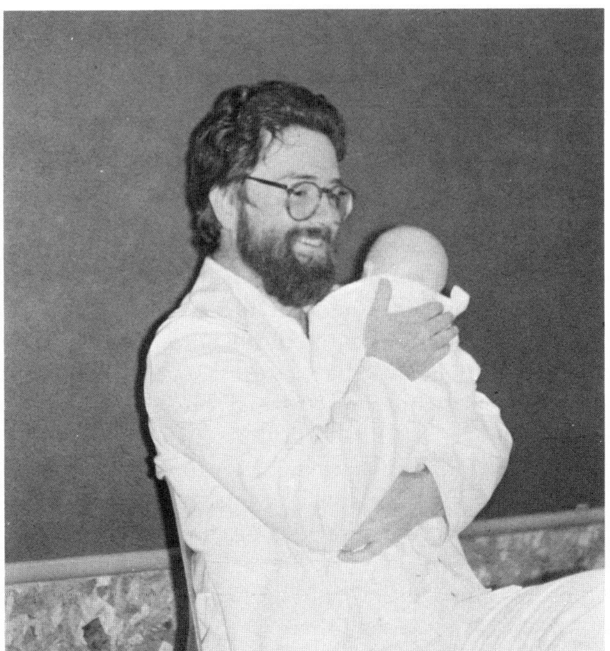

Figure 19.9
Burping the infant.

of breast pumps available for the mother if she wishes to express milk for a feeding when she will not be present. Cadwell (1980) explores the pros and cons of several breast pumps and suggests that evaluation should be based on the following factors: availability, sterility, capacity of the pump, power source (electric or hand), cost, and portability (for working mothers). Breast pumps may also be rented. If breast milk is to be stored, it should not be kept in plastic bottles since antibodies tend to cling to the sides of the bottle. It is important to remind the mother that breast milk removed by any means will be replenished. Sometimes breast-feeding mothers are concerned about leaving their infants, but nurses know that mothers who have to be separated from ill infants maintain lactation. Motivation to breast-feed is undoubtedly the critical factor.

Maternal attitudes about breast-feeding were explored in a research article by Arafat et al. (1981). The research looked at trends in breast-feeding over the last 30 years in an attempt to verify the claim that the decline in breast-feeding has been reversed. The study also looked at ethnicity, religious orientation, and marital status; it also explored occupation and income and the effect of income level on mothers' practices in infant feeding. Sociocultural factors such as mother–child relationships, mother–partner relationship, and mother relationship with her own mother were addressed. There were 441 people in the study.

The research presented some interesting data that are useful for nurses. This New York City survey showed a decline in breast-feeding since 1940; it seems that the proportion of breast-feeding mothers has stabilized at 50%. In this sample, 60% of the mothers who were breast-fed themselves also breast-fed their children. The data in this study indicate that even if the mother breast-feeds the first child she is likely to switch to the bottle with subsequent children. This survey also showed that only 33% of black mothers reported breast-feeding as opposed to 55% white and 67% Hispanic. Marital status was not significant; just as many unmarried as married mothers breast-fed. Mothers in the lowest and four top-income brackets are much more likely to breast-feed than mothers in middle-income brackets. The decision on whether to breast-feed or not seems to be largely the woman's; secondary influences are mate, friends, health care personnel, relatives, and the media. The fact that the mother herself was breast-fed seems to be the factor that increases the chance that she will in turn breast-feed her child. Breast-feeding mothers believed it was more nutritious and emotionally healthier for the child, as well as natural; they also expressed the feeling that it brings mother and child closer. Only half of the breast-feeding group saw it as more economical.

On the other hand, bottle-feeding mothers are less positive about their attitudes toward the benefit of bottle-feeding. In general, they see bottle-feeding as more convenient and that breast-feeding would interfere with work requirements. The substance of this research seems to reflect the view that mothers, whether they choose to breast-feed or not, tend to see the practice as advantageous and that breast-fed neonates have a better chance of avoiding infection and digestive problems. The fact that even breast-feeding mothers tend to bottle-feed subsequent children makes us wonder about social inhibitors that may be present in American society. Lack of role models, which are evident in many other cultures, may be a significant factor. As in so many other facets of maternity nursing, nurses need to examine their own values, be knowledgeable about the pros and cons of each position, and then assist and support their patients in decision making.

POSTPARTUM COMPLICATIONS

There are several broad categories of complications of the postpartum, including both physiologic and psychosocial concerns. It is the nurse's role to be aware of etiologic and predisposing factors and of signs and symptoms of these complications, as well as of appropriate nursing interventions.

Puerperal Infections

Historically, *puerperal infection* (infection of the genital tract associated with childbearing, usually occurring within the first 10 days postpartum) was the cause of many maternal deaths. It was not until Oliver Wendell Holmes (1843) showed that the epidemic nature of childbirth fever could be traced to poor aseptic techniques on the part of nurses and physicians that people became aware of the etiology of the problem. Semmelweiss (1847) pointed out that the cause of puerperal infection was directly related to the fact that physicians were examining patients vaginally without proper hand washing. Unfortunately, his findings were largely ignored and it was not until after the work of Pasteur and Lister that aseptic technique was used and mortality lessened. With the advent of antibiotics and bacteriologic culturing, treatment of puerperal fever improved considerably. In the nineteenth and twentieth centuries, streptococcal epidemics were active, but with the discovery and use of sulfonamide, control of this organism occurred. Unfortunately, other organisms came to the front.

In the 1950s, the incidence of puerperal infection was reported to be 2–8%; in some selected populations it was as high as 40–50% (Huff & Pauerstein, 1979). Puerperal infection can be caused by anaerobic (not using oxygen) or aerobic (using oxygen) bacteria and usually is a mixed infection containing both anaerobic and aerobic bacteria. The most common organisms are anaerobic streptococci, aerobic streptococci, *Bacteroides* species, and *Escherichia coli.* Sometimes the following organisms are involved: *Staphylococcus aureus, Clostridia,* and Gram-negative organisms.

Predisposing factors of puerperal infection include women who have had prolonged rupture of the membranes, cesarean birth, trauma, or anemia (see Chapter 22). The vagina and cervix of approximately 70% of healthy women contain pathogenic bacteria, and once the membranes are ruptured (before rupture of the membranes the uterine cavity is essentially sterile), infection is possible. Other factors that can provide portals for infection are the placental site, operative site, episiotomy, lacerations, or abrasions.

If a genital tract infection spreads and involves the lymphatic system, pelvic cellulitis or peritonitis can occur. The most common sites for pelvic abscesses are the uterine ligaments, subdiaphragmatic space, or Douglas's cul-de-sac. The relationship between infection and internal fetal monitoring is debated in the literature, but any monitored patient, especially one who subsequently has a cesarean birth, should be watched closely.

Chorioamnionitis (clinical infection of the fetal membranes and amniotic fluid) is caused in most cases by ascent of bacteria from the cervix and vagina after spontaneous rupture of the membranes. It is possible to have organisms cause a chorioamnionitis and even fetal death with the membranes intact. The organisms involved are the same as those causing puerperal infection.

Localized infections can also occur during the postpartum period and are usually related to the episiotomy or lacerations of the vagina, perineum, or vulva. The process of incisional infection after cesarean birth is characterized by a reddened, tender area at the site of the incision followed by purulent material draining from the wound.

Early detection and management of an infectious process results in a quicker resolution of the underlying problem. The Joint Committee on Maternal Welfare defines *puerperal morbidity* as a temperature of 100.4°F (38.0°C) or higher–if taken at least 4 times daily by mouth on any two of the first 10 days postpartum, excluding the first 24 hours after delivery. It is not unusual for the temperature to be elevated the first 24 hours because of exhaustion and dehydration. For example, if a woman had a temperature of 100.4°F on the second day after delivery and a temperature of 100.6°F on the third day, she would be considered morbid or infected, and the source of the infection would have to be sought.

Physical examination of an infected woman may elicit complaints of discomfort, anorexia, low grade fever, or malaise. Symptoms of severe infection include elevated temperature (101–103°F), chills, anorexia, extreme lethargy, rapid pulse, and localized pain. Diagnosis of the infection site is determined by physical examination, blood work, urinalysis, and cultures. Culturing any discharges or urine helps to identify the causative organism. Subjective data will also assist in determining where the infection is occurring. For example, if the woman has pain when urinating and voids frequently in small amounts, a urinary tract infection is suspected and urine culture undoubtedly would be ordered. When endometritis is suspected, a urine culture is also often done to rule out asymptomatic urinary tract infection. If the nurse smells foul lochia when caring for the woman (or sometimes just walking into the room), endometritis is suspected.

The goals of nursing care in puerperal infection are to promote healing and to educate the woman about the infection and the personal hygiene measures necessary to alleviate the immediate problem and to prevent future infection. Antibiotic therapy is instituted quickly following cultures, and, if the infection is severe, combination antibiotic therapy may be started to cover a broad range of potential Gram-positive or Gram-negative organisms. The newborn of a nursing mother who is on antibiotic therapy should be assessed for signs of thrush. Treatment with antibiotics often destroys the normal oral flora, and a *Candida albicans* (thrush) infection can occur. When this occurs, breast-feeding is discontinued. The mother may wish to continue to pump breast milk and resume breast-feedings later.

Sometimes pelvic cellulitis or peritonitis results in abscesses that require surgical intervention to drain or remove retained or necrotic placental fragments. The nursing roles are to assist the physician with any procedures, ascertain that infected materials are disposed of properly, and administer any ordered drugs, antibiotics, or analgesics. If puerperal infection becomes severe, in addition to antibiotic therapy and possible surgical intervention, position of the patient, hydration, blood transfusions, and oxytocics may be part of the therapy. A sitting position, or semi-Fowler's, improves drainage of the lochia and may deter upward extension of the infection from the pelvis. Fluid intake of 3,000–4,000 ml is often instituted; to achieve this intake, parenteral fluids are often administered. Diet should consist of foods with high caloric and vitamin content that are easy to digest. Adequate rest and sleep are necessary, and pain relief should be provided. Oxytocics may be given to keep the uterus contracted and to prevent extension of bacteria or toxins through the uterine wall. Oxytocics may also ease passage of clots or pieces of tissue. Blood transfusions are used to help increase the patient's resistance. Women with puerperal infections should be isolated from other maternity patients. Ongoing, frequent assessment of vital signs and all signs and symptoms of the infection, as well as routine postpartum assessment by the nurse are all crucial.

In summary, the progression of puerperal infection begins most often in the uterus and is called endometritis, or an inflammation of the uterine lining. Initially, the woman complains of chills, has a moderate temperature elevation, and may have a relaxed and tender uterus. If the infection progresses and involves the lymphatics or bloodstream and spreads to the connective tissues around the uterus, it is called parametritis, or pelvic cellulitis. Symptoms then progress to severe chills, fever, rapid pulse, and generalized malaise. The final and severe progression is a peritonitis infection, including the peritoneum, which can lead to generalized systemic infection of the whole body. Symptoms include pain, abdominal distention, vomiting, chills, fever, rapid pulse, restlessness, and anxiety. When the infection progresses to this extensive state, the woman is extremely ill; therefore, the nurse's responsibility is to prevent puerperal infection. Cleanliness and aseptic technique are stressed in the section on basic postpartal care, and every principle discussed in that section is important in preventing puerperal infection.

Venous Thrombosis or Thrombophlebitis

Recall that under normal conditions in the human body, a balance exists between the coagulation and fibrinolytic systems. During pregnancy, the balance tilts in the direction of coagulation, which is nature's way of preparing for delivery. Clotting factors, particularly fibrinogen and platelets, increase during the puerperium, which in itself predisposes to clot formation. Slowing of blood flow in the legs, especially after cesarean birth, contributes to clot formation.

According to some research, suppression of lactation by estrogen contributes to risk of thrombus formation (Cooper, 1976). In addition, all of the following factors may contribute to the risk of thromboembolism: maternal age, high parity, operative delivery, obesity, toxemia, a history of thromboembolitic disease, and familial tendency.

Thrombosis occurs in both superficial and deep veins; superficial vein involvement is considerably more common than deep vein involvement.

Prevention of venous thrombosis is best accomplished by early ambulation. A woman who for any reason has to remain in bed for a period of time needs to be instructed about and helped with active and passive leg exercises. The knee gatch on the bed should not be elevated as this can impede venous return and compound or contribute to the problem.

The symptoms that usually appear in lower extremity puerperal thrombophlebitis are sudden onset of leg pain, edema, and increased skin temperature. Homan's sign is positive; that is, while holding the woman's knee flat, dorsiflexion of the foot causes pain in that leg. Peripheral pulses may decrease, and the leg may be pale and cool. Treatment may include hot moist packs, TED (elastic) stockings, and anticoagulant therapy. Although heparin does not dissolve the clot, it may prevent further clot formation; heparin is not excreted in breast milk and, therefore, can be safely administered to breastfeeding mothers. The greatest threat from thrombophlebitis is pulmonary embolism. Symptoms of pulmonary embolism are sudden onset of dyspnea, sweating, pallor, cyanosis, and hypotension. Increased jugular pressure may signal pulmonary emboli. Chest pain, along with the woman saying, "I am going to die," should alert the nurse. The almost prophetic verbalization is an ominous sign. X-ray films and electrocardiograms are not always reliable. Even if pulmonary embolism is only suspected, treatment should be instituted and the patient transferred to a medical intensive care unit.

Mastitis

Mastitis is the inflammation of breast tissue by pathogenic organisms and should be differentiated from localized inflammation of the breast from a blocked milk duct. The causative organism in mastitis is usually *S. aureus,* but *Bacteroides* can sometimes cause abscess around the areola. The source of the infection can be the hands of the mother or caretaker, as well as from the nose or the mouth of the infant. People who care for infants and mothers need to be especially careful with hand washing techniques. If cracks, or fissures, of the nipples are present, it is relatively easy for the organism to ascend into the breast tissue. Milk stasis provides an ideal medium for the growth of organisms.

The symptom is a warm, hardened, tender area most often in the upper, outer quadrant of the breast. Heat, antibiotics, and analgesics are all part of the treatment; a milk sample is sent for culture and sensitivity (to see which antibiotic is effective). Nasal cultures can be done to assist in identifying potential carriers. Frequent breast-feeding (which eliminates stasis of milk) usually prevents mastitis.

A controversy exists as to whether breast-feeding should be continued or not if mastitis occurs. Those on the pro side contend that if the milk contains bacteria, it also has the antibiotic to treat it. The con side says breast-feeding should cease since a cycle of reinfection—milk-to-infant to-breast to-mother to-milk—is perpetuated. Sudden cessation of feeding can cause caking, which is painful and contributes to severe engorgement and pain. If breast abscesses form, surgical intervention may be required and breast-feeding inhibited.

Breast infection can occur any time during lactation; it is not unusual for it to occur as late as 3–4 weeks postpartum. A well mother experiences chills and fever and a lobe of the breast becomes tender and painful. Fortunately, with antibiotic therapy the condition is usually rapidly resolved.

Cystitis

The bladder and urethra always suffer some degree of trauma and stretching during delivery, which causes mucosal edema and hyperemia. Slight lesions of the bladder (that are apt to occur), catheterization, or residual urine are factors that may contribute to cystitis. After the baby is born there is a temporary loss of bladder tone that makes the mother unaware of how full her bladder is, which can result in overdistention, incomplete emptying of the bladder, or residual urine—all predisposing factors to cystitis. If the urethra has been traumatized, voiding may be difficult or impossible.

Prevention of cystitis is, of course, the best treatment, and assessment of the mother for a full bladder or residual urine is the key. Overdistention is avoided by observation in the early postpartum period and draining the bladder once with a straight catheter, if necessary. If overdistention is recurrent or occurs after the first 24 hours, a Foley catheter is often used as the physician may wish to leave the catheter in place. Residual urine (urine left in the bladder after voiding) that is greater than 100 cc is often a criteria for leaving an indwelling catheter in place. Protocol for postpartum catheterization also often requires that when 900–1,000 cc are siphoned off, the catheter should be left in place and clamped. This protects the bladder, and rapid intra-abdominal decompression is prevented. If the patient has no ill effects after 1 hour, the catheterization is completed. Any time a woman is catheterized in the postpartum period, a urine specimen is sent for a culture; the tip of the catheter may be cultured also. Vital signs before and after the procedure, as well as the woman's response to the procedure, should be charted.

Symptoms of cystitis include frequency, urgency, dysuria, hematuria, and costal vertebral angle (CVA) tenderness. Treatment, in addition to antibiotics (after urine culture), includes forcing fluids and ambulation to assist fluid mobilization. There is no reason to discontinue breast-feeding, and interaction with her newborn may prevent the mother from focusing on her cystitis, as well as promote mother–infant attachment.

Hematomas and Hemorrhage

The criterion for postpartum hemorrhage has traditionally been set at any bleeding greater than 500 cc in the first 24 hours after delivery. Normal blood loss after vaginal delivery is approximately 300–400 cc. There is some feeling that this figure is low and needs revision (Willson & Carrington, 1979). Postpartum hemorrhage is classified as early or late.

Early postpartum hemorrhage is generally caused by uterine atony or lacerations of the genital tract. Careful observation and assessment of vaginal bleeding, often by counting the perineal pads used, are important. A *boggy uterus,* one that does not stay contracted without constant massage, is atonic. Recall that the uterus is a muscle and exhaustion of this muscle can result in atony. Predisposing factors to hemorrhage include overdistention of the uterus (multiple birth, hydramnios), overmassage (overstimulation of a muscle causes it to relax), precipitous or prolonged labor, and general anesthesia. The usual treatment for hemorrhage is continuous infusion of fluids and oxytocin. If the woman has a normal blood pressure, either ergonovine or methylergonovine may be administered intramuscularly. If oxytocic drugs are not effective or if retention of a placental fragment is suspected, curretage and initiation of prophylactic antibiotics are done.

If late postpartum hemorrhage—hemorrhage occurring anytime after the first 24 hours—happens, it is most often a week or more after delivery, after the woman has gone home. Therefore, the woman is instructed to call the physician if bright red bleeding occurs after she is home. The treatment is the same as for early hemorrhage—oxytocic drugs and curettage if retained placental fragments are the cause.

Hematomas, as a result of injury to a blood vessel, develop in the connective tissue of the vulva or under the vaginal mucosa. Hematomas may occur in spontaneous or forceps deliveries. Since the soft tissue in the vagina and vulva offer little resistance, 250–500 cc of blood can collect rapidly. The woman complains of severe pain in the perineal or rectal area. When the hematoma is external, it is seen as a unilateral bulging at the introitus or involving the labia. However, hematomas can occur higher in the vagina, where they are not readily visible and require careful inspection. Large hematomas can develop rapidly and may require surgical intervention to evacuate the clot and restore hemostasis.

One other rare but extremely serious cause of postpartal hemorrhage is placenta accreta, which is abnormal penetration of the trophoblast into the uterine wall. Complete placenta accreta will not separate from the uterine wall and no bleeding occurs, but incomplete or partial accreta (because complete separation cannot occur) can result in profuse bleeding. Manual extraction may be required. Placenta accreta can result in catastrophic hemorrhage; hysterectomy is often necessary.

Psychosocial Complications

Attachment behaviors and the reciprocity of the neonate–mother–father are discussed in Chapter 17, and the factors that contribute to successful parenting are explored in Chapter 18. Maladaptive attachment patterns and neurotic and psychotic complications do sometimes occur postpartally, and the nurse needs to assess these factors.

In the postpartum period the nurse is in an ideal position to collect data and observe the interactions of the family. Behaviors such as feeding, eye contact, talking to the infant all should be noted and recorded. As mentioned earlier, anticipatory guidance and positive reinforcement do much to promote the desired attachment process.

Psychiatric problems encountered in the postpartum period are rarely serious, but approximately 70–80% of postpartum women experience some depression (Danforth, 1977). Sometimes this depression is referred to as the *postpartum blues;* symptoms include crying and the woman saying something such as, "I really just can't help myself." Usually the crying and depression is self-limiting, but occasionally serious psychiatric problems occur. Many factors can contribute to the stress of coping postpartally: planned or unplanned pregnancy, marital status, pre-existing personality patterns, breast-feeding, perineal discomfort, and hormone imbalance. Full-blown psychoses after pregnancy and delivery are usually related to other causes, with pregnancy serving as a precipitating factor. If prolonged evidence of poor attachment (not holding or feeding the neonate) or examples of coping dysfunction continue, referral for psychiatric assistance is appropriate. As described earlier in the chapter, major physiologic and psychosocial changes are taking place in the postpartum period, and it is important that the nurse detect any complications early so that quick and effective intervention can be started.

SUMMARY

This chapter described and discussed physiologic characteristics that occur in the postpartum period. Changes specific to the reproductive tract, ovarian function, and urinary and gastrointestinal tracts were explored. Adaptation related to the breasts, body weight, vital signs, and endocrine status were presented. Psychosocial characteristics were described, and the phases of taking-in, taking-hold, and letting-go were introduced.

The next section described postpartum nursing management and reviewed assessment procedures and appropriate nursing interventions in many areas. For example, vital signs, breast care, perineal care, ambulation, sleep, and exercise appropriate for postpartum women were described.

Nursing interventions useful for helping accomplish the postpartal maternal tasks were presented. Interventions relating to the mother and her postpartum recovery progress were stressed. The parent education section reinforces the use of teaching–learning principles presented in Chapter 2.

The next section discussed nursing management and intervention for the bottle-feeding or breastfeeding mother. Pros and cons of breast versus bottle were discussed briefly, and a research study looking at maternal attitudes about infant feeding and implications for nursing were shared.

The last section of this chapter discussed assessment and treatment of complications that occur during the postpartum period. Conditions such as puerperal infection, mastitis, cystitis, hemorrhage, and psychosocial complications were summarized.

REFERENCES AND READINGS

Affonso, D. D. Nursing Pieces: A Study of Postpartum Feelings. *Birth Fam J* 4:159, 1977.

Arafat, I., Allen, D., Fox, J. E. Maternal Practice and Attitudes Toward Breastfeeding. *J Obstet Gynecol Neonatal Nurs* 10(2):91, 1981.

Bard, B. Nurses' Messages About Breastfeeding. *Am J Nurs* 81(8):1491, 1981.

Bull, M. J. Change in Concerns of First-Time Mothers After One Week at Home. *J Obstet Gynecol Neonatal Nurs* 18(5):391, 1981.

Caldwell, K. and Tibbetts, E. Selecting the Right Breast Pump. *Am J Mat Child Nurs* 5(4): (July/August), 1980, pp. 262–264.

Cooper, K. Thrombosis and Embolism in Obstetrics. *Nurs Mirror* 142:65, 1976.

Danforth, D. N. (Ed.) *Obstetrics and Gynecology*. Hagerstown, Md.: Harper & Row, 1977.

Davidson, N. REEDA: Evaluating Postpartum Healing. *J Nurs Midwifery* 19:7, 1974.

Doucette, J. S. Is Breastfeeding Still Safe for Babies? *Am J Matern Child Nurs,* 3(6):345, 1978.

Gorrie, T. M. A Postpartum Evaluation Tool. *J Obstet Gynecol Neonatal Nurs* 8:41, 1979.

Grams, K. E. Breastfeeding: A Means of Imparting Immunity. *Am J Matern Child Nurs* 3(6):340, 1978.

Grassley, J., Davis, J. Common Concerns of Mothers Who Breast-feed. *Am J Matern Child Nurs* 3(6):347, 1978.

Henderson, K., Newton, L. Helping Nursing Mothers Maintain Lactation While Separated from Their Infants. *Am J Matern Child Nurs* 3(6):352, 1978.

Huff, R. W., Pauerstein, C. J. *Human Reproduction: Physiology and Pathophysiology.* New York, John Wiley & Sons, 1979.

Levine, N. H. Family-Centered Maternity Units—Fact or Fiction? *J Obstet Gynecol Neonatal Nurs* 9(2):116, 1980.

Marechi, M. P. Postpartum Follow-Up Goals and Assessment. *JOGN* 8(4):214, 1979.

Maslow, A. H. *Motivation and Personality* (2nd ed.). New York: Harper & Row, 1970.

Mercer, R. T. The Nurse and Maternal Tasks of Early Postpartum. *Am J Matern Child Health Nurs* 6(5):341, 1981.

Perez, A., Vela, P., Masnilk, G. S., Potter, R. First Ovulation After Childbirth. *Am J Obstet Gynecol* 114:1041, 1972.

Petrowski, D. D. Effectiveness of Prenatal and Postnatal Instruction in Postpartum Care. *J Obstet Gynecol Neonatal Nurs* 10(5):386, 1981.

Pritchard, J. A., MacDonald, P. C. *Williams Obstetrics* (15th ed.). New York: Appleton-Century-Crofts, 1976.

Riordan, J., Countryman, B. A. Basics of Breastfeeding, Part II: The Anatomy and Psychophysiology of Lactation. *J Obstet Gynecol Neonatal Nurs* 9(4):210, 1980.

Riordan, J., Rapp, E. Pleasure and Purpose: The Sensuousness of Breastfeeding. *J Obstet Gynecol Nurs* 9(2):109, 1980.

Rising, S. The Fourth Stage of Labor: Family Integration. *Am J Nurs* 74(5):870, 1974.

Rubin, R. Maternal Touch. *Nurs Outlook* 11(11):828, 1963.

Rubin, R. Basic Maternal Behavior. *Nurs Outlook* 9(11):683, 1961a.

Rubin, R. Puerperal Change. *Nurs Outlook* 9(12):753, 1961b.

Sharman, A. Menstruation After Childbirth. *J Obstet Gynaecol British Commonwealth,* 58:440, 1951

Tanner, L. M. *Developmental Tasks of Pregnancy, Current Concepts of Clinical Nursing.* Anderson, E. H. (Ed.) St. Louis: C. V. Mosby, 1969, Vol. 2.

Tibbetts, E., Cadwell, H. Selecting the Right Breast Pump. *Am J Matern Child Nurs* 5(4):262, 1980.

Turnbull, A. C. et al. Antenatal and Postnatal Thromboembolism. *Practitioner* 206:727, 1971.

Wietchetek, W. J. et al. Puerperal Morbidity and Internal Fetal Monitoring. *Am J Obstet Gynecol* 119:230, 1974.

Willson, J. R., Carrington, E. R. *Obstetrics and Gynecology* (6th ed.) St. Louis: C. V. Mosby, 1979.

Zuspan, F. P., Goodrich, S. Metabolic Studies in Normal Pregnancy, I: Nitrogen Metabolism. *Am J Obstet Gynecol* 100:7, 1968.

UNIT FIVE

REPRODUCTIVE RISK

INTRODUCTION

Reproductive risk is a health problem of considerable magnitude throughout the world today. Much progress has been made, however, toward reducing the incidences of maternal mortality and morbidity and of neonatal and infant deaths. Maternal and infant mortality rates reached lowest recorded figures in 1980 (see Chapter 3). However, infant mortality in the United States remains higher than in many other industrialized countries.

The maternity nurse plays a key role in assessing and treating reproductive at risk conditions. The nurse is the principal health educator for both healthy expectant parents and those at reproductive risk. Maternity and perinatal nurses are the primary sources from which the family at reproductive risk receives therapeutic and emotional support. The nurse is the link between the hospitalized neonate, who has suffered reproductive damage, and that infant's family.

Nursing management of reproductive risk conditions often requires a knowledge and skill base that supercedes beginning maternity nursing practices; however, all maternity nurses should be able to recognize potential and real reproductive risk conditions and to make sound judgments about the health care of these consumers, such as whether to provide nursing care or to refer the person to more specialized care. Unit Five consists of six chapters that provide basic information about reproductive risk to students of maternity nursing.

Chapter 20, "Families at Reproductive Risk," examines the scope of reproductive risk and factors that predispose the pregnant woman and her family to risk. Categories of reproductive risk are discussed; special attention is given to risk associated with or deriving from psychosocial, genetic, biophysical, and economic concerns. The cost of reproductive risk is presented from the vantage of financial and human expenditures. Assessment of reproductive risk addresses the use of clinical, biochemical, electronic, sonographic, and radiologic modalities for diagnosing reproductive risk conditions. Particular attention is given to the types of information to which the nurse should attend in taking a health history; observations that can be made by the nurse; and the ways in which the nurse uses and gives meaning to data relevant to diagnosing and treating risk conditions. The chapter closes with a statement of general nursing responsibilities for health care of pregnant families at reproductive risk.

Chapter 21, "Maternal Disorders and Problems During Pregnancy," discusses a variety of risk conditions from the perspective of the pregnant or newly delivered woman. Major risk conditions such as hypertensive disorders, bleeding, diabetes, heart disease, and infections receive the most attention; however, other risk conditions, such as anemia and respiratory problems, are included. The pregnant woman and her unborn child are considered as a unit in which a condition arising from one affects the other.

Chapter 22, "Abnormal Labor," contains information about dysfunctional labor, operative obstetrics (cesarean section and forceps delivery), and emergency delivery. Induction, augmentation of labor, and management of the delivery of a woman with a multiple gestation are also discussed. Anesthesia is covered. Special attention is given to the impact of abnormal labor on the woman and the fetus, as well as on the neonate immediately after birth. The focus of the chapter is on how the nurse uses information about abnormal labor to provide safe comprehensive care for the woman and her family during this stressful event.

Chapter 23, "Fetal–Neonatal Disorders," includes conditions or problems associated with gestational age: prematurity, low birth weight, postterm infants. Respiratory distress syndrome receives considerable attention. Metabolic problems, such as hypoglycemia and hypocalcemia, and hematologic disorders, such as hyperbilirubinemia, anemia, and polycythemia, are also discussed. Common infectious disorders and selected minor disorders are included. The focus of Chapter 23 is on the nursing management of the neonate as a new human life and as a member of a family.

Chapter 24, "Inheritance and Its Legacy: Genetic Disorders," presents inherited conditions. Prenatal genetic diagnosis is explained, and the more common genetic disorders, such as chromosomal aberrations, single gene defects, autosomal dominant, recessive, and X-linked transmission, are discussed. Selected multifactorial disorders are presented. Genetic counseling and ethical considerations are discussed. The role of the nurse in providing care for families who have potential for a child with congenital disorders or whose child is born with congenital disorders is emphasized.

Chapter 25, "Reproductive Psychosocial Disorders," is concerned with a significant contemporary health problem. The chapter looks at some important areas of concern, such as maternal drug and alcohol use and its effect on the unborn/newborn, spouse and parental abusive behaviors, and postpartum depression. Other psychosocial disorders, including maternal vomiting disorders during pregnancy (hyperemesis gravidarum), psychosomatic infertility, false pregnancy (pseudocyesis), abnormal cravings, and aversions are briefly discussed. The role of the nurse in early detection of psychosocial disorders, as well as the importance of concerned nursing care of the patient and family experiencing a disorder of such a socially sensitive nature are emphasized.

BEHAVIORAL OUTCOMES

Upon completion of the study of this unit, you should be able to:

- ▲ List the leading causes of reproductive risk
- ▲ Describe the scope of reproductive risk in the United States in regard to incidence and population affected
- ▲ Explain the use of five contemporary modalities important for the assessment of reproductive risk conditions
- ▲ Describe three ways in which a nurse participates in assessment of reproductive risk
- ▲ Describe the pathophysiologic basis for two major maternal risk conditions during each of the periods of pregnancy, labor, and recovery
- ▲ Explain the scientific basis for nursing care of two major reproductive risk conditions during each of the periods of pregnancy, labor, and recovery
- ▲ Describe four factors that contribute to fetal/neonatal risk
- ▲ Explain the nursing management of three neonatal disorders
- ▲ Explain the genetic basis for three inherited disorders
- ▲ Describe two modalities used for genetic diagnosis
- ▲ Explain the relationship between maternal drug or alcohol intake and fetal/neonatal well-being
- ▲ Describe two other psychosocial pathologic conditions and related nursing care

20

FAMILIES AT REPRODUCTIVE RISK

A family can be said to be at reproductive risk whenever a pregnancy within that family poses a threat to the health and well-being of any member of the family, particularly the pregnant woman and her unborn child. In other words

> *The expectant family, specifically the pregnant woman and fetus, is placed in jeopardy of such dimensions that achievement of the goal of reproductive health is rendered unlikely. This jeopardy is usually the result of a combination of circumstances or variables. It may arise from pre-existing conditions or occur as a result of pregnancy. The threat may be of maternal, fetal, familial or societal origins or a combination of all four.*
>
> *Butnarescu, 1978, p. XXVII*

This chapter discusses levels, categories, factors, and economic and human costs of reproductive risk. Attention is given to the use of clinical skills and biochemical and technologic modalities, such as electronic monitoring, sonography, and radiologic techniques, that are helpful and often necessary for the diagnosis of existent risk conditions or factors that can place the pregnant woman, fetus/neonate, and family in jeopardy of poor pregnancy outcome.

LEVELS OF RISK

Reproductive risk includes all levels of threat and incorporates the concepts of high-, moderate-, and low-risk pregnancies that frequently appear in writings on the problems associated with a pregnancy that is complicated by biophysical or psychosocial factors. The extremes of high and low risk require precise, meaningful definitions. Since there is no universal agreement about what constitutes high, moderate, and low risk, we will view reproductive risk from a somewhat different perspective, that being the extent of the damage with which the woman or family is threatened. Reproductive risk can then be examined as a continuum ranging from minimal damage to death.

When the family is at *minimal risk*, there is increased vulnerability to the usual risks associated with pregnancy. The pregnant woman often requires short-term medical management, and there is a good prognosis for all concerned (mild nutritional anemia in the pregnant woman; transitory hypoglycemia in the newborn). *Moderate risk* describes the family where usual risks associated with pregnancy are aggravated either because of pre-existing conditions, such as obesity, maternal age, or genetic-related conditions, or because of problems that arise from the pregnancy, such as urinary tract infection, mild hypertension, or transitory depression. The pregnant woman and her family must deal with an increased number of variables that threaten their physical and emotional stability. The problems arising can be managed, and no permanent damage is usual for mother, fetus/neonate, or family.

Maximal risk occurs when the numbers and intensity of the threat(s) place the pregnant woman and/or the fetus/neonate at grave risk of severe damage or death during pregnancy, labor, recovery, or the neonatal period. The likelihood of the family unit becoming debilitated because of the physical, emotional, and economic stresses placed on it is increased. (maternal diabetes, heart disease, genetic disorders, respiratory distress in the newborn).

You can remember these levels easily by associating the degree of threat with the extent of damage: the lesser the threat the better the outcome; the more serious the threat the graver the outcome. Table 20.1 summarizes the various levels of reproductive risk. Breaking down reproductive risk into levels enables the nurse and other health care providers to place the pregnant family into an appropriate perspective for determining needs and setting priorities for health care.

CATEGORIES OF RISK

Reproductive risk can also be viewed by looking at categories representing the factors that created the threat and at what will have the greatest impact by the threat. Most threats to health outcome for pregnancy can be classified as having psychosocial, genetic, biophysical, or economic origins.

Biophysical factors originate with the maternal, fetal, or neonatal body systems or impact on the functioning of these systems. *Psychosocial* factors arise from or affect interpersonal relationships, social climate and environment, emotional and mental responses, and culture. *Genetic* variables result in congenital anomaly or interfere with normal development or function of the fetus/neonate and can be traced to inheritance or early embryonic development. *Economic* factors contribute to the monetary expenditure by the family for matters associated with reproductive risk.

These four categories are not discrete—as presented here for learning purposes—but are usually interrelated. The risk factors are organized according to when these categories—in regard to reproduction—are most likely to be a threat to pregnancy and its outcome. (See Tables 20.2–20.5.) Other chapters in Unit Five elaborate on many of these factors or introduce others. A family is rarely at reproductive risk because of the presence of a single factor. More often reproductive risk occurs because of a combination of threats.

The pregnant woman and her fetus are a *unit* in which there is a symbiotic relationship; any threat to the well-being of the mother is likely to have a direct or indirect effect on the fetus. For example, when the maternal circulation is altered for any reason, such as vasoconstriction, the maternal blood pressure will increase in order to meet cardiovascular demands of the mother's body. Impaired maternal circulatory function can decrease the transport of nutrients and oxygen to the fetus. In such a situation, both the mother and fetus are in jeopardy (see Chapter 21). The dependence of a pregnant woman on drugs and alcohol will influence the well-being of her unborn child (see Chapter 25). Some threats are of fetal origin, such as problems associated with maternal–fetal blood incompatibility. In some cases the mother will be at greater risk and in other cases the infant will be. A good rule to remember is that whenever the mother is in serious jeopardy, the fetus will also be in peril.

Pregnancy occurs within the context of some type of family unit. When a member, or members, of that unit is threatened, in this instance the pregnant woman and fetus, the family is likely to experience increased stress and economic hardship. The family may be the source of the threat, as in genetic risk, or there may be a reciprocal interchange between the family and the pregnant woman much as there is between the woman and fetus. Pregnancy may be aggravated by family factors; or pregnancy may cause increased stress in the family that in turn affects the way in which the woman responds to the pregnancy thus creating a cycle of threat.

TABLE 20.1
LEVELS OF REPRODUCTIVE RISK

Characteristics of Reproductive Health	*Minimal Risk*	*Moderate Risk*	*Maximal Risk*
Biophysical and psychosocial adaptation to pregnancy is apparent	Increased vulnerability because of the usual risks associated with pregnancy. There is distortion in one or more of the characteristics of reproductive health that necessitates increased supervisory and short-term therapy during prenatal period.	There is an increase in the number of variables during the prenatal period that can contribute to damage to one or more members of the pregnant unit. There is a distortion in or increment of the usual risks associated with pregnancy.	The increment in number of variables contributing to reproductive risk or the intensity of existing variables are such that the pregnant unit (mother/fetus) is placed at great risk of damage or death at any point during pregnancy, labor, or recovery.
Present maternal and family health status is good. Functioning is maintained within normal limits. Growth and development of the fetus is congruent with gestational age. Neonatal adaptation to extrauterine life is apparent through biophysical and psychosocial behavior.	No maternal or family history of serious illness with residual damage, genetic disorder, or obstetric problem.	History of illness, genetic disorder, or obstetric problem is able to be managed or controlled through diagnosis and therapy during the prenatal period without major damage to the pregnant unit.	History of illness, genetic disorder, or obstetric problem of such magnitude that residual damage to the pregnant unit is likely and extensive damage or death is a probability.
Coping patterns are working as seen by the behavior of the pregnant woman and her family. Communications systems are open and effective. Support systems are used by the pregnant family in an effective and satisfying way.	There is a possibility for alterations in family and economic stability, but there is a history of capability for coping by the woman and family.	Stress is increased to the point that professional support and short-term therapy are necessary to restore family equilibrium; limited evidence of damage to the pregnant unit or family.	Stress is increased to the point that family stability and coping or economic stability is absent or disrupted; coping patterns are not working; damage to the mother/fetus and family is likely; long-term professional support and therapy are necessary.
The pregnancy is planned. Prospective parents demonstrate willingness to take on parenting role responsibilities.	Attitude toward the pregnancy is uncertain. Apprehension concerning assumption of a parenting role is discernable.	Attitude toward pregnancy is equivocal. Anxiety concerning assumption of parenting role is demonstrated through verbal/nonverbal communication.	There is overt and covert rejection of the pregnancy. Denial of the parenting role is evident.
The pregnant woman and her family are motivated to learn about pregnancy and parenting.	Pregnant woman or her family requires educational, diagnostic, and supervisory prenatal care in order to adapt to the fact of pregnancy.	There is increased need for educational, diagnostic, and supervisory, as well as therapeutic professional care.	Sustained educational, supervisory, and therapeutic professional care is necessary.

Source: Butnarescu, G. F., Tillotson, D. M., Villarreal, P. P. *Perinatal Nursing Vol. 2. Reproductive Risk.* New York: John Wiley & Sons, 1980. Used with permission.

TABLE 20.2
GENERAL FACTORS THAT PREDISPOSE TO REPRODUCTIVE RISK (CATEGORIZED ACCORDING TO POINT OF ORIGIN OR IMPACT)

Biophysical	*Psychosocial*	*Genetic*	*Economic*
MATERNAL Structural anomalies ▲ Uterus ▼ Morphology ▼ Position ▼ Poor muscle tone ▼ Incompetent cervix ▲ Pelvis ▼ Abnormal size ▼ Abnormal shape ▼ Fractures ▲ Skeleton ▼ Pronounced lordosis ▼ Pelvic joint ▼ Dislocations Pathophysiology and pathology ▲ Heart disease ▲ Chronic hypertension ▲ Kidney disease ▲ Blood disorders ▲ Diabetes mellitus ▲ Chronic infections ▲ Malignancy ▲ Immunologic disorders ▲ Tuberculosis Malnutrition ▲ Anemia ▲ Obesity ▲ Underweight Poor gynecological history ▲ Abnormal menstrual cycles ▼ Irregular ▼ Anovulatory ▼ Menorrhagia	MATERNAL History of psychopathology ▲ Neuroses ▲ Psychoses ▲ Depression ▲ Emotional disorders related to pregnancy, birth, or recovery History of sociopathology ▲ Abusive behavior patterns ▲ Drug dependence or addiction ▲ Alcohol dependence or addiction ▲ Promiscuity Mental or social disability Speech or communication disorders Habitual smoking Residence ▲ High altitude ▲ Exposure to pollutants ▲ Radiation ▲ Rural or inner city FAMILY History or presence of psychosocial pathology among family members Migrant or mobile family life-styles Poor interpersonal relationships Poor communication patterns Poor education patterns Unusual social life-styles	MATERNAL Blood type and Rh Congenital anomalies Height under 5 ft Age ▲ Under 18 years old ▲ Over 35 years old Race: nonwhite FAMILY History of inheritable disorders	FAMILY Economically disadvantaged ▲ Inadequate income ▲ Poor housing ▲ Inadequate food ▲ Poor education ▲ More likely to be nonwhite ▲ Limited or no health insurance Affluent ▲ Increased incidence of divorce ▲ Frequent drug or alcohol use ▲ Older age at first pregnancy

▼ Menorrhalgia
▼ Metrorrhagia
▲ Uterine pelvic or breast tumors
▲ Endometritis
▲ Endometriosis
▲ Pelvic inflammatory disease (PID)
▲ Infertility

Poor obstetric history

▲ Abnormal clinical course of pregnancy, labor, or recovery
▲ Previous poor pregnancy outcome
▼ More than two abortions
▼ Stillbirth
▼ Neonatal death or abnormality
▲ High parity: five or more pregnancies

FAMILY

Parental history of infertility or chronic illness among family members

TABLE 20.3
FACTORS DURING PREGNANCY THAT PREDISPOSE TO REPRODUCTIVE RISK (CATEGORIZED ACCORDING TO POINT OF ORIGIN OR IMPACT)

Biophysical	*Psychosocial*	*Genetic*	*Economic*
MATERNAL High parity (five or more pregnancies) Nutritional status ▲ Iron deficiency ▲ Folic acid deficiency ▲ Limited or no weight gain ▲ Excessive weight gain Pathophysiology ▲ Pregnancy-induced hypertension ▲ Chronic hypertension with superimposed pregnancy-induced hypertension ▲ Gestational diabetes ▲ Infections of any etiology ▲ Factors that predispose to hemorrhage ▼ Abruptio placenta ▼ Placenta previa ▼ Blood clotting disorders Excess uterine distention because of ▲ Fetal size ▲ Multiple gestation ▲ Hydramnios ▲ Tumor Ectopic pregnancy Uterine rupture ▲ Blood disorders ▲ Disorder in any maternal system MATERNAL/FETAL Abnormal placental development, function, or position Hydramnios Oligohydramnios Premature rupture of the membranes (PROM)	MATERNAL Alcohol abuse during pregnancy Drug abuse during pregnancy Marital status ▲ Unmarried ▲ Divorced Emotional disorders related to pregnancy Inadequate, delayed, or absent prenatal care Adverse environmental factors such as ▲ Teratogens ▲ Iatrogenic practices Emotional trauma Hyperemesis gravidarum FAMILY Unusual family life-styles Unplanned or unwanted pregnancy Major family stresses or disruptions Abusive behaviors directed at the pregnant woman Unsafe cultural or ethnic practices PROFESSIONAL Depersonalized health care services Inadequate prenatal supervision Indiscriminant use of technology, drugs, radiation Inconsistent prenatal supervision No constant health care personnel Inadequate provision for prenatal consumer education	MATERNAL Age at conception ▲ Under 18 years ▲ Over 35 years Multiple gestation Parabiotic twins Transmissible inherited disorders PARENTAL/FETAL Maternal–fetal blood incompatibility ▲ Rh− mother; Rh+ fetus ▲ ABO incompatibility Paternal transmitted inherited disorders FETAL Abnormal fetal development	FAMILY Inadequate income to support needs of pregnancy Hospitalization during pregnancy Inadequate food

Prolonged ruptured membranes
Feto–pelvic disproportion
Missed abortion
Multiple gestation
Physical trauma

FETAL

Intrauterine growth retardation
Uterine infection
Umbilical cord anomaly or compression
Premature labor: 38 weeks
Prolonged pregnancy: 42 weeks
Abnormal fetal position, presentation, or lie

FAMILY

Presence of communicable diseases within family

TABLE 20.4
FACTORS DURING LABOR THAT PREDISPOSE TO REPRODUCTIVE RISK (CATEGORIZED ACCORDING TO POINT OF ORIGIN OR IMPACT)

Biophysical	*Psychosocial*	*Genetic*	*Economic*
MATERNAL Latent or transient hypertension Intrapartal pre-eclampsia Hemorrhage Dysfunctional labor Precipitate labor and delivery Infection Prolonged labor (in any stage) Uterine tetany Dehydration Lacerations during birth MATERNAL/FETAL Cephalo–pelvic incompatibility Abnormal fetal size ▲ Less than 2,000 gm ▲ More than 4,000 gm Abnormal fetal position, presentation, or lie Abnormal fetal response to labor ▲ Tachycardia ▲ Bradycardia ▲ Hyperactivity ▲ Absence of fetal activity ▲ Scalp pH less than 7.25 ▲ Meconium-stained amniotic fluid	MATERNAL Apathy, withdrawal, or disinterest in labor or its outcome Inadequate support resources FAMILY Alternative birth styles without professional supervision Separation of family from laboring woman Death or damage of the fetus diagnosed during labor PROFESSIONAL Iatrogenic practices ▲ Medical or elective induction of labor ▲ Intrusive procedures ▲ Indiscriminant use of drugs, technology, anesthesia ▲ Operative procedures (cesarean section, forceps, vacuum extraction) ▲ Trauma during labor and delivery Inadequate supervision during labor	FETAL/ NEONATAL Previously undiagnosed congenital abnormalities	Routine use of sophisticated technology for healthy laboring women Cost of hospitalization

SCOPE OF REPRODUCTIVE RISK

Reproductive risk is a major health issue in the United States today. It is not only a personal and family problem but also a national concern. Before we can come to grips with the problem of reproductive risk as a nation, however, we must examine our own values and beliefs concerning the social welfare of all Americans and the right of all people to have access to health care services.

Any woman of childbearing years is a potential victim of a threat that can place her at risk for poor pregnancy outcome. Certain population groups are more vulnerable to risk associated with pregnancy than are others. In the United States, the largest population at greatest risk is the population least able to afford health care—the poor, nonwhite Americans. A major political controversy revolves around who should be responsible for seeing that health care is accessible to and affordable by all peopie.

The maternity nurse can begin to understand the magnitude of the problem of reproductive risk by seeking answers to questions such as

- ▲ Who are the populations at risk?
- ▲ Why are these people at reproductive risk?
- ▲ Which risk conditions are most prevalant?
- ▲ What is being done to decrease the incidence of reproductive risk?

Information about the incidence of reproductive risk, like other health problems, is usually reported in terms of four demographic characteristics: socioeconomic status, race, age, and residence.

TABLE 20.5
FACTORS AFTER BIRTH THAT PREDISPOSE TO REPRODUCTIVE RISK (CATEGORIZED ACCORDING TO POINT OF ORIGIN OR IMPACT)

Biophysical

MATERNAL

Birth trauma
- ▲ Lacerations of reproductive tract
- ▲ Pelvic hematomas

Hemorrhage as a result of
- ▲ Uterine atony
- ▲ Retained placenta or membranes
- ▲ Birth trauma
- ▲ Disseminated intravascular coagulation

Infection of any etiology, especially
- ▲ Uterine
- ▲ Urinary tract
- ▲ Breasts

NEONATAL

Premature birth
Postmature birth
Low birth weight of any etiology
- ▲ Less than 2,500 gm

Large for gestational age
- ▲ More than 4,000 gm (particularly with a maternal history of diabetes)

Birth trauma
Hypothermia
Hyberbilirubinemia
Hypocalcemia
Acidosis (pH less than 7.25)
Hypoxia
Hypoglycemia
Respiratory distress of any etiology
Polycythemia
Seizures and/or tetany
Persistant vomiting
Absence of stools or urine
Abdominal distention
Generalized cyanosis
Sluggish or absent weight gain

Psychosocial

MATERNAL

Separation from family or significant other for any reason
Depression
Withdrawal
Disinterest in infant
Early discharge from hospital without access to health care
Conception within 2–30 months from this delivery

MATERNAL/NEONATAL

Environment of labor and delivery rooms (cold, bright lights)
Separation of mother and infant

NEONATAL

Placement in incubator or isolette for extended periods of time
Inadequate social stimulation during long-term hospitalization
Poor response to social stimuli
Any indication of failure to thrive

FAMILY

Isolation of mother and infant from family support
Inadequate home preparation for receiving infant
Inadequate preparation of parents for parenthood
Stress associated with neonatal death or anomaly
Limited access to therapeutic or rehabilitative health care services for mother or infant

PROFESSIONAL

Iatrogenic practices, such as
- ▲ Poor environment for labor and delivery
- ▲ Resuscitative procedures causing trauma to the neonate
- ▲ Indiscriminant use of drugs and technology for mother and/or infant

Hospital routines that are nonsupportive to mother–infant–family relationships
Inadequate provision for parent education

Genetic

NEONATAL

Gross genetic anomalies
Subnormal mental capacity of genetic origin
Subnormal physical capacity of genetic origin
Generalized or specific genetic anomaly

Economic

FAMILY

Long-term hospitalization of mother or infant
High-cost therapeutic and rehabilitative regimens for mother or neonate
Inadequate income to support needs of mother or child
High costs of health care and special programs needed by the damaged mother or neonate

Socioeconomic Status

Socioeconomic status contributes to the potential for reproductive risk. This is borne out in statistics that reveal the extent of risk problems among the poor compared with the middle-income and affluent populations. The poorer population is more likely to be *nutritionally deprived*, and malnutrition is associated with low birth weight infants. These infants are less likely to survive extrauterine life than are the infants of higher birth weight.

> *The birth weight of an infant, simple as it is to measure, is highly significant in two important respects. In the first place, it is strongly conditioned by the health and nutritional status of the mother, in the sense that maternal malnutrition, ill-health and other deprivation are the most common causes of retarded fetal growth and/or prematurity, as manifested in low birth weight (LBW). In the second place, low birth weight is, universally and in all population groups, the single most important determinant of the chances of the newborn to survive and to experience healthy growth and development.*
>
> *WHO, 1980, p. 197*

Low birth weight (LBW) is not restricted to infants born in the United States. Close to 21 million LBW infants are born each year throughout the world. Many of these infants do not survive the first few weeks of life.

The poorer members of society are generally more prone to nutrition-related disorders during pregnancy, such as iron deficiency anemia and malnutrition. These conditions in turn cause the pregnant woman to be more susceptible to infections and hemorrhage.

Indigent populations do not have money for private health care. Although there are many public facilities that provide health care for poor citizens, there are not enough to serve the number of people needing them. Many facilities are located in urban areas, leaving the rural poor without available care facilities. The poor, like many other groups, do not place a high priority on health care services that are designed to prevent illness or to maintain health, such as prenatal services. Therefore, poor pregnant women are less likely to seek early prenatal care than are more affluent pregnant women.

The poor marry earlier, have more children, and have them closer together. Age at first birth is closely related to age at marriage. Many women from poor populations marry before they complete high school or shortly thereafter; middle-income and affluent women go on to college and often delay marriage until they are into their twenties.

Access to family planning information makes a difference in the number of children born to any family. For many years poor citizens had unequal access to family planning information and contraceptives since these were distributed to the public principally through private medical services. Efforts by interested consumers, professional groups, and politicians brought social welfare to the public mind as a governmental responsibility during the 1960s, and some reproductive health services were provided for the nation's poor.

Medicaid now provides public support of health care for the indigent pregnant population, and family planning services are available through public funding. In 1970 the Family Planning Services and Population Research Act was passed, which provided public money for the establishment of family planning projects and services. In 1973 the United States Supreme Court determined that elective abortion within the first 90 days of pregnancy was legal. Federal monies were used to provide elective abortion services to indigent women from that time through 1977. During the period 1966–1976, fertility among indigent women decreased considerably. A major contributing factor for this decrease was cited as the availability of family planning information, the use of contraceptives, and the planning of pregnancies by more poor women.

During this same period, there was a significant reduction in maternal and infant mortality, two indices for determining the scope of reproductive risk. Morris et al. (1975) reported that infant mortality rates alone decreased 27% between the years 1965–1972. This was attributed to changes in maternal age at first pregnancy and birth order of the infant—changes made possible because of access to family planning information and contraceptives. Neonatal mortality, however, remains almost 3 times as great among the poor as among the affluent population. Maternal mortality rates, too, are higher for poor than for affluent women. Miller (1975) estimated that 600,000 poor women needed maternity care and public programs provided for the needs of only 130,000 of these women, leaving a significant health care deficit for pregnant women from poor families. This deficit remains today a contributing factor to reproductive risk among the nation's poor population.

The affluent population is not without reproductive risk problems. Malnutrition of young women is not limited to the poor population, even though it is more prevalent there. Neither is pregnancy at extreme ends of the reproductive years only a problem of the poor. Some unique reproductive risk problems are emerging that are predominantly associated with the wealthier or middle-income groups in the United States—problems related to drug and alcohol abuse (see Chapter 25). Increasingly, alcoholism, like drug use, is beginning in the junior high and high school years. Drug and alcohol use has been, particularly since the 1960s, and continues to be a major health problem in the United States. During the past 20 years the health care provider has seen an increase in the incidence of drug and alcohol dependence among pregnant women and its corresponding effect on their infants. Drug and alcohol problems are seen among the poorer populations, but with lesser frequency.

Race

In most cases, race, per se, is not a major contributing factor to reproductive risk. Some genetic disorders are racially transmitted, but they do not constitute a large percentage of congenital risk conditions (see Chapter 24). Race has been associated with clinical course of labor, particularly delivery, in that a woman pregnant by a man of the same race seems to have fewer problems with pelvic dystocia during labor than does a woman pregnant by a man of a different race. These problems are essentially a result of incompatible skeletal structure of the fetus and the mother's pelvis.

Race, in association with other factors such as socioeconomic level, education, and age at first pregnancy, presents a clear dichotomy regarding the incidence of many reproductive risk conditions. Risk pregnancy is more likely to occur in the nonwhite population than in the white. Between 1968 and 1975, maternal mortality rates for the black woman in the United States was 48.1; for the white woman it was 13.1 (Rochat, 1981). Today, maternal mortality rates are down for both groups; however, the maternal mortality rate for nonwhite women is more than double that for Caucasions. Perinatal mortality, too, is higher among the nonwhite population. Since birth weight is associated with the quality of maternal health, particularly the nutritional status, this finding is not surprising for reasons mentioned earlier.

Age

Women at either end of the reproductive years (15 years and under; 35 years and older) tend to be at greater risk than women between the years of 16 and 34. Factors other than age contribute to age-related reproductive risk. The very young pregnant girl is more likely to be unmarried, malnourished, and with an unplanned pregnancy that she may be neither physiologically nor psychosocially ready to handle. This can result in numerous problems during pregnancy and labor, as well as place her at risk in regard to parenting activities. The older pregnant woman faces risk for different reasons. She faces increased likelihood of genetic disorders, such as Down's syndrome (see Chapter 24). She may be more prone to physical disorders such as hypertension. If she is diabetic, her diabetes will often be more difficult to control later in her reproductive years. Labor may be more problem prone for the older pregnant woman, especially if she is experiencing a first pregnancy. Maternal mortality is two times as great for women under 15 years and five times as great for women over 35 years as for women between 16 and 34 years (Rochat, 1981).

Reproductive risk conditions tend to repeat with each pregnancy. The young adolescent primigravida at risk is likely to become a multigravida at risk. The older woman who had earlier risk pregnancies will be more vulnerable to risk with each subsequent pregnancy. Early diagnosis and treatment of risk pregnancy, whatever the woman's age, may help prevent a future risk pregnancy or help decrease the intensity or magnitude of its threat.

Age at pregnancy can also contribute to increasing the family stress and decreasing the family's ability to cope with the pregnancy and to give the pregnant woman the support she needs. This is particularly true if the pregnancy is unplanned and the woman is either very young or nearing the end of her reproductive years and has grown children. The years 18 through 29 are considered by many to be the physically optimal years during which a woman should have a child; however, once more, age alone does not determine how well a woman undergoes the experience of pregnancy.

Residence

Place of residence may contribute to reproductive risk. For example, pregnant women who have cardiopulmonary problems may find that higher altitudes aggravate their problems.

Women who live in rural areas have fewer options for specialized health care. Health care in some inner cities has been evaluated as being of poorer quality than that available in the suburbs. Also, affluent sections of a city may have better facilities than poorer sections. The reasons given for these inequities include inadequate monies to maintain quality services and failure to attract adequate numbers of qualified health care personnel, especially physicians and nurses, to certain facilities.

Maternal mortality rates are slightly higher for white and nonwhite women who live in rural areas. Factors other than place of residence probably contribute to this reported incidence, most prominently socioeconomic level, age of the women who live in rural areas (they tend to be somewhat older than women in the city, particularly the rural nonwhite woman), decreased availability of health care, and incomplete reporting of statistics concerning maternal morbidity and mortality in the nonmetropolitan areas.

Without a doubt, the scope of the problem of reproductive risk is great. Many efforts have been made to deal with this problem, both in the United States, as well as in other parts of the world, during this century. Some risk conditions result from controllable factors, such as ignorance, inadequate health care, and unplanned pregnancies. These are the areas where health care efforts are paying dividends through consumer education, improved maternal health, particularly maternal nutrition, early assessment and diagnosis of conditions that can be treated, genetic counseling, and accessible, affordable health care services such as prenatal supervision, family planning, increased research into reproductive risk, improved technology, and better education for health personnel.

COST OF REPRODUCTIVE RISK

Cost is generally viewed only in economic terms—expenditures of money to purchase something. Reproductive risk frequently involves large expenditures of money by the family at risk, as well as society as a whole. But reproductive risk is also costly in nonmaterial terms—human cost. Human expenditures may be greater than material costs in both scope and duration for damage to or loss of a life requires personal expenditures that are not readily measured. *Cost of reproductive risk* is defined here as the expenditure of personal or public resources to meet the economic, social, and emotional demands imposed on the woman, the family, and society by events arising from human reproduction.

Monetary Cost

The proper medical management of many reproductive risk conditions requires the use of sophisticated technology, such as ultrasonography, electronic monitoring of mother and fetus, and biochemical studies. This technology is costly in terms of initial purchase price, maintenance, and personnel. Such *material,* or *monetary, costs* to the private physician or institution are eventually passed on to the consumer as health care costs for services provided. Some risk conditions not only require use of sophisticated technology, they may also require long-term hospital care for the pregnant woman and, later, her infant. Even without extensive technological management, hospitalization costs have been steadily rising since the end of World War II. In 1976, the cost of having a baby (without complications) and providing for that child during the first year was approximately $2,300.00 (Williams, 1976). Presently, with inflation, that cost easily exceeds $3,000.00. The cost of having a baby with a risk pregnancy can range from a few dollars to hundreds of thousands of dollars.

Pomerance et al. (1978) found the costs of care for 75 infants born weighing 1,000 gm or less at birth to average $14,236 per nonsurvivor (range $72–124,627) and $40,287 per survivor (range $10,744–106,050). Such costs were only for hospital care; physicians' fees were not included. Today costs would, most likely, exceed these figures. Much of the cost is related to the duration of hospital stay needed by small or premature infants (average length of hospitalization for surviving infants in Pomerance's study was 89 days).

Butterfield (1977) found that the average stay in hospitals for small babies was 75 days with a cost of care ranging from approximately $15,000 to more than $100,000 (again, not including physicians' fees).

Most families cannot bear such costs without some type of assistance, usually public funds from state and national programs, local efforts such as the United Way Fund, or foundations such as the National Foundation—March of Dimes. Private insurance coverage usually has been inadequate to meet the costs of reproductive risk. In some cases, however, insurance coverage has been increased to include selective aspects of reproductive risk. The irony is that those people that are most vulnerable to reproductive risk—the indigent population—are least likely to have adequate, if any, insurance coverage.

The functional burden of reproductive risk is devastating to most families experiencing such an event. The costs are eventually borne by society through taxes to support necessary health care programs for risk pregnancy and its sequelae such as long-term custodial care for infants who need it. Citizens' voluntary contributions to foundations and other organizations is another way that society indirectly bears the cost of reproductive risk. Society also contributes to reproductive health care costs (and health care generally) through supporting educational programs to prepare physicians, nurses, and other health care personnel to provide safe services. In 1980–1981 the estimated cost to the state for educating one student physician and one student nurse per year in a state university was approximately $25,000 and $10,000, respectively. (These figures do not include cost to the student.)

Numerous other less prominent costs are also a part of reproductive risk: drugs, expenses associated with travel to and from health care services, special procedures, and so on. Without question, reproductive risk and its related demands impose a financial burden on the woman, the family, and, ultimately, society.

Human Cost

All costs associated with reproductive risk impact on the person in some way. However, there is no deeper personal payment than *human cost,* that cost extracted because of stress, trauma, and loss from potential or real poor pregnancy outcome. The birth of a child is anticipated and valued in every society. It is usually a happy event that evokes joy among the family members and close friends.

The death of a child—even in its fetal stage—elicits strong emotions and feelings, especially those of guilt, frustration, anger, and loss. Aside from the impact of the death of a child on its family, society may have lost a potentially productive member.

Death to a badly damaged fetus/baby has its advantages for it is real and final; it is an event that the parents and relatives can face and accept (and most do). Damage of a mother or child, on the other hand, may remain as a constant reminder of a pregnancy that failed in some way.

Stress is a part of daily living, and stress in regard to healthy pregnancy is a normal occurrence. Whenever a pregnancy is complicated in some way, stress experienced by the pregnant woman and her family is increased. *Anxiety* about the outcome of the pregnancy is one way in which stress is demonstrated. It is not uncommon for a woman experiencing a healthy pregnancy to worry about herself and her unborn child.

The normal fears about death or an abnormal child are exaggerated in a pregnancy that is at risk. This anxiety may manifest itself through the woman's preoccupation with self, pregnancy, and her unborn child. Numerous questions, concerns, and comments by the pregnant woman may be addressed to the nurse. Janis (1958, 1965) calls this "work of worry" and sees it as a healthy manner of coping with stress in most cases. The nurse needs to be alert to indicators that such a preoccupation has become unhealthy or even morbid. The woman may also express anxiety about the pregnancy through *exaggerated fantasies* about the death of herself and her child or about the child being grotesquely malformed. *Anger* that this has happened to her is also a usual part of a woman's anxiety about risk pregnancy. The family, too, may experience anxiety about the pregnant woman and unborn child. On the one hand, they may overprotect the pregnant woman; on the other, they may ignore her concerns.

The opposite of verbalized anxiety about the pregnancy is *denial* that there is a problem. Refusal to talk about the risk condition or to report symptoms such as decreased fetal activity is common. Poor compliance with prenatal appointments or therapeutic regimens may also be associated with or arise from denial.

Guilt about what she or her partner did to cause the risk threat is another manifestation of anxiety. Expectant parents tend to blame themselves or each other for problems associated with pregnancy. Risk pregnancy is a major stress on a marriage and a family.

Reproductive risk imposes stress by causing *disruption or change in the usual family life-style.* The disruption may be minimal and handled within the family, or it may be extensive resulting in disolution of the family through separation, divorce, or, in some cases, desertion of the family by one or the other spouse. The stable, mature family will most likely be able to cope with disruption, but most families will require some degree of support and reassurance by the physician and nurse. Some factors that predispose to disruption or change are:

- ▲ Long-term hospitalization of the pregnant woman (a particular problem if there are young children at home).
- ▲ Inability of the woman to perform her usual tasks related to her home or to her work. This requires that her role be taken on by someone else, either a family member or an outside helper.
- ▲ The addition to the family of a damaged infant whose requirements for time, attention, and monetary outlay may be great, diverting attention and consideration away from other family members. There is a significant incidence of abusive behavior directed toward the infant by parents and siblings, especially if the infant is grossly abnormal or has remained in the hospital for a prolonged period of time after birth.
- ▲ Family priorities and goals may need to be adjusted, first, during the pregnancy and, later, after the child has been born.

Reproductive casualty is another facet of human costs of reproductive risk. This *casualty* may take the form of trauma to the mother, infant, or both, which may arise from iatrogenic sources such as intrusive procedures performed for diagnosis or therapy, drugs, or operative procedures such as cesarean section or forceps delivery. Infection that occurs as a result of diagnostic or therapeutic practices, associated with the risk condition is another type of physical trauma. While the mother and infant are most directly affected by such trauma, the family is also affected by the stress induced by such trauma, as well as by the financial burden associated with the reason for or treatment of the trauma.

Reproductive loss—death of mother and child or damage that prevents their functioning as productive members of society—represents another category of human cost as a result of reproductive risk. This *loss* may occur because of disease or physical disorder, or it may occur because of a psychosocial deprivation such as failure of the mother or family to accept responsibility for care of the infant or, ultimately, failure of the family to survive the assault of reproductive risk on the family as an intact unit.

The human cost of reproductive risk is most likely far greater than what can be presently envisioned by health professionals who probably have a sporadic rather than sustained contact with the family at risk. The long-range effects of reproductive risk on the mother, child, and family have not been studied extensively, although some longitudinal research on premature, low birth weight, and mentally and physically disabled infants has been reported or is ongoing.

CLINICAL ASSESSMENT AND NURSING IMPLICATIONS

Clinical assessment of reproductive risk refers to information primarily obtained from physical examination (observation, palpation, percussion, auscultation) and measurement. Many of the assessment modalities discussed in this section are important in the detection of problems, but confirmation that assessment is within normal limits is in itself reassuring to patients.

Pelvic and Breast Examinations

Both pelvic and breast examinations are discussed in Chapter 26. The nurse's role during these examinations is to decrease embarrassment and fear, to provide an opportunity for discussion, to describe the procedure and its purpose, and to encourage asking of questions and expressing of concerns. Although the nurse who prepared as a clinical specialist may perform the initial as well as subsequent examinations, it is more common that the physician examines and the nurse assists as well as acts as patient advocator and educator. Reproductive tract and breasts examination involve intimate parts of the anatomy associated with sexuality and reproduction; thus the psychosocial implications of the data collected is usually very personal. Strategies for climate setting and history taking are discussed more completely in Chapters 9, 14, and 26.

Abdominal Examination

Abdominal examination in the first trimester of pregnancy reveals minimal information, but it provides significant data throughout the rest of the antepartum period. Recall that the measurement of fundal height (McDonald's maneuvers) provides ongoing important assessment data and that after the twentieth week of gestation fundal height, measured in centimeters, corresponds to weeks of gestation (see Fig. 20.1). Fundal height measurement can alert the examiner to inaccurate menstrual history, large- or small-for-gestational-age infant, multiple gestation, fetal anomalies, or hydramnios, to cite some examples. (See Chapter 12.)

Leopold's maneuvers (Fig. 20.2) also provide critical data in suspected risk pregnancies. Multiple gestation, fetal abnormality, and maternal pathology can be detected in some cases. Degree of extension or flexion of the head can be determined by the skilled observer. Information about presentation, lie, and position of the fetus, as well as descent into the maternal pelvis can be obtained by examination using these four maneuvers (see Table 12.2, Chapter 12, for procedure). During the latter part of pregnancy the uterus is sensitive to digital examination, and abdominal examination may elicit uterine contractions. These contractions should be evaluated in terms of strength and duration, as well as maternal and fetal responses.

Measurement

MATERNAL AND FETAL VITAL SIGNS

Maternal and fetal vital signs should be assessed at each prenatal visit (see Chapter 12). Maternal blood pressure that indicates a 30-mm increase in systolic or a 15-mm increase in diastolic over the normotensive baseline blood pressure of the woman is significant in regard to potential problems and signals the need for further evaluation (see Chapter 21). Similarly, a mean arterial pressure greater than 90 mm in the second trimester and greater than 100 mm in the third trimester is significant and should alert the nurse to screen the patient for other indications of hypertensive disor-

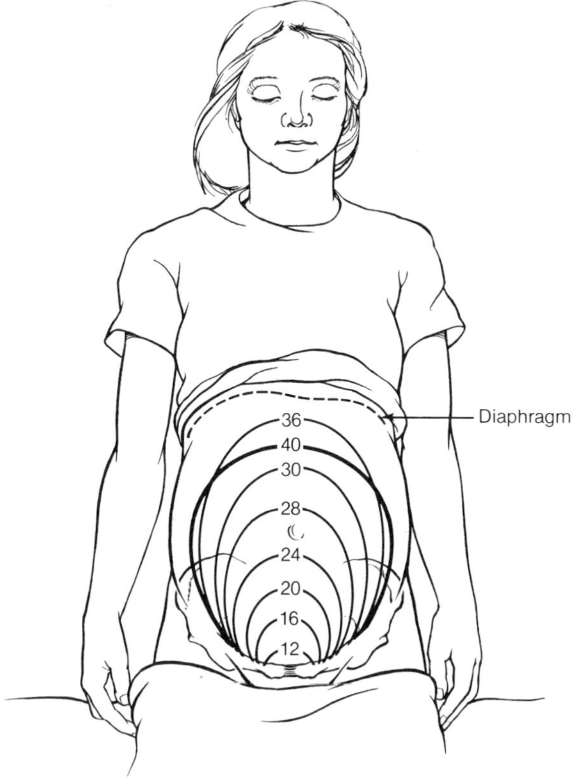

Figure 20.1
Fundal height corresponding to weeks of gestation.

ders such as proteinuria or edema. Recall that the mean arterial blood pressure remains unchanged during the first trimester (Chapter 12), decreases during the second trimester, and slowly increases during the third trimester and labor. The nurse needs to keep in mind other factors that affect blood pressure such as physical activity, maternal position in which the blood pressure is taken, time of day, and evidence of physiologic or psychosocial stress.

Fetal heart beat is useful in assessing fetal well-being, as well as in confirming pregnancy and validating gestational age. It is taken and recorded at each prenatal visit and monitored for rate (120–160, normal limits), rhythm, and quality. The rate tends to decrease as age increases; however, marked decelerations are usually ominous and related to fetal stress. Electronic fetal monitoring as an assessment modality in suspected risk conditions is discussed later in this chapter.

ASSESSMENT OF FETAL MOVEMENT

Assessment of fetal movement (also called fetal activity determination, FAD) can also be used to indicate fetal well-being. Fetal activity becomes apparent to most women during the eighteenth to twentieth week of gestation (quickening). Notation by the mother of daily fetal movement has been shown to be a reliable index of fetal activity and is used as an adjunct to clinical assessment of fetal well-being. The nurse needs to be alert to a mother's casual comment such as, "the baby doesn't seem to move as much these days," since this may be an early clue to a problem. There is a correlation between diminished fetal movement and fetal jeopardy (Sadrovsky, 1973). See Table 20.6, Protocol for Use of Daily Fetal Movement Count (DFMC) and Figures 20.3 and 20.4 for forms for recording the information.

MATERNAL WEIGHT

Maternal weight is recorded at each prenatal visit since it provides information about normal or abnormal response to pregnancy, retention of extracellular fluid, fetal growth, and dietary habits. As with other measurements, weight gain is most useful when compared with baseline prepregnant weight and weight recorded on previous visits. Re-

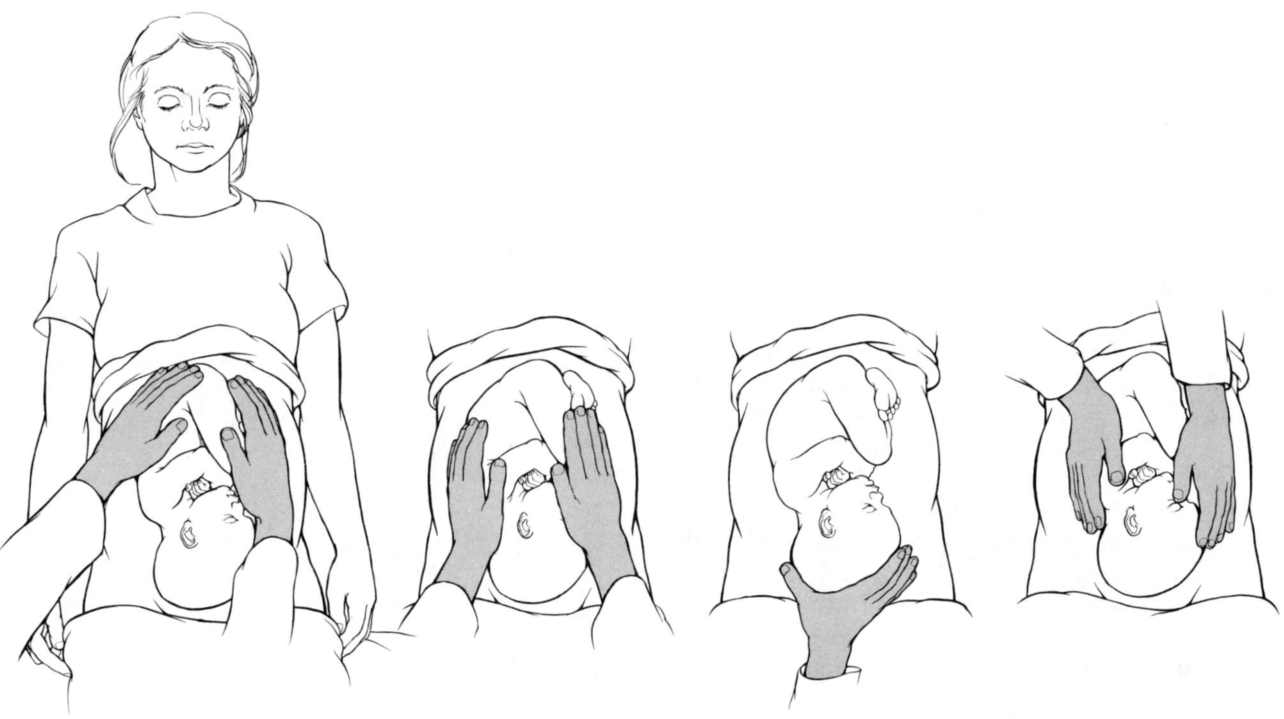

Figure 20.2
Leopold's maneuvers.

call that severe weight restriction is not recommended in pregnancy. A weight gain of 25–30 lbs is desirable for the neonate's weight to be adequate.

Additional External Observations

Pretibial, ankle, hand, or facial edema should be assessed. Varicosities in the legs or anal area should be evaluated. Although pooling of the blood in the lower torso and legs is common in pregnancy, thrombophlebitis can occur, and signs of inflammation should be assessed. Any lesions on the woman's body should be noted, recorded, and described. This is of particular concern in the diabetic woman and in cases of suspected battering or abuse.

Psychosocial Factors

Data need to be collected regarding psychosocial factors—communication and learning. One way is by observing the woman's attire carefully. From such observations certain inferences or nursing diagnoses can be made and subsequently validated. For example, if the woman who always comes to the office or clinic clean and neat with makeup on and hair attractively arranged appears one day in sloppy attire and a bit unkempt, the nurse may guess that she has had a crisis, is depressed, or maybe just got up late and did not have time to do her usual preparation for the visit. The point is that the nurse mentally notices a behavior change and can follow up with appropriate therapeutic communication techniques to determine if indeed the woman is depressed, for example, and then intervene appropriately.

TABLE 20.6
PROTOCOL FOR USE ON DFMC

Beginning at the 29th week of pregnancy, the mother is requested to count and record daily fetal movements (following instruction and practice) according to directions on the form provided for this purpose (see Fig. 20.3). The DFMC recordings are then transferred from the mother's daily record sheet to a graphic form at the time of each prenatal visit. In this way a record of the DFMC baseline is established for that particular fetus (see Fig. 20.4).

The mother is instructed to report a cessation or significant decrease ("movement alarm signal") of fetal movements according to the predetermined criteria. For example, if the DFMC is less than 10 for the counting period (one hour), the mother is instructed to

1. Continue the count for another six hours unless 10 or more movements occur in any one-hour period. During this time she may change her activity level and may stimulate the fetus by gentle abdominal palpation, as instructed, in order to elicit a fetal movement response.
2. If the mother is not satisfied that acceptable fetal movement has occurred during that time, she should report her concern.
3. The presence of an acceptable DFMC should then be established to the satisfaction of both mother and examiner either by external electronic fetal monitoring or by abdominal palpation of movements in conjunction with assurance of fetal heart sounds. Mother may then resume the usual schedule of DFMC recordings if not contraindicated.
4. If developing fetal distress is indicated by assessment technique, the attending physician can determine subsequent action

Source: Hoffmaster, J. E., Fetal Movement as an Indicator of Fetal Well-Being. *Perinatal Press* 6:75, 1978. Used with permission.

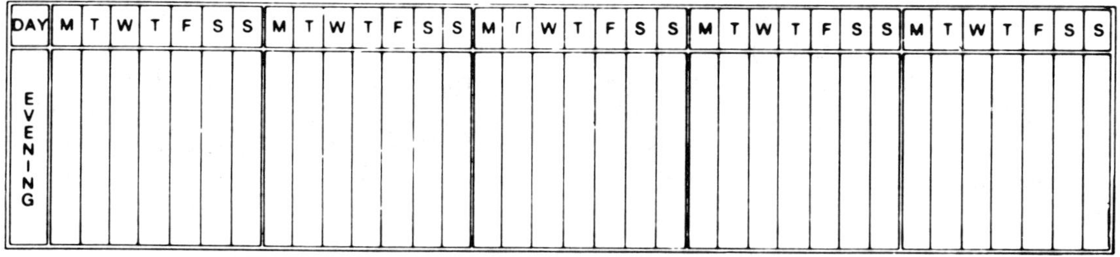

NAME ______________________ DATE COUNT STARTED ______________________

Please lie down on your left side for one hour each day after evening meal and count the number of times you feel the baby move during that period; write the number of movements in the proper space below. Count every movement (kicks, turns, rolls, flutters by the baby); if there are a group or series of movements that seem to "run together" without a break or pause between them, count this as just one movement. Bring this sheet with you for each clinic visit. (If you have been admitted to the hospital, the nurse and/or physician will review this sheet each day.)

You are requested to call this number at any hour to discuss any specific changes or counts of the baby's movements—as instructed previously; also, call at any time that you have any particular concern.

DAY	M	T	W	T	F	S	S	M	T	W	T	F	S	S	M	T	W	T	F	S	S	M	T	W	T	F	S	S	M	T	W	T	F	S	S
EVENING																																			

Figure 20.3
Daily Fetal Movement Count Form. *Source:* Hoffmaster, J. E., Fetal Movement as an Indicator of Fetal Well-Being. *Perinatal Press* 6:75, 1978. Used with permission.

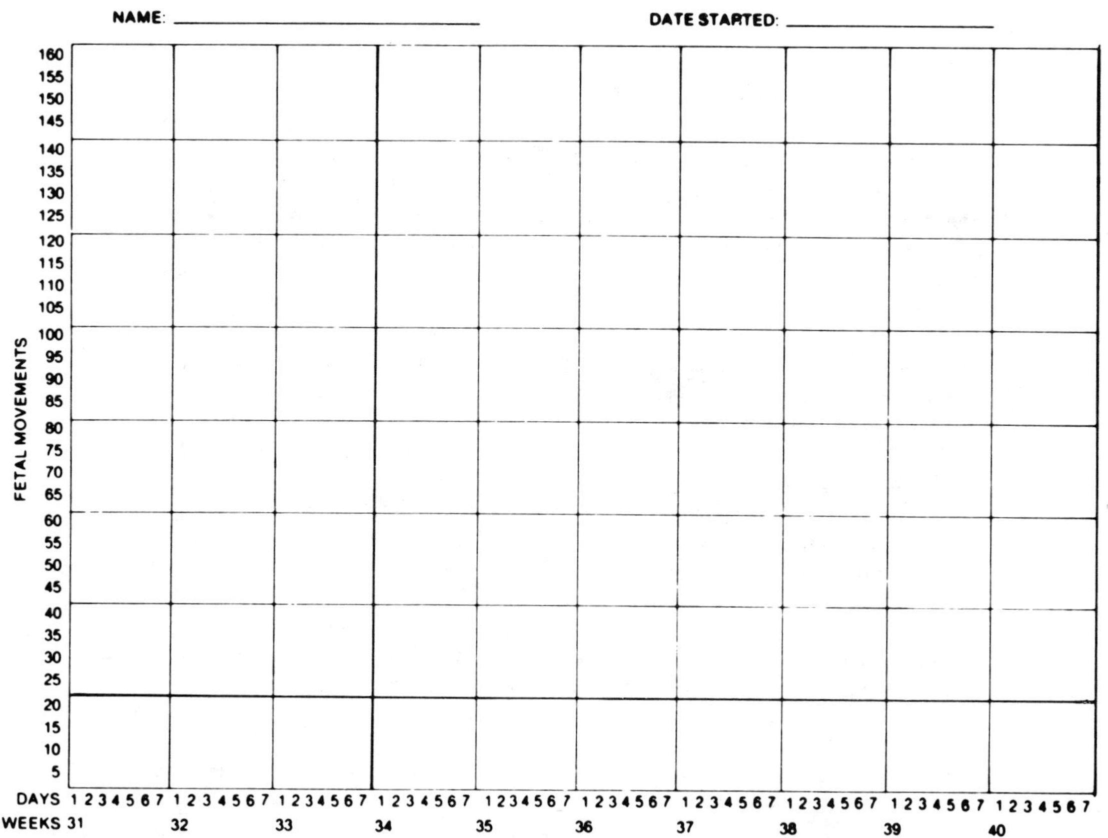

Figure 20.4
DFMC Baseline. *Source:* Hoffmaster, J. E., Fetal Movement as an Indicator of Fetal Well-Being. *Perinatal Press* 6:75, 1978. Used with permission.

Interaction among family members, if the woman is accompanied on her visits, may give important information about the family's attitude toward the pregnancy. Both verbal and nonverbal communication needs to be assessed. Psychosocial risk can occur at anytime in the antepartum period, and psychosocial stress can lead to or contribute to biophysical stress with subsequent risk to mother or fetus. Learning is affected by anxiety, and if the woman is stressed, perception is narrowed and ability to learn is decreased. Evaluation of learning can be done by asking the patient to review what was discussed on the previous visit.

BIOCHEMICAL EVALUATION

Laboratory Studies

Laboratory studies that are significant for the maternity nurse are listed in Table 20.7. Specific procedures for these studies are not included as some may vary from laboratory to laboratory; some laboratory values are generally agreed upon and these values are included.

DIAGNOSTIC ULTRASOUND

Ultrasound (also *ultrasonography* or *sonography*) is the use of sound pulses transmitted through the maternal abdomen via a transducer; these sound waves are partially reflected as they encounter tissue boundaries such as body organs. The returning waves are picked up by the same transducer and appear on a cathode ray oscilloscope as a visual image (Campbell, 1974). This image can be photographed and studied. Sound echoes are visually displayed in several modes (ways).

- ▲ ***Mode A (Amplitude Modulation).*** Used for measurement of the distance between points. Echoes are seen as vertical spikes on a horizontal time base.
- ▲ ***Mode B (Brightness Modulation).*** Used to assess uterine contents. The transducer moves across the abdomen at different angles. Echoes are seen as spots of light that merge to form a two-dimensional visual image (Figs. 20.5, 20.6).
- ▲ ***Mode M (Real Time).*** Technique where multiple echograms are rapidly recorded and viewed on the same screen. This adds the element of movement to the two-dimensional picture. For example, you can visualize the fetus sucking a thumb in utero.

Diagnostic ultrasound is noninvasive and painless (Fig. 20.7). However, the procedure can be frightening, so a careful explanation should be given regarding the procedure, process, and purpose. Except when locating the placenta before amniocentesis, the woman is scanned with a full bladder, which allows the sonographer to see the relationship of bladder to vagina and other organs. The procedure takes approximately 20–30 minutes (or less). The woman is placed in a supine position and the abdomen is covered generously with mineral oil, which is the contact medium for the transducer. If the woman is in late stage of pregnancy, the nurse should be alert for signs of supine hypotensive syndrome. The sonography technician slowly scans both longitudinally and transversely and thereby obtains a picture of the contents of the uterus (Figs. 20.8, 20.9). If the physician is present, the results are shared immediately; if the physician is not present, information may be withheld until physician interpretation can be shared. Serial sonography at 2-week intervals is sometimes done to assess fetal growth on an ongoing basis. The uses of ultrasound during the various stages of pregnancy are as follows.

Early pregnancy assessment for:

- ▲ Embryonic maturity and growth
- ▲ Embryonic demise
- ▲ Multiple pregnancy
- ▲ Missed abortion
- ▲ Hydatid mole
- ▲ Ectopic pregnancy
- ▲ Abdominal pregnancy
- ▲ Coexisting tumors
- ▲ Detection of IUDs

TABLE 20.7
LABORATORY STUDIES (MATERNAL–FETAL)

Study	*Purpose*	*Significance*
Blood studies: Type Rh	Determination of maternal and paternal blood group and Rh factor to ▲ Identify type and Rh combinations that may predispose to reproductive risk ▲ Plan ahead for available blood if needed by mother or fetus/neonate at any point during or following pregnancy See Chapters 21 and 23	*Rh* Woman presensitized by previous pregnancy or blood transfusion to the Rh antigen may have Rh antibodies in her system that can cause hemoagglutination in an Rh+ fetus. In some instances, nonsensitized women pregnant by Rh+ men and carrying Rh+ fetus may develop antibodies to Rh antigen during current pregnancy. Blood group O female, pregnant by group A, B, AB male has the potential for development of ABO incompatibility. The pathophysiology and clinical manifestations are similar to those of Rh incompatibility (hemolytic disease of the newborn). Hemorrhage of the pregnant woman should always be considered. Knowledge of female blood type expedites transfusion therapy if and when needed. Intrauterine fetal or neonatal blood transfusion is sometimes necessary. Knowledge of maternal blood type and Rh is essential.
Serology	Detection of syphilis in the pregnant woman Provide diagnostic basis for early treatment of syphilis	Syphilis, detected and treated before 16–18 weeks fetal age, will usually result in a nonaffected neonate because of the failure of the spirochete to cross the placental barrier during the first trimester of pregnancy. Failure to diagnose and treat syphilis during the first 20 weeks of pregnancy will likely result in a diseased neonate. Serology should be repeated during pregnancy for ▲ Patients with previous diagnosis and treatment ▲ Patients who admit to sexual activity with more than one partner during the pregnancy ▲ Patients who come from a population known to be at risk for venereal disease
Hematocrit Hemaglobin	Determination of presence of anemia in the pregnant female. Hematocrit is a test for determining the percentage volume of erythrocytes in centrifuged oxalated whole blood. It is faster and less expensive than measurement of hemoglobin levels and may be preferred. Provide baseline information for direction to do other anemia studies such as	A number of women in the reproductive years have an iron deficient or nutritional anemia. This may be aggravated or first noted during pregnancy. Chronic anemia places both mother and fetus/neonate at risk and has been associated with prematurity and infants of low birth weight. Hematocrit of 30 mg% or less or a hemoglobin of 10–11 gm/100 mL or

Study	Purpose	Significance
	▲ Blood indices ▲ Serum iron content and binding capacity ▲ Folate levels ▲ Sickle cell studies	less should alert the examiner to potential for anemia. Hemoglobin of 10 gm/100 mL is true anemia.
White blood count differential	Diagnosis of ▲ Infection ▲ Blood abnormalities such as leukemia	Normal increase in WBC during pregnancy and a further increase during labor ▲ Leukocytes ▾ 5,000–12,000 normal during pregnancy ▾ 5,000–25,000 normal during labor ▲ Excess of these values likely indicates infectious process ▲ Less than 5,000 should be investigated for possible blood disorders Differential examination of WBC ▲ Polymorphonuclear granulocytes ▾ Neutrophiles ▾ Eosinophiles ▾ Basophiles ▲ Mononuclear cells ▾ Monocytes ▾ Lymphocytes Increase or decrease in specific WBC provides assistance with specific diagnosis Increase in neutrophiles considered to be normal Caution should be exercised to not treat this normal increase in WBC with antibiotics
Antibody studies Atypical	Determination of presence of maternal antibodies to isoantigens that may cause hemolytic disease in the newborn, for example, Rh antigen	Reveals presence of previously unknown sensitization to isoantigens Provides guidelines for management of sensitized woman and fetus during and following pregnancy ▲ Repeat titres during pregnancy in conjunction with serial amniocentesis to determine damage to fetus ▲ Family planning counseling regarding future pregnancies for women with positive titres ▲ Direct antibody titres on neonate after birth when indicated

TABLE 20.7 (continued)

Study	*Purpose*	*Significance*
Rubella	Determination of woman's immune status regarding rubella (German measles)	Rubella—clinical or subclinical case during early pregnancy—can cause significant damage to the developing fetus. Live-born neonates may have severe congenital malformations, for example, eye disorders such as cataracts, heart defects, auditory defects, central nervous system defects. Immunization should be given to women in the childbearing years *only if pregnancy can be prevented* for a minimum of 2 months. All women who have received rubella vaccine or who report having had German measles should have a rubella screening before pregnancy (1:10 = + titre).
Plasma estriol (See also urine studies)	Obtain serial measurements of estriol to ▲ Determine adequacy of placental functioning and fetal well-being ▲ Aid in decisions regarding time and method for delivery of a stressed fetus	Estriol production is greatly increased during normal pregnancy (1,000×) and is one indicator of healthy functioning of the placental–fetal unit. Estriol levels fall whenever the placental–fetal unit is in jeopardy because of problems such as ▲ Pregnancy-induced hypertension ▲ Diabetes ▲ Partial separation of placenta ▲ Some fetal anomalies ▲ Renal and cardiovascular disease Estriol production increases gradually but consistently throughout pregnancy. Day-to-day variations in levels are normal. The following, however should be considered reasons for serious concern. ▲ A decrease of 35–50% below a previously reported value ▲ A persistent gradual decrease of less than 35% below previously reported values ▲ A decrease below 12 mg after the thirty-fourth week of gestation Levels below 4 mg after the thirty-fourth week are ominous and usually incompatible with life.
Serial urinary estriol	See plasma estriol	High amounts of estriol are excreted in the urine, making serial urinary estriol measurements a relatively easy method of obtaining information about placental–fetal functioning and well-being. The guidelines mentioned in the section on plasma estriol apply to urinary estriol measurements as well. Urinary estriol levels have been

Study	Purpose	Significance
		shown to be a valid and usually reliable way for obtaining information that aids in the management of pregnancies at risk. It has been reliable for predicting early fetal stress in conditions such as hemolytic disease of the newborn, as well as the other conditions mentioned in the section on plasma estriol. Excretion of urinary estriol can be altered by a number of factors. ▲ Impaired placental or fetal functioning ▲ Pathology or pathophysiology of the maternal kidney
Estriol/creatinine (E/C) ratio	Determination of impaired renal function often associated with hypertensive disorders and diabetes Assess placental function and fetal well-being	Creatinine clearance is increased during pregnancy. Renal impairment resulting in decreased creatinine clearance also causes a decrease in estriol clearance. E/C ratio may be used to determine accuracy of 24-hour urine studies. Short collection periods should be avoided since they are less accurate than the 24-hour E/C ratio.
Fetal capillary blood sampling for ▲ pH[a] ▲ Pco_2 ▲ Po_2 ▲ O_2 saturation Hematocrit[a]	Determination of fetal acid–base status during labor to diagnose fetal asphyxia See Chapter 23	All infants are mildly asphyxiated during labor causing acidosis because of tissue hypoxia and CO_2 retention. Capillary pH may not be representative of central circulation. Should be done serially since a spot sample alone may be misleading or may provide inadequate information about fetal asphyxia stress and fetal coping. Lack of agreement about normal values for fetal capillary blood; however, the following are widely used as guidelines for the limits of normal ▲ pH >7.25 (range 7.20–7.30) ▲ $Pco_2 < 60$ mm Hg ▲ Base excess > -8 mEq/L
Glucose	Determination of hypoglycemia or hyperglycemia Determination of CHO metabolic disorders such as diabetes (see Chapter 21)	Normal nonpregnant range is 80–120 mg/mL; ideal pregnant range is 70–100 mg/mL Most glucose is reabsorbed in the renal tubules. Glycosuria is present in about 30% of pregnant women and is probably related to ▲ Decreased renal threshold for glucose ▲ Increased resistance to insulin ▲ Increased destruction of insulin because of levels of HCS (human chorionic somatommatropin also known as human placental lactogen, HPL)

TABLE 20.7 (continued)

Study	*Purpose*	*Significance*
		Dipstick or other spot checks should be performed at each prenatal visit. Indications of excess excretion of glucose should alert the nurse to the need for blood sugar assessments. Glucose readily passes the placenta and, therefore, it is important that maternal blood sugar stay within normal limits (normoglycemic) so that the fetus is not subjected to a fluctuating hyperglycemic and hypoglycemic environment.
Urine studies Bacteria	Diagnosis of urinary tract infections, particularly pyelonephritis	From 4 to 7% of pregnant women have asymptomatic bacteriuria during the first trimester. Approximately 25% of these women will develop acute pyelonephritis; 30% will have underlying chronic pyelonephritis; 25–30% may have bacteriuria after pregnancy. Method of specimen collection of urine greatly influences bacteria count. Clean midstream urine specimen for culture and sensitivity in the first trimester should be done and repeated in second and third trimesters. Attitudes toward use of antibiotic therapy vary. More than 100,000 organisms per milliliter on urine culture is usually requires use of antibiotics. Postpartal urine culture is advised at 6 weeks for women having asymptomatic bacteriuria because of increased incidence of renal problems postgestationally.
Protein (albuminuria)	Determination of renal pathology usually associated with pregnancy-induced hypertension (see Chapter 21).	Protein is normally reabsorbed in the kidney glomerulus. Presence of >1 gm/24 hour of protein in urine indicates renal disorder of some type. Measurement of urinary protein is a simple procedure if done by dipstick and should be performed at each prenatal visit (1+ or more on a clean catch urine specimen is significant). 24-hour urine specimens should be done if dipstick readings are positive for protein. Presence of proteinuria should alert the nurse to assess patient blood pressure levels and evidence of generalized edema carefully. Generalized edema in the absence of proteinuria and hypertension is likely physiologic rather than pathologic.

[a] Because of size of blood sample, priority is usually given to these measurements.

Source: Adapted from Butnarescu, G. F., Tillotson, D. M., Villarreal, P. P. *Perinatal Nursing: Vol. 2, Reproductive Risk.* New York: John Wiley & Sons, 1980, pp. 48–57. Used with permission.

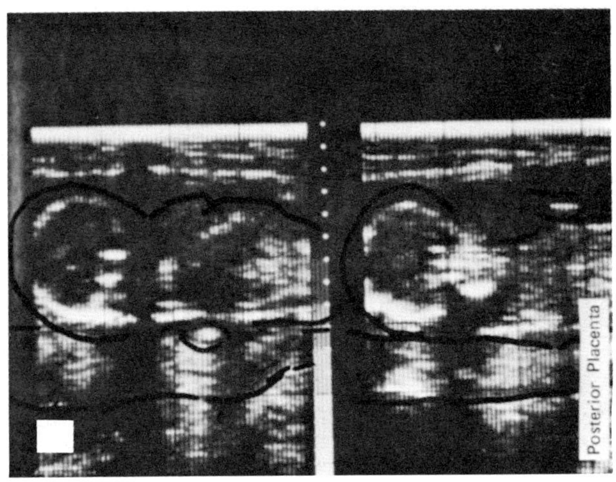

Figure 20.5
Sonographic representation of fetus at 20-weeks gestation. *Source*: Butnarescu, G. F., Tillotson, D. M., Villarreal, P. P. *Perinatal Nursing: Vol. 2. Reproductive Risk*. New York: John Wiley & Sons, 1980. Used with permission.

Midpregnancy assessment for:

- ▲ Fetal maturity and growth rate
- ▲ Measurement of or parietal diameter to date pregnancy
- ▲ Neural tube anomalies
- ▲ Hydramnios, oligohydramnios

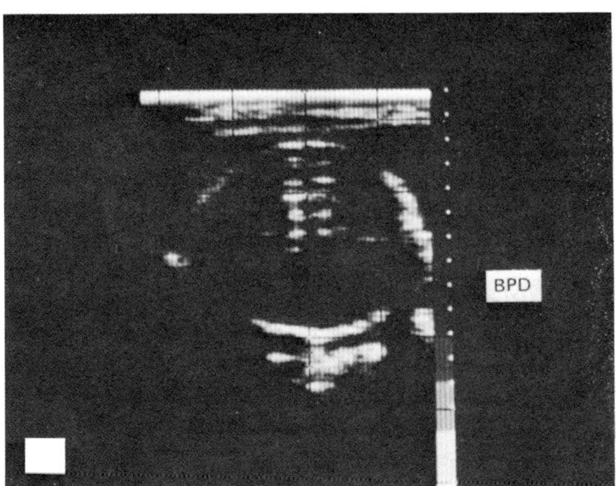

Figure 20.6
Sonographic representation of biparietal diameter of fetus at 31 weeks. *Source*: Butnarescu, G. F., Tillotson, D. M., Villarreal, P. P. *Perinatal Nursing: Vol. 2. Reproductive Risk*. New York: John Wiley & Sons. 1980. Used with permission.

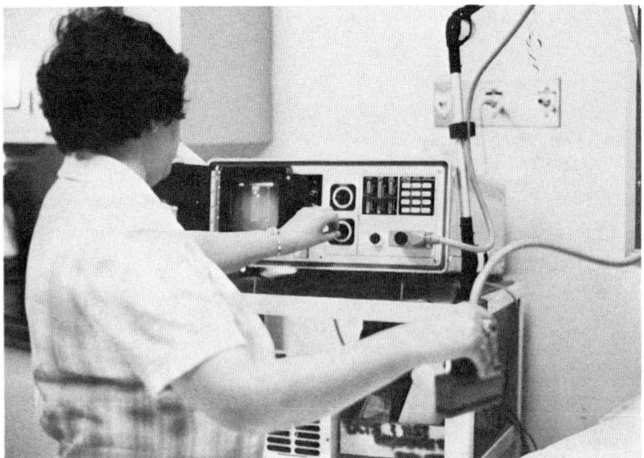

Figure 20.7
Ultrasound equipment and wand used by technician.

- ▲ Multiple pregnancy
- ▲ Intrauterine death
- ▲ Localization of placenta before amniocentesis

Late pregnancy assessment for:

- ▲ Placenta previa
- ▲ Presentation and position of fetus
- ▲ Fetal growth rate and size
- ▲ Fetal respiratory movement (Patrick, 1978)

Puerperium assessment for:

- ▲ Involution of uterus
- ▲ Possible retained products of conception

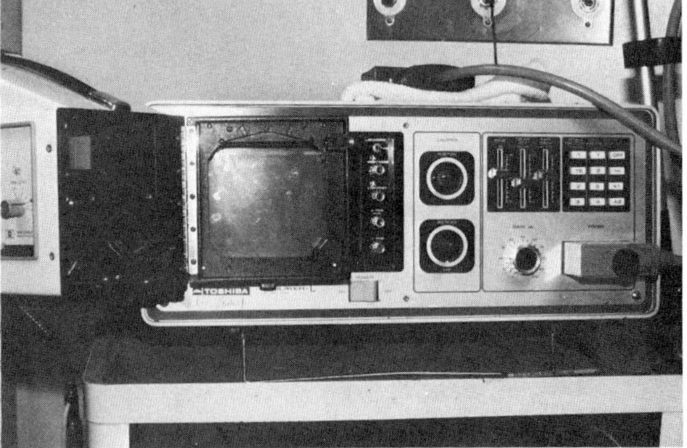

Figure 20.8
Close up of sonography screen on which picture is displayed. Camera at left swings over and can photograph screen.

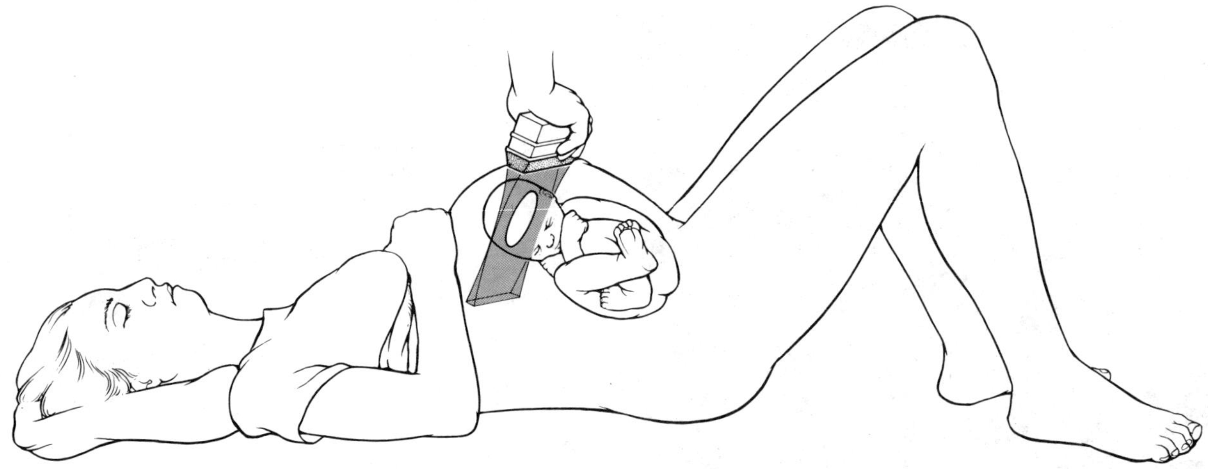

Figure 20.9
Illustration of transducer being applied to the mother's abdomen and reflecting biparietal diameter.

RADIOLOGIC ASSESSMENT

X-ray examination is rarely used today except for assessment of pelvic measurement (pelvimetry) in late pregnancy. Information regarding size and shape of the pelvis, as well as abnormal presentation, can be helpful when labor is prolonged or not progressing satisfactorily.

AMNIOTIC FLUID ANALYSIS

Amniocentesis

Amniocentesis—puncture of the amniotic sac through the abdominal and uterine wall to obtain a sample of fluid—is a relatively simple and safe procedure when done with knowledge and skill. Amniotic fluid analysis provides information about fetal maturity, fetal distress (presence of meconium), the extent to which Rh immunization has progressed, chromosomal analysis (see Chapter 24), and presence of open neural tube defect (α-fetoprotein—AFP—analysis). Amniocentesis is rarely done earlier than 12–14 weeks; when it is done before the period of viability, it is usually to detect genetic anomalies that can provide parents with data for decision making. Ideally, before amniocentesis ultrasound is used to visualize the contents of the uterus and help the procedure. Complications of amniocentesis are rare (less than 1%) but can include trauma, hemorrhage, and infection. The mother needs to be informed of the risk, and an operative permit is usually signed.

Preparation of the woman for amniocentesis involves:

- ▲ Informing the woman about the procedure
- ▲ Ascertaining that the woman voids before the procedure
- ▲ Positioning the woman in a supine position with legs extended
- ▲ Monitoring fetal heart rate
- ▲ Cleansing the lower abdomen with an antiseptic agent

A local anesthetic is used before insertion of the needle (often 4 in., 20–22-gauge spinal needle), and approximately 20 cc of fluid is withdrawn and placed in container that protects it from light. This is critical if analysis includes Rh immunization analysis as bilirubin is altered by light and analysis becomes useless. After the procedure the woman should be advised to report any unusual happenings such as fluid leakage, discomfort, or change in fetal activity. Both maternal and fetal vital signs are taken before and after the procedure and should be repeated at least 2 times during the first hour after the procedure.

Amnioscopy

Amnioscopy is a procedure for visualizing the color, depth, and composition of the amniotic fluid. The procedure is indicated when fetal assessment is necessary, in conditions such as postmaturity, fetal hypoxia (indicated by meconium-stained fluid) or pre-eclampsia. As with any procedure, the woman and her family should be told about the purpose, process, and outcome.

The woman is placed in a dorsal lithotomy position and draped. Pelvic examination is done to determine effacement, dilatation, and presentation. Fetal and placental position are often determined by ultrasound before the procedure. A sterile *amnioscope* is inserted (size depends on dilatation); when the tip is in the cervical canal the obturator is removed and a light source is attached to the distal end permitting visualization of the amniotic fluid. Gross fetal anomalies may also be seen. The procedure is most often done in the last month of pregnancy.

Amniography

In *amniography*, a contrast medium (dye) is inserted into the amniotic sac and radiographs are taken. Such conditions as twins, fetal anomalies or death, and placental localization can be determined. Fetal gastrointestinal disorders can sometimes be diagnosed as the fetus swallows the amniotic fluid containing the dye. Because ultrasound is available, this assessment modality is less often used.

Important tests regarding fetal maturity and fetal well-being are summarized in Table 20.8. All of these amniotic fluid studies need to be understood by nurses, especially if they care for the at risk maternity woman. The nurse's understanding and interpretation of these studies for the mother has a direct affect on her well-being, which indirectly affects the fetus.

STRESS AND NONSTRESS TESTING

Two other tests for fetal well-being are important for the maternity nurse to know; both are forms of antepartum monitoring to test for fetal compromise. The first to be developed was a *stress test*, the *oxytocin challenge test* (OCT) (also called *contraction stress test* CST), and the other is the *nonstress test* (NST) sometimes referred to as *fetal acceleration determinations* (FAD).

Oxytocin Challenge Test

The OCT is a method of evaluating the respiratory function of the placenta and is useful in evaluating woman with suspected placental insufficiency or those whose estriol values may be low and difficult to evaluate. OCT can afford additional data that will help the physician determine appropriate intervention. OCT can be done on an outpatient basis by a nurse familiar with electronic fetal monitoring and interpretation of fetal monitor strips. The procedure takes about 2 hours. The woman needs to empty her bladder, is confined to bed, and the external fetal monitor is attached. Low doses of intravenous oxytocin are given until three contractions are produced in a 10-minute period. If placental function is adequate, the fetus remains oxygenated and no late decelerations occur; the test is then classed as a negative OCT. A negative OCT is generally a reliable indicator that the fetus will do well in the week following the test. Fetal demise within a week of OCT is less than 1% (Evertson, et al., 1978). Freeman (1975) classifies OCTs as positive if consistent late deceleration occurs with most contractions and suspicious if intermittent late decelerations occur. A negative OCT has much more prognostic value as it is a good indicator that placental support is adequate and premature intervention can be avoided. A negative test also implies that the fetus can withstand the stress of labor.

The OCT has several disadvantages. Although false-negative test results are rare, false-positive test results are usual—late decelerations during the OCT without late decelerations in labor (Weingold et al., 1975). In addition, the test is time consuming and involves expensive equipment and personnel for a period of 2–3 hours. Since there is always the risk of premature labor, it is not used when labor is contraindicated (Cooper et al., 1975).

Nonstress Testing

As OCTs were analyzed further it was discovered that the risk of fetal distress during labor was

TABLE 20.8
AMNIOTIC FLUID LABORATORY ANALYSIS

Study	*Purpose*	*Significance*
Fetal maturity studies Cytology	Determination of the presence of fat cells in the amniotic fluid	Fetal cells (probably squamous) increase as pregnancy progresses. These cells are covered with a fatty substance, possibly vernix. When they are stained with 1% Nile blue sulfate, they turn orange. The nearer to term gestation, the greater the percentage of cells that stain orange. ▲ <1% orange cells appear prior to 34 weeks ▲ 1–20% appear 34–38 weeks ▲ 20–50% appear 38–40 weeks ▲ >50% appear postterm (Brosens, 1966) Respiratory distress is usually not seen if the fat cell count exceeded 10% (Nelson, 1969).
Shake test (foam stability test)	Determination of fetal lung maturity	Based on the ability of surfactant in the amniotic fluid to form bubbles in the presence of ethanol (Clements, 1972). Exact amounts of 95% ethanol, isotonic saline, and amniotic fluid are shaken for 15 seconds. If a ring of bubbles persists on the surface of the liquid after 15 minutes, shake test is positive and fetal lung is mature. Extremely high—false negative; extremely low—false positive.
ratio (L/S ratio)	Determination of fetal lung maturity through assessment of the phospholipid and lecithin—the surfactant essential for fetal and neonatal pulmonary function	Lecithin can be found in the amniotic fluid and is believed to be of lung origin. By the thirty-fifth week gestation, the L/S ratio should be 2:1 or greater. Maternal hypertension, narcotic addition, intrauterine growth retardation (IUGR), and so on have been associated with increased L/S ratio. Maternal diabetes and hemolytic disease of the newborn and respiratory distress syndrome may be associated with decreased L/S ratio.
Creatinine	Determination of fetal maturity through the assessment of fetal renal functioning	Amniotic fluid creatinine rises with the maturity of the fetal kidney and is particularly evident during the third trimester. Normal pregnancy concentration >2.0 mg/100 mL equals gestational age 37+ weeks (43). Caution: In some conditions creatinine levels can be misleading. ▲ *Overestimation* of fetal maturity can occur in conditions such as maternal renovascular disease, diabetes, toxemias.

Study	Purpose	Significance
		▲ *Underestimation* of fetal maturity may occur where there is diminished renal plasma flow with a decreased creatinine level, for example, fetal asphyxia, Rh isoimmunization, IUGR
Fetal well-being Bilirubin	Determination of optical density (OD) of the amniotic fluid to assess levels of bilirubin in the amniotic fluid. This test may be an accurate measurement of fetal maturity in the absence of disease; but it is also a measurement of fetal well-being, especially in relation to problems generated by Rh isoimmunization.	Amniotic fluid (OD) levels by the 36+ weeks gestation are near zero if bilirubin metabolism is normal since bile pigments decrease as pregnancy advances. If there is a disorder of bilirubin metabolism or in the presence of isoimmunization, greater amounts of bilirubin are produced and appear in the amniotic fluid.
Meconium	Determination presence of meconium in the amniotic fluid	Meconium, present in the amniotic fluid, is abnormal and usually indicates fetal distress since it is associated with fetal hypoxia. Meconium in association with fetal heart rate deceleration and/or fetal capillary blood pH <7.25 presents a grave prognosis for the fetus/neonate. Anytime the nurse is aware of meconium in the amniotic fluid, she or he should take measures to assess fetal heart rate patterns, particularly if this is noted during labor or with prematurely ruptured membranes.
Vaginal amniotic fluid Nitrazine test	Determination of rupture of membranes through the analysis of vaginal secretions mixed with amniotic fluid	Amniotic fluid is alkaline in nature, while vaginal secretions and urine during pregnancy are acid. Determinations of alkalinity of secretions may be indicative of ruptured membranes. Nitrazine paper, when exposed to the vaginal fluid, will become dark blue if the substance is alkaline, yellow if the substance is acid.
Fern test		Amniotic fluid will form a fernlike pattern when dried on a clean slide and examined microscopically. Presence of blood or meconium in the sample will distort the microscopic picture.
Nile blue sulfate		Fetal cells in the amniotic fluid will stain orange when amniotic fluid vaginal secretions are mixed with 1% Nile blue sulfate (see fetal maturity studies). Prematurely ruptured membranes place the fetus at risk for infections such as chorioamnionitis. Ruptured membranes may also predispose to premature onset of labor.

Source: Butnarescu, G. F., Tillotson, D. M., Villarreal, P. P. *Perinatal Nursing: Vol. 2, Reproductive Risk.* John Wiley & Sons, 1980, pp. 62–64. Used with permission.

greatest if there was lack of fetal heart rate (FHR) acceleration with fetal movement and if baseline variability was less than 10 beats per minute (Fox et al., 1976; Brady & Freeman, 1977). This led to the development of the nonstress test that evaluates accelerations with fetal movement and reactivity of the FHR baseline without using oxytocin. The external fetal monitor and positioning of the patient are the same as with the OCT. However, this test requires no intravenous therapy and can be done in less than an hour, although it does require trained personnel to be in attendance at all times. The FHR is recorded for 20–40 minutes with the maternal blood pressure taken every 10 minutes. The classification of reactive and nonreactive patterns is as follows (Nochism et al., 1978).

REACTIVE PATTERN

The FHR exhibits at least four episodes of acceleration of at least 15 beats per minute lasting 15–20 seconds after fetal movement. See Figure 20.10.

NONREACTIVE PATTERN

The FHR exhibits fewer than four accelerations following fetal movement, or FHR accelerations of fewer than 15 beats per minute, and lasting fewer than 15 seconds. See Figure 20.11.

If the woman has a nonreactive stress test, the fetus should be evaluated further by OCT, sonography, estriol determinations, or amniocentesis. Any risk condition such as hypertension, diabetes, infection, prematurity, or postdates, are indicators for nonstress testing. This test seems to continue to be a good indicator of fetal well-being and is used frequently in risk assessment because of relative ease of the procedure and apparent low risk to the patient.

NURSING RESPONSIBILITIES

The maternity nurse can contribute to the control and management of the problem of reproductive risk in a number of ways.

- Participation in the development and implementation of programs to educate the consumer about the indicators of reproductive risk, family planning options, family life and

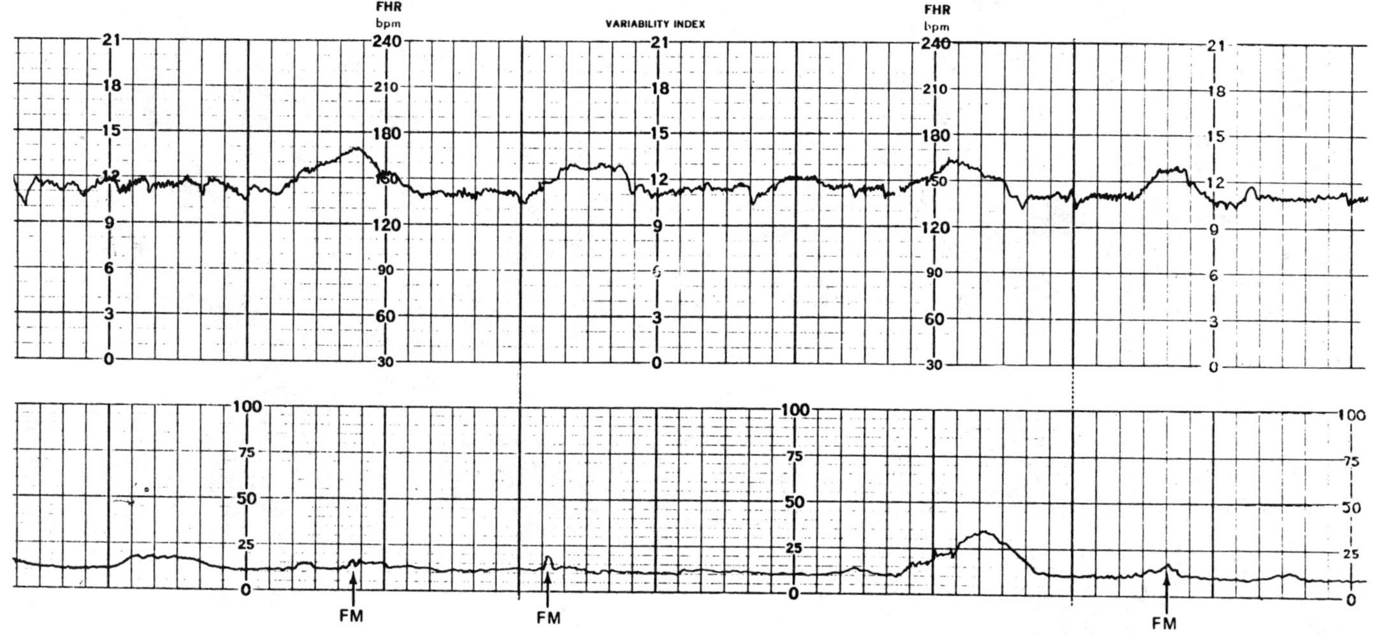

Figure 20.10
Reactive nonstress test. *Source:* Butnarescu, G. F., Tillotson, D. M., Villarreal, P. P. *Perinatal Nursing Vol. 2. Reproductive Risk.* New York: John Wiley & Sons. 1980. Used with permission.

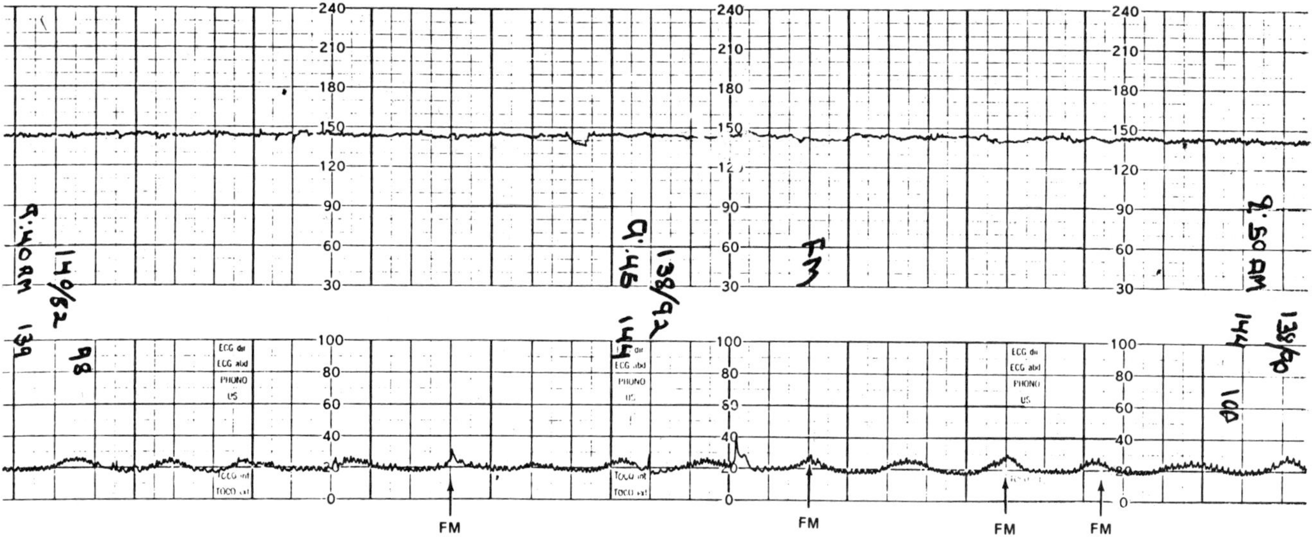

Figure 20.11
Nonreactive nonstress test. *Source:* Butnarescu, G. F., Tillotson, D. M., Villarreal, P. P. *Perinatal Nursing Vol. 2. Reproductive Risk.* New York: John Wiley & Sons. 1980. Used with permission.

sex education for young people, and preparation of the woman and family for pregnancy, childbirth, and parenthood

- ▲ Early detection of reproductive risk in the population and conditions that predispose to risk pregnancy among persons approaching or in the childbearing years
- ▲ Prevention of progression in severity of diagnosed risk conditions through conscientious and comprehensive nursing management of pregnant women during all phases of their reproductive experience
- ▲ Concern with the human aspects of reproductive risk and sensitivity to the demands risk places on the woman and family
- ▲ Use of an accurate theory base to make sound judgments about the nursing care of families at risk
- ▲ Participation in intradisciplinary and interdisciplinary efforts to combat the problem of reproductive risk

The maternity nurse is a key health professional in the prevention, detection, and management of conditions that place the childbearing family in jeopardy of a traumatic reproductive experience or a poor pregnancy outcome. The knowledgeable and skilled maternity nurse is often the pregnant woman's and her family's greatest ally.

SUMMARY

This chapter discussed the scope of the problem of reproductive risk in the United States today. Populations at greatest risk, such as poor nonwhite citizens, and other vulnerable groups were addressed. The financial and human costs of reproductive risk associated with poor pregnancy outcome and risk generally were viewed. Assessment of reproductive risk was approached through discussion of clinical assessment to include pelvic, breast, and abdominal examination. Special attention was given to the nurse's use of information collected from the patient and the significance of measurements such as maternal and fetal vital signs. A tool and a protocol for assessing fetal movement were presented. The significance of edema and varicosities and their relationship to risk conditions were mentioned. Psychosocial factors and the impact of these on risk conditions were restated. Biochemical evaluation followed; laboratory studies important to selected risk problems and the significance of these tests were presented in table form.

The chapter also discussed ultrasound, amniocentesis, amnioscopy, and amniography. A table presented the tests done on amniotic fluid and their relationship to fetal maturity and fetal well-being. The last section of the chapter discussed stress and nonstress testing both of which can be used to further assess fetal well-being. Electronic monitoring of mother and fetus was also included.

The chapter closed with a statement of broad nursing responsibilities for the prevention, detection, and management of reproductive risk; this topic is developed further in subsequent chapters in this unit.

REFERENCES AND READINGS

Adamsons, K., Fox, H. A. (Eds.) *Preventability of Perinatal Injury*. New York: Alan R. Liss, 1975.

Aubrey, R. H., Rouke, J. E., Cuenca, V. G., Marshall, L. D. The Random Urine Estrogen/Creatinine Ratio: A Practical and Reliable Index of Fetal Welfare. *Obstet Gynecol* 46:64, 1975.

Berendes, H. W. The Epidemiology of Perinatal Injury, in Adamsons, K., Fox, H. A. (Eds.), *Preventability of Perinatal Injury*. New York: Alan R. Liss, 1975, pp. 1–33.

Berkowitz, R. L., Hobbins, J. C. Ultrasonography in the Antepartum Patient, in Bolognese, R. J., Schwartz, R. H. (Eds.), *Perinatal Medicine: Management of the High Risk Fetus and Neonate*. Baltimore: Williams & Wilkins, 1977, pp. 85–112.

Berry, L. G. Age and Parity Influences on Maternal Mortality: United States, 1919–1969. *Demography* 14(3):297, 1977.

Brady, P., Freeman, R. K. The Significance of the Fetal Heart Rate Reactivity with a Positive Oxytocin Challenge Test. *Obstet Gynecol* 59:689, 1977.

Brosens, I., Gordon, H. The Estimation of Fetal Maturity by Cytological Examination of the Liquor Amnii. *J Obstet Gynecol British Commonwealth* 73:88, 1966.

Brown, J. B. The Value of Plasma Estrogen Estimation in the Management of Pregnancy. *Clin Perinatol* 1:273, 1974.

Butnarescu, G. F. *Perinatal Nursing: Volume I, Reproductive Health*. New York: John Wiley & Sons, 1978.

Butnarescu, G. F., Tillotson, D. M., Villarreal, P. P. *Perinatal Nursing: Volume II, Reproductive Risk*. New York: John Wiley & Sons, 1980.

Butterfield, L. J. Can Society Afford to Save These Babies? *Contemp Obstet Gynecol* 10:110, 1977.

Campbell, S. The Assessment of Fetal Development by Diagnostic Ultrasound. *Clin Perinatol* 1:507, 1974.

Carrington, E. R. Biochemical Monitoring of the Fetus, in Bolognese, R. J., Schwartz, R. H. (Eds.), *Perinatal Medicine Management of the High-Risk Fetus and Neonate*. Baltimore: Williams & Wilkins, 1977, pp. 56–65.

Chase, H. C. (Ed.) A Study of Risks, Medical Care and Infant Mortality. *Am J Public Health* (Supplement) 63:1, 1973.

Clements, J. A., Platzker, A. C., Tierney, D. F., et al. Assessment of the Risk of Respiratory Distress Syndrome by a Rapid Test for Surfactant in the Amniotic Fluid. *New Engl J Med* 286:1077, 1972.

Cooper, J. M., Soffronoff, E. C., Bolognese, R. J. Oxytocin Challenge Test in Monitoring High Risk Pregnancies. *Obstet Gynecol* 53:27, 1975.

Dryfoos, J. G. The United States National Family Planning Program, 1968–74. *Stud Fam Plann* 7(3):80, 1976.

Dubois, D. R. Indication of an Unhealthy Relationship Between Parents and Premature Infants. *J Obstet Gynecol Nurs* 4:21, 1975.

Duvall, E. *Marriage and Family Development* (5th ed.). Philadelphia: J. B. Lippincott, 1977, p. 209.

Effer, S. B. Biochemical and Biophysical Indices of Fetal Risk. *Clin Perinatol* 1:161, 1974.

Evertson, L. R., Gauthier, R. J., Collin, J. V. Fetal Demise Following Negative Construction Stress Tests. *Obstet Gynecol* 51:671, 1978.

Ford, K. Socioeconomic Differentials and Trends in the Timing of Births. DHHS No. (PHS) 81–1982, Hyattsville, Md: United States Department of Health and Human Services, February 1981.

Fox, H. E., Steinbrecher, M., Ripton, B. Antepartum Fetal Heart Rate and Uterine Activity Studies: I Preliminary Report of Accelerations and the Oxytocin Challenge Test. *Am J Obstet Gynecol* 126:61, 1976.

Freeman, R. K. The Use of the Oxytocin Challenge Test for Evaluation of Uteroplacental Function. *Am J Obstet Gynecol* 121:481, 1975.

Gilberg, A. L. The Stress of Parenting. *Child Psychiatry Hum Dev* 6:59, 1975.

Gordeuk, A. Motherhood and a Less than Perfect Child. *Matern Child Nurs J* 5:57, 1976.

Hoffmaster, J. E. Fetal Movement as an Indication of Fetal Well Being. *Perinatal Press* 2:75, 1978.

Hon, E. H., Khazin, A. F. Observations on Fetal Heart Rate and Fetal Biochemistry: I. Base Deficit. *Am J Obstet Gynecol* 105:721, 1969.

James, L. S. Fetal Blood Sampling. *Clin Perinatol* 1:141, 1974.

Janis, I. L. *Psychological Stress.* New York: John Wiley & Sons, 1958.

Janis, I. L. Psychodynamics of Stress Tolerance, in Klausner, S. Z. (Ed.). *The Quest for Self-Control: Classical Philosophies and Scientific Research.* New York: Free Press, 1965.

Kinch, R. A. H., Schiff, D. Carbohydrate Metabolism in Normal and Diabetic Pregnancy, in Goodwin, J. W., Godden, J. O., Chance, J. O. (Eds.), *Perinatal Medicine.* Baltimore: Williams & Wilkins, 1976, pp. 383–394.

Lilienfeld, A. M., Parkhurst, E. The Study of the Association of Factors of Pregnancy and Parturition with the Development of Cerebral Palsy: A Preliminary Report. *Am J Hygiene* 53:262, 1951.

Lincoln, R. The Select Committee Reports. *Fam Plann Perspect* 11(2):101, 1979.

Lubchenco, L. O., Horner, S. A., Reed, L. H., et al. Sequelae of Premature Birth—Evaluation of Premature Infants at 10 Years of Age. *Am J Dis Child* 106:101, 1963.

Miller, C. A. Health Care of Children and Youth in America. *Am J Public Health* 65(4):355, 1975.

Morbidity and Mortality Weekly Report. Childbearing and Abortion Patterns Among Teenagers—United States, 1978. *Morbidity and Mortality Weekly Report* 30(49):611, 1981.

Morris, N. M., Udry, J. R., Chase, C. L. Shifting Age—Parity, Distribution of Births and the Decrease in Infant Mortality. *Am J Public Health* 65(4):359, 1975.

Naeye, R. L., Blanc, W. A. Influences of Pregnancy Risk Factors on Fetal and Newborn Disorders. *Clin Perinatol* 1:187, 1974.

Nelson, G. H. Amniotic Fluid Phospholipid Patterns in Normal and Abnormal Pregnancies. *Am J Obstet Gynecol* 105:1072, 1969.

Nochism, D. J., Turbeville, J. S., Terry, J. E., Petrie, R. H., Lundy, L. E. The Non-Stress Test. *Obstet Gynecol* 51:419, 1978.

Patrick, J. E., Fetherston, W., Vick, H., Voegelin, R. Human Fetal Breathing Movements and Gross Fetal Body Movements at Weeks 34–35 of Gestation. *Am J Obstet Gynecol* 130:693, 1978.

Pearse, W. H. Doctors and Patients in Obstetrics and Gynecology, The Next 15 Years. *Am J Obstet Gynecol* 125:361, 1976.

Pomerance, J. J., Ukrainski, C. T., Ukra, T., Henderson, D. H. Cost of Living for Infants Weighing 1,000 Gms. or Less at Birth. *Pediatr* 61:908, 1978.

Prechtl, H. F. R. Neurological Sequelae of Prenatal and Perinatal Complications. *Br Med J* 34:763, 1969.

Robson, J. S. Proteinuria and the Renal Lesion in Preeclampsia and Abruptio Plancentae, in Lindheimer, M. D., Katz, A. I., Zuspan, F. P. (Eds.), *Hypertension in Pregnancy*. New York: John Wiley & Sons, 1976, pp. 61–73.

Rochat, R. W.. Maternal Mortality in the United States of America. *WHO Stat Quart* 34(1):2, 1981.

Rosoff, J. I. Blocking Family Planning. *Fam Plann Perspect* 13(3):125, 1981.

Sadovsky, E., Yaffer, H. Daily Fetal Movement Recording and Fetal Prognosis. *Obstet Gynecol* 41:845, 1973.

Schneider, J. M. Perinatal Laboratory Evaluations: Part I: Routine Prenatal Maternal Assessments. *Perinatal Press* 1:3, 1977.

Select Panel for the Promotion of Child Health. *Better Health for Our Children: A National Strategy* (The Report of the Select Panel for the Promotion of Child Health, 1980. To the United States Congress and the Secretary of Health and Human Services. Vol. I: Major Findings and Recommendations). DHHS No. 79-55071. Washington, D. C.: Department of Health and Human Services, 1980.

Stickle, G., Ma, P. Some Social and Medical Correlates of Pregnancy Outcome. *Am J Obstet Gynecol* 127:162, 1977.

Tietze, C. Maternal Mortality (excluding Abortion Mortality). *WHO Stat Rep* 30(4): 312, 1977.

Towell, M. E. Fetal Acid–Base Physiology and Intrauterine Asphyxia, in Goodwin, J. W., Godden, J. O., Chance, G. W. (Eds.), *Perinatal Medicine*. Baltimore: Williams & Wilkins, 1976, pp. 187–208.

Weingold, A. B., de Jesus, T., O'Keefe, J. Oxytocin Challenge Test. *Am J Obstet Gynecol* 123:466, 1975.

WHO. The Incidence of Low Birth Weight: A Critical Review of Available Information. *WHO Stat Quart* 33(3): 197, 1980.

Williams, C. How Much Does a Baby Cost? *Redbook* (April) 1976.

Willis, W. Perinatal Loss: Socioeconomic Factors. *J Obstet Gynecol Nurs* 6:44, 1977.

Wilson, D. R. Renal Function in Pregnancy, in Goodwin, J. W., Godden, J. O., Chance, G. W. (Eds.), *Perinatal Medicine*. Baltimore: Williams & Wilkins, 1976.

21

MATERNAL DISORDERS AND PROBLEMS DURING PREGNANCY

Maternity nurses need the information they have learned in their basic behavioral and natural sciences courses plus the ability to apply selected content from medical–surgical nursing, psychiatric nursing and community health nursing in order to help maternity patients at risk. For example, a pregnant woman with diabetes requires the nurse to combine what she knows about diabetes with what she knows about pregnancy; a pregnant woman with a rheumatic heart with mitral valve damage requires a nurse with certain knowledge to apply that knowledge for intervention. Caring for the at-risk maternity client with multiple factors involved requires true internalization of the nursing process in order to assess and intervene appropriately. In any complicated pregnancy, the risk of death or damage to the fetus, mother, or both must be assessed and reassessed throughout the course of pregnancy and the childbirth experience.

This chapter focuses on medical–surgical conditions (drug abuse and other psychosocial disorders are discussed in Chapter 25). Conditions are divided here into those existing before pregnancy and those arising from the pregnancy; nursing implications for the more prevalent risk conditions are included.

PRE-EXISTING CONDITIONS THAT COMPLICATE PREGNANCY

Cardiac Disease

Approximately 1% of all pregnant women have heart disease. The usual underlying pathophysiology is rheumatic heart disease, but other causes, such as congenital malformation, can also be the basis. Diagnosis is based on history, physical examination, cardiac X-ray photos, and electrocardiographic (EKG) recordings. There are several pregnancy-induced changes that mimic cardiac disease. They are fatigue, edema, dyspnea, cardiac enlargement, EKG changes, and murmurs, all of which can occur in normal pregnant women. Functional heart disease needs to be ruled out when these symptoms appear. In other words: Is it a normal pregnancy-induced change or is it heart disease?

Ideally, the diagnosis of heart disease is made before pregnancy, but this is not always the case. Once heart disease is diagnosed, the woman's health team should include a cardiologist as well as an obstetrician.

Prognosis during pregnancy for the cardiac patient correlates with the functional classifications established by the New York Heart Association criteria, which are as follows.

▲ ***Class I.*** Patients with cardiac disease that does not limit activity. Ordinary physical activity does not cause discomfort. The patients have no symptoms of cardiac insufficiency nor do they have anginal pain.

▲ ***Class II.*** Patients with cardiac disease that produces slight limitation of activity. The patients are free from symptoms while at rest, but ordinary activity is accompanied by undue fatigue, palpitation, dyspnea, or anginal pain.

▲ ***Class III.*** Patients with cardiac disease that produces marked limitation of activity. Less than ordinary activity is accompanied by fatigue, palpitation, dyspnea, or anginal pain.

▲ ***Class IV.*** Patients with cardiac disease that prevents them from carrying out any activity without discomfort. Symptoms of cardiac insufficiency or anginal pain are present at rest, and any activity increases them.

In general, class I and II cardiac patients do well during pregnancy; class III patients usually require bed rest throughout the pregnancy; and class IV patients are in cardiac failure at rest so both fetal and maternal mortality is high. Recall that the blood volume increases 30–40% during pregnancy, and it is easily understandable that congestive heart failure is the big concern. *The most likely time for the pregnant woman to go into heart failure is 28–32 weeks gestation,* the time at which the blood volume peaks. Other likely times for decompensation are discussed later in this section. Since increased blood volume cannot be controlled, management of the pregnant cardiac patient is aimed at preventing heart failure.

Antepartum management includes:

▲ ***Rest.*** Have rest periods each morning and afternoon and 10 hours rest in bed at night.

▲ ***Infection.*** Avoid crowds and areas where exposure to infection is high. If infected, treat vigorously with antibiotics.

▲ ***Diet.*** Excessive weight gain and abnormal fluid retention should be avoided. Normal weight gain and minimal sodium intake, however, is appropriate.

▲ ***Anemia.*** Correct and prevent anemia since it increases cardiac output. Iron supplements should be given.

▲ ***Medications.*** Besides iron and vitamin supplements, anticoagulant, digitalis, and antibiotics may be necessary. Heparin is the anticoagulant of choice as it does not cross the placenta. Penicillin prophylaxis may be used.

▲ ***Antepartum Visits.*** Weekly visits throughout pregnancy. At each visit, cardiac status is assessed. Signs of heart failure include cough (an unexplained cough is the *early sign* of cardiac decompensation), dyspnea, edema, heart murmurs, palpitations, and rales.

▲ ***Psychological Support.*** Reduction of any stress factors occurring in the family. Information and anticipatory guidance regarding the pregnancy reduce anxiety.

Intrapartum management includes:

▲ ***Monitoring.*** Monitor fetal and maternal blood pressure, pulse, and respirations. These vital statistics should be taken every 15 minutes. Pulse and respirations are very significant —pulse increases to 110 and a respiratory increase of 24 in the first stage of labor usually indicates that failure will occur.

▲ ***Pulmonary Assessment.*** Note and report dyspnea or cough, and auscultate for rales at the lung bases.

▲ ***Reduce Exertion and Conserve Energy.*** Position in semi-Fowler's and side-lying positions to promote oxygenation.

▲ ***Medications.*** Prophylactic antibiotics are usually started in labor to prevent infection (such as subacute bacterial endocarditis). Medications include oxygen by mask, diuretics if fluid retention occurs, sedatives or analgesics if indicated, and digitalis if signs of cardiac decompensation occur.

▲ ***Analgesia and Anesthesia.*** Vaginal delivery is preferred unless there is obstetric reason for cesarean birth. Caudal or epidural (see Chapter 22) is preferred as each can be started in active phase of first stage and reduce stress associated with pain, anxiety, and increased muscular activity.

- ▲ ***Reduce Bearing Down Efforts by Shortening Second Stage.*** Pudendal block, low forceps.
- ▲ ***Alert Other Health Team Members.*** Pediatrician, cardiologist, nursery, and postpartal nurses, and others as necessary.

Postpartum management includes:

- ▲ ***Assessment of Postdelivery Adaptation.*** Rapid fluid shifts, diaphoresis, and diuresis can increase cardiac output, and cardiac decompensation can occur.
- ▲ ***Hospital Stay.*** Longer hospital stay until cardiac function is restored.
- ▲ ***Attachment.*** Minimal personal and infant caregiving activities. Allow infant to be held and seen but nurse should assist with infant caretaking and maternal grooming.
- ▲ ***Ambulation.*** Progressive, as determined by cardiac status.
- ▲ ***Intake and Output.*** Monitor daily weight carefully to assess fluid balance. Use stool softeners to avoid straining.
- ▲ ***Discharge Planning.*** Referral, education, and assessment of home situation and needed support. Education regarding resumption of sexual activities and contraception information.
- ▲ ***Psychosocial Support.*** Reinforce coping and supportive roles of significant others.

SUMMARY OF CARE OF THE PREGNANT CARDIAC PATIENT

Key concepts in care of the pregnant cardiac are that cardiac decompensation is most likely to occur in the antepartum period, 28–32 weeks, when blood volume peaks. Other peak times of decompensation are during labor, immediately postpartum, and after the mother returns home since, if she feels well, it is easy for her to do too much. The goals of management are to conserve energy, allay anxiety, and prevent cardiac failure. If anticoagulants are used, the drug of choice is heparin since it does not cross the placenta. Ideally, delivery is vaginal with regional or local anesthesia and low forceps used to minimize bearing-down efforts in the second stage. Care taking by the mother postpartally should be assumed slowly and only if cardiac function is adequate. If the pregnancy is managed well and outcome is favorable, the course of the woman's heart disease and her life expectancy should not be altered.

CHRONIC HYPERTENSION

(See section on hypertensive disorders later in this chapter.)

Diabetes

Diabetes mellitus and pregnancy fall into two general categories; the overt or known diabetic and the gestational diabetic—the woman who develops diabetes during pregnancy. Once diabetes is diagnosed, the management of the pregnant diabetic is the same, whether overt or gestational. Diabetes and pregnancy have unique effects on each other, which is important for the maternity nurse to understand.

EFFECTS OF PREGNANCY ON DIABETES

During pregnancy three things occur physiologically that increase the need for insulin.

- ▲ The growing fetus requires insulin, that is, physiologic requirements increase.
- ▲ Human placental lactogen (HPL)* produced by the placenta induces lipolysis, increases free fatty acids, and inhibits cellular uptake of glucose; insulin becomes less effective.
- ▲ Placental insulinase (enzyme) causes increased degradation of insulin (breaks down).

Because of these three physiologic events, the need for insulin in *all* pregnancies increases, which is why pregnancy is in itself diabetogenic (causing diabetes).

DIAGNOSIS OF DIABETES

The *overt diabetic* is easy to identify as she is the person who has diabetes before she becomes preg-

*Also know as human chorionic somatomammotropin (HCS).

nant. The *gestational diabetic*, the person who develops diabetes after she becomes pregnant, is diagnosed by oral glucose tolerance test (OGTT). In some areas of the United States, all pregnant women are screened for diabetes. Most women, however, are evaluated for gestational diabetes when one of the following is noted (Huff, & Pauerstein 1979).

- ▲ ***Postobstetric History.*** Unexplained stillbirth, nursery death, child with anomalies, or infant over 9 lb or past history of gestational diabetes
- ▲ ***Family History.*** Diabetes in one close relative (parent or sibling) or two distant relatives
- ▲ ***Physical Exam.*** Obesity, weight gain of 20 lb in first half of pregnancy, polyhydramnios, or recurrent monilial vaginitis
- ▲ ***Laboratory Report.*** Glycosuria on two or more occasions or elevated postprandial (after a meal) blood sugar

When diagnosing the gestational diabetic by OGTT, most institutions use O'Sullivan et al. (1973) criteria in which the OGTT is considered positive if two of the patient's blood sugar values are elevated above the levels given below or if one blood sugar value was exceeded in two successive tests.

- ▲ Fasting 90 mg/100 mL
- ▲ One hour 165 mg/100 mL
- ▲ Two hours 145 mg/100 mL
- ▲ Three hours 125 mg/100 mL

The nurse needs to know that for 2 or 3 days before the OGTT, the woman is told to eat a high-carbohydrate diet, for example, one or two candy bars a day. On the morning of the test, if the fasting blood sugar is greater than 140 mg/100 mL, the test is canceled as it may be dangerous and the diagnosis of gestational diabetes is clear. If below 140 mg/100 mL, the woman is given 100-gm oral drink of glucose, and blood sugar determinations are obtained at 1, 2, and 3 hours. It is customary to check for glycosuria at the same time blood sugar determinations are made. Many times, if OGTT is normal early in pregnancy, the test is repeated after the twenty-eighth week of pregnancy since the diabetogenic effect of pregnancy increases as pregnancy continues.

CLASSIFICATION OF DIABETES

As with overt diabetics, once a gestational diabetic is diagnosed she is classified according to the duration and severity of disease and the need for insulin. *White's* (1978) *classification* of diabetes is shown in Table 21.1; this table also relates fetal survival to classification.

The other classification of importance to the maternity nurse is *Pedersen's* (1977) *prognostically bad signs in pregnancy* (*PBSP*). White's classification is based on factors present in the mother before pregnancy. Pedersen's classification calls attention to factors that become evident during pregnancy, which include:

- ▲ ***Polynephritis.*** The development of polynephritis can influence premature labor. Checking for asymptomatic bacteriuria during the antepartum period is critical (see Chapter 12).
- ▲ ***Ketoacidosis.*** The most serious effect of ketoacidosis is intrauterine death. Weekly blood sugars (postprandial and fasting) and urine testing can alert the nurse to impending acidosis. Frequent hospitalization for regulation of insulin if biophysical or psychosocial stressors are evident becomes important.
- ▲ ***Toxemia.*** Incidence of toxemia is 25%, and of those, 25% have fetal loss (Huff, 1979). Assessment for signs of toxemia is critical.
- ▲ ***Neglectors.*** Pedersen uses the term *neglectors* to encompass the group of clients who do not follow prescribed regimens. He relates this to socioeconomic status, intelligence, or lack of proper information. Frequently, these women are unable to accept a diagnosis of diabetes mellitus; rapport with the health care team is critical for good management.

The important things to remember about White's and Pedersen's classifications are:

- ▲ The higher the letter (A, B, C, etc.), the more severe and longer standing the diabetes.
- ▲ Class A diabetics do not require insulin. Gestational diabetics who require insulin are then reclassified as class B diabetics.
- ▲ All classifications after class A require insulin.
- ▲ Once any of Pedersen's PBSP appears, the risk of death or damage to the fetus increases.

TABLE 21.1A
CLASSIFICATION OF DIABETES IN PREGNANT WOMEN

Class of Diabetes	*Fetal Survival (%)*
Class A: Chemical diabetes	100
Class B: Maturity onset (age over 20 years), duration under 10 years, no vascular lesions	67
Class C: Age 10 to 19 years at onset of 10 to 19 years' duration, no vascular lesions	48
Class D: Under age 10 at onset or over 20 years' duration or calcification of vessels of legs or hypertension or benign retinopathy	32
Class E: Calcification of pelvic arteries	13
Class F: Nephropathy	3

Source: White, Priscilla. Classification of obstetric diabetes. *American Journal of Obstetrics and Gynecology* Jan. 15, 1978, p. 229. Used with permission.

TABLE 21.1B
UPDATE OF CLASSIFICATION OF DIABETES IN PREGNANT WOMEN

*Class**	*Criterion*
C_1	Age 10 to 19 years at onset
C_2	10 to 18 years' duration
D_1	Under age 10 years at onset
D_2	Over 20 years' duration
D_3	Benign retinopathy
D_4	Calcified vessels of legs
D_5	Hypertension
E	No longer sought
F	Nephropathy
G	Many failures
H	Cardiopathy
R	Proliferating retinopathy
I	Renal transplant added by Tagatz and colleagues of the University of Minnesota

*Classes A and B are the same as in Table 21.1A.

Source: White, Priscilla. Classification of obstetric diabetes. *American Journal of Obstetrics and Gynecology* Jan. 15, 1978, p. 229. Used with permission.

These two international classifications enable the maternity nurse to process data and to set goals for the management of the diabetic pregnancy.

EFFECTS OF DIABETES ON PREGNANCY

There are maternal, fetal, and neonatal complications from diabetes superimposed on pregnancy.

- ▲ ***Maternal.*** Acidosis, hydramnios, toxemia, infection, dystocia
- ▲ ***Fetal.*** Increased morbidity, congenital anomalies, hyperbilirubinemia, LGA, stillborn, or death
- ▲ ***Neonatal.*** Large infant—"big baby" (BB), hyperbilirubinemia, hypoxia, respiratory distress syndrome, hypoglycemia (see Chapter 23)

Blood sugar control of the pregnant diabetic is critical, and insulin requirements increase in 70% of all patients after the twenty-fourth week of gestation (Willson & Carrington, 1979). Carbohydrate metabolic control is affected by several factors: vomiting, which can lead to acidosis; the higher concentration of ketone bodies (the accelerated starvation mechanism of pregnancy); hormonal changes (especially placental, which increase insulin requirements); and the lowered renal threshold for glucose. The latter necessitates that insulin adjustment should not be made on the basis of urine testing but only by blood sugar determination. Also, remember that glucose crosses the placenta but insulin does not, a key concept that has great significance for the fetus and neonate and is discussed in Chapter 23.

Overall effects of diabetes on pregnancy include increased incidence of toxemia and hydramnios. The cause of the hydramnios is unknown; because hydramnios and toxemia are frequently seen together, vascular factors are suggested. Apart from the complications of metabolism, acidosis, and coma, problems of pregnant women who are diabetic and nondiabetic are similar, except in the former problems occur more often.

MANAGEMENT OF THE PREGNANT DIABETIC

The management of diabetic women who are pregnant requires a team effort; goals include individualized care, strict metabolic control, liberal hospitalization for complications, monitoring of fetal environment to detect intrauterine distress before death or damage occurs, prevention of iatrogenic prematurity, and special care for the neonate after delivery.

Antepartum management includes:

Baseline Data

- ▲ Evaluation of cardiovascular status
- ▲ Evaluation of renal status
- ▲ Ophthalmologic examination
- ▲ Accurate assessment of gestational age (sonography, FHR, uterine size, fetal activity)
- ▲ Evaluation of socioeconomic factors (risk pregnancy management can be costly)
- ▲ Weekly prenatal visits to include routine prenatal checks—fundal height, urine, weight—*plus* FBS, and postprandial blood sugar
- ▲ Intensive education regarding diet, insulin, and what to expect throughout the pregnancy
- ▲ Monthly urine culture
- ▲ Diabetic diet—2,000–2,400 calories/day; weight gain of 25 lb desired
  - ▾ Protein 1.5–2 gm/Kg
  - ▾ Carbohydrate 200–500 gm
  - ▾ Fat 70–80 gm
- ▲ Three meals and three snacks per day
- ▲ Insulin administration to maintain FBS: ↓90 mg—preferably 60–80 mg/mL; 2-hour postprandial not greater than 145 mg/mL
- ▲ Fractional urine testing of woman for sugar and acetone; glucose tested by testape or dipstick (not Clinitest, which tests for sugars other than glucose)
- ▲ Insulin readjustment according to blood sugars only (urine testing is rough guide)
- ▲ Insulin may be required more than once a day (divided doses)
- ▲ Fetal growth and maturity studies, such as, estriols, serial ultrasound, amniocentesis, CST, or NST (see Chapter 20), as indicated
- ▲ Liberal hospitalization for complications; routine hospitalization about 34–37 weeks until delivery
- ▲ Psychosocial support in any identified areas of need; blood sugar levels are influenced by psychological stress

Intrapartum management includes:

- ▲ Vaginal delivery preferred.
- ▲ Induction with oxytocin may be initiated if biochemical and biophysical monitoring indicates delivery time is optimum. (Physician's decision regarding induction balances the risk of intrauterine death against the risk of neonatal death.)
- ▲ Insulin dosage on day of delivery reduced one-half to one-third—blood sugar monitored during labor. If insulin is required during labor, regular insulin (short acting) should be used.
- ▲ Intravenous therapy to provide route for medication if necessary. Also intravenous (IV) fluids should include dextrose to provide energy needed for labor.

- ▲ Electronic fetal monitoring, capability for scalp pH desirable.
- ▲ Psychosocial support from nurse and significant others.
- ▲ Regional anesthesia for delivery.
- ▲ Pediatrician should be alerted.
- ▲ Allow opportunity for mother–infant bonding if infant is stable.

Postpartum management includes:

- ▲ Careful observation of blood sugar value and insulin coverage. (Recall that the physiologic basis for increased insulin—baby and placenta—is no longer there. Most overt diabetics revert to prepregnant insulin requirements, and gestational diabetics no longer require insulin.
- ▲ Intravenous therapy is usually continued 24 hours postpartum.
- ▲ Fractional urines are checked for sugar and acetone.
- ▲ Education regarding infant care, intergestational health care, and family planning should be initiated (see Chapter 26).

SUMMARY OF CARE OF THE PREGNANT DIABETIC

A key concept to remember in the care of the pregnant diabetic is that all pregnancies have a diabetogenic effect because of physiologic events related to fetal growth and placental maintenance of that growth. Insulin needs are increased, and successful outcome depends on strict metabolic control that is individual for each woman. An interdisciplinary health care team is essential to provide optimal care for mother and infant. Insulin, not oral hypoglycemics that may be teratogenic, is required during pregnancy, and blood sugar levels are assessed carefully throughout the pregnancy. Since glucose passes the placenta but insulin does not, the aim of management is to maintain the mother in a normoglycemic range. Ideally, delivery is vaginal, and postpartal recovery to prepregnant insulin requirements is rapidly accomplished. In general, pregnancy does not add hazards to the long-term effects of diabetes such as vascular changes; aggravation of pre-existing vascular disease is reported in the literature as 3% of the population (Pedersen, 1977). As with class III and IV cardiacs, diabetic pregnant women who are class C or D or higher run a much higher risk of poor outcome.

Thyroid Disease

Normal pregnant women demonstrate changes in thyroid function that can be interpreted as hyperthyroidism. Recall that normally during pregnancy the thyroid gland enlarges because of hyperplasia and increased vascularity, and the basal metabolic rate (BMR) increases 25% because of metabolic activity of the placenta and fetus. The fetus manufactures its own thyroid stimulating hormones (TSH); maternal TSH does not cross the placenta. This situation is analagous to the fetus of the diabetic mother; that is the fetus manufactures its own insulin since maternal insulin does not cross the placenta. Thyroid dysfunction is not a common complication of pregnancy, but it is an important one to recognize and manage. It is generally classified into hypothyroidism and hyperthyroidism.

DIAGNOSIS OF THYROID DISEASE

Usually diagnosis of thyroid disease is made by clinical assessment with laboratory data confirming the findings.

HYPOTHYROIDISM

Hypothyroidism occurs in approximately 1 in 20,000 pregnancies. Seventy percent of these women are anovulatory, and if conception occurs, there is a high incidence of abortion. Clinical signs of hypothyroidism are decreased BMR, enlarged thyroid gland, fatigability, myxedema, cold intolerance, dry skin, and headache. Laboratory findings in hypothyroidism indicate that the free thyroxin index is decreased; in pregnancy it usually remains normal (same as nonpregnant). If a woman who is on thyroid medication becomes pregnant, her dosage should be increased and an evaluation of her need for thyroid hormone should be done after delivery. Radioactive iodine uptake studies cannot be done on a pregnant woman as iodides cross the placenta and are picked up by the fetal thyroid.

HYPERTHYROIDISM

Signs and symptoms of thyrotoxicosis are the same as in the nonpregnant woman and include:

- ▲ Resting heart rate over 100 beats/min
- ▲ Eye findings, that is, staring, exophthalmus
- ▲ Nervousness, palpitation, tremor, heat intolerance, muscle weakness, and personality changes
- ▲ Weight loss—important in pregnancy as weight gain used as a guide for adequate treatment

The incidence of hyperthyroidism varies from 1 in 500 to 1 in 2,500. If undiagnosed and untreated, the hyperthyroid woman is at risk for toxemia, premature labor, and developing heart failure or thyroid storm (thyrotoxic crisis). Symptoms of thyroid storm include extremely high temperature, tachycardia, sweating, dehydration, and heart failure. Mortality rate is 25%.

Treatment of hyperthyroidism during pregnancy can be medical or surgical. Unfortunately, although treatment is necessary, none is ideal. Thioureas (propylthiouracil and methimazole) are the usual drugs used, but therapeutic effects of these drugs may not be noted for 4–6 weeks. Thioureas also pass the placenta, which can lead to development of fetal goiter (can be large enough to obstruct airway) or a neonate born hypothyroid or mentally retarded. It is, therefore, critical to use the lowest effective dosage in order to prevent fetal problems. Surgical intervention can be done in the first or second trimester and is sometimes indicated. Most of the literature suggests medical management at the lowest possible dose and surgical management only if the former is not effective.

COMPLICATIONS ARISING BECAUSE OF PREGNANCY

Bleeding During Pregnancy

Bleeding complications during pregnancy can be divided into early, or first and second, trimester bleeding and late, or third, trimester bleeding. The two major conditions that result in bleeding late in pregnancy are placenta previa and abruptio placentae. Early bleeding is usually a result of *abortion,* which is defined as termination of a pregnancy before the twentieth week of gestation when the fetus weights approximately 400 gm. Abortion (the lay term is miscarriage) can be spontaneous or induced (brought on intentionally) and can be further differentiated into legal and illegal (performed by an individual not approved by the law). Induced abortion is discussed in Chapter 26; spontaneous abortion is discussed in this chapter.

Spontaneous Abortion

Causes of *spontaneous abortion* include both fetal and maternal factors. Etiologic factors include:

- ▲ Defective ovum or sperm
- ▲ Defective nidation
- ▲ Maternal disease such as infection or nutritional deficiencies
- ▲ Abnormalities of the reproductive organs
- ▲ Physical trauma
- ▲ Endocrine problems
- ▲ Blood group incompatibility
- ▲ Psychogenic factors

The precipitating cause of abortion, whatever the underlying etiology, is the death or failure of the embryo to develop normally. As the embryo fails, there is a reduction in estrogen and progesterone production by the trophoblasts. Once the hormone level falls, the uterus becomes irritable, and eventually contractions occur and the products of conception are expelled in whole or in part. Sometimes incompetent cervix is a factor in abortion, particularly second trimester abortion, and is discussed in this chapter. Abortions are further divided into the following classifications.

Classification of Abortion

- ▲ ***Threatened Abortion.*** Unexplained bleeding that usually ceases in 1–2 days or increases, and is followed by uterine cramps and partial or complete expulsion of the products of conception.
- ▲ ***Inevitable Abortion.*** As is implied by the name, an irreversible process of uterine evacuation has begun, the internal cervical os is dilated, and bleeding and cramping increase until the products of conception are passed.

- ▲ ***Incomplete Abortion.*** Not all of the products of conception have passed, but the os is dilated and partial evacuation has taken place.

- ▲ ***Complete Abortion.*** All products of conception are passed, and no treatment is required.

- ▲ ***Missed Abortion.*** A fetal death in which the products of conception have not evacuated the uterus. Diagnosis to ascertain that the diagnosis is correct is important (e.g., no FHT, pregnancy test is negative). Early missed abortion can be treated by surgical intervention (see Chapter 26). Second trimester missed abortion and intrauterine fetal death (IUFD) are treated by initiating labor (see induced abortion, Chapter 26).

- ▲ ***Habitual Abortion.*** Abortion in three or more consecutive pregnancies. Treatment of habitual abortion depends on correction of physical or nutritional deficiencies. If no hormonal or organic cause is demonstrated, some women benefit from preconceptual psychotherapy aimed at resolving psychic conflict that can be contributory.

Treatment of Abortion and Nursing Implications

Treatment, of course, depends on the type of abortion and the evaluation of the progress of uterine evacuation. If bleeding is active, treatment usually involves restriction of activities, bed rest, no coitus, and sometimes sedation. If persistent bleeding or incomplete passage occurs, hospitalization, IV therapy, and dilatation and curettage or vacuum curettage may be necessary. Psychosocial support is critical as almost all mothers feel sadness or sometimes anger. Negative feelings about the pregnancy may result in the mother feeling guilty, blaming herself for not being normal, or punishing herself for some wrong doing.

If the basis for habitual abortion is incompetent cervix, this can often be corrected by a surgical procedure called Shirodkar operation (circlage procedure). The weakened cervix is closed by purse-string suture that remains in place until vaginal or cesarean delivery is imminent.

Ectopic Pregnancy

Ectopic refers to something that occurs outside of its usual place. A pregnancy that results from implantation of the fertilized ovum at a site other than the endometrial lining of the uterine cavity is described as an *ectopic pregnancy.* Ectopic pregnancy is *not* synonomous with extrauterine pregnancy although the two terms are frequently used interchangeably. Ectopic pregnancy may also develop from other uterine sites such as the cervix and interstitial part of the oviduct. (You will recall that the interstitial part of the fallopian tube passes through the uterine myometrium; hence it is more a part of the uterus than of the tube.) The fertilized ovum may also implant outside of the uterus (*eccyesis*) in a site such as the oviduct, ovary, or abdomen. The most common site of extrauterine pregnancy is the oviduct, which accounts for 90–95% of all ectopic pregnancies.

INCIDENCE

The incidence of ectopic pregnancy varies with the series of cases being reviewed. However, the reported incidence ranges from 1 ectopic pregnancy for every 30 infants born to 1 for every 300 infants born (Huff & Pauerstein, 1979). The incidence of ectopic pregnancy has increased during the past decade to a rate of 2.1 ectopic pregnancies per 100,000 live births (Huff & Pauerstein, 1979). There is an association between socioeconomic status and ectopic pregnancy. The incidence is highest in the indigent black population.

Ectopic pregnancy occurs whenever there is a condition that interfers with normal implantation of the fertilized ovum. The most frequent conditions are those that deter the transport of the fertilized ovum through the oviduct to the uterus. Conditions such as tubal infections, anomalies, or tumors are frequent causes. Iatrogenic factors such as tubal surgery with resultant adhesions can also block passage of the blastocyst. Certain techniques to prevent pregnancy such as elective abortion, intrauterine devices (about 15 million women worldwide are estimated to use IUDs), and tubal sterilization are believed to predispose to ectopic pregnancy. Ectopic pregnancy is believed to occur in some instances because of the proliferation of endometrial tissue to sites outside of the uterus (*endometriosis*). This tissue may attract the implantation of the blastocyst. Such tissue has been found in the tubal mucosa of an oviduct where an ectopic pregnancy has occurred, however, infrequently. This association has been described but not yet proven.

Occasionally, ectopic pregnancy will result from transabdominal migration of the ovum after fertilization. This delayed transport provides time for the blastocyst while it is still in the tube to develop more fully than it normally would, thus becoming ready for implantation before reaching the uterine cavity.

TYPES OF ECTOPIC PREGNANCIES

Implantation of the fertilized ovum in the oviduct accounts for 90–95% of all of the ectopic pregnancies (Fig. 21.1). Of all tubal pregnancies, about one-third are caused by tubal inflammatory diseases, frequently of gonococcal etiology. Before the widespread use of penicillin to treat gonorrheal infection of the tubes (*salpingitis*) the tubes became blocked resulting in sterility. Penicillin has enabled gonorrheal infections to be treated before they reach the oviducts or before they result in decreased tubal patency. Women who earlier would not have become pregnant may now add to the incidence of tubal pregnancies. About 60% of tubal pregnancies occur in the ampulla or fimbriated part of the oviduct, another 25% implant in the isthmus, and about 5% lodge in the interstitial part of the tube (Page et al., 1976).

When the fertilized ovum implants, the invasive action of the trophoblasts are believed to weaken the tubal structure predisposing it to rupture as the conceptus enlarges. Such a rupture will either extrude the embryo into the peritoneal cavity, or if the ampulla is the site of implantation, the embryo is likely to be expelled through the fimbriated end of the tube because of pressure from a hematoma formed when the conceptus separates from the tubal wall. Ectopic abortion from the tube usually occurs between the sixth and twelfth week of gestation. Some trophoblastic tissue may remain in the wall of the tube contributing to intraperitoneal hemorrhage.

Primary abdominal pregnancy, which is rare, develops within the peritoneal cavity rather than in association with the oviduct or adjacent structures such as the broad ligament (Pritchard & MacDonald, 1976). Occasionally, the blastocyst will be extruded from the tube and implant on some abdominal structure. Such *secondary abdominal pregnancies* have gone to term gestation and have resulted in the birth of a live infant. However, this too, is uncommon. Implantation of the blastocyst on a vital organ can cause serious damage to or death of the mother. Abdominal pregnancy at anytime predisposes to intraperitoneal abortion and hemorrhage.

The *cervix* is another site for ectopic pregnancy although such an occurrence is rare and usually does not progress beyond the twentieth week of gestation. Painless vaginal bleeding is a usual clinical finding. *Ovarian ectopic pregnancy* can also occur, and there are recorded cases of delivery of a term viable fetus.

One of the most dangerous sites for ectopic pregnancy is the *interstitial part of the fallopian tube.*

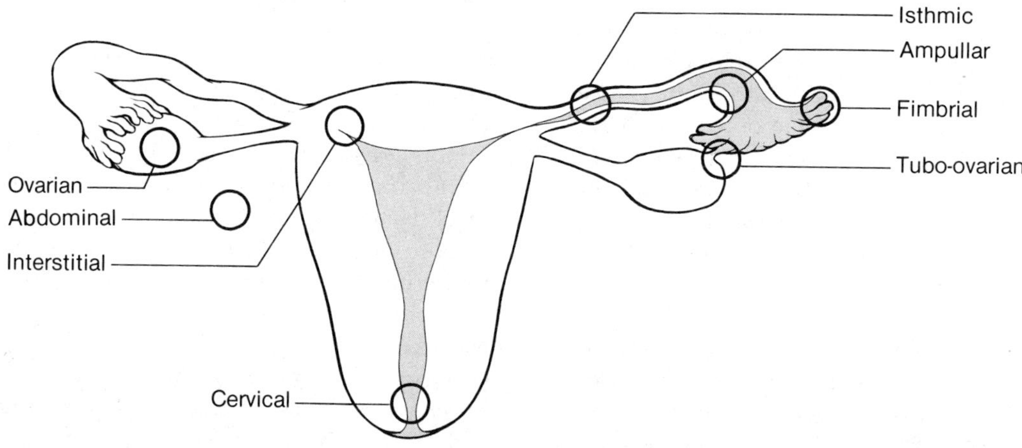

Figure 21.1
Sites for ectopic pregnancies.

Pregnancy in this area is concealed and diagnosis may be missed. Rupture of interstitial ectopic pregnancy often results in extensive hemorrhage because of the proximity of major maternal vessels in the uterus to the interstitial part and generalized uterine vascularity. These pregnancies may progress to 8–16 weeks of gestation before rupture.

CLINICAL PICTURE

Ectopic pregnancy in any site predisposes to maternal hemorrhage. Until such hemorrhage and associated pain and bleeding are evident, diagnosis of ectopic pregnancy is not made. Even in the presence of symptomatology, diagnosis may be missed. The classic symptoms of tubal ectopic pregnancy include:

- ▲ Severe lower abdominal pain usually confined to the lower right or left quadrant of the abdomen. This pain, which is a result of hemorrhage, from the ruptured ectopic pregnancy, is intense and sharp.
- ▲ Vertigo.
- ▲ Abdominal tenderness on palpation and exquisite pain on vaginal examination.
- ▲ Observation or palpation of a bulging posterior vaginal fornix resulting from accumulation of blood.
- ▲ Palpation of a soft mass lateral to the uterus on vaginal examination.
- ▲ Referred pain to the shoulder resulting from the rise of free blood in the peritoneal cavity to the diaphragm where the phrenic nerve is irritated. The right shoulder is most often affected.
- ▲ Symptoms of shock may be present; however, most women are normotensive with early ectopic rupture. Tachycardia or bradycardia may be the only early indicators of hemorrhage.

Ectopic pregnancies arising from sites other than the tube may be more difficult to diagnose for their symptomatology may vary. The most reliable adjunct to the diagnosis of ectopic pregnancy is an accurate history.

DIAGNOSIS

Tubal pregnancy is frequently confused with conditions such as salpingitis, twisted ovarian cyst, ruptured corpus luteum, or appendicitis. A differential diagnosis may be difficult to make, costing the woman precious minutes during which her life may be in jeopardy. An erroneous clinical diagnosis is not uncommon. The immunochemical pregnancy test is positive about 50% of the time. If it is positive, it will confirm that a pregnancy exists but will not aid in identifying the site of the pregnancy. Such a test relies on the presence of adequate amounts of circulating HCG; for these levels to be adequate, there must be viable trophoblastic cells close to maternal vascular channels where the hormone can be picked up and circulated. Such is often not the case in ectopic pregnancy.

Culdoscopy, culdocentesis, and laparoscopy may also be helpful in determining the presence of ruptured tissue or blood. Culdoscopy and culdocentesis can be performed transvaginally by entry of the scope or needle into the peritoneal cavity via Douglas's cul-de-sac in the posterior vaginal fornix and the pregnancy visualized or blood aspirated.

In some instances, clinical symptoms of pregnancy may be present; however, the amenorrhea of normal pregnancy may be replaced by vaginal spotting that serves to cloud diagnosis further. This clouding is particularly true with cervical ectopic pregnancy. Breast enlargement may also be present in ectopic pregnancy.

In a review of 4,000 cases of ectopic pregnancies, the following breakdown of symptoms was found (Huff & Pauerstein, 1979).

- ▲ Abdominal pain—96%
- ▲ Shoulder pain—17%
- ▲ Amenorrhea—76%
- ▲ Abnormal vaginal bleeding—83%
- ▲ Fainting—21%

TREATMENT

The treatment of ectopic pregnancy is designed to control hemorrhage and to save the woman's life. A laparotomy is performed as soon as diagnosis is made. Occasionally a *hysterectomy* will be necessary, but most often removal of the affected tube (*salpingectomy*) or of the tube and ovary (*salpingo-oophorectomy*) will suffice. If maternal vital organs are involved, treatment options may be limited and prognosis is grave.

PROGNOSIS

Ectopic pregnancy accounted for about 6% of maternal deaths over the past decade. Most of these maternal deaths were a result of hemorrhage. The risk of maternal death from ectopic pregnancy is about 1 death for every 800 ectopic pregnancies.

Ectopic pregnancy, particularly tubal pregnancy, tends to reoccur. About one-third of women who have had an ectopic pregnancy will deliver a living child from a subsequent normal pregnancy. There is an increased incidence of abortion among women with a history of ectopic pregnancy.

The death of the embryo/fetus is almost certain in an ectopic pregnancy. Where the embryo is extruded into the abdominal cavity, it may become mummified or be reabsorbed by the mother's body and never be recovered.

Placenta Previa and Abruptio Placentae

Although we will discuss placenta previa and abruptio placentae separately, the contrast between them will also be presented since being able to relate them improves recall of both. These are the two main conditions seen in last trimester bleeding and are important for the maternity nurse to recognize and understand.

PLACENTA PREVIA

The pathophysiology underlying *placenta previa* is that of an abnormally implanted placenta. The fertilized ovum implants low in the uterus in the vicinity of the internal os. In the course of labor as the cervix effaces, separation of the placenta occurs. There are three types of placenta previa—low placental implantation, partial placenta previa, and total placenta previa (Fig. 21.2). The total or complete previa is the most serious, causing early and often profuse hemorrhage.

Placenta previa occurs in about 1 in 200 pregnancies; the incidence is greater as age and parity increase. Past history of placenta previa or low segment cesarean section also increases the incidence of placenta previa. The classic sign of placenta previa (which occurs in 80% of the cases) is *painless vaginal bleeding*.

According to Huff and Paurestein (1979), the most accurate way to diagnose placenta previa is

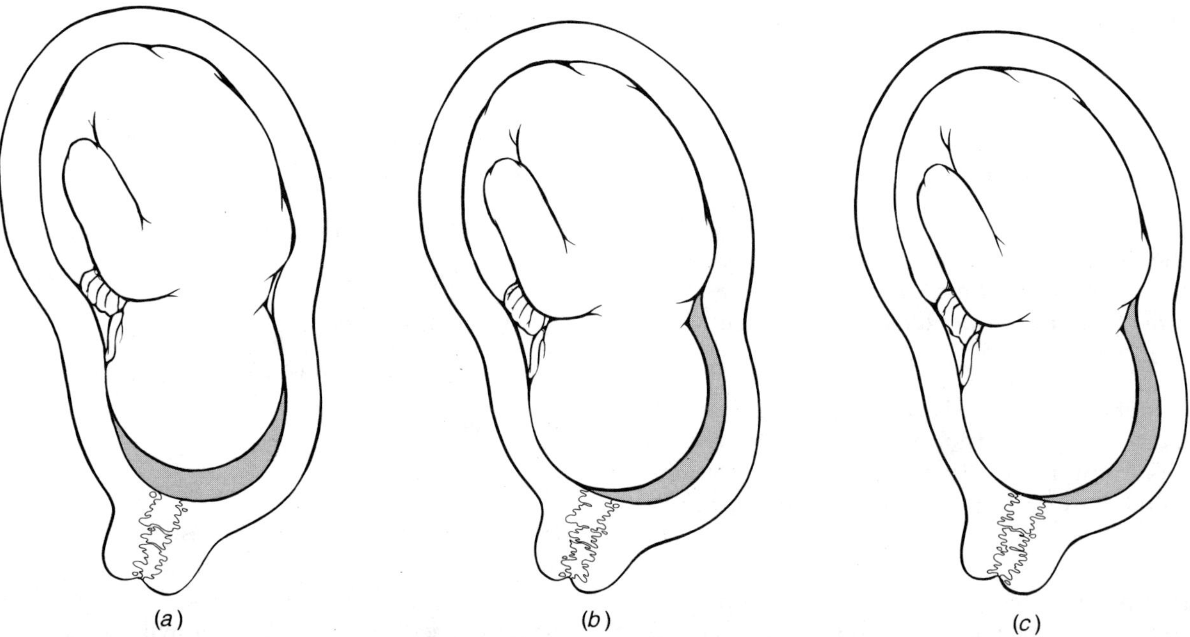

Figure 21.2
Placenta previa. (*a*) Complete; (*b*) partial; (*c*) marginal.

by direct method, that is, by inserting a finger at or near the cervix and palpating the placenta. However, this is never done unless the patient is in an operating room with blood ready and all preparations made for cesarean section since hemorrhage can be profuse. This is often referred to as a *double set up*. The nurse sets the woman up for vaginal examination and preparations for immediate cesarean are made at the same time. Other methods of diagnosing previa are amniography, x-ray, with or without contrast medium, and ultrasound. Since ultrasonic localization of the placenta is 95% accurate, it is used most often for diagnosis.

Maternal mortality from placenta previa was reduced in the 1920s when cesarean delivery and blood transfusion became part of the treatment protocol. Focus today is on improving fetal mortality, which is usually a result of prematurity. Management focuses on delaying delivery until the fetus is able to survive outside the uterus. Care of the mother depends on gestational age of the fetus, the amount of bleeding, and when the first episode of bleeding began. Characteristically, the first bleeding episode is scant, and if no rectal or vaginal examination is done (no nurse should ever do a rectal or vaginal examination on any bleeding maternity patient) the bleeding usually subsides spontaneously. Delivery, depending on the type of previa, may be vaginal since the head of the fetus can sometimes act as a tamponade. In marginal placenta previa, cesarean section may be done.

ABRUPTIO PLACENTAE

In contrast to placenta previa, which is an abnormally implanted placenta, *abruptio placentae* is a normally implanted placenta that lets go, or separates, between the twentieth week and the birth of the neonate. The incidence of placental abruption varies from 0.7 to 2.0%. Premature separation of the placenta can be either partial or complete, and hemorrhage can be either overt (visible) or concealed (hidden or occult). When the placenta lets go in the center there is bleeding, but clot formation is occurring retroplacentally so no bleeding is seen. If the placenta separates and the blood escapes from beneath the placenta and dissects the membrane off the uterine wall, the blood flows through the cervix resulting in external bleeding.

In Pritchard's (1970) study of 201 women, he found positive etiologic relationship to the following.

- ▲ Maternal hypertension (47% had diastolic blood pressure over 90)
- ▲ High parity (a para 7 had 3 times the incidence of a para 3 and 6 times of a para 0)
- ▲ Past incidence of abruptio (30-fold increased chance of severe abruption in a woman who had one previously)

Clinical manifestations include vaginal bleeding and pain. Approximately 20% of women with abruptio placentae have no visible bleeding; of the 80% who have visible bleeding, there can be more concealed than apparent blood loss. This situation gives rise to the symptom that shock may be out of proportion to blood loss, which is not actually true, but it may be out of proportion to visible blood loss. The abdominal pain can be described as "labor pains," uterine tenderness, or uterine tetany (contracted and boardlike). Overall perinatal loss with abruptio placentae is as high as 50% in some series.

Traditionally, blood loss in placental abruption is underestimated, and blood pressure and pulse rate are not reliable indicators. Central venous pressure monitoring and urinary output monitoring are the most useful guides to correcting hypovolemia.

Management of women with placental abruption includes blood and intravenous fluids to replace circulating blood volume. If the fetus is alive and in no distress, vaginal delivery is attempted. If the fetus is dead, vaginal delivery is indicated as well. However, if the fetus is in distress, cesarean delivery may be indicated. Electronic fetal monitoring, as well as monitoring fluids and output of the mother, is critical. Coagulopathy (see disseminated intravascular coagulation, DIC) is a common complication of abruptio placentae, although it is more likely to occur if the fetus has died. DIC is always a secondary condition, so the management is to treat the underlying condition, which in this case is the pregnancy. The goal of management is to deliver the woman as quickly as possible, replacing fluids, and blood volume that will also replace clotting factors. Use of heparin in DIC, secondary to placental abruption, is not recommended (Pritchard, 1970).

Contrast of Symptoms of Abruptio Placentae and Placenta Previa

The contrast of the symptoms of these two last trimester bleeding problems is presented below from Willson and Carrington (1979) and should be committed to memory. Recalling the underlying pathophysiology of these two conditions and remembering the symptoms of each will allow the maternity nurse to be able to differentiate and subsequently intervene swiftly and effectively.

Abruptio Placentae	*Placenta Previa*
The bleeding is accompanied by pain	The bleeding is painless.
The blood usually is dark.	The blood is bright red.
Signs of shock may be out of proportion to visible bleeding.	Observed bleeding and signs of shock are comparable.
The first bleeding is usually profuse.	Bleeding is usually slight at the onset.
The uterus is firm, tender and tetanically contracted.	The uterus is soft, not tender, and may be contracting.
The fetus may be difficult to feel, and fetal heart tones may be absent or irregular.	The fetus can be felt easily, and fetal heart tones usually are present.
The placenta cannot be felt.	The placenta may be felt.
The patient may have toxemia, but the blood pressure may be low because of excessive bleeding.	There is no evidence of toxemia.
The urine may contain protein, or the patient may be anuric.	The urine usually is normal.
A clotting defect may be present.	The blood usually clots normally.

Source: Wilson, J. R., Carrington, E. R. *Obstetrics and Gynecology* (6th ed.). St. Louis: C. V. Mosby, 1979.

Nursing Care of the Antepartum Patient with Vaginal Bleeding

Medical treatment of the bleeding patient focuses on controlling the bleeding, replacing the lost blood, and emptying the uterus. Nursing care of any bleeding antepartum patient revolves around the general principles described below, remembering that the underlying pathophysiology and the point in the pregnancy both influence intervention. For example, one of the obvious differences between early and late antepartal bleeding is that with the former, the fetus is frequently not viable. The nurse needs to be alert to the general signs of hemorrhage remembering that in obstetrics blood pressure and pulse changes are not always the early indicators. Cool, clammy extremities, thirst, and anxiety may first alert the nurse to impending hypovolemic shock. General nursing measures should include:

- ▲ No vaginal or rectal exam.
- ▲ Start intravenous fluids (most institutions have a standing order for this) using at least an 18-gauge needle (adequate for blood).
- ▲ Do a clot observation test. When the IV is started, draw blood, place approximately 5 cc in a clean test tube, and label with woman's name and the time. If the blood fails to clot (5–7 minutes) or the clot is unstable, a clotting defect can be anticipated. This is a quick method of making an initial assessment; more definitive coagulation studies should follow.
- ▲ Withhold food and fluids.
- ▲ Type and cross match for at least 1,000 cc of blood.
- ▲ Monitor intake and output.
- ▲ Test urine for glucose and protein.
- ▲ Administer oxygen as necessary.
- ▲ Evaluate blood loss—measure or weigh blood-soaked pads.

- ▲ Ascertain if adequate and key personnel are available. (Surgery may be necessary.)
- ▲ Reassure and inform the woman and family by word and deed.

Disseminated Intravascular Coagulation

Disseminated intravascular coagulation (DIC) is a secondary event encountered in obstetrics, as well as in many medical–surgical conditions, and occurs when the factors opposing and favoring clotting become deranged. *Acute DIC* (*chronic DIC* is less common in obstetrics) is characterized by development of a shock state and is a clinical emergency. The DIC syndrome is sometimes called *defibrinogenemia* and *fibrinopenia*. *Consumption coagulopathy*, another term used, is descriptive of the clinical picture—bleeding and consumption of clotting factors. Instead of coagulation taking place within the confines of a platelet plug (recall the delicate balance that normally exists in the human body between coagulation and fibrinolysis), it occurs in a disseminated or scattered fashion throughout the vascular system.

The basic pathophysiology is secondary to a host of diseases and diverse etiologic factors that cause the release of procoagulant substances in the blood, for example, bacterial toxins, thrombosis-producing placental tissue, and amniotic fluid. Two major events occur—microthrombosis in the peripheral circulation and the development of a coagulation defect because the clotting factors are consumed (used up). This results in an initial state of hypercoagulability followed by hypocoagulability (as clotting factors are consumed). The laboratory test that is most diagnostic is for the presence of fibrin breakdown products (FBP)*; other laboratory tests that are significant are for decreased fibrinogen and platelets and for prolongation of the thrombin time.

Stress plays an important role in DIC as it is a primary activation of fibrinolysis. It may be helpful to recall that the capillary system in the adult exceeds 100,000 miles. If you can picture the amount of blood clot in the capillary system, it is not difficult to realize that clotting factors are used up faster than they are replaced. The patient's bleeding is a result of the above factors plus the fact that the reticuloendothelial system fails to keep pace (cannot clear fibrin) and the cycle perpetuates itself. In summary, the pathophysiologic process is:

- ▲ DIC is always secondary to some other pathologic process.
- ▲ DIC is a serious bleeding disorder occurring because of a hypercoagulable state.
- ▲ Extensive capillary thrombosis leads to platelet and clotting factor depletion.
- ▲ Simultaneous events occur
    - ▾ Arterial hypotension
    - ▾ Opening of A–V shunts
    - ▾ Capillary blood stagnation
    - ▾ Acidosis
    - ▾ Capillary thrombosis
- ▲ Stress associated with DIC increases fibrinolytic activity.
- ▲ Lysis of the formed microclots occurs as the fibrinolytic system is activated.
- ▲ Fibrin breakdown products appear.

In obstetrics, delivery usually removes the cause of the DIC and hemostasis is resumed. The use of heparin in the maternity woman, except in cases of IUFD, is contraindicated since the possibility of a residual heparin load in the postpartum woman with multiple bleeding sites (placental, cervical trauma) is a great risk.

Management of DIC and specific maternity complications includes the following (Coopland, 1976).

1. Abruptio placentae
    - ▾ Rupture membranes to initiate labor and theoretically reduce pressure on the retroplacental clot, which may be infusing clot-producing substances into the maternal circulation.
    - ▾ Transfuse liberally with fresh whole blood, fresh frozen plasma, or packed red blood cells (blood loss is frequently underestimated in abruptio placentae).

*Also called fibrin degradation products (FDP); fibrin split products (FSP).

- Deliver as quickly as possible (cesarean section may be indicated in cases of disproportion because DIC is progressing or renal function is deteriorating).

2. Intrauterine fetal death, also known as the "dead fetus" syndrome
   - Coagulation studies once IUFD is suspected (especially if more than 3 weeks).
   - Treat with heparin 24–48 hours before operative intervention (allows for clearance of FBP and for hemostasis to re-establish).
3. Amniotic fluid embolism
   - Renal cortical necrosis and bleeding diasthesis common if patient survives the pulmonary assault.
4. Gram-negative endotoxemia
   - Remove focus of infection.
   - Administer antibiotics.
   - Blood transfusion.
   - Steroids.
5. Pre-eclampsia–eclampsia
   - Laboratory studies may indicate hypercoagulability.
   - Prophylactic administration of heparin in selected cases (reverses thrombocytopenia and increased levels of FBP and improves placental function as evidenced by increased urinary estriol output) (Heine, 1977).

NURSING MANAGEMENT OF THE WOMAN WITH DIC

Nursing care is key to successful patient outcome in DIC. Since predisposing factors include hypotension and shock, early signs are often detected by the nurse and should be treated vigorously with blood and fluid replacement. Monitoring of urine output (30–60 cc/hr) and respiratory function must be done in order to detect regression or improvement of the syndrome.

The alert maternity nurse can prevent DIC by being alert for signs of subacute DIC. Evidence of thrombocytopenia, petechiae under the skin, and decreased hematocrit with no clinical bleeding are all suspicious signs. Before acute clinical bleeding is observed, the nurse sometimes notes a previous intravenous site that oozes and does not clot; this can be significant. Scrutiny of laboratory reports, assessment for clinical signs of DIC, and assessment of the patient's stress level are all critical. Excellent nursing care along with correction of the underlying cause of DIC can make the difference in a successful outcome.

Anterior Pituitary Necrosis

Anterior pituitary necrosis, which occurs postdelivery and is called *Sheehan's syndrome*, is preceded by hypovolemic shock, DIC, or severe puerperal infection. The pituitary gland, which is enlarged in pregnancy, is susceptible to hemorrhage, thrombosis, infection, and subsequent necrosis in the postpartum period. If a sizable portion of the anterior lobe is destroyed, gonadatropic, adrenal, and thyroid functions are depressed. Hormone replacement is essential. Maternity nurses who encounter a patient with DIC need to be alert for this syndrome.

Hydatidiform Mole

Hydatidiform mole is a neoplastic proliferation of the trophoblast in which terminal villa are transformed into vesicles that are filled with clear viscid material. It is usually benign, but it has malignant potential. Although, hydatidiform mole is relatively uncommon in the United States (1 in 2,000–2,500 pregnancies), it is fairly common in the Orient (1–200). The etiology is unknown, but the pathology involved is that the fertilized ovum deteriorates and the chorionic villi change into a mass of clear, grapelike vesicles that resemble tapioca. Unless the typical grapelike vesicles are passed, most patients with moles are treated for abortion. Clinical symptoms include:

- A uterus that is larger than expected for duration of pregnancy
- Nausea and vomiting
- Brownish-red discharge
- Fullness and thinning of the lower uterine segment
- Early diagnosis of toxemia before 24 weeks

Laboratory findings may reveal proteinuria; and hematocrit and hemoglobin values as well as RBCs are decreased. Human chorionic gonadotropic (HCG) may be elevated as much as 1–2 million IU in 24 hours. Normal value at 10 weeks of gestation is about 400,000 IU. Fetal heart tones, of course, cannot be heard. A positive diagnosis can be made by ultrasound.

Management includes evacuation of the uterus as soon as the diagnosis is made. Willson and Carrington (1979) suggest that women over 35 may be candidates for total abdominal hysterectomy as malignant potentialities of hydatidiform moles are greater in older women. Every woman who has been diagnosed as having a hydatidiform mole should be watched until the physician is certain that malignant trophoblastic disease did not occur.

Choriocarcinoma

Choriocarcinoma is the highly malignant trophoblastic tumor that can follow hydatidiform mole, abortion, or even normal pregnancy. One-third to one-half of choriocarcinomas are preceded by hydatidiform moles, but only 20% of the latter have malignant tenderness (Willson & Carrington, 1979). Forty percent of choriocarcinoma follow abortion and fewer follow term pregnancy and delivery. In choriocarcinoma, bleeding usually increases as more tissue is destroyed. Unfortunately, the first evidence of a problem may be caused by symptoms of metastasis to the lungs or brain.

Before the availability of chemotherapeutic drugs, 80–85% of women with choriocarcinoma died within a year. With drug therapy, the overall remission is about 75%, and if the disease is treated early, may be as high as 90%. Women who have been treated are checked monthly for a year after the gonadotropin concentration has returned to normal.

Hypertensive Disorders

Hypertensive disorders can arise before, during, or immediately after pregnancy; in some texts they are referred to collectively as the *toxemias of pregnancy*. From 7 to 10% of all pregnancies are complicated by hypertension—one-half of which is pre-eclampsia and one-half is chronic hypertensive disease. The American College of Obstetricians and Gynecologists proposes the following classification.

- ▲ Pre-eclampsia–eclampsia
- ▲ Chronic hypertension
  - ▾ Essential
  - ▾ Secondary
  - ▾ Chronic hypertension with superimposed pre-eclampsia–eclampsia
  - ▾ Late or transient hypertension

PRE-ECLAMPSIA–ECLAMPSIA

Pre-eclampsia is a clinical syndrome of unknown etiology occurring after the twentieth week of gestation; it is characterized by hypertension, edema, and/or proteinuria. The differential diagnosis between pre-eclampsia and *eclampsia* is made on the basis of seizure. Once the woman convulses, she is eclamptic. Pre-eclampsia is more common in nulligravidas; predisposing factors include diabetes mellitus, multiple gestation, hydatidiform mole, renovascular disease, pre-existing hypertension, and malnutrition.

Pathophysiologic changes occurring with the progression of pre-eclampsia are:

- ▲ ***Arteriolar Spasm.*** Generalized arteriolar spasm that results in decreased peripheral resistance and decreased flow to vital organs (perfusion ↓).
- ▲ ***Major Fluid Shifts.*** Intravascular fluid moves to the extravascular space resulting in generalized edema, a rising hematocrit, and rapid weight gain.
- ▲ ***Sodium Retention.*** Sodium increase accompanies increase in total water but is proportionately less than water increase.
- ▲ ***Decreased Renal and Uterine Blood Flow.*** Acute vasospasm causes a decrease in renal blood flow and uterine blood flow, which accounts for higher intrauterine fetal death rate and fetal distress during labor.
- ▲ ***Decreased Renin and Aldosterone Levels.*** How this affects the progression of the disease is unclear.
- ▲ ***Decreased Estrogen and Progesterone.*** Again, how this hormonal decrease affects the pathophysiology of pre-eclampsia is unclear.
- ▲ ***DIC.*** Evidence that DIC occurs in relation to pre-eclampsia–eclampsia (see section on DIC this chapter).

Detection and management of the pre-eclamptic woman is aimed at prevention of convulsions. The only cure for pre-eclampsia is delivery; if the mother's condition remains stable and if the fetal health as determined by tests of fetal well-being (see Chapter 20) remains good, the pregnancy is allowed to continue until the fetus is mature. If the mother's condition worsens, induction of labor and/or cesarean birth is indicated. Pre-eclampsia is classified as mild or severe.

Mild Pre-eclampsia (Any two of these three symptoms indicates the woman is pre-eclamptic.)

- ▲ ***Hypertension.*** Blood pressure of 140/90 or 30 mm Hg increase in systolic or 15 mm Hg increase in diastolic. The levels must occur on two occasions at least 6 hours apart to be an indication of hypertension. (A baseline blood pressure is critical in order to assess this symptom accurately for if the woman has a baseline pressure of 90/60, a change to 120/75 is indicative of hypertension).
- ▲ ***Edema.*** Sudden weight gain of greater than 2 lb a week.
- ▲ ***Proteinuria.*** Excretion of 500 mg or more in 24 hours (trace, 1+ dipstick).

Severe Pre-eclampsia

- ▲ ***Hypertension.*** Blood pressure of 160/100 or higher (systolic over 200 mm Hg usually indicates chronic hypertensive disease).
- ▲ ***Edema.*** Marked weight gain and edema of face and hands.
- ▲ ***Proteinuria.*** Excretion of 5 gm in 24 hours (3 + 4+ dipstick).
- ▲ ***Later Signs.*** Concentrated urine, oliguria; headaches, dizziness; visual disturbances; hyperreflexia; epigastric pain (alarming sign that may herald seizure).

Eclampsia

- ▲ Convulsions with no other apparent reason or pathology.

Antepartum management of the pre-eclamptic woman includes the following.

- ▲ Early detection during prenatal care. The earliest sign is the edema, which is evidenced by weight gain.
- ▲ No salt or diet restrictions; *no* diuretics (dietary or salt restrictions do not help pre-eclampsia and may have serious side effects such as hyponatremia or hypokalemia).
- ▲ Bed rest at home if the condition is mild. Woman is encouraged to be in left lateral Sims' position to improve circulatory status and aid in reversing fluid shift.
- ▲ Evaluation of maternal and fetal vital signs (fetal well-being studies)
- ▲ Education regarding toxemias of pregnancy and the need for rest.
- ▲ Assessment and maintenance of balanced diet.
- ▲ Psychosocial support.
- ▲ Hospitalization if bed rest at home does not result in improvement of edema.

Intrapartum management of pre-eclamptic patient includes the following.

- ▲ Vaginal delivery unless fetal distress or other obstetric indications occur.
- ▲ Administer magnesium sulfate to prevent seizures if signs of pre-eclampsia persist.
- ▲ Protocols for magnesium sulfate can be either IV or intramuscular (IM). Initial dose IM 10 gm (50% solution) followed by 5 gm every 4 hours; initial dose IV 4 gm (10% solution); continuous IM 1–2 gm per hour (see discussion regarding magnesium sulfate later in this chapter).
- ▲ Have antidote for magnesium sulfate (calcium gluconate) at bedside.
- ▲ Monitor intake and output. Once magnesium sulfate therapy is started, a Foley catheter should be inserted in order to be able to assess hourly output.
- ▲ Test urine for protein hourly.
- ▲ Monitor maternal and fetal vital signs (may include electronic monitoring).
- ▲ Assess progress of labor.

- ▲ Reduce stimuli in environment that may trigger convulsion.
- ▲ Maintain seizure precautions (tongue blade, suction, oxygen).
- ▲ Maintain safety measures (side rails).
- ▲ Maintain central venous pressure monitoring if indicated.
- ▲ Assess for abruptio placentae.
- ▲ Keep patient's family informed.

Postpartum management of pre-eclampic–eclamptic patient includes the following.

- ▲ Maintain magnesium sulfate therapy until danger of convulsion has passed (may be 24–48 hours postpartum).
- ▲ Perform all routine postpartum assessments including vital signs, fundal measurement, and lochia.

Magnesium sulfate therapy. Magnesium sulfate ($MgSO_4$) is the drug of choice to prevent eclamptic seizures. It is a cerebral depressant that reduces neuromuscular irritability—magnesium replaces calcium at the myoneural junction. $MgSO_4$ relaxes all muscles, and respiratory depression or arrest is a dreaded side effect. For this reason IV calcium gluconate is kept at the bedside. When $MgSO_4$ is administered IV, it causes burning, and patients will say that they feel on fire; it also can cause nausea. $MgSO_4$ must be administered slowly, and it is important to forewarn the woman about the side effects and reassure her that they are only temporary. Intramuscular $MgSO_4$ is also very painful. It should be given deep IM and Z track. The needle should be changed after drawing up the medication and before injecting the woman as the medication is necrotic to the tissues. $MgSO_4$ dosage should never be repeated without checking the following three criteria.

- ▲ Deep tendon reflex (knee jerk present)
- ▲ Urine output greater than 30 cc/hr
- ▲ Respiratory rate greater than 12–14 per minute

Nursing care of the pre-eclamptic–eclamptic patient, as in the other at risk conditions described in this chapter, requires knowledge and skill.

CHRONIC HYPERTENSION

Chronic hypertension is diagnosed by history of hypertension before pregnancy or before the twentieth week of gestation. If the woman is not seen until late in her pregnancy, it is sometimes impossible to determine if the diagnosis is pre-eclampsia or chronic hypertension.

In general, chronic hypertensive women are older and are more often parous. The hypertension is often essential (unknown), but it may be secondary to chronic pyelonephritis, diabetic nephropathy, and so on. Although the fetus of the chronic hypertensive mother often suffers intrauterine growth retardation (IUGR), most mothers do well (85%).

CHRONIC HYPERTENSION WITH SUPERIMPOSED PRE-ECLAMPSIA–ECLAMPSIA

About 15% of chronic hypertensive women develop superimposed pre-eclampsia. It is diagnosed when there is increase in the hypertension (30 mm Hg systolic and 15 mm Hg diastolic) and sustained proteinuria and edema. The pre-eclampsia in these women tends to occur earlier and progress more rapidly. These women are frequently very ill (contributing to this is age and general poor health) and require expert nursing care.

LATE OR TRANSIENT HYPERTENSION

Late or transient hypertension is defined as the occurrence of hypertension only late in pregnancy, in labor, or in the postpartum woman who was normotensive. No proteinuria or edema is noted, and the hypertension usually disappears in 10 days. It is postulated that these women may have latent essential hypertension or mild pre-eclampsia.

Rh Isoimmunization

Erythroblastosis fetalis, or hemolytic disease of the newborn, is discussed in Chapter 23. The most important factor in maternal management of Rh isoimmune disease is diagnosis. If the mother is Rh negative, an indirect Coombs' test should be done to ascertain presence of any antibodies. (If the father is negative, no problems will occur. It is the situation with an Rh+ father and an Rh− mother that is of concern.) Sensitization occurs when Rh positive cells enter the circulation of the Rh negative person. The most common time for this to occur is at delivery (fetus is Rh+), but it can also occur with abortion, ectopic pregnancy, amniocentesis, fetal–maternal transfusion during pregnancy, or after incorrectly cross-matched blood transfusion.

If the mother is assessed as having antibodies, she is followed throughout the pregnancy with titers. Once the mother's titer is 1:32 in the first sensitized pregnancy or 1:16 in any subsequent pregnancy, amniocentesis is done to evaluate the risk to the fetus. Concentration of bilirubin and other breakdown products from the lysed fetal RBCs can be detected in amniotic fluid by spectrophotometry. Analysis of this data is the basis for intervention or intrauterine transfusion (see laboratory studies in this chapter).

Fortunately, in the 1960s treatment of Rh sensitization for most women became prevention. D-immune globulin (Rhogam) has been available since 1968 and is highly effective in preventing sensitization. Rhogam prevents the antibodies from forming. Candidates to receive Rhogam are Rh negative women with no indication of sensitization as evidenced by indirect Coombs' test and who have:

- ▲ Delivered an Rh positive infant
- ▲ Received an Rh positive blood transfusion
- ▲ Had a spontaneous abortion or ectopic pregnancy
- ▲ Had amniocentesis in the second trimester in which bleeding occurred

Rhogam provides only passive immunity and must be repeated after each potentially sensitizing event.

ABO INCOMPATABILITY

Most hemolytic diseases of the newborn are caused by ABO incompatabilities between mother and fetus, but fortunately these are not usually severe and are readily managed in the newborn (see Chapter 23).

Other Medical Conditions Complicating Pregnancy

Neurologic conditions, such as epilepsy, myasthenia gravis, and multiple sclerosis, are mentioned only briefly since they are less frequently encountered. It is important to remember that many times maternity nurses must apply what they know about a particular medical–surgical condition to what they know about pregnancy and then plan the care for the particular woman.

Epilepsy is totally unpredictable in its effect on pregnancy. If anticonvulsant drugs need to be used, the possibility of congenital anomalies and/or intrauterine growth retardation is greater than normal. Pregnancy in patients with myasthenia gravis and multiple sclerosis, though not totally predictable, seems to be well tolerated.

Surgical Conditions Complicating Pregnancy

Appendicitis and intestinal obstruction occurring during pregnancy will not resolve without surgical intervention; prognosis is usually satisfactory but is dependent on the stage and status of the pregnancy. Attacks of gallbladder disease, on the other hand, may be responsive to medical management and surgical intervention can be delayed. Again, application of knowledge about the particular medical or surgical problem to the individual pregnant woman and her pregnancy will direct the treatment modality that is optimal for her and the fetus.

Malignant melanomas, although rare during pregnancy, must be treated surgically according to protocols for nonpregnant patients. Although placental metastasis of malignant melanoma has been reported, transmission to the fetus is rare (Friedman & Mc Mahon, 1960).

Infections Complicating Pregnancy

PYELONEPHRITIS—ACUTE AND CHRONIC

Acute *pyelonephritis* and upper urinary tract infections usually occur late in the second or early in the third trimester. The incidence is 1–3% of all pregnant women; once pyelonephritis occurs, it tends to recur in subsequent pregnancies. The infection can be a descending one, that is, organisms from the adjacent colon invade the kidney.

Symptoms may be obscure initially, but within 2–3 days pain becomes severe and radiates downward to the pelvis or groin area, temperature rises, and the woman often has chills. As the infection continues, dysuria, frequent, cloudy urine, and hematuria can follow. When infection peaks, the fever can swing from a high of 104–106°F (40–41°C) to a low of 97–98°F (36–37°C). The patient appears very ill, and palpation of kidney areas causes excrutiating pain. Diagnosis is confirmed by culturing a catheterized urine specimen, and the antibiotic treatment is begun. Fluid intake should be at least 3000 ml per day unless the patient is vomiting, in which case parenteral fluids are instituted. In addition to antibiotic treatment of the infection, a urinary antiseptic may be ordered. Analgesics, codeine, aspirin, or Demerol can be used to control pain, depending on the severity and the stage of the pregnancy. Although pyelonephritis is more often seen postpartum, it does occur in the antepartum woman.

Acute pyelonephritis, if inadequately treated, may not be completely eradicated and recurrent attacks may occur and the infection becomes chronic. In time this can result in tissue damage and impaired kidney function. Chronic pyelonephritis complicates pregnancy since acute attacks are likely to occur and permanent damage can result. Women who have chronic urinary tract infections are often treated prophylactically during pregnancy. If renal function is impaired and blood pressure is elevated, pregnancy may be contraindicated.

RESPIRATORY INFECTIONS

Pregnant women are more susceptible to the common cold and upper respiratory infection than are nonpregnant women. Symptomatic treatment is in order, and there is no evidence to suggest that the usual viruses that presumably cause the common cold have teratogenic effects. Pneumonia was a more serious problem during pregnancy before antibiotics, and although antibiotics will not influence the influenza virus, antibiotic therapy may reduce the severity of the complications.

OTHER INFECTIOUS DISEASES

There are infectious diseases that pregnant women are susceptible to that do not affect the pregnancy and, unfortunately, some that have serious deleterious effects. Table 21.2 shows some infectious conditions and their maternal symptoms and fetal effects. (See also Chapter 27.)

TABLE 21.2
MATERNAL INFECTION IN PREGNANCY

Agent	*Maternal Effects*	*Fetal–Neonatal Effects*
Cytomegalovirus (CMV)	Virus carried for life, probably in infectious form Subclinical or mild onset in most adults Usually no maternal warning of symptoms Sexually transmitted	Intrauterine or neonatal death Premature delivery Severe generalized disease CNS disease; microcephaly Impaired uterine growth Hemolytic anemia and jaundice Hepatosplenomegaly
Herpes genitalis [Herpes simplex virus (HSV) II]	Infection recurs throughout lifetime Triggered by infection, stress Virus lies dormant in sensory nerve ganglia (more severe in pregnancy)	Abortion, premature birth Transplacental infection rare Neonatal infection includes mild infection with a few skin

TABLE 21.2 (continued)

Agent	*Maternal Effects*	*Fetal–Neonatal Effects*
	Genital herpes at delivery indication for cesarean birth Usually involves external genitalia, vagina, and cervix Painful vesicles that drain and become ulcerations Fetus affected via maternal genital tract Indications that if acquired during adolescence may lead to invasive carcinoma in middle age Frequency of intercourse; number of partners are factors	lesions or viremia, severe generalized disease Neonatal infection Mortality rate high
Varicella (chicken pox) (virus)	Characteristic skin lesions Shingles (in some instances) Clinical course mild to severe In some cases disseminated epidemic type may cause maternal or fetal death	Chorioamnionitis—septicemia Congenital or neonatal varicella—rare, mortality high Premature delivery
Rubeola (virus)	Uncommon during pregnancy because of childhood immunity If present, clinical symptoms mild to severe May cause abortion; premature labor	Perinatal death Congenital or neonatal measles
Influenza (virus)	Increased incidence during pregnancy Clinical course mild to severe	Abortion; premature labor Congenital malformation Anencephaly
Mumps (virus)	Clinical course mild to severe Parotitis Fever	Abortion; premature birth Stillbirth Congenital anomalies
Coxsackie B (virus)	Clinical manifestations rarely seen in mother	Fetal death Congenital malformations Meningoencephalitis or myocarditis
Polio (virus)	Clinical symptoms mild to severe Women affected in first trimester tend to abort	Perinatal death Growth retardation Congenital or acquired poliomyelitis
Variola (small pox) (virus)	Rare because of vaccinations Clinical symptoms mild to severe Abortion; premature labor Postpartal hemorrhage common	Death Abortion Intrauterine infection
Hepatitis (virus)	Clinical symptoms mild to severe Treatable with supportive therapy Liver failure is potential concern	Fetal anomalies Abortion Neonatal hepatitis
Serum hepatitis (hepatitis B)	May be transmitted sexually	Intrauterine fetal death Infection occurs during birth

Agent	Maternal Effects	Fetal–Neonatal Effects
Listeria (bacteria)	Urinary frequency or dysuria Enteritis Fever Abortion or premature labor Amnionitis Placentitis Treatable with penicillin	Death—mortality rate high Generalized disease Delayed infection (meningitis)
Gonococcus (bacteria)	Mother often symptom free Postnatal complications include salpingitis, dermatitis, and arthritis if disease is untreated	Prematurity Ophthalmia neonatorum by direct infection
Group B streptococcus (bacteria)	Amnionitis Puerperal sepsis Septicemia	Septicemia Meningitis Mortality rate high
Tuberculosis (bacillus)	Mild-to-severe clinical symptoms depending on type, maternal resistance, therapeutic maternal response	Premature birth Congenital infection rare
Syphilis (spirochete)	Varies with stage of infection May be asymptomatic Chancre Rash	Midtrimester abortion Congenital syphilis Septicemia Skin lesions Anemia Jaundice Periostitis
Toxoplasmosis (protozoa)	Headache, malaise Often asymptomatic Associated with cat feces, raw meat	Death rate high Hydrocephalus Microcephalus Mental retardation Cerebral calcification Hepatosplenomegaly
Malaria (protozoa)	Clinical symptoms mild to severe—chills, fever Associated with tropical climates Severity of disease determines therapy Abortion Premature labor Recurrence of disease postpartum	Impaired intrauterine growth Neonatal infection SGA Choroquine toxicity—retinal damage—death
Pyelonephritis (bacteria)	Acute urinary tract infection Chills and fever Tenderness of kidney May be asymptomatic Incidence higher in women with diabetes, dystocia	Prematurity Sulfonamides may cause jaundice, hemolytic anemia Nitrofurantoin—megoblastic anemia

SUMMARY

Chapter 21 presented a comprehensive review of major maternal risk conditions. The discussion was divided into those conditions pre-existing and complicating pregnancy and those conditions arising from pregnancy.

Cardiac disease, diabetes mellitus, and thyroid disease were described. Underlying pathophysiology and nursing and medical management of the patient antepartum, intrapartum, and postpartum were included. This was followed by a section on bleeding problems occurring during pregnancy. Early pregnancy bleeding and abortion were defined, and types of abortion were discussed. Ectopic pregnancy, including incidence, pathophysiology, sites, symptoms, and nursing implications were extensively described.

The next section of the chapter was a discussion and differentiation of the two major conditions resulting in late or third trimester bleeding—placenta previa and abruptio placentae. Underlying pathophysiology and relationships to other pregnancy complications such as hypertension were described. Nursing protocols and management of any bleeding antepartum patient were enumerated.

Disseminated intravascular coagulation was defined and its pathophysiology and relationships to specific obstetric conditions were described. The significance of the nursing role in DIC was stressed. Sheehan's syndrome and hydatidiform mole were mentioned.

Hypertensive disorders in pregnancy was given considerable attention. Classification of hypertension and nursing and medical management throughout pregnancy were described. The use of magnesium sulfate therapy and nursing responsibilities related to administration of this drug were stressed.

Rh isoimmune disease and ABO incompatability were thoroughly discussed. Other medical and surgical conditions complicating pregnancy such as epilepsy and appendicitis were reviewed briefly.

The last section focused on infection and pregnancy. Pyelonephritis and respiratory infection were described. Many other infections, some of which have serious implications for the fetus, were presented in Table 21.2.

REFERENCES AND READINGS

Assali, N. *Pathophysiology of Gestation: Fetal Placental Disorders, Vol. II.* New York: Academic Press, 1972.

Bahr, J. Rising Perinatal Infections, Herpes Virus Hominis Type 2 in Women and Newborns. *Am J Matern Child Nurs* 3(1):16, 1978.

Butnarescu, G. F., Tillotson, D. M., Villarreal, P. P. *Perinatal Nursing: Volume 2, Reproductive Risk.* New York: John Wiley & Sons, 1980.

Chesley, L. C. Hypertensive Disorders of Pregnancy, in Hellman, L. M., Pritchard, J. A. (Eds.), *Williams Obstetrics* (14th ed.). New York: Appleton-Century-Crofts, 1970.

Coopland, A. T. The Hemostatic Mechanism and Its Disturbances in Pregnancy, in Goodwin, Godden, Chance (Eds.), *Perinatal Medicine.* Baltimore: Williams & Wilkins, 1976.

Dove, S. L., Davies, B. L. Catharsis for High-Risk Antenatal Inpatients. *Am J Matern Child Nurs* 4(2):96, 1979.

Edwards, M. S. Venereal Herpes: A Nursing Overview. *J Obstet Gynecol Nurs* 7(5):7, 1978.

Friedman, W. L., McMahon, F. J. Placental Metastasis: Review of the Literature and Report of a Case of Metastatic Melanoma. *Obstet Gynecol* 16:550, 1960.

Gabbe, S. G. et al. Management and Outcome of Pregnancy in Diabetes Mellitus Classes B to R. *Am J Obstet Gynecol* December 1, 1977.

Heine, D. L. Disseminated Intravascular Coagulation: Evaluation of Therapeutic Approaches. *Sem Thromb Hemostas* 3:4, 1977.

Huff, R. W., Pauerstein, C. J. *Human Reproduction: Physiology and Pathophysiology*, New York: John Wiley & Sons, 1979.

Jones, M. B. Hypertensive Disorders of Pregnancy. *J Obstet Gynecol Nurs* 8(2):92, 1979.

Morrison, J. C. Heparin Therapy for Disseminated Intravascular Coagulopathies. *Perinatal Press* 5(1):10, 1981.

O'Sullivan, J. B. et al. Screening for High Risk Gestational Diabetic Patients. *Am J Obstet Gynecol* [illegible] 1973.

Pedersen, J. *The Pregnant Diabetic and Her Newborn* (2nd ed.). Baltimore: Williams & Wilkins, 1977.

Pritchard, J. A. Genesis of Severe Placental Abruption. *Am J Obstet Gynecol* 108:22, 1970.

Pritchard, J. A., MacDonald, P. C. *Williams Obstetrics* (15th ed.). New York: Appleton-Century-Crofts, 1976, pp. 551–581.

Tichy, A., Ching, D. Placental Function and Its Role in Toxemia. *Am J Matern Child Nurs* 4(2):84, 1979.

Vice, L. J. Touching the High Risk Obstetrical Patient. *J Obstet Gynecol Neonatal Nurs* 8(5):294, 1979.

White, P. Classification of Obstetric Diabetes. *Am J Obstet Gynecol* 229, 1978.

White, P. Pregnancy Complicating Diabetes. *Am J Med* 7:609, 1949.

Willson, J. R., Carrington, E. R. *Obstetrics and Gynecology* (6th ed.). St. Louis: C. V. Mosby, 1979.

22

ABNORMAL LABOR

Abnormal labors extend beyond the maximum duration time of normal labor, which is 24 hours. In some of the literature, multiparous labor extending beyond 18 hours is considered prolonged. Difficult labor is referred to as *dystocia* and can be caused by ineffective uterine contractions (powers), abnormalities in size or position of the fetus (passenger), or alteration in the structure of the birth canal (pelvis). Many texts refer to abnormal labor as a problem of the 3 Ps: powers, passengers, or pelvis.

This chapter discusses dystocia, induction of labor, premature labor, operative obstetrics, anesthesia, multiple births, and emergency delivery. The nursing interventions that are appropriate during any of these labor complications are incorporated into the discussions.

DYSTOCIA FROM UTERINE DYSFUNCTION

Recall that in normal labor contractions occur regularly, last only a few seconds initially, and increase in frequency and intensity. The outcome of normal uterine contractions is progressive cervical dilatation and delivery of the neonate. Uterine dysfunction is suspected if the early contraction pattern does not assume a normal pattern within a few hours. The contractions may be as uncomfortable as in normal labor, but they are less effective in dilating the cervix.

Caldeyro et al. (1950) divides uterine dysfunction into two types.

- ▲ Weak contractions with a normal gradient
- ▲ Incoordinate uterine action

In the first type of uterine dysfunction, there is slow but progressive dilatation; in the second, contractions may be initiated by both pacemakers, allowing several areas of myometrium to contract without synchronization (see Chapter 16). In fact, the contraction wave may spread upward (inverted gradient). This type of asynchronous contraction is ineffective in retracting and dilating the cervix.

Clinically, the woman with dystocia exhibits an abnormal latent or active phase of cervical dilatation (see Chapter 16). Recall that during normal labor the upper part (fundus) of the uterus contracts and the lower part is relaxed and at the peak of a contraction, the fundus cannot be indented with a finger. In abnormal labor, not only is the duration less but the uterus is less firm and can be indented with a finger. Because of the uncoordinated uterine muscle activity, the lower part does not retract, and the cervix remains thick and undilated. Instead of the presenting part being applied tightly against the cervix, it hangs down ahead of the presenting part. Abnormal labor can be easily recognized when cervical dilatation is being plotted on a normal labor curve graph.

Latent Phase Dysfunction

Normally, the mean time for latent phase is 7.26 hours for primigravidas and 4.14 hours for multigravidas. Prolonged latent phase is anticipated when the time extends 2 hours beyond the mean time.

Active Phase Dysfunction

Active phase mean times are 3.7 hours for primigravidas and 2.6 hours for multigravidas. There are two dysfunctional active phase patterns.

▲ ***Slow Slope Active Phase.*** Cervix is dilating steadily but at a slower rate than normal

▲ ***Active Phase Arrest.*** Progress ceases before dilatation is complete

Recall that dilatation in normal labor progresses steadily during the active phase; abnormalities should be recognized early. Slow slope active phase is dilatation less than 0.7 cm/hr in primigravidas and less than 1.1 cm/hr in multigravidas. Active phase arrest is diagnosed when dilatation does not change during a 2-hour period.

Etiology of Uterine Dysfunction

Uterine dysfunction is a complication principally of primigravidas and is not usually seen in subsequent labors; no specific cause is known. Prolonged latent phase is sometimes attributed to too early administration of analgesia, although evidence seems to indicate that analgesia can increase an abnormality already existing but probably does not cause it. Active phase arrest is almost always a sign of *cephalopelvic disproportion* (CPD), a condition in which the fetal head cannot pass through the mother's pelvis. There is some evidence that there are psychogenic factors in prolonged labor; the mother who is dependent or who has intense guilt feelings about sex and pregnancy may unconsciously delay labor.

The effects of prolonged labor include increased incidence of infection, perinatal mortality, and postpartum hemorrhage. Exhaustion and dehydration can occur with prolonged labor. Although management of latent and active phase dysfunctional labor may differ, both require evaluation, protection against infection, sedation, and hydration.

After evaluation has established prolonged latent phase and CPD has been ruled out (usually by x-ray), a sterile vaginal examination is done to determine dilatation, effacement, and station. At this time an amniotomy may be done as this can be followed by improved contraction pattern. Once the membranes are ruptured, the commitment for delivery is made. If normal labor is not established within 1 hour after amniotomy (see oxytocin induction in this chapter), the usual next step in medical management is to augment the labor with oxytocin.

Slow slope active phase does not respond significantly to either amniotomy or oxytocin. If labor progression is slow but the rate of dilatation seems to indicate that the woman will deliver in 24 hours or a little longer, no intervention is needed. If time is extended significantly, cesarean birth is indicated.

Active phase arrest requires vaginal examination and x-ray film of pelvimetry to either establish or rule out CPD. The physician then decides either to rupture membranes and augment if it looks as though the pelvis will be adequate or to perform a cesarean section if it does not.

Constriction Ring Dystocia

A *constriction ring* is a tetanic annular contraction of smooth muscle that can occur at any level in the uterine wall. Diagnosis is established by passing the hand into the uterine cavity and feeling the ring. Clinically it should be suspected when contractions are irregular and uncoordinated. Cesarean section is often indicated.

Pathologic Retraction Ring (Brandl's Ring)

Brandl's ring occurs during obstructed but otherwise normal labor. The ring occurs at the junction of the active upper uterine segment and the inactive lower uterine segment. Because of the obstruction, the descent of the fetus is stopped. In contrast to constriction ring dystocia, which is the *cause* of the obstruction, Brandl's ring is the *result* of the obstruction. The lower segment becomes increasingly thin and can rupture. Since disproportion is usually the cause, cesarean birth is indicated to prevent rupture of the uterus.

DYSTOCIA BECAUSE OF FETAL DISORDERS

Dystocia Because of Fetal Size

Conditions in which a big baby may be anticipated are:

- ▲ Large parents
- ▲ Maternal diabetes

Normally, the pelvis will accommodate infants weighing between 4,000 and 4,500 gm; if uterine contractions are effective, vaginal delivery will follow. Sometimes shoulder dystocia occurs (head delivers but broad shoulders of the infant are unable to pass the inlet), which requires skill in manipulation by the physician as the infant must be delivered quickly to alleviate chest compression. It is hoped that big babies or CPD will be suspected by dysfunctional labor patterns and diagnosed by pelvimetry early so that a decision regarding the optimal delivery method can be made.

Dystocia from Developmental Anomalies

Hydrocephalic (enlarged head) infants usually result in prolonged labor as the head is too large to enter the inlet. Vaginal delivery is sometimes possible by puncturing an enlarged ventricle and withdrawing fluid. This allows the skull bones to collapse and labor proceeds normally. Other developmental anomalies, such as Siamese twins, may also present problems.

Dystocia from Abnormalities in Position and Presentation

The infant can present in a variety of positions, some of which make vaginal delivery virtually impossible (Fig. 22.1). In any case of abnormal position or presentation, early diagnosis before the mother or her uterus becomes fatigued is critical. In most cases of transverse lie (shoulder presentation) and severely deflexed head cesarean section is indicated. Careful assessment is made by the physician and, depending on the mother's pelvic measurements and fetal size, manipulation such as flexing the head sometimes can be attempted.

Occiput posterior positions, on the other hand, rarely require cesarean delivery. Almost all infants rotate to the anterior position or deliver in the posterior position without difficulty. Posterior labor is often related to the shape of the bony pelvis. If the transverse diameter of the inlet is narrow and the anteroposterior diameter is lengthened (as in an android pelvis), the head must descend with its long axis in an anteroposterior diameter and is quite likely to descend in a posterior oblique position. No interference in labor is indicated as long as labor is progressing within normal time limits.

DYSTOCIA BECAUSE OF PELVIC CONTRACTION

Anatomic and physiologic foundations for reproduction are found in Chapter 4; review of its content will promote understanding of pelvic dystocia.

Effects of Contracted Pelvis—Antepartum

Because pelvic measurements are decreased, the fetus is usually carried high and lightening is less likely to occur.

Effects of Contracted Pelvis—Intrapartum

In general since lightening is less likely to occur, abnormal presentations and positions occur more often in women with contracted pelves. Deflexed attitudes of the head, shoulder presentation, and compound presentation occur 2–3 times more often (Willson, 1979). Consequently, if delivered vagi-

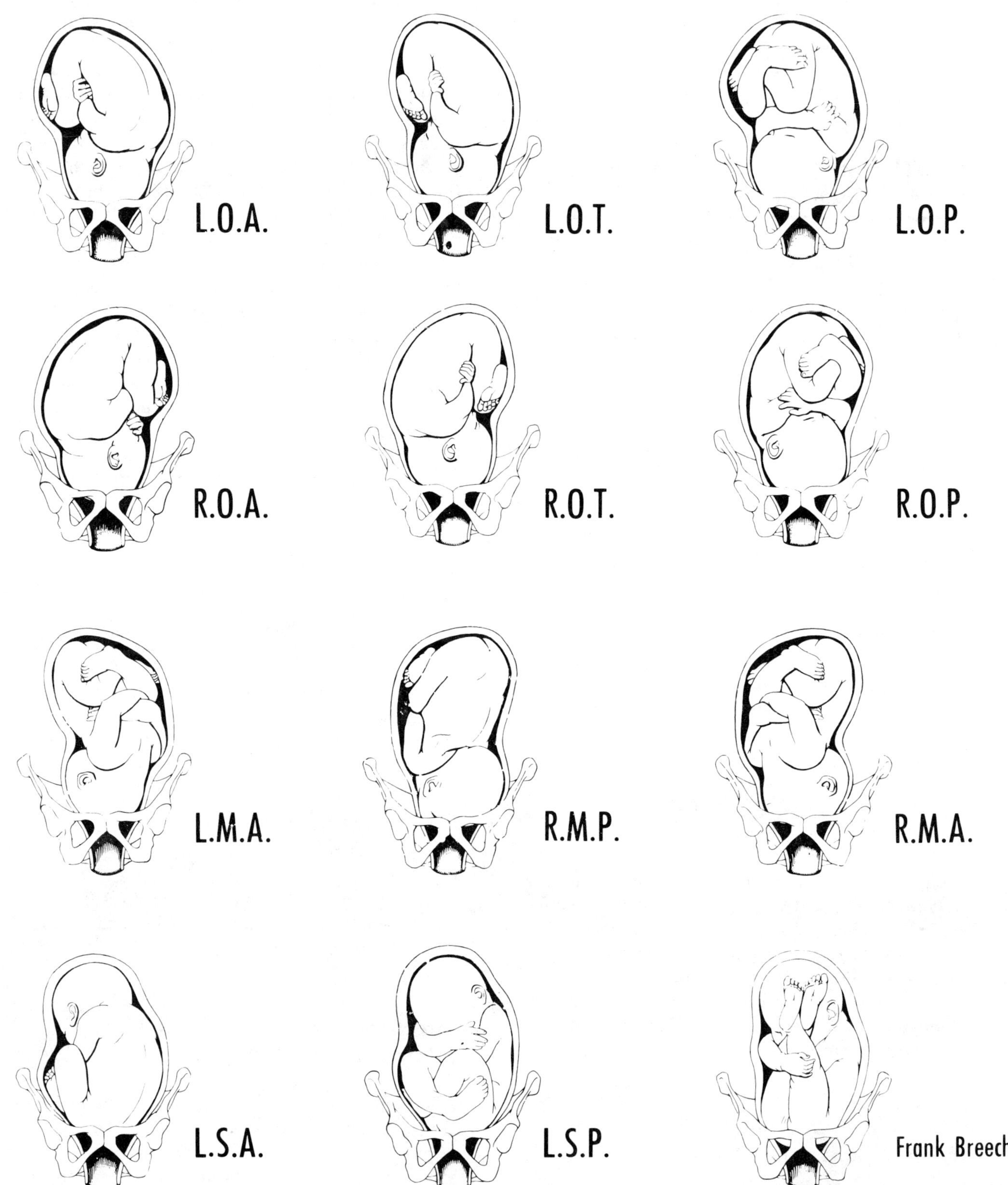

Figure 22.1
Abnormal lie and presentation. *Source:* Ross Laboratories. Used with permission.

nally, these women are prone to soft tissue injury, postpartum hemorrhage, and infection, and fetal injury can occur.

Mechanisms of Labor with Contracted Pelvis

Alterations in the fetal trip down the birth canal may occur as a result of a contracted pelvis. In some instances, contracted pelves are similar to normal growth types and the mechanism of labor is like that which occurs normally. Possible deviations related to pelvic types are:

- ▲ ***Gynecoid Pelvis.*** The head must flex at a higher level and mold more. All diameters are reduced; therefore, resistance may be met at all levels of the birth canal.
- ▲ ***Platypelloid Pelvis.*** The main alteration in measurement is anteroposterior diameter of the inlet. Therefore, delay in first stage and early second stage can occur. Transverse arrest both high (head near the ischial spines) and deep (station +2) can occur.
- ▲ ***Android Pelvis.*** Since the anterior inlet is wedge shaped and the posterior is flattened, the head often descends in oblique occiput posterior position and the delivery may be occiput posterior.
- ▲ ***Anthropoid Pelvis.*** Occiput posterior positions are common. The transverse diameter of the pelvis is reduced the entire length of the birth canal so the head often delivers without rotating.

Management of Contracted Pelvis

Abnormal pelves for management purposes can be divided into two groups—inlet contraction and midpelvic or outlet contraction. Abnormal labor should be anticipated in women with reduced pelvic diameters or in women who have had dystocia in previous pregnancies. If the fetal head is still floating at term, inlet disproportion should be suspected.

INLET CONTRACTION

When the anteroposterior (AP) diameter is less than 10 cm or the transverse diameter is less than 12 cm, inlet contraction is diagnosed. Although labor progression and outcome are dependent to a large extent on the obstetric conjugate, pelvic configuration, size, and position of the infant and the effectiveness of the uterine contractions are all factors.

Most women with minimal inlet contraction can deliver vaginally; therefore, a trial of labor is permitted. Within 8–10 hours, if contractions are occurring regularly, the physician can assess if the inlet contraction has been overcome. Amniotomy is usually done since sometimes intact membranes will prevent the head from descending. There is always a danger of prolapsed cord if the head is high, and assessment of fetal heart rate before, during, and after amniotomy is critical. If the disproportion is minor, oxytocin augmentation may be used. If progress is not continuous, cesarean section is indicated. In contrast to primigravidas, multigravidas with contracted pelvic inlets sometimes have tumultuous labors, and uterine rupture becomes a concern. Nursing measures include all of the biophysical, psychosocial, and behavioral assessment characteristics included in Chapter 16. In abnormal labor, the nurse must integrate the implication of the labor problem with normal labor and adapt the nursing process to the individual woman.

MIDPELVIC OR OUTLET CONTRACTION

Lower pelvic adequacy cannot be assessed completely; therefore, trial labor is less satisfactory than in inlet contraction. If the head descends beyond +2, vaginal delivery is usually possible as the head can be turned manually or by forceps.

OXYTOCIN INDUCTION OF LABOR

Oxytocin induction of labor is useful in women with complications that may worsen if the pregnancy is allowed to continue. In normal pregnancy, oxytocin induction is not necessary.

Indications for oxytocin induction include:

- ▲ Pre-eclampsia–eclampsia
- ▲ Chronic hypertension
- ▲ Bleeding complications

- ▲ Premature rupture of the membranes (PROM)
- ▲ Diabetes mellitus
- ▲ Rh sensitization
- ▲ Recurrent pyelonephritis
- ▲ Repeated intrauterine fetal death

Contraindications for oxytocin stimulation include:

- ▲ Cephalopelvic disproportion
- ▲ Fetal distress
- ▲ Previous uterine surgery (see section on cesarean birth)
- ▲ Overdistended uterus
- ▲ Grand multiparity

Technique for Oxytocin Induction

Oxytocin is always administered with caution since it is always unknown how responsive the uterus will be to the drug. An intravenous infusion is started (often 5% dextrose) in the woman's vein. A needle from a second liter of fluid, in which 10 units (1 ml) of oxytocin has been added, is connected through an infusion pump into the tubing of the already started infusion. This set up is known as a *piggy back*. Since oxytocin has a *half-life* (time required for drug to be metabolized) of 3–6 minutes, this intravenous setup allows for the oxytocin infusion to be stopped immediately if necessary and the initial infusion to be kept running and the vein to be kept open.

Oxytocin should be administered in dilute solutions and should always be infused by a controlled pump that is unaffected by needle size, flow of the vein, or drop size. The dosage of oxytocin is calculated in milliunits (mU). If 1 ml of oxytocin (10 IU or 10,000 mU) is added to 1,000 ml of 5% dextrose, each 0.1 ml of solution contains 1 mU of oxytocin. For induction of labor at term, an infusion rarely exceeds 16 mU/min. Dosage necessary to initiate induction of labor may be as low as 1 mU/min, and the pump is set to deliver that amount. If the uterus does not contract in 15–20 minutes, the dosage is increased 2 mU/min at 15-minute intervals until the contractions are 2–4 minutes apart and lasting 40–60 seconds (intrauterine pressure on the internal monitor 50–70 mm Hg). The total dosage of oxytocin in any one uninterrupted period should be limited. Oxytocin has an antidiuretic effect, particularly when administered in electrolyte-free fluids over a long period of time. During induction intake, output should be monitored closely; this is true of any intrapartum patient.

Nursing Management of the Patient During Oxytocin Induction

During oxytocin induction the patient *must at no time be left unattended*. Fetal heart rate, mother's vital signs, and frequency and intensity of uterine contractions as well as resting period between contractions should be recorded every 15 minutes. At no time should a contraction exceed 90 seconds, and the resting period between contractions should be at least 2 minutes. If signs of stress appear during oxytocin induction, the critical nursing intervention is to shut off the oxytocin infusion and open the plain solution flow and *then* report immediately to the physician. As mentioned earlier, oxytocin has a half-life of 3–6 minutes, so when in doubt shut off oxytocin and notify the physician.

Ideally, patients undergoing oxytocin induction are monitored by an internal electronic monitor (see Chapter 16) so that nurses have technology to assist them. Evidence of fetal hypoxia as noted by late decelerations or an increase in uterine resting tonus can alert the nurse to compromise of the uteroplacental circulatory exchange. The resting pressure as monitored by intrauterine catheter should not exceed 15–20 mm Hg. As noted in Chapter 16, normal resting pressure is between 6 and 15 mm Hg. Figure 22.2 shows a fetal monitor recording during oxytocin stimulation (note elevated resting pressure) and a prolonged variable deceleration caused by oxytocin stimulation.

Remember that machines are only tools to assist in the care of the patient, and their value depends on intelligent use. The wise nurse will continue to auscultate the fetal heart rate and palpate the contraction periodically. Behavioral observation of the woman for pain, extreme restlessness, apprehension, and so on also gives clues to a hypertonic contraction. Assessment of the patient's expectations, as well as explanations regarding the procedure of induction and the equipment being used

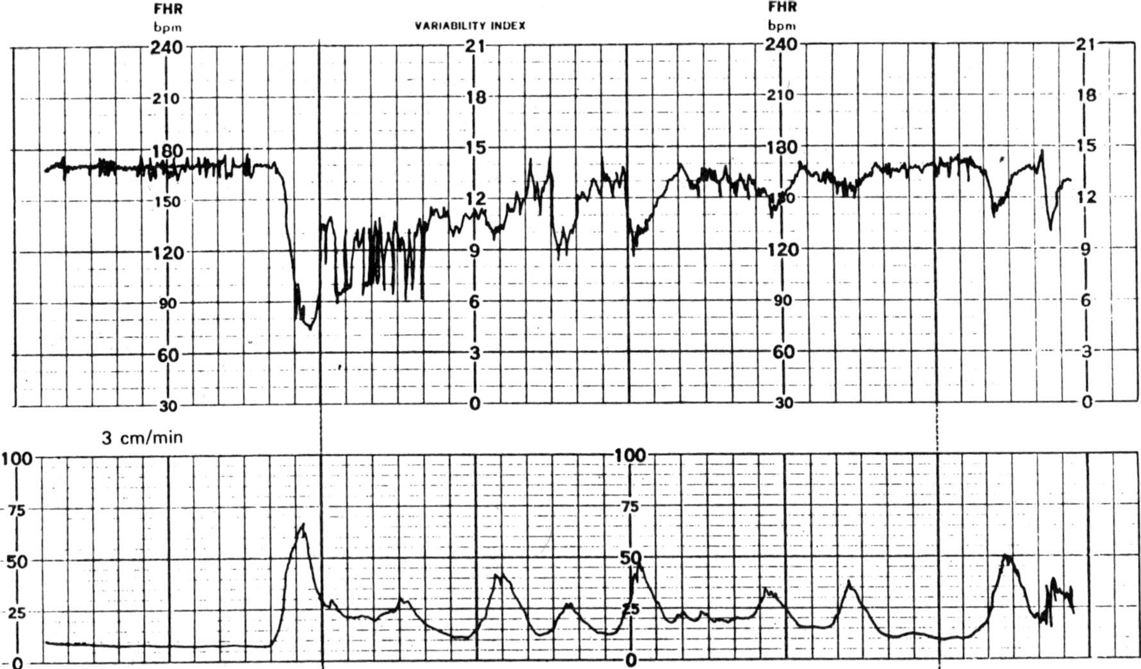

Figure 22.2

Uterine hyperstimulation and prolonged variable deceleration caused by oxytocin stimulation. *Source:* Butnarescu, G. F., Tillotson, D. M., Villarreal, P. P. *Perinatal Nursing Vol. 2. Reproductive Risk.* New York: John Wiley & Sons, 1980. Used with permission.

lessens anxiety by reducing fear of the unknown. It may be very reassuring to a mother to know that the "noise" is her baby's heart beat. By keeping the mother informed, the nurse not only reassures her but may facilitate the induction. An informed person is more relaxed, has less discomfort, and is cooperative. In turn, this allows for increased uterine efficiency and less resistance to descent of the baby so that the goal of induction—safe delivery for mother and child—can be met.

Augmentation of Labor

Augmentation of labor means stimulation of labor that started spontaneously but progressed unsatisfactorily (Cibils, 1965). Oxytocin is the drug most often used to stimulate labor. Implications and management have been discussed earlier in this chapter.

Dystocia problems that may benefit from augmentation have been discussed. It is important for the nurse to remember that in augmented labor, sensitivity to oxytocin is greater than it is during induction, and lower infusion rates of oxytocin are necessary (Cibils, 1965).

PROSTAGLANDIN INDUCTION OF LABOR

Prostaglandins (PG) are unsaturated fatty acids derived from prostanic acid. Two prostaglandins used for induction of labor are PGE_2 and $PGF_{2\alpha}$. Evidence is accumulating that endogenous prostaglandin plays a role in spontaneous labor. It will be interesting to see the future role of prostaglandins in the *induction of labor.*

Technique and Uses of Prostaglandin Induction

$PGF_{2\alpha}$, when given orally, causes considerable gastrointestinal upset, therefore, PGE_2 is used almost exclusively for oral induction of labor. (Both drugs can be administered intravenously.) Side effects of both $PGF_{2\alpha}$ and PGE_2 are gastrointestinal upset and venous erythema. Both have a low incidence of uterine hypertonus and no known adverse fetal or neonatal effects. However, oxytocin is still the drug of choice for women at term because of the uncomfortable side effects of prostaglandins. Prostaglandin is, however, the method of choice for termination of pregnancy in intrauterine fetal death (IUFD) (Thiery, 1977). Intravaginal suppositories seem to prepare the unripe cervix, and spontaneous explusion of the fetus follows.

PREMATURE LABOR

Labor that occurs after the twenty-eighth and before the thirtieth week of gestation resulting in an infant of less than 2,500 gm is called *premature labor*. Incidence of prematurity in the United States is about 7%. Two-thirds of infant deaths are attributable to prematurity. Although maternal, placental, and fetal causes can be identified, they account for about one-third of premature births; in approximately two-thirds of the births, no definite cause is identified. Iatrogenic reasons for prematurity are thought to be responsible for 9% of preterm babies. The significance of a premature birth is that the neonate developmentally is not ready for adaptation from intrauterine to extrauterine life (see Chapter 23). Moreover, the parents are usually unprepared, so the implications for intervention by nurses are many.

Maternal Problems Relating to Premature Labor

The following conditions are frequently associated with premature birth.

- ▲ Pre-eclampsia–eclampsia
- ▲ Renal disease
- ▲ Cardiovascular disease
- ▲ Traumatic accidents
- ▲ Abdominal surgery
- ▲ Incompetent cervix
- ▲ Excessive smoking
- ▲ Untreated hyperthyroidism
- ▲ Drug addiction (heroin)
- ▲ Infection
- ▲ Orgasm
- ▲ Age—young teenager; women over 35

Fetal Problems Relating to Premature Labor

The following fetal conditions are associated with premature birth.

- ▲ Transplacental infection (rubella, toxoplasmosis)
- ▲ Multiple pregnancy
- ▲ Hydramnios
- ▲ Premature rupture of the membranes
- ▲ Congenital adrenal hyperplasia

Placental Problems Relating to Premature Labor

The following placental disorders are associated with premature birth.

- ▲ Placental separation
- ▲ Abnormalities of the placenta
- ▲ Genetic abnormalities

Suppression of Premature Labor

Suppression of premature labor currently involves a variety of drugs that are often administered by nurses; therefore, nurses are responsible for knowing the drugs' pharmacologic action and side effects to mother or fetus and whether the mother may be given the drugs.

Before learning the main pharmacologic agents appropriate for management of premature labor and nursing care related to their use, it is important to note that there are some conditions in which it is *not* desirable to stop labor, for example, severe pre-eclampsia–eclampsia, abruptio placentae, fetal anomalies incompatible with life, fetal demise, and chorioamnionitis. When a woman is admitted who is in premature labor, it is critical that a decision about medications to suppress labor be made quickly, as these drugs are most effective when administered when premature labor first begins.

ETHANOL (ALCOHOL)

Ethanol has been used for a long time and can inhibit labor for 24–48 hours if membranes are intact and the cervix is less than 4-cm dilated. During therapy, blood ethanol levels can range from 0.12 to 0.16%. Since inebriation legally exists when the concentration is 0.10%, the nurse caring for a patient receiving ethanol for premature labor is dealing with an inebriated woman. The family and patient should be informed that the patient will appear drunk and may exhibit nausea, vomiting, crying, disorientation, slurred speech, and poor muscle coordination. Safety needs of the patient are a priority concern.

Ethanol inhibits gluconeogenesis; therefore, hypoglycemia is a concern. It also inhibits antidiuretic hormone (ADH) and promotes diuresis so hydration of the patient is important. Headaches are often a side effect postinfusion.

Since alcohol crosses the placenta, blood concentration in mother and fetus are approximately the same. If the infant is born, he or she may exhibit lethargy, apnea, poor muscle tone, or abnormal reflexes. Ethanol therapy should not be used in recovered alcoholics or women with liver disease or diabetes.

BETA-ADRENERGIC STIMULANTS

Three beta-adrenergic receptor stimulants are used to suppress labor: isoxsuprine hydrochloride (Vasodilan), ritodrine (Youtopar), and terbutaline (Bethine). As a group, these drugs cause the uterus to relax. When therapy is instituted, electronic fetal monitoring is used; after therapy, it is important to palpate the uterus to see if contractions have resumed.

Side effects include hypotension and compensatory tachycardia due to the fact that beta II receptors cause vasodilation in the smooth muscle of the vascular system. Maternal heart rate increases 30–50 beats per minute, but blood pressure should not fall below 90/60. Vital signs are taken every 10–15 minutes until 1 hour after the infusion is completed. If severe hypotension or tachycardia occurs, the drug is stopped, the mother is placed in Trendelenburg's position, and intervention to support hypotension is begun. Prevention of hypotension indicates using hypertonic or isotonic solutions intravenously and placing the woman on her left side. Other symptoms are nausea, sweating, drowsiness, and headache. Beta II stimulation enhances glycogenolysis; hyperglycemia can also occur and needs to be monitored.

Fetal side effects of beta-adrenergic receptor stimulants relate to the mother's problems. If the mother is hypotensive, fetal bradycardia can occur. Fetal heart rate deceleration usually is mild. Metabolic effects of hyperglycemia require that the preterm infant's glucose level be assessed carefully. If labor is successfully suppressed by the beta-adrenergic stimulants, the mother may be discharged on an oral maintenance dose. The mother needs to be told of side effects and have explicit, written directions regarding the medication she is to take. Weekly visits for assessment of fetal heart rate and drug therapy protocol are necessary.

MAGNESIUM SULFATE

Magnesium sulfate ($MgSO_4$) has labor-inhibiting properties and can be used to suppress labor, although its use in pre-eclampsia is much more evident. Precautions and nursing care for the woman in premature labor receiving $MgSO_4$ would be the same as those discussed in Chapter 21 for hypertensive disorders. Magnesium toxicity must be assessed regularly by monitoring urine output, deep tendon reflexes, and maternal respiratory rate.

OPERATIVE OBSTETRICS

Operative obstetrics includes episiotomy, forceps delivery, vacuum extraction, and cesarean delivery.

Episiotomy

An *episiotomy* is an incision made in the perineum to enlarge the vaginal orifice for the following reasons.

- ▲ Prevent tearing of the perineum
- ▲ Prevent stretching of the muscles supporting the bladder or the rectum
- ▲ Reduce time and stress of second stage (cardiac patient, persistent fetal bradycardia)
- ▲ Enlarge vagina for manipulation (breech, forceps)

TYPES OF EPISIOTOMIES

Median, or *midline,* episiotomy is probably the most often used; the incision is from the vagina directly toward the rectum. Advantages are that the incision heals easily, is easily repaired, and causes less discomfort for the woman. A disadvantage is that extension of the incision can involve the rectal sphincter (third degree) or the anal canal (fourth degree). Fortunately, with good surgical repair and primary healing sphincter tone is resumed.

A *mediolateral* incision is made to the right or to the left of the vaginal orifice at approximately a 45 degree angle. Mediolateral episiotomy is used when posterior extension may occur, for example, with a very large baby. Disadvantages are that healing is slower, blood loss is greater, and the incision is more uncomfortable since it cuts across muscle fibers. The advantage is that it prevents rectal involvement, although a third-degree laceration can still occur.

Forceps Delivery

Indications for the use of forceps involve both maternal and fetal considerations. Maternal indications include:

- ▲ Cessation of progress in second stage of labor (inadequate contractions)
- ▲ Abnormal position of fetus because of minor degree of pelvic contraction
- ▲ Shorter second stage (cardiac patient, hypertensive or hemorrhaging patient)

Fetal indications include:

- ▲ Prolapsed cord
- ▲ Fetal distress during second stage

TYPES OF FORCEPS

Although there are hundreds of different obstetric forceps dating back to 1625 when they were invented, only five major types are used today.

- ▲ ***Simpson's.*** Outlet forceps
- ▲ ***Kielland's.*** Rotational forceps with a pelvic curve (for example, in posterior delivery it would be used to rotate for OP to OA)
- ▲ ***Barton's.*** Rotational forceps without pelvic curve but with a deep posterior and short anterior blade (used for rotating OP to OA)
- ▲ ***Tarnier's.*** Axis-traction forceps (designed to assist infant down birth canal)
- ▲ ***Piper's.*** Used to help deliver head in breech

PREREQUISITES FOR FORCEP DELIVERY

Forceps should be used by the experienced physician when the following conditions exist.

- ▲ No cephalopelvic disproportion
- ▲ Head is engaged
- ▲ Membranes are ruptured
- ▲ Fully dilated cervix
- ▲ Empty bladder

An episiotomy is usually performed before forceps application, and pudendal anesthesia may be used (see section on anesthesia later in this chapter).

CLASSIFICATION OF FORCEPS IN RELATION TO STATION

The level of forceps used relates to the fetal station. In general, the higher the forceps the more difficult the application. (see Chapter 16).

- ▲ ***Low Forceps Extraction.*** Head deeply engaged or on pelvic floor. Used if mother is unable to use her secondary powers (abdominal muscles) or if uterine contractions become ineffective (minimal risk to mother or infant).
- ▲ ***Mid-Forceps Extraction.*** Head is at ischial spines. Contraindicated unless clear-cut reason to terminate labor. Sometimes used when second stage has exceeded 2 hours. Oxytocin augmentation is preferred. Cesarean section preferred to traumatic mid-forcep application.
- ▲ ***High Forceps Extraction.*** High forcep deliveries are not justified. Cesarean section is preferred.

Nursing responsibilities during forceps delivery are to take and record the fetal heart rate and to assist the physician. Assessment of the neonate immediately post-forceps delivery is often the purvue of the nurse.

Vacuum Extraction

The *vacuum extractor* is basically a suction cup attached to a handle; it is applied to the baby's head and used in vertex deliveries to exert traction or to help rotation. It was originally conceived to reduce the damage caused by forceps. Indications for use are the same as for low forceps. The device must be used by a trained operator as careless use can be traumatic. It is widely used in Europe. Neonates who have had a vacuum extractor applied may have ecchymosis and swelling in the shape of the suction cup.

CESAREAN DELIVERY

Cesarean delivery is an operative method by which the infant is delivered through incisions in the abdominal and uterine walls. The 1974 rate of cesarean delivery was reported at 12.2% by Pritchard and MacDonald (1976). It is suggested that electronic fetal monitoring has increased the incidence of cesarean births, but monitoring has also allowed for recovery of the fetus in utero or at least stabilization of a stressed fetus. Electronic surveillance has allowed surgical intervention to occur at a more optimal time.

Maternal Indications for Cesarean Delivery

Conditions that often result in cesarean delivery include the following.

▲ Dystocia

▲ Placenta previa

▲ Abruptio placentae

▲ Hypertensive diseases

▲ Herpes type 2 infection

▲ Malposition of the fetus (transverse lie)

▲ Previous cesarean birth

▲ Uterine operations

▲ Abnormal labor

▲ Trauma

Fetal Indications for Cesarean Delivery

Fetal indications for cesarean delivery include the following.

▲ Prolapsed cord

▲ Abnormal fetal heart pattern

▲ Growth retardation

▲ Breech presentation

▲ Diabetes mellitus

▲ Compound presentations

Types of Cesarean Deliveries

It is important to remember that there are two main incisions—abdominal and uterine—and that there are five principal types of procedures (see Fig. 22.3).

▲ ***Classic Cesarean Delivery.*** Vertical incision through skin and uterus. Simplest procedure and can be done rapidly. Also indicated in shoulder or in some placenta previas.

▲ ***Low Cervical or Lower Segment Cesarean Delivery.*** Transverse incision through the visceral peritoneum. Incision is behind the bladder—seepage from uterus is reduced and postpartum peritoneal infection is less likely.

▲ ***Peritoneal Exclusion Cesarean Delivery.*** Low cervical cesarean delivery with suture of the parietal peritoneum to the transversely incised visceral peritoneum before incision through the lower uterine segment. An outside route for drainage of fluid is established. Since the use of antibiotics, this procedure is used less often.

▲ ***Extraperitoneal Exclusion Cesarean Delivery.*** Technically difficult and bladder and ureteral injuries are more common. Value is limited although it may be used in grossly infected patients.

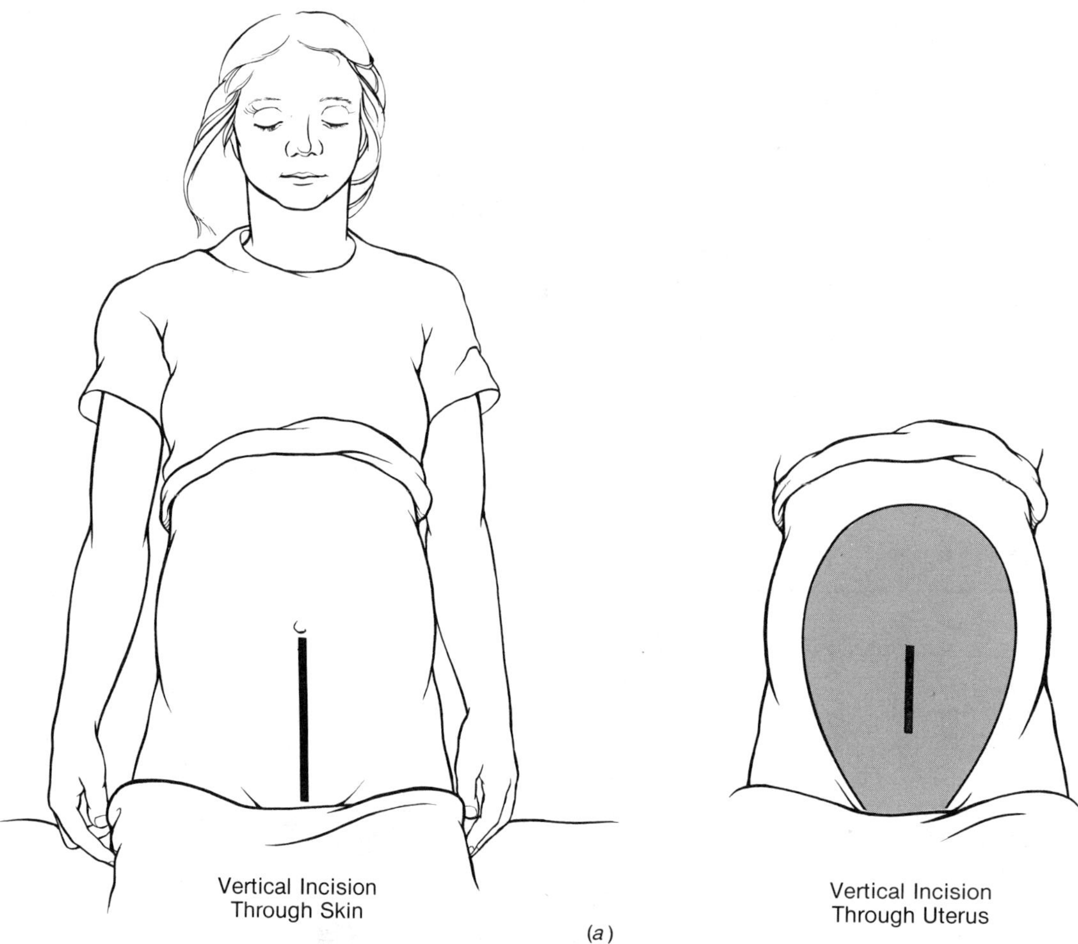

Figure 22.3
Types of cesarean deliveries. *(a)* Classic cesarean delivery.

- ▲ ***Cesarean Hysterectomy.*** Total or subtotal hysterectomy may be performed, usually after classic cesarean delivery. Indications are placenta previa, placenta accreta, or uterine myomas or if the placenta will not separate at operation.
- ▲ ***Postmortem Cesarean Delivery.*** When the mother dies and the fetus is thought to be viable, a cesarean delivery may be done within 5–10 minutes of the mother's death. Delivery of a viable infant who survives is not common because of either hypoxia or immaturity.

Repeat Cesarean Deliveries

It is now more common to allow a mother with low horizontal incisions of the uterus and skin to deliver vaginally in a subsequent pregnancy. Needless to say, evaluation of the woman and assessment of the reason for the previous cesarean delivery are critical. Many women who have previously delivered by cesarean birth do so subsequently; only if the woman labors in a center where cesarean delivery can be done quickly should trial of labor be considered.

Nursing Management of a Woman Undergoing Cesarean Delivery

The nurse plays a significant role in the preparation of the woman for cesarean delivery and her postoperative care. Preparation includes:

- ▲ Obtain laboratory data.
- ▲ Type and cross match two units of blood.

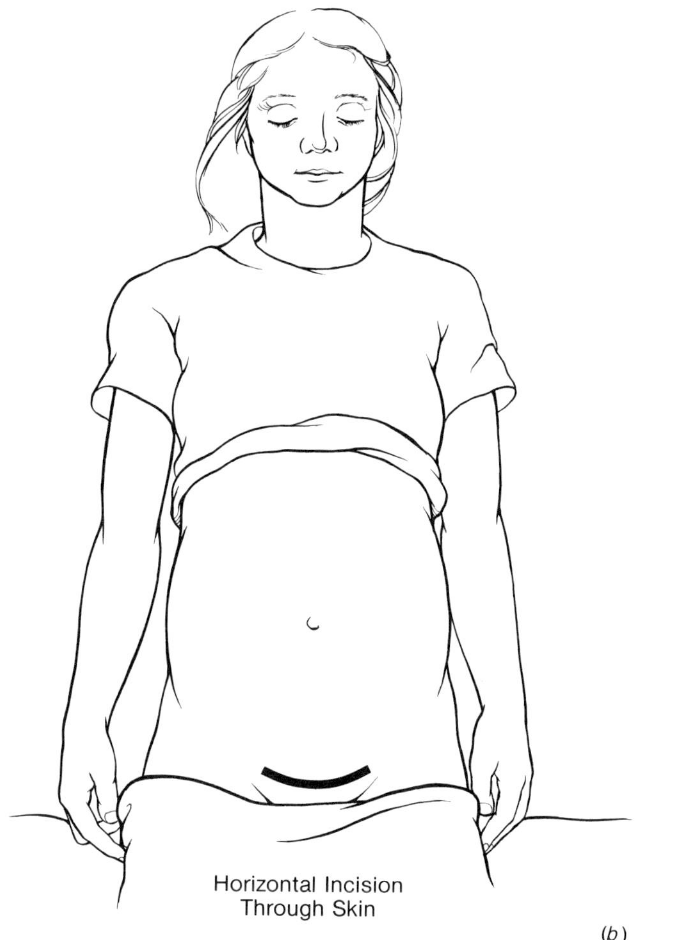

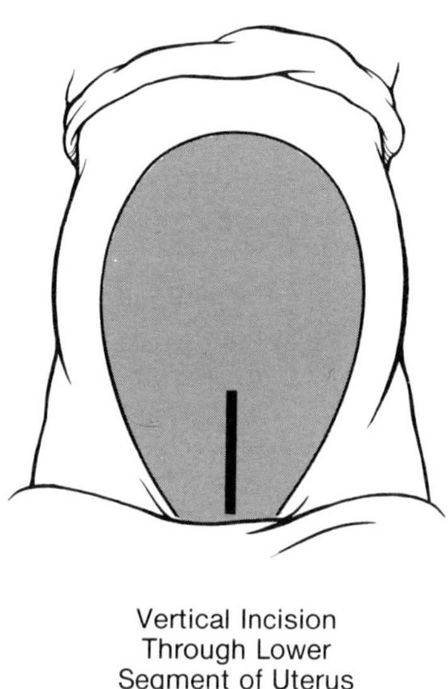

(b)

Figure 22.3 (continued)
(b) Low cervical cesarean delivery.

- ▲ Assure adequate fluid balance.
- ▲ Insert a Foley catheter.
- ▲ Administer preoperative medications.
- ▲ Start an intravenous infusion.
- ▲ Complete routine preoperative care (operative permit, jewelry, contact lenses).
- ▲ Notify family members and keep them informed.

Postoperative care includes:

- ▲ Assess fundus (should be palpated; it is, therefore, important for the nurse to know what type of incision was made).
- ▲ Prevent cardiopulmonary problems (cough, turn, deep breath).
- ▲ Monitor fluid intake and output.
- ▲ Auscultate for bowel sounds (distention can be a problem).
- ▲ Perform all routine postpartal care (fundal checks, lochia, breast).
- ▲ Administer medications as ordered (analgesics, oxytocics, antibiotics).
- ▲ Promote attachment process (opportunity to see and hold infant as soon as possible).
- ▲ Provide emotional support.

More attention has been given to the psychosocial aspects of cesarean birth in recent years. Many parent education classes are including information about cesarean delivery. However, there is always some grief reaction, and the nurse needs to antici-

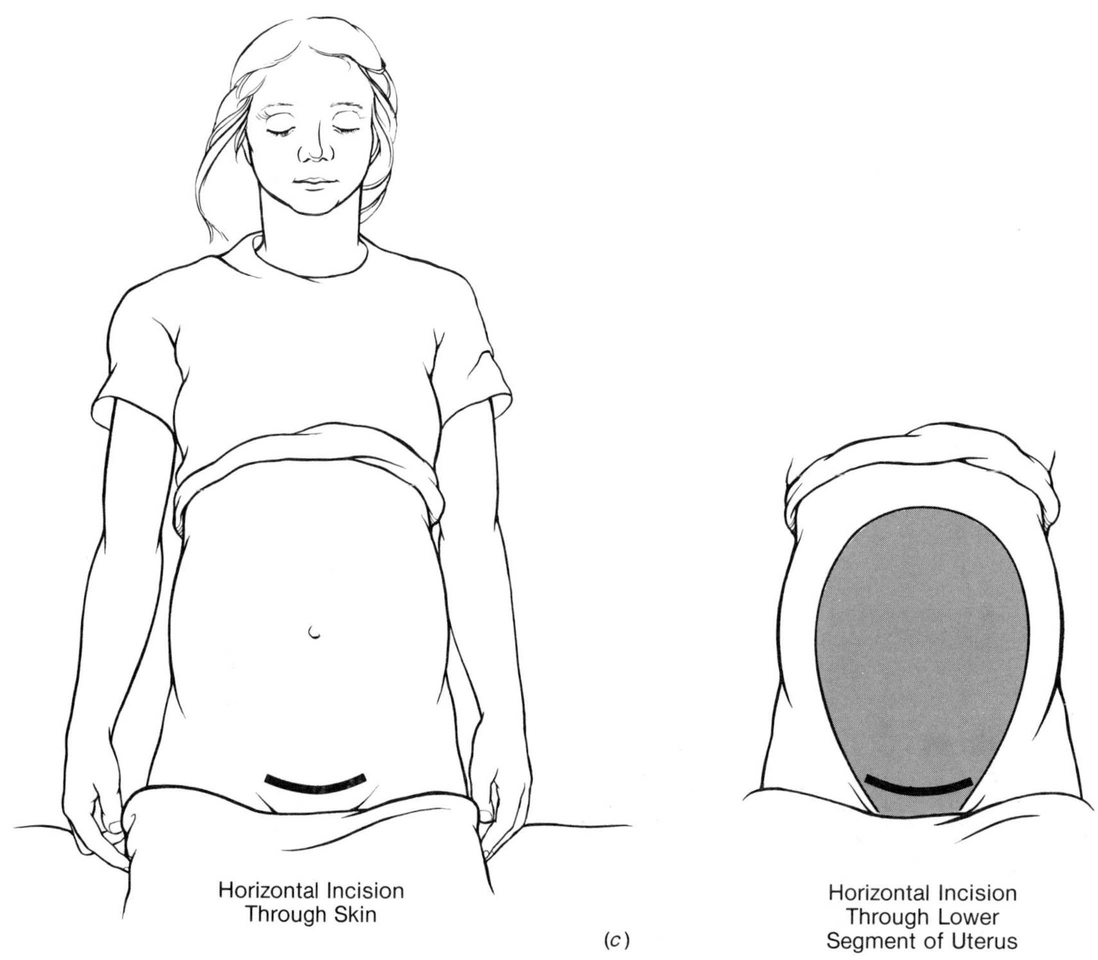

22.3 (continued)
(c) Low cervical cesarean delivery.

pate this and intervene appropriately. The mother who has had a cesarean delivery is both a surgical and a maternity client and the nurse needs to keep this in mind. It is important that the *birth,* even though it be by cesarean section, be noted and that mother become part of family-centered maternity care.

BREECH DELIVERY

Breech positions occur in about 3.5% of all deliveries of infants weighing more than 2,500 gm (5½ lb). *Breech delivery* is a baby whose position is a longitudinal lie in which the buttocks alone or the buttocks and some portion of one or both lower extremities descends through the birth canal first. Types of breech positions are illustrated in Figure 22.4. The frank or single breech represents two-thirds of all breech deliveries.

Etiology of Breech Delivery

The capacity of the fundal area is decreased when the placenta implants in the cornua, leaving the head in the fundus to fit better and the buttocks to remain lower in the uterus. Repeated breech pregnancies lead to the suspicion of uterine anomalies such as bicornate uterus. Other causative factors are multiparity, hydramnios, multiple pregnancy, fetal anomalies, or low implantation of the placenta. The most common causes of infant mortality

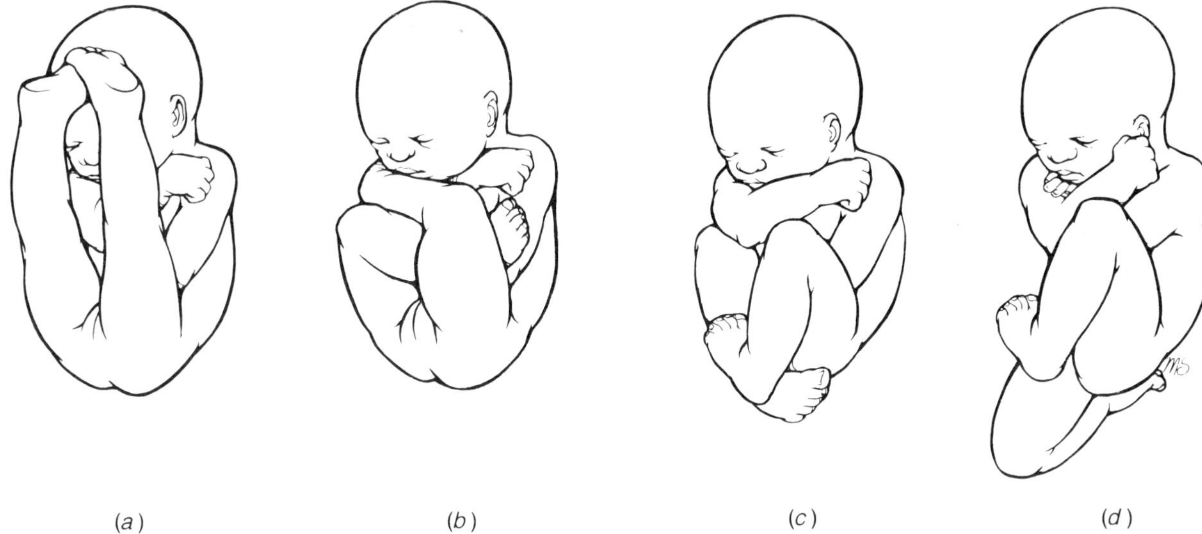

Figure 22.4
Types of breech deliveries. (*a*) Frank breech; (*b*) complete breech; (*c*) incomplete (foot below buttocks); (*d*) incomplete (knee below buttocks).

are associated with vaginal delivery of the breech and include the following:

- ▲ Anoxia from delay in delivery or prolapsed cord (occurs 10 times more often than in vertex) (Morley, 1967)
- ▲ Injuries—intracranial hemorrhage, fractures of spine and spinal cord injury, rupture of liver, spleen, adrenals
- ▲ Complications of prematurity
- ▲ Developmental anomalies

Diagnosis of Breech

The diagnosis of breech can often be made by abdominal examination and confirmed by vaginal exam, x-ray photos, or ultrasound.

Mechanism of Labor

The cervix dilates in multigravidas and primigravidas at the usual rate (same as vertex) if contractions are normal. The presenting part often remains high, above the ischial spines, until complete dilatation is reached. The mechanisms of labor in breech are shown in Figure 22.5.

Nursing Care of Breech Delivery

The nursing care of the breech baby and mother is essentially the same as in vertex labor, except that the FHR is located at or above the umbilicus. The labor is sometimes longer as the presenting part may not help dilate the cervix as well as the head.

Incidence of prolapsed cord is higher, and the nurse needs to be alert to this possibility (Fig. 22.6). Meconium from the vaginal introitus is more common in breech delivery because of pressure on the fetal abdomen and is not necessarily an indication of fetal distress.

Parents are always concerned when told that the baby is breech and require reassurance and explanation. They should be kept informed of the progress of labor. At the time of delivery, the nurse can anticipate that in addition to routine supplies, Piper's forceps may be needed. Neonatal resuscitation equipment and adequate personnel should be available.

A conservative approach to breech delivery has recently developed, and consultation and more liberal use of cesarean delivery are the trend. Breech presentation is frequently an indication for cesarean birth in primigravidas; it indicates cesarean birth in multigravidas with fetuses larger than 3,360 gm (7½ lb), especially if labor is not effective or if complications arise.

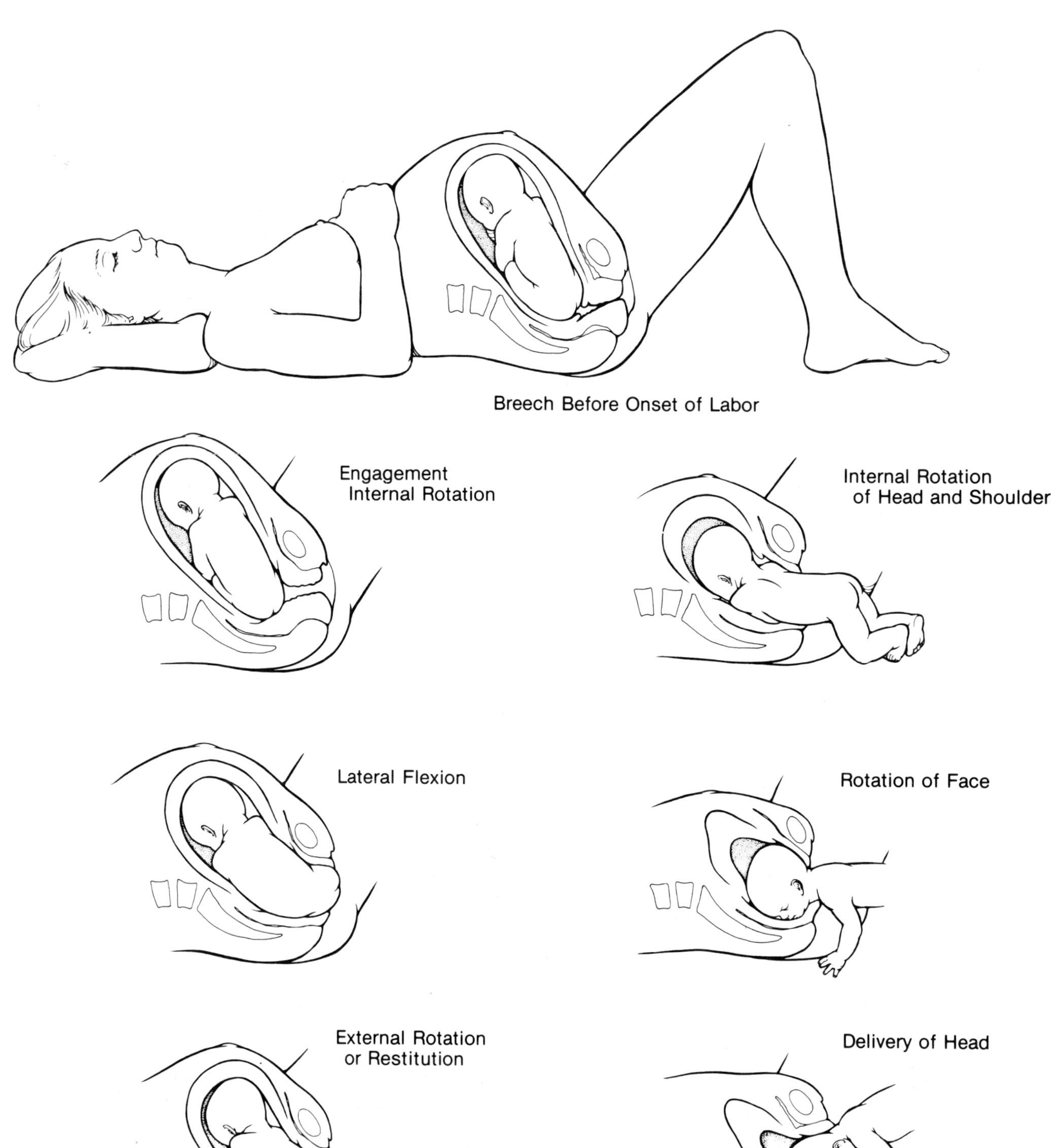

Figure 22.5
Breech: Mechanisms of labor.

ANESTHESIA

Anesthesia includes two main categories—inhalation anesthesia and regional anesthesia. Inhalation anesthesia is sometimes requested by women who want to be asleep; currently it is rarely used, except for cesarean section. The important implication of general or inhalation anesthesia is that the agent (usually cyclopropane) crosses the placenta rapidly and can cause fetal depression. The obstetrician and nurse should be prepared for delivery before anesthesia is started.

Regional Anesthesia

Conduction, or *regional,* anesthesia in obstetrics is administered to relieve pain and includes the following types of anesthesia:

- ▲ Caudal
- ▲ Epidural
- ▲ Paracervical
- ▲ Pudendal
- ▲ Simple infiltration
- ▲ Spinal

Caudal, epidural, or paracervical anesthesia can be used in the active phase of the first stage of labor; the other forms are used in second stage before delivery. The drugs used are *caine* drugs and can be Pontocaine, Novocain, lidocaine, procaine, Nesacaine, Xylocaine, or Murcaine. The important fact to remember about any of the caine drugs is that hypotension can be a side effect. Both blood pressure and fetal heart rate need to be monitored carefully. Nursing actions to correct hypotension include increasing IV fluids, positioning the woman on her side, and administering oxygen by mask or nasal cannula. The advantages and disadvantages of the various types of anesthesia, as well as a brief discussion of each method, follow.

Paracervical (Uterosacral) Block

In the *paracervical block* a dilute anesthetic (often procaine) is injected into the cervix at the 9 o'clock

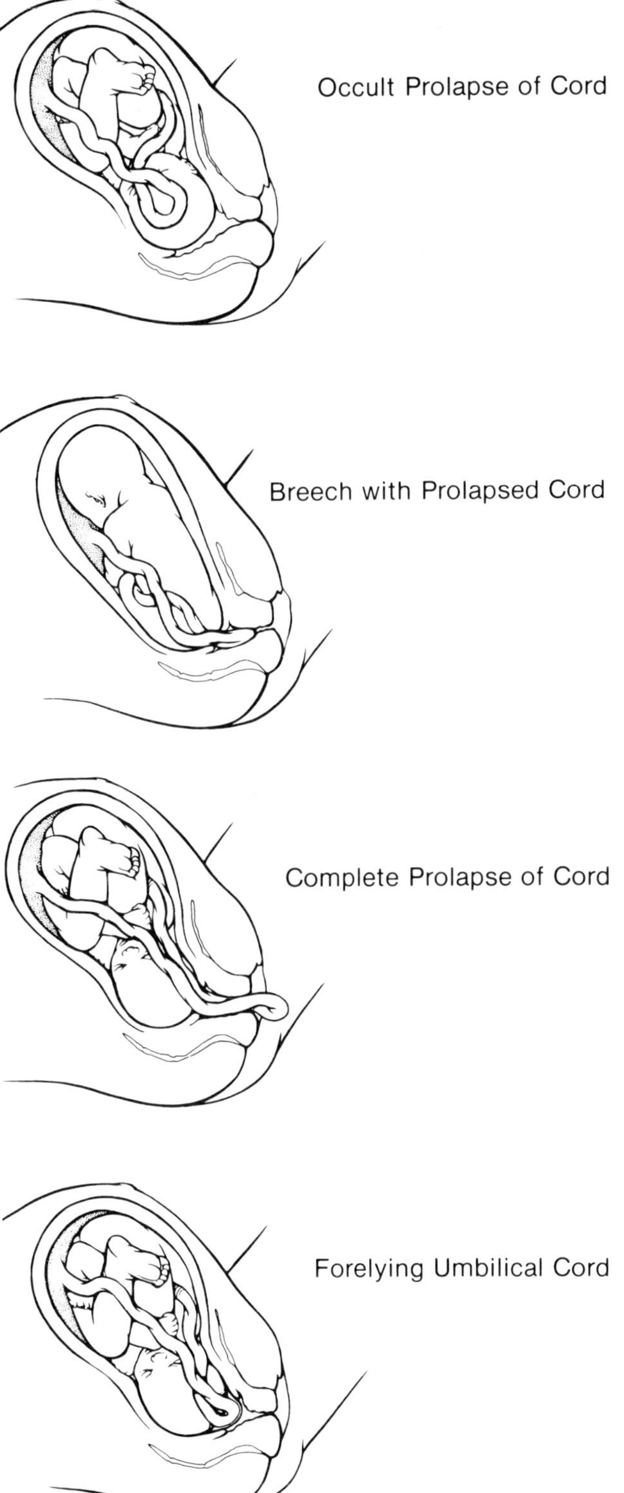

Figure 22.6
Types of prolapsed cord.

and 3 o'clock positions. Pain relief lasts approximately 1 hour; the injection can be repeated if necessary. Anesthesia affects the lower uterine segment and cervix, as well as the upper third of the vagina—no perineal anesthesia. Usually the injection is first done at approximately 5-cm dilatation, and it can be repeated until transition (8 cm). The fetus can be affected and may exhibit bradycardia. An example of a fetal monitor strip showing prolonged deceleration after paracervical block is shown in Figure 22.7. Paracervical block is not recommended in labor although it is useful in abortion.

Pudendal Block

Once the presenting part is through the cervix, vaginal and pudendal stretching occurs. The *pudendal block,* which is anesthetic administered beneath the inferior median border of the ischial tuberosity, will anesthetize the pudendal nerves. This type of anesthesia is injected via a long needle inserted through a trumpet guide, which is inserted into the vagina. It provides anesthesia for the vaginal and perineal area and is often used before episiotomy.

Epidural and Caudal Anesthesia

Epidural or caudal anesthesia, which is an extrathecal (outside the spinal canal) injection between a lumbar interspace or caudally, provides excellent anesthesia and is often used in the active phase of the first stage of labor.

Advantages are that fetal distress is rare, mother is alert, good relaxation results, and only partial motor paralysis occurs. Blood loss is minimal and headache is rare since the spinal canal is not entered. This method offers continuous, prolonged anesthesia and analgesia. A disadvantage is that the procedure must be done by a trained person.

The woman is positioned on her side and the needle and a fine plaster catheter are inserted into

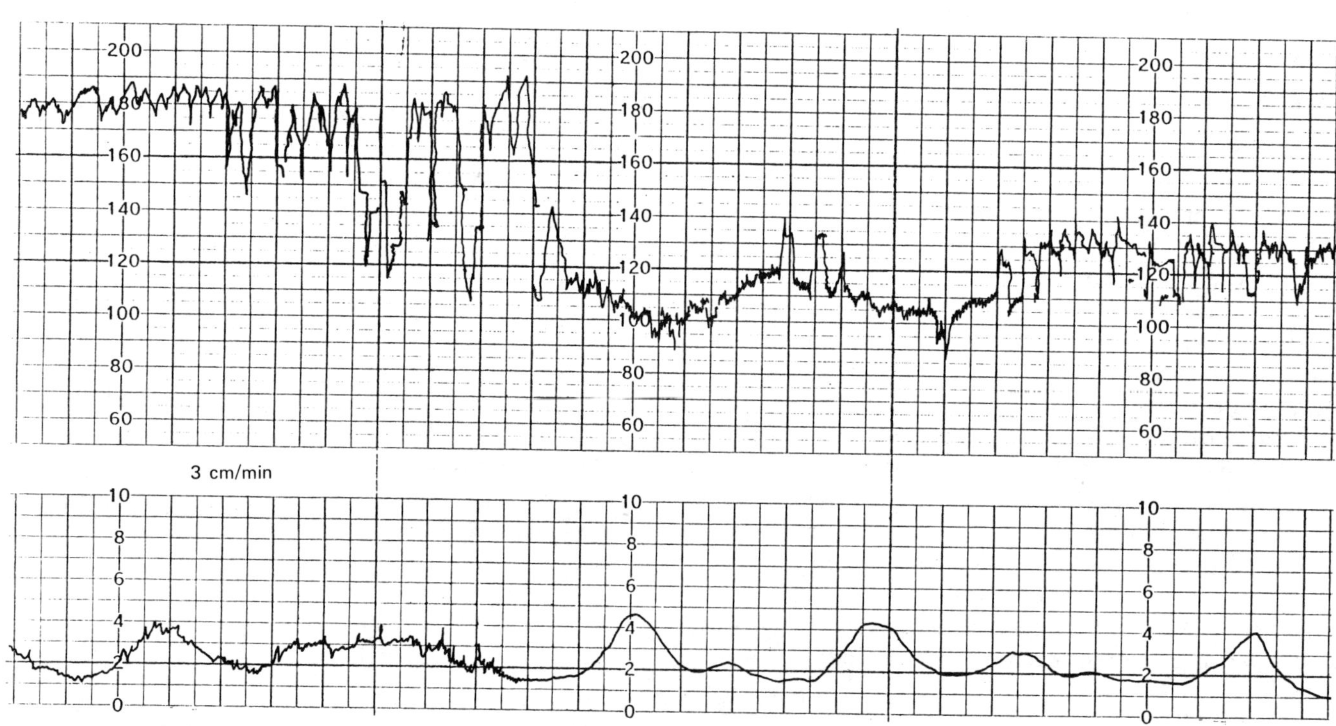

Figure 22.7
Prolonged deceleration following a paracervical block. *Source:* Butnarescu, G. F., Tillotson, D. M., Villarreal, P. P. *Perinatal Nursing Vol. 2. Reproductive Risk.* New York: John Wiley & Sons, 1980. Used with permission.

the caudal canal. After correct placement is verified, the needle is removed and the catheter is taped securely in place and the woman remains on her side. This allows for repeated doses of medication to be given. Blood pressure should be taken and recorded every 5 minutes initially; maternal and fetal vital signs should be taken every 15 minutes subsequently. The nurse must continue to monitor the labor carefully as the mother is basically unaware of uterine contractions. During second stage the mother will need direction and encouragement to push; low forceps are required to complete delivery.

Spinal Anesthesia (Saddle Block)

In contrast to epidural or caudal anesthesia, *spinal anesthesia* is intrathecal (into the spinal canal) and is used during late first stage or early second stage. Anesthetic effects last from 1 to 2 hours.

Advantages of spinal anesthesia are that there is excellent muscle relaxation, the mother is awake, and no other anesthetic agents are needed. Disadvantages include hypotension, increased tendency for bladder or uterine atony, loss of voluntary pushing efforts (low forceps needed for delivery), and postnatal headache.

The medication is administered at L4 or L5 with the woman sitting on the side of the delivery table or bed. The nurse stands in front of the woman and coaches her. Once the drug is injected, the woman is returned to the supine position and given a pillow beneath her head so that the drug will not go up the spinal canal and affect respiration. Blood pressure, pulse, respiration, and FHR must be checked and recorded every 5 minutes. If signs of hypotension or fetal distress occur, nursing actions are giving oxygen to the mother, increasing IV fluids, and manually displacing the uterus laterally, which allows for improved venous return. Postpartum care is similar to that of a surgical patient who has received spinal anesthesia. Neurologic evaluation of level of anesthesic is important. Intake and output and fundal and lochia assessment should be done every 15 minutes or more often if there is any indication of complications. The woman must remain supine for 8 hours to prevent spinal headache; fluids should be encouraged.

MULTIPLE PREGNANCY

Multiple pregnancy occurs relatively frequently in humans; twins occur in approximately 1 in 99 conceptions in North America. Twins are either dizygotic (double ovum or fraternal) or monozygotic (single ovum or identical). (See Chapter 11.)

Monozygotic twins are a random occurrence, whereas dizygotic twins are an autosomal recessive trait carried by daughters of mothers of twins. The likelihood of twinning also increases with maternal age. Nearly 70% of twins are dizygotic. Maternal morbidity and perinatal morbidity and morality are increased in multiple pregnancy when compared to single births, largely because of medical and obstetric complications.

Maternal Problems in Multiple Pregnancy

The greater occurrence of maternal problems related to multiple gestation requires that the nurse be alert to possible complications. Problems can include:

- ▲ Hypertension
- ▲ Abortion
- ▲ Anemia
- ▲ Hydramnios
- ▲ Placenta previa

Problems occurring during labor can include:

- ▲ Uterine dysfunction (overdistention)
- ▲ Abnormal fetal presentations (see Fig. 22.8)
- ▲ Premature labor
- ▲ Placental abruption

Fetal Complications in Multiple Pregnancy

All of the following can affect the fetus in a multiple birth:

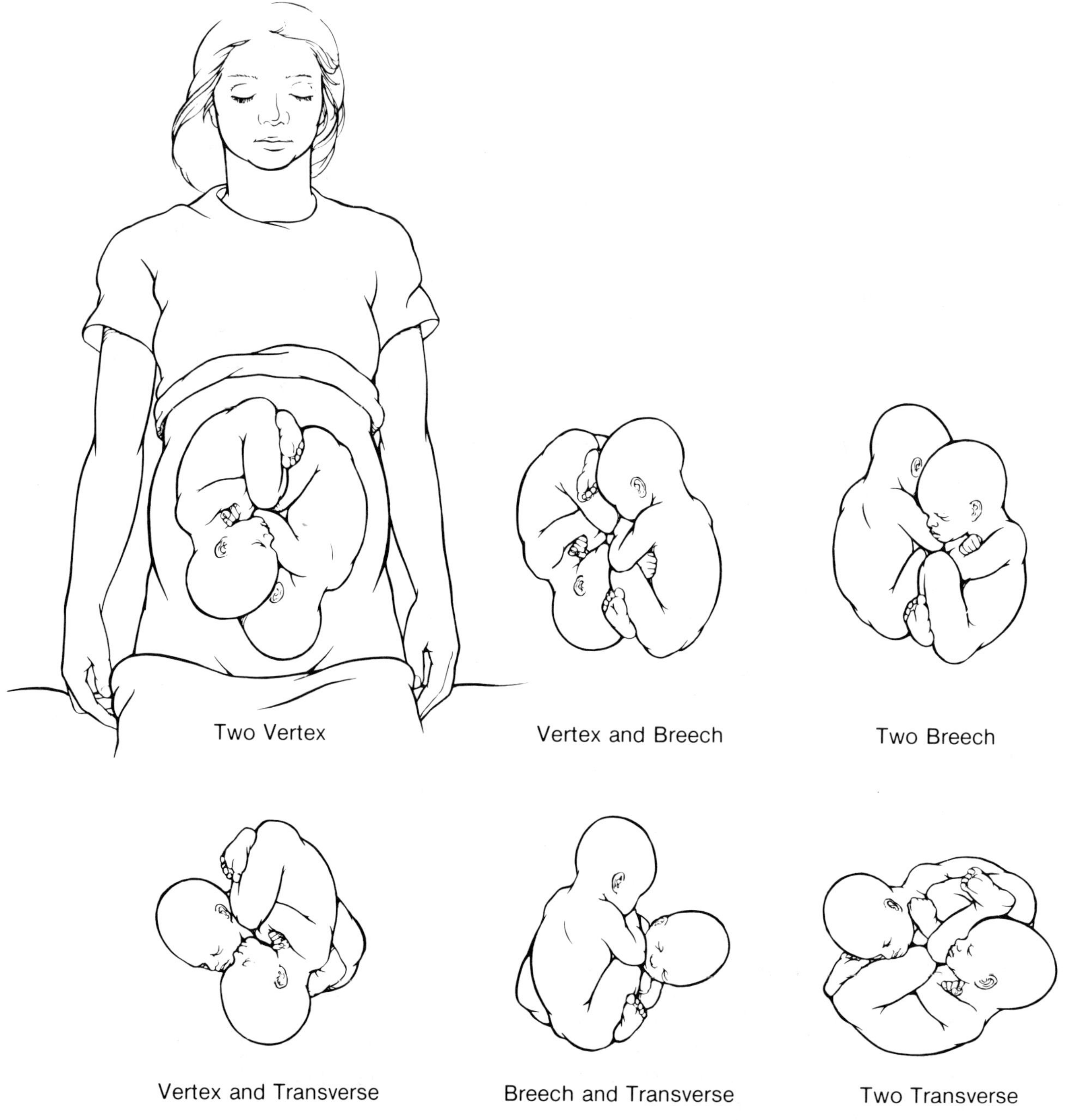

Figure 22.8
Twin delivery.

▲ Each twin and placenta weighs less than a single pregnancy.

▲ Monochorionic placentas with artery-to-artery anastomosis can occur (one twin is overperfused, hypervolemic, and polycythemic; the other twin is hypovolemic and exhibits intrauterine growth retardation).

▲ Congenital malformations.

▲ Prematurity and associated RDS are more common. (See Chapter 23.)

Nursing Management of Multiple Pregnancy

Antepartum management includes:

- Prenatal visits at least every 2 weeks
- Dietary supervision
  - 300 calorie increase daily over single pregnancy requirements
  - Protein increase to 1.5 gm/kg
  - Iron supplement 60–80 mg
  - Vitamin supplements
  - Weight gain 18 kg (40 lb)
- Prevention of backache resulting from overdistention
  - Maternity girdle
  - Selected exercises
  - Supportive leotards
- Scheduled daily rest periods in left lateral position to increase uterine and kidney perfusion

Intrapartum management includes:

- Admission at first sign of labor
- Limit analgesic (infants may be premature)
- Monitor both (or all) fetuses—sometimes can use combination of external and internal monitoring
- Monitor mother's vital signs and labor pattern
- Watch for prolapsed cord
- No oxytocin to mother until all infants are delivered
- Careful identification of each baby and placenta
- Vaginal or cesarean delivery depending on fetal status
- Prepare equipment for two infants
- Personnel needed to care for each new arrival

Postpartum management includes:

- Continued assessment of mother for hemorrhage
- Psychologic support of mother and family
- Attend to physiologic needs of mother, including rest
- Continue all routine postpartal procedures—vital signs, fundal assessment, lochia
- Provide opportunity for maternal–infant bonding

Mothers of twins or other multiple births are often overwhelmed, even if they are prepared for more than one infant. The astute nurse carefully assesses the woman biophysically and behaviorally and meets the needs she identifies. Anticipatory guidance of the highest order is important for this new mother for all of the variables are at least doubled. (See Chapter 18.)

EMERGENCY DELIVERY

Knowing what to do in an emergency delivery wherever it may occur is by heritage a nurse's role. Historically, nursing students had to deliver a certain number of infants on their own in order to graduate. Although opportunity to deliver an infant is not a scheduled event in undergraduate curricula today, the unwritten rule is that in an emergency, the nurse will know what to do.

The Required Knowledge Base

What knowledge is needed? Certainly the mechanism of labor and the average duration of each stage are necessary fundamentals. The nurse should be able to picture a labor graph mentally and, by assessing the woman and using communicative, physical, and behavioral clues, determine how long she has been in labor and approximately how dilated she is. If sterile equipment is not available, vaginal examinations are not performed. Recall that particularly in transition the woman gives numerous clues as she reaches full dilatation (see Chapter 16).

Nursing Actions as Delivery is Imminent

Providing the mother with a physically and psychologically safe experience is the goal in emergency delivery. It is very important to get the mother's attention, to assure her that you are there and can help her, and to ask her to help you by following your directions. Having her cooperation will be key to your success, and talking her through what is occurring will help you organize yourself. The mother is frightened (and you may be too), but giving her the message that you are in control will focus both of you on the "what to do."

HOSPITAL EMERGENCY DELIVERY

If the emergency delivery occurs in the hospital, an emergency delivery pack is probably prepared, and the nurse can ask auxillary personnel to retrieve it. Sterile contents of the pack are:

- ▲ A drape to place under the woman's buttocks
- ▲ Gauze squares to clean the infant's face and mouth
- ▲ Bulb syringe
- ▲ Two clamps to use before cutting the cord
- ▲ Scissors
- ▲ Cord clamp for the infant's cord
- ▲ Baby blanket
- ▲ Gloves

If there is time, a hand scrub should be done. But the most important thing is to be sure the mother is attended. If in the delivery room, be sure that you do not "break" the table but leave it extended. As the baby crowns, the nurse tells the mother to pant and says something like: "I can see the baby's head and it won't be long. But it's important that you not push, so open your mouth and pant. You're doing very well. I am right here and everything is fine." If the amniotic sac is intact, wearing sterile gloves, tear the sac at the back of the head and pull the membrane off. Place the flat of your hand (with fingers toward the rectum) against the baby's head gently. This way you can control the head and slow the advance as the maternal tissue accommodates. Depending on the mother's tissue resistance, she may have several contractions with the head visible at the introitus. After the forehead is out, the rest of the head comes out easily and you can feel, with the other hand, for the cord around the neck. If there is a nuchal cord, slip the cord over the baby's head. If the cord is tight and cannot be moved, place two clamps on the cord, cut between the clamps with the sterile scissors, and unwind the cord from the neck.

Allow restitution and external rotation to occur on its own, which it will. Place palms of your hands over the baby's ears and apply gentle downward pressure until you see the anterior shoulder indicating that it has passed the symphysis pubis. Direct the baby's movement upward and, as the body emerges (the mother can push after the shoulders are free), slide your hand along the back cradling the buttocks in one hand and the head and back in the other. Hold the head lower than the trunk, place the baby on the mother's abdomen, and allow her to hold her infant. The priorities then are to:

- ▲ Clear the airway and dry the baby
- ▲ Clamp the cord and cut at 1 minute of age

The mother's body is a reliable heat source; cover the baby's head to prevent heat loss. The mother can be encouraged to nurse, and even the nuzzle of the baby against the breast will cause oxytocin to be released. Both the weight of the infant on the abdomen and the oxytocin release stimulates uterine contractions. Remain alert for signs of placental separation, being certain not to pull on the cord. Placental separation is heralded by lengthening of the cord, a gush of blood from the introitus, and the fundus rising in the abdomen and becoming globular in shape. After these signs appear, the mother can be instructed to push and the placenta is delivered. The cord clamp is placed slightly away from the infant's abdomen as it will dry and shrink in size.

After delivery of the placenta, check the fundus, which may be gently massaged to stimulate contractions and decrease bleeding.

Record keeping is important, and the following data should be recorded:

- ▲ Position of fetus
- ▲ Presence of cord around neck or not
- ▲ Time of delivery

- ▲ Apgar score (1 minute and 5 minutes)
- ▲ Sex of baby
- ▲ Time of placental delivery
- ▲ Appearance and intactness of the placenta
- ▲ Mother's condition
- ▲ Any medications given to mother or baby

The physician checks the mother and infant upon arrival. The infant may be transferred to the nursery, depending on protocols in the institution. Resumption of routine postpartal care or newborn care continues; this includes vital signs, bonding, fundal check, breast-feeding, and praise for the mother's efforts. Mother and infant should be identified before being separated.

OUT OF HOSPITAL BIRTH

The process of delivery out of the hospital is the same as in the hospital except that no sterile equipment is available. Therefore, the cord is not cut and baby and placenta are not separated. The cord will clot naturally. The placenta can be wrapped in newspaper and the mother and infant can be transported to an emergency room where the cord is cut as soon as sterile equipment is available.

Infant heat loss needs to be provided against when a delivery occurs outside the hospital (as well as inside the hospital), and this can involve measures such as skin-to-skin contact with the mother and providing a covering for mother and infant. Drying the head and body to prevent heat loss is also very important.

Mother–infant interaction is stimulated by pointing out the newborn's behavior and appearance. The interaction with the infant helps alleviate the fear of the delivery experience as the mother realizes that everything is all right. Although reassurance and praise from the nurse during and after the delivery are important, the realization that the infant has arrived and is well is the best reassurance. Fortunately, most emergency deliveries are uneventful.

SUMMARY

This chapter discussed several facets of abnormal labor, including dystocia, induction of labor, and premature labor. Nursing responsibilities of the woman receiving medications to suppress labor were included.

Operative obstetrics included forceps delivery, episiotomy, and cesarean birth. Types of cesarean deliveries and fetal and maternal care were described. Anesthesia, particularly types of regional anesthesia, used in obstetrics was explored. Advantages and disadvantages of caudal, epidural, paracervical, and pudendal anesthesia were discussed. Breech delivery and multiple pregnancies were discussed. Mechanism of labor in a breech presentation and types of twinning were described and illustrated. The last section of the chapter discussed emergency delivery inside the hospital and outside of the hospital. Step-by-step nursing responsibilities and priorities regarding emergency delivery were given.

REFERENCES AND READINGS

Burden, T. R., Peter, J. B., Merkatz, I. R. Rilotrine Hydrochloride: A Betamimetic Agent for Use in Preterm Labor. *J Am Coll Obstet Gynecol* 56(1):1, 1980.

Bells, B. Nursing Considerations: Administering Labor-Suppressing Medications. *Am J Matern Child Nurs* 5(4):252, 1980.

Butnarescu, G. F., Tillotson, D. M., Villarreal, P. P. *Perinatal Nursing: Volume 2, Reproductive Risk.* New York: John Wiley & Sons, 1980.

Caldeyro, R., Alvarez, H., Reynolds, S. R. M. A Better Understanding of Uterine Contractility Through Simultaneous Recording With an Internal and a Seven Channel External Method. *Surg Gynecol Obstet* 91:641, 1950.

Cibils, L. A. Enhancement and Induction of Labor, in Aladjem, S. (Ed.) *Risks in the Practice of Modern Obstetrics* (2nd ed.). St. Louis: C. V. Mosby, 1965, Chap. 6.

Friedman, E. A. *Labor: Clinical Evaluation and Management* (2nd ed.) New York: Appleton-Century-Crofts, 1978.

Huff, R. W., Pauerstein, C. J. *Human Reproductive Physiology and Pathophysiology.* New York: John Wiley & Sons, 1979.

Jennings, B. Emergency Delivery: How to Attend One Safely. *Am J Matern Child Nurs* 4(3):148, 1979.

Jensen, M. D., Benson, R. C., Bobak, I. M. *Maternity Nursing* (2nd ed.). St. Louis: C. V. Mosby, 1981.

Merkatz, I. R. A Retrodine Update. *Perinatal Press* 5(4):47, 1981.

Morley, G. W. Breech Presentation: A 15 Year Review. *Obstet Gynecol* 30:745, 1967.

Pritchard, J., MacDonald, P. C. *Williams Obstetrics.* New York: Appleton-Century-Crofts, 1976.

Thiery, M. et al. A Comparison of Buccal (Oromucosal) and Oral Prostaglandin E_2 for the Elective Induction of Labor. *Prostaglandins* 14(2), 1977.

Thiery, M., Amy, J. J. Spontaneous and Induced Labor: Two Roles for Prostaglandins, in Wynn, R. M. (Ed.) *Obstetrics and Gynecology Annual.* New York: Appleton-Century-Crofts, 1977.

Willson, J. R., Carrington, E. R. *Obstetrics and Gynecology* (6th ed.). St. Louis: C. V. Mosby, 1979.

23

FETAL–NEONATAL DISORDERS

Jean A. Foster

Across the United States—in hospitals and homes; in doctors' offices; in clinics and birthing centers; and, occasionally, in ambulances and taxicabs—3 million babies were born last year. These infants were delivered by doctors, nurses, midwives, fathers, policemen, or neighbors, and the majority of them arrived healthy and remarkably problem-free. Despite the enormous adaptation required in their transition from intrauterine to extrauterine life, most babies continue to pass the first test of their lives as independent human beings successfully.

Health care professionals dedicated to caring for neonates recognize that the improved health status and perinatal care of childbearing women have enhanced an event that has occurred successfully more often than not for centuries. Thus, support, encouragement, and guidance are the most common interventions provided to these infants and their families.

But what about the other infants—the minority of babies born each year with a problem or problems, the one out of 20 who are born prematurely, the one out of 12 who begin life with an anomaly or defect? It is to this group of infants that the team of care givers commit the greatest proportion of their time, energy, and expertise (Fig. 23.1).

This chapter describes some of the conditions that characterize a high-risk infant and discusses the therapy, treatment, and nursing care required by that infant. The content of the chapter provides the beginning practitioner with an overview.

HEALTH CARE SPECIALISTS AND FACILITIES FOR THE CARE OF HIGH-RISK NEONATES

The field of *neonatology* has expanded markedly since its inception about 20 years ago. At one time everything from ventilators to medication dosages to ostomy bags were simply "trimmed up" or "scaled down" for use with sick babies; then research and practice began to demonstrate the need for an approach to the neonate as a unique human being. Subsequently, specialized care regimens, supplies, and equipment designed expressly for the newborn infant appeared (Fig. 23.2). Today, in fact, it is not unusual to find entire companies devoted to the production of neonatal care products and the professional literature swelling with journals and textbooks on neonatal special care.

Specialization has also occurred within the health care professions. The physician caring for a sick newborn is often a *neonatalogist*—a pediatrician

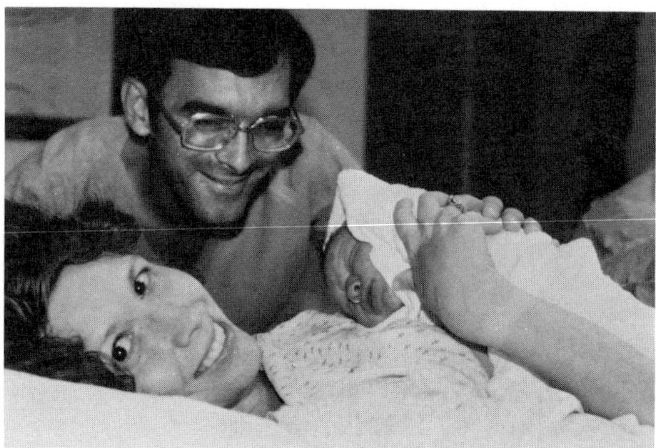

Figure 23.1
When a risk condition is present, its severity does not always require separation of the infant from its family.

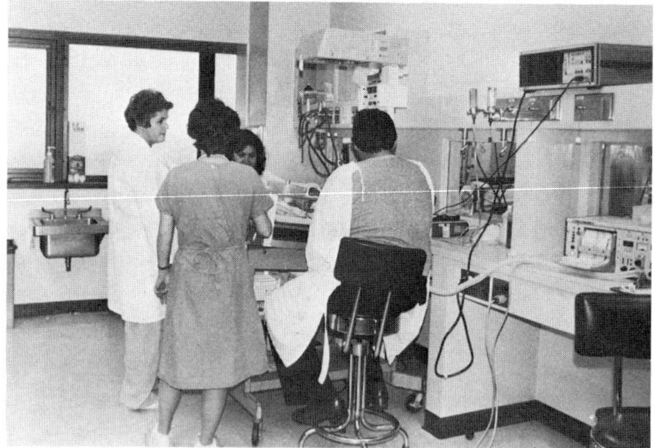

Figure 23.3
Perinatal team at infant's cribside.

who has had additional training in caring for critically ill neonates. Expanded nursing roles, such as neonatal nurse specialists and neonatal nurse clinicians, have developed (Fig. 23.3). Other members of the multidisciplinary team caring for the infant may include a perinatal social worker, a neonatal nutritionist, an infant development specialist, or a neonatal respiratory therapist. The multidisciplinary approach to care is certainly exemplified here.

Obviously, not every hospital or facility that delivers newborns has such a comprehensive team of specialists available. Realistically, the high cost of providing these services and the limited number of specially trained personnel available have necessitated a more efficient approach to the provision of neonatal special care. In 1976, the Committee on

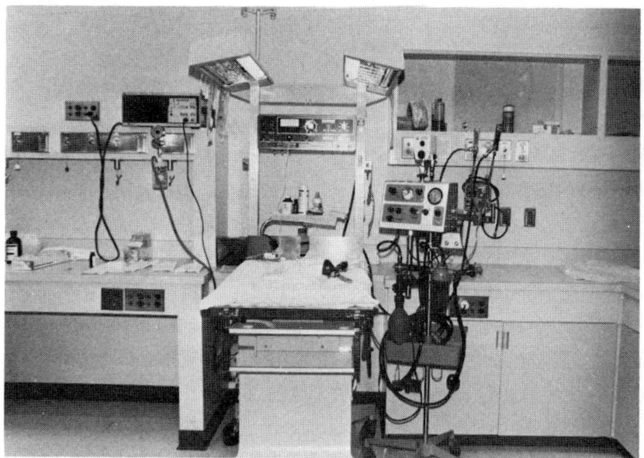

Figure 23.2
Equipment for managing a high-risk neonate.

Perinatal Health published *Toward Improving the Outcome of Pregnancy*, which described a systematic solution to the personnel and economic problems described above: *regionalization.* Regions are medical service areas defined by the population base they serve and the services that this population requires. Each region includes multiple Level I facilities, which deliver care to low-risk patients; several Level II facilities, which attend to the medium-risk patients; and one or two Level III facilities, where the specialists described earlier are concentrated to deliver care to the high-risk patients.*

For regionalization to succeed, two important processes must be well developed. First, an effective and efficient referral network for patients within the region, including mechanisms for the transmission of information, for consultation, and for transportation of patients, must be operational. Critically ill infants may be moved from a Level I to Level III facility so that they may have the advantage of the special services available there. Once the critical nature of their illnesses are past, the infants may be transferred back to a Level II or Level I facility to recover closer to home and family at a more economic price.

Additionally, for regionalization to succeed, continuing education must be made available to personnel at the Level II and Level I facilities. This so-called outreach education is generally considered to be the responsibility of the specialists at the Level

*Although only neonates are discussed here, the regionalization concept is a perinatal one and applies to high-risk mothers as well.

III facility. Information regarding new techniques and knowledge, procedures for stabilization of infants before transport, and so forth, are shared with the care givers at the Level I and Level II facilities.

Regionalization has been put into practice in varying degrees in different areas; the impact has been felt by patients, families, and care givers. The decrease in perinatal mortality and morbidity can, in part, be attributed to this systematic approach to care. On the other hand, families have experienced great economic expense at the hands of Level III facilities and equally great emotional expense at being separated by long distances from their critically ill infants. Care givers are continually looking for creative ways to deal with these problems. Whether or not the regionalization concept will survive the transition from ideal theory to realistic application remains to be seen.

The roles of nurses involved in caring for neonates with problems are as varied in depth and breadth as are the problems themselves. The staff nurse in the Level I nursery must be able to identify potentially harmful situations, to stabilize critically ill infants in preparation for transport to Level II or III facilities, and, in some cases, to transport the patients personally to the next facility. In Level II and III nurseries, staff nurses must have in-depth knowledge regarding the many problems of the critically ill neonate as well as sophisticated technical skills for dealing with the proliferation of technologic aids available for neonatal intensive care (Fig. 23.4). Also, many Level III nurseries have developed transport programs that involve expanded role neonatal nurse clinicians who have additional skills in intubation, chest thoracotomy, x-ray film interpretation, and so forth. And finally, many follow-up programs for neonatal intensive care patients (NICP) include primary health care nurse practitioners who follow the growth and development of these at risk patients in hospitals, homes, and clinics.

In spite of the varied nature of these nursing roles, there are several common attributes of all of these nurses. The nursing process, or problem-solving approach, is second nature to them. Rapid assessment and interpretation of data from multiple sources, knowledgeable planning, and skillful intervention, evaluation, and renewal of the cycle occur repeatedly in their practice. Additionally, nurses of neonates at risk recognize the uniqueness of their tiny patients—the very small scales of treatments, the low dosages of medications, the incredibly narrow margin of error. Failure of others to realize this uniqueness has led to neonatal nurses being very protective of their patients. Consulting health workers must demonstrate their awareness of the special needs of the neonate before the neonatal nurses will relax their vigilant appraisals of interlopers' every move. Finally, parents are very important people to neonatal nurses and sensitivity to parent–infant interactional needs is always present. Recognizing that they are caring for a *family*, staff members in neonatal intensive care units almost universally allow parents to visit 24 hours a day (Fig. 23.5). With accessibility to their infants, parents are encouraged to touch and hold their infants as soon as possible, to call or be called frequently if separated by distance from the

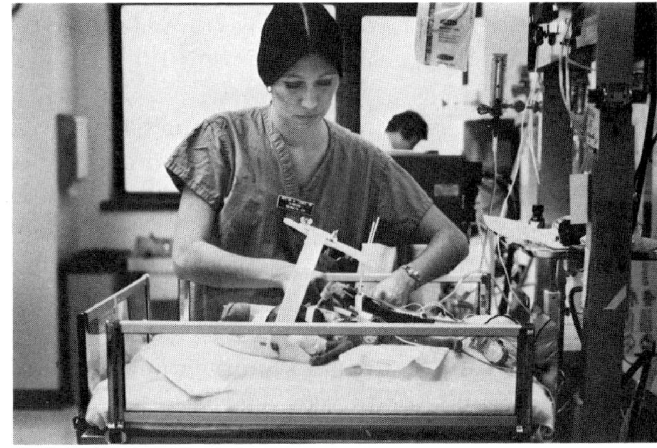

Figure 23.4
Nurse with high-risk neonate.

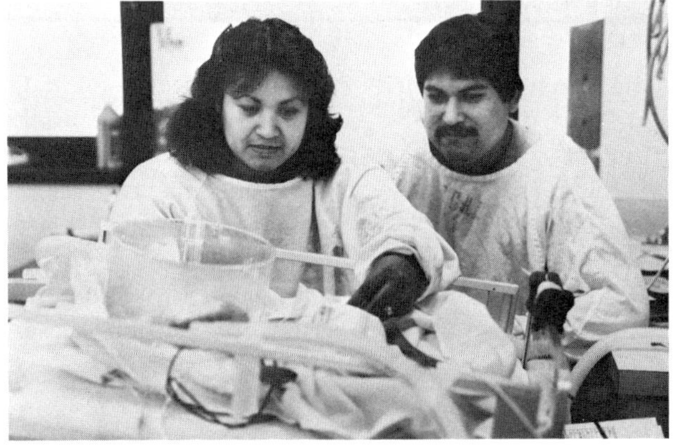

Figure 23.5
Family with sick neonate.

neonatal intensive care unit (NICU), and to be involved in decision making regarding the care and management of their infants.

The health care team of professionals caring for neonates at risk—newborns who are potentially or actually ill—knows that its most important actions are anticipation and prevention. Subjective and objective information about the patient is available prenatally, at delivery, and postnatally, and none of it can afford to be ignored or disregarded. When problems are anticipated and interventions planned before problems occur, successful resolution is much more frequently the result.

PRENATAL RISK FACTORS

Reproductive risk factors have been discussed at length in earlier chapters. Whether they be social, medical, and/or obstetric, and whether they occur before conception, prenatally, or at delivery, the effects of the maternal–fetal history upon the subsequent condition of the neonate are profound. Chapter 20 discusses some of these risk factors and their possible effects on the fetus and newborn.

In most labor and delivery units it is common practice to notify nursery personnel when an at risk infant is expected. Often the nursery nurse or doctor is present at the delivery so that anticipated problems can be dealt with immediately.

NEONATAL PROBLEMS THAT PRESENT AT DELIVERY

The attendant, whether an obstetric or neonatal nurse or doctor, who cares for the neonate at the time of delivery is responsible for immediate assessment of the newborn infant in four critical areas.

- ▲ Establishment and maintenance of adequate cardiorespiratory function (prevention of asphyxia)
- ▲ Assessment of gestational age
- ▲ Observation for evidence of birth trauma
- ▲ Observation for major gross physical anomalies

The Infant Who Experiences Asphyxia

In utero, the fetus is dependent upon an effective placental–fetal circulation for oxygenation. At birth, as described in Chapter 11, the neonate is required to establish his or her own cardiopulmonary functioning to sustain life. If either system is unsuccessful and the supply of oxygen to the baby interrupted, *asphyxia* may be the disasterous outcome. Prolonged *hypoxia* leads to cardiovascular failure and metabolic and respiratory acidosis. If unchecked, the brain and other vital organs sustain permanent damage. Obviously, timely and effective intervention are essential if the infant is to survive this insult intact.

Any event in fetal life that interrupts the supply of oxygen may lead to asphyxia. Common predelivery events include placenta previa, abruptio placentae, nuchal cord with compression, and maternal overmedication. Fetal distress may be noted by fetal heart tones greater than 160 or fewer than 120 beats per minute, irregular fetal heart tones, or passage of *meconium* in utero (meconium-stained amniotic fluid).

Once delivered, the infant's respiratory effort, heart rate, color, and muscle tone are the best indicators of his or her status. The Apgar score (Chapter 17) is the most practical and efficient systematic manner in which to make an emergency assessment.

Any infant with an Apgar score of 2 or less at 1 minute is severely asphyxiated and immediate intervention to establish adequate oxygenation is required. The infant's airway should be suctioned quickly and positive pressure ventilation with oxygen should be started. Ventilation may be mouth to mouth, bag to mask, or bag to endotracheal tube if an attendant skilled in intubation is present. (Effective bag and mask ventilation is much preferred to prolonged attempts at intubation by inexperienced persons.) It is hoped that the infant will respond with improved color and activity and with a heart rate greater than 100 beats per minute. If not, the administration of sodium bicarbonate or epinephrine and closed chest cardiac message are indicated.

An infant having an Apgar score of 3–6 at 1 minute is generally mildly-to-moderately asphyxiated. Improvement is usually noted after brief suctioning and positive pressure bag-to-mask ventilation with oxygen. Infants with Apgar scores of

7–10 rarely require resuscitative intervention other than bulb syringe suctioning of the nasopharynx.

Long-term prognosis for asphyxiated infants can be predicted based upon their 5-minute Apgar scores since the degree of asphyxia still present at 5 minutes is represented by this score. In general, 5-minutes scores of 0–3 are associated with higher neonatal mortality and neurologic morbidity in survivors. Prompt and effective intervention is of the essence.

Other than the treatment described above, nursing consideration should be given to the ready availability and proper functioning of supplies, equipment, and medications needed for resuscitation in the delivery room. There is *never* an excuse for delaying the resuscitation of an infant while a proper-sized endotracheal (ET) tube or laryngoscope bulb are being located.

Sometimes during resuscitation of an infant, the attendants' overvigorous response can be harmful rather than helpful. Prolonged nasopharyngeal suctioning, in addition to delaying the supply of oxygen to the infant, may have the effect of causing reflex bradycardia and/or apnea and should be avoided. Excessive pressure or too rapid positive pressure ventilation may complicate the resusciative efforts by producing pneumothorax. Some manufacturers of infant resuscitation equipment, in an effort to prevent this complication, have produced a bag that "cuts out" if maximal pressure is exceeded. Unfortunately, many care givers do not understand this mechanism and believe that *more* pressure is required to work the bag. The simple solution to this unnecessary situation is for all personnel attending births to familiarize themselves thoroughly with the equipment available.

As was discussed in Chapter 17, the thermoregulatory capabilities of newborn infants are limited. In the case of a compromised infant, the maintenance of a warm, dry environment during resuscitation is imperative.

Meconium aspiration often accompanies asphyxia. As noted earlier, passage of meconium in utero is a sign of fetal distress. When an infant presents with meconium-stained amniotic fluid or is covered with meconium at birth, rapid, meticulous laryngotracheal suctioning under direct visualization by laryngoscope should be performed *before* the infant breathes or positive pressure ventilation is begun. As soon as possible, the stomach contents should also be aspirated into a specimen (De Lee) trap so that regurgitation and inhalation do not occur.

If meconium-stained amniotic fluid reaches the terminal airways, aspiration pneumonia and severe respiratory disease often result. Pneumomediastinum and pneumothorax are commonly seen, along with extremely poor oxygenation as a result of cardiopulmonary shunting. Most infants with meconium aspiration pneumonia require mechanically assisted ventilation. Further treatment is symptomatic while waiting for the natural pulmonary defenses to clear the lungs of debris. This process may be accelerated by carefully administered percussion and postural drainage (Fig. 23.6). Since these infants are often postmature and small for gestational age, they should also be observed for hypoglycemia. Central nervous system disorders with long-term sequelae are not uncommon.

Nursing attentiveness to vital signs and overall clinical condition cannot be overstressed in the care of infants with meconium aspiration. The nurse

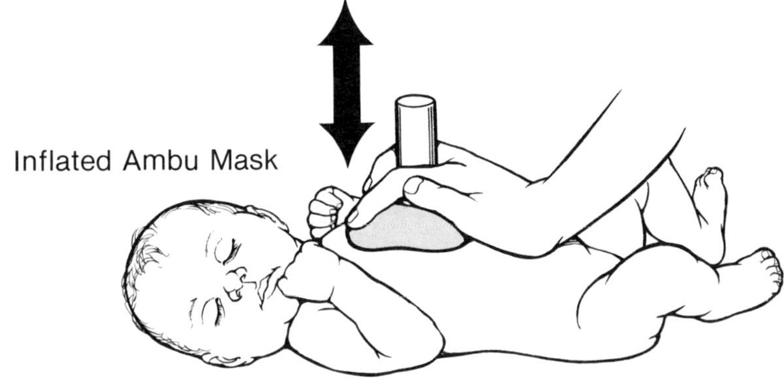

Figure 23.6
An illustration of percussion of an infant's chest to loosen secretions. The inflated mask protects the infant from bruising soft tissue injury.

who is caring for the patient, usually on a one-to-one basis, must be vigilant to the slightest change in patient status so that intervention may be undertaken at the earliest possible moment.

The Infant Who Is Inappropriate in Size or in Gestational Age

In Chapter 17 a detailed discussion of gestational age assessment was presented. Why be concerned with an infant's gestational age? Because the infant's behavior, susceptibility to various complications, and eventual outcome are all a function of both size and gestational age. This important step of gestational age assessment in anticipatory care will be most valuable in identifying potential problems if it is accomplished as soon as possible after delivery of the infant.

Table 23.1 lists the possible complications for infants of inappropriate size or gestational age. The disorders are described in more detail later in this chapter. Two types of infants inappropriately grown for gestational age merit discussion at this time.

The small for gestational age (SGA) baby with *intrauterine growth retardation* (IUGR) is an infant whose weight falls below 10% on intrauterine growth charts. Such infants, who are also known as *small for dates* or *dysmature,* are often characterized at birth as looking like a starving little old man. Their scalp hair is sparse, and the sutures on their heads are widely spaced because of impaired bone growth. With their brow furrowed, they often ap-

TABLE 23.1
ASSESSMENT OF GESTATIONAL AGE

Problems Associated with Specific Gestational Age Groups

1. Premature infants
   - ▲ Hyaline membrane disease
   - ▲ Apnea
   - ▲ Inability to maintain adequate temperature
   - ▲ Hypoglycemia
   - ▲ Difficulty feeding (may need gavaging)
   - ▲ Intracranial hemorrhage
   - ▲ Hypocalcemia
   - ▲ Infection
   - ▲ Jaundice
2. SGA infants
   - ▲ Hypoglycemia
   - ▲ Hypocalcemia
   - ▲ Asphyxia at birth
   - ▲ Meconium aspiration
   - ▲ Polycythemia
   - ▲ Other problems related to the etiology of the infant's poor growth (e.g., congenital anomalies)
3. Postterm infants
   - ▲ Hypoglycemia
   - ▲ Fetal distress
   - ▲ Neonatal asphyxia
   - ▲ Meconium aspiration pneumonia
   - ▲ SGA
4. LGA infants
   - ▲ Hypoglycemia
   - ▲ Birth trauma with resultant central nervous system problems

pear worried. Their skin is dry, cracked, and peeling; it hangs loosely in folds over their bodies because of muscle wasting and absence of subcutaeous fat. Their abdomens appear sunken or scaphoid, and their umbilical cords are small, thin, dry, and yellowed (see Fig. 23.7).

Although many factors have been associated with IUGR, clearly identifiable causes remain obscure. It is generally accepted that the growth retardation is a result of either cellular hypoplasia (diminished number of cells with normal amounts of cytoplasm in each cell) or decreased cellular size with accompanying decrease in the amount of intracellular cytoplasm.

Infants with IUGR are at risk for asphyxia and meconium aspiration at birth, as well as for the development of other disorders such as hypoglycemia, hypocalcemia, and hypothermia in the neonatal period. Nursing management is aimed at observation for, prevention of, and symptomatic treatment for these disorders.

Prognosis for IUGR infants remains somewhat unclear. Obviously, for those infants with a serious, overlying congenital anomaly or syndrome, the outlook is not favorable. But for those infants where etiology is indeterminate, prognoses differ from author to author and researcher to researcher. While some evidence suggests that increasing percentages of minimal brain dysfunction, electroencephalogram (EEG) abnormalities, speech deficits, and educational difficulties are present in IUGR infants as they grow up, other data indicate that IUGR infants and their same weight, but premature, counterparts have similar growth and developmental potentials. Significant research into this problem and its sequelae is ongoing.

In contrast to a SGA infant, the *infant of a diabetic mother* (IDM) who is *large for gestational age* (LGA), is fat and cherubic, but often less mature than would be expected for the gestational age (see Fig. 23.8). The delivery is frequently traumatic because of the infant's size. The major complication encountered by the infant is hypoglycemia in the first few hours of life.

It is generally believed that elevated levels of maternal blood glucose are responsible for the infant's size and predisposition to hypoglycemia. The stimulus of high levels of glucose causes pancreatic hyperplasia and hyperinsulinemia in the fetus. Given this internal environment, the infant grows excessively and accumulates large amounts of fat. At birth, the maternal glucose supply is cut off, but continued production of insulin leads to marked hypoglycemia. Management includes frequent measurement of blood glucose levels in the infant during the first hours of life and early feedings and/or administration of intravenous dextrose. The excessive production of insulin usually slows down in the first day or so and no further sequelae are noted. Infants of diabetic mothers are, however, inexplicably at significantly higher risk for many congenital anomalies, especially congenital heart disease. Close observation and assessment for signs and symptoms of other problems is, therefore, important.

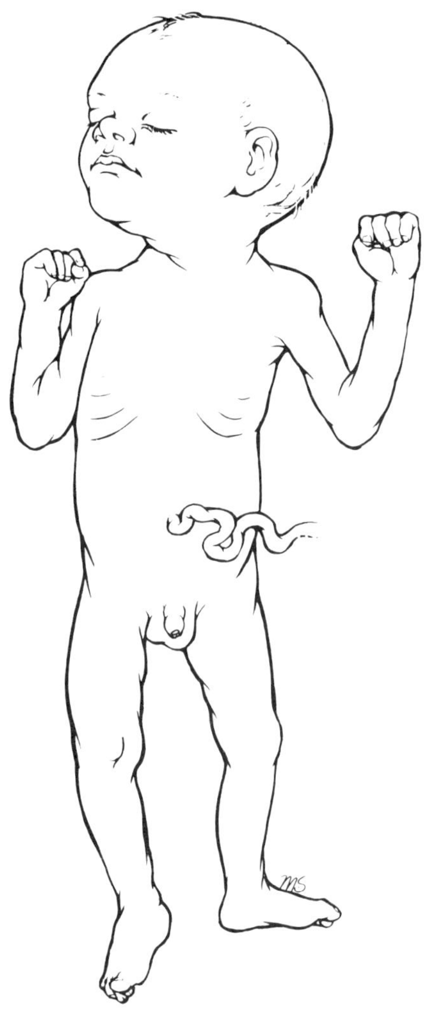

Figure 23.7
An intrauterine growth retarded baby, small for gestational age, with characteristic loose skin folds, sparse scalp hair, scaphoid abdomen, and small, thin umbilical cord.

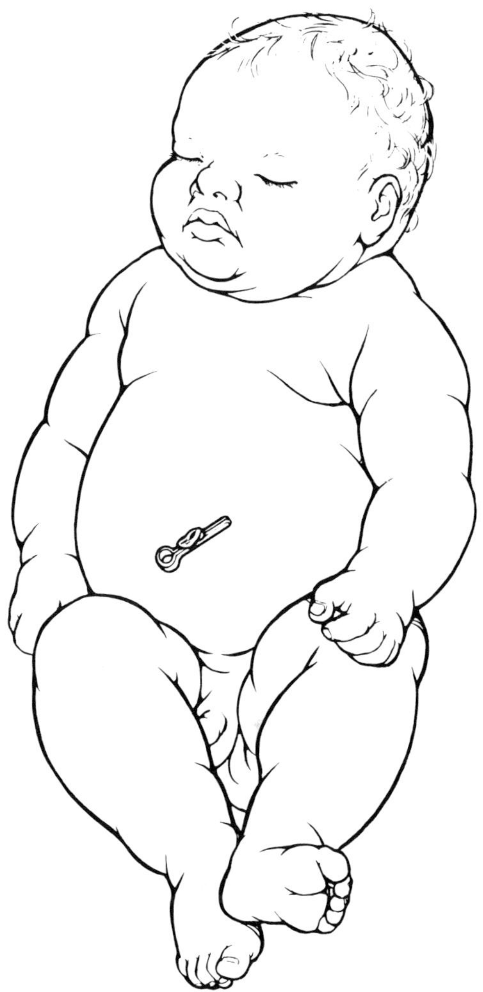

Figure 23.8
Large for gestational age infant with characteristic chubby, cherubic appearance.

The Infant Who Sustains Physical Birth Trauma

The transition from intrauterine to extrauterine life for a neonate is marked not only by physiologic adjustments but also by a physical journey. Many factors influence the infant's successful navigation of womb to world, including position in utero before and during labor and at delivery, the length and effectiveness of labor, size in relation to the bony and soft birth canals, and elements surrounding the birth itself. Surprisingly few infants are injured during this remarkable transition; those who are generally recover with little or no intervention from care givers. Although a few injuries are serious enough to warrant treatment, birth injuries are rarely fatal.

Caput succedaneum, edema of the scalp, results from pressure of the fetal head against the dilating cervix. Similarly, swelling of the buttocks and/or extremities may occur in breech presentations. In both cases, impaired venous return in the affected area may also cause localized petechiae or ecchymoses. These signs of difficult or prolonged labor are present at birth and disappear in 2–3 days. They are rarely pathologically significant, although they may contribute to hyperbilirubinemia.

The neonate's head may also appear misshapen as a result of *molding* (Fig. 23.9). Because of the incompletely fused sutures of the cranium, the neonate's head is able to be gradually shaped to fit through the birth canal. Generally, the head appears elongated in an anterior-to-posterior dimension.* Restoration of normal cranial appearance by 2–3 days is expected.

Cephalhematoma, a collection of blood as a result of rupture of blood vessels between the skull and overlying periosteum, is also evidenced by an altered scalp contour. However, unlike caput succedaneum, it appears gradually over the first few hours of life, becoming larger until the second or third day when the bleeding stops. Cephalhematoma is circumscribed by the outline of the cranial sutures and is usually noted over one or both parietal bones. Occasionally, an x-ray film shows linear skull fractures beneath a cephalhematoma. No treatment, however, is indicated, and a hematoma itself usually disappears by 1 month of age. Some periosteal thickening may be apparent for several years. Again, hyperbilirubinemia may be worsened by breakdown of the accumulated blood.

The effects of pressure against the bony pelvis or of forceps are often visible as *abrasions of the skin* or *pressure necrosis* of the subcutaneous fat. These injuries are most frequently seen in the facial area and often are referred to as *forceps' marks*. Their resolution in 2–3 days is usually without incident.

Subconjunctival hemorrhages are ruptures of scleral capillaries as a result of changes in intracranial pressure during delivery. They appear as bright red halos around the irises of the eyes. They also disappear in 2–3 days and are unremarkable clinically.

Fractures as a result of difficult labor and/or de-

*Occiputal–frontal circumference (OFC) (head circumference) may be less at birth than at 3–4 days because of molding.

livery are not uncommon. As mentioned earlier, *linear skull fractures* may underlie cephalhematoma and are asymptomatic unless cerebral blood vessels have been damaged also, resulting in subdural hematoma. "Ping pong ball" fractures, or *depressed skull fractures*, are indentations of the cranial bone, which may occur after prolonged pressure of the fetal head on the bony pelvis or after improper application of forceps. Most of the time these fractures heal without intervention. Infrequently, the bony depression causes the underlying brain to become compressed and surgical elevation of the fracture is required.

The most common *long bone fractures* occur in the upper extremities, most frequently in the middle third of the *clavicle* (Fig. 23.10). Shoulder dystocia during delivery is the usual cause. Asymmetry of the upper extremities during Moro reflex and limited spontaneous movement of the affected side

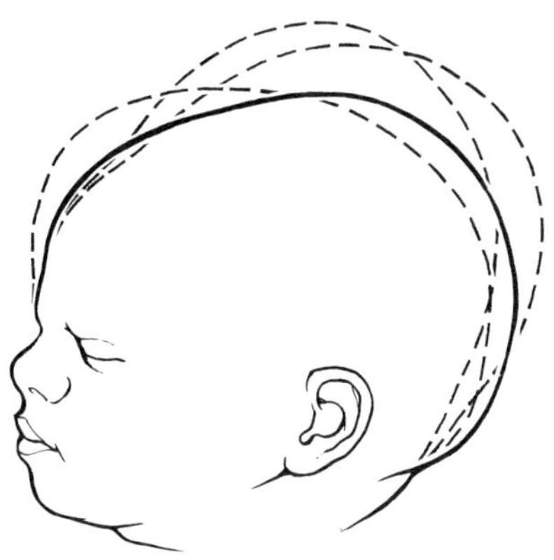

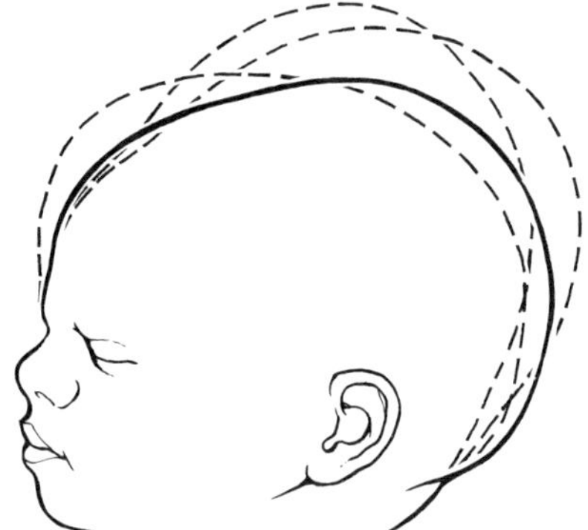

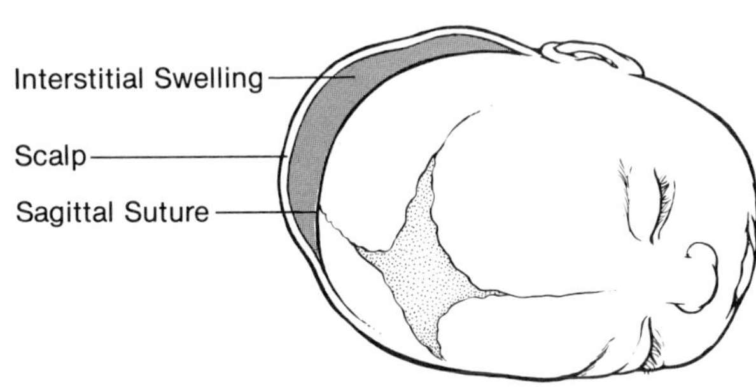

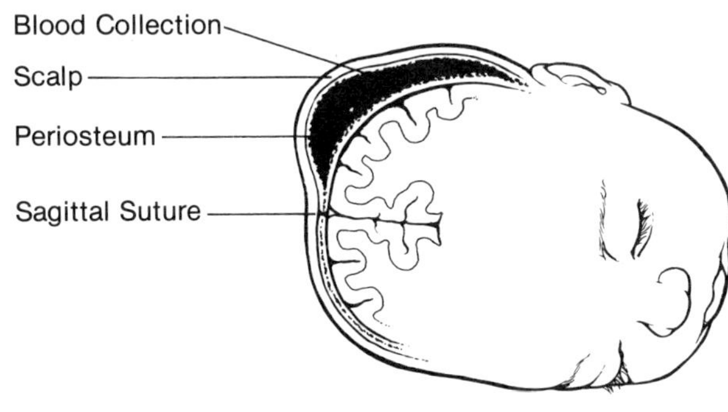

Figure 23.9
(*a*) Molding. The solid line is the normal shape of an infant's head; the broken lines show possible misshapen head; (*b*) Caput succedaneum; (*c*) cephalhematoma. An illustration of the differences between caput succedaneum and cephalhematoma. Edema in caput is external to the periosteum and would be noted crossing the suture line, while cephalhematoma is delineated by the suture line.

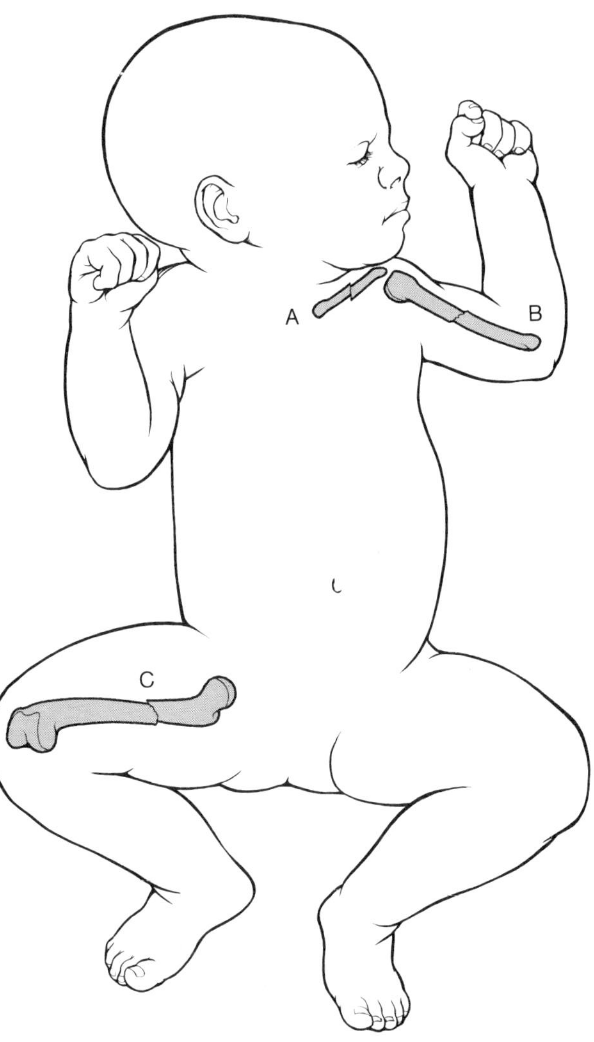

Figure 23.10
Common sites for neonatal fractures. (*a*) Clavicle; (*b*) humerus; (*c*) femur.

are noted. *Humeral fractures* result in even more evidence of diminished motion and pain in the affected side. As may be expected, the incidence of these fractures is greater with larger babies, particularly those weighing over 4,000 gm. Fractures of the *femur* occur infrequently and usually follow difficult breech deliveries. Redness, swelling, or discoloration of the thigh accompanied by limited spontaneous movement are noted.

Clavicular fractures are treated by careful handling—no other immobilization is required. In cases of fractured humerus or femur, the affected limb may be splinted and/or wrapped with a supportive bandage.

Transient paralysis may occur as a result of injuries to nerves during labor and delivery. *Brachial plexus palsy* resulting from injury to or edema of the brachial plexus of nerve trunks located in the infant's neck may follow stretching of the neck in either routine or traumatic deliveries. Symptoms are immediately apparent and include limited mobility of the upper extremity on the affected side, asymmetrical Moro reflex response, and dangling of the affected extremity when the infant is held up. At rest, the infant's arm lies close to the body, elbow straight and palm face down. In general, the paralysis disappears in a few weeks, although occasionally it is permanent. Treatment regimens of positioning have been described; however, careful handling and passive range of motion are likely to be the most effective interventions.

Diaphragm paralysis as a result of severe *brachial plexus injury* is noted by the additional complication of respiratory distress in an infant already observed to have brachial plexus palsy. Although many cases resolve in a few weeks to 1 year, careful positioning and feeding are required to prevent pneumonia. Rarely is surgical fixation of the diaphragm indicated.

Facial paralysis, evidenced by asymmetry of the face during crying, is the result of pressure on the facial nerve just below and behind the ear lobe. Again, pressure against the maternal bony pelvis or misapplication of forceps are the culprits. The infant's mouth, in particular, may present difficulties as its lack of muscle tone unilaterally makes effective sucking impossible. Time and care must be taken when feeding these infants; jaw, cheek, and chin support is necessary. Facial paralysis usually disappears in just a few days.

Central nervous system damage, as a result of labor and delivery, fortunately occurs infrequently. *Intracranial hemorrhage,* usually subdural, may occur as a result of rapid expansion and compression of the fetal head, particularly during precipitous delivery. Signs and symptoms are those of increased intracranial pressure, such as tense, bulging fontanel, widely separated suture lines, absent or diminished reflexes, bradycardia, tachypnea, hypotension, lethargy or irritability, hyperemesis, high-pitched cry, and eventually seizures and coma. Depending on the location of the hemorrhage, subdural taps through the fontanel may relieve the symptoms transiently. Unfortunately, prognosis is not good. *Spinal cord injury* during breech delivery may, depending upon the level of the insult, result in total or partial paralysis. Again, prognosis is very poor. Fortunately, improved obstetric management has made this a rare injury.

Nursing care of infants who have sustained birth trauma is generally passive in nature. Gentle handling and nonspecific relief of symptoms with positioning, feeding techniques, and so on, have been noted above. Perhaps the nurse's most important role is one of educator. Parents require simple explanations, demonstrations, and reassurances that most of these evidences of difficult labor and delivery will disappear without intervention.

The Infant with a Major Physical Anomaly

Those present during the delivery of a newborn—doctors, nurses, parents—are the first to observe any obvious physical anomalies. Etiologically, these defects may occur as a result of embryologic error, genetic inheritance, or a combination of both. Some of the more common birth defects are discussed below.

Cleft lip and/or *palate* results from the incomplete fusion during embryologic development of the facial processes. The defect may range in severity from merely a dimple in the chin to complete, bilaterally clefted lip and palate. While the initial appearance of the infant may be grotesque, reconstructive surgery is quite successful and markedly improves the baby's appearance. Lip repairs are usually done by the rule of 10s—when the infant is 10 weeks old, weighs 10 lb, and has a hemoglobin of at least 10. Waiting for this period of time allows for tissue growth to occur so that more is available with which to work during repair. Waiting also provides an opportunity to observe the infant for any other anomalies. Palate repairs are usually done when the baby is 12–15 months old.

The major care and treatment consideration with infants who have cleft lips and/or palates is feeding. Numerous, specially designed nipples and other apparati are available that supposedly make feeding easier. However, the mother–infant relationship benefits from normalization of feeding, that is, the absence of unusual appearing devices. By holding the infant in an upright position and using either a soft premie nipple with an enlarged cross cut or a double nipple system, the majority of infants can be fed effectively if provided with chin and cheek support (Fig. 23.11). Occasionally, an obturator or dental prosthesis is recommended to assist in alignment of the structures in the infant's mouth. If an appliance is used, care should be taken to clean it and the infant's mouth meticulously after each feeding. Also the mouth should be observed carefully for any signs of pressure or breakdown.

Meningomyelocele is a midline neural tube defect whereby the spinal cord and meninges have herniated through a defect in the vertebrae to the outside of the spinal column. Since the defect occurs early in embryologic life, the nerves contained in the cele have grown randomly and without any order; thus, there is no innervation below the level of the defect. As a result, meningomyelocele is usually accompanied by orthopedic and genitourinary complications and obstructive hydrocephalus.

The first issue to be addressed in the treatment of meningomyelocele is whether or not to intervene. Depending upon the projected degree of impairment and brain damage that has occurred or may occur, as well as upon the individual philoso-

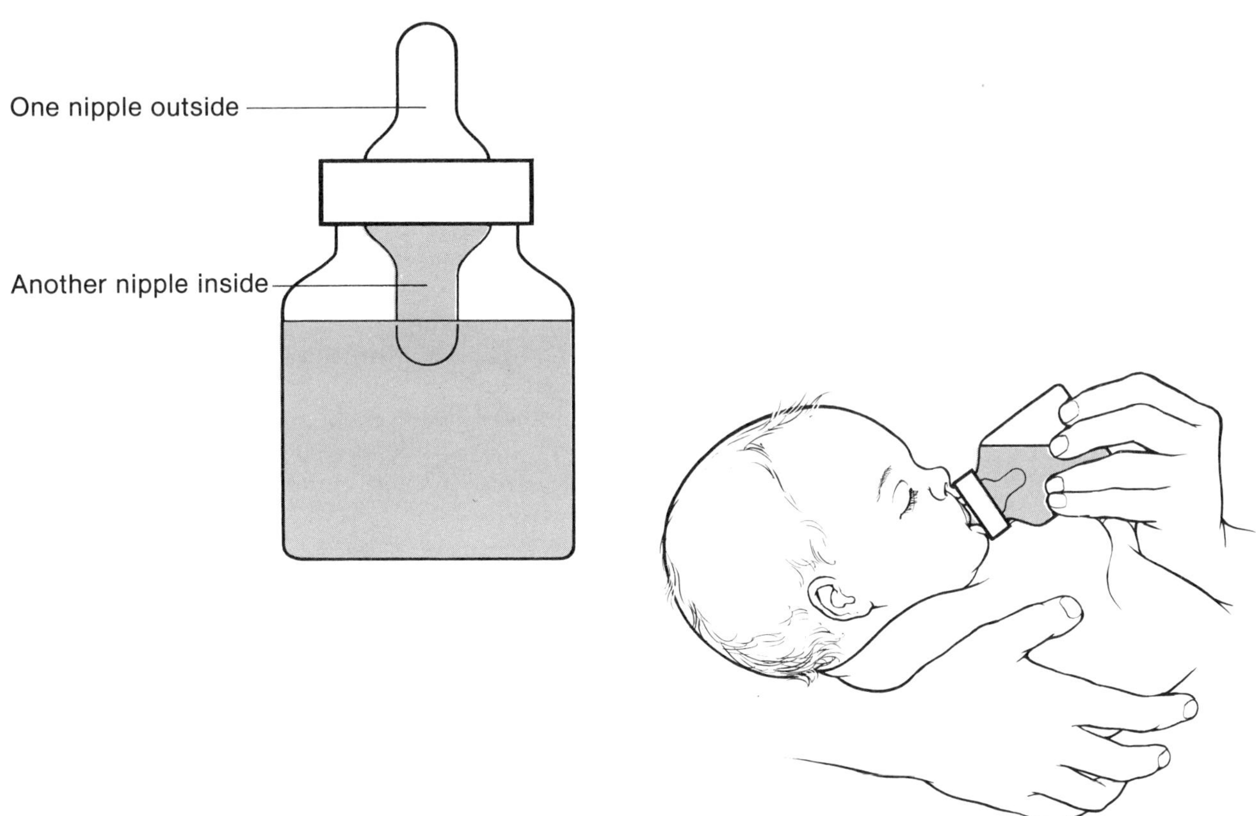

Figure 23.11
Feeding an infant with cleft lip and palate. The double nipple system for feeding an infant with a cleft lip and/or palate. Before feeding the infant, the bottle is inverted and the *outer* nipple repeatedly squeezed until the *inner* nipple fills completely with formula. After this, slight pressure on the *outer* nipple will result in the formula being released.

phies of the persons involved, some doctors, nurses, and parents believe that a nonaggressive approach of providing nutritional support without surgical intervention is best. Others believe that closure of the defect and aggressive management of infection, hydrocephalus, and so on are indicated. It goes without saying that disagreement exists, and that this is one of the most highly charged moral, ethical, and legal issues in health care today.

Assuming the medical–surgical intervention is selected, nursing care of the infant begins preoperatively with the protection of the cele. In the delivery room, sterile saline soaks should be placed over the sac so that it is protected and kept moist. The infant should be placed in a prone position. Postoperatively, the incision line should be protected carefully from contamination, especially from feces. Again, the infant is maintained in a level, prone position, even during feedings, to prevent any strain on the surgical site. Elevating the infant's entire body on a large role of blankets or pads so that the hips may be flexed and abducted will help to prevent hip dislocation and walking problems later in life. Most infants with meningomyelocele have atonic bladders, and credé of the bladder every 2–3 hours is indicated. Since hydrocephalus is a frequent complication, ventriculoperitoneal shunting will usually be accomplished during the initial hospitalization, as well.

Congenital hydrocephalus—abnormally large head size as a result of excessive accumulated cerebral spinal fluid and subsequently enlarged ventricles—is associated with brain atrophy. When present at birth, hydrocephalus carries a poor long-term prognosis. The infant's head appears smooth and shiny with prominent vessels, the forehead is particularly prominent, and the eyes exhibit the classic "setting sun" sign. Without intervention, signs of increased intracranial pressure appear as the infant's condition deteriorates—irritability, then lethargy; respiratory distress; hyperemesis; and eventually signs of neurologic damage: seizures and coma. Despite shunting to alleviate spinal fluid accumulation and intracranial pressure, permanent damage has usually occured and mental retardation is not uncommon.

Initially, nursing care of the infant with hydrocephalus may be directed at confirming diagnosis. Measurement of OFC at birth and serially for days afterward will help document whether or not the infant's head size is abnormal and growing. With infants whose heads are already large, skin care to prevent pressure sores and breakdown of skin is important since the infant may not be able to lift and turn the head. This is especially important if a shunt has been placed under the surface of the scalp. Also, care should be taken when holding the infant to support the head and neck.

Microcephaly and *anencephaly* are characterized by head sizes that are markedly smaller than normal and are generally associated with brain growth arrest or retardation of some degree. Frequent causes are radiation, viral infections such as rubella or cytomegalovirus, and some genetically acquired syndromes. Developmental prognosis is poor. Care takers who are pregnant (doctors, nurses, technicians, etc.) should not care for these infants if viral infection is suspected.

Gastroschisis and *omphalocele* are defects whereby the contents of the abdomen (usually intestines, sometimes liver, pancreas, and other organs) are found at birth outside the abdominal wall. Embryologically, the two defects differ in that omphalocele results from failure of the midgut to migrate back into the abdomen from the umbilical stalk, while gastroschisis represents a simple failure of the musculature of the abdominal wall to close completely. Consequently, omphalocele has a much higher association with other anomalies, particularly gastrointestinal. The herniated intestines of omphalocele may be covered with the amniotic membrane of the cord, or the membrane may have ruptured, leaving the intestines floating in the amniotic fluid. In gastroschisis, the intestines are never covered.

In the delivery room treatment of the exposed bowel consists of covering it with sterile saline soaks. Surgical intervention is undertaken as soon as possible. If the defect is small, the repair may be completed at once. If the defect is large, the abdominal cavity is not capable of accepting the intestines without severe respiratory compromise, so a staged repair (step by step) is performed. In either case, prolonged inability of the infant to feed by mouth is not unusual, and intravenous hyperalimentation is provided.

Imperforate anus is the congenital absence of a gastrointestinal outlet—the anus. Embryologically, failure of the primitive urogenital sinus and cloaca to differentiate have occurred. High and low types of imperforate anus have been described depending upon the relationship of the blind rectal pouch to the levator muscles. Frequently, there is a fistula from the rectal pouch to the perineum such as the rectovaginal fistula seen in a high percentage of female infants. In the absence of a fistula, emergency colostomy is indicated. Definitive corrective surgery is aimed not only at externally connecting the rectum but also at providing continuence in that new connection.

Ambiguous genitalia are often apparent at birth and may be the result of embryologic, hormonal, metabolic, or genetic errors. The multiplicity of causes and treatments will not be explored here. However, crucial management of the infant with ambiguous genitalia is sharing the information with the parents, which begins in the delivery room.

For most parents, the first question asked upon delivery of their newborn is: "Is it a girl or boy?" Certainly it is incredibly difficult for the doctor or nurse in attendance to answer: "We don't know." We are certainly aware of the embarrassment and confusion that this answer and the delay in sexual assignment will cause the family. However, these difficult circumstances are much preferred to the devastating and heartbreaking situation of sexual *reassignment* once chromosomal, anatomic, and physiologic determinations have been made.

Musculoskeletal anomalies of various degrees are readily apparent at the time of birth. At one extreme is *congenital amputation*—the absence of the infant's arms, legs, or both. Such deformities may result from teratogenic agents ingested by the mother during pregnancy (e.g., Thalidomide during the 1960s), constricting bands of amniotic membrane, or other unknown mechanisms. Rehabilitative adaptation through use of prostheses is the course of treatment.

Talipes equinovarus, clubfoot, may occur alone or i· conjunction with other anomalies such as meningomyelocele. Depending upon the severity of the deformity, treatment may range from passive range of motion to successive casting, bracing, and possible surgical intervention.

Polydactyly, the presence of extra digits, may be associated with certain syndromes or may occur as in isolated deformity. If no bone is present in the extra digit, the usual treatment is to tie off the digit with silk suture and wait for it to necrose and fall off in a few days. Surgical intervention is required for cases where bone involvement is present.

Nursing care for the infant with a major physical anomaly, other than the specific interventions discussed above, is centered around parent education and preparation. It has been well documented that parents of deformed babies experience a grieving reaction at the loss of the "perfect" child that they had imagined. When we couple this grief with the multitude of questions and concerns that they have about their infant, it is not difficult to understand that such parents require special supportive attention. This support may take the form of repeated, honest answers to their questions, information about available parent groups, or pictures and other graphic demonstrations of the eventual outcome that their child will attain. At some point early in the experience, it is helpful if the nurse explains the roles of the many members of the health care team who intervene with the infant since this is particularly confusing to many parents. Preparation of the family for repeated rehospitalizations may also be indicated.

NEONATAL PROBLEMS THAT PRESENT IN THE NURSERY

Infants identified as high risk because of prenatal factors and labor and delivery experiences are usually transferred from the delivery room to an intensive care or observation nursery. Infants presumed to be healthy and at low risk are cared for in a minimal care nursery or at the mother's bedside. In either situation, care takers, particularly nurses, must be alert for the signs and symptoms of neonatal problems. Skilled assessment of subtle changes in the infant's behavior or condition is the key to successful early intervention.

Given the variable problems that may afflict neonates, nursing care and management for sick newborns is remarkably consistent. Certain specific interventions are mentioned in the ensuing discussion of neonatal problems. However, overall considerations for all sick newborns should include the following.

▲ ***Assurance of a Thermally Neutral Environment*** (Fig. 23.12). Even in emergency situations, the maintenance of warmth and humidity is crucial since cold stress may exacerbate an infant's poor condition or undo or prevent successful therapy. Numerous devices such as overhead warmers, incubators, and heat shields are available. Many of these devices have servocontrol mechanisms that allow the machine to adjust to the baby's temperature.

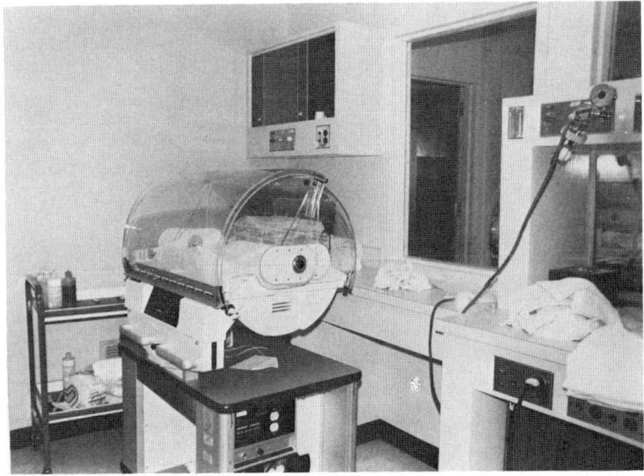

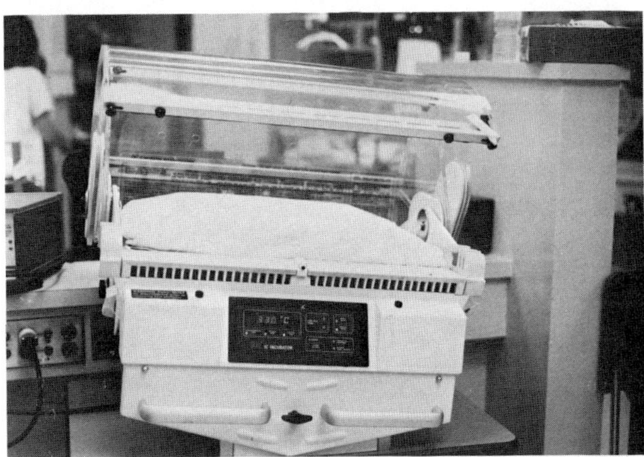

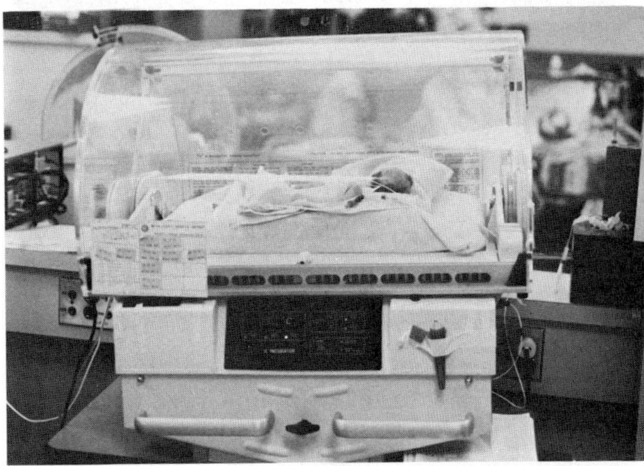

Figure 23.12
Isolette.

▲ ***Close Attention to Vital Signs.*** Gradual, subtle changes in temperature, heart and respiratory rates, and blood pressure may be the earliest signs of impending crises. If such changes are noted, they provide care givers with extra time to anticipate, prevent, or treat the problems. Reliable mechanical means for measuring these parameters, designed specifically for neonates, are available.

▲ ***Careful Measurement and Monitoring of Intake and Output.*** It is often surprising to nonneonatal care givers that the measurement and recording of ½ cc of blood, 5 cc of urine, or 2 cc of intravenous fluid are of utmost importance in the management of neonates. However, since the total blood volume of the newborn is only about 80 cc/kg of body weight, it is easy to see that seemingly minute amounts of fluid in or out can make a substantial impact on the infant's condition. Nursing strategies include weighing diapers, using controllers or pumps on all IV fluid administration, limiting the amount of fluid "hanging" in a soluset to 2-hour's worth, and recording all blood withdrawn.

▲ ***Continuous Scrutiny for Signs of Change in Condition.*** The nursing assessment that an infant "doesn't look right" is one of the most respected. Whether this represents intuition or subconscious observation of clinical signs is not important; further investigation and confirmation of impending problems are indicated.

▲ ***Protection of Skin and Mucous Membrane Integrity.*** Skin and mucous membrane breakdown often leads to infection, complicating the already tenuous course of the high-risk infant. Meticulous care to the sites of IVs, skin electrodes, transcutaneous oxygen monitor electrodes, and nasal and endotracheal tubes is required. Furthermore, limited use of tape is preferred.

▲ ***Encouragement of Parent Involvement and Interaction with the Sick Neonate.*** As described by Klaus and Fanaroff (1973), the early establishment of an affectionate, emotional bond between parent(s) and infant may have an impact on later growth and development of healthy relationships. Encouraging parents to touch their infants, to bring in cards or toys to place on their beds, or to clothe their babies in their own shirts and gowns will promote attachment of parents and infant (Fig. 23.13). It should be remembered that the family may also include siblings, grandparents, and so on, and an effort to include these people in family-centered care is recommended.

The Infant with Respiratory Distress

During the prenatal months, the developing fetus's organ systems grow and mature in preparation for independent, postnatal functioning. Many of the major organs actually begin working before the infant is delivered—the heart pumps blood, the kidneys produce urine, and so on. One notable exception to this "practice run" is the lungs. During prenatal life, the fetal lungs bear little resemblance in function to their postnatal activities. Gaseous exchange is handled completely by the fetal–placental circulation. The changes undergone by the respiratory system at birth are substantial (see Chapter 17). It is not surprising that the majority of problems exhibited by neonates, particularly in the first few hours of life, are respiratory in nature. In fact, most of the morbidity and mortality in this period are as a result of respiratory disease.

The infant experiencing respiratory distress is readily identifiable in the newborn nursery by certain characteristic signs.

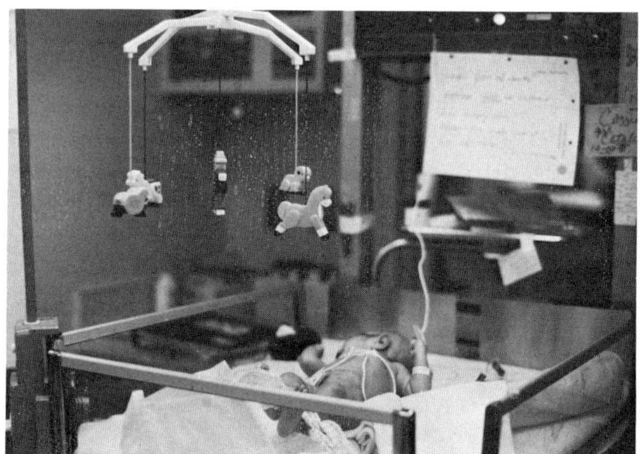

Figure 23.13
Mobile in crib in neonatal intensive care unit.

- ▲ ***Increased Respiratory Rate (Tachypnea).*** The respiratory rate of the healthy newborn who is not crying is 48–60 breaths per minute. The distressed infant may breathe 70–80 or even 100 times per minute.
- ▲ ***Nasal Flaring.*** The nares of the infant dilate visibly with each breath.
- ▲ ***Expiratory Grunting.*** At first this sound may be audible only with a stethoscope. As the distress becomes more severe, grunting may be heard with the naked ear.
- ▲ ***Chest Retractions.*** As the infant works harder and harder to breathe effectively, the chest begins to show visible evidence of the struggle. At first, subcostal, xiphoid, and mild intercostal retractions appear. Later, marked intercostal, sub- and suprasternal, and clavicular retractions become noticeable.
- ▲ ***Cardiovascular Compromise.*** Tachycardia and eventual bradycardia, cyanosis, and hypotension are observed.
- ▲ ***Asynchronized "See Saw" Chest Movement Interrupted by Periods of Apnea.***

Whenever a neonate exhibits signs of respiratory distress, attendant care givers should initiate two activities simultaneously—respiratory support to alleviate distress and prevent further deterioration and immediate investigation into the cause of the infant's distress.

Respiratory support to a distressed infant begins with the assurance of a clear and patent airway by positioning and suctioning the infant's airway. Sometimes improvement will be seen after this simple step. If not, judicious administration of oxygen either into the ambient environment or by assisted ventilation (bag and mask, bag and endotracheal tube, ventilator, etc.) is indicated. Since respiratory distress is worsened by low blood pH, care should be taken to avoid cold stress and to treat metabolic/respiratory acidosis.

Concurrently, the search for the cause of the respiratory distress should begin immediately. Obviously, any condition that interferes with airway patency, alveolar/capillary exchange of gases, cardiovascular or neurologic functioning, or diaphragm and chest wall movement may result in or contribute to respiratory distress. Thus, the etiologies are substantial in number. The more common entities are discussed below.

RESPIRATORY DISTRESS SYNDROME (HYALINE MEMBRANE DISEASE)

Respiratory distress syndrome (RDS) is the most common problem encountered in the neonatal intensive care unit and accounts for the most number of deaths. It is almost exclusively a disease of premature infants and is characterized by a series of events within the lungs that probably begins with an inability of the alveoli to remain inflated because of diminished amounts of surfactant. *Surfactant* is a lipoprotein substance present in the mature lung, lining the surface of the alveoli and preventing their collapse on expiration. Thus, as air is expelled from the lungs, the surfactant exerts a counteractive pull on the alveoli, keeping them partially expanded and inflated.

Surfactant appears in the fetal lungs at about 23–24 weeks gestation but is not present in sufficient amounts until 36–37 weeks. In its absence or diminished presence, alveolar collapse occurs after each of the infant's respirations. The struggle to reinflate the lungs, as evidenced by the previously described signs, will ultimately fail and atelectasis will result.

Other factors that complicate this disease process are as follows.

- ▲ ***Decreased Pulmonary Compliance.*** The stiffness of the lungs means that the infant must work harder and exert more pressure to inflate the lungs.
- ▲ ***Decreased Pulmonary Blood Flow (Vasoconstriction).*** Reduced blood flow to the alveoli leads to ischemia, which further impairs the lung's ability to perform gaseous exchange.

Impaired gaseous exchange results in systemic accumulation of carbon dioxide, hypoxia, and acidosis. Since these conditions contribute to further ischemia and vasoconstriction, the cycle is self-defeating.

RDS usually presents in the first few hours of life. In addition to the signs previously described, severe hypotension and shock may be observed. Definitive diagnosis is usually based on the characteristic reticulogranular appearance of the chest x-ray film, which reflects the areas of atelectasis. Also, as expected, arterial pH and PO_2 levels are decreased.

The treatment of infants with RDS specific to their lung diseases is dependent upon the severity of the clinical condition (see Fig. 23.14). In less severe cases, the administration of ambient O_2 by oxyhood is sufficient. Other infants may require continuous positive airway pressure (CPAP), a mechanical means of exerting pressure back into the lungs at the end of expiration in order to keep the alveoli partially inflated. CPAP may be administered by endotracheal tube or nasal prongs, with or without oxygen. Infants most severely affected will require endotracheal intubation and mechanical ventilation, sometimes with very high peak pressures.

All patients receiving oxygen therapy have their arterial oxygen tension levels measured and monitored at frequent intervals. In this way, adequacy of treatment can be ensured while the development of chronic lung changes (bronchopulmonary dysplasia) or retinal blindness (retrolental fibroplasia) is avoided. An arterial PO_2 maintained between 50 and 90 mm Hg is appropriate.

Nursing care of the infant with severe RDS involves suctioning the endotracheal tube to ensure patency, closely observing for signs of sudden deterioration that may signify pneumothorax, and frequently collecting blood specimens for assessment of oxygenation. These patients usually have umbilical arterial catheters and care must be taken with these lines to prevent clotting, hemorrhage, and introduction of infection.

The course of uncomplicated RDS is generally increasing severity over the first few days, with a peak at the third day. This is followed by improvement during the fourth to sixth day. Prognosis is still guarded for several weeks, however, until full recovery has occurred.

TRANSIENT TACHYPNEA OF THE NEWBORN (RDS, TYPE II)

Unlike RDS, transient tachypnea of the newborn (TTN) is generally seen in term infants. Mild respiratory distress as evidenced by tachypnea, but without the more severe symptoms, is noted. X-ray film findings are completely different than those with RDS and suggest the presence and slow absorption of amniotic fluid. Oxygen by hood is the only treatment that is usually required (Fig. 23.15). The disease ordinarily runs an uncomplicated 4–5-day course.

PNEUMOTHORAX

Term infants experiencing moderate signs of respiratory distress such as cyanosis, tachypnea,

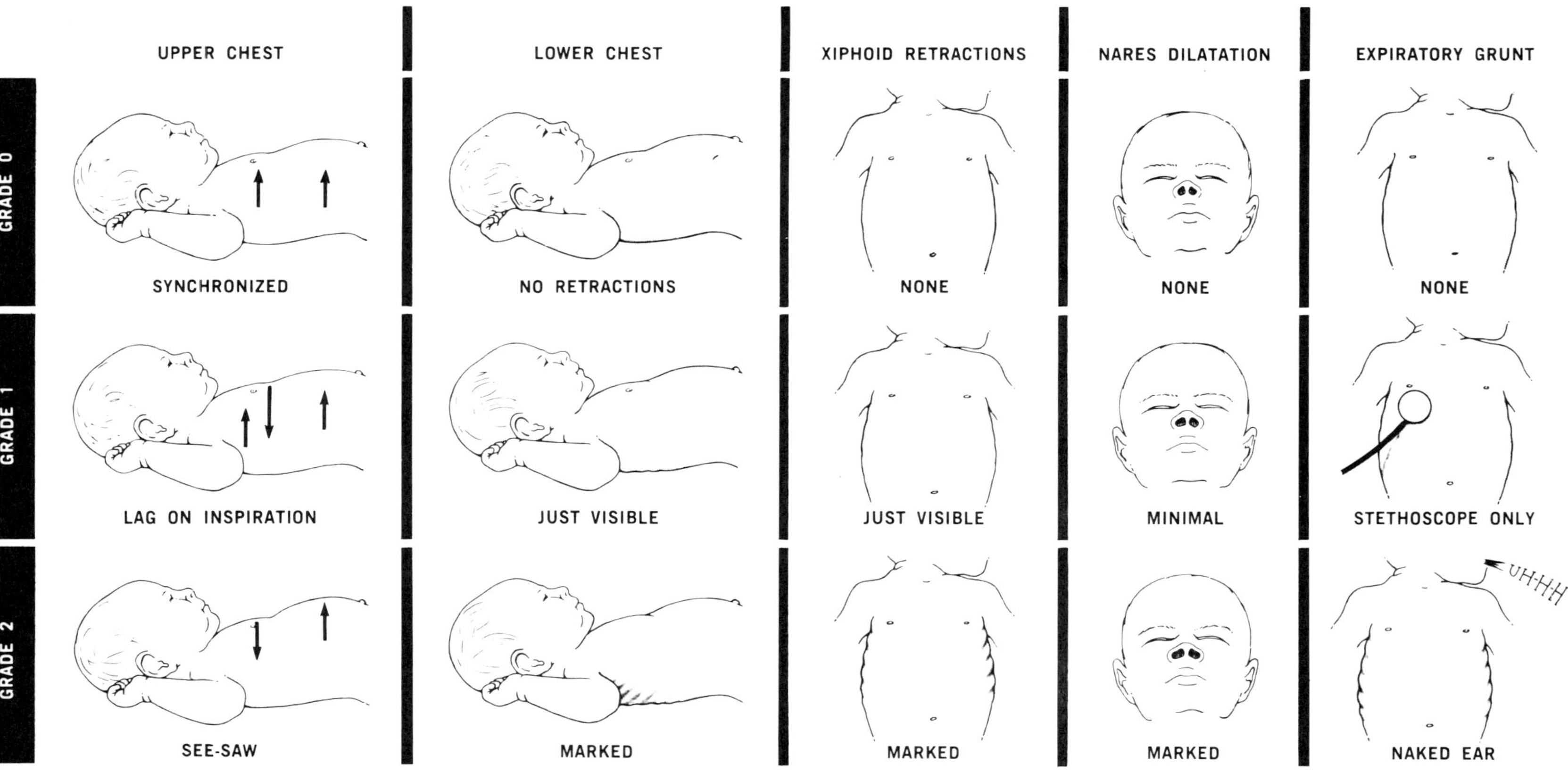

Figure 23.14
Evaluation of respiratory status. This index is designed to provide a continued evaluation of the infant's respiratory status. An index of respiratory distress is determined by grading each of five arbitrary criteria; chest lag, intercostal retraction, xiphoid retraction, nares dilatation, and expiratory grunt. The "retraction score" is computed by adding the values (0, 1, or 2) assigned to each factor that best describes the infant's manifestation at the time of a single observation. A score of 0 indicates no respiratory distress; a score of 10 indicates severe respiratory distress. *Source:* Silverman, W. A., Anderson, D. H. *Pediatrics* 17:1, 1956. Used with permission.

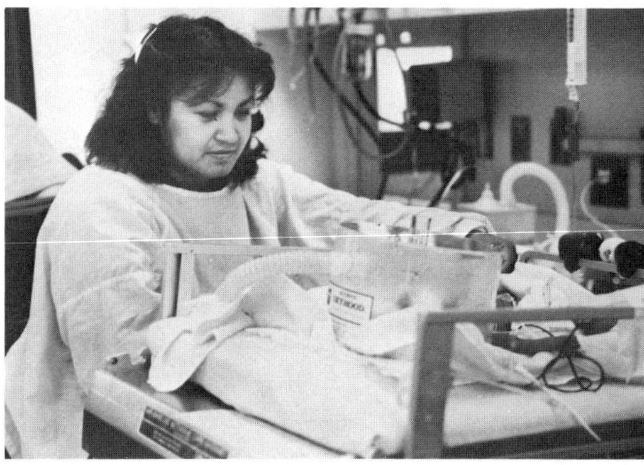

Figure 23.15
Oxyhood.

grunting, and nasal flaring sometimes demonstrate pneumothorax on x-ray films. Possibly because of high intrathoracic pressures during the first few minutes of life, although sometimes because of a complication of meconium aspiration or mechanical ventilation, pneumothorax is treated differently depending on the overall clinical condition of the infant. Otherwise healthy term newborns may absorb all the air if placed in 100% oxygen for a short period of time. If this fails or if the infant is premature or has suffered meconium aspiration, placement of a chest tube to suction is required.

DIAPHRAGMATIC HERNIA

Respiratory distress in the infant with a sunken, scaphoid abdomen whose heart sounds are displaced to the right side of the chest is characteristic of diaphragmatic hernia, a congenitally acquired disease. Since about three-fourths of the defects occur on the left side of the diaphragm, intestines are found in the left chest cavity while the heart is pushed to the right. Immediate recognition, x-ray film confirmation, and surgical intervention are required for the infant to survive.

The Infant with Cardiovascular Disease

Heart disease in infants occurs almost exclusively as a result of congenital heart defects of embryologic origin. In the neonatal intensive care unit, mortality from *congenital heart disease* (CHD) is second only to problems associated with premature birth.

The human heart is a marvelously complex organ that, when properly designed, provides life-sustaining circulation of blood throughout the body. Embryologic development of this incredible pumping system is complicated, however, involving numerous twists, turns, divisions, and degenerations (see Chapter 11). Suprisingly, most infants are born with normal hearts. In about 7 in 1,000 births, however, developmental errors result in CHD.

Since fetal circulation and respiration are uniquely shared by the mother (placenta) and infant, CHD rarely is noted prenatally. Heart disease may be noted immediately after birth or may develop gradually over several hours or days. Characteristic of the infant with CHD are cyanosis and/or congestive heart failure.

In an earlier time, infants with CHD were referred to as *blue babies*. Indeed, the phrase *blue blooded* as a description of royalty and well-born persons acknowledges the fact that historically, the consanguinous marriages of the high society resulted in a very high proportion of infants with cyanotic CHD. Today, cyanotic lesions account for about two-thirds of the congenital heart defects seen in infants.

Cyanosis in infants is observable in varying degrees as a result of its several causes. *Acrocyanosis* is duskiness of the hands and feet soon after birth because of the sluggish circulation of the infant's polycythemic blood. *Peripheral cyanosis* is observed as dark blue or dusky coloration of the skin, mucous membranes, lips, and nail beds.

As discussed in the preceding section, cyanosis may denote respiratory distress of pulmonary etiology. Differentiation of this cyanosis from that of cardiac origin is important in determining diagnosis and treatment. Two observations of the infant are helpful in making this discrimination. First, an infant with respiratory disease and cyanosis usually improves with crying; an infant with heart disease and cyanosis becomes increasingly blue with any energy expenditure such as crying, feeding, stooling. Second, the administration of oxygen to infants with respiratory disease usually improves their color. Infants with CHD, however, remain cyanotic. This easily done preliminary diagnostic procedure is frequently performed in the nursery and is called a *shunt study*. This name refers to the fact that cyanosis in CHD is a result of shunting of blood from the right to the left sides of the heart and is unresponsive to oxygen.

Not all congenital heart disease in infants presents with cyanosis, though. Since acyanotic lesions involve a left-to-right shunt within the heart, signs of heart failure are evidence of pathology. Early signs include tachypnea (respiratory rate over 60 breaths per minute), tachycardia (apical pulse greater than 160 beats per minute), retractions, grunting, nasal flaring, and diaphoresis. As mentioned with cyanosis, these signs are usually exacerbated by feedings, crying, and so forth. Edema and hepatosplenomegaly are later occurring signs and imply more significant failure.

Other signs of congenital heart disease in infants include murmurs of varying magnitude and indications of diminished cardiac output such as poor peripheral pulses, mottled skin and hypotonia.

Diagnosis of CHD that is suspected by clinical observation is confirmed by x-ray film, EKG, or sonography. Definitive identification of the cardiac lesion by cardiac catheterization has become common practice in the last 10–15 years as the techniques and procedures associated with it have been perfected. Also, improvement in cardiothoracic surgery has occurred, and many of the infants with CHD undergo either palliative or corrective open or closed heart operations. The risks of attempting cardiac catheterization and heart surgery on a small neonate are significant. Still, the procedures have improved outcomes as well as decreased mortality.

Some congenital heart disease is managed medically, usually with digoxin (Lanoxin) and furosemide (Lasix). The combination of a diuretic and an agent to improve cardiac efficiency is particularly useful with acyanotic defects with accompanying heart failure. The drugs are often used postoperatively as well.

Figures 23.16 *a–f* illustrate the common types of cyanotic and acyanotic heart defects seen in infants. Nursing care for neonates with CHD begins with early assessment and identification of symptoms. Especially during feedings, the infant may demonstrate circumoral cyanosis, diaphoresis of the forehead, and early exhaustion with tachypnea.

Preoperative care includes attention to the infant's postcardiac catheter needs. Although the umbilical artery may be used, sometimes the femoral artery is punctured to pass the catheter, in which case observation for extravascular bleeding is called for. Femoral and pedal pulses should also be checked regularly. Vital sign monitoring at least hourly is indicated.

Postoperatively, most infants require one-to-one, nurse-to-patient care for at least 24 hours as they are generally on ventilators and need constant monitoring of vital signs, especially blood pressure, intake and output, arterial oxygen levels and chest tube patency and function. Careful calculation and administration of Lanoxin and Lasix, whether used postoperatively or for medical management, is imperative. Since dosages may be so small as to be measured at 0.05 cc or less, most nurses prefer to double check their preparation of the drug with another professional. Heart rate in neonates of less than 100–110 beats per minute should be brought to the physician's attention since this may be a sign of digoxin toxicity. Other signs include irritability and emesis. Serum levels may be checked for appropriateness of Lanoxin therapy.

Attention to the needs of the family of an infant with CHD is similar to that described in Chapters 17 and 18. Parents need extensive education and preparation, in addition to a sensitive and supportive attitude as they adjust to the birth of their baby with a defect. Before discharge, instructions in administering medications, in recognizing signs of heart failure or increasing distress, and in feeding the infant (which may include naso- or orogastric tube feedings) are indicated. Frequent follow-up and repeated hospitalization are common.

The Infant Who Is Jaundiced

Almost every newborn can be expected to show the yellow-tinged skin color characteristic of hyperbilirubinemia. While in most cases, the transient elevation of bilirubin causes no serious problems or sequelae, in a small percentage of infants hyperbilirubinemia may cause serious brain damage (kernicterus) if untreated.

Bilirubin, a by-product of red blood cell (RBC) breakdown, is present in the blood in two forms: 90% of it occurs as unconjugated, or indirect, bilirubin; 10% is conjugated, or direct, bilirubin. Indirect bilirubin resulting from RBC hemolysis is carried to the liver bound to albumin in the blood. In the liver, the bilirubin is first bound to liver proteins and then conjugated by an enzyme (glucuronyl transferase) into direct bilirubin, which is excreted in bile into the intestine. Some of this direct bilirubin is in turn excreted in the stool. However, the newborn is peculiarly able to reabsorb bilirubin from the intestine because of the presence of another enzyme (bilirubin glucuronidase), which unconjugates the bilirubin and allows it to be reabsorbed. Any event or process that impacts this metabolism can increase the circulating bilirubin: increased numbers of RBC being hemolyzed (such as following severe bruising or cephalhematoma), decreased albumin available to bind and carry the bilirubin (such as occurs with administration of some medications that bind with albumin), immature or ineffective liver function, impaired excretion of bile from the liver, or delay in passage of stool from the intestines.

Jaundice may be classified as either physiologic or pathologic. *Physiologic jaundice* is defined as occurring in otherwise healthy newborns with levels of unconjugated bilirubin not exceeding 12.0 mg% and levels of conjugated bilirubin not exceeding 1–1.5 mg%. Typically, the course for term infants is jaundice appearing after 24 hours of age, peaking at 3–4 days, and disappearing by 6–7 days.

Premature infants' bilirubin peaks somewhat later, at about 5–6 days. It is important, however, that the assumption of physiologic jaundice not be made until all other possible causes are considered and eliminated. Furthermore, *visible jaundice and/or elevations of bilirubin greater than 10 mg% on the first day of life is always pathologic.* Causes of neonatal jaundice include the following:

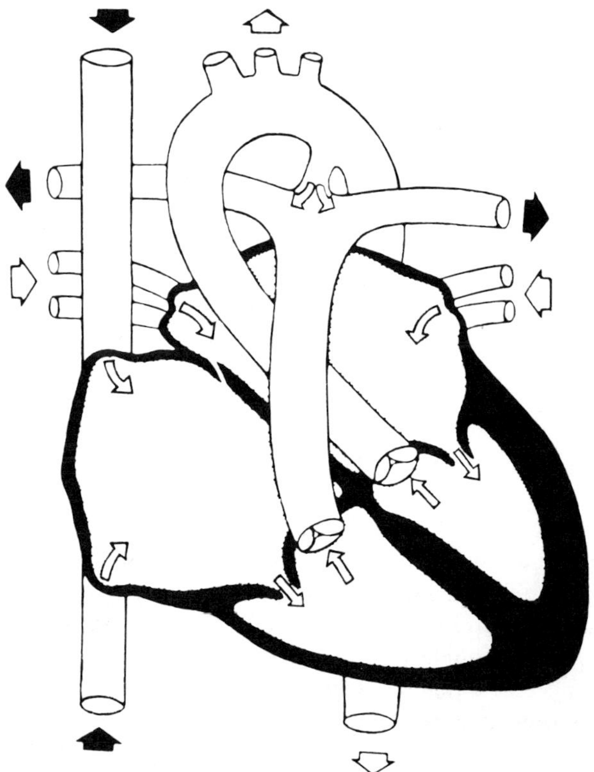

Figure 23.16*a*
Patent ductus arteriosus. Patent ductus arteriosus is the persistence of the vascular communication, which short-circuits the pulmonary vascular bed and directs blood from the pulmonary artery to the aorta during fetal life. Functional closure of the ductus normally occurs soon after birth. If the ductus remains patent after birth, the direction of flow through the ductus is reversed from that in the fetal state, flowing instead into the pulmonary artery.

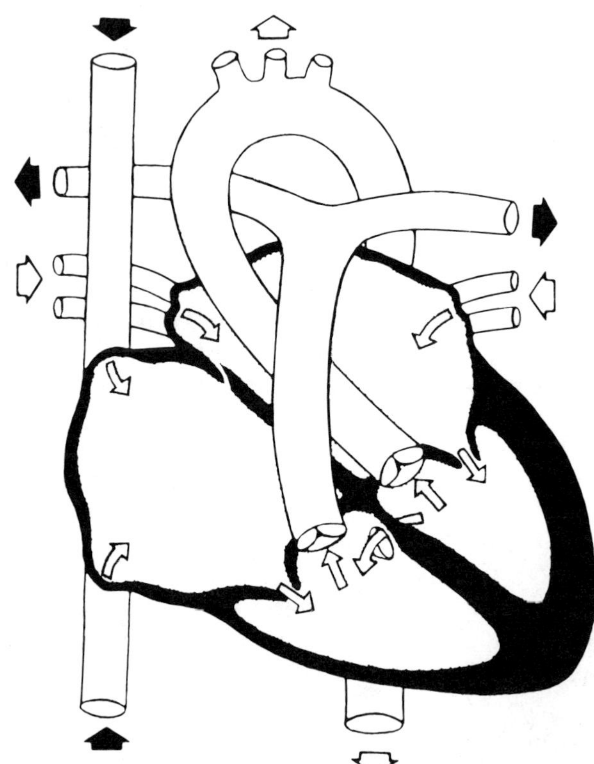

Figure 23.16*b*
Ventricular septal defect. Ventricular septal defects can occur anywhere in the ventricular septum but most commonly involve the membranous portion of the septum. Occasionally, more than one defect is present. Blood is shunted from the left to the right ventricle because of the normal pressure differential between these two chambers. Size of the defect is more important than location. Clinical and laboratory features, treatment, and natural history vary with size of the ventricular septal defect.

- Hemolytic disease of the newborn
- Polycythemia
- Abnormality of red blood cells
- Petechiae, ecchymosis
- Hematoma
- Hemorrhage
- Intraventricular hemorrhage
- Infection (sepsis)

One of the most commonly encountered is hemolytic disease of the newborn.

Hemolytic Disease of the Newborn

Hemolytic disease of the newborn, which is also called isoimmune disease or erythroblastosis fetalis, is characterized by fetal and/or neonatal RBC hemolysis by antibodies produced by the mother's blood. Rh incompatibility, the more well known but less frequently seen hemolytic disease occurs when an Rh negative mother has an infant with Rh positive blood. If the mother receives any Rh positive blood (transfusion with mismatched blood, abortion of previous Rh positive fetus, delivery of previous Rh positive infant), then her own Rh

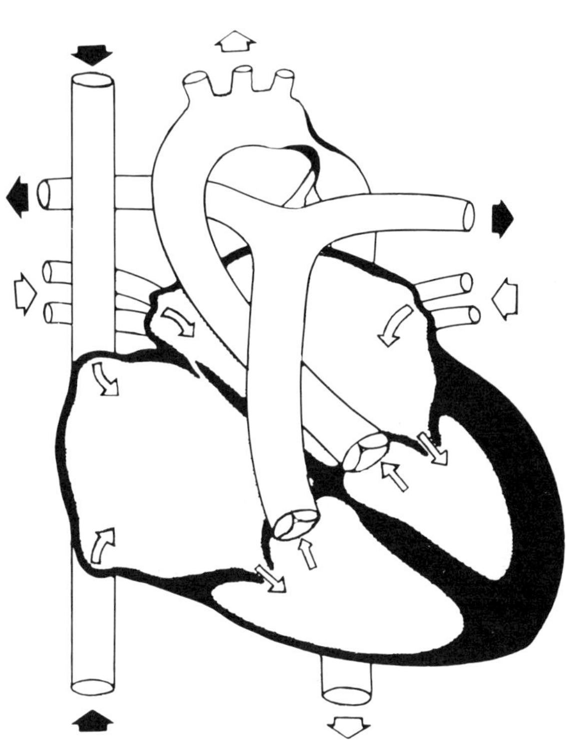

Figure 23.16*c*
Coarctation of the aorta. Coarctation of the thoracic aorta consists of a narrowed aortic lumen before, at, or just beyond the entrance of the ductus arteriosus. When located proximal to the ductus, the coarctation is often associated with a long, narrowed area (hypoplastic segment) and additional intracardiac defects, such as a bicuspid aortic valve. Coarctation of the abdominal aorta occurs rarely. It usually involves the origins of the renal arteries but may involve other arteries and is more common in females.

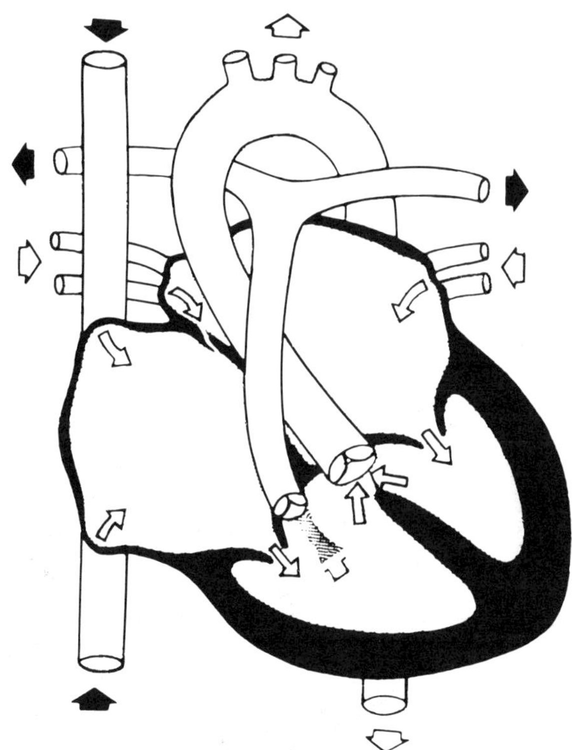

Figure 23.16*d*
Tetralogy of fallot. Tetralogy of Fallot includes four conditions: (1) Pulmonary stenosis; (2) ventricular septal defect; (3) overriding aorta; and (4) hypertrophy of the right ventricle. It is the most common cardiac malformation causing cyanosis in patients older than 2 years of age. Severity of symptoms depends primarily on degree of pulmonary stenosis. The obstruction can be located in the outflow area (infundibulum) of the right ventricle, at the pulmonary valve leaflets, at the pulmonary valve ring, the pulmonary arteries, or any combination of these.

negative blood synthesizes anti-Rh antibodies. In subsequent pregnancies, these antibodies are passed to the fetus where they attack and destroy RBCs and cause anemia and elevated bilirubin levels. These effects can be eliminated if the mother receives Rhogam after every pregnancy or abortion. This medication is designed to destroy the anti-Rh antibodies in the mother's blood so that future pregnancies will not be affected.

ABO Incompatibility

ABO incompatibility occurs more frequently than Rh/incompatibility (about 2 to 1) with a generally less severe course. Since anti-A and anti-B antibodies are naturally present in type O mothers' blood, the passage of antibodies from an O mother to an A or B baby can occur in the first pregnancy. The same symptoms of anemia and hyperbilirubinemia are noted, but with markedly less severity.

The diagnosis of isoimmune disease is confirmed by a positive direct or indirect Coombs' test. The direct Coombs' test measures the presence of antibodies attached to neonatal RBCs. However, the specific type of antibody cannot be determined unless an indirect Coombs' test, or antibody titer, is performed on the maternal blood. Naturally, the knowledge of both maternal and neonatal blood types will aid in anticipating hyperbilirubin problems.

Treatment of hyperbilirubinemia depends upon

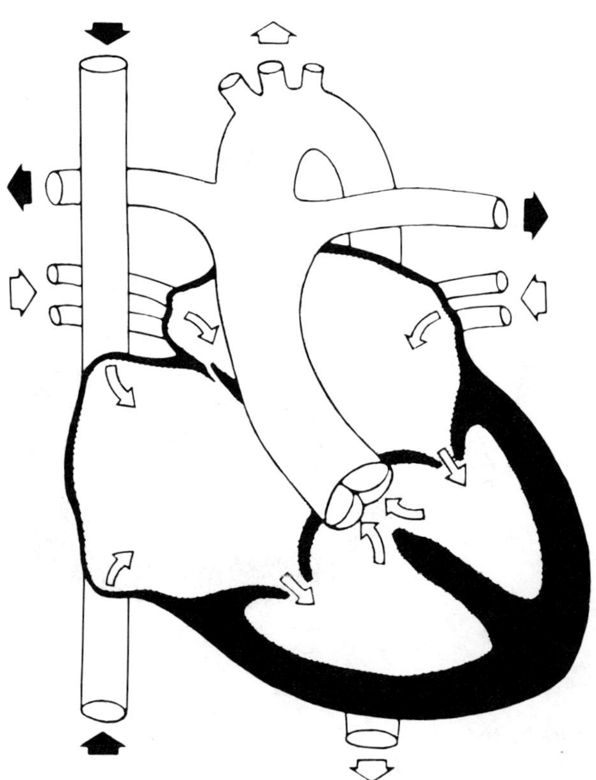

Figure 23.16*e*
Truncus arteriosus. In truncus arteriosus, a single arterial vessel arises from the heart and gives origin to the coronary arteries, pulmonary artery, and aorta. The truncus overrides an associated ventricular septal defect and receives blood from both ventricles. These abnormalities result from failure of normal septation and division of the embryonic truncus into an aorta and pulmonary artery.

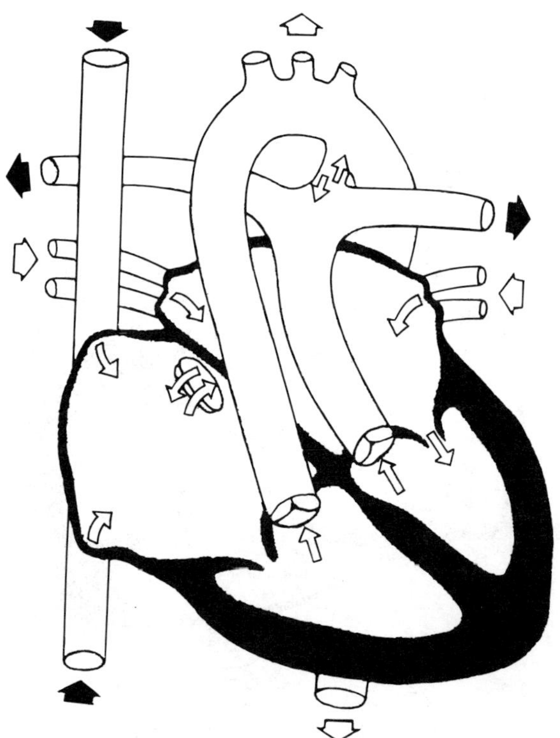

Figure 23.16*f*
Complete transposition of the great vessels. Because of the embryologic and anatomic complexity of the spectrum of defects included under this heading, there has not been general agreement on terminology and definition. However, the usual form, discussed here, can be described as a malformation in which the aorta originates from the right ventricle and the pulmonary artery from the left ventricle, the aorta arising anterior to the pulmonary artery.

its cause and its severity. Phototherapy for lower levels of bilirubin has been popular as a treatment since it is noninvasive (Fig. 23.17). However, bililites are not without their own disadvantages. Since the lights work by breaking down the bilirubin into other by-products, some concern has been expressed regarding the effects of these unknown by-products on the infant. Also, infants frequently have loose stools, hypo- or hyperthermia, and eventual dehydration if not closely managed. Nursing responsibilities include watching for these complications, as well as providing protective eye coverings for the infant to prevent corneal damage.

Treatment of severe hyperbilirubinemia is generally double-volume exchange transfusion with adjunct phototherapy. In the exchange transfusion, small amounts of neonatal blood are withdrawn through an umbilical venous catheter and replaced with equal amounts of fresh whole blood. The process is repeated over and over again until the total amount of blood used is equal to twice the estimated blood volume of the infant.

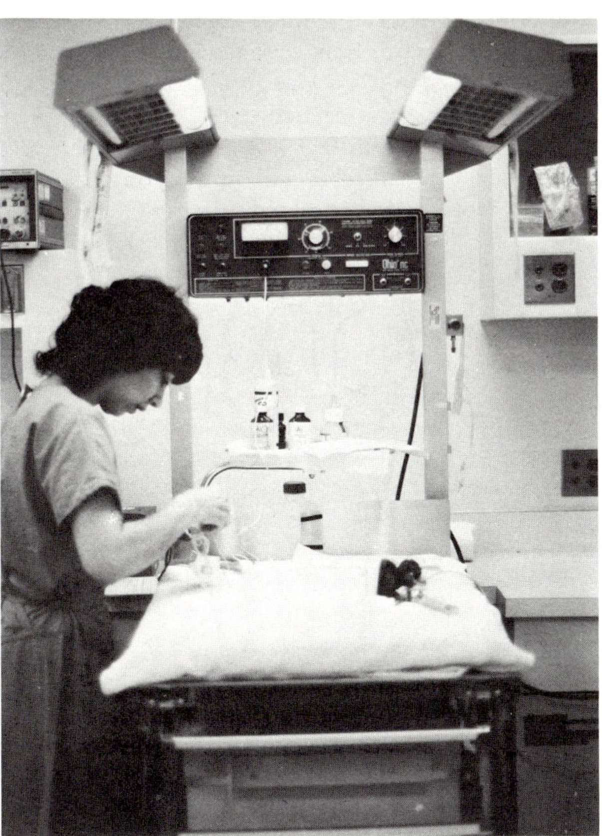

Figure 23.17
Bilirubin light.

During an exchange transfusion, the infant should be monitored closely by the nurse. The vital signs should be taken and recorded with every exchange of blood. Even though the blood being administered is warmed, temperature fluctuations as well as respiratory and circulatory distress may be observed. It is important that the infant be observable during the procedure so care should be taken not to cover the infant completely with drapes. Depending on the type of anticoagulant used in the blood, signs of hypoglycemia and hypocalcemia such as jitteriness and falling blood glucose may be noted.

Untreated jaundice with high levels of indirect bilirubin may eventually result in passage of free bilirubin into the brain, causing irreversible damage. This condition is called *kernicterus,* and, fortunately, it does not occur much today because of improved prevention, diagnosis, and treatment of hyperbilirubinemia. Indeed, most infants recover from hyperbilirubinemia without sequelae. However, if brain damage does occur, the prognosis is uniformly morbid.

The Infant with Jitteriness or Seizures

Neuromuscular manifestations of disease in neonates are considerably different from those seen in older children and adults. Classic tonic/clonic, grand mal convulsions, petit mal, and Jacksonian seizures are rarely observed. Instead, the neonate's immature neurologic system produces seizure activities such as rapid, nystagmoid eye movements, chewing and swallowing motions, color changes, respiratory arrest/apnea, generalized muscle rigidity or flaccidity, or myoclonic seizures.

Myoclonic seizures are fairly common and may be either generalized or focal. Focal seizures are observed as irregular jerking of an extremity or other body part for a sustained interval. Although similar clonic jerking is also seen in jitteriness, the two entities should not be confused as their significances differ. In seizures, the back and forth movement is irregular while the jittery movement is regular and rhythmic. *The seizing extremity will continue to move if immobilized while the jittery extremity will quiet.* Finally, jitteriness usually follows some stimulation; seizures, on the other hand, occur without stimulus.

Generalized myoclonic seizures resemble Moro reflex response, although, as in the case of focal seizures, the stimulus of neck flexion or startle has not been present.

Myoclonic seizures may occur singly or in series. If an infant with generalized seizures does not recover consciousness between successive episodes or if any seizure lasts for more than 15–20 minutes, the infant is regarded as suffering from status epilepticus. Brain anoxia will almost certainly occur if treatment is not initiated.

Jitteriness in the neonate may indicate hypoglycemia or hypocalcemia or it may have no identifiable cause. Seizures, a more serious manifestation of disease, have a variety of causes, including metabolic imbalances, neurologic injury or infection, and drug withdrawal. Treatment is based upon the etiology of the problem.

METABOLIC IMBALANCES

Hypoglycemia is the most common metabolic complication observed in the neonate. As mentioned repeatedly in this chapter, many infants are at risk for hypoglycemia, including premature infants, SGA babies, infants of diabetic mothers, and infants experiencing hypoxia and/or cold stress. To prevent the later developing onset of seizures as a result of hypoglycemia, any infant at risk, as well as any infant observed to be jittery, should have serial blood glucose levels checked. In general, glucose levels less than 45 mg% in term or premature infants indicate the need for immediate intervention: IV administration of 10% dextrose water. The glucose levels should be monitored until stabilization at an acceptable point occurs. Administration of 25% dextrose IV (50% dextrose is never used with neonates because of its hypertonicity) in other than an emergency resuscitative effort is definitely contraindicated. Since the infant's insulin response will be excessive and rebound hypoglycemia of much greater dimension will result, this cycle of mismanagement can only get worse.

Hypocalcemia may occur in premature infants, infants of diabetic mothers, asphyxiated infants, and erythroblastotic infants receiving exchange transfusion with blood preserved with the anticoagulant citrate. Decreased serum calcium levels (less than 7–10 mg%) are noted when infants are jittery, apneic, or edematous or when they experience abdominal distention and feeding difficulties. Prevention of Ca^{2+} depletion is the best therapy; infants at high risk should receive calcium supplementation in their IV fluids or feedings, with serum levels followed at least daily.

Blood specimens for glucose or calcium levels are frequently obtained by puncturing the heel of the infant and filling capillary tubes with the ensuing blood. Proper technique in carrying out this procedure is important to ensure accurate results as well as to prevent injury to the infant's heel. The use of knife blades to puncture the skin is especially discouraged. Proper site selection (see Fig. 23.18), aseptic technique, and the use of an appropriately sized lancet will reduce the incidence of complications.

NEUROLOGIC INJURY OR INFECTION

Etiologically, seizures may occur in infants who have suffered perinatal asphyxia, cerebral birth trauma, or meningitis/encephalitis. Congenital anomalies and syndromes also may cause neurologic complications and seizures. Usually therapy includes anticonvulsants, most commonly phenobarbital and Dilantin. Low dosages are begun and are then increased until therapeutic levels (absence of seizure activity) are reached.

Infants with neurologically induced seizure disorders are often discharged on anticonvulsants so nursing intervention is aimed at parental education. The family must be taught how to measure and

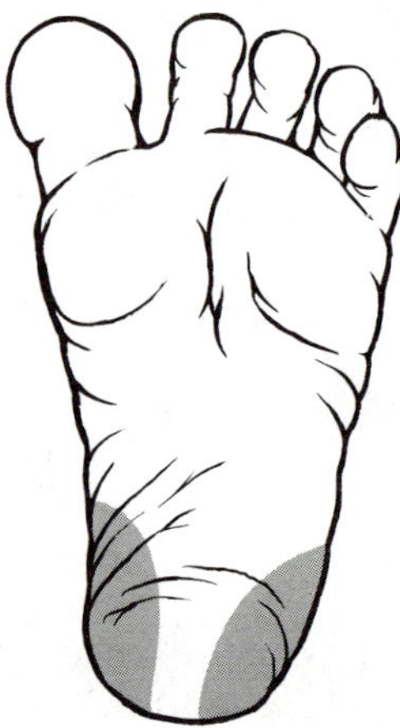

Figure 23.18
Heel sites for drawing blood in the neonate. The shaded areas indicate locations for puncturing an infant's heel for peripheral capillary blood samples.

administer the drugs and the signs and symptoms of inadequate amounts of medication; the importance of keeping clinic or doctor's office visits so that dosage adjustments can be made as the infant grows needs to be emphasized.

The approach of care givers to the family of a neurologically impaired infant should generally be one of cautious, realistic optimism. Of course, in some cases of profoundly pathologic disease, the prognosis for even marginal development is poor, and this information should be shared with the family in simple, sensitive terms, preferably by the physician. But in the majority of cases, eventual potential cannot be predicted based upon the neonate's short course of disease. The possibility of partial or full recovery cannot be totally disregarded.

DRUG WITHDRAWAL

The infant of a mother who has been dependent on or who has abused drugs or alcohol will most certainly experience withdrawal within a few hours to 1 day after birth. Early signs of jitteriness, irritability, and high-pitched cries will be apparent, along with the classic signs of excessive yawnings and sneezing. If untreated, the infant will develop diarrhea, vomiting, dehydration, respiratory distress, and convulsions. Untreated drug withdrawal in infants may result in death. Treatment protocols involving the use of phenobarbital or paregoric in gradually tapered dosages are sucessful in 1–2 weeks.

Nursing intervention with infants of drug-dependent mothers involves early recognition of symptoms and provision of a quiet, nonstimulating environment for the infant. Coordination with social services and public health nursing for follow-up is imperative.

The Infant with Gastrointestinal Problems

Evidence of feeding problems such as choking, emesis, and large aspirants coupled with failure of a newborn to pass stools is a strong indication of gastrointestinal (GI) problems. Since the nurse is most closely involved with the feeding of infants, she or he is most likely to be the first care giver to recognize the signs of GI distress. Causes of GI problems include congenital anomalies, complications of other disease processes, and, unfortunately, iatrogenic complications. Some of the more common etiologies follow.

TRACHEOESOPHAGEAL FISTULA WITH ESOPHAGEAL ATRESIA

Abnormal connections between the trachea and esophagus are the result of embryologic failure of the foregut to differentiate into two parts. The most commonly seen tracheoesophageal fistula (TEF) is upper esophageal atresia with lower esophageal fistula into the trachea.

The infant usually presents with a history of polyhydramnios. In the delivery room, excessive mucus in the nose and mouth may be noted. When the first attempt is made to feed the infant, he or she regurgitates immediately, choking and coughing. The abdomen becomes progressively distended because of passage of air across the fistula and into the stomach. Additionally, gastric juices from the stomach may follow the same route in the opposite direction with resultant respiratory distress. Confirmation of suspected TEF based on these signs may be made by attempting to pass a catheter through the nose or mouth into the stomach. If TEF is present, the catheter will meet the obstruction and not be passed into the stomach. Radiologic confirmation is also possible. Surgical repair is required and, unless other complications exist, is done promptly.

Preoperative management of infants with TEF includes keeping the head of the bed elevated at least 30 degrees to decrease the chances of aspiration of stomach contents, suction to the blind esophageal pouch to prevent aspiration of mucus and saliva, and IV therapy. Oxygen administration may be needed for respiratory distress. Postoperative care is nonspecific with the exception of closely guarded nothing by mouth (NPO) status. Most infants have a gastrostomy, and feedings are given through this tube until healing of the surgical site is assured. Sometimes dilations are performed to ease stenosis at the site of repair. Complete recovery is generally attained.

GASTROINTESTINAL TRACT OBSTRUCTIONS

Partial or complete obstruction of the small or large intestine is evidenced in the neonate by four classical signs: history of polyhydramnios, vomiting of bile-stained fluid, abdominal distention, and failure of the infant to pass meconium in the first 24 hours of life. GI obstruction in infants may be a result of embryologic events, neurogenic impairments, or unknown functional causes.

Embryologically, the midgut may malrotate as it re-enters the abdominal cavity from the umbilical stalk (see Chapter 11). Malrotation leads to stenosis and/or atresia of the small intestine with great regularity, and surgical correction is required. Postoperatively, these infants may present challenging feeding problems, especially if large portions of intestine were resected (short gut syndrome). Repeated attempts at feeding with many different formulas may be required while the infant is supported nutritionally with hyperalimentation and lipid therapy.

The absence of ganglion cells in the large intestinal walls prevents the colon from expelling stools. This disease, known as *Hirshsprung's disease,* requires surgical intervention—the resection of the aganglionic portion of the bowel. If only a small section is involved, eventual pull through of the colon to the anus may be possible. If much or all of the colon is involved, then permanent colostomy or ileostomy must be performed.

Meconium plug, a dehydrated mass of meconium that obstructs the bowel, is diagnosed by barium enema and is frequently relieved by the same procedure. The cause is unknown.

Nursing care of infants with GI obstructions begins with prompt recognition of signs and symptoms. General, nonspecific pre- and postoperative care are delivered. Since many of the surgical interventions include placement of temporary or permanent ostomies, attention to skin care and stool collection is an essential component of care planning. Parent education and preparation for the care of permanent ostomies may include referral to an enterostomal therapist or ostomate club.

NECROTIZING ENTEROCOLITIS

The diagnosis or even the suspicion of necrotizing enterocolitis (NEC) is one of the most dreaded by care givers of premature infants. While the prognosis has improved in recent years, NEC remains a medical and surgical emergency in the neonatal intensive care unit.

NEC is characterized by damage to the intestinal wall mucosa as a result of ischemia, probably because of factors such as hypoxia, shunting of blood away from the gut during hypoxic episodes (diving duck phenomenon), and hypotension. The cause of NEC remains unclear, but certain factors predispose an infant to NEC, including prematurity, asphyxia, shock, respiratory distress, sepsis, inappropriate formula feedings (excess volume, hyperosmolar), and patent ductus arteriosis (PDA).

The cardinal signs of NEC are well known to neonatal care givers: abdominal distention, increased gastric residuals, grossly or occultly bloody stools, general deterioration in conditions noted by hypotension or episodic apnea, and the subjective assessment that the infant "doesn't look right." Confirmation of diagnosis may be made with x-ray films of the abdomen, demonstrating pneumatosis (free air in the walls of the intestines).

Immediate treatment includes cessation of oral feeding and institution of IV therapy, placement of nasogastric tube to suction, and initiation of antibiotic administration. Further than this, treatment is directed toward observing for and treating the complications of NEC: respiratory distress, hypovolemic shock, metabolic acidosis, thrombocytopenia (DIC). Medical management is continued unless perforation or peritonitis is suspected or the infant is unresponsive to treatment and deteriorates further. Surgical intervention involves the resection of necrosed bowel and the placement of one or more ostomies. Surgical complications, especially adhesions, are common later in the neonatal period.

Research into the causes of NEC and attempts to identify improved treatment regimens are ongoing. At this time, the most effective way to improve the outcome of the infant with NEC is to recognize the disease as early as possible so that treatment may begin.

The Infant with an Infection

Infection in the neonatal period has long been the subject of close consideration by infant health care professionals. In earlier times, much attention was given to the prevention of epidemic infections such as respiratory disease or diarrhea in the nursery. Extreme measures of isolation included minimal handling of the infant and exclusion of all visitors, including the infant's parents, from the nursery. Recently, however, it has been demonstrated that not only is this enforced separation not necessary, it may also impair the relationship between infant and parents. Furthermore, evidence exists that demonstrates that the single most effective means for preventing contamination of infants within the nursery is strict, meticulous hand washing by all who come into contact with the infant. As stated earlier, most neonatal intensive care units encourage parents and even siblings to visit regularly, and when properly supervised, this visitation has *not* led to increased infections.

In utero, during delivery, and in the neonatal period, the infant is susceptible to most common pathogenic micro-organisms. However, the infant's response to these organisms is often much different from that of the older child or adult. Additionally, the infant's defense mechanisms against infection are poorly developed and as a consequence the typical early response of localized inflammation is rarely seen. Instead, pathogenic organisms may spread rapidly and systematically before nonspecific signs of illness begin to appear. Thus, the key approaches to care of the infant with an infection are prevention, early identification, and immediate and appropriate therapy.

Prevention of infection in the unborn or newborn infant may be as simple as effective hand washing in the nursery or as far-reaching as communitywide immunization of school children against rubella. In either situation, the infant's best protection against the sequelae of infection is never to contract the infection in the first place. The preventative approach cannot be overstated.

Early identification of fetal–neonatal infection is made difficult by the nonspecific signs and symptoms the infant may exhibit. The exception to this is in cases of congenital viral infection, where characteristic signs including small size for gestational age, malformations, microcephaly, jaundice, petechiae, and other systemic (often neurologic) signs of infection are usually present. Other than this, it is generally the nurse who is caring for a seemingly healthy baby who closely observes the appearance and behavior and notes that the baby "doesn't look right," or "doesn't act right." This subjective assessment may reflect subtle, barely detectable changes in color, activity, muscle tone, feeding behavior, and/or responsiveness to stimuli. Other signs may include inability to maintain temperature (usually hypothermia), abdominal distention/vomiting/large gastric aspirants, respiratory distress, and jaundice. Usually, an infant presenting the described clinical picture, especially if accompanied by a suspicious history such as premature rupture of membranes, is a candidate for immediate investigation.

As mentioned earlier, the neonate demonstrates poor localized response to infection. Thus, the site of infection may be difficult to determine and hence the responsible organism difficult to detect. Consequently, the infant must undergo culturing of all likely sites of infection. This process, known as a *septic workup,* usually includes culturing of cerebral spinal fluid via lumbar puncture, urine via suprapubic bladder tap, stool via rectal swab, umbilical cord, gastric aspirant, and blood. Additionally, chest x-ray films and complete blood count are indicated, as well as an antibody titer screen (TORCH, *t*oxoplasmosis, *r*ubella, *c*ytomegalovirus, *h*erpes, screen) if congenital viral infection is suspected.

A septic workup is important diagnostically. Unfortunately, it involves much manipulation—poking and proding of the infant. The nurse caring for the infant should be alert for signs of worsening condition especially during the procedures described above. Positioning of the infant should not impair respiration nor accessibility for constant observation.

Treatment of infection in the neonate is centered around antibiotic and, more recently, antiviral and antifungal therapy. Specific dosage regimens for preterm and term infants based upon their weight and age have been developed and are constantly being revised and updated. The nurse administering antimicrobial therapy to a neonate should know the current dosage recommendations, the desired and undesired effects of the medications, and the proper technique for intravenous, intramuscular, and oral administration to infants. Maintenance of appropriate blood levels of antibiotics is crucial to treatment of infection, and the nurse's knowledgeable, timely, and technically complete administration of medication is imperative.

Isolation of an infected infant is generally accomplished in an incubator, with strict adherence to hand washing, gowning, and gloving (if indicated). Parents should be encouraged to interact with their infant just as they would if the baby were not infected. Supportive care such as temperature regulation, intake and output monitoring, and careful assessment of vital signs are important in the care of high-risk infants.

Long-term prognosis for infants with infections depends upon the site of the infection, type of organism, and effectiveness of treatment. On one end of the continuum, the congenitally infected infants described earlier have a high incidence of mortality and morbidity. Fortunately, on the other hand, many septic infants undergo antibiotic therapy successfully with no sequelae.

SUMMARY

This chapter discussed disorders of the newborn. It began with a discussion of health care personnel and facilities for the care of high-risk infants. Perinatal risk factors were enumerated. The chapter was then divided into an elaboration on neonatal conditions, which present at delivery and neonatal conditions, which arise in the nursery. The former included asphxia, meconium aspiration, and SGA and LGA infants. This was followed by a discussion of infants who sustained birth trauma including fractures and paralysis. The next section discussed physical anomalies such as cleft lip and palate, meningomyelocele, hydrocephalus, gastroschisis, and other gastrointestinal and musculoskeletal anomalies. Nursing implications and care were included with each neonatal condition.

The chapter continued by discussing neonatal conditions that arise in the nursery. Many broad categories of conditions, such as the infant with respiratory distress, the infant with cardiovascular disease, the infant with jitteriness or seizures, metabolic imbalances, and neurologic injury, and the infant with gastrointestinal problems, were described.

The last section discussed the infant with an infection. Throughout the chapter assessment by the nurse and early detection of problems in order to institute treatment modalities early was emphasized. The minimal margins of safety with these tiny and special humans were stressed, and the role of the nurse in continuing to improve the outcome for the sick neonate was emphasized.

REFERENCES AND READINGS

American Academy of Pediatrics. *Standards and Recommendations for Hospital Care of Newborn Infants.* (6th ed.). Evanston, Ill: The American Academy of Pediatrics, 1977.

American Nurses Association. Congenital Cardiac Defects. *Am J Nurs* 78:255, 1978.

Avery, G. B. (Ed). *Neonatology.* Philadelphia: J. B. Lippincott, 1975.

Bliss, V. J. Nursing Care for Infants With Neonatal Necrotizing Enterocolitis. *Am J Matern Child Nurs* 1:37, 1976.

Dingle, R. E. et al. Continuous Transcutaneous O_2 Monitoring in the Neonate. *Am J Nurs* 80:890, 1980.

Generra, S. Necrotizing Enterocolitis: Detecting It and Treating It. *Nurs* 80:52, 1980.

Harrison, L. K. Making a Good Thing Better: The Regionalization of Neonatal Intensive Care Units. *J Obstet Gynecol Neonatal Nurs* 4:49, 1975.

Hazle, N. An Infant Who Survived Gastroschisis. *Am J Matern Child Nurs* 6:35, 1981.

Hill, S. The Child With Ambiguous Genitalia. *Am J Nurs* 77:810, 1977.

Klaus, M., Fanaroff, A. *Care of the High-Risk Neonate.* Philadelphia: W. B. Saunders, 1973.

Korones, S. B. *High Risk Newborn Infants: The Basis for Intensive Care Nursing.* St. Louis: C. V. Mosby, 1972.

Luke, B. Maternal Alcoholism and Fetal Alcohol Syndrome. *Nurs'77* 77:1924, 1977.

National Foundation—March of Dimes. *Toward Improving the Outcome of Pregnancy.* New York: The Foundation, 1976. (Recommendations for the Regional Development of Maternal and Perinatal Health Servives.)

Porth, C. M., Kaylor, L. E. Temperature Regulation in the Newborn. *Am J Nurs* 78:1691, 1978.

Schriener, R. L. (Ed). *Care of the Newborn.* New York: Raven Press, 1981.

Sullivan, R., Foster, J., Schreiner, R. L. Determining a Newborn's Gestational Age. *Am J Matern Child Nurs* 4:38, 1979.

24

INHERITANCE AND ITS LEGACY: GENETIC DISORDERS

Patricia A. Farrell

The fact that genetics is the study of heredity has, until recently, generated little interest among most health care professionals. It is only within the past few years that this course of study has been included in the medical school curriculum. Unfortunately, few nursing programs today include more than a minor review of the subject.

The importance of genetics to health care in general and to reproductive health care in particular should become evident when you take into account the amount of fetal wastage and the number of *congenital* abnormalities thought to have a genetic basis. Consider, for example, that more than 15 million Americans suffer, to a varying degree, the effects of birth defects and as many as 80% of these defects are attributable to genetic involvement. A significant number of the affected are infants and children, who account for more than one-third of all pediatric admissions to hospitals. At least 33% of all conceptions terminate as spontaneous abortions, and chromosomal abnormalities are thought responsible for 50% of these. Consider also that about 3% of the United States population is mentally retarded and of those so affected, at least 60% are thought to result from a genetic component. For these reasons, a working knowledge of genetic transmission and its potential outcome is essential to nursing practice.

To appreciate the nature of problems associated with the transmission and expression of genetic information you must have an understanding of the hereditary process. The normal physiology of inheritance has been previously described and a review of that discussion would be helpful to understanding the concepts presented here (see Chapter 6).

It is now generally accepted that most of the information necessary to control cellular activities such as replacement of various body cells and reproduction of the species is found in genes located on the cell's *chromosomes*. Depending upon the underlying cause or causes of the problem, genetic disorders may be broadly categorized as chromosomal, single gene, and multifactorial.

CHROMOSOMAL ABERRATIONS

The technologic explosion in the field of genetics during the past quarter of a century, but particularly during the past decade, has provided sophisticated methods for studying the chromosomal makeup of human cells (Fig. 24.1). Although the peripheral blood lymphocyte is the cell most frequently examined, similar studies may be performed on cells from bone marrow, amniotic fluid, and various organs or tissues. Analysis of a sufficient number of cells (about 30) will usually yield a *karyotype*—a standard display of the number, size, and shape of the chromosomes from a somatic cell—of the person that can help confirm or rule out a chromosomal defect.

Chromosomal aberrations may be numeric or structural. The shorthand used to describe a karyotype begins with the total number of chromosomes found in the cell and is followed by the sex chromosome complement. 46,XX and 46,XY are the notations for normal female and male karyotypes, respectively. When an aberration is found, the defect is described through use of standard symbols, some of which are listed in Table 24.1. The notation 46,XX,4p−, for example, would indicate a female with the correct number of chromosomes but with a portion of the small arm of chromosome number 4 missing.

Until 1956, it was generally held that there were 48 human chromosomes. However, improved laboratory techniques during the 1950s led to the discovery that in the germ cells (sperm and egg) there are 23 single chromosomes while in the somatic cells the 23 are paired for a total of 46 chromosomes. Problems can occur when a person's cells contain more or less than the normal number of chromosomes (*aneuploidy*) as there is then an imbalance of genetic information. Aneuploid states may arise during *meiosis* or *mitosis* and are thought to occur primarily as a result of anaphase lag or *nondisjunction* (Fig. 24.2). These events usually lead to a single (monosomy) or triple (trisomy) representation of one of the chromosomes.

In 1959, approximately 90 years after Down's syndrome was first described, researchers found that condition to be associated with the presence of an extra number 21 chromosome (trisomy 21). In most cases the karyotype is 47,XX,+21 or 47,XY,+21. More than 50% of those diagnosed as having Down's syndrome exhibit flattened occiput and facial features, hypotonia, slanted palpebral fissures, short, broad hands and fingers, and short limbs. As a result of advances in medical treatment, particularly in the area of cardiac disease, and of the trend toward home care, the life expectancy for those with Down's syndrome has increased significantly over the past three decades. Down's syndrome, though by no means the only aneuploid condition, is the one most frequently observed.

Other autosomal trisomies described during the decade following the 1950s involve chromosomes number 13 and number 18. Congenital heart defects are signficant in both Patau's (trisomy 13) and Edwards' (trisomy 18) syndromes, and the prognosis for both is extremely poor with minimal survival beyond 1 year. Also common in these syndromes are rocker-bottom feet, micrognathia, overlapping flexed fingers, and feeding difficulties. Polydactyly, microphthalmia, and cleft lip and palate are more prevalent in Patau's syndrome.

There are a number of syndromes that involve aneuploidy of the *sex chromosomes*. Turner's syndrome, also known as a *gonadal dysgenesis*, is a *monosomic* condition (45,XO) in which female patients with primary amenorrhea are found to be infertile, and most exhibit short stature, webbed neck, and shieldlike chest with small nipples. On the other hand, trisomy X syndrome (47,XXX) patients generally have a normal appearance, are frequently fertile and, if so, usually produce offspring with no chromosomal abnormality. Although rare, cases of tetrasomy X (48,XXXX) and pentasomy X (49, XXXXX) have been described. For the majority of these patients, mental retardation is a common feature.

Klinefelter's syndrome patients (47,XXY) are infertile males. Many are tall in stature and have poorly developed secondary sexual characteristics. Most are of normal intelligence and half exhibit enlarged breast development (gynecomastia) after puberty.

Like the 47,XXX females, most males with a 47,XYY karyotype appear normal, are usually fertile, and in most cases father chromosomally normal children. However, a number of studies suggest that the association between aggressive and criminal behavior and 47,XYY individuals is significant (Thompson & Thompson, 1980).

Occasionally, chromosomal studies will reveal that a person has two or more karyotypes or distinct cell lines, which is called *mosaicism* (Fig. 24.3). Up to 10% of patients with Turner's syndrome have 45,XO/46,XX karyotypes while 5% have 45,XO/47,XXX (Yunis, 1977). Mosaicism results from nondisjunction or anaphase lag during embryonic development, and the ratio of one cell line to the other depends on how early in development

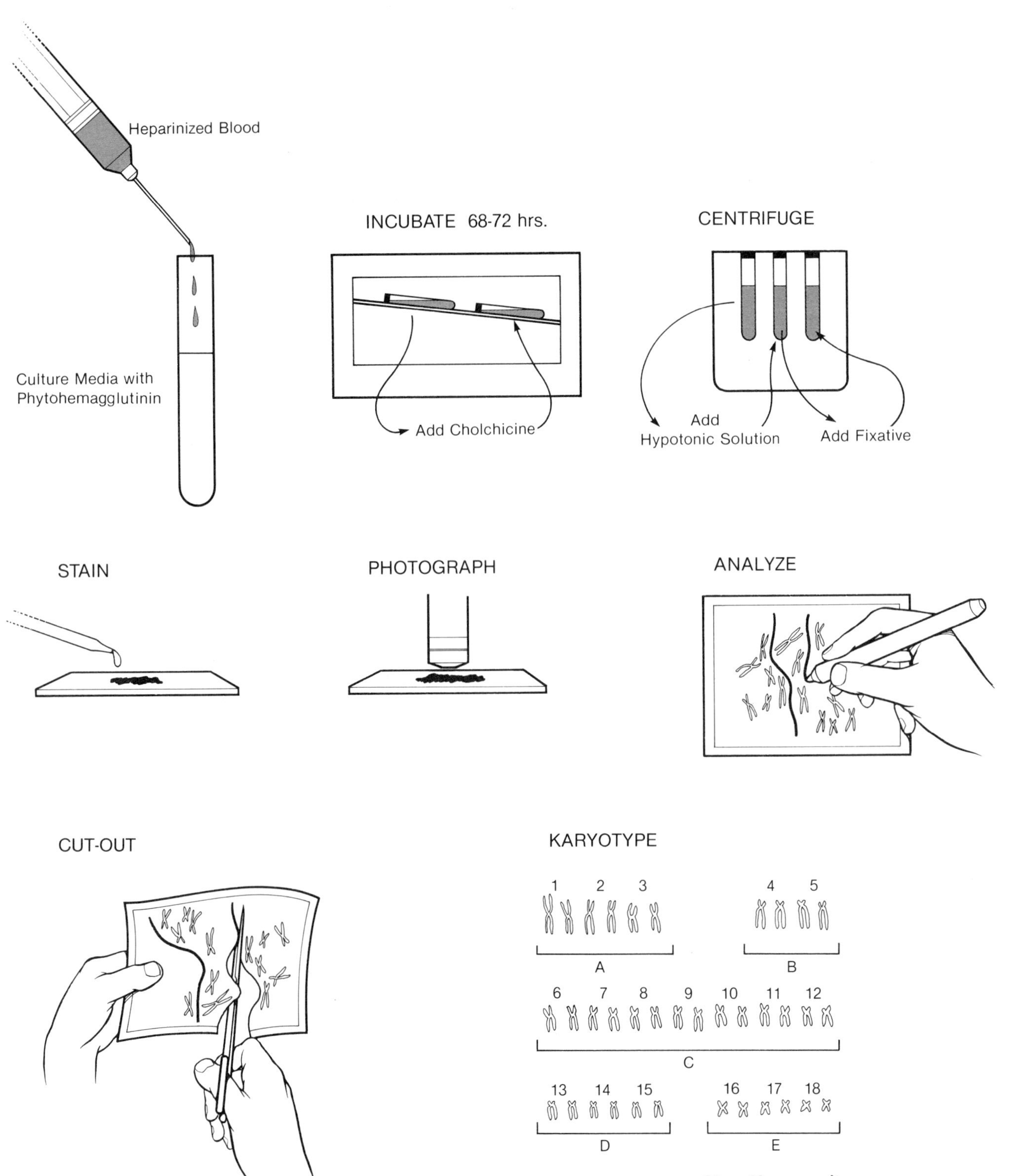

Figure 24.1
Chromosomal analysis procedure.

TABLE 24.1
PARTIAL LIST OF KARYOTYPE SYMBOLS

Chromosomes 1–22	Autosomes
X, Y	Sex chromosomes
45, 46, 47, and so on	Total number of chromosomes in cell (includes sex chromosomes)
XX	Normal female sex complement
XY	Normal male sex complement
p	Short arm
q	Long arm
t	Translocation
i	Isochromosome
r	Ring

the event occurs. Mosaic states can occur with any of the chromosomal aberrations, whether numerical or structural.

Structural

In addition to extra or missing whole chromosomes, an imbalance of genetic information can also result when the structural integrity of the chromosome is altered. A number of *syndromes* associated with deletions or rearrangements of chromosomal material following breakage have been described. A *deletion* of the long arm of one of the number 18 chromosomes (18q− syndrome) produces features that include seizures, hypotonia, mental retardation, hypoplastic genitalia, and congenital heart defects. The aberration in cri-du-chat syndrome (5p−) is a deletion of a portion of the short arm of one of the number 5 chromosomes. Affected infants usually have a weak but shrill catlike cry, microcephaly, hypertelorism, strabismus, micrognathia, and low-set ears. Formation of a ring by the number 5 chromosome (5r) can produce the same syndrome.

Of the other kinds of rearrangements, *translocations* and *isochromosomes* are noted more frequently (Fig. 24.4). Translocations occur when material from one chromosome is relocated to another nonhomologous chromosome. The impact of a rearrangement depends on the amount of genetic material lost or gained in the process. A physically normal female with a 45,XX,t(14;21) karyotype has a balanced translocation that, if passed on, can create an unbalanced 46,XX,t(14;21) karyotype in her child. It is important to note that although the mother has only 45 chromosomes, she has all chromosomes represented, whereas her child, with 46 chromosomes, has three representations of the number 21 chromosome and is therefore afflicted with Down's syndrome. The child's features would be the same as those associated with the 47,XY,+21 karyotype. Rearrangements may also occur be-

Anaphase Lag

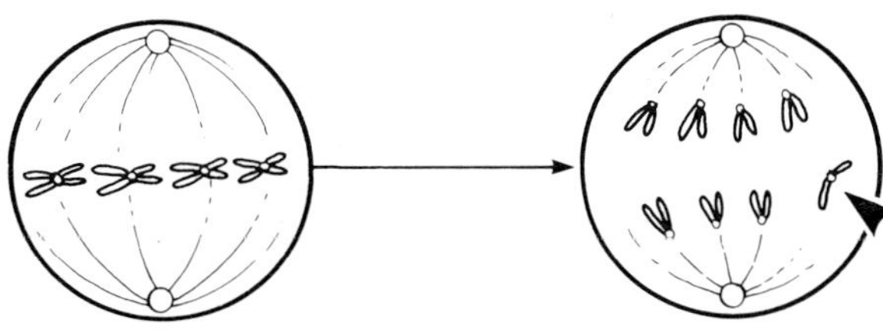

Nondisjunction

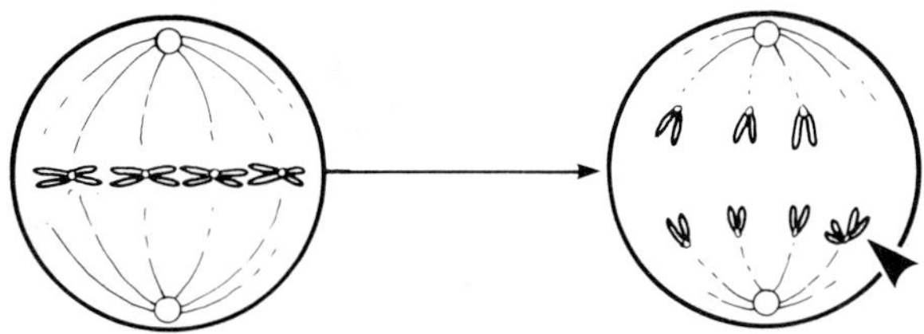

Figure 24.2
(*Top*) Anaphase lag; (*bottom*) nondisjunction.

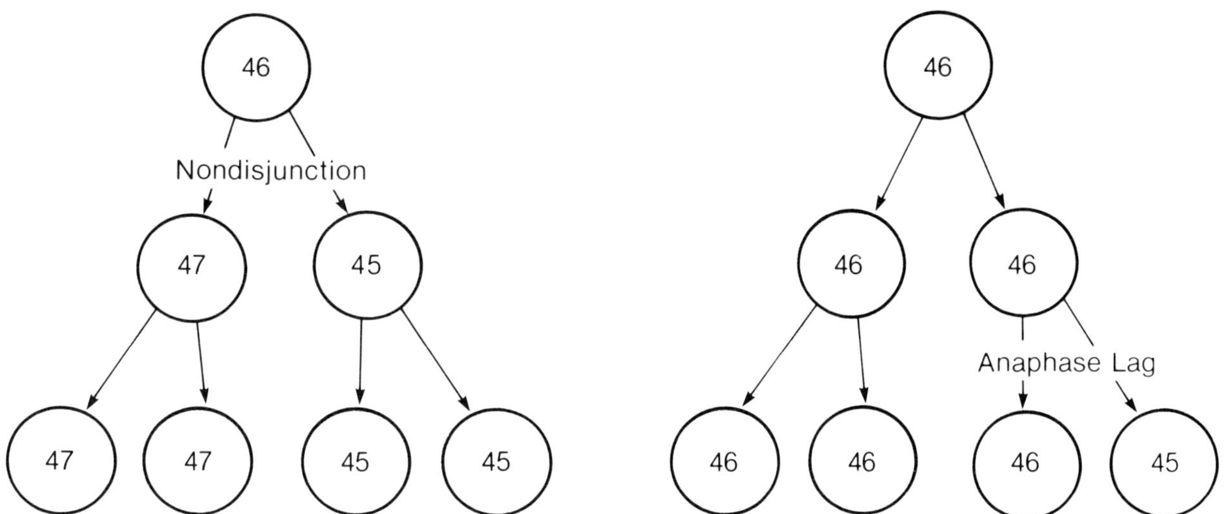

Figure 24.3
Mosaicism.

tween any of the other *autosomes* or sex chromosomes, and it is interesting to note that approximately 10% of couples who frequently miscarry have balanced translocations of one type or another (Fitzsimmons & Fitzsimmons, 1980).

If during cell division a chromosome erroneously divides transversely so that the short and long arms are separated from one another, an isochromosome may be formed. Between 15 and 20% of all females who exhibit features that are common to

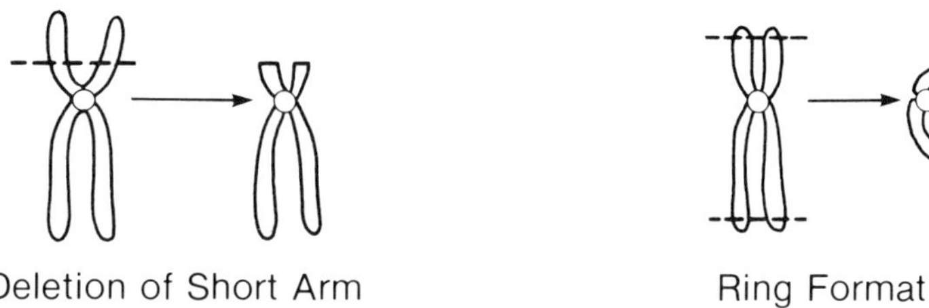

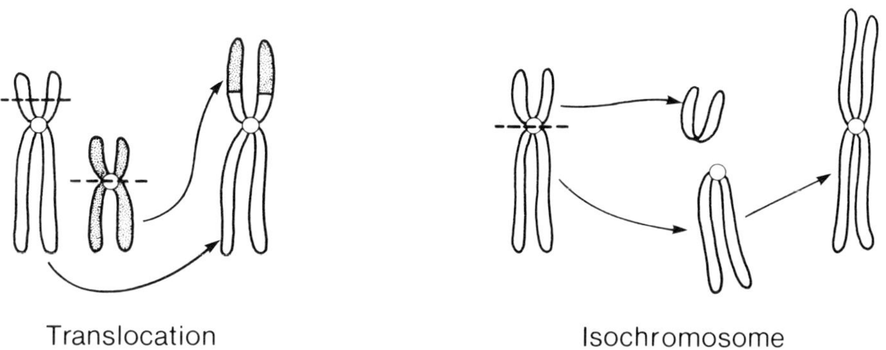

Figure 24.4
(*a*) Deletion of short arm; (*b*) ring formation; (*c*) translocation; (*d*) isochromosome.

Turner's syndrome have a 46,XXqi karyotype where there is a genetic imbalance because of the single X chromosome short arm and the triple set of X chromosome long arms. (Thompson and Thompson, 1980). Also pertinent is that of those whose karyotypes show this particular isochromosome, at least 66% are mosaics with 45,XO/46,XXqi cell lines.

In females each of the normally structured X chromosomes carries identical information. Males, however, normally have only one X chromosome, and its genetic information has little or nothing in common with that carried on the much smaller Y chromosome. This seeming inequity has been explained by the Lyon hypothesis, which notes that in somatic cells only one X chromosome is active. Each additional X chromosome is inactivated and can be demonstrated in laboratory preparations of buccal mucosa cells as a condensed chromatin mass known as the *Barr body*. It is important to note that a Barr body study alone does not accurately establish the *phenotypic* sex of an individual but does establish the number of X chromosomes in the cell. Cells from people with a 46,XX (female) or a 47,XXY (male) karyotype will have a Barr body, while those with a 46,XY (male) or a 45,XO (female) karyotype will not. Early in embryonic development X inactivation is a random process, so that in some cells the maternal X will be active while in other cells the paternal X will be active.

SINGLE GENE DEFECTS

Each person has two sets of genes: one set on the 23 chromosomes provided by the mother and the matching set on the 23 chromosomes provided by the father. *Genes*, which are *DNA* code segments responsible for synthesis of *polypeptide* chains, work in pairs. If both genes in a pair are alike, the person is said to be *homozygous* for that gene; if the genes are unalike, the person is said to be *heterozygous*.

Despite the fact that protein synthesis occurs in another part of the cell (*cytoplasm*), the DNA gene codes controlling this process do not leave the *nucleus* (Fig. 24.5). When a polypeptide is to be manu-

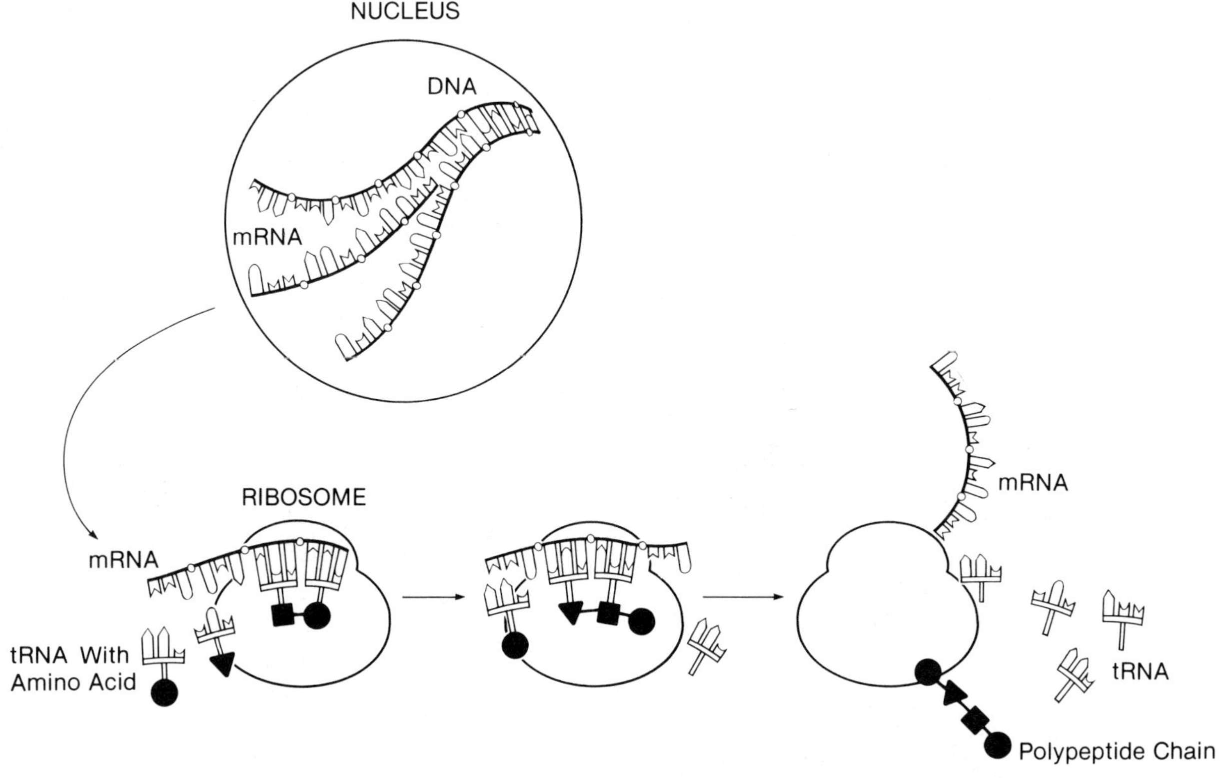

Figure 24.5
Protein synthesis.

factured, the appropriate segment of DNA "unzips" allowing one of the strands to act as a template from which a strand of messenger RNA (mRNA) can be formed. Through specified bonding, the nitrogenous bases on the DNA strand dictate the sequence of the RNA bases, which, after migration to *ribosomes* in the cytoplasm, will direct the protein chain's amino acid sequence. Base *triplets* provide the code that specifies amino acid positions in the chain. A gene may be altered by a change in its structure, for example, a substitution of one nitrogenous base for another. The change in the DNA strand will in turn affect the triplet code of the mRNA *transcribed* from it and in many cases alter the amino acid sequence of the polypeptide chain into which it is *translated*. Such gene changes are known as *mutations* and may produce obvious clinical effects.

More than 250 different hemoglobin (Hb) abnormalities in which the defect is a single amino acid substitution in either the alpha (α) or beta (β) chains that make up this molecule have been described. One of these abnormal molecules, designated HbS (normal Hb is HbA), is found in patients with sickle cell anemia, a disease often fatal in early childhood (Fig. 24.6). Red blood cells of people homozygous for the mutant gene have a tendency, when oxygen tension is low, to become sickle shaped, making their passage through the blood vessels difficult at best. As may be expected, the abnormally shaped cells cause obstructions that result in ischemia and severe pain in the areas of the body where the impactions occur. Other symptoms of this sickling disease, which occurs primarily in the black population, include anemia and jaundice. The mode of transmission is autosomal *recessive* as described later in this chapter.

Traits that are determined by single gene pairs may be dominant or recessive. If the trait is expressed in both the heterozygous and homozygous states it is *dominant*; if the trait is only expressed in the homozygous state it is *recessive*. When the gene pair in question is located on any of the numbered chromosomes it is autosomal; if the gene pair is found on the X chromosome it is X linked. In general, dominant diseases are more frequently observed yet milder in effect than recessive ones and usually involve defects that are structural in nature. On the other hand, many recessive conditions manifest themselves as errors of metabolism.

AUTOSOMAL DOMINANT TRANSMISSION

The chance that the child of a parent with an autosomal dominant disorder will be similarly affected is 1 in 2 (50%) if the parent is heterozygous and 1 in 1 (100%) if the parent is homozygous (usually very severe or lethal). The history or *pedigree* of a family with an autosomal dominant trait will often reveal that each generation has one or more affected members and that there is a relatively equal number of affected males and females (Fig. 24.7). Children of unaffected family members will also be unaffected, and most often the severity of the features, called *expressivity*, varies among those affected.

Tuberous sclerosis, a multisystem disease, is a good example of variable expression. The major symptoms of the disorder include epilepsy, mental retardation, and adenoma sebaceum, but other features may also be present. Though growth proceeds normally, seizures are often noted in early childhood, and impairment of mental development may range from moderate to severe. Regardless of how mildly affected, the person with tuberous sclerosis has a 50% chance of passing on the abnormal gene, and the recipient child may be more

Hemoglobin A +HIS—VAL—LEU—LEU—THR—PRO—[GLU]—GLU—LYS

Hemoglobin S +HIS—VAL—LEU—LEU—THR—PRO—[VAL]—GLU—LYS

Figure 24.6
Partial beta chain of the hemoglobin molecule.

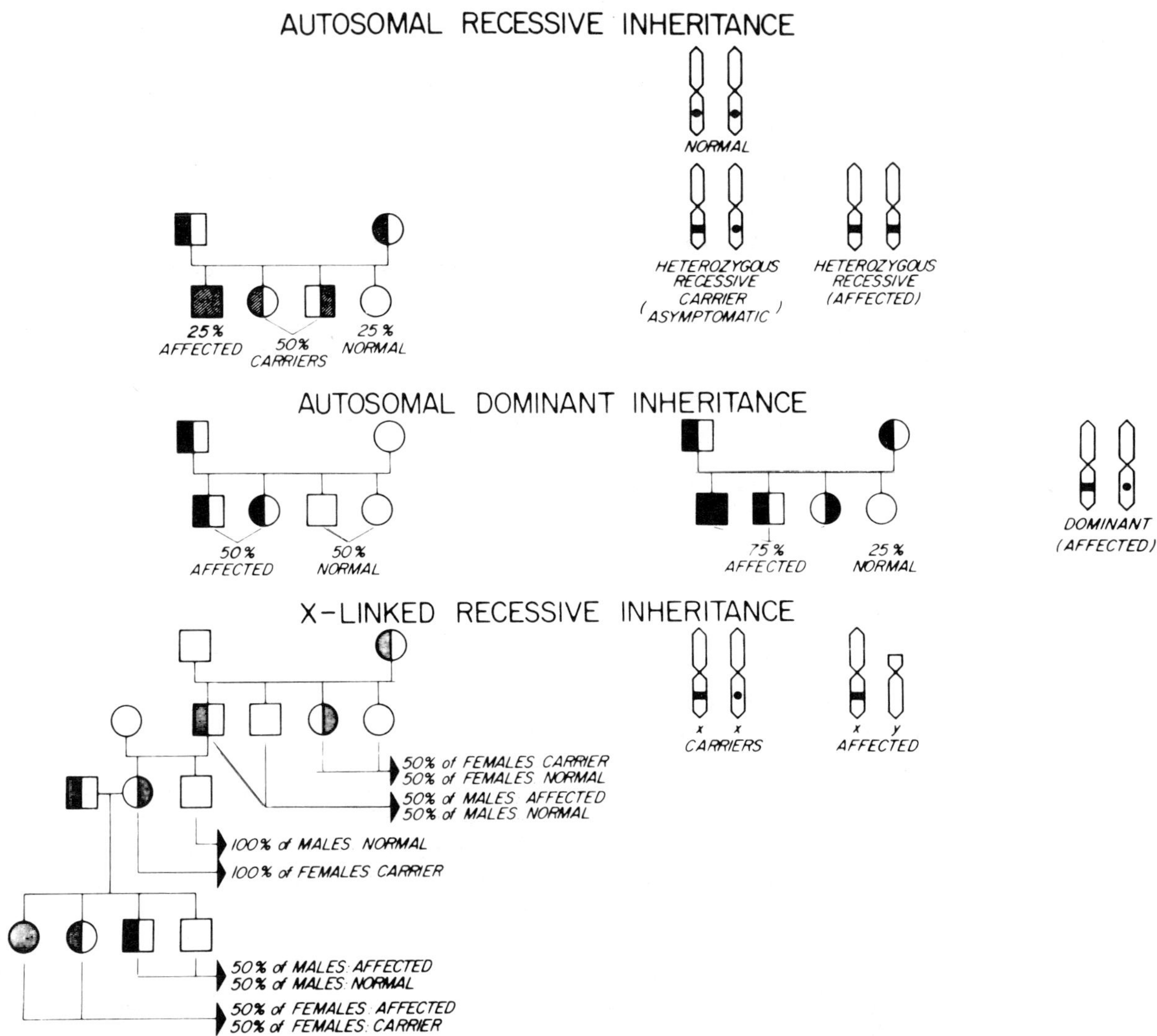

Figure 24.7
Types of inheritance: autosomal recessive; autosomal dominant X-linked. *Source*: Huff, R., Pauerstein, C. (Eds.). *Human Reproduction: Physiology and Pathophysiology*. New York: John Wiley & Sons, 1979. Used with permission.

severely impaired than the parent.

More than 1,400 genetic defects have been identified where the suspected mode of inheritance is autosomal dominant (McKusick, 1978, p. xiv). Among the more commonly seen autosomal dominant conditions are Marfan's syndrome and Huntington's chorea. Elongated thin extremities (dolichostenomelia), spider fingers (arachnodactyly), and subluxated lenses (ectopia lentis) are common features of Marfan's syndrome. Prognosis is variable and usually dependent upon the occurrence of dissecting aneurysms of the aorta that may present in either early childhood or quite late in life.

Characterized by choreic movements and psychiatric symptoms, Huntington's chorea has a progressive course that lasts 10–20 years. Although it can vary, the first symptoms usually appear between 35 and 40 years of age. It is unfortunate that by the time most people learn of their condition they already have a family and may have transmitted the disorder to their children.

AUTOSOMAL RECESSIVE TRANSMISSION

As noted before, features associated with autosomal recessive traits are generally not expressed in people heterozygous for the abnormal gene. These people are, however, unaffected carriers of the disorder. If only one parent is a carrier then the child has a 1 in 4 (25%) chance of receiving an abnormal gene from each parent and will, therefore, express the defect. The stylized pedigree of an autosomal recessive defect shows that males and females may be affected equally and that the disorder generally appears among siblings but not their parents or offspring. As relatives are more likely to carry similar mutant genes, *consanguinity* of the parents is often a factor in bringing the two abnormal genes together in the child.

Many autosomal recessive disorders are classified as inborn errors of metabolism because components essential for maintaining normal passage of nutrients through various metabolic pathways may be abnormal or deficient. The assumption is that a normal gene will facilitate production of the enzyme that acts upon a specific nutrient to convert it to another product. If the gene is abnormal, the enzyme may not be available and the metabolic process will therefore be blocked. Each stage in a metabolic pathway is controlled by a specific enzyme, and blocks that occur at different stages in the pathway can produce a variety of disorders.

Phenylketonuria (PKU) is an autosomal recessive disorder characterized by the affected person's inability to convert the amino acid phenylalanine to tyrosine because of a deficiency of the liver enzyme phenylalanine hydroxylase. Severe mental retardation is the major feature of this condition, and it is thought to be caused by metabolites produced from the breakdown of phenylalanine through an alternate pathway. PKU is detected through newborn screening programs that are mandatory in most of the 50 states. Once identified, affected people are treated by restricting intake of foods containing phenylalanine, thereby helping to minimize the mental impairment.

A number of autosomal recessive diseases are found to be more prevalent among certain populations. For example, Tay-Sachs disease, although occasionally found in other groups, primarily affects descendants of the Ashkenazi Jews of Eastern Europe. A disorder of lipid metabolism, Tay-Sachs results from a deficiency of the enzyme hexosaminidase A and is characterized by postnatal developmental retardation. Diagnosis can be confirmed on opthalmologic examination by the presence of a cherry red spot in the macula. Affected people appear normal at birth but by 4–6 months psychomotor retardation is evident and blindness, seizures, and hypotonia soon follow. Death usually occurs before the fourth year.

Just as sickle cell anemia is more prevalent among the black population, cystic fibrosis, for which the specific defect is unknown at this time, mainly affects Caucasian children. In this condition pancreatic enzyme deficiencies interfere with normal digestion and absorption. As a result of the generalized involvement of the exocrine glands there is abnormal secretion production, and the excessively high sweat electrolyte levels can lead to heat prostration. Chronic pulmonary disease is common in cystic fibrosis, and although the life expectancy for males is greater than females, most affected individuals die by age 20.

X-LINKED TRANSMISSION

Genes carried on the X chromosomes, like those on autosomes, are also responsible for traits that are dominant or recessive, but the preponderance of X-linked disorders are recessive. For dominant traits, if the affected parent is female, half her sons and daughters can be similarly affected; if the affected parent is male, half his daughters and none of his sons can be affected. Children of unaffected female carriers of an X-linked recessive disorder have a 50% chance of receiving the abnormal gene; if they do, the daughters will also be unaffected carriers but the sons will be affected.

Classic hemophilia, though relatively rare, is perhaps the best known of the X-linked recessive diseases because of its impact upon the royal families of Europe (Fig. 24.8). The defect in this disorder appears to be an abnormal protein molecule (Factor VIII), which is a component in the clotting process. The affected person exhibits excessive bleeding because of an unusually prolonged clotting time. Severe arthritis may also be present as a result of

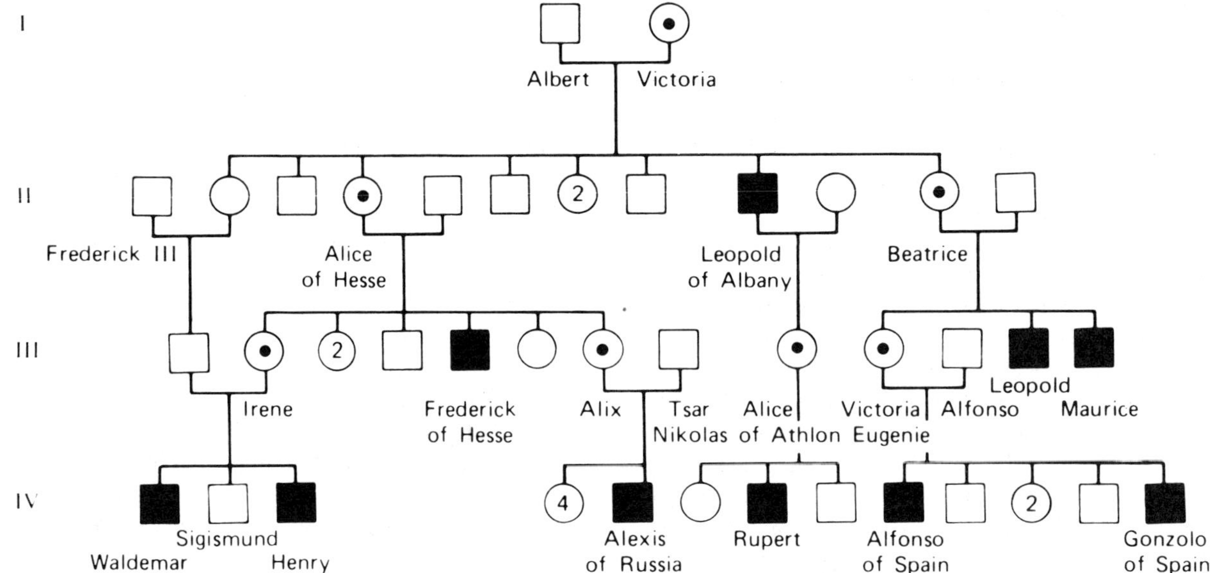

Figure 24.8
Pedigree of hemophilia A in royal families. *Source:* Nora, J., Fraser, F. C.: *Medical Genetics: Principles and Practice* (2nd ed.). Philadelphia: Lea and Febiger, 1982. Used with permission.

hemorrhage into the joints. Survival depends upon successful limitation of the frequency and severity of bleeding episodes.

Duchenne muscular dystrophy is an X-linked recessive form of one of the largest groups of muscle diseases affecting children. The onset of symptoms, which include a tendency to fall, clumsiness in walking, pseudohypertrophy, especially of the calf muscles, and generalized progressive decline in muscle function, is usually between 3–5 years of age. Survival beyond age 20 is rare.

MULTIFACTORIAL DISORDERS

There are a number of disorders in which the inheritance pattern is not as clearly defined or evident as it may be for chromosomal aberrations or single gene defects. When a trait results from the interaction and small additive effects of factors, such as environmental agents and/or several genes, the transmission is said to be multifactorial. In these cases it may be difficult to ascertain if and to what extent environmental agents facilitate expression of genetically controlled traits. Much of the variation noted among family members can be attributed to *multifactorial inheritance.*

The distribution of a multifactorial disorder in the population generally follows the bell-shaped, or normal curve (see Fig. 24.9). Therefore, a small percentage of the general population will be affected because it possesses all or most of the genes collectively responsible for a certain disorder. When there are affected members within the same family, however, the normal curve shifts so that a greater percentage of the family population is susceptible to the disorder as it is most likely to have received a large number of the genes in question. Classic examples of multifactorial disorders include cleft lip and palate and the neural tube defects.

Although cleft lip (CL) with or without cleft palate (CL/P) is a feature often seen as part of a number of syndromes of either chromosomal or single gene origin, the majority of cases exhibit multifactorial inheritance. This disorder results from the failure of the lateral palantine processes to fuse at about the seventh week of fetal development (Fig. 24.10). This fusion requires that the processes move from a lateral position on either side of the tongue to a horizontal position above it. Timing is critical and success of this maneuver depends upon a number of factors including the position and size of the tongue, the width of the head, and the size of the lateral processes when

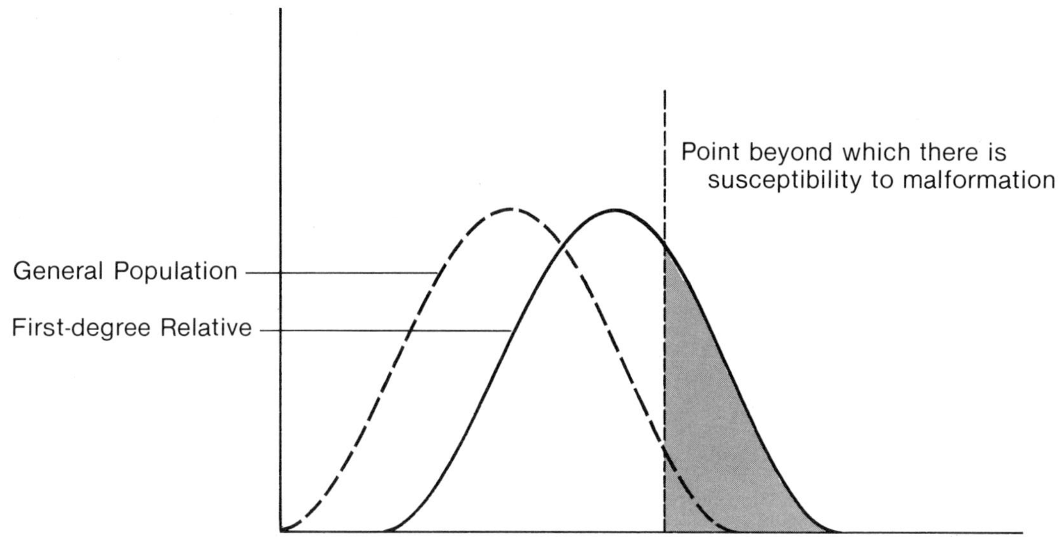

Figure 24.9
Susceptibility of general population and first-degree relatives to multifactorial disorders.

they reach the horizontal position. In most cases the defects can be surgically corrected.

Anencephaly and spina bifida are the two common classifications of neural tube defects. Failure of the neural tube folds at the cranial end of the neural plate to fuse and form the midbrain results in anencephaly. Life expectancy for affected people is several hours at best. The spina bifidas result from failure of the two halves of the vertebral column to fuse. The term spina bifida refers to vertebral or neural defects of the spinal column, which are commonly found in the sacral, lumbar, and lower thoracic regions. These lesions range in severity from those that are covered with skin to those in which the neural tube is exposed (Fig. 24.11).

Besides developmental disorders, there are a number of diseases thought to demonstrate multifactorial inheritance. The familial pattern evident in diabetes mellitus and the increased risk to subsequent offspring when more than one family member is already affected makes this type of inheritance likely. Other disorders thought to be the result of interacting multifactors include hypertension, peptic ulcers, epilepsy, mental retardation, and some of the psychoses.

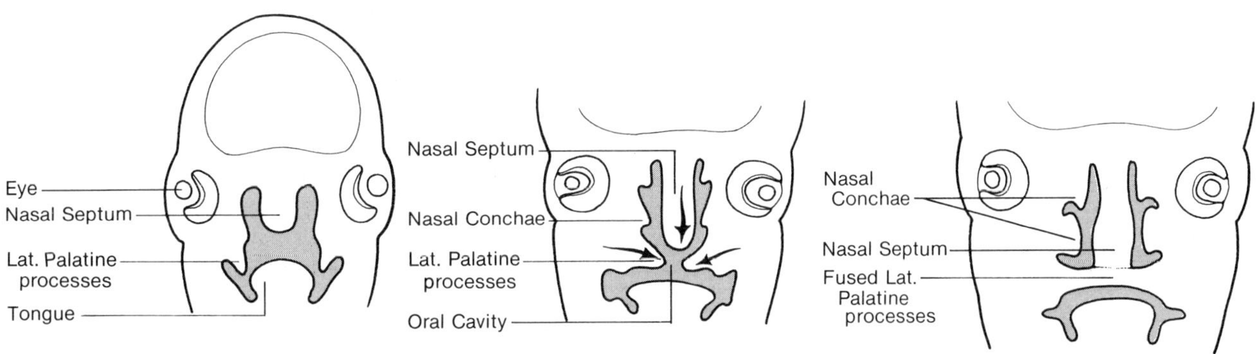

Figure 24.10
Formation of palate.

It has become increasingly apparent that exposure of the fetus to a number of environmental agents, known as *teratogens*, during the early weeks of development can have a profound effect upon that development. These teratogens include radiation; drugs and chemicals like Thalidomide, anticonvulsants, and alcohol; and infectious agents like the German measles virus and cytomegalovirus. When teratogens are involved, the extent, if any, of genetic involvement is unknown, but it is interesting to note that many fetuses exposed to these same agents, possibly in larger doses, are not affected. It has been suggested that the mother's genetic makeup may facilitate detoxification of the teratogen rendering it harmless to the fetus.

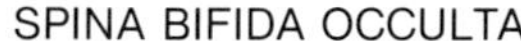

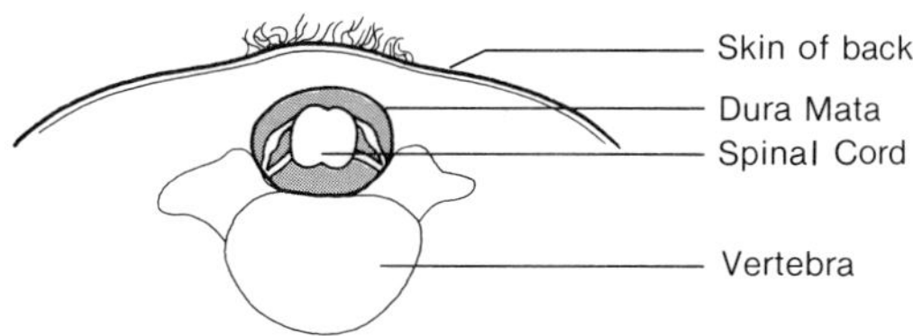

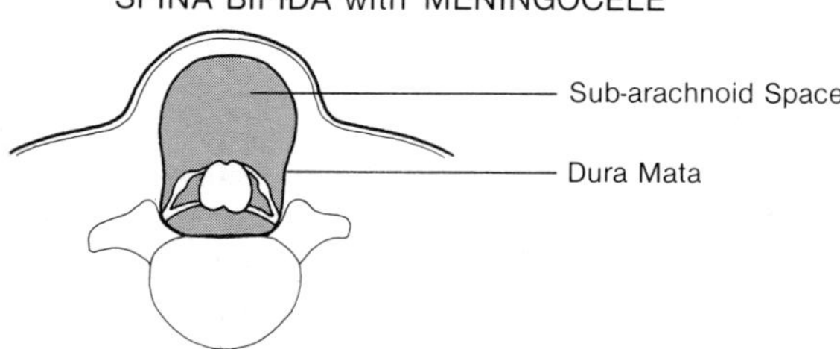

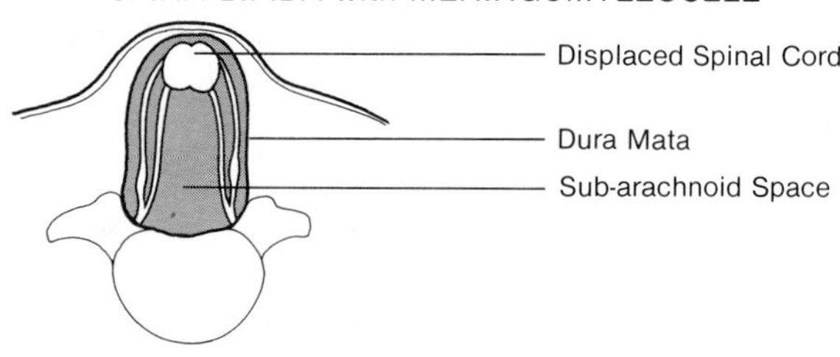

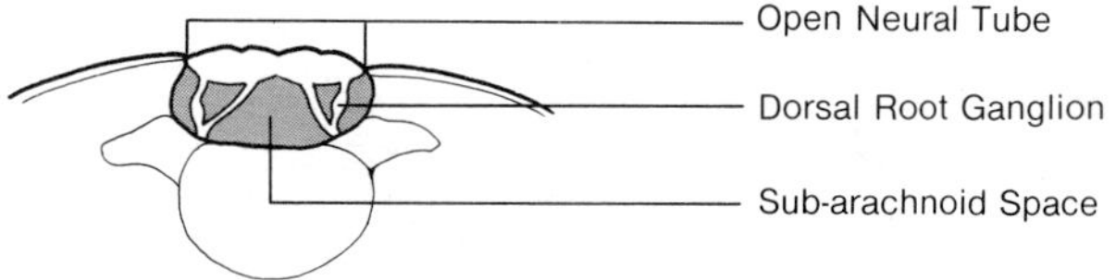

Figure 24.11
Common types of spina bifida.

GENETIC COUNSELING

Along with normal curiosity as to the sex of their unborn child, parents are primarily concerned with its health and general lack of flaws. The birth of an abnormal child is one of the main reasons parents seek genetic counseling. They want to know what happened, why it happened, and if it can happen again. Others who may desire counseling include couples unable either to achieve conception or to carry a pregnancy to term or people who are aware of an identified genetic disorder within the family and want to know the risks to their children. Genetic counseling is the communication process designed to answer questions about these problems. This type of counseling should only be undertaken by health care professionals with expertise in the field of clinical genetics.

Perhaps the single most important aspect of genetic counseling is an accurate diagnosis. As with other clinical entities, genetic diagnosis is determined by a family history (often presented in the shorthand pedigree form), a complete physical examination (autopsy reports of deceased family members), and appropriate laboratory tests. Many nurses today are members of interdisciplinary teams that provide genetic counseling. By using their skills in physical assessment and family history gathering, nurses can contribute immeasurably to the diagnosis-determining process. Once the diagnosis is established, the risk for recurrence can be estimated.

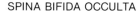

As part of the physical examination, a study of dermal ridge and flexion crease patterns (*dermatoglyphics*) of the hands and feet can sometimes provide a clue to the diagnosis of chromosomal disorders. Evidence provided by dermatoglyphic configuration similarities among members of the same family, especially twins, suggests a genetic determinant, and it is therefore reasonable to assume that deleted or *duplicated* genes can alter these patterns. Because dermatoglyphics formation is generally complete by the ninteenth week of fetal life, the presence of abnormal patterns suggests the disorder's causative factor was operating during early fetal development. A common example of dermatoglyphic response to a chromosomal aberration can often be found in Down's syndrome (Fig. 24.12).

Thanks to recent improvements in techniques such as ultrasonography, amniocentesis, and fetoscopy there are a number of genetic diseases that can be detected prenatally (see Table 24.2). Gross fetal abnormalities like anencephaly can be observed through use of ultrasound equipment (See Chapter 20). Amniocentesis, generally performed between the fourteenth and sixteenth weeks of pregnancy, provides a source of cells from which chromosomal karyotypes and some biochemical levels of the fetus can be determined. Advances in fiberoptics combined with development of the fetoscope now permits direct visualization of the live fetus in utero and the recording of this examination on videotape.

Armed with an accurate diagnosis, a full knowledge of the disease entity involved, and prognosis and recurrence risks, the counseling team can then set about answering questions for those concerned. Counselors must consider the wide range of emotions people can experience when faced with the knowledge that they or their offspring may not be genetically sound. Once these emotions have been dealt with and pertinent questions have been answered, the couple is better prepared to make decisions concerning the affected family member and whether or not to risk future pregnancies.

TABLE 24.2
PARTIAL LIST OF DISORDERS THAT CAN BE DETECTED PRENATALLY

Chromosomal aberrations (numerical or structural)
Tay-Sachs disease
Niemann-Pick disease
Hunter's syndrome
Neural tube defects
Lesch-Nyhan syndrome
Pompe's disease

ETHICAL CONSIDERATIONS

As medicine and science continue to broaden the base of genetic knowledge, nurses will have to

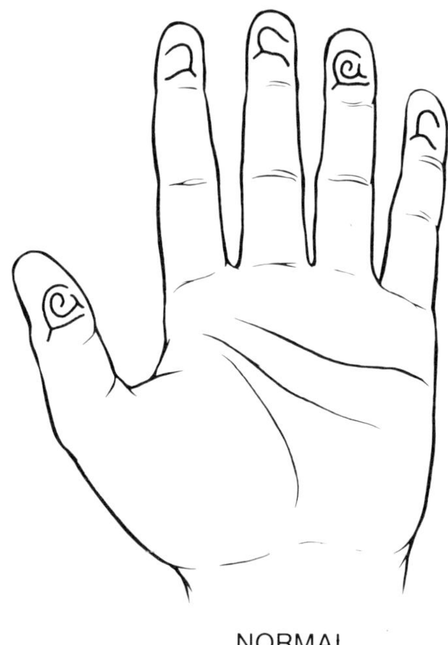

NORMAL

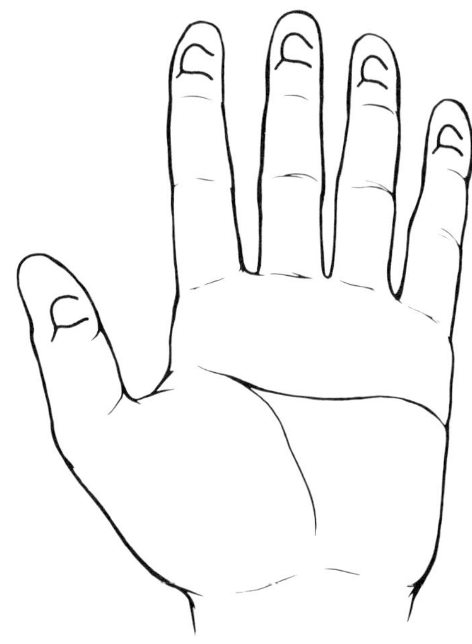

DOWN'S SYNDROME

Figure 24.12
Dermatoglyphic patterns.

consider professionally, and perhaps personally, a number of the legal, ethical, and moral issues being raised: Should genetic engineering experiments be regulated? If so, by whom? If not, how will abuses be controlled? Should society, who will most likely bear the financial burden of institutionalization of the affected person, have any recourse when a woman, determined to be carrying a severely handicapped fetus, elects not to abort? Should the decision to sterilize a mentally retarded person come from the parents, physicians, society, or only from the incapacitated person concerned? There are no simple answers to questions associated with genetic progress for each situation must be considered in light of the personal circumstances. To be able to make informed decisions about these and other questions, nurses must be aware of the potential influence genetics can exert on almost every aspect of life.

NURSING CARE

Genetic disorders in a child, particularly those that were undiagnosed prenatally, can have a devastating effect on the parents. The parents are often unable to take in all the careful explanations of cause and effect that professional personnel are ready to give them. Before they see the child, parents may have exaggerations about the child's appearance, which may or may not be borne out in reality. Should facts be withheld from the parents, they are likely to lose trust in people who misled them when they are confronted with their genetically defective child.

Parents often experience a feeling of loss when they have other than the perfect child for which they have prepared. The nurse must be able to transfer understandings about grief and loss to the care of these families. Guilt feelings are prominent at this time, and the parents are likely to blame themselves, together or individually. The nurse frequently hears the question, "What did I (we) do to cause this?"

In the case of inherited disorders, prevention of the recurrence of a similar disorder with another pregnancy is the best course to follow. Education is a most important component of prevention. Many birth defects, such as those of teratogenic or iatrogenic origins, can be prevented. Education should stress the health of both parents, especially good nutrition and avoidance of habits that can be harmful to the unborn such as the use of drugs, alcohol, and cigarettes. Health providers must be made cognizant of the need to protect the pregnant woman and her unborn child from unnecessary procedures or treatments that may prove harmful. Education for family planning can help ensure that childbirth can occur in the prime reproductive years rather than too early or too late. Education for pregnancy and parenthood should begin during the school years, and information about genetic disorders should be a part of such education. However, educational programs should not be limited to the young, but should also be available to people throughout their reproductive years.

Genetic screening is a means for determining, before conception, the potential for inherited disorders or for detecting a defective fetus after conception. Diagnostic studies mentioned earlier, as well as those discussed in Chapter 20, provide much useful information about the potential of the fetus for having a genetic disorder. The nurse can encourage genetic screening by educating others about its availability and about the indications for genetic screening procedures. Nurses can be involved in publicizing programs and in recruiting high-risk populations into the screening process.

Prenatal supervision with careful attention to avoidance of harmful procedures, critical observation and reporting of significant symptomatology, and accurate and detailed prenatal history-taking is an essential adjunct to prevention or detection of genetic abnormalities.

Genetic counseling, discussed earlier, should be encouraged for families who have borne a defective child or who have a family history of genetic disorders.

The nurse should be informed about resources available to those considered to be at risk because of genetic disorders. Public and private resources such as mental retardation and birth defects programs are available in most states.

SUMMARY

Genetic disorders are one of humankind's most tragic legacies. However, much has been and continues to be done to prevent genetic disorders and to diagnose early those so afflicted and to rehabilitate them. This chapter addressed mechanisms of chromosomal aberrations and autosomal and X-linked dominant and recessive transmission and has discussed some of the more prevalent disorders arising from chromosomal, single gene, and multifactorial inheritance. Genetic counseling and ethical issues related to genetic advancements were discussed. Nursing care was addressed.

REFERENCES AND READINGS

Bergsma, D. (Ed.) *Birth Defects: Atlas and Compendium.* Baltimore: Williams & Wilkins, 1974. (Published for The National Foundation—March of Dimes.)

Fitzsimmons, J. S., Fitzsimmons, E. M. *A Handbook of Clinical Genetics.* London: William Heinemann Medical Books, 1980.

Goodman, R. M. (Ed.) *Genetic Disorders of Man.* Boston: Little, Brown, 1970.

Goodman, R. M., Gorlin, R. J. *Atlas of The Face in Genetic Disorders.* St. Louis: C. V. Mosby, 1977.

Gorlin, R. J., Pindborg, J. J., Cohen, M. M., Jr. *Syndromes of the Head and Neck.* New York: McGraw-Hill, 1976.

Kelly, P. T. *Dealing with Dilemma: A Manual for Genetic Counselors.* New York: Springer-Verlag, 1977.

McKusick, V. A. *Mendelian Inheritance in Man* (5th ed.). Baltimore: The Johns Hopkins University Press, 1978.

McKusick, V. A., Claiborne, R. (Eds.) *Medical Genetics.* New York: HP Publishing Co., 1973.

Moore, K. L. *The Developing Human: Clinical Oriented Embryology.* Philadelphia: W. B. Saunders, 1973.

Nagle, J. J. *Heredity and Human Affairs* (2nd ed.). St. Louis: C. V. Mosby, 1979.

Nora, J. J., Fraser, F. C. *Medical Genetics: Principles and Practice.* Philadelphia: Lea & Febiger, 1974.

Stevenson, A. C. *Genetic Counselling* (2nd ed.). Philadelphia: J. B. Lippincott, 1976.

Thompson, J. S., Thompson, M. W. *Genetics in Medicine* (3rd ed.). Philadelphia: W. B. Saunders, 1980.

Whaley, L. F. *Understanding Inherited Disorders.* St. Louis: C. V. Mosby, 1974.

Yunis, J. J. (Ed.). *New Chromosomal Syndromes.* New York: Academic Press, 1977.

25

REPRODUCTIVE PSYCHOSOCIAL DISORDERS

Physical disorders that place a pregnant woman, her unborn child, and her family at reproductive risk are familiar to most maternity nurses because of their widespread prevalence. Reproductive psychosocial disorders, however, may be overlooked or overshadowed by physical problems or they may be ignored by the nurse who feels ill prepared to deal with the individuals and families experiencing such disorders. Some psychosocial disorders have stimulated concern and attention for a number of years—postpartum depression is one such problem. Recently, however, other psychosocial disorders have been reported as having a particularly detrimental effect on pregnant women and their offspring. Drug abuse, including alcohol and nicotine, has received attention by the media as well as in professional journals during the past 20–25 years. Whether a problem has been long recognized or recently identified, the maternity nurse should be aware that psychosocial disorders are prevalent in contemporary childbearing families. The maternity nurse who is alert to indicators of psychosocial disorders, may well be the first health professional to detect the presence of such a problem for a pregnant woman. Further, the nurse may be the key health provider to give sensitive, supportive health care.

This chapter addresses selected psychosocial disorders of both long-standing and recent concern. These disorders are divided into three major categories: disorders that arise from drug abuse, from abusive behavior, and from psychogenic origins. Some of these disorders have their origins before conception as pre-existing conditions that are aggravated by pregnancy; others seem to be tied much more closely with pregnancy as the precipitating factor. Drug abuse and abusive behaviors have only recently been recognized by the health care world as contributing to poor pregnancy outcome and problems with parenting. Psychogenic disorders have been recognized by medicine for a longer period of time. However, all of these disorders have potential for harm to mother, infant, or both and as such place them along with their family at reproductive risk.

DRUG ABUSE

Drug abuse is defined here as the improper use of drugs and may take the form of *addiction, dependence,* or *habituation* (see Table 25.1). The use of drugs,

TABLE 25.1
DRUG ADDICTION, DEPENDENCE, AND HABITUATION

	Addiction[a]	*Dependence*[a]	*Habituation*
Definition	Periodic or chronic state of *intoxication* that results from repeated consumption of a drug (WHO, 1957)	A *physical* or *psychologic* state that occurs because of repeated, periodic, or continual consumption of a drug (WHO, 1963)	Repeated consumption of a drug because of a desire for the effects of the drug that is not associated with urgent physical or psychologic compulsion
Characteristics (Ferguson, 1975; Eddy, 1965)	Compulsion to take the drug as evidenced by overpowering desire or need Acquisition of the drug by whatever means necessary Increased dosage with use Physical and psychologic dependence with the appearance of physical symptoms on withdrawal	Drug specific characteristics that vary with the drug taken Characteristics are described as drug dependence of the morphine type; drug dependence of the alcohol type	Absence of physical compulsion to take the drug Dosage levels that do not increase with use No physical withdrawal symptoms Some psychologic dependence associated with desire for feelings of well-being
Impact	Adverse impact on the person, family, society, and, in the event of pregnancy, on the unborn child	Related to the drug-specific dependence Can have a detrimental effect on the person, the family, society, and the unborn	Major impact on the person and those closest to him or her If a pregnant woman, likely to have an adverse impact on the unborn

[a] *Terms are sometimes used interchangeably.*

whether obtained by prescription, or across the counter, or by illegal methods, is increasing almost everywhere making drug use a widespread phenomena in all parts of the world. Drugs have historically been used for religious, therapeutic, analgesic, social, and other reasons by almost all known civilizations. Growing numbers of pregnant women are among the users of legal and nonlegal drugs, making drug use a major reproductive health problem in the United States.

Legally, a *drug* is defined as "any substance, vegetable, animal or mineral used as a medicine," [Carroll Perfumers v. State Ind., 7 N.E. (2d 970, 1972)]. Sociologically, the definition is broadened to include not only medicines, but any chemical substance that enhances feelings of physical and mental well-being. This broader definition permits the inclusion of hundreds of agents used by the person. The toxic effects of many drugs today are not completely known. The information about the effects of such drugs on the unborn child is even more incomplete.

The specific causes of drug abuse are not always apparent. There is universal agreement that drug abuse occurs because of a combination of factors that arise from both physical and psychosocial origins. Most of these predisposing or causative factors tend to spring from stimuli originating with

- ▲ ***Personal Characteristics.*** Age, idiosyncratic physical response to certain drugs, emotional instability or personality maladjustments (e.g., neuroses and personality disorders), curiosity, and the need to experiment.
- ▲ ***Life-style.*** (Including relationships with associates, particularly peer groups, and the influ-

ence of their values and pressures.) Use of drugs for social intercourse, relaxation, and pleasure. Boredom arising from absent or unclear responsibilities and goals, excess leisure time, or religious and spiritual purposes, affiliations, or requirements.

▲ ***Environment.*** There is a high incidence of drug use and juvenile crime found among adolescent men who come from crowded, urban areas where poverty is rampant; parental supervision and discipline are absent or inconsistent; and peer group, cliques, or gangs abound. These young people are often school dropouts, unemployed, and often unemployable. Increasingly, young women are becoming a part of such a profile; many of these women find themselves pregnant. The poverty in the inner city environment is not the only origin of drug abuse. Middle-income and affluent families also produce significant numbers of drug users. Drug use, particularly alcohol, in schools is increasing and penetrating the lower grades as well as the high school level. Drug use among young women is tied to sexual promiscuity that often results in pregnancy or reproductive-related health problems.

In spite of the associations between drug abuse and the factors just described, there is really little that is definitive about the cause of drug use and abuse among the population generally.

Drug use is of concern in regard to pregnancy because of the possibility—even likelihood—of adverse effects on the unborn child. Drugs have been shown to cause extensive damage to the pregnancy resulting in spontaneous abortion or even stillbirth of a fetus who has reached viability. Drugs have caused teratogenic disorders in the newborn—both congenital malformations and other physical disorders. The pregnant addict will compromise not only her own physical, emotional, and social well-being but that of her child as well. The alcohol-dependent woman places her unborn child in danger of serious mental and physical disorders, not to mention the stress and trauma suffered by herself and her family. The effect of drugs on the unborn was dramatically demonstrated for the public in 1962 with the recognition of the association between the use of a drug called Thalidomide. by pregnant women and the resultant gross abnormalities found in their offspring. Thalidomide was promptly removed from the market place in some countries, and its use was prohibited in the United States. Since that time an increased awareness of drugs and their effects on the unborn has emerged; subsequent research on drugs has confirmed this concern and raised questions in the minds of health providers and consumers alike concerning the use of drugs during pregnancy. In spite of what is known, drug use is still a widespread health problem that is of particular interest to maternity nurses and their clients.

Drug use and pregnancy can be examined by looking at the impact of drug consumption on the pregnant woman and her unborn or newborn infant. Given the right combination of factors, drug use for medicinal or social reasons could, at any time, become drug abuse with all of its associated problems. The following discussion however, will be limited to the effects of drugs on the maternal–fetal unit.

Drug Consumption for Medicinal Purposes

American families indulge in considerable self-treatment by the use of myriads of drugs that can be purchased without prescription in drugstores, supermarkets, convenience stores, airports—almost anywhere the shopper chooses to buy. If a headache persists, take aspirin or an aspirin substitute; plagued by an allergy, take an antihistamine; bothered by a head cold, use a cold medicine, cough syrup, or combination drug to relieve all symptoms. This reliance on drugs to provide comfort is so prevalent in the United States today that few people consider what they are taking or how the preparation will affect them. The American public regularly consumes expectorants, analgesics, antiemetics, leftover prescriptions, antacids, coffee, tea, tobacco, and alcohol as a part of daily living activities. Most people, if asked, would deny that they habitually use drugs. In a strict sense most Americans do not habituate to one drug but are much more ecumenical in their use of drugs. The effects of most of these drugs are not completely known in spite of rigid national food and drug laws. The teratogenic effects of drugs on the unborn child are still being studied.

Salicylates (aspirin and aspirin compounds) have been reported to be associated with congenital malformations (McNeil, 1973; Nelson & Forfar, 1971). Aspirin is found in almost every home in the United States, and aspirin substitutes, about which even less is known, are replacing the use of aspirin in some instances. Salicylates have also been associated with gastrointestinal tract bleeding in the adult; this effect on the unborn is still under investigation. The salicylates are only one group of drugs that are known or suspected to cause teratogenic damage to the unborn. Other drugs are dangerous as well.

Doering and Steward (1978), in a study of 168 pregnant women, showed that all of these women had taken a minimum of two different drugs and that 93.4% of them had taken five or more drugs, with an average of 11 different drugs taken during pregnancy. Stortz (1977) reported that in a sample of 100 hospitalized women during the postpartum period, 97% reported use of at least one nonprescription drug before becoming pregnant and 88% used at least one drug during pregnancy. These women were mature young adults from socioeconomically middle-class backgrounds and most likely are representative of many other young women.

The public also relies on prescription drugs such as analgesics (many of which contain various amounts of narcotics), tranquilizers, barbiturates, and antibiotics most of which have the potential for becoming abused drugs (see Table 25.2). Jokes have been made about the amount of drugs taken by women in the United States—they take tranquilizers to calm them down, amphetamines or other stimulants to pep them up; their purses resemble a medicine chest. These, of course, are generalizations, but the nurse must remember that the use of prescription drugs, particularly tranquilizers, is widespread, which is a serious matter when the women are of childbearing age.

Drug Use for Psychosocial Reasons

Drugs are often used as an adjunct to social activity or as a palliative for stress. Smoking and drinking alcoholic beverages have long been a part of social events. Alcohol and tobacco advertising is designed to make the products appear exciting and attractive. One brand of cigarettes presents a subtle, but appealing invitation to the "liberated" woman to show her independence by smoking their brand of cigarettes.

Despite the fact that in the 1960s the Office of the Surgeon General brought the hazards of smoking to the public's attention and major federal restrictions were imposed on advertising practices for tobacco products, a large number of Americans have continued to smoke, many of whom are women and some of whom are pregnant. Although all cigarettes are required to carry a statement warning that cigarette smoking may be dangerous to a person's health, studies have repeatedly shown that fear of adverse health effects does not deter smoking among most of the population.

Pregnant women who smoke tend to deliver infants that are low birth weight (Greenwood, 1979). Fielding (1978) found that infants of women smokers weigh 150–250 gm less than infants of nonsmokers; perinatal mortality was 27% higher and fetal death from placenta previa and abruptio placenta was increased among infants of smokers when compared to infants of nonsmokers. Women who smoke tend to have an increased incidence of abortion (Kline et al., 1977). Congenital anomalies are more prevalent among infants of mothers who smoke (Himmelberger et al., 1978). These are just some of the findings about the relationship between smoking and poor pregnancy outcome. The literature abounds with data supporting smoking as a health hazard, especially to the unborn child.

The association between alcohol consumption by pregnant women and fetal ill health was first reported in the sixteenth century. Recently, the use of alcohol, *in any quantity*, by pregnant women has come into question. Jones et al. (1973) brought the problem to the attention of the public when he reported a pattern of fetal anomalies among women who consumed alcohol during pregnancy. This neonatal profile showed intrauterine and postnatal growth retardation, cardiac problems, joint anomalies, and mental deficiency and has become widely known as *fetal alcohol syndrome* (FAS) (see Table 25.3). Subsequent research has associated FAS with the amounts of alcohol consumed by the pregnant woman. The consumption of 3 oz of 95–100% ethyl alcohol per day places the fetus at risk (Henahan, 1977). This amount converts into two to five drinks per day (depending on the composition and strength of each drink). Whether it is the alcohol itself that causes this problem or the nutritional deficiency that accompanies alcoholism is not certain. It is known, however, that alcohol crosses the placenta in about the same concentrations as

TABLE 25.2
USE OF PRESCRIPTION PSYCHOACTIVE DRUGS, ILLEGAL DRUGS, AND ALCOHOL IN WOMEN 18–34 YEARS OF AGE

Drug	*Number*	*Percent Using One or More Other Psychoactive Drugs*	*Percent Using Alcohol*	
			Regular	*Heavy*
Narcotic analgesics Darvon, Talwin	1,000,000	15%	50%	10%
Minor tranquilizers Valium, Librium	750,000	15%	40%	15%
Barbiturates Seconal, Tuinal	585,000	33%	50%	10%
Stimulants and hunger suppressants Dexedrine, Dexamyl, Preludin	675,000	25%	90+%	50%
Prescription narcotics Demerol, Dilaudid	125,000	33%	25%	5%
Prescription antidepressants Elavil, Tofranil	100,000	50%	20%	10%
Alcohol	3,240,000 (daily)			
Marijuana	446,000			
LSD or other hallucinogens	130,000	"Hidden" users not known to treatment or enforcement systems		
Cocaine	100,000			
Heroin	90,000			

Source: Butnarescu, G. F., Tillotson, D. M., Villarreal, P. P. *Perinatal Nursing Vol. 2. Reproductive Risk.* New York: John Wiley & Sons, 1980. Used with permission.

does maternal blood, making alcohol the likely offender because of the effect of acetaldehyde, a by-product of alcohol metabolism (Rawat, 1978). Since the precise amounts of alcohol that causes FAS are unknown and safe drinking levels are difficult to establish, it was recently recommended that women who are pregnant avoid all alcoholic beverages during pregnancy.

Some women are more than occasional smokers. Smoking habituation, when a woman smokes more than one pack of cigarettes per day, is increasing among women. Chain smoking has been associated with high stress and stress-related activities. As more women move into stress-related positions in the work world, their health profiles, with all of the related problems, are beginning to resemble more closely those of their men counterparts. Smoking habits may very well be a part of this general trend. As working women delay pregnancy and parenthood until careers are well established, the possibility of stress-related habits such as smoking take on new and more serious meanings.

Alcohol dependence is a major health problem among women in the United States. It carries with it social, emotional, and physical problems of major dimensions for the woman and her family, as well as her unborn fetus. Some of these women will be unsuccessful with pregnancy and are at risk for poor parenting practices. Alcohol is a great destroyer of families in America. When the woman, who is the central figure in the family of childbearing age, is affected by the problem of alcohol dependence, the jeopardy to the family is likely to be intensified.

The management of drug-related problems and pregnancy is prevention; however, efforts toward prevention of many psychosocial disorders of this nature have fallen short of their goals. This should not discourage health professionals such as the maternity nurse from making as vigorous an effort to prevent the problem as an effort to treat and rehabilitate people who are victims of the disorders.

Drug Addiction and Pregnancy

Addiction of a person to any drug at any age is a tragedy since drug addiction can destroy the soul of a person, debilitate the family, and damage the body of a person often beyond physical, emotional, or social rehabilitation. Pregnancy superimposed on the problem of drug addiction adds another dimension for it introduces the developing fetus into the picture and places the fetus at maximal risk for intrauterine as well as extrauterine survival. Of all women who are drug addicts, 5% are dependent on heroin or methadone and the other 5% may be dependent on other drugs such as other narcotics or barbiturates.

Carr (1977) characterizes the drug-dependent woman as:

- ▲ Coming from an unstable family background where the family is not intact or is dysfunctional.
- ▲ Frequently a victim of sexual abuse by a male parent or family member. Histories often reveal rape or prostitution as well.
- ▲ Having a poor self-concept and low self-esteem. She is unlikely to trust or even to be able to trust.
- ▲ Tending to use drugs to escape from reality or to relieve emotional pain. More than one drug is frequently used. (The use of multiple drugs is more a characteristic of women than of men drug abusers.) Barbiturates, tranquilizers, and alcohol are used more often among middle-class and affluent women; narcotics are used more often among poorer women. The need to acquire the drug is overpowering, and 20% of drug-dependent pregnant women have been prostitutes, have had positive serology at the time of pregnancy, and have been in jail or involved in some type of criminal offense (Rementeria & Marrero, 1977).

The addict who is pregnant may view the pregnancy as a positive part of her life and try to break the drug habit during this time. Finnegan (1977) has suggested that the pregnancy reinforces a woman's need to feel that she is capable of doing something worthwhile.

There is an increased incidence of biophysical and psychosocial disorders with drug addiction and pregnancy. Nutritional deficiency is a major problem for both mother and fetus. Infectious diseases, particularly venereal diseases, are more prevalent. There is an increased chance of abortion, stillbirth, toxemia, fetal growth retardation, premature labor, and complications of labor (Weisman, 1977).

Management of the pregnant addict closely follows therapy for anyone who is drug dependent; however, the effects of therapy on the fetus is always a concern, and therapy must make adaptations to accommodate this consideration. The pregnant addict is unlikely to be able to assume responsibility for infant care giving without assistance from the nurse and other professional personnel since the addict is basically a dependent personality with high anxiety levels and expectations to fail in whatever she undertakes.

The infant of the drug-addicted mother enters the extrauterine environment with the problems associated with drug addiction superimposed on the usual physiologic and environmental adjustments to be made after birth. The infant may present narcotic withdrawal symptoms such as irritability, generalized hyperactivity, and tremors. Sleep disturbances may be apparent, and poor weight gain after birth is common (see Chapter 23).

Management of Drug Abuse and Pregnancy

The management of pregnant women who have unknowingly taken drugs harmful to themselves or their unborn child, as well as of those who are drug abusers, depends largely on the nature and extent of their drug use or habit. Some general guidelines follow.

Attempts should be made to prevent the problem to whatever extent possible given the complexity of factors that created the problem in the first place. Obviously, nurses cannot remedy all of the prevalent social ills that are associated with drug abuse or a culture that uses drugs as a part of normal living. The nurse can, however, inform

TABLE 25.3
CLINICAL FEATURES OF FETAL ALCOHOL SYNDROME

Incidence	*Identified Abnormality*	
50% or more of children	Prenatal and postnatal growth retardation Mental retardation Fine motor dysfunction Microcephaly Short palpebal fissures	Maxillary hypoplasia Joint anomalies Altered palmar crease pattern Cardiac anomalies
10–50% of children	Epicanthus folds Strabismus Ptosis of eyelids	Pectus excavatum Hemangiomas Ear anomalies
Fewer than 10% of children	Microphthalmia Cleft palate	Small nails Hirsutism

Source: Data from Jones, K. L. et al. Patterns of Malformation in Offspring of Chronic Alcoholic Mothers. *Lancet* 1:1267, 1973.

people by speaking to appropriate groups about the impact of and sequelae to drug abuse. Further, the nurse can participate in the designing and implementing of educational services for prospective parents to help them understand the dimensions of the problem. The nurse can also work to see that such educational services are accessible to those people in greatest need.

The nurse should use assessment skills and knowledge about drug use and abuse to aid in early detection of drug-related problems of women who are or could become pregnant.

It is important to approach the woman with a drug problem and her family—if accessible—with sensitivity. The nurse cannot empathize with the problems being experienced, but the nurse can comprehend the nature and scope of these problems and draw upon the best interpersonal skills to provide support and promote self-esteem rather than act in a punitive or disapproving manner.

When necessary, the nurse should be prepared to set limits for the woman with a drug problem who may be unable to do so for herself and to help with realistic goals that can be reached so that success rather than failure becomes possible for the woman and those closest to her.

The nurse needs to be knowledgeable about and supportive of the medical regimen planned for the woman during the antepartal, intrapartal, and postpartal periods. If the pregnant woman or neonate is on a drug withdrawal program, the nurse should be alert to withdrawal symptoms and the stresses and demands confronting either or both clients.

Successful mother–infant bonding is crucial to the mother's success in her parenting role. She needs to feel that she is capable of caring for her infant.

The nurse has to be prepared to help the woman with grief work if the infant is severely damaged or stillborn. Guilt is prominent among parents, particularly the mother, any time there is a problem with the infant. This guilt may be increased if the mother associates a personal habit or event for which she is responsible as contributing to the problem.

The nurse should identify and promote the use of patient support systems such as family, friends, and relatives if they are available. When necessary, the nurse must help the woman establish new support networks. Remember that the drug-addicted woman does not usually have visible family members available; and even if they are accessible, they may not be the most appropriate resources to provide the needed support. Where family members are available and involved, they may be experiencing considerable stress, and they may need support from the nurse and other health professionals, as well as does the mother. All medical, social, and legal resources need to be explored and appropriate referrals made and consultations provided. Collaboration with interdisciplinary groups is an essential part of nursing for the woman who is pregnant and a drug abuser or addict.

The goals for care of the pregnant woman in regard to drugs are complex and can be summarized as follows.

- ▲ Make every effort to inform the public about drugs and their effect on pregnancy and the unborn child
- ▲ Support the pregnant woman and her infant through the best possible professional nursing care
- ▲ Participate in and support medical therapeutic regimens planned for the woman throughout pregnancy and recovery
- ▲ Participate in rehabilitation and follow-up where indicated
- ▲ Be patient with and tolerant of the woman during her pregnancy and recovery period

The ultimate goal is to *prevent the problem for families of the future.*

ABUSIVE BEHAVIOR

Physical abuse of one person by another is *not* a recent social event. Throughout history human beings have perpetrated crimes of violence against one another. Authorities tell us that most crimes of personal violence are directed toward a person who is known to the assailant. In all societies 25–67% of homicides take place within the family; in 1975, 25% of the murders in the United States were reported as occurring in the home (FBI Uniform Crime Report, 1975). Potentially 50% of all women will become *battered women* at some time during their lives (Fleming, 1979). Battering of children by parents has also been present in society throughout history. *Wife abuse,* battering of the female spouse or mate by the male, often goes hand in hand with *child abuse* by either or both of the parents.

Efforts are underway today to increase understanding about the dynamics of violent abusive behavior. Research is being done by a number of disciplines, including some of the health professions. Attempts to encourage reporting of abusive behavior, particularly spouse and child abuse, are seen through provision of legal protection and anonymity both to those who report such incidents and to the victims of the attack.

Wife beating is defined as a deliberate violent act that intends to bring about physical injury to the victim through actions, by the assailant. It may take the form of a severe beating with the hands or a weapon, or biting or choking. Wife beating is believed to be more prevalent than official records indicate. It has been called the most underreported crime in the United States, with one beating estimated to take place every 15 seconds (FBI Uniform Crime Reports, 1975). Emergency room records show that 20% of their cases are related to wife abuse and more than two-thirds of assault cases are wives. These facts are both alarming and frightening, especially since most of the public is unaware of the scope of the problem.

Myths about wife abuse abound and include beliefs such as:

- ▲ The problem is insignificant in terms of numbers of victims
- ▲ Women provoke the assault
- ▲ Battering is limited to certain minority groups
- ▲ Batterers have inherited their violent personalities
- ▲ Batterers are psychopaths
- ▲ The woman could help herself if she wanted to

These statements have been shown to be inaccurate and misleading. Contrary to such widespread beliefs, it is known that:

- ▲ The problem is of significant dimensions as mentioned earlier.
- ▲ Most assaults are difficult to anticipate, and provocation, if present, is not clear.
- ▲ Wife abuse is found in all socioeconomic strata, age groups, and educational levels with no particular ethnic or social group showing an af-

finity for the practice. Affluent groups can often conceal the problem more easily than can their poorer counterparts.

- ▲ Battered women are rarely the provokers of assault and are usually unprepared for the timing and the violence of the assault.
- ▲ Violent behavior is learned and is believed to represent an acting out of frustrations and rage that may arise from a variety of stressful sources.
- ▲ While personality disorders have been described among men who are batterers, there is no definite association of the characteristics of these men with psychopathology.
- ▲ The abused woman often perceives few options open to her, especially if there are young children in the family. She may not have a place to go or the economic means to leave and support herself and her family. In some instances, she is not physically able to remove herself from the home. Relatives, friends, and community sources such as the clergy and the police may not be willing to become involved. The woman is often made to feel that she, not her mate, is the person at fault.

Victims

There are multiple *victims* of the violence associated with wife abuse. The woman is both physically and emotionally traumatized and the children (or child) in the family are at risk for abuse by the father during the acute stage of the violence or by the mother who may direct her rage and frustration toward them.

The Battered Pregnant Woman

Abuse of pregnant women by their mates is a health problem of significant dimensions. Like wife battering in general, physical abuse of the pregnant woman has received little attention until the past few years. Such an assault places both the pregnant woman and her unborn child (and any other children) in jeopardy of bodily harm and extensive psychologic trauma. They are also at risk because of the increased chance of repetition of the attack and because of inadequate economic, supportive, and emotional resources (Sammons, 1981). The children of the woman are at risk since about 25% of wife abusers are also child abusers (Johnson, 1979) and about one-third of battered women abuse their children (Walker, 1979). The emergency room or maternity nurse is often the first health professional seen by the *battered pregnant woman* seeking help. The decisions made by the nurse and the nurse's response to both the woman and her problem play a large part in whether or not health care will be effective.

The factors that cause a man to attack his pregnant mate are not entirely clear. Several possibilities have been mentioned. The wife batterer is described as a jealous man who wants to keep his mate to himself. This same jealousy may be directed, consciously or unconsciously, toward the unborn fetus. Anything that takes his mate's attention away from himself may cause anger and resentment and ultimately the rage of attack. The emotional changes in a woman as a result pregnancy that make her more egocentric and introverted may add to the resentment felt by her mate. He may feel that he is being deprived of her attention to his needs, particularly his emotional and sexual needs (see Chapters 12 and 14). Pregnancy may also demand major adjustments in roles and relationships within the family that may be intolerable to the abusive man. Hendrix et al. (1978) suggests that the abuse may represent an overt or covert desire to destroy the pregnancy and rid himself of the competition from and responsibility for another person. He may see himself as "bad" and not want another person such as himself to be born (Walker, 1979; Sammons, 1981). Whatever the reason, pregnancy has been identified as one of nine precipitating factors to abusive behaviors (Roy, 1977).

Wife battering has been characterized as a process that consists of three components or stages (Walker, 1979): (1) the period during which rage and frustrations intensify in the man (the tension-building stage); (2) the actual violent event (acute battering incident); and (3) a conciliatory stage during which the man gives and the woman accepts kindness, contrition, remorse, even loving behavior and he promises that the abusive behavior will not be repeated. These stages have relevance for planning nursing care for the battered pregnant woman.

The abused pregnant woman may remain in seclusion at home for days following the attack; or, if her symptoms warrant it, she may go to the emergency room of a hospital. Usually, a battered pregnant woman reports for a prenatal appointment with abrasions, bruises, swollen face, and so on. She either explains these as the result of an accident or offers no explanation at all.

Sammons (1981) describes the emotional symptoms of the battered pregnant woman that are associated with Walker's stages of this abusive syndrome. These symptoms provide excellent guidelines for recognizing the problem or potential problem. During the tension-building stage the nurse should pay attention to complaints such as "chest pain, choking sensations, hyperventilation, gastrointestinal symptoms, pelvic pain, conversion reactions, allergies, backache, headache, or hypertension" (p. 248). After the attack the nurse should be alert "to a history of serious bleeding injuries; to evidence of broken bones, particularly of the head, extremeties, pelvis, or vertebrae; to burns; and to bruises or lesions, particularly of the abdomen, which may result in antepartal hemorrhage or premature labor" (p. 248).

Nursing care of the battered pregnant woman, like that of the woman drug abuser, must reflect a caring, nonpunitive, sensitive attitude. This requires that the nurse not only be knowledgeable about the problem but also understand personal values and attitudes about abusive behavior. The nurse needs to remember that the woman is not only physically abused, she is also emotionally battered. The pregnant woman is frightened and angry; her self-image is poor and her self-esteem is low; she feels isolated, dependent, insecure, and is unable to trust even those who are trying to help her. She needs to know that the nurse accepts her, as she is, without judgment and without unnecessary, inquisitive probing.

Nursing care should be directed toward the achievement of four goals.

- ▲ Protection of the woman, her unborn, and her children from further harm
- ▲ Promotion of self-esteem and a positive self-image
- ▲ Facilitation of decisions about her problem and its resolution during the period of pregnancy
- ▲ Planning for her future, particularly after the birth of her child

Protection of the battered pregnant woman depends, to a large extent, on what the woman is willing to accept. Some helpful measures that the nurse can provide are as follows.

- ▲ The nurse can furnish information about protective resources (shelters, safe houses, refuges) if the woman wishes to leave her home. If she returns to her home, the nurse can provide her with information about resources that she can contact in the likelihood that another attack occurs (crisis lines, women's shelters, hospitals, police).
- ▲ If the woman indicates that she is willing to accept help, the nurse can make referrals to legal, financial, and psychologic counseling resources.
- ▲ The nurse can provide careful prenatal supervision, including physical, supportive, and educative care. Assessment of fetal well-being, as well as maternal response to the assault and related stress, is important. If there is evidence of abdominal injury, it is particularly important to note changes in fetal vital signs and daily fetal movement patterns. When the woman decides to remain in her home, her mate can be invited to participate in the prenatal care. This gives the nurse the opportunity to help them with education and anticipatory guidance and to encourage them to seek family or individual counseling. The nurse must be careful not to react to the man in a punitive or angry manner, but rather to accept him as a part of a unit in need of help. The nurse can help the couple to prepare for the stresses associated with childbirth and with early parenthood. This is of particular importance if the couple is expecting its first child. If there are other children at home, the nurse can help the parents learn strategies for managing both the new infant and the older children and to identify resources upon which they can rely for support and assistance. The woman who leaves her

mate will need guidance and information about resources to help her manage as a single parent. She may also want information about her legal rights. Financial assistance is usually needed, and she should be made aware of resources such as Medicaid and women's, infants', and children's nutrition programs (WIC).

Another important nursing responsibility is to help the battered pregnant woman promote self-esteem and feelings of self-worth. The nurse can do this by:

- Accepting the woman as she is—where she is in her life at the moment. If she is in crisis, her coping capabilities will be diminished. She will only be able to attend to the problem at hand. The nurse can help her set short-term goals that can be reached, thereby promoting success rather than failure. Little successes are very important since they say "I can succeed, and I am worthy of success."
- Correcting misconceptions such as those that place the blame for the incident on the woman rather than on her mate. The nurse can provide the woman with facts that she can attend to rather than overwhelm her with too much information.
- Allowing her to express feelings of anger about her problem and her mate while helping her to maintain a realistic perspective—all men are not abusers.

It is difficult for the battered pregnant woman to make decisions about herself and her unborn child, but she must make such decisions often fairly quickly. The principal immediate decision concerns whether to leave her home and seek shelter elsewhere or to take her chances with her mate. Many women will remain in the situation for a number of reasons: responsibility for other family members; lack of financial resources; criticism by relatives and friends; the children need a father; no where to go; no way of supporting herself; optimism that her mate will change. Leaving is far from easy. The woman who does leave often leaves immediately after the abusive incident. She will need help with shelter, food, clothing (since many incidents of wife abuse take place during the night, she may have fled in her nightgown or robe), and money. The resources mentioned earlier may help her through this period. She will also need to make decisions about whether or not to take legal action such as pressing criminal assault charges, to institute divorce proceedings, or to request legal protective measures. (The legal rules governing these options differ from state to state, and the nurse will need to be knowledgeable about those existing in the state of practice.) The nurse can help the woman make decisions by:

- Informing her of the options open to her. Feelings of futility are common with the battered woman, who may believe that there is little or no hope for her.
- Accepting whatever decision she makes as being the best she can do under the circumstances whether or not the nurse agrees with that decision. Nurse disapproval will increase feelings of conflict and frustration. The woman does not need the additional stress associated with this.

Plans for the future will need to be made as soon as the woman is able to attend to them. She should not be rushed into long-range planning while she is still in crisis. When the woman is ready, the nurse can help her with the following.

- *Anticipatory guidance* in the areas of most need such as postpartal recovery, child care, and future employment.
- Education, particularly in regard to resources that she may rely upon to help her after the birth of her child.
- Reassurance, which is perhaps one of the most needed nursing strategies as the woman looks ahead to her future. She is used to expecting failure, and apprehension about whether or not she can succeed as a single parent is quite common. If she remains with her mate, then fear of future abusive incidents will be present. Helping both partners to use counseling resources after the birth of the child is appropriate.

The battered pregnant woman needs consistent, high-quality physical, emotional, and social health care. The nurse may be an effective resource not only in the role of care giver during the pregnancy, childbirth, and recovery periods, but also in the roles of teacher, counselor, friend, intermediary between the woman and other health professionals, and coordinator of all necessary health care services.

PSYCHOGENIC DISORDERS

In 1980 the American Psychiatric Association recommended that the psychiatric community adopt a new classification for mental conditions and disorders—*Diagnostic and Statistical Manual of Mental Disorders* (DSM-III) (APA, 1980). The DSM-III reordered existing conditions into a classification that is believed to be more clinically accurate and relevant. Because much of the literature still contains the older, more traditional classification, both old and new terms are used here to help you comprehend what is being discussed.

Many conditions previously labeled *neuroses* are now categorized as *anxiety disorders* because of their common symptoms such as exaggerated motor tension, autonomic hyperactivity, apprehension, and hyperattentiveness. Some previous psychoses are now included under *schizophrenic disorders, psychotic disorders not elsewhere classified,* and *paranoid disorders.* Manic–depressive states are now known as *affective disorders.*

Medical and nursing management of anxiety, schizophrenic, and affective disorders are included in most psychiatric nursing texts and are not repeated here except for basic information needed by the maternity nurse.

Psychogenic disorders associated with pregnancy and childbirth constitute a small percentage of disorders that place the pregnant woman, her unborn, and her family at reproductive risk. However, such problems do exist, and the maternity nurse will be a care provider for many women with these problems. The nurse can be a helpful adjunct to the health team through participation in early identification of symptoms that indicate emotional disorders; the nurse is also a primary supportive person for the women, infant, and family during such periods of stress.

Psychogenic disorders that appear as episodes aggravated by the pregnancy exist, in most cases, before conception. Even though they often present severe clinical symptoms during or especially after childbirth, they are pre-existing conditions to pregnancy. Three categories of psychogenic disorders are briefly discussed here: anxiety states (neuroses) particularly depression, schizophrenia, and manic–depressive reactions (one of several affective disorders).

In the past, the term neuroses has been used as a general classification for nonpsychotic mental disorders. Its classification change to an anxiety state better describes its symptoms including phobias, obsessions, depression, hysteria, and hypochondria, all of which appear to have their bases in acute anxiety. An anxiety state can occur at anytime during pregnancy or the first postpartal year (Kaij & Nillson, 1972). It may occur in various degrees of severity and tends to be more apparent during the first trimester and latter part of the third trimester, as well as during the postpartum period. The etiology of such episodes is not certain. However, the episodes have been associated with deep-seated conflicts about feminine identity and self-image and with stresses associated with pregnancy and the responsibilities of parenthood.

Many "normal" behaviors during pregnancy and recovery closely resemble aspects of anxiety symptoms. The nurse needs to be able to differentiate between symptoms that are usual for the period of pregnancy and symptoms that are indicators of an exaggerated response on the part of the woman. For example, nausea (morning sickness), fatigue, and emotional lability are seen during early pregnancy in a significant number of pregnant women (see Chapter 12). Exaggeration or prolongation of any of these symptoms, such as persistent nausea accompanied by vomiting, despondency, or deep depression, is not usual in normal pregnancy and is often a symptom of various degrees of anxiety. Such symptoms can become progressively more severe and result in emotional debilitation for the woman. During the last month of pregnancy apprehension about labor, birth, and impending parenthood is usual; fear of outcome for self and infant is normal. Preoccupation with death and extreme anxiety unrelieved by information and reassurance is again a symptom of neurotic behavior.

Childbirth thrusts the woman into confrontation

with motherhood when she may be neither physically nor mentally completely prepared for it. Depression is a common response of new mothers during the postpartum period. This *postpartum depression,* commonly known as *after baby blues* or *postpartum blues,* is considered to be a normal occurrence among about 70–80% of newly delivered women. It is associated with events related to the childbirth and early parenthood experiences such as fatigue, rapid physiologic readjustment, and apprehension concerning the immediate care-giving responsibilities of parenthood rather than with prepregnancy psychogenic states. Characteristically, postpartum depression has its onset between the third and tenth day after birth with symptoms of crying without apparent cause mixed with almost giddy euphoria. It is a transitory condition, not prognostic of emotional disorders to come.

The following clinical incidents are illustrations of postpartum blues. A newly delivered mother, just discharged from the hospital, called the nurse on the postpartum unit who had cared for her after delivery. The mother was crying loudly and exclaiming: "I don't know why I'm calling you because I know why I'm crying, but I can't stop crying. I just burst into tears at everything, even if my husband smiles at me." Another new mother commented jokingly amid tears as she cuddled her baby: "He's so beautiful, but I feel just like a star of a Broadway play replaced by the understudy on opening night." This young mother, nevertheless, demonstrated caring, sensitive attention to her baby. Had this self-centered attitude been seen in her behaviors toward her infant, you would need to assess for other symptoms that could be more serious in regard to mother–infant relationships. You can separate usual behavior from unusual neurotic symptomatology if careful attention is given to the woman's response to events in regard to the intensity and duration of the behavior, the subjective rather than objective nature of her behavior, the degree of functional disability, and the number of symptoms. Behavior that appears in any way unlike that expected of healthy, newly delivered women should be reported to appropriate health professionals; in some cases referral needs to be made for psychiatric evaluation.

Anxiety disorders in pregnancy are usually treated according to their presenting symptomatology. Occasionally, drugs will be used for the woman who is severely depressed, but in most instances psychotherapy is the treatment of choice.

Psychoses is the name given to many mental disorders that result in prolonged behavior distortions that range from clouding of consciousness, in varying degrees, to complete withdrawal from reality. *Postpartum psychosis* is the emergence of psychotic behavior during pregnancy or after childbirth. The name comes from the fact that a large number of psychotic episodes occur during the postpartum period. Specifically, postpartum psychosis refers to the onset of a psychosis during the first six months after delivery. Psychosis can, however, occur during pregnancy, particularly during the third trimester.

Symptoms of postpartum psychosis, which may be mild or extreme usually come on suddenly; the nature of the symptoms varies considerably. Symptoms that have been described include the following.

- ▲ Clouding of consciousness ranging from slight disorientation to violent, severe delirium
- ▲ Various degrees of general anxiety, apprehension, and confusion
- ▲ Occasional hallucinations (of all types) and delusions
- ▲ Exaggerated dependency with unrealistic demands made on the nurse and particularly the family
- ▲ Preoccupation with the infant, accompanied by concerns about how the infant will disrupt relationships with husband; violent behaviors directed toward the infant are rare
- ▲ Preoccupation with motherhood and its responsibilities; fear of death or malformation related to pregnancy and birth, which may be present or unreal

More than 50% of symptoms associated with psychosis are affective in nature, hence the reclassification of conditions such as manic–depressive states as affective disorders. Psychotic illness is difficult to diagnose in the absence of a good psychiatric history since etiology is often unclear and complex. The stresses of pregnancy childbirth, and motherhood, superimposed on a personality that is vulnerable to such stress, may combine to play a role in the onset of psychotic episodes. Some factors have been associated with pregnancy or postpartum psychoses, for example, age, parity, marital status, but none of these explain fully the reason for the problem.

Schizophrenia is the major psychotic disorder associated with pregnancy. *Schizophrenia* is a complex psychotic disorder in which thought patterns, feelings, moods, and general behavior are altered in such a way that the person is unable to perceive self realistically or to communicate with and relate to others rationally. Symptoms may be extreme distortions in thought and behavior, in which the person is out of step with the real world, or lesser distortions, in which the person may experience some anxiety, depression, confusion, or social withdrawal. Schizophrenia knows no age restrictions, but it occurs predominantly in young adults. Less than 2% of the total population suffers from this disorder; however, this translates to about 4 million citizens who have schizophrenia (Kramer, 1978). Some of these people are women in their childbearing years.

An acute schizophrenic episode may occur during the reproductive experience, and when it does it is most likely to be in the postpartum period. The symptoms may range from mild feelings of paranoia and inadequacy regarding parenthood and its responsibilities to complete withdrawal from reality. The cause is not known, but it has been associated with personality characteristics (shy, retiring, immature, even infantile personality patterns), as well as disorders of cerebral metabolism.

Schizophrenia is treated with a combination of therapies, including antipsychotic drugs such as chlorpromazine (Thorazine), electric shock therapy (EST), and psychotherapy. The major nursing responsibilities for the woman experiencing such a disorder is paying careful attention to her symptomatology and reporting and referring her to appropriate health professionals for diagnosis and care. Support of and reassurance to the family is crucial since they are faced not only with the woman's illness, but with the care of the infant as well. Specific nursing care for the woman depends upon the symptoms that she is presenting and the therapy used. If she is in an acute state, then she is likely to be removed from the maternity service and placed in the hands of those best prepared to care for her. If her symptoms are mild, then she may remain with the maternity nurse who then must be prepared to be alert to sudden changes indicating worsening condition.

Manic–depressive states also occur during pregnancy, childbirth, and recovery. Manic reactions tend to be seen most often in younger women, while depression is more common overall. These reactions may occur anytime from third trimester of pregnancy on. Their incidence is greatest during the first postpartum month, but they are also seen as early as 3–6 days or as late as 6 months after delivery. In the manic state the woman will exhibit symptoms of hyperactivity such as exaggerated movements, agitation, and general excitement. The woman may show complete or partial unconcern about personal hygiene, disinterest in food and drink, or physical and emotional exhaustion. Problems associated with poor fluid intake, such as dehydration, may occur. The depressive state varies from mild, sporadic crying to extreme symptoms of anxiety, despondency, fatigue, and deep depression. Depression is differentiated from postpartum blues by the intensity, duration, and number of symptoms.

Manic–depressive states are treated according to symptomatology. Use of central nervous system depressants such as phenothiazine drugs (promethazine hydrochloride—Phenergan) that have a sedative effect is common. Lithium carbonate, a psychotherapeutic agent specifically for manic–depressive patients, is also used to control manic episodes. It may also be used prophylactically if diagnosis is definite. EST is still used for some patients, especially those with severe symptoms. Psychotherapy is recommended for these patients as an essential aspect of their care. Depressive states are treated with antipsychotic drugs such as trifluoperazine hydrochloride (Stelazine). These drugs offer a more potent and prolonged activity than drugs such as Thorazine. Maximum effect is usually apparent within 2–3 weeks after onset of therapy. Once more nursing care is related to presenting need and involves careful observation, reporting, and data collection. Reassurance and support of both the patient and family are essential. Education of the family in the care of the infant may also be indicated since the family is likely to experience frustration and apprehension.

Several themes permeate nursing care of women with psychogenic disorders. These include early detection of symptoms through careful observation and history taking and reporting of these symptoms to appropriate personnel. It is crucial to reassure and support the woman, as well as the family. The prognosis for the woman depends on the condition. The development of the children born to these women has not been clearly described in terms of problems that they may face. The genetic characteristics of psychogenic disorders have been mentioned, but it is not definitive.

SUMMARY

Psychosocial disorders do occur in association with pregnancy, and those disorders most likely to be encountered by the maternity nurse were discussed in this chapter. The use of drugs, alcohol, and tobacco and their effects on pregnant women were covered. Abusive behaviors, particularly battering of pregnant women by their mates, is a problem increasingly encountered by the nurse and was dealt with extensively. Finally, attention was given to three conditions of psychogenic origin—anxiety states, particularly postpartum depression, schizophrenia, and manic–depressive affective disorders. The chapter closed with a brief statement of major responsibilities for the nurse in regard to care for women and their families experiencing psychosocial disorders.

REFERENCES AND READINGS

American Psychiatric Association. *Diagnostic and Statistical Manual of Mental Disorders* (3rd ed.). New York: The American Psychiatric Association, 1980.

Black, H. C. *Black's Law Dictionary* (4th ed.). St. Paul, Minn.: West Publishing, 1957.

Butnarescu, G. F., Tillotson, D. M., Villarreal, P. P. *Perinatal Nursing: Volume 2, Reproductive Risk.* New York: John Wiley & Sons, 1980.

Carr, J. N. Psychological Aspects of Pregnancy Childbirth and Parenting in Drug Dependent Women, in Rementeria, J. L. (Ed.), *Drug Abuse in Pregnancy and Neonatal Effects.* St. Louis: C. V. Mosby, 1977, Chap. 7.

Chambers, D., Hunt, L. G. Drug Patterns in Pregnant Women, in Rementeria J. L. (Ed.), *Drug Abuse in Pregnancy and Neonatal Effects.* St. Louis: C. V. Mosby, 1977, Chap. 6.

Chertok, L. The Psychopathology of Vomiting of Pregnancy, in Howells, J. G. (Ed.), *Modern Perspectives in Psycho-Obstetrics.* New York: Brunner/Mazel, 1972, Chap. XIII.

Davidson, S. Smoking and Alcohol Consumption: Advice Given by Health Professionals. *J Obstet Gynecol Neonatal Nurs* 10:256, 1981.

Doering, P. L., Steward, R. B. The Extent and Character of Drug Consumption During Pregnancy. *JAMA* 239(9):843–846, 1978.

Eddy, N. Drug Dependence: Its Significance and Characteristics. *Bull WHO* 32:721, 1965.

Federal Bureau of Investigation. Uniform Crime Reports, 1975.

Ferguson, R. W. *Drug Abuse Control.* Boston: Holbrook Press, 1975.

Fielding, J. E. Smoking and Pregnancy. *New Engl J Med* 298(6):337–339, 1978.

Fleming, J. B. *Stopping Wife Abuse.* New York: Doubleday, 1979.

Gibbs, R. S., Gibbs, C. E. *Ambulatory Obstetrics: A Clinical Guide.* New York: John Wiley & Sons, 1979.

Greenwood, S. G. Warning: Cigarette Smoking is Dangerous to Reproductive Health. *Fam Plann Perspect* 11:196, 1979.

Henahan, J. Mom's Couple of Drinks a Day May Produce an Abnormal Child. *Med News* 1:1, 1977.

Hendrix, M. J., Lagodna, G. E., Bohem, C. A. The Battered Wife. *Am J Nurs* 78(4):650–653, 1978.

Himmelberger, D. U., Brown, B. W., Cohen, E. N. Cigarette Smoking During Pregnancy and the Occurence of Spontaneous Abortion and Congenital Abnormality. *Am J Epidemiol* 108(6):470–479, 1978.

Johnson, S. H. *High-Risk Parenting: Nursing Assessment and Strategies for the Family at Risk.* Philadelphia: J. B. Lippincott, 1979.

Jones, K. L. et al. Patterns of Malformation in Offspring of Chronic Alcoholic Mothers. *Lancet* 1:1267, 1973.

Kaij, L., Nillson, A. Emotional and Psychotic Illness Following Childbirth, in Howells, J. G. (Ed.), *Modern Perspectives in Psycho-Obstetrics.* New York: Brunner/Mazel, 1972, Chap. XX.

Kline, J. et al. Smoking: A Risk Factor for Spontaneous Abortion. *New Eng J Med* 297:793, 1977.

Kramer, M. Population Changes in Schizophrenia, 1970–1975, in Wynne, C. L., Cromwell, R. L., Matthysse, S., et al. (Eds.), *The Nature of Schizophrenia: New Approaches to Research and Treatment.* New York: John Wiley & Sons, 1978.

Lieberknecht, K. Helping the Battered Wife. *Am J Nurs* 78:654, 1978.

Loebl, S., Spratto, G., Heckheimer, E. *The Nurse's Drug Handbook (3rd ed.).* New York: John Wiley & Sons, 1982.

McNeil, J. R. The Possible Teratogenic Effects of Salicylates on the Developing Fetus. *Clin Pediatr* 12:347, 1973.

Morgan, A. J., Morgan, M. D. *Manual of Primary Mental Health Care.* Philadelphia: J. B. Lippincott, 1980.

Nelson, M., Forfar, J. Associations Between Drugs Administered During Pregnancy and Congenital Abnormalities of the Fetus. *Br Med J* 1:523, 1971.

Pizzey, E. *Scream Quietly or the Neighbors Will Hear.* Middlesex, England: Penguin Books, 1974.

President's Commission on Law Enforcement and Administration of Justice. *The Challenge of Crime in a Free Society.* Wash. D.C.: U.S. Government Printing Office, 1968.

Pritchard, J. A., MacDonald, P. C. *William's Obstetrics* (16th ed.). New York: Appleton-Century-Crofts, 1981

Rawat, A. K. Fetal Alcohol Syndrome: Metabolic Abnormalities. *Ohio State Med J* 74(2):109–111, 1978.

Rementeria, J. L., Lotongkhum, L. The Fetus of the Drug-Addicted Woman, in Rementeria, J. L. (Ed.), *Drug Abuse in Pregnancy and Neonatal Effects.* St. Louis: C. V. Mosby, 1977, Chap. 1.

Rementeria, J. L., Marrero, G. Drug Addicted Family (Mother, Father and Infant): Some Sociomedical Factors, in Rementeria, J. L. (Ed.), *Drug Abuse in Pregnancy and Neonatal Effects.* St. Louis: C. V. Mosby, 1977, Chap. 22.

Roy, M. (Ed.) *Battered Women: A Psychosociological Study of Domestic Violence.* New York: Van Nostrand Reinhold, 1977.

Sammons, L. N. Battered and Pregnant. *Am J Matern Child Nurs* 6:246, 1981.

Stortz, L. V. Unprescribed Drug Products and Pregnancy. *J Obstet Gynecol Neonatal Nurs* 6:9, 1977.

Walker, L. *The Battered Woman.* New York: Harper & Row, 1979.

Weisman, I. Drug Abuse and the Law, in Rementeria J. L. (Ed.), *Drug Abuse in Pregnancy and Neonatal Effects.* St. Louis: C. V. Mosby, 1977, Chap. 24.

Wilson, H. S., Kneisl, C. R. *Psychiatric Nursing.* Menlo Park, Calif.: Addison-Wesley, 1979.

UNIT SIX

WOMEN'S HEALTH

INTRODUCTION

The primary focus of this book is on the events immediately surrounding pregnancy; these events, however, actually account for only a small portion of a woman's life. Given the fact that the average woman's reproductive life span is approximately 38 years (menarche to menopause) and the average family size is 2–3 children, this means the woman spends about 2 years in the maternity phase, or 5% of her reproductive life actually pregnant. Therefore, the aspects relating to the well-being of the woman during her nonpregnant years is of major importance. It is through the concepts of health promotion and health maintenance that completeness of women's health care can be provided.

Chapter 26, "Health Maintenance for Women," focuses on the details of the complete gynecologic examination with emphasis on breast and pelvic examinations. The existing contraceptive control methods, which are important in that they allow women to plan their pregnancies in synchronization with their individual life goals and their family lifestyles, are included in the chapter. Induced abortion is dealt with from a technical, rather than psychologic standpoint. The failure of present-day contraceptive methods, the reality of human error, and the right to freedom of choice are important factors that allow induced abortion to be considered a component of health maintenance for women.

Chapter 27, "Reproductive-Related Health Care Problems of Women," deals with the most common reproductive-related health care problems of women. Dysmenorrhea which for many years has left a physical and psychologic mark on millions of women, and sexually transmitted diseases which may cause women minor irritating symptoms to life-threatening and life-long diseases, are discussed. An abnormal Pap smear is a concern and dread for many women. The chapter deals with consequences of an abnormal Pap test and explains how therapy can reduce the anxiety and fear that women tend to suppress regarding this matter. The battle of a couple to conceive and attain parenthood can be a frustrating and emotionally depleting experience. The chapter helps nurses to appreciate how therapy may make the months of waiting and trying more tolerable for an infertile couple or individual.

BEHAVIORAL OUTCOMES

Upon completion of the study of this unit, you should be able to:

- ▲ Describe the components of a complete gynecologic examination
- ▲ Discuss the existing contraceptive methods in relation to mechanism of action, advantages and disadvantages, and effectiveness
- ▲ Describe the nurse's role in the provision of contraceptive methods
- ▲ Name the appropriate abortion techniques for first and second trimester induced abortions
- ▲ Discuss the advantages, disadvantages, and complications of each abortion method
- ▲ Describe the interrelationships between prostaglandin inhibitors and dysmenorrhea
- ▲ Identify the common sexually transmitted diseases
- ▲ Discuss clinical symptoms of sexually transmitted diseases and the appropriate choice for treatment
- ▲ Discuss the relationship between Pap smears, colposcopy, and cryosurgery

- ▲ Describe the basic components of a complete infertility evaluation
- ▲ Describe the nurse's role in providing care to women with common reproductive-related health problems

26

HEALTH MAINTENANCE FOR WOMEN

Linda G. Staurovsky

During the past years, a number of factors have had a bearing on the delivery of health care to women (see Chapter 2). The most significant of these is the women's health movement, which is an outgrowth of the women's liberation movement of the late 1960s. Marieskind (1979) categorized the work of the women's health movement into three main areas: (1) changing consciousness level of women through consciousness-raising groups and self-help courses where women gain knowledge about their bodies and learn they can control their own lives; (2) providing health-related services by establishing alternate clinics where the woman (client) actively participates in the delivery of health care; and (3) attempting to change delivery of care in traditional health institutions. Women, as consumers, are expressing dissatisfaction with the health care system and demanding changes. Changes are evolving, but more need to be made.

Nurses can play an instrumental role with respect to clients' rights by being a client advocate and by effecting changes in the delivery of health care. In order for nurses to help meet the demands that women are making, the nurse must take a more active role in the provision of primary, or interconceptional, care. Varney (1980) states that the term *interconceptional* technically refers to the time between pregnancies, but in practice this period has come to mean the primary health care of women between menarche and menopause.

The majority of women enter the health care system because of health needs related to their reproductive system. It is primarily pregnancy and the need for contraception that cause women to seek assistance from a physician, nurse-midwife, or nurse practitioner regarding their obstetric or gynecologic needs. Oftentimes women use these health providers as their sole source of care.

The recognition of these factors stresses the need for nurses to be thoroughly knowledgeable about health assessment, particularly gynecologic assessment. As in any setting, the assessment combines data obtained from client history, physical examination, and laboratory studies. This data base allows for planning intervention and implementing care. To assist in this endeavor, this chapter will focus on the components of the gynecologic examination, on family planning methods, on abortion techniques, and on the nurse's role in providing these aspects of care to women.

GYNECOLOGIC EXAMINATION

The complete *gynecologic examination* involves an evaluation of the total woman (Hofmeister, 1971). A thorough approach is necessary to truly define the health status of a woman. Being alert to the fact that other than for a yearly gynecologic examination some women do not have any preventive health care, the components of the examination should consist of the woman's health history, physical examination, and diagnostic studies.

Woman's History

Using basic communication and interviewing skills, the nurse or other health care provider can begin the examination by obtaining a complete history. The initial history sets the stage for future care. Therefore, particular attention should be given to thoroughness and details, otherwise relevant data may be missed. Such information may not come to the surface until a gynecologic problem exists or other medical problem that is unrelated to the gynecologic examination or pregnancy is detected.

The major history categories include personal identification information, chief complaint or reason for seeking care, history of present illness, past medical history, family history, personal and social history, and review of systems. (For a detailed outline of health history at a glance, see Berger & Fields, 1980.)

For the woman who has a specific gynecologic complaint, the history-taking should be related to history of present illness. The gynecologic history, in addition to the items outlined, should also include investigation of *dysmenorrhea* (pain during menstrual periods) and use of tampons or sanitary pads; vaginal, uterine, or tubal infections and treatment; and contraception presently and previously used and reasons for discontinuation. The obstetric history should elaborate on each pregnancy by detailing the type of delivery, length of gestation, length of labor, birth weight and condition of infant at birth, and any complications that occurred during the antepartum, intrapartum, or postpartum period. If the woman experienced an abortion, information should be obtained about whether it was spontaneous or induced, the length of gestation, therapeutic measures after a spontaneous abortion or method used for induced abortions, and any complications.

Physical Examination

With the completion of the history taking, preparation of the client for the ensuing physical examination should be made. The components of the physical examination, as well as *laboratory examination* or diagnostic tests to be performed, are reviewed. Before proceeding, the nurse should be assured that the client has been adequately informed, has had ample opportunity to have her questions answered, and has been able to express any fears or anxieties. The actual examination begins with measurement of the woman's height, weight, and blood pressure; a urinalysis and hematocrit are routinely obtained. The general aspects of the physical examination will not be discussed as there are numerous texts that address them in detail. However, inspection and palpation of the neck for cervical adenopathy or thyroid enlargement is essential as a variety of gynecologic problems can be related to abnormal thyroid function. Fundamental to any examination is the inspection, palpation, percussion, and auscultation of the chest and auscultation of the heart.

The breast examination is a mandatory part of every gynecologic examination. It is the responsibility of nurses and physicians to encourage, teach, and evaluate the woman in the performance of breast self-examination.

Breast Examination

Breast examination should begin at puberty and be done at periodic intervals thereafter for the rest of the woman's lifetime. *Puberty* is the time when the mammary glands begin to develop and become ready for their functional role in childbearing. Both *self-examination* of the breast and periodic examination by the nurse or physician should become a part of ongoing health assessment practices (Fig. 26.1). The purposes of breast examination are to assess breast development; to diagnose breast pathophysiology, such as inflammation or abnormal tumor growth, particularly carcinoma; and to evaluate the breast during and after pregnancy to determine its readiness for supplying food for the newborn infant.

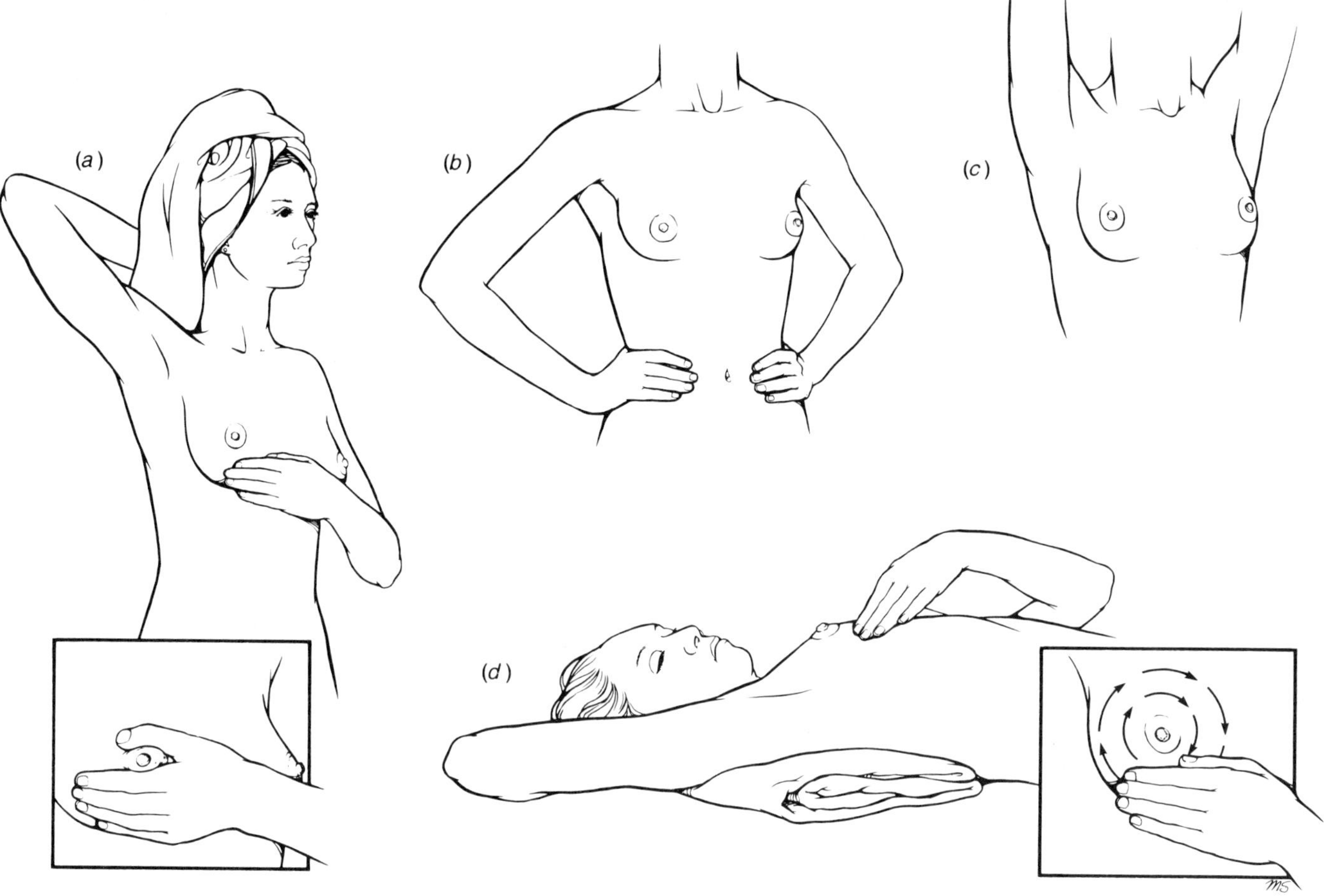

Figure 26.1
Breast self-examination. (*a*) Breast palpated in standing position with arm and shoulder raised. Insert shows compression of areola to express any discharge from nipple. (*b*) Symmetry of breast observed with hands on hips. (*c*) Symmetry is observed with arms raised above head noting any dimpling or retraction. (*d*) Breast is examined in a supine position with shoulder elevated by small pillow or folded towel and arm abducted. Insert depicts scheme of palpation to ensure all aspects of breast are examined.

The breasts are examined using the techniques of inspection and palpation with the client assuming five different positions during the examination (see Fig. 26.2):

- ▲ Sitting with arms at the sides
- ▲ Sitting with arms lifted overhead
- ▲ Sitting and bending forward with the breasts hanging loosely
- ▲ Sitting with hands placed on and pushing into the hips while contracting the pectoral muscles
- ▲ Lying flat on the back with arms abducted. The breasts are observed with the woman assuming all of these positions before palpation (Fig. 26.2). The following observations should be made:

- ▾ ***Symmetry.*** The location and appearance of the two breasts on the anterior chest wall should correspond closely in regard to level, size, shape, and nipple placement.
- ▾ ***Tone.*** The breasts of a young woman who has not borne a child are likely to appear as firm, globular mounds. With repeated pregnancies, as well as with aging or obesity, the breasts may become pendulous with rupture of the connective tissue that attaches the breasts to the muscle beneath them

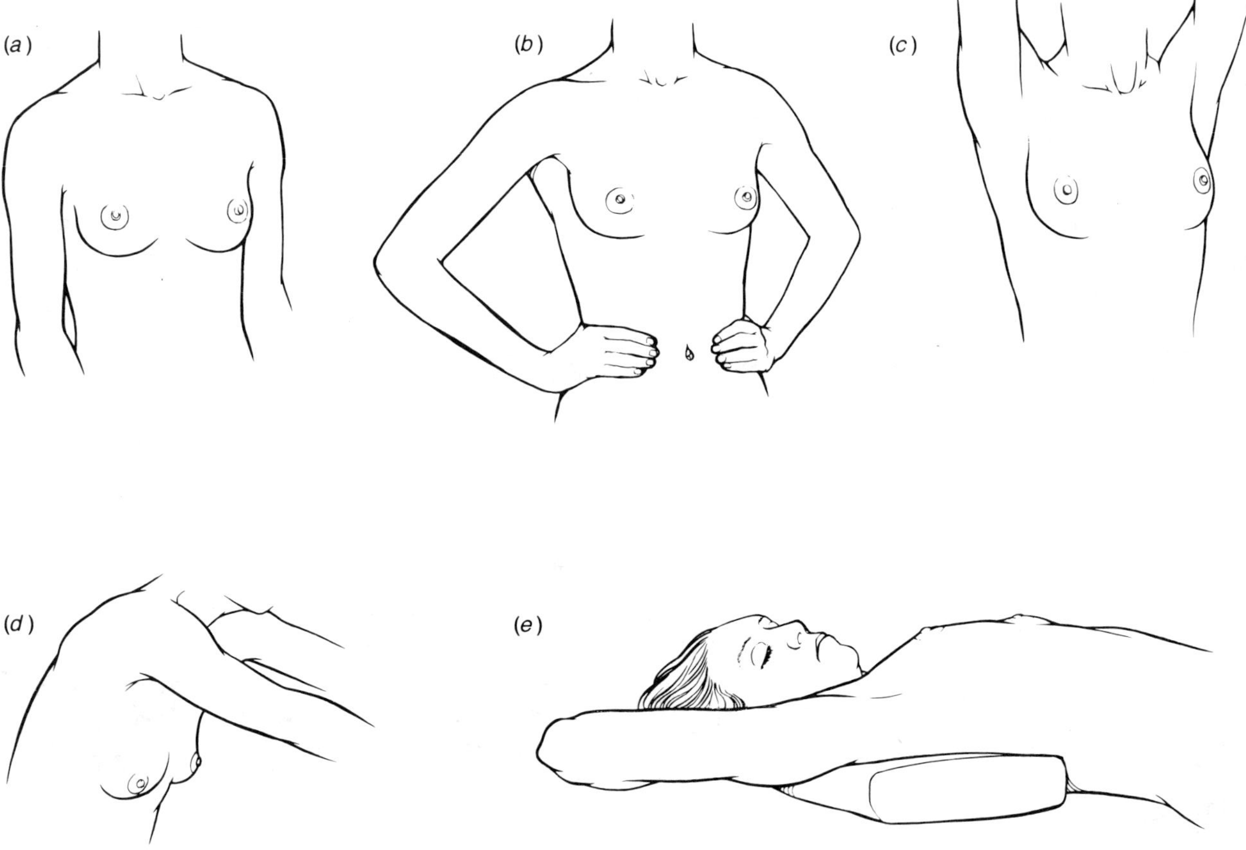

Figure 26.2
Positions assumed by woman for examiner evaluation. (*a*) Sitting with arms at the sides; (*b*) sitting with hands placed on and pushing into the hips; (*c*) sitting with arms lifted overhead; (*d*) sitting and bending forward with breasts hanging loosely; (*e*) lying flat on the back with arm abducted.

(pectoralis muscle). Edema, as well as skin tone, should be noted.

- ***Skin.*** Skin texture and color should be noted. Healthy breast skin, except for the areola and nipple, will be smooth. Condition of the skin and any unusual markings, such as hyperpigmentation, or growths, such as moles, should be noted. Breasts that have been stretched as a result of pregnancy or obesity may show tiny ruptures in the elastic fibers. These may appear as pinkish marks or may lighten with time to a silvery white. They are called *striae.* Sometimes vascular patterns will be visible below the skin surface. This is particularly true during pregnancy when there is increased vascularity of the breasts. Redness or other signs of inflammation are significant.

- ***Lesions.*** Any breast lesion or growth is abnormal and should be observed and reported. Discharge from the nipple occurs during pregnancy and sometimes in women who have been pregnant. This discharge, called *colostrum,* is a semitransparent, yellowish discharge with no odor. It is easy to differentiate from a purulent or other discharge associated with pathology.

- ***Hair.*** The hair that is present on the breasts of most women is fine, of light color, and usually not noticeable. Hair amount and distribution patterns that are abnormal should be noted.

- ***Retraction or Dimpling.*** The puckering or indentation of the skin of the breast is indicative of tissue change below the surface of

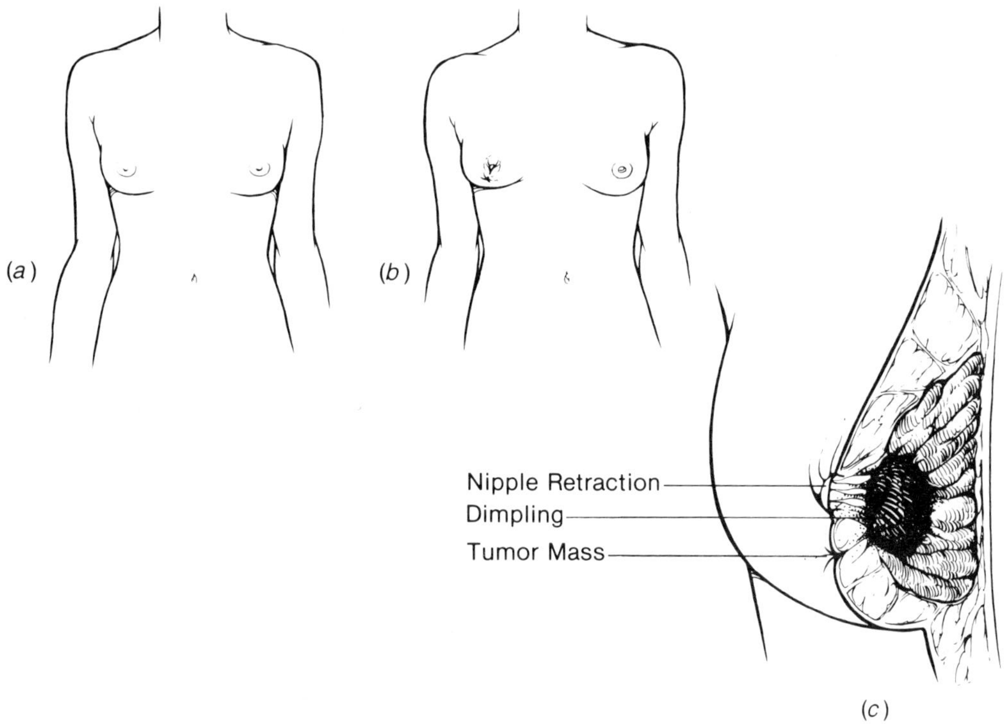

Figure 26.3
Breast observations. (*a*) Symmetry of breasts on anterior chest wall; (*b*) retraction or dimpling noted on right breast; (*c*) external observation of retraction and dimpling as a result of internal tumor mass.

the skin and is frequently the result of an invasive process. It should be noted and reported immediately.

Palpation of the breasts and axillae is done to determine presence, degree, and location of tenderness and to locate any breast masses. The time at which palpation is performed is significant. During the luteal phase of the menstrual cycle and pregnancy, levels of progesterone are high. You will recall that progesterone acts to promote the development of the lobular system of the breasts, causing the breasts to feel nodular on palpation where ordinarily breast tissue would be consistent and smooth. Should any growth be felt on palpation, the following characteristics should be noted and reported:

- ▲ ***Location.*** Report location according to breast quadrant.
- ▲ ***Size.*** Size is a subjective assessment. Where size cannot be precisely estimated, an analogy to something familiar, such as the diameter of a dime, can be made. Whenever possible, precise estimations should be made and recorded in centimeters.
- ▲ ***Shape.*** Shape is another subjective assessment. All breast masses do not have a definitive shape. If shape is discernible, it should be reported as round, ovoid, irregular, or flat. Again, an analogy may be helpful, but caution is advised in that analogies may be misleading.
- ▲ ***Discreteness.*** The presence of both vague and definitive margins should be assessed and associated with the shape of the mass. Margins are usually described either as sharp and clearly defined or as irregular.
- ▲ ***Consistency of the Mass.*** There are only two categories of consistency (degree of firmness): soft/hard and solid/cystic.
- ▲ ***Mobility.*** Is the mass fixed or movable?
- ▲ ***Appearance of the Skin Over the Mass.*** Presence of dimpling and puckers of the skin, as mentioned earlier, are quite important. Any erythema should also be noted.

▲ ***Pain or Tenderness.*** The woman's perception of discomfort should be obtained before palpation. She is asked about pain or tenderness in terms of sharp/dull; minimal/moderate/severe; sustained/transient. The woman should also be questioned about the time and frequency of occurrence and whether or not it is in association with any particular activity or event.

Assessment of the breasts during pregnancy and lactation should take into account the changes that occur during these periods, as well as increase awareness of any problems and conditions that are associated with these changes (see Chapters 12 and 19).

The inspection, auscultation, percussion, and palpation of the abdomen should be performed before the pelvic examination. For further details about abdominal examination, refer to the discussions of assessment during pregnancy in Chapters 9 and 12.

Pelvic Examination

The pelvic examination includes four basic parts: (1) inspection and palpation of the external genitalia, (2) speculum examination, which provides for visualization of the vaginal walls and cervix, (3) bimanual examination, which is a combination of vaginal and abdominal palpation, and (4) a rectovaginal abdominal examination. The examiner will require gloves, adequate lighting, and a stool in order to perform the examination.

EXTERNAL GENITALIA

With the woman in lithotomy position and appropriately draped, the pelvic examination starts with the inspection of the *external genitalia,* which include the mons verneris, labia majora and minora, clitoris, vaginal introitus, and perineal region. General observations begin with the presence or absence of pubic hair and the pattern of distribution. On the average, hair begins to appear about 1 year before menarche and takes approximately 2.7 years to reach the adult pattern of hair distribution (Emans & Goldstein, 1977). The normal pattern of distribution is an inverted triangle with the hair covering the mons veneris and spreading to the medial surface of the thighs (see Chapter 8).

Close inspection of the vulva should be performed to ascertain normalcy of development. The clitoral size should not exceed 2 cm in length and 1 cm in width. The labia majora and minora are basically symmetrical. Asymmetry would be considered an abnormal finding and would warrant further investigation. The asymmetrical appearance may be indicative of a variety of problems that may include tumors, cysts, infections, edema, or trauma.

The vulva is observed for any signs of pathology, including lesions, erythema, inflammation, edema, lacerations, cysts, masses, hyperpigmentation, white epithelium, ulcerations, varicosities, pubic lice, and discharge. When a discharge is present, the color, amount, odor, and consistency should be noted. Previous perineal surgery may be evidenced by the presence of a scar and should be noted.

With inspection completed, the examiner proceeds to palpation of Skene's and Bartholin's glands. Neither set of glands is normally visible or palpable. Skene's glands lie posterior and lateral to the urinary meatus at approximately the 5 and 7 o'clock positions. The gloved index and middle fingers are inserted palmar side up beneath the meatus to palpate for enlargement of Skene's glands. Positive palpation is usually indicative of infection. A technique called *stripping the urethra* can be performed at this time to detect any urethral discharge (Fig. 26.4). This can be accomplished by positioning the fingers as previously mentioned for palpation of Skene's glands, providing upward pressure to compress the urethra as the fingers are withdrawn. Erythema of the meatus or discharge from the urethra is abnormal and warrants further investigation.

Bartholin's glands are located posterolaterally behind the labia majora with the duct openings just outside the lateral margin of the vaginal introitus at approximately the 4 and 8 o'clock positions. The index finger is inserted inside the vagina with the thumb on the outside of the labia majora; the area is then palpated between the fingers, down the side, across the perineum, and on the opposite side (Fig. 26.5). Palpation of the glandular mass and presence of discharge or pain is considered abnormal. Both Bartholin's and Skene's glands can often become infected by the gonococcal organism, although other organisms may be the causative factor as well (Huff & Pauerstein, 1979) (Fig. 26.6). Further details regarding treatment of sexually transmitted diseases and other infections are in Chapter 27.

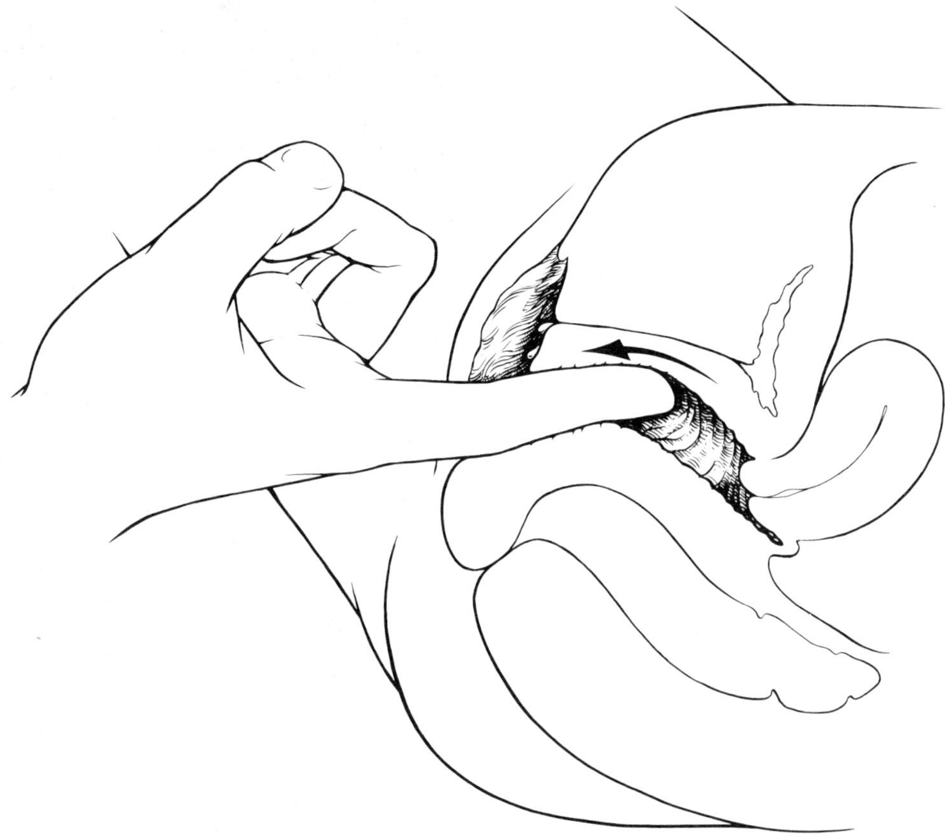

Figure 26.4
Technique of stripping or milking the urethra.

The final inspection of the external genitalia is to detect any support deficiency or poor perineal muscle tone. Place the index and middle finger palmar surface down and firmly exert pressure against the perineal body as the woman bears down or coughs. The anterior vaginal wall is observed for evidence of a cystocele, a hernia of the bladder. This will be noted if the anterior vaginal wall bulges downward and outward.

The posterior vaginal wall is evaluated with the fingers separated and the woman bearing down. A bulging upward and outward of the posterior vaginal wall is because of a rectocele, a herniation of a part of the rectum into the vagina.

SPECULUM EXAMINATION

The *speculum* is either a metal or plastic instrument that is used to visualize the vaginal walls and the cervix (Fig. 26.7). It is comprised of two blades; the anterior blade has a thick piece that allows the blades to be separated, and the posterior blade has a handle for easier manipulation. While the basic design of all specula are the same, there are variations in size and shape of the blades.

The Graves's speculum is the most commonly used and is available in three sizes; small (infant), medium (regular), or large. The speculum size used is dependent on the size of the introitus and the size and length of the vaginal canal of each woman. The regular Graves's speculum is the most frequently used speculum for women who are sexually active or who are parous. The large size may be used in a woman who is a grand multipara, has poor vaginal wall tone, or is obese. While the infant Graves's speculum should always be available, it is infrequently used, except in some prepubutal girls, because the length of the blades is inadequate.

For the virginal woman or the sexually active teenager, Huffman's or Pedersen's speculum is the most appropriate. The blades of these specula are narrower, straighter, and flatter than the Graves. The narrow blade speculum allows for good visu-

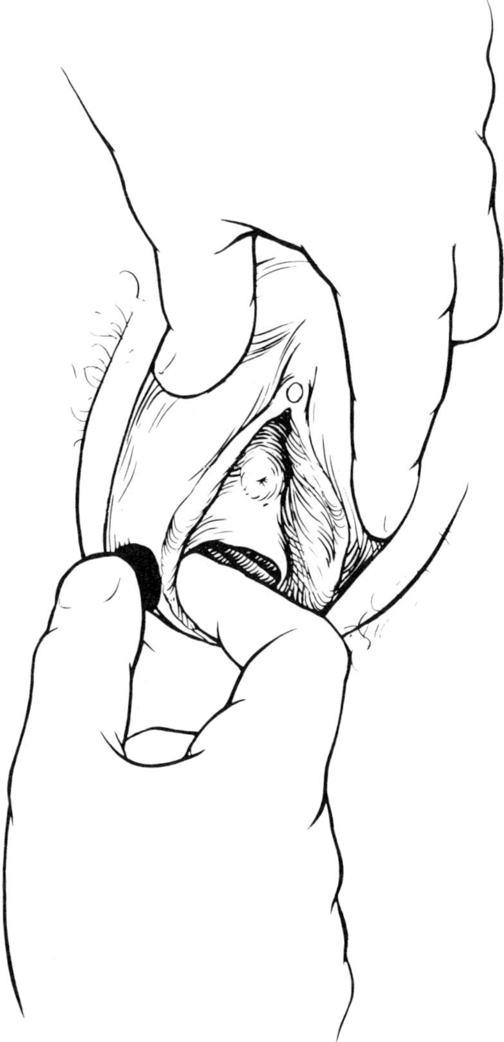

Figure 26.5
Palpation of Bartholin's gland.

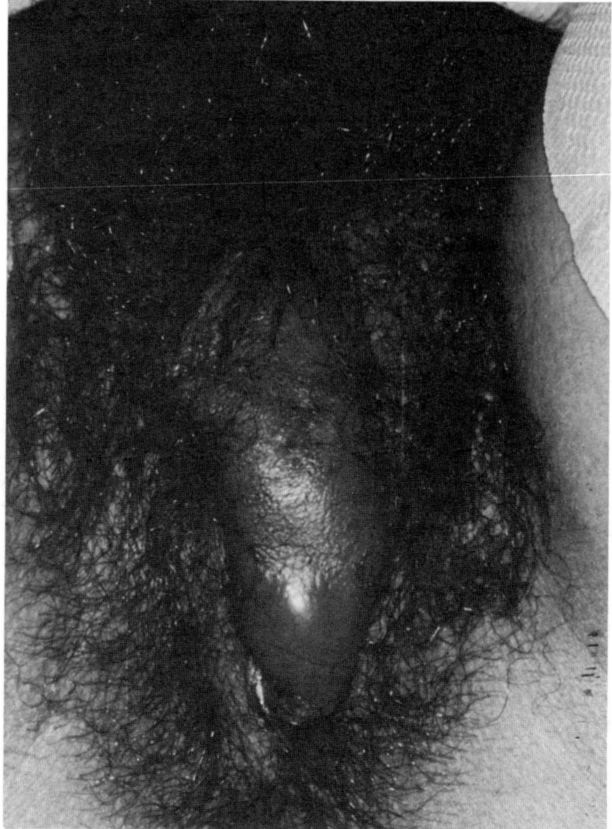

Figure 26.6
Infected Bartholin's gland.

alization of the cervix without difficulty in cases where the hymen is intact or the vaginal opening is small. Based on the gynecologic and obstetric history, as well as on observation, the examiner should be able to select the appropriate speculum that will minimize the discomfort for each woman.

If any diagnostic studies are to be performed, the speculum should be lubricated with warm water before insertion. The examiner firmly depresses the perineal body with two fingers as the speculum is inserted in a downward and backward direction the full length of the vagina (Fig. 26.8). Once inserted, the blades of the speculum are opened by depressing the thumbpiece and exposing the cervix and vaginal walls.

In visualizing the cervix, the color, position, size, and shape are determined. A careful inspection is made for growths, lesions, discharge, eversion, and signs of inflammation or infection. The significance of color can be reviewed in the section in Chapter 12 relating to signs of pregnancy (*Chadwick's sign*). The position of the cervix can be helpful in determining the position of the uterus. Usually, the cervix is located posterior, in the distal end of the vagina since the normal position of the uterus is anteflexed or anteverted superior to the bladder (Fig. 26.9). A cervix located anteriorly is correlated with a retroverted uterus. A cervix may be positioned right or left because of reproductive tract congenital anomalies, pelvic masses, or adhesions. The normal variations in the size and shape of the cervix will depend on the age of the woman and her parity. The external os (the visible opening of the cervix) in the nulliparous woman appears

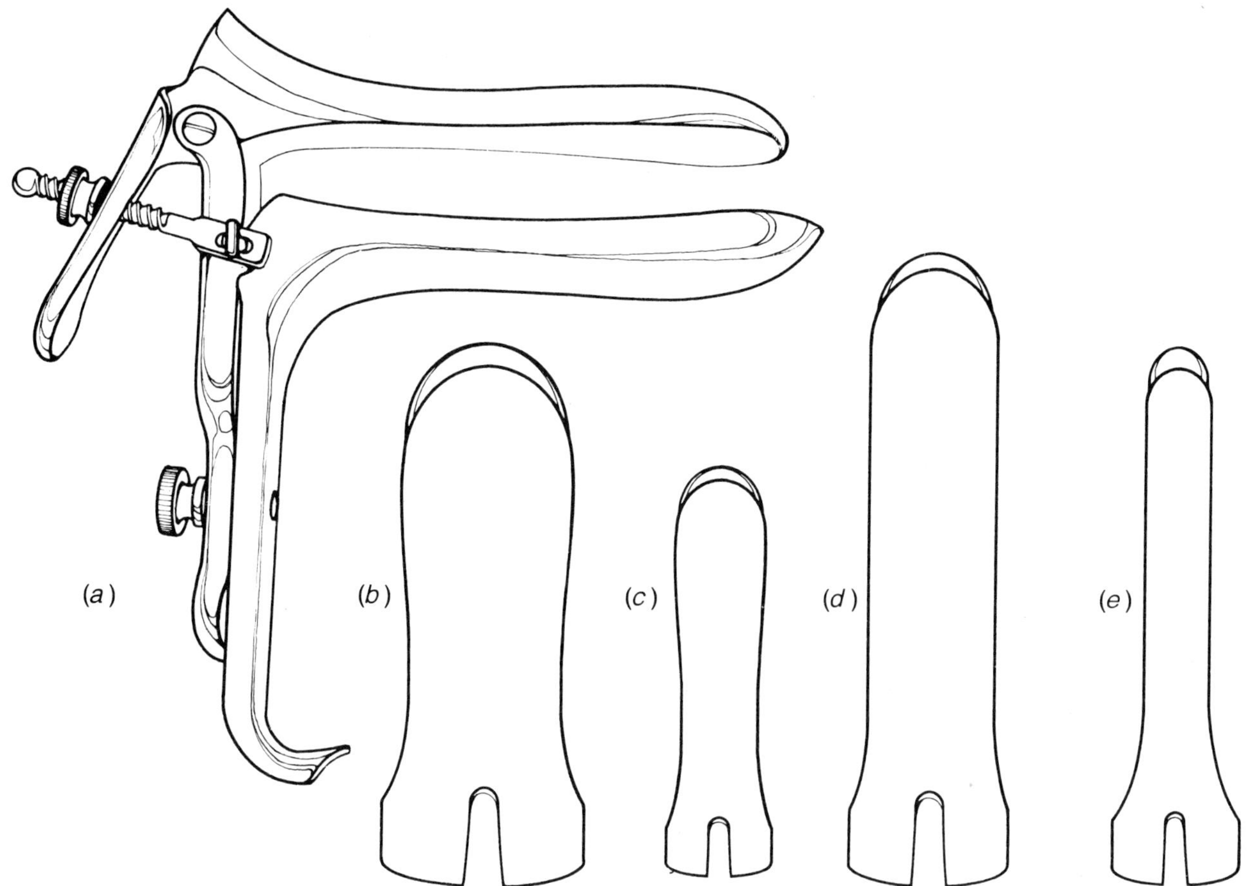

Figure 26.7
Speculum shape and size. *(a)* lateral view of regular Graves speculum; *(b)* regular Graves speculum blades; *(c)* infant Graves speculum; *(d)* Huffman's speculum blades; *(e)* Pedersen's speculum blades.

small, regular, and either circular or oval (Fig. 26.10). However, once the cervix has undergone marked dilatation, the external os converts into a transverse opening that is irregular in shape with dimpling or grooves noted around the edges, particularly at the 3 and 9 o'clock positions. The presence of any growths or lesions requires further diagnostic evaluation to determine the precise cause. With respect to discharge, the determination of cervical versus vaginal origin requires close observation. Inflammation or infection of the cervix may be accompanied by some type of discharge or other identifiable characteristic. Infections of the reproductive tract will be discussed in greater depth in Chapter 27. Cervical eversion occurs when the endocervical tissue composed of columnar epithelium extends onto the ectocervix replacing the squamous epithelium. It is important to remember that the point at which the columnar epithelium and the squamous epithelium interface is known as the *squamocolumnar junction* and that it is usually at the external os. However, when an eversion is present, the squamocolumnar junction may appear at various distances from the external os. This is important to recognize when obtaining the Papanicolaou smears.

Observations of the vagina and vaginal walls include inspection for color, discharge or bleeding, inflammation or infection, growths or lesions, and abnormal tissue formation. The normal color of the vaginal walls in the nonpregnant state is pink, and in pregnancy or other situations when there is increased vascularity to the area, the color is bluish. Noting any signs of inflammation or infection will

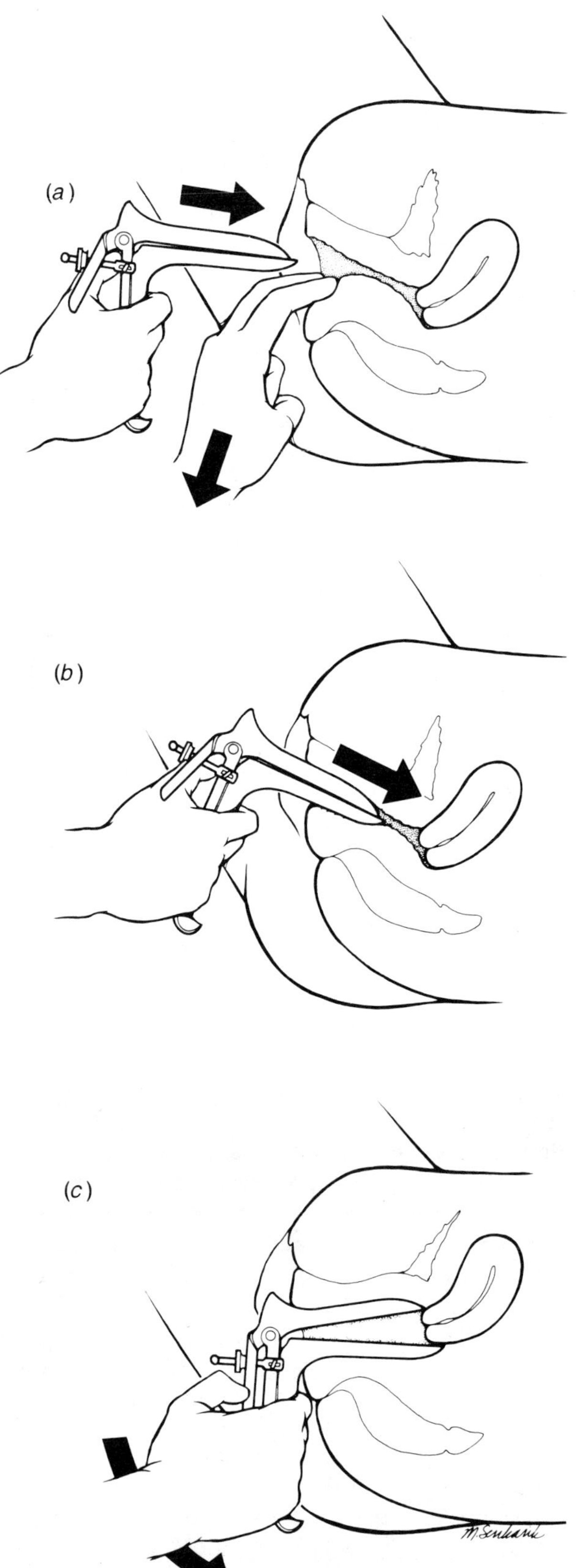

warrant further diagnostic tests to validate the causative organism and the institution of appropriate therapy. The presence of growths, lesions, or abnormal tissue formation may necessitate a tissue biopsy. As the speculum is removed, the blades are held slightly open so that the anterior and posterior vaginal walls can be observed falling together in front of the speculum blades.

BIMANUAL EXAMINATION

The purpose of the *bimanual examination* is to determine, by palpation, the size, shape, and position of the *internal genitalia,* or reproductive organs, and to identify any abnormalities or growths that are present. The bimanual examination is a systematic palpation of the vagina, cervix, uterus, and *adnexal* areas (fallopian tubes and ovaries).

The bimanual examination is performed by inserting the lubricated index finger, or index and middle fingers, of either the examiner's right or left hand into the vagina (Fig. 26.11). The other hand is placed on the abdomen above the symphysis pubis and creates counterpressure during the internal examination. As the fingers are inserted into the vagina, the walls are palpated for any cysts, nodules, masses, or growths. These are abnormal findings that may not have been detected by visualization during the speculum examination. With the fingers inserted the length of the vagina, the examiner locates the cervix and feels all aspects of the cervix, including the areas of the vaginal fornices. The position of the cervix is reconfirmed as to anterior, posterior, midplane, midline, deviated right or left. The size and shape are confirmed by palpation. The consistency is evaluated as to firm (nonpregnant) or soft (pregnant). The *ectocervix* is normally smooth; with an eversion, nabothian cyst (retention cyst) or other abnormal growths or lesions, the surface may feel rough and irregular. In pregnancy, it is important to evaluate the dilatation of the cervix; this is discussed in Chapters 12 and 16. The last critical maneuver in the examination

Figure 26.8
Technique for speculum insertion. (*a*) Perineal body is depressed as speculum blades are inserted; (*b*) speculum is inserted in a downward, backward direction the full length of the vagina; (*c*) Speculum blades are opened by depressing thumbpiece. Cervix is brought into clear view by moving handle toward the perineum.

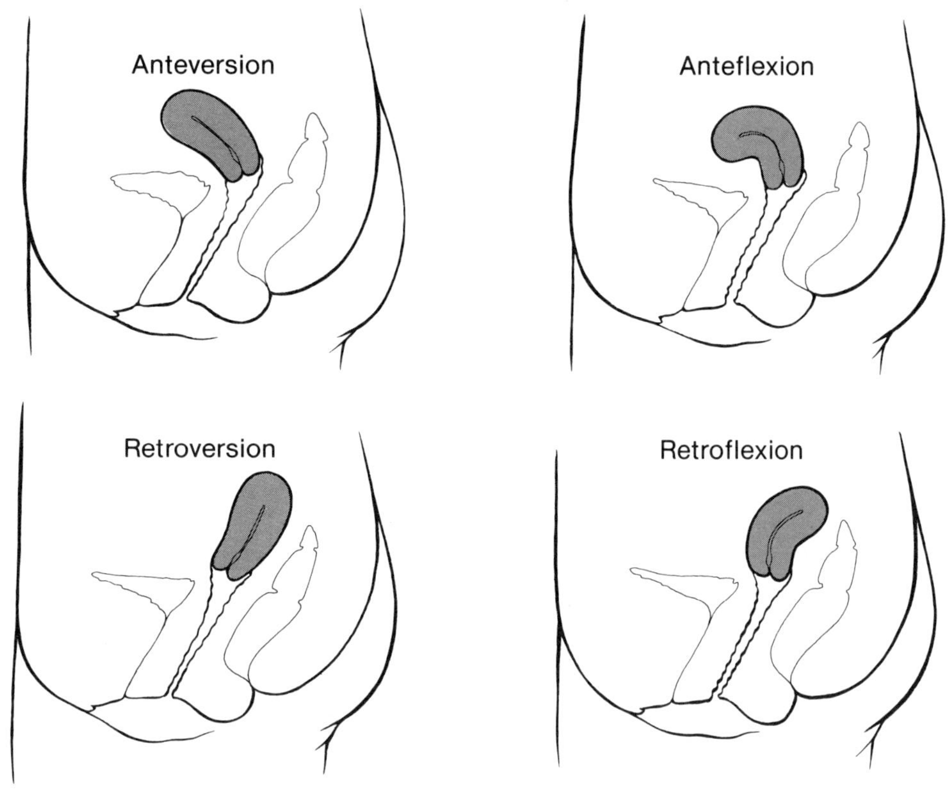

Figure 26.9
Uterine positions.

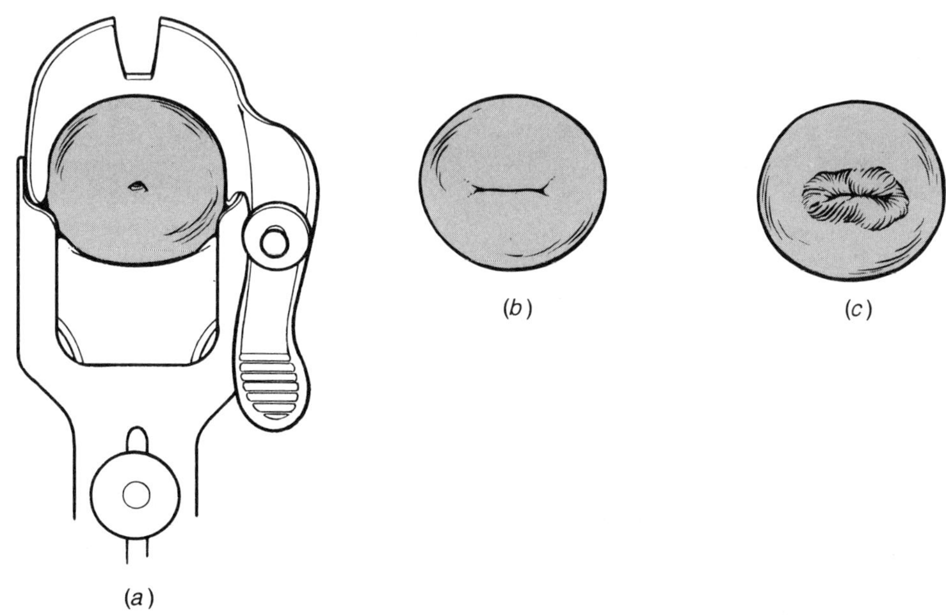

Figure 26.10
Cervical characteristics. *(a)* Nulliparous cervix—circular external os; *(b)* multiparous cervix—longitudinal slit or external os; *(c)* cervical eversion.

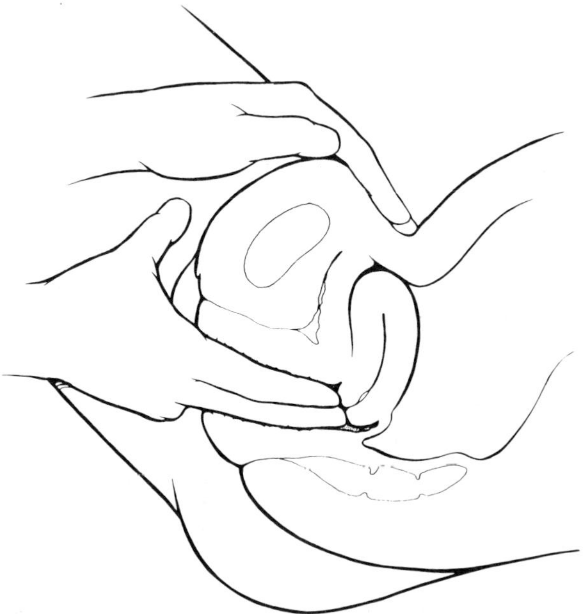

Figure 26.11
Bimanual vaginal examination with one hand in vagina and other hand compressing the abdomen.

of the cervix is to move the cervix from side to side and front to back. The woman is observed for signs of pain or tenderness during this manipulation; such signs would be indicative in cases of a pelvic inflammatory disease or ruptured ectopic pregnancy.

The next part of the examination is palpation of the uterus by entrapping it between the abdominal and vaginal hands. First, the position of the uterus is determined (see Fig. 26.9). The usual position is one of anteflexion, although variations of anteversion, retroflexion, or retroversion can occur and be asymptomatic. Variations in the position of the uterus may also be associated with a number of symptoms including backache, dysmenorrhea, dyspareunia (pain on intercourse), and infertility. Along with the uterine position, the location is determined and is usually midline. A lateral deviation may be indicative of pelvic adhesions or pelvic masses.

The uterus should be mobile in an anterior–posterior direction. Fixation of the uterus can occur if adhesions form after surgery or pelvic infection. The woman should not experience any tenderness or pain with movement of the uterus. If this symptom is present, pelvic inflammatory disease is suspected.

The size and shape of the uterus can, for the most part, be easily palpated during the bimanual examination. The specific dimensions of the uterus are given in Chapter 4 for nonpregnant states and in Chapter 12 for the stages of pregnancy. The examiner should have an idea of the anticipated uterine dimensions from the woman's history. In the assumed nonpregnant woman, a uterine size larger than expected can be attributed to one of two primary causes: pregnancy (if of childbearing age) or benign or malignant tumors. In the pregnant woman, finding a fundal height greater than expected for the gestational age would lead the examiner to considerations such as hydatidiform mole, multiple gestation, incorrect dates, or polyhydramnios.

The shape of the uterus is usually described as an inverted pear. Remember, a change in the shape of the uterus will vary its size or dimensions but an increase in size may not alter its shape. Variations in uterine shape can be primarily attributed to uterine tumors, pregnancy, or congenital abnormalities.

Congenital abnormalities, depending on the degree of failure of the müllerian ducts to fuse, may cause variations in the shape of the uterus that may be mild to severe. Some of the variations as a result of congenital malformations are illustrated in Figure 27.16. The milder forms of malformation may not be detected on bimanual examination. There can be a complete duplication with the formation of a double cervix and a vaginal septum. If the palpation of the uterus indicates a congenital malformation, revisualization, by speculum, of the cervix and vagina should be performed to re-evaluate the normalcy of development in these areas.

The consistency of the uterus is determined during this aspect of the examination. Generally, the nonpregnant uterus is firm while the pregnant uterus is soft in early gestation (*Hegar's sign*). Softening may also be present during the normal postpartum involution and in some pathologic conditions where tumors are developing.

The bimanual examination continues with the palpation of the adnexal area. The examiner places the fingers of the vaginal hand in either the right or left lateral fornix while the abdominal hand is placed in the central area of the corresponding lower abdominal quadrant. The fingers of the two hands are brought together and moved in a downward midline direction allowing the tissue to slip between the approximated fingertips. During this movement, the tissue lying between the two hands is palpated primarily by the fingers in the vagina. After completing the procedure on one side, the same maneuvers are performed on the opposite side.

The adnexal areas are palpated to determine the normalcy of the ovaries and tubes and to detect any abnormal masses, tenderness, or pain in the area. Inability to palpate precisely the specific organs in the adnexal area denotes a normal finding. Even the experienced examiner may frequently find it difficult to locate the organs in the normal state because of position and/or amount of adipose tissue (Varney, 1980). When the normal ovaries are palpated in the adult woman, they are smooth, almond shaped, and approximately 2.5–5.0 cm in length, 1.5–3.0 cm in width, and 0.5–1.5 cm thick (Pritchard & MacDonald, 1981). The normal ovary is tender to touch, and the woman will experience a twinge as it slips through the fingers. Therefore, to avoid undue discomfort to the woman, the ovary should not be trapped between the examining fingers.

The fallopian tubes are not palpable in the normal state. Ectopic pregnancy or tubal infections can cause tubal enlargement that would be palpable. Another finding that should alert the examiner is the palpation of an arterial pulse in the adnexal area, which is indicative of an ectopic pregnancy (Malasano, 1981). The palpation of any adnexal masses is considered abnormal and requires further diagnostic evaluation.

The bimanual examination is completed with the thorough evaluation of the adnexal area; the fingers are then withdrawn from the vagina.

RECTOVAGINAL ABDOMINAL EXAMINATION

The rectovaginal abdominal examination should be a part of every pelvic examination. The purposes of the rectovaginal abdominal examination are to confirm the findings of the bimanual examination regarding the uterus and adnexae, explore the *pouch*, or *cul-de-sac of Douglas*, examine the rectovaginal septum, evaluate the rectal sphincter tone, and palpate for hemorrhoids or other abnormal masses of the rectum.

Before beginning the rectovaginal abdominal examination, apply additional lubrication to the index and middle fingers. The index finger is reinserted into the vagina, while the middle finger is inserted into the rectum (Fig. 26.12). The opposite hand is placed on the abdomen above the symphysis pubis to apply counterpressure, as in the bimanual examination.

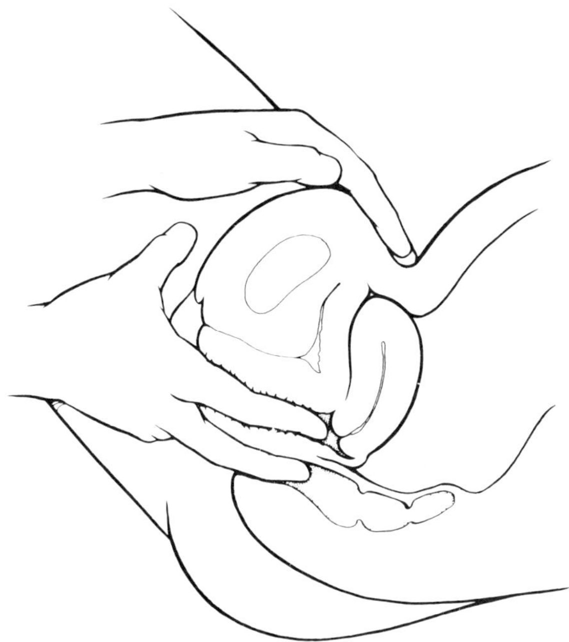

Figure 26.12
Rectovaginal, abdominal examination.

During this aspect of the examination the posterior wall of the uterus can be better evaluated. Nodularities may be present in cases of endometriosis (see Chapter 27). If the uterus is retroverted, the body and fundus can now be palpated. The adnexae are re-evaluated and further delineation may be possible by palpation through the pouch of Douglas. As with other components of the pelvic examination, any findings of masses or any eliciting of pain is significant and warrants further investigation. Having completed the examination bilaterally, the fingers are gently removed, and the perineum is cleaned of excess lubricating jelly.

Diagnostic Tests

Obtaining the various smears or cultures may not be the direct responsibility of the nurse; however, the nurse should know how the procedures are performed in order to promote client understanding. *Papanicolaou (Pap) smear* and a *gonococcal (GC) culture* are done first. Depending on the client's complaints and/or pelvic examination findings, *wet preparations (wet preps)* for vaginal infections, biopsies, or other cultures may be obtained. All of the samples for these tests will be obtained during the speculum examination.

PAPANICOLAOU SMEARS

The Papanicolaou smears provide cervical cellular samples that can be evaluated for abnormalities by the cytopathologist. Despite all the technologic advances, the Pap test is still the best screening device that is available for detecting cervical abnormalities. There are variations as to the recommended sites and techniques of obtaining samples, the method of submitting samples on a slide or slides, and the method of fixation. The following is one suggested procedure for Pap smear sampling (Fig. 26.13).

Two sites are recommended for sampling: the *endocervix* and the cervix (ectocervix), with each sample being placed on a separate slide. The endocervical smear is obtained by inserting a sterile cotton-tip applicator moistened with normal saline in the cervical canal. The applicator is rotated at least one complete turn and withdrawn. Upon removal, the material from the applicator is rolled across the slide and labeled "endocervical." It is important to be careful to deposit sampled material from all areas of the applicator. Immediately, the slide is sprayed thoroughly with a fixative or is placed in a jar containing fixative solution. The important fact to remember regarding the fixation of the sample is if the cellular material starts to dry or dries before being fixed, the cells will become distorted in appearance and the cytopathologist will have difficulty interpreting the normalcy or abnormalcy of the cells.

The cervical smear is obtained using a wooden spatula. The sample of cellular material must be obtained from the squamocolumnar junction. Depending on the location of the squamocolumnar junction, either the notched or rounded end of the

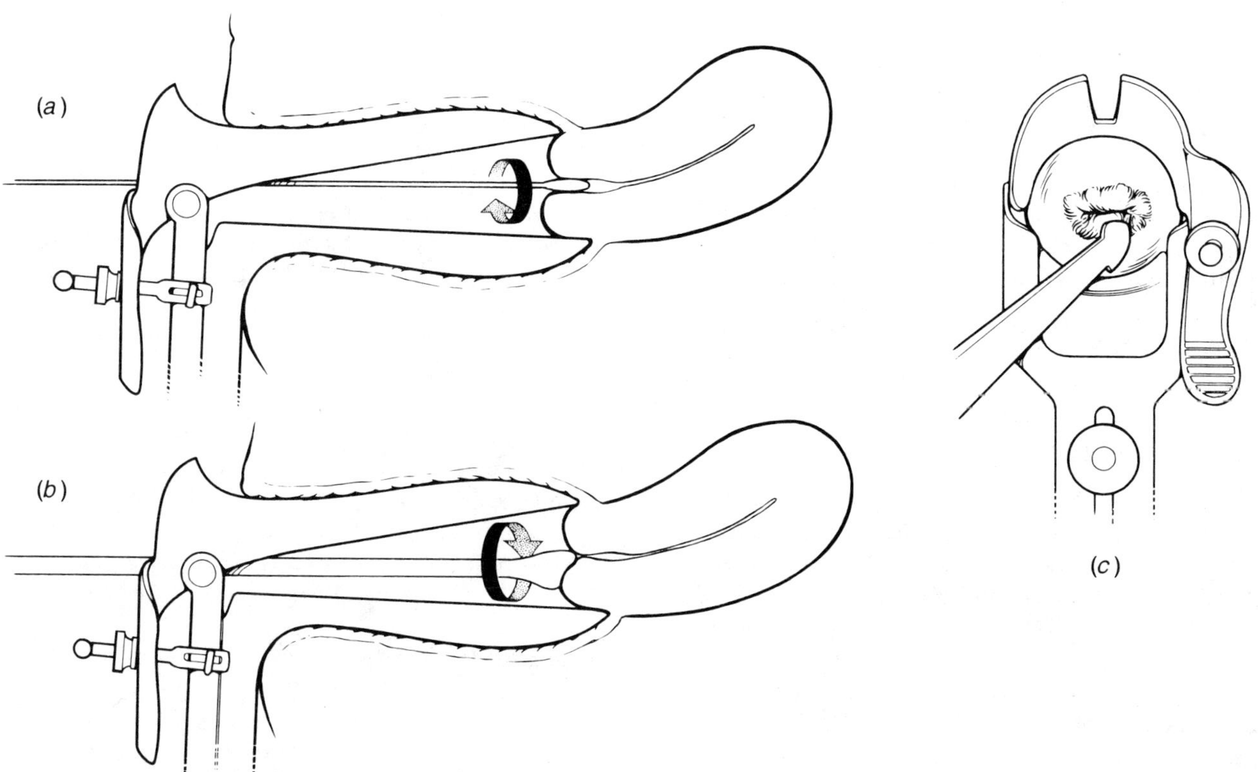

Figure 26.13
Papanicolaou smear. (*a*) Endocervical smear is obtained with a cotton-tipped applicator; (*b*) cervical scraping using wooden spatula; (*c*) cervical sampling in presence of cervical eversion.

spatula will be used. If the squamocolumnar junction is at the external os or a short distance out from the os, the notch is placed in the cervical opening and the spatula is rotated 360 degrees. If the squamocolumnar junction is a wider distance out from the os than the width of the spatula or is at irregular distances from the cervical os, the rounded end of the spatula should be used to obtain a 360-degree sample from all areas of the junction. The material from the end of the spatula is spread on the slide labeled "cervical" by making one stroke down the slide. Care should be taken to avoid a thick deposit of material. If this occurs, a light stroke of the spatula can remove the excess or provide a more even distribution of material. If the smear is too thick or an inadequate sample is obtained, the Pap smear will be useless. As with the endocervical smear, the cervical smear must be fixed with the same amount of haste and in the same manner.

The Pap smear can be obtained at any time throughout the menstrual cycle. During menstrual flow, however, it is more difficult to obtain an adequate cellular sample, and interpretation of results may be more difficult because of an abundance of menstrual flow obscuring the specific cervical cells. It is important to ascertain that the woman has not douched or used any vaginal medication or vaginal contraception within 24–48 hours before having the Pap smear (Fogel, 1981; Hawkins & Higgins, 1981).

The reporting of the Pap test results has been traditionally in numerical classes I–V (see Table 26.1). More recently, the reporting is done in three broad categories (normal, borderline, positive cancer) with a written interpretation or description of the microscopic findings by the cytologist. This approach is replacing the numerical class system since it is believed to provide a more accurate clinical picture. A more detailed discussion of follow-up of abnormal Pap smears is presented in Chapter 27.

GONOCOCCAL CULTURE

To obtain a gonococcal culture (GC), a dry, sterile, cotton-tipped applicator is inserted into the endocervical canal and gently rotated. For best results, the examiner should be certain that the applicator comes in contact with the sides of the canal and remains in the canal for approximately 30 seconds. After the applicator is removed, a Thayer–Martin medium culture plate is streaked by rolling the cotton-tip on the medium in a Z pattern over a large portion of the plate. This will allow for maximum distribution and transfer of the cultured material onto the culture surface. The gonococcus organism prefers an anaerobic environment; therefore, the culture plates must be incubated in a carbon dioxide environment. Clinical laboratories should be consulted regarding special directions for taking, storing, and handling culture plates. Also available are *transgrow bottles,* which are transport media charged with carbon dioxide. As with other cultures, the GC culture will be evaluated at 24 and 48 hours to determine the presence of the gonococcal organism.

WET PREPARATIONS FOR VAGINAL INFECTIONS

In the presence of symptomatic vaginal discharge, wet preparations (wet preps) are performed to document a vaginal infection caused by *Trichomonas vaginalis, Candida albicans,* or *Hemophilus vaginalis.* (The specifics of vaginal infections will be discussed in Chapter 27.) The wet preps are obtained

TABLE 26.1
PAPANICOLAOU CLASSIFICATIONS

Traditional	*Recent*
Class I Negative—normal	
Class II Atypical cells—not suggestive of malignancy	Negative
Class III Atypical cells—suspicious of malignancy	Borderline
Class IV Probable malignant cells	
Class V Definite malignant cells	Positive cancer

during the speculum examination using a wooden spatula or a cotton-tipped applicator moistened with saline. A sample of the vaginal discharge is obtained from the posterior fornix and/or the vaginal walls. This specimen sample is first mixed with one drop of saline on a glass slide and then with one drop of 10% potassium hydroxide (KOH) on another slide. A coverslip is placed on each slide. The wet preps are now ready to be examined under the microscope with low and high power. The characteristic microscopic findings of the aforementioned vaginal infections are shown in Figures 27.5 and 27.6.

Nursing Interventions

The nursing interventions focus on client education and comfort and on assisting with the pelvic examination. In many settings, the professional nurse now performs the complete gynecologic examination. The assumption of these expanded responsibilities, however, does not preclude the continuation of other identified roles. The main goal of the nurse is to help the woman view the pelvic examination in a positive light and experience the examination with minimal or no discomfort.

As the nurse begins to address the area of client education, it is well to remember the basic principles of teaching and learning (see Chapter 2). It is of primary importance to determine the client's level of knowledge before embarking on a teaching plan. Furthermore, the focus of client education can take many directions, depending upon the nurse's assessment of client needs. The woman who presents herself for a gynecologic examination may have teaching needs related to fears and anxieties, the details of the examination, information about her body structure and function, or instructions on relaxation techniques.

Whether or not this is a woman's first gynecologic examination, the nurse should investigate the woman's feelings regarding pelvic examination, either from past experiences or hearsay. These feelings may be so intense that some women do not seek care, delay in routine gynecologic care, or only seek care when symptoms can no longer be tolerated. These emotional considerations need to be explored to enable the woman to have a more positive approach to this area of health care. Unlike other aspects of a physical examination, the pelvic examination is often dreaded and feared for a variety of reasons.

Women may view the pelvic examination as *uncomfortable* because of the position or as *embarrassing* because of exposure of the perineal area. A significant number of women also associate pain with the pelvic examination. The woman may feel vulnerable because of lack of any control over the invasive aspect of this examination. Furthermore, fears may be enhanced by a lack of knowledge about what the examination entails or a fear of the outcome. These are only some of the factors that may contribute to women's unease with the gynecologic examination.

The woman, regardless of age, should be informed of what to expect during the entire visit. The nurse should carefully explain, in terms the woman will understand, what is involved in a pelvic examination. The following outline of the gynecologic examination can be used as a guide.

1. Inspection and palpation of external genitalia
   - A. Mons veneris
   - B. Labia majora and minora
   - C. Clitoris
   - D. Urethra and Skene's glands
   - E. Vaginal introitus
   - F. Bartholin's glands
   - G. Perineal area—support deficiencies
2. Speculum examination
   - A. Visualization of the cervix
   - B. Visualization of the vaginal walls
   - C. Pap smear
   - D. GC culture
3. Bimanual examination—palpation of
   - A. Vagina
   - B. Cervix
   - C. Uterus
   - D. Fallopian tubes and ovaries
4. Rectovaginal abdominal examination
   - A. Confirm previous findings (uterus and adnexae)
   - B. Evaluate cul-de-sac of Douglas
   - C. Explore the rectal area (rectovaginal septum and rectum)

The explanation about the examination provides an opportunity to teach the woman about her body and health in general. If this is the woman's first examination or if she has never been offered the option, show her the equipment that will be used during the examination, allow her to handle it if she desires and explain its purposes. As the examination is in progress, the nurse should reinforce what is occurring and what is to happen next. The examiner should be elaborating on the findings, correlating them to normalcy or pointing out the abnormal aspects and their significance. All of these explanations should help the woman relax, reduce her fears and anxieties, and provide her with a good foundation for a positive experience.

Promoting the comfort of the woman begins by providing her with the opportunity to empty her bladder before starting the examination. If a prolonged period of time has elapsed between voiding and the start of the examination, the nurse should reassess the woman's need to urinate. Aside from the fact that it is uncomfortable for the woman to be examined with a distended bladder, it is also more difficult for the examiner to palpate the internal pelvic organs.

It is the responsibility of the nurse to be certain that all equipment necessary for the examination is readily available in the examining room. To show what this has to do with client comfort, we will present the following illustration. The woman is placed in lithotomy position, the speculum is inserted, and the examiner requests a drop of KOH be placed on a slide. The KOH is in the utility room down the corridor. The delay in obtaining the KOH either prolongs the period of time the speculum is kept in the vagina or, if it is removed, necessitates a second insertion. There is no doubt that this will influence the comfort level of the woman. To avoid such situations, it is important that the following basic equipment for the pelvic examination be available.

- ▲ Various sizes of specula
- ▲ Gloves
- ▲ Equipment for Pap smears (slides, fixative, wooden spatula, cotton-tipped applicators)
- ▲ Materials for GC culture (cotton-tipped applicators, Thayer–Martin culture plate)
- ▲ Wet prep supplies (slides, coverslips, 10% KOH, saline, wooden spatula or cotton-tipped applicator)
- ▲ Lubricant

The nurse should verify with the examiner before beginning the examination if any additional equipment will be needed based on the woman's history or chief complaint.

Properly draping and positioning a client can make a significant difference in her perceived and actual comfort. The technique of draping a woman for pelvic examination is illustrated in Figure 9.2. The placement of the drape across the woman's knees should be done in such a manner so as not to obscure the woman's/examiner's visual contact. It is important for the examiner to be able to observe the woman's reactions to the examination. From the woman's point of view, draping in this fashion may promote better relaxation and may enhance communication during the examination process. In some circumstances, the woman may prefer not to be draped at all. If this is her preference, then it is certainly acceptable.

To promote maximum comfort of the woman on the examination table, it is recommended that her head be elevated to a 30–45 degree angle (Hamilton & Dodge 1981; Schrag, 1978). The degree of elevation also facilitates eye-to-eye contact. The woman's arms should be placed across her chest or alongside her body to help her abdominal muscles relax. With the traditional metal stirrups, the woman may wish to wear her shoes for greater comfort. Various forms of padding have been added to the metal stirrups, from simply covering them with a pair of socks to adding sponge foam covered with a washable polyester fleece (Olson, 1981). With the woman supine and her feet in the stirrups, the nurse should assist her in maneuvering to the end of the table until her buttocks are extended slightly beyond the table's edge. Once the examination is completed, the nurse should instruct the woman to slide up the table before assisting her to a sitting position using good body mechanics. These factors have been shown to increase the woman's comfort. One other consideration regarding the examining table is its placement in the room. Whenever possible, the foot of the table should *not* be facing the door. The fear of someone barging through the door as the woman lies exposed on the table may interfere with her ability to relax.

During the examination itself, there are interventions that can aid the woman's comfort and relaxation. First, the examiner should reinforce that the examination will be performed gently and that if any discomfort is experienced, this should be reported. The woman needs to be instructed in relaxation and breathing techniques before the examination and supported in doing these throughout the examination. The pain associated with the pelvic examination has true origin either in an examiner who is rough (inexcusable) or a woman who is tense and has her perineal muscles contracted. The woman who concentrates on breathing in through her nose and out through her mouth (abdominal or chest breathing) in a slow regular fashion will not be able to contract her perineal muscles simultaneously during any portion of the pelvic examination. Hence, there will not be any increase in pain or discomfort as a result of a contracting muscle against an opposing force.

The technique of relaxation elaborated on for use in labor and delivery can be used during pelvic examination. The woman's state of relaxation can be maintained by forewarning her that she will feel the examiner touching her, pressure with the insertion of the speculum, stretching as the blades of the speculum are opened, pressure with insertion of the fingers in the vagina and rectum, and as if she is having a bowel movement with removal of the finger from the rectum. For the woman who is extremely tense and apprehensive about the insertion of the speculum, some examiners will offer and allow the woman to insert the speculum herself. This may not be an acceptable option for all women, but it should not be overlooked for those who could benefit from this technique.

The nurse can further assist with the pelvic examination by having a speculum available that is at body temperature, not metal cold. This can be accomplished in a variety of ways: running warm water over it, which will also aid as a lubricant; holding it in the hands; placing it near a warm light bulb in the examining lamp; or having it rest on a heating pad set on a low temperature. A warmed speculum is greatly appreciated by every woman.

It is essential for the nurse to use all of these procedures, especially if the examiner is intent on the medical aspects of the examination. Remember that the woman's attitude toward future examinations will be influenced by the nurse's consideration of her as an individual, by the nurse's ability to communicate and assist in comfort measures, and by the nurse's capabilities to assess and perceive accurately client needs.

Mirror Pelvic Examination

The *mirror pelvic examination* (MPE) is an option that should be available and offered to women during their routine gynecologic examination. The mirror can be a hand-held type that the woman or nurse can hold during the examination of the perineum, external genitalia, vagina, and cervix. With women who have participated in an MPE, favorable and positive attitudes were generally expressed in regard to the addition of this technique to the routine gynecologic examination. The advantages of the MPE as a health education technique have been identified as increasing women's knowledge about their bodies, aiding in relaxation during the procedure, and reducing fears about present and future examinations (Liston & Liston, 1978). The MPE is not for every woman, but it should be the woman's choice to accept or decline its use during the examination.

Self-Examination

The concept of pelvic self-examination is presented because some women are engaged in this practice. It evolved as women strove to attain newer heights of self-awareness and self-control. Factors, such as dissatisfaction with the traditional gynecologic care, pain associated with pelvic examinations, and the depersonalization of care, helped to promote this concept. The woman is taught to inspect the external genitalia, insert the speculum, and visualize the cervix. The original theory was that the woman would be able to recognize subtle changes in her body that are indicative of progression to abnormal states. It is important to emphasize that self-care should not be a substitute for regular gynecologic examinations by a physician or nurse practitioner. Furthermore, the concept of self-care, if taken to an extreme, can be hazardous to the health of the woman.

CONTRACEPTION CONTROL

General Considerations

The dilemma facing couples seeking *contraception control* is the fact that the ideal contraceptive has neither been discovered nor is it on the horizon of those methods being researched. An ideal contraceptive is one that is 100% effective, without side effects or contraindications, easy to understand, simple to use, readily available, inexpensive, not connected closely with intercourse, and without permanent effects. Present methods may meet some of these conditions but none comes close to fulfilling all of the criteria. Therefore, couples are faced with making personal choices based on an advantage–disadvantage ratio. When the nurse provides contraceptive counseling, her responsibility centers around helping couples weigh the advantages and disadvantages of each contraceptive method so that they may decide which one, with its disadvantages, is most appropriate for them.

Whether or not a couple chooses to employ some contraceptive method can be influenced by sociocultural factors, religious beliefs, social class, and physical and psychologic reasons. Therefore, the nurse involved in contraceptive counseling must (1) recognize that choosing a contraceptive method is a family affair that, for maximum efficacy, requires both partners' acceptance of the method, and, when possible, both partners should be present for the counseling session; (2) assess the woman's/couple's knowledge of the available methods; (3) assist the woman/couple in selecting an appropriate method by providing information on how methods work and are used, on the advantages and disadvantages, on costs, on effectiveness, and on potential side effects; (4) ascertain the couple's reason for using contraceptives; (5) obtain a complete history; and (6) assist with or perform the physical examination to determine if any contraindicated reasons for a given method exist.

Most reasons couples give for using contraceptives are based on prevention of an unplanned pregnancy or unwanted children. Sexually active people who are unmarried may not want to have children yet they do not wish to abstain from intercourse. Newly married couples may wish to prevent pregnancy in order to have time to adjust to the marriage partnership. Other couples may simply make the decision that they do not wish to reproduce at the present time or ever for a variety of personal reasons. A vast majority of families employ contraceptive control to limit the number of children and to have the children at desired intervals. There are certain circumstances that would cause a pregnancy to be hazardous to the health of the woman or would result in a child with a birth defect or hereditary disease. In these situations, the maintenance of health and prevention of diseases are the primary incentives for contraception control.

Recently, a change in trends has been seen in the selection of specific contraceptive methods. While the oral contraceptive pill is still the most widely used, there has been a decline in its popularity over the past 5 years. The use of the diaphragm and, more recently, of the cervical cap has increased. A number of recent studies of women university students has demonstrated a significant rise in diaphragm use in the university population to the degree that it is almost equal to or surpassing the use of oral contraceptives (Ayvazian, 1981; Berlin et al., 1979). The various intrauterine devices (IUD) have remained fairly constant in percentage of overall use. It appears that a definite correlation between the age of the woman and her contraceptive choice exists. Women in their late teens or early twenties still prefer oral contraceptives, while women in their late twenties prefer the diaphragm.

This correlation of age and contraception choice leads us to a special area of consideration related to the contraceptive counseling of the adolescent. Generally, adolescents are aware of availability of contraceptive methods; however, they are lacking in overall contraceptive knowledge. Adolescents have also shown lack of motivation concerning contraceptive use (Burbach, 1980). This poses significant problems in advising a specific method for the adolescent because, with the exception of the IUD, all methods require high motivation in use to be effective. The IUD is not the contraceptive method of choice for adolescents because of associated high infection rates (Rebbie, 1978). The counseling of the adolescent, therefore, requires that adequate time be given for the teaching–learning process regarding contraceptive knowledge and that the adolescent assumes responsibility for the choice of method, which is necessary with a client of any age.

The effectiveness of a contraceptive method is dependent on a number of factors. There is always the potential for human error as a result of improper use of a technique or lack of motivation. A method may fail because of inherent failure risks or defects in the method. Therefore, the effectiveness of any given method can be based on theoretical effectiveness in comparison to clinical effectiveness. Clinical effectiveness takes into account those failures related to human error. Effectiveness is reported either as percentages successfully using a method or as the pregnancy rate (considered failure of a method) per 100 woman years of exposure. The latter figure is derived from the formula

$$\text{Pregnancy rate} = \frac{\text{number of pregnancies} \times 1{,}200 \text{ months}}{\text{women observed} \times \text{months of exposure}}$$

The *number of pregnancies* refers to the exact number of pregnancies observed in a given population during a given time using a given contraceptive method, regardless of the outcome of the pregnancy. The *1,200 months* is derived by multiplying 100 times 12 months and is equivalent to the number of months in 100 years. The *women observed* equals the number who have used a given contraceptive method for a given period of time; the period of time is designated as the *months of exposure*. For example, the pregnancy rate of 100 couples who have used a contraceptive method for 6 months with 5 pregnancies resulting is derived as follows.

$$\text{Pregnancy rate} = \frac{5 \times 1200}{100 \times 6} = \frac{6000}{600} = 10$$

The effectiveness, as calculated from this method, would be a pregnancy rate of 10 per 100 woman years. It is important to understand this concept as most of the literature reports effectiveness in this manner.

With these basic considerations in mind, each of the contraceptive methods will be discussed in greater depth. The mechanism of action, client instructions, side effects, advantages/disadvantages, and effectiveness will be specified for the various methods. The methods of contraception control can be grouped under five major headings: (1) natural family planning methods, (2) chemical methods, (3) mechanical methods, (4) hormonal methods, and (5) permanent methods.

Natural Family Planning Methods

The natural family planning methods are so designated because they require only a thorough understanding of the normal physiologic processes of the male and female reproductive tracts. A high degree of motivation is also necessary for the users of these methods.

COITUS INTERRUPTUS

Coitus interruptus, or withdrawal, depends on the man's perception or sensation that ejaculation is imminent. At this time, the penis is withdrawn from the vagina so that ejaculation occurs outside the vagina and away from the woman's genital area. While the man may be successful in withdrawing his penis before ejaculation, it still may not have been soon enough. Pre-ejaculatory fluid originating from Cowper's glands may contain sperm that have been deposited in the vagina. Although millions of sperm are ejaculated, it only takes one for conception.

Coitus interruptus is one of the oldest techniques and is reported to be the most widely used method in the world today (Fogel & Woods 1981; Martin, 1978). Coitus interruptus does not produce any direct physical side effects, although over a long period of time it may have psychologic repercussions on both partners.

The advantages to the method are that there is no cost, it can be used when other methods are not available, there is no need to seek medical evaluation before implementing the method, and there are no physical side effects.

The disadvantages are that it requires a great deal of self-control on the part of the man to withdraw at precisely the right moment. It places both men and women under stress since they fear that withdrawal will not be appropriately timed, which thereby interferes with achieving full satisfaction from the sexual experience. The major disadvantage, however, is that withdrawal is not very effective. It has an effectiveness rate of 20–25 pregnancies per 100 woman years, or a success rate of 70–80%.

RHYTHM METHODS

The *rhythm method* is no longer one specific method but contains a variety of methods that can be used singularly or in combination with one another. The rhythm methods are now identified as the (1) calendar method, (2) temperature method, (3) ovulation method, or (4) combination method. The basic purposes of these methods are to predict, or detect, the time of ovulation. The primary focus of all of these methods is identification of the woman's *safe period* when she may engage in intercourse versus her *unsafe period* when she could conceivably become pregnant and must abstain from sexual intercourse. There are two basic assumptions that preface the theoretical working of these methods. The first assumption is that the ovary expels only one ovum per cycle or if multiple, it is simultaneous and that the ovum survives for 24–48 hours. The second assumption is that the sperm remain viable in the female reproductive tract for a period of 48–72 hours. Taking these two assumptions into consideration, there will be a minimum of 5 days during each menstrual cycle when the couple will need to abstain from intercourse to prevent pregnancy. However, the last statement is true only if the woman has a consistent, precise, regular pattern of menstrual cycles. Few women, if any, will be so regular that they will establish an exact number of days recurring in each cycle without deviating a few days over the course of their reproductive years. The variation in the number of days of a woman's menstrual cycles will ultimately increase the theoretical number of unsafe days and increase the number of days that abstinence must be practiced.

Calendar Method. The *calendar method* assumes that ovulation occurs 14 days before the onset of the next menstrual cycle with a plus or minus variation of 2 days. Therefore, the ovulatory days are 12–16 of the menstrual cycle. Because of the 48-hour survival of the ovum and the possibility of fertilization during this time, an additional 2 days are added onto day 16, making it now 18. Because of the survival time of the sperm, day 11 is also considered an unsafe day, making unsafe days 11–18. A woman who has a regular cycle, regardless of the number of days, will have 8 days per cycle of potential fertility.

In order to enhance the accuracy of the rhythm method, it is recommended that the woman keep an exact menstrual history for a minimum of 6 months and preferably 1 year before using rhythm as a contraceptive method. This will document the variations in cycle length for the particular woman. Once this information is obtained, she must then subtract 18 days from the shortest cycle and 11 days from the longest cycle to determine her safe and unsafe days. For example, a woman's menstrual history record shows the shortest cycle is 23 days and the longest cycle is 30 days. Subtracting 18 from the shortest cycle (23 − 18 = 5) provides her with the first fertile day, day 5, after the start of a menstrual period. Subtracting 11 from the longest cycle (30 − 11 = 19) provides her with the last fertile day, day 19, after the start of a menstrual period. Therefore, the woman with the above menstrual history has potential fertile days during each menstrual cycle from day 5 to day 19, during which she must abstain from intercourse if rhythm is her contraceptive method.

A major disadvantage of this method can be illustrated with the same menstrual history by adding the data that the woman's menses usually lasts 4 days. This means that upon completion of her menstruation on day 4, she immediately enters her fertile period until day 19. This, coupled with a short cycle of 23 days, leaves the woman with only 3 days when she is either safe or without a menstrual discharge. The potential of so few safe days makes this an undesirable method for many couples.

Basal Body Temperature Method. The *basal body temperature method* (BBT) requires a woman to obtain her BBT upon awakening each morning before any activity of any kind and to keep an accurate record. For increased accuracy, a BBT thermometer should be used; it can be purchased at most drugstores. The advantage of this thermometer over a standard one is it is scaled so 0.1°F reading can be obtained. The method of taking the temperature can be oral or rectal (rectal may be more accurate). Regardless of the method chosen, it should be stressed that the site should be constant and not changed once the method is initiated. The recommended length of sleep before taking the BBT varies from 2–3 hours (Fogel, 1981) to 5–6 hours (Varney, 1980).

The BBT method is based upon the body's physiologic response to progesterone. At the time of ovulation, the release of progesterone causes a sustained rise in temperature from 0.5 to 1.0°F in the basal body temperature. Occasionally, the rise in temperature is preceded by a drop in BBT; however, this is not predictive. A sustained rise for 3 consecutive days indicates that ovulation has occured and the unsafe period has passed (Fig. 26.14). By using only the BBT method, intercourse

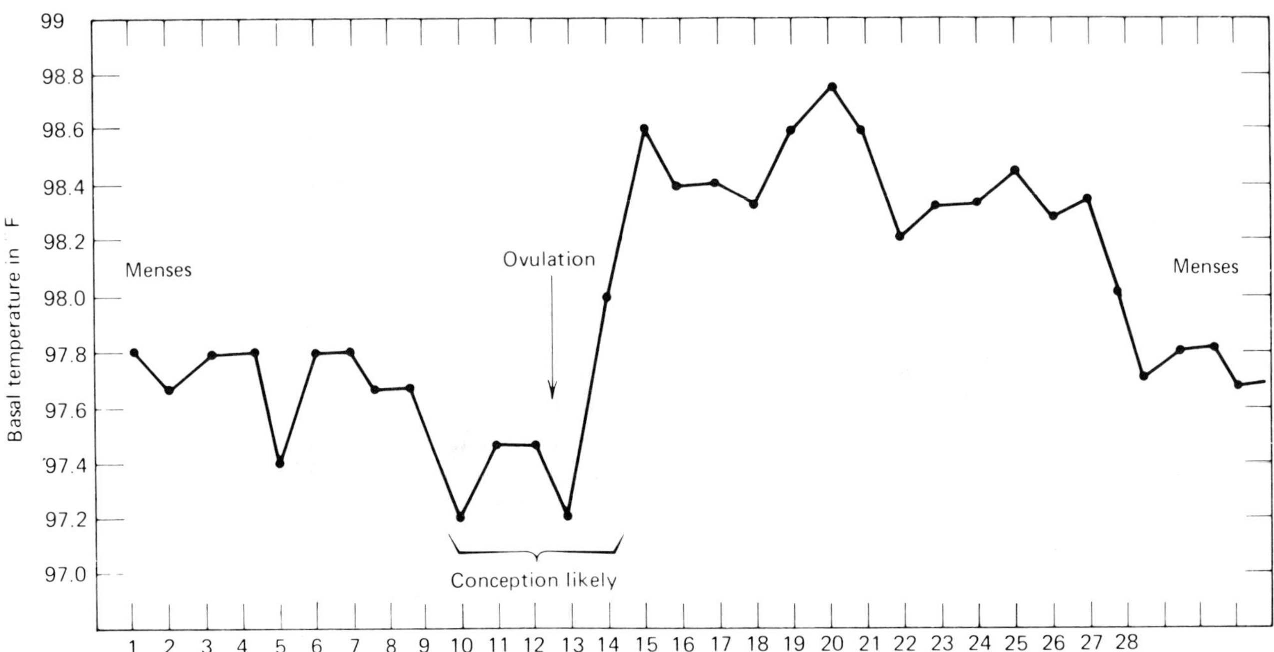

Figure 26.14
Basal body temperature method. Safe days for intercourse after 3 days of sustained temperature elevation. *Source:* Sloane, E. *Biology of Women.* New York: John Wiley & Sons, 1980. Used with permission.

is restricted to the second half of the cycle when the temperature has remained elevated for the minimum number of days. This can be viewed as a disadvantage of the method along with the need for a high level of motivation for the woman to take her BBT daily. Another disadvantage is that factors such as illnesses, medications, altered sleep pattern, air conditioning, and electric blankets can affect the BBT and provide invalid temperature recordings.

Ovulation Method. The *ovulation method,* sometimes referred to as the Billing's method in honor of the obstetrician–gynecologist who first began teaching this method, is based upon the fact that characteristic changes occur in cervical mucus during the menstrual cycle. The changes in the cervical mucus are estrogen triggered and can be catergorized into four patterns.

- ▲ ***No or Very Little Secretion of Mucus.*** This occurs immediately after menstruation for a varying number of days. The longer the cycle, the longer the number of days with no or little mucus. These are referred to as the *dry days* and are considered safe (Elder, 1978).
- ▲ ***Sticky Mucus.*** The second phase involves a mucus that is cloudy white or yellowish in color and sticky in consistency. This type of mucus is present during some preovulatory days, which is the beginning of the unsafe period.
- ▲ ***Fertile Mucus.*** Fertile mucus, also known as type E or spinnbarkheit, is clear, slippery, lubricative, and stretchy (Fig. 26.15). (For more information see Chapter 27, section on infertility.) This type of mucus has been compared to raw egg white because of the similarity in consistency and in glossy appearance. The volume of mucus increases significantly, and this time is referred to as wet days. Type E mucus is observable immediately before and after ovulation. The day that this type of mucus seems most pronounced in terms of identified characteristics is considered to be the peak day. The day of ovulation is thought to occur some time within 24 hours surrounding the peak day. The 3 days after the peak day are included in the unsafe days.
- ▲ ***Infertile Mucus.*** Infertile mucus, also known as type G (see Fig. 26.15), predominates in the

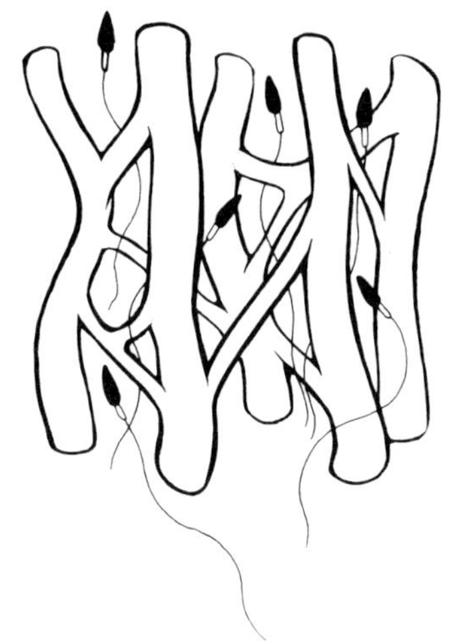

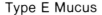

Type E Mucus

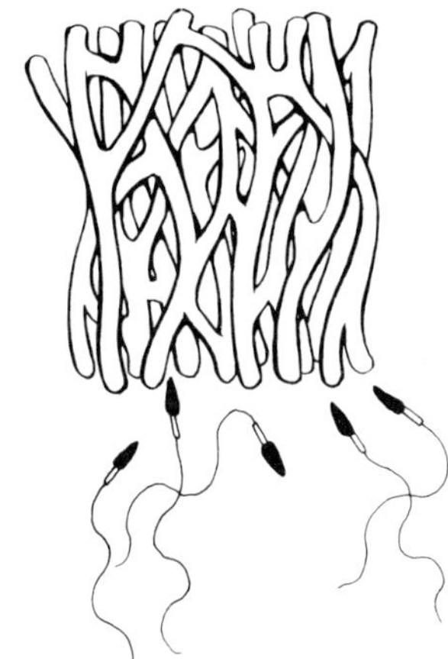

Type G Mucus

Figure 26.15
Cervical mucus types and sperm penetration.

> second half of the cycle as the progesterone levels rise. This mucus has a drier quality, decreases in volume, loses its elasticity, and becomes cloudy and sticky. The appearance of type G mucus is correlated with the fourth day after the peak fertile type mucus appears and heralds the beginning of the safe days. (Elder, 1978)

In instructing couples about the ovulation method, it is necessary to emphasize that the woman must learn to detect, identify, and evaluate the changes in her cervical mucus by being aware of the degree of dampness around the vaginal introitus and by digital examination of the mucus. Accurate records must be kept that identify the type of mucus and the day of the menstrual cycle. The woman may require 1 month, 6 months, or more time to become proficient at this method. Abstinence should be practiced, especially during the first half of the cycle, until the woman has determined her pattern and recognition of changes with some degree of certainty. Further, intercourse should *not* be performed during the menstrual cycle since if the menstrual flow is prolonged, it may mask the production of fertile mucus. With this method intercourse is permitted on the evening of dry days following that day's observation. Intercourse is permitted only every other night on dry days as the seminal discharge may mask the onset of fertile mucus the day after intercourse.

The ability of the woman to ascertain the changes in her cervical mucus and the continuous monitoring that is necessary in relation to awareness, observations, examinations, as well as the record keeping, require a very high level of motivation. This can be viewed as the major disadvantage of this method.

Combination Method. The *combination method* may use any or all of the previously described methods in addition to the woman recognizing other signs or symptoms that may be associated with varying stages of her menstrual cycle. Some women experience *Mittelschmerz,* which is a pain in the lower abdomen that may occur in conjunction with spotting or breakthrough bleeding at the time of ovulation. Mood changes and sexual desire may fluctuate in cyclic patterns associated with significant happenings in the menstrual cycle. The calendar and BBT methods can be combined. Using this combination, the first fertile day is calculated on the basis of the calendar method, subtracting 18 from the shortest cycle; the last fertile day is determined by the BBT method. If you add to this the detection of cervical mucus changes, you will greatly increase the reliability of determining your safe versus unsafe period.

The potential for side effects in these natural methods, aside from pregnancy, is nonexistent. There are advantages and disadvantages that can be generalized for all of the rhythm methods. The advantages are (1) little or no expense, (2) not discouraged by the Roman Catholic church, (3) makes the woman more aware of her bodily functions, (4) requires cooperation and open communication between sexual partners, and (5) is reversible. The disadvantages are (1) takes time to gather the necessary information before method can be used safely, (2) periods of imposed abstinence may be unacceptable, (3) high degree of motivation by both partners is necessary, and (4) high failure rate.

The failure rate of the rhythm method has a wide range depending on the method or combination of methods used, the regularity of the woman's cycles, the length of time taken to gather data before instituting the method, and the ability and motivation of the couple to abstain during unsafe days. The rhythm methods are not feasible during the postpartum period, lactation, menopause, illnesses, after discontinuation of oral contraceptives, or with women who have irregular menstrual cycles.

CHEMICAL METHODS

The *chemical methods* of conception control include douching and use of spermicidal agents in the form of foams, creams, jellies, or vaginal suppositories.

Douching. The inclusion of *douching* under chemical methods of contraception control is on the basis that some people believe it is effective in preventing pregnancy. Contrary to these opinions, douching with a vinegar or other type solution does *not* destroy or wash the sperm from the vagina. Basically, the douching process cannot occur soon enough to overcome the physiologic process of sperm penetration. The presence of sperm has been detected within 90 seconds of ejaculation in the cervical mucus and within 3–5 minutes in the fallopian tubes (Kuczynski, 1980). While it is generally accepted that douching is *not* an effective contraceptive control method, it is not considered to be hazardous. Douching with unconventional solutions or equipment, however, can be very hazardous and detrimental. These practices, which have been reported to occur in the teenage population, should be strongly discouraged.

Spermicidal Preparations. Spermicidal preparations are chemical combinations of active and inert ingredients. The active ingredient is the spermicidal agent that immobilizes and kills the sperm. The inert ingredient is the vehicle for dispensing the spermicidal agent; it also provides bulk to the spermicidal preparation so that the active ingredient can be spread over the cervical os and upper vagina. The motile sperm must pass through the spermicidal preparation in order to gain entrance into the uterine cavity. In so doing, they are immobilized and destroyed by the active ingredient.

Spermicidal preparations are available in foam, cream, jelly, or vaginal suppository forms. The choice of the substance is a personal one. When spermicidal preparation is used as the primary means of contraception control, the most popular form is foam. The foam looks and feels like shaving cream; it comes in an aerosal can with a plastic reusable applicator (see Fig. 26.16). The applicator allows for a measured dose of spermicidal foam to be administered. The cream and jelly are spermicidal preparations that can be used alone or, if designated, in conjunction with a diaphragm. The cream and jelly are less frequently used as the primary means because women say they are messier than the foam. The cream and jelly are available in tubes that also have the necessary measured-dose applicator. In using foam, cream, or jelly, the applicator should be completely filled with the spermicidal preparation. The applicator is inserted the full depth of the vagina and is withdrawn approximately ½ inch before depressing the plunger and dispensing the spermicidal preparation. Vaginal suppositories also contain active spermicidal and inert ingredients. The suppositories are available as a melting or as an effervescing suppository; the type depends on the inert base.

The melting suppository has a melting point slightly below body temperature and a melting time of approximately 10–15 minutes. A disadvantage of this type of suppository is the melting point, which in warmer climates will necessitate it being stored in a cool place or refrigerated. The 10–15-minute time period needed for the suppository to dissolve may also be considered a disadvantage. Some couples find this delay a significant interruption in the sexual act, while others incorporate the suppository insertion as part of foreplay with no adverse affect in spontaneity.

The effervescing suppository bubbles and dissolves when moistened by vaginal secretions. It takes approximately 10 minutes for it to effervesce completely. In the normal process of the suppository's effervescing action, a small amount of heat is generated and perceived by the woman. The disadvantage of this suppository type is the complaint

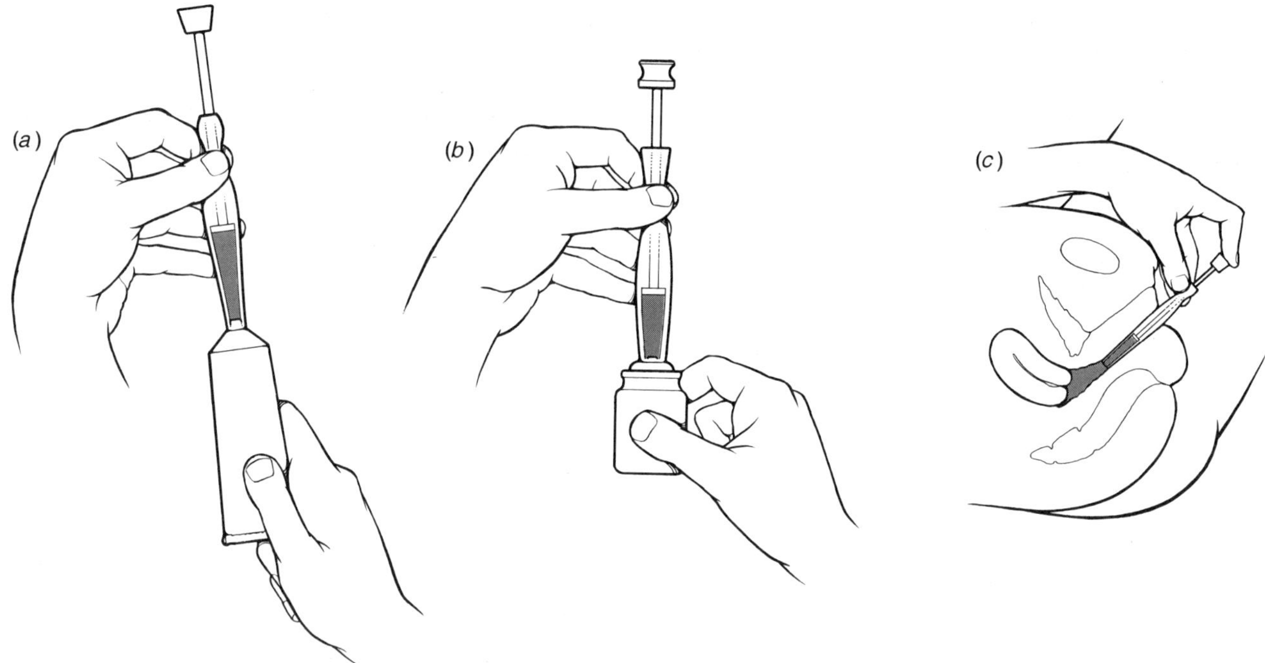

Figure 26.16
Spermicidal agents. (*a*) Cream or jelly spermicides available in tubes with applicator; (*b*) foam spermicide in an aerosol can must be held upright for proper filling of applicator; (*c*) Lying down, the applicator is inserted the length of the vagina; is withdrawn 1/2 inch; the plunger is depressed dispersing the foam at the cervix.

by both women and men of the heat sensation causing significant vaginal and penile discomfort and irritation.

Regardless of the suppository type, the technique for insertion is identical. The women or her partner manually inserts the suppository in the vagina, using a finger to push it as deeply into the vagina as possible. Once the suppository has dissolved, the mechanism of action is the same as for other spermicidal preparations; it forms a barrier that the sperm must penetrate and in so doing are immobilized and destroyed. Women should be advised not to confuse the hygienic vaginal suppositories, which do not have a contraceptive action, with the vaginal spermicidal suppositories.

General instructions for spermicidal preparations include the following.

- ▲ Fill the applicator as directed. With the foam preparation, the can should be shaken well before filling the applicator.
- ▲ Insert the spermicidal agent *no more* than a half-hour before intercourse. Lie in the supine position and direct the applicator in a downward and backward direction into the vagina. Once the spermicidal preparation is inserted, do not get up and walk around since its effectiveness will be lessened by the preparation draining down the vagina away from the cervix. If you must get up and move around or more than a half-hour has passed, another applicator of spermicide should be inserted. The motto here is "be prepared." Have several containers of spermicidal preparations strategically located to be prepared, as well as to have an extra on hand in case one becomes empty.
- ▲ Insert the applicator the full depth of the vagina, then withdraw it ½ inch, then depress the plunger to disperse the spermicidal agent.
- ▲ Additional applications are necessary if intercourse is repeated.
- ▲ Do not douche for 6–8 hours after the last sexual intercourse. (Douching is not generally necessary nor should it be encouraged. However, you must evaluate if this is a practice of the woman and instruct appropriately.)

▲ Double the dosage for women who have had three or more children. Two applicators of the spermicide should be inserted initially and each time thereafter.

The potential side effects with spermicidal preparations are allergic reactions and irritation of the vagina or penis. Recent concern has been expressed regarding adverse fetal effects when spermicidal agents are used after conception but before diagnosis of pregnancy. While the data at this time is not conclusive, it is recommended that you review the literature for the most up-to-date findings.

The major advantages of spermicides is that they are readily available without the need of a physician's prescription. They are relatively easy and safe to use. Their effect is local, and they are without major side effects. They are used only as needed and partners can share in the responsibility. They are also relatively inexpensive.

The major disadvantages are that they are messy and that they must be used so close to the time of intercourse. The couple may feel that the spontaneity of the sexual act is interrupted by this method and sexual satisfaction is decreased by an annoying drainage. For the couple who engage in oral–genital sex, the spermicidal preparation may interfere with this practice since it has an unpleasant taste. The insertion of the spermicide would have to be done after oral–genital sex, but before penile–vaginal penetration to avoid this drawback.

The effectiveness of spermicides is 15–30 pregnancies per 100 woman years. With conscientious use, the method is successful about 75% of the time. The effectiveness of this method can be increased if used in combination with other contraceptive measures like the condom or diaphragm.

MECHANICAL METHODS

Although the *mechanical methods* of contraception control are devices that are primarily used by the woman, this is the one category that has an acceptable method for male contraception. The mechanical methods of contraceptive control are (1) condom, (2) diaphragm, (3) cervical cap, and (4) intrauterine devices.

Condom. The *condom* is the mechanical method that has been available for male use for centuries. Condoms are made of latex rubber or processed collagenous tissue (lamb cecum, also referred to as natural skin condoms). The latex rubber condom is the major type used in the United States and accounts for the common terminology, *rubber*, being used synonomously for condom. This rubber or skin sheath is unrolled over the erect penis to serve as a receptacle for the semen, thereby preventing the deposit of the ejaculate into the vagina.

The condom comes in two basic designs: plain-end and nipple-end condoms. The advantage of the nipple-end condom is that there is a preformed small pouch to receive the semen after ejaculation. When using the plain-end condom, the user must provide space for the semen. This is done by grasping ¼–½ inch of the end of the condom, thereby creating an air-free pouch or space that extends beyond the glans (Fig. 16.17). This technique of applying the plain-end condom is necessary in order to reduce the risk of breakage during intercourse and to leave room for the ejaculate. Other adaptations to the condom design include lubricated or nonlubricated, ribbed or nonribbed, and a variety of colors.

The proper use of the condom includes some important details that should be discussed with the couple using this method. The most important aspect is the application of the condom upon the penis when erection has occurred. This should be done before any contact with the female genitalia and should not be delayed until the man perceives that ejaculation is imminent. Instruction should be provided regarding the technique for creating a pouch when using the plain-end condom. Immediately after ejaculation and before erection is lost, the penis should be withdrawn from the vagina while holding onto the condom at the base. By grasping the condom, you can prevent the possibility of it slipping off inside the vagina and avoid the leakage or spillage of semen over the top. The last aspect of instruction is that a new condom must be used for each sexual act.

The advantages of the condom are that it is readily available without prescription or medical consultation and relatively inexpensive. The skin condoms are 2–3 times more expensive than the latex rubber condoms. Condoms are simple to use and do not have any known side effects. The condom not only provides a barrier for the sperm, but also a barrier for sexually transmitted diseases. The condom may be used as an adjunct method with spermicides, in cases of questionable intrauterine device expulsion or missed oral contraceptives, or

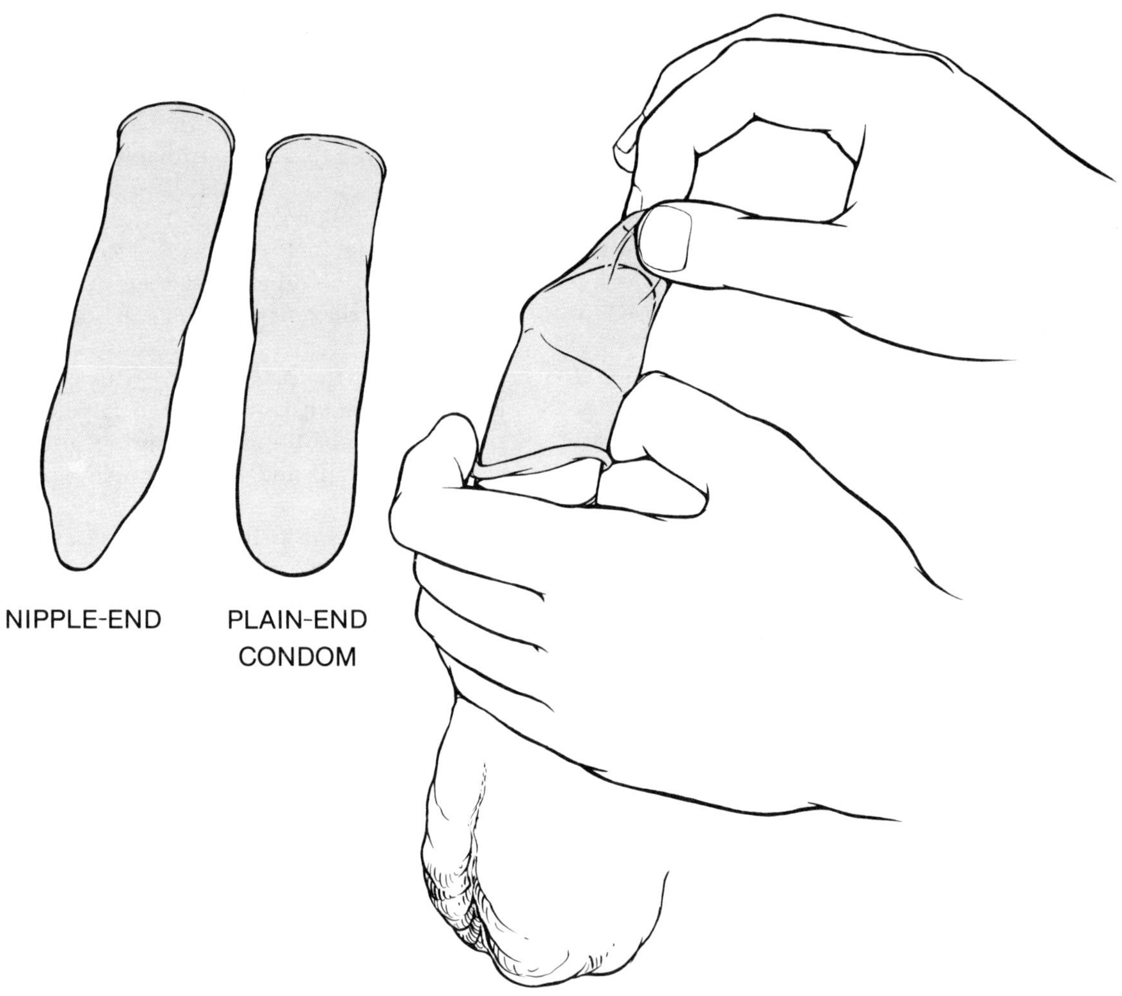

Figure 26.17
Nipple-end and plain-end condom designs. Proper application of the plain-end condom requires the 1/2-inch extended beyond the glans to provide a pouch or space for the collection of the ejaculate.

as an alternate to the diaphragm, allowing the couple to alternate responsibility in their contraceptive practices.

The disadvantages most frequently cited are the interruption of lovemaking and reduction of sensations during intercourse by both partners. In *Consumer Report* (1979), the following reasons were given for not using the condom: always aware of presence, fear of slipping off, prompt withdrawal necessary, does not stay on, and difficult to put on. The problem of discharge or leakage of semen into the vagina is a disadvantage that can be reduced by proper instruction. There is also a federal government quality control of condom production in the United States that provides some reassurance regarding defective or broken condoms. As a prophylactic measure, couples using the condom may wish to have a spermicidal preparation available for immediate use in those infrequent cases when a condom breaks, spillage of semen occurs, or there is failure to apply the condom.

The effectiveness ranges from three pregnancies per 100 woman years to 15 pregnancies per 100 woman years. The effectiveness is advertised to be 99% when used in conjunction with a spermicidal foam (Crooks & Baur, 1980).

Diaphragm. The *diaphragm* is a latex rubber, dome-shaped device with a spring rim similar in shape to half of a tennis ball. The diaphragm functions as a contraceptive control method by two means: (1) the device blocks the passage of sperm from the vagina into the cervix and uterine cavity (barrier) and (2) the device serves as a container for keeping spermicidal cream or jelly in contact with the external cervical os (receptacle). Thus, the diaphragm is not only a mechanical method but is used in conjunction with a chemical method.

The concept of the diaphragm as a contraceptive method has also been around for many centuries. The acceptance of the diaphragm has been increasing as women are becoming more aware and more concerned about subjecting their bodies to adverse or potential side effects of oral contraceptive pills and intrauterine devices. The diaphragm seems to be most popular with women in their late twenties (Ayvazian, 1981).

Diaphragms vary in size and construction of the rim portion (Fig. 26.18). The sizes range from 50 to 110 mm in diameter, increasing in increments of 5 mm. The majority of women use diaphragms in the 70–80 mm range. Variations in normal anatomy, muscle tone, and patient dexterity will influence the decision as to what type of diaphragm is prescribed.

There are three diaphragm spring constructions in the rim that are widely used: coil, flat, and arcing. The purpose of the spring is to return the diaphragm to its original shape and to help provide a good fit. The coil-spring diaphragm contains a spiral metal spring in circumference of the rim. When the device is compressed for insertion it folds in one plane or a straight line. This particular device would be more likely to have improper insertions in a woman with a very posterior cervix. The device is particularly suited for women with normal size and contour of the vagina, strong vaginal muscles, and a deep arch behind the symphysis pubis.

The flat-spring diaphragm has a flat metal band in the rim. This device is appropriate for women with the same characteristics as for the coil spring, with the exception of being more suitable for women with a shallow arch behind the symphysis pubis. This diaphragm also folds in a single plane.

The arcing-spring diaphragm is a combination of the coil-spring and the flat-spring diaphragms. Because of the double metal spring in the rim, this diaphragm is held properly in place by the strong pressure of the double springs. Therefore, women who have some degree of relaxation of the vaginal walls such as cystocele (bulging of urinary bladder into the vagina) or mild uterine prolapse would be candidates for this style of diaphragm. When compressed for insertion, this diaphragm forms an arc that easily follows the posterior direction of the vagina. For women who have a very posterior cervix, there is less likelihood that an improper positioning of the diaphragm will occur with the arcing-spring type. The disadvantage of this type diaphragm is the need for the fitting to be precise. If the diaphragm is a little too large, excess pressure (because of the double spring) can be exerted against the walls and urethra causing pain or difficulty in voiding.

There are two points to emphasize concerning the proper fitting of a diaphragm: (1) the normal placement of the diaphragm and (2) the changes that occur in the vagina during sexual response. (See Chapters 7 and 14 for details.) When properly placed, the diaphragm completely covers the cervix with the posterior rim encircling the cervix and being stabilized in the posterior fornix. The anterior rim is lodged upward behind the symphysis pubis, while the lateral edges fall into the lateral fornices and maintain contact with the vaginal walls. During coitus with insertion of the penis, the diaphragm is compressed anteriorly against the vaginal wall while covering the cervical os.

A woman can be fitted for a diaphragm by a physician, nurse-midwife, family planning nurse practitioner, or another properly trained nonphysician. Before examining the woman, she should be provided the opportunity to empty her bladder. The correct size of the diaphragm is determined by measuring the distance of the vaginal canal from the posterior aspect of the symphysis pubis to the posterior vaginal fornix (Fig. 26.19). The examiner inserts the middle and index finger into the vagina until the tip of the finger rests in the posterior fornix. The fingers are then elevated against the pubic bone. The point at which the symphysis pubis touches the index finger is marked by the tip of the thumb on the same hand. The fingers are then withdrawn with the thumb maintaining its position against the index finger. The appropriate size fitting diaphragm or ring is the one that extends from the tip of the middle finger to the tip of the thumb. The fitting diaphragm or ring is then inserted into the woman's vagina to confirm the size. As a double check, the next smaller and larger

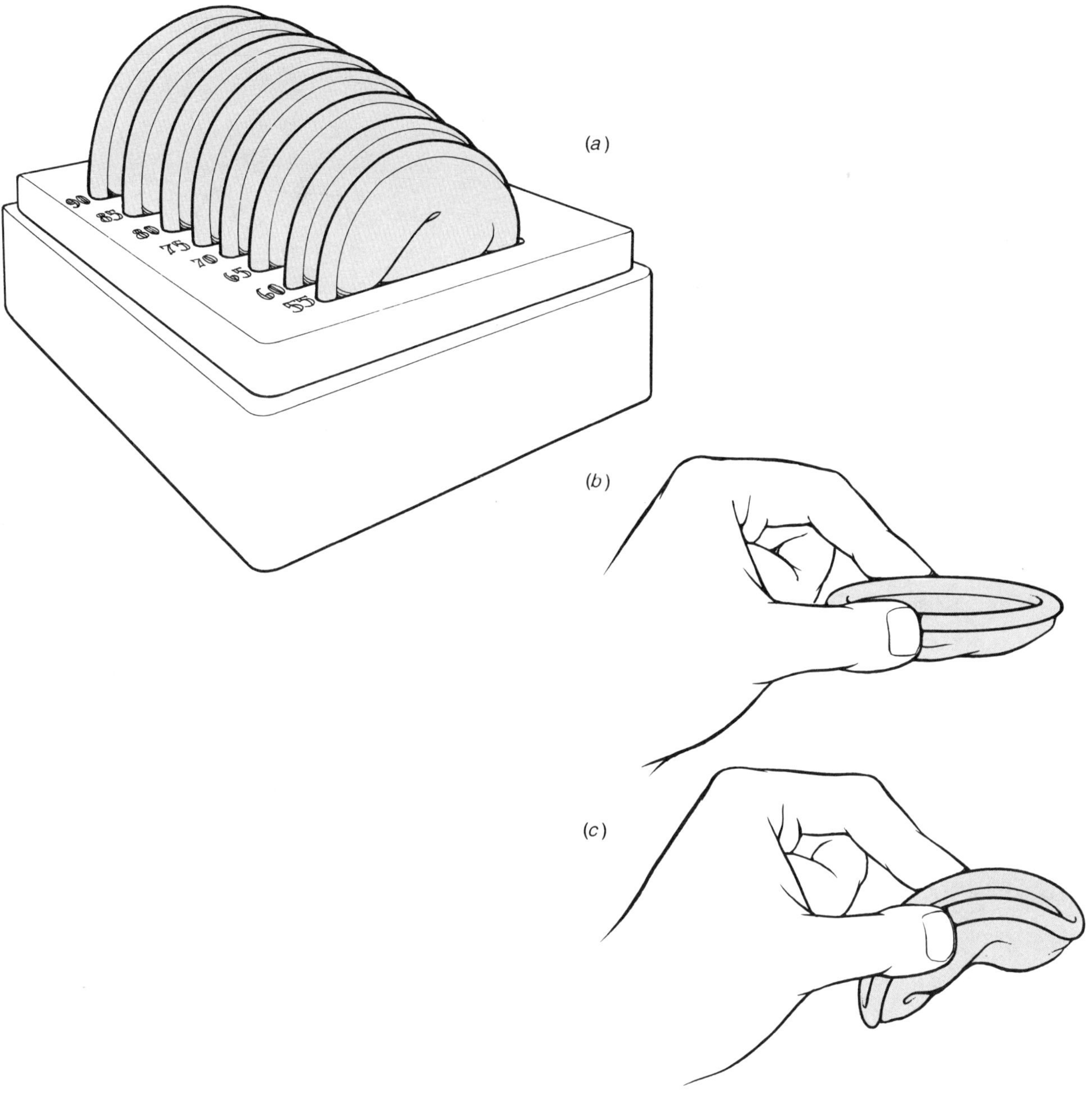

Figure 26.18
Diaphragms. (*a*) Fitting rings or diaphragms; (*b*) flat and nonarcing diaphragm folded for insertion; (*c*) arcing-spring diaphragm folded for insertion.

sizes from the identified size should be inserted into the vagina before a final choice is made. After this procedure, the woman can be advised of the prescribed size.

An improperly fitted diaphragm will have decreased effectiveness (Fig. 26.20). A diaphragm that is too small may slip out of place leaving the cervical canal unobstructed, or it may drop away from the cervix as the upper vagina expands or enlarges with sexual stimulation. A diaphragm that is too large may allow for insertion of the penis anterior to it, thereby leaving the cervix uncovered. One that is too large may also unfold improperly and/or cause discomfort (dyspareunia) for the woman. When a properly fitted diaphragm is in place, neither partner should be aware of its presence.

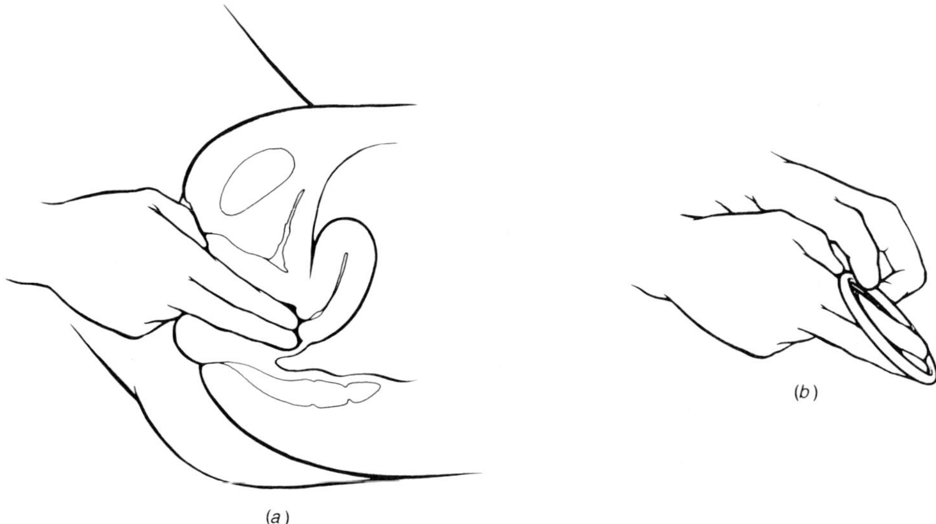

Figure 26.19
Technique of diaphragm fitting. (*a*) Vaginal examination allows for measuring the distance between the posterior fornix and the posterior aspects of the symphysis pubis; (*b*) the proper size diaphragm is selected by choosing the one that extends from the tip of the finger to the marked portion of the thumb.

While the diaphragm fit is a prime factor in influencing effectiveness, the most important aspect related to effectiveness is the client teaching that is done and the time allocated to having women practice under the supervision of the teacher (nurse). The teaching process may begin with validation that the woman has an understanding of the basic anatomy of the reproductive system. The techniques for proper insertion, removal, and use are then discussed with the woman (Fig. 26.21). Before inserting the diaphragm, the woman should place approximately one teaspoon full of spermi-

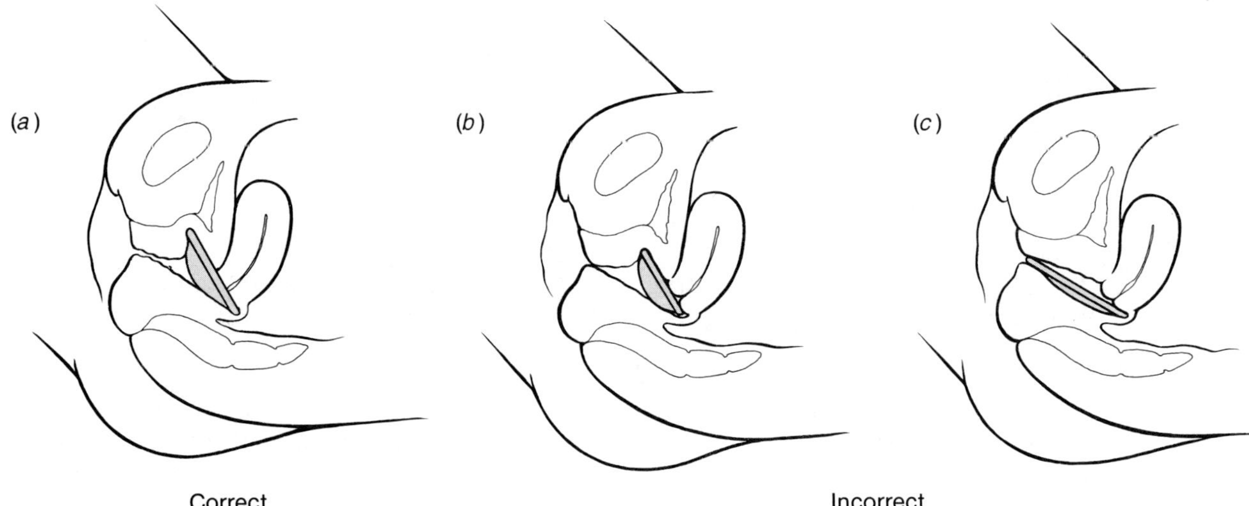

Figure 26.20
Results of diaphragm fitting. (*a*) Correct fit and proper placement; (*b*) incorrect fit—diaphragm is too small and not properly fitting in posterior fornix; (*c*) incorrect fit—diaphragm is too large and not properly fitting behind symphysis pubis.

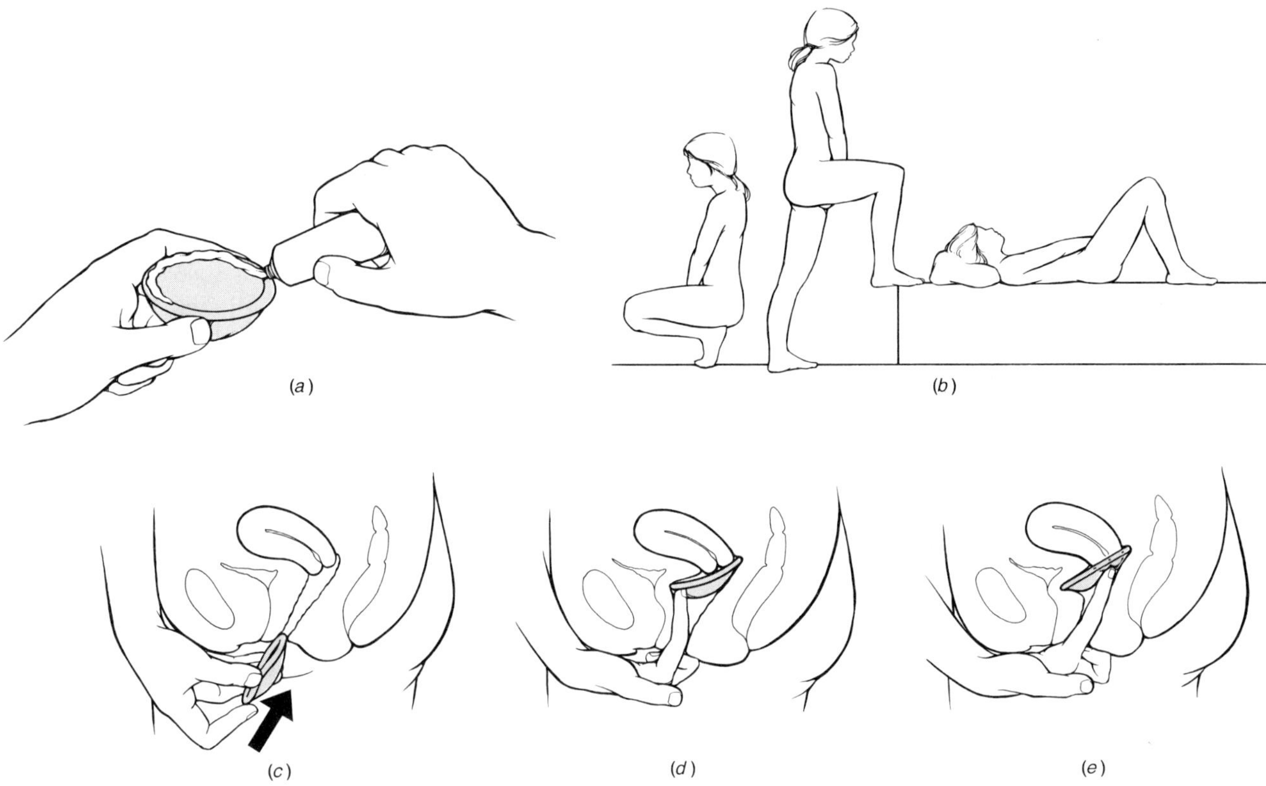

Figure 26.21
Sequence of diaphragm insertion. *(a)* Spermicidal cream is applied to rim and inner aspects of diaphragm; *(b)* three positions women may assume for the diaphragm insertion; *(c)* diaphragm is compressed and inserted the length of the vagina; *(d)* with the posterior rim in the posterior fornix the anterior rim is pressed upward behind the symphysis pubis with the index finger; *(e)* proper placement is determined by palpation of the cervix covered by the diaphragm.

cidal cream or jelly in the cup of the diaphragm and spread a thin layer of the spermicide around the inner rim of the diaphragm. The use of the spermicide in this manner will destroy any sperm that may gain entrance underneath the diaphragm. The general rule is that the diaphragm should *always* be used with a spermicide. It may be emphasized that the objectionable messiness attributed to spermicides by some couples is not a factor when used with the diaphragm. Remind the couple that the diaphragm acts as a container to keep the spermicide in place against the cervix.

The woman may then insert the diaphragm manually or with an inserter. Generally, the inserter, or as it is sometimes called the introducer, is used infrequently. The inserter is unnecessary if adequate time is provided for client education. For insertion, the woman may assume one of four positions, whichever seems the most comfortable (see Fig. 26.21): (1) sitting on the edge of a chair, (2) lying flat on her back with knees bent, (3) squatting, or (4) propping one leg up on a chair, stool, or toilet seat. The woman proceeds to compress the edges of the diaphragm together using her index and middle fingers and her thumb. She may need to practice this aspect of insertion as the diaphragm may be quite slippery around the edges if the spermicide has been spread excessively. If the woman attempts to rush the insertion, the diaphragm may spring from her hand causing a considerable if not total disruption to the lovemaking. The other hand separates the labia as the diaphragm is inserted into the vagina in a posterior direction. Once it is inserted as far as it will go, the woman reaches into her vagina with her index finger and presses the anterior rim of the diaphragm upward behind the symphysis pubis bone. With her finger still in the vagina, the woman checks the diaphragm placement by palpating the cervix with her finger. The cervix should be covered by the dome and palpable through the rubber of the diaphragm. Some couples incorporate diaphragm insertion as part of foreplay with the partner sharing responsibility for inserting it and checking the position.

The diaphragm is removed by inserting the index finger in the vagina and grasping the diaphragm rim that is behind the symphysis (Fig. 26.22). Care must be taken during the removal process not to tear or puncture the diaphragm. When the diaphragm is at the introitus, it can be grasped by the thumb and index finger and be completely withdrawn. After giving the woman these instructions, she should be allowed ample time to practice inserting, checking position of, and removing the diaphragm in privacy, but with assistance available. The woman should repeat this process until she develops confidence in her ability to insert and assess the correct position of the diaphragm accurately. Accomplishing this, the woman then inserts the diaphragm and has the professional examiner (physician or nurse) examine the position of the diaphragm to validate the correctness of her technique. An estimated 30–45 minutes should be allotted in order for this fitting–teaching process to take place (Bradbury, 1975).

There are additional instructions that need to be provided regarding use and care of the diaphragm. The diaphragm can be inserted any time before intercourse. If inserted more than 2 hours before intercourse, an additional application of spermicide should be used at the time of intercourse. If multiple episodes of intercourse occur, an application of the spermicidal agent *must* be administered without removing the diaphragm before each coitus. Also, the position of the diaphragm should be rechecked before further penile penetration to ascertain that the diaphragm was not dislodged during the thrust of the previous sexual act. It is also necessary to evaluate the position of the diaphragm if a vibrator was used during foreplay. As with the penis, a vibrator could displace the diaphragm and reduce the effectiveness.

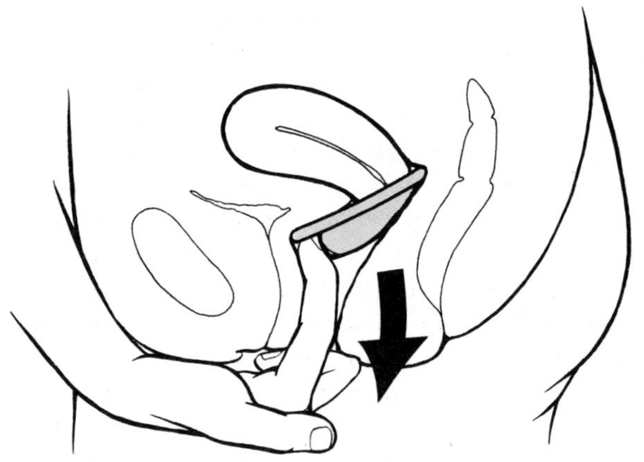

Figure 26.22
Diaphragm removal. Index finger grasps anterior lip and pulls the diaphragm downward and outward.

After the final act of intercourse, the diaphragm should remain in place for 6–8 hours. This measure will virtually guarantee that no viable sperm remain in the vagina. Douching during this time is definitely contraindicated; if desired, it should be done after the 6–8-hour time period has elapsed.

It is estimated that with proper care, a diaphragm can last from 2 to 3 years. Manufacturer's recommendations should be adhered to regarding care of the diaphragm. The usual procedure is to wash the diaphragm with warm water and a mild soap. It should then be thoroughly dried and returned to its container. Some sources suggest dusting the diaphragm with cornstarch or an unscented talcum powder. The necessity of this beyond the cleaning procedure is open to question.

Periodically, the diaphragm should be inspected for tears, holes, or other signs of deterioration. This can be done by careful inspection of the dome and the edge where the dome and rim meet. The diaphragm can be held up to a light to detect small pinhole perforations or filled with water and observed for leaking.

At the time of the woman's annual gynecologic examination the size of the diaphragm should be reassessed. The woman should also be advised of factors that can alter diaphragm size and require refitting. The virginal woman should have her diaphragm size re-evaluated after the first few weeks of sexual relations because of a possible stretching of her vaginal muscles. A gain or loss of 15 lb or more, pelvic surgery, childbirth, or second trimester abortion all may require a change in diaphragm size.

With the diaphragm there are definite physical and psychologic contraindications. Anatomic conditions such as severe cystocele, very poor vaginal muscle tone, complete uterine prolapse, certain congenital abnormalities of the reproductive tract like vaginal septum, and use immediately postpartum before complete involution are all contraindications to the use of a diaphragm. The psychologic contraindications include the woman who is repulsed by or has an aversion to handling her genitals or self-examination. Obviously, if a woman is not able to learn proper insertion and usage techniques, another contraceptive method must be considered.

The fact that the diaphragm has few side effects may be considered its most important advantage. A rare allergic reaction to the rubber by either partner and vaginal irritation related more to the spermicide are the extent of side effects attributed to the diaphragm. Other advantages of the diaphragm are (1) only need to use it at times of anticipated or expected intercourse, (2) use can be somewhat removed from sexual act, thereby not interfering with spontaneity, (3) does not interfere with sexual sensations as neither partner should be aware of its presence, and (4) reasonable cost considering the projected 2–3 year life span of the diaphragm. Another advantage is that the diaphragm will catch menstrual flow, enabling couples to have intercourse during a woman's period if desired.

The disadvantages include (1) must be fitted by a professionally trained individual, which necessitates an office or clinic visit and raises the cost, (2) must remember to carry and have it available at all times, (3) must be used in combination with spermicide, which is objectionable to some couples because of messiness, (4) need for high motivation, and (5) possible aversion to self-examination. The effectiveness reflects in part the disadvantages of this method. The theoretic effectiveness is two to three pregnancies per 100 woman years use. In actual practice, however, this rises to 20–25 pregnancies per 100 woman years use.

Cervical Cap. The *cervical cap* is still being studied in the United States. Under the Medical Device Act of 1976, the cervical cap has been restricted by the FDA to clinical investigation studies to determine its safety and efficacy (Willis, 1981). A brief discussion of the cervical cap will be given; however, we advise you to review the literature for recent changes in status.

The cervical cap is a small thimble-shaped rubber device that fits over the cervix (Fig. 26.23). The cervical cap is held in place by suction as compared to the springs associated with the diaphragm. The instructions for use are similar to those given for the diaphragm. The cap is filled to one-third capacity with a spermicidal agent and inserted anytime before intercourse. To insert, the woman either squats or raises one leg on a chair. The cap is pushed along the posterior wall of the vagina and pressed onto the cervix with the inserting finger. It is necessary to check that the cervix is covered completely by the cap. After intercourse, the cervical cap must remain in place at least 8 hours. Douching is not recommended until after the cap is removed. The cap can be removed by grasping and tilting the rim away from the cervix to break the suction. The cap is pulled off the cervix and

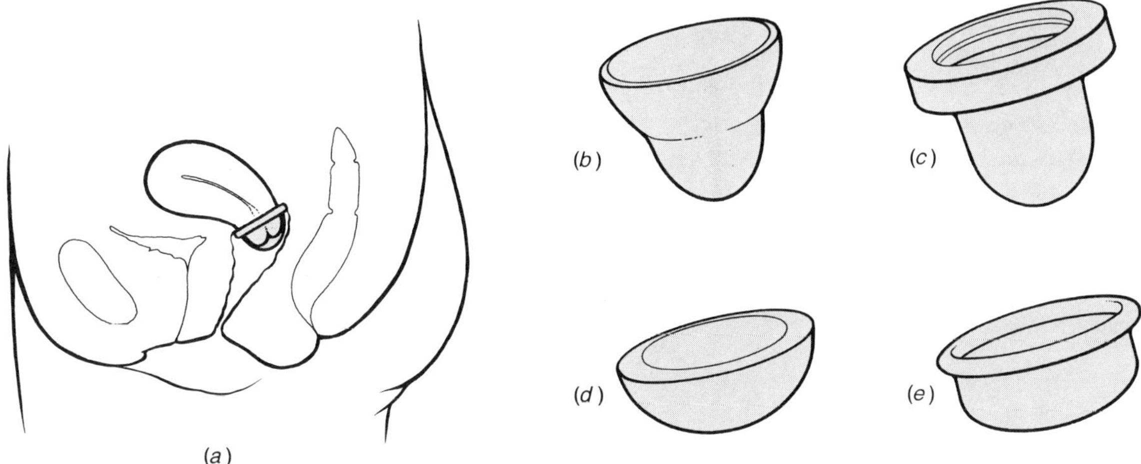

Figure 26.23
Cervical cap placement and types. (*a*) Proper position of cervical cap; (*b*) venule cap; (*c*) cervical cap; (*d*) dumas cap; (*e*) dutch cap.

out of the vagina. The cap should be washed with mild soap and water and dried thoroughly.

The advantages to the cap are: (1) it can be left in place longer than the diaphragm (several days to a complete menstrual cycle), (2) poor vaginal muscle tone is not a deterrant to the method, (3) there is no difficulty with urethra or bladder pressure, and (4) less spermicide is used, therefore there is less cost and less mess (Capiello & Grainger-Harrison, 1981). Disadvantages include (1) allergic reaction, (2) difficulty with learning insertion and removal, (3) 60–90 minutes required for initial fitting–teaching session, (4) not all women can be fitted, and (5) lack of health personnel trained in this technique (Canavan & Lewis, 1981). The effectiveness is unknown and is being investigated. The cervical cap appears to have its place in the contraceptive world; however, it is far from perfect and has some definite drawbacks.

Intrauterine Devices. The technology of *intrauterine devices* (IUD) continues to evolve as varying shapes, sizes, and combinations of materials are evaluated and judged to improve its efficacy. The present design of IUDs falls into two major categories: nonmedicated and medicated (Fig. 26.24). The Lippes Loop is the best known example of a nonmedicated device. There are two substances incorporated either on or into the medicated device that are released into the uterine environment. One substance is copper, and an example of such a device is the Copper 7 (Cu 7). The other substance used and released in the uterine cavity is progesterone, and the device is called the Progestasert. A brief description of each of these popular IUDs follows.

The *Lippes Loop* is as an S-shaped device made of flexible polyethylene plastic. This device was the first to have barium added to the plastic to allow for x-ray film detection; this concept has been incorporated into all IUDs. The Lippes Loop has a plastic string attached to the lower portion that extends from the uterine cavity out through the cervix into the vagina. The purpose of the string is to provide a way to validate the presence of the IUD and to have an easy way for removing the device. The Lippes Loop is available in four sizes identified as A, B, C, and D. The two smaller sizes, A and B, are infrequently used because of high pregnancy and expulsion rates. The C and D size Loops are suited for the parous woman but not for the nulligravida or nulliparous woman.

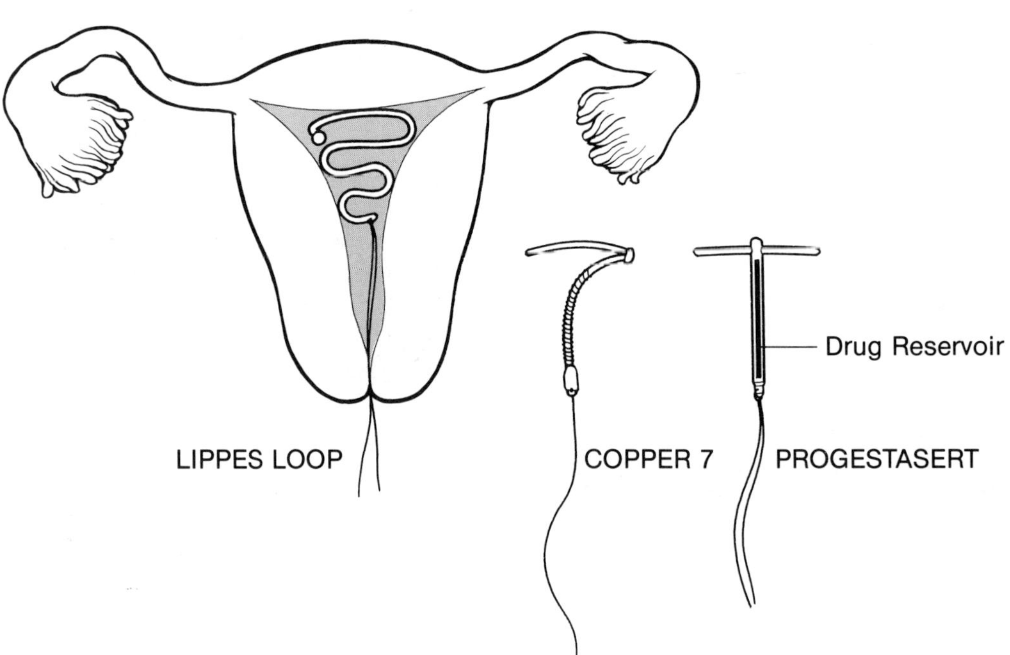

Figure 26.24
Intrauterine device. Placement and examples of the three basic types: nonmedicated, copper, and medicated.

The *Copper 7*, more commonly referred to as the Cu 7, is a polypropylene plastic device in the shape of a 7 that has a fine copper wire wrapped around the vertical arm (G. D. Searle & Co., 1977). It has a single thread attached to the vertical arm. The Cu 7 is available in one size and has been used by nulliparous women without difficulty, which is a distinct advantage over the Lippes Loop. In order for maximum efficacy, the Cu 7 must be replaced every 3 years.

The *Progestasert* is a hormone-releasing IUD in the shape of a T. The Progestasert is an ethylene/vinyl acetate copolymer (EVA), which has a drug reservoir in the vertical shaft (Alza Corp., 1976). The drug reservoir contains 38 mg of progesterone in a silicone oil base with barium for radiopacity. The EVA surrounding the drug reservoir controls the diffusion of the hormone into the uterine cavity at a rate of 65μg per day. The amount of hormone released exerts only a local effect and does not interfere with ovulation. The Progestasert must be replaced or changed annually because of a reduction in the drug reservoir. This is its major disadvantage. During a year of use, the Progestasert system delivers a total of 24 mg of progesterone. Two nylon monofilament threads extend from the base of the vertical arm.

The precise mechanism of action of IUDs is unknown, but several theories have been proposed. While no single theory explains the action, a combination of existing theories or a yet undetermined hypothesis may eventually prove to be the mode of action. The theory that seems to provide the best explanation is that of a foreign body interferring with the normal environment. The contraceptive action is the result of a local sterile inflammatory reaction caused by the presence of the foreign body in the uterus. This, in essence, promotes a bad environment which is not conducive to implantation of the ovum.

The addition of copper may cause an even greater inflammatory response. The detailed product information for the Cu 7 (Searle & Co., 1977) states the hypothesis that copper placed in the uterus interferes with normal enzyme action thereby preventing implantation of the fertilized ovum. It is also speculated that the copper may affect sperm motility and thereby exert a spermicidal effect. Two other properties that may have a significant bearing on the addition of copper to IUDs are a reduction in uterine contractility in the presence of a low concentration of copper ions and the inhibiting effect of copper on the gonococcus organism in laboratory experiments.

The progesterone-releasing IUD mechanism of action is also unknown. The theoretical considerations are (1) locally produced alterations in the endometrium interfere with sperm survival, (2) alteration of the cervical mucus blocks sperm passage or is hostile to sperm, and (3) alteration of the endometrium is nonconducive to implantation (Porter & Waife, 1978). While the theories exist regarding possible mechanism of action, further research will need to be done to confirm the precise manner in which the IUD is able to provide contraceptive control.

An IUD should not be inserted before a complete history and pelvic examination have been performed to rule out any possible contraindications. Absolute contraindications to an IUD are known or suspected pregnancy, known or suspected cervical or uterine malignancy, acute or chronic pelvic infections, history or presence of valvular heart disease, or presence of congenital malformations of the reproductive tract (particularly those affecting the uterine cavity). Relative contraindications of IUD insertion are conditions or situations that could potentially be aggravated or worsened by an IUD insertion. Women with a history of dysmenorrhea (painful menstruation), menorrhagia (heavy or excessive menstrual flow), metrorrhagia (bleeding between periods or irregular intervals), ectopic pregnancy, acute cervicitis, or anemia fall into the category of relative contraindications and require special consideration and evaluation before implementing the IUD as a contraceptive method.

Women may be advised that an IUD can be inserted at any time during the menstrual cycle. The optimal time for insertion, however, is during menstruation because you can be relatively certain that the woman is not pregnant, the cervix is softer and slightly open, and bleeding and cramps associated with the IUD insertion will be less bothersome during menstruation. Insertions can also be performed in the immediate postpartum period (first few days, no more than 4 days after delivery) or immediate postabortion period.

The equipment needed to insert an IUD includes the IUD itself, speculum, single-toothed tenaculum, sponge forceps, uterine sound, scissors, sterile gloves, antiseptic solution, and cotton balls. The actual insertion technique will vary depending on the IUD selected; however, there are basic steps that occur in all insertions. The nurse should be familiar with these steps in order to inform the woman what is going to occur, to tell her what sensations she will have, and to support her during the insertion procedure.

The vaginal speculum is inserted and the cervix is cleansed with an antiseptic solution such as benzylkonium chloride or iodine. The woman will experience a cold, wet sensation and slight pressure during the cleansing process. The cervix is then grasped with the tenaculum and gentle traction is applied to straighten the curve of the uterus. With the application of the tenaculum, the woman will experience a pinching sensation and slight pain or a cramping of the uterus. The uterine cavity is then gently sounded to determine exact depth and direction of the cavity. This will cause the uterus to contract or cramp. The IUD is loaded into the inserter using sterile technique; the inserter is then placed in the cervical canal and the IUD is deposited in the uterine cavity. The uterus may again contract causing the woman pain or discomfort. After the IUD is in place, the string is cut to an appropriate 3-cm length. The instruments are removed; pressure with a cotton ball may need to be applied to the cervix after removal of the tenaculum to control bleeding. The insertion procedure is now complete; however, it is recommended that the woman remain supine for 5–10 minutes until cramping has subsided. It is also true that some women experience faintness if they try to stand up too soon after insertion. Providing time for the body to adjust to the invasive procedure that has just been done by remaining supine will usually prevent the fainting episode.

There are side effects and complications associated with IUDs. Bleeding and pain are the most common side effects reported and are the reasons most frequently given for discontinuing the method. The insertion of an IUD will cause a change in menstrual flow for most women. It can be anticipated that menstrual bleeding will be heavier and last longer and that spotting may occur between periods. The type of IUD used will cause some variations in these changes; however, the woman should be advised to expect these changes as a general rule. The bleeding tends to be heaviest during the first three periods after insertion; it then tends to taper off.

The pain or cramping associated with the IUD is a result of the uterus contracting to expel the foreign body. As stated earlier, the woman should be forewarned that this will occur, that it will be most severe the first few minutes after insertion, that it will rapidly subside, and that it may reoccur at the time of menstruation. Pain and cramping can be minimized by gentle insertion techniques and selection of an appropriate size and type IUD. The tolerance of the discomfort can be increased by client teaching and advanced notice that this discomfort will occur. Reports of pain are most severe during the first 3 months after insertion, with decreasing symptoms and, in some cases, complete alleviation of the symptoms. A mild analgesic such as aspirin or one of the newer prostaglandin inhibitors should suffice in providing adequate relief for most women.

The complications that can occur with an IUD are expulsion, perforation, pregnancy, or pelvic infection. Expulsion is the most frequently occurring complication and obviously places the woman at greater risk for pregnancy. The contractions of the uterus can cause the IUD to be either expelled partially to the lower uterine segment and varying degrees of the cervical canal or expelled completely. Expulsions occur most often during the first 3 months; thereafter the expulsion rate declines significantly. The occurrence of IUD expulsions is directly related to the type of device, size of the device, age and parity of the woman, and skill of the person inserting the device.

The expulsion is most serious if it is not noticed by the woman. It is estimated that 20% of the explusions are not detected until a pregnancy results or a routine examination reveals the absence of IUD strings. This points out the need to teach woman to check for the IUD string, which should be done immediately after the IUD is inserted so that the woman knows what the normal or expected palpation will be. During the initial visit it is also necessary to help the woman perfect her palpation of the strings. The woman should be advised that if no string is felt, there is the possibility of complete expulsion, retraction of the string into the uterine cavity, or missed palpation of the string. If the firm plastic part of the IUD is palpated at the cervix, she may be experiencing a partial expulsion. If any of the above situations are encountered, the woman should assume that she is not protected and either refrain from intercourse or use another form of contraception until validation of IUD placement can be properly made.

The risk of uterine perforation is present with all IUD insertions. There are many factors that contribute to this, including type of device, size, technique of insertion, anatomic characteristics, and most important the skill of the practitioner performing the insertion. A careful, gentle insertion and being absolutely positive of uterine size and position will reduce the potential of perforation.

The perforation can be the result of the uterine sound or the IUD insertion. The site of perforation can vary, but the most frequent and significant type is the fundal perforation. In these cases, the IUD passes through the myometrium and is deposited in the abdominal cavity. This may happen at the time of insertion or there may be a delayed perforation. In a delayed perforation, the device has been partially inserted into the myometrium and the process is completed by uterine contractions.

The signs and symptoms of a perforation are not always clear. Sometimes a sharp severe pain at the time of insertion may be suggestive of a perforation, but the pain is certainly not conclusive. Whenever there is a missing IUD string, perforation should be considered, as well as expulsion and pregnancy. The suspicion of a perforation necessitates a thorough evaluation; the nurse should be aware of such evaluations in order to counsel and support the woman through this experience.

The steps in determining the location of the possible IUD perforation include pelvic examination, probing the cervical canal and uterine cavity, and x-ray filming. A confirmation of an IUD perforation gives rise to the issue of treatment, which is controversial. The basis of treatment will be predicated on two factors: the type of IUD and whether the woman is experiencing any symptoms. If the woman is asymptomatic and the device was a nonmedicated type, the decision to leave in place may be a realistic and appropriate choice of management as serious complications have resulted from attempting to remove a misplaced IUD. On the other hand, the copper or medicated devices that have perforated the uterine wall are best removed surgically because potential affects of the device on surrounding tissues are unknown.

Pregnancy, as with any other contraceptive control method, can occur with IUDs. The effectiveness of the IUDs is related to the type of device and the length of time the method has been used. Porter and Waife (1978) illustrate this point by providing Lippes Loop pregnancy rates as 3.2 per 100 woman years for the first year of use compared to 0.9 per 100 woman years after 6 years of continuous device use. In general, the theoretic effectiveness of IUDs is 1–3 pregnancies per 100 woman years and the actual effectiveness is 5–10 pregnancies per 100 woman years.

The prime aspect with respect to IUDs and pregnancy is the importance of removing the device in cases of suspected or confirmed pregnancy. The result of leaving the device in place can be a serious intrauterine infection, sepsis, that has led to maternal deaths in a few cases. There is also the potential of spontaneous abortion with removal of the device. The risk of spontaneous abortion is 50% in women with the device in utero as compared to 25–30% in women who have had the device removed and 10–15% in normal pregnancies. These facts along with the fact that there is a 70–75% possibility of the pregnancy going on to term should be presented to the woman. Counseling the woman regarding her choices and assisting her in making a decision about whether or not to continue the pregnancy is an intricate role and responsibility of the nurse.

Last and perhaps the most serious complication associated with IUDs is pelvic inflammatory disease (PID) or pelvic infection. Recent studies have demonstrated that the type of IUD and the length of time used are significant factors related to infection rates in IUD users. Women using the nonmedicated devices have a significant increase of risk of infection as compared to women using the copper devices (Duguid et al. 1980). The degree of infection may range from a mild pelvic infection to severe PID with tubo-ovarian abscess. The symptomatology will vary according to the extent of the infection. General symptoms of fever, lower abdominal tenderness or pain, pelvic tenderness and pain, and dyspareunia in IUD users should warrant a more thorough examination, possible removal of the IUD, and treatment with appropriate antibiotics. The responsibility of family planning personnel to advise women of the potential complications of IUDs and the associated symptoms is paramount so that when necessary, women can seek immediate medical care and therapy can be instituted without delay.

Some aspects of client education have been incorporated into the discussion of side effects and complications. Other aspects of client education are elaborated upon here. During the initial visit, after the IUD has been inserted, the woman should be taught how to check the IUD string, making sure she performs the procedure successfully before leaving the medical facility (Fig. 26.25). The steps

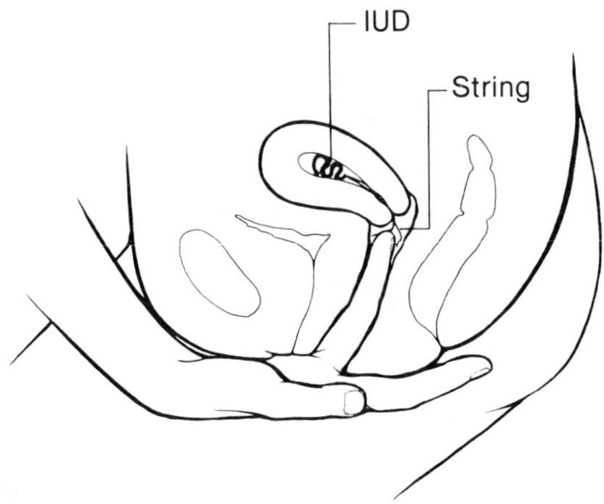

Figure 26.25
Woman checking placement of IUD by inserting middle finger in vagina and palpating strings of IUD coming from cervical canal.

for checking the placement of the IUD and palpation of the strings are (1) wash your hands and assume a squatting, sitting, or one leg elevated position; (2) insert your index or middle finger deep into the vagina locating the cervix (the cervix feels like the tip of the nose); (3) feel for the strings that should be protruding from the cervical os (note that you do not feel any of the rigid or firm plastic part of the IUD). This procedure provides the woman with a baseline normalcy to compare with checks she will perform at home. There is no set frequency or time for checking for the strings. However, it is advisable for women to check at least once every 1–2 weeks during the first 3 months when the expulsion rate is at its peak. Thereafter, the woman should check for IUD placement and string palpation after each menstrual period. If the woman palpates anything out of the ordinary, she should seek medical advice and use an alternate contraceptive method until confirmation of IUD placement is made. In line with the high expulsion rates in the first 3 months, the woman may be advised to use foam or condoms during this time for added protection against pregnancy. Some couples have incorporated the checking of IUD strings as part of foreplay in lovemaking. The use of tampons or douching is not contraindicated for IUD users.

Yearly examinations should include a Pap smear and IUD check. The Cu 7 and Progestasert will need to be replaced every 3 years and 1 year, respectively. The woman should be advised of the side effects and complications and the actions to be taken by her in case of their occurrences. It should be restressed that if pregnancy occurs, removal of the device must be performed without delay to ensure the health of the woman.

When the decision is made to discontinue the use of the IUD, the removal will need to be performed by skilled medical personnel. As with the insertion, the most advantageous time for removal is during a menstrual period; however, this is not essential. The removal is usually a simple procedure involving a speculum examination. The string of the IUD is grasped with a sponge forcep or other similar instrument, and with steady firm traction, the IUD is removed. The woman may experience some cramping during the removal procedure and some spotting for a day or two after if she is not already having menstrual flow.

The advantages of the IUD are: (1) once inserted no contraceptive concern or thought is needed before intercourse, (2) the IUD can be used for a number of years without adverse effects, and (3) once inserted there is not a high level of contraceptive motivation required. The disadvantages are: (1) self-examination for string check may be objectionable to some women, (2) side effects and complications as previously outlined are a significant factor, (3) a specially trained person must perform the procedure, and (4) the cost of the device, including a fee for the examination and insertion, is usually high.

HORMONAL METHODS

The *hormonal contraceptive methods* include those methods that arise from a basic understanding of the male and female physiologic reproductive cycles, (see Chapters 4 and 5). There are male oral contraceptives that are in the research phase of development. It is hoped that they will prove to be safe, effective, and acceptable and without many side effects. The existing methods, however, are for female use and are commonly referred to as *oral contraceptives* (OCs) or *the pill.* The two basic types of OCs are the combined pills and the minipills. Each of the combined pills contains a form of two synthetic hormones—estrogen and progestin—in varying dosages. The minipills contain only small doses of synthetic progestational substances.

The mechanism of action of oral contraceptives is to (1) inhibit ovulation, (2) alter the endometrium, and (3) effect changes in the cervical mucus.

The inhibition of ovulation occurs by interfering with the normal hypothalamic–pituitary–ovarian axis (Chapter 5). Estrogen suppresses the follicle-stimulating hormone (FSH), most likely at the hypothalamic level. This suppression causes a failure of the follicle to develop and be extruded on a monthly basis. The progestin component allows the release of the luteninizing hormone (LH). The effect on the endometrium is related to the progestin by causing premature maturation of the glandular epithelium (Chez, 1976). In addition, the action of the synthetic progesterone causes the perpetuation of the hostile-type cervical mucus (type G) that is resistant to sperm penetration and that normally occurs during the second half of the menstrual cycle.

The combined OCs attempt to mimic the natural hormonal and uterine responses but block the ovarian response by preventing ovulation. The minipills (progestin only) do not necessarily inhibit ovulation, but they do have an affect on the endometrium and the cervical mucus. The fact that ovulation is not suppressed limits the usefulness of the minipill to those people who have experienced estrogen-related problems in the combined OCs but wish to continue using a hormonal form of contraception.

There are approximately 20 combined and three minipill brands of OCs available in the United States. Table 26.2 lists some minipills used today. Both the minipills and the combined pills contain one of five progestin compounds: norethindrone, norethindrone acetate, norgestrel, ethynodiol diacetate, or norethynodrel. The estrogenic, androgenic, and progestational effects vary from one brand to another according to the particular progestin incorporated into the OC. The combined pills are composed of one of the five progestins mentioned, as well as one of two synthetic estrogens—mestranol and ethinyl estradiol. The dosage of the synthetic estrogen varies according to the brand; it is either 20, 30, 35, 50, 80, or 100μg. Those pills containing 50μg of synthetic estrogen are presently the most commonly prescribed. The recent thoughts regarding potency of these two estrogenic compounds is that they are equivalent (Chez, 1976).

TABLE 26.2
MINIPILLS AND PROGESTIN COMPOUND

Minipills	*Progestin Compounds (mg)*
Micronor	Norethindrone 0.35
Nor-Q.D.	Norethindrone acetate 0.35
Ovrette	Norgestrel 0.75

Table 26.3 lists some of the more common brands of combined pills with their estrogen and progestin compounds. It is important to note the differences in compounds and dosages used in these brands. Another important aspect to note is in those brands that are followed by a fraction, that is, Ortho-Novum 1/80, the numerator refers to the dosage of the progestin while the denominator refers to the dosage of the estrogen.

Knowledge about the estrogenic and progestational compounds is important to the clinician prescribing the pills and to the nurse when counseling women regarding their choice of oral contra-

TABLE 26.3
COMBINED PILLS WITH PROGESTIN ESTROGEN TYPE AND DOSAGE

Pill	*Progestin (mg)*	*Estrogen (μg)*
Brevicon	Norethindrone 0.5	Ethinyl estradiol 35
Enovid E	Norethynodrel 2.5	Mestranol 100
Loestrin 1/20	Norethindrone acetate 1.0	Ethinyl estradiol 20
Ortho-Novum 1/80	Norethindrone 1.0	Mestranol 80
Ovral	Norgestrel 0.5	Ethinyl estradiol 50

ceptives and when advising women who are experiencing side effects from a pill, which may be alleviated by changing the estrogen/progestin ratio.

The contraindications for the use of OCs can be broken down into absolute and relative. The absolute contraindications are (1) thrombophlebitits or thromboemoblic disorders (past or present history), (2) cerebral vascular or coronary artery disease (past or present history), (3) carcinoma of the breast or reproductive system (known or suspected), (4) estrogen-dependent neoplasia (known or suspected), (5) pregnancy (known or suspected), (6) undiagnosed abnormal vaginal bleeding, and (7) impaired liver function or history of hepatitis. The relative contraindications are (1) hypertension, (2) migraine headaches, (3) diabetes—family history, gestational history, or present history, (4) past or present history of any cardiac, breast, renal, gallbladder, or thyroid disease, (5) depression, (6) lactation, (7) asthma, (8) epilepsy, (9) varicose veins, (10) chloasma, (11) sickle cell disease or trait, (12) acute phase of mononucleosis, (13) extreme obesity, and (14) surgery scheduled within 4 weeks. The list of relative contraindications is rather extensive, and a thorough history and complete examination

TABLE 26.4
MAJOR ORAL CONTRACEPTIVE SIDE EFFECTS AS RELATED TO HORMONAL ALTERATIONS

Estrogen Excess	*Progestin Excess*
Nausea/vomiting	Tiredness/fatigue
Headaches	Depression
Fluid retention (breast, pelvic extremities)	Breast tenderness
	Decreased libido
Hypertension	Hypertension
Weight gain	Weight gain
Irritability	Acne
Chloasma	Amenorrhea
Estrogen Deficiency	*Progestin Deficiency*
Early cycle bleeding	Late cycle bleeding
Decreased libido	
Nervousness/irritability	
	Androgen Effects
	Increased libido
	Acne
	Hirsutism

of any woman would be necessary before initiating the OC method. A woman with any of the relative contraindications should be told about the increased risks and advised to consider the use of contraceptive methods other than the pill.

The side effects of OCs are attributed to either an excess or a deficiency of estrogen or progestin and often mimic symptoms that occur in women premenstrually or during pregnancy or that accompany other gynecologic disorders. Given these facts, it is obvious that the potential side effects are quite numerous. The development of any undetermined symptom in a woman taking oral contraceptives probably can be attributed to a side effect of the OCs. The major reported side effects are nausea, depression, weight gain, headache, and irregular bleeding. These tend to manifest themselves most frequently during the first 3 months of hormonal therapy and diminish significantly if not completely thereafter. If symptoms persist beyond 3 months, an alteration or change of pills is probably necessary. Table 26.4 gives a more complete listing of side effects according to the suspected hormonal problem.

While there is a general consensus that certain symptoms are a result of an excess or a deficiency of a particular hormone, it is also true that the symptom of deficiency in one woman may be the symptom of excess in another woman because of variations in hormone production and metabolism. Because of all of these variables, we suggest that you refer to a pharmacologic text for complete details of OC side effects.

The relationship of OCs to severe complications such as thrombophlebitis, cancer, or myocardial infarcts remains controversial. A survey by the Royal College of General Practitioners reported in *Population Reports* (1975) identified increased incidences in urinary tract infections, hypertension, gallbladder disease, superficial and deep thrombosis of the leg, chloasma and cardiovascular disease among OC users as compared to non-OC users. Despite this report, *Current Concepts in Contraceptive Treatment* (1980) states that there is no validity or correlation between OCs and monilia vaginitis, cancer, infertility, delayed menopause, or impaired growth in teenage users. While there are studies to support a definite risk for thromboembolism and cerebrovascular problems, there are other studies that have found no actual increased incidence of these conditions in pill users compared to controls.

There is an increased risk factor for women who

are OC users and are over 35 and are cigarette smokers. The combination of heavy cigarette smoking and OCs leads to an increased risk of cardiovascular problems, mainly heart attacks and strokes. There is, however, no reported increased risk of cardiovascular problems to OC users who are nonsmokers, regardless of age. The studies, therefore, support the fact that smoking is hazardous to your health when not taking oral contraceptives. However, in women between the ages of 35 and 40 other risk factors such as diabetes and hypertension may contribute to myocardial infarctions when combined with OCs. Therefore, the general trend is to discontinue use of OCs in women when they become 40 years old. With all of the conflicting reports and data, the nurse counseling women in the method of contraceptive control should advise them that there may be increased risk of diseases such as thrombophlebitis, cholelithiasis, hypertension, and myocardial infarctions, even though the data supporting this are very controversial.

The physiologic advantages to OCs are (1) regulation of menses, (2) decrease in menstrual flow (periods of shorter duration and scantier flow), (3) decrease in endometriosis, and (4) reduction of dysmenorrhea (painful menstruation). If a woman desires contraception, as well as relief from dysmenorrhea, oral contraceptives could be an appropriate choice (Goodwin, 1980). The fact that taking the pill is unrelated to the act of intercourse is a definite advantage. Other advantages are (1) no messiness, (2) no interference with foreplay, (3) no periods of abstinence, and (4) no fear of device expulsion. The oral contraceptive pill is essentially 100% effective when used properly. In clinical use, however, there is a failure rate of 4 to 10 pregnancies per 100 woman years of use.

The disadvantages are the numerous side effects and potential complications previously mentioned. The need to have a complete physical examination before obtaining a prescription for the pills necessitates preplanning the implementation of this method. Some women have difficulty taking pills or remembering to take them as scheduled. In all situations even when intercourse is infrequent, the oral contraceptives *must* be taken daily as directed in order to be effective when needed.

The nurse's role in client instructions can greatly enhance the effectiveness of this method since the majority of failures are a result of human error in not adhering to the proper method of pill taking.

Client teaching should include the proper method for taking the pill, what to do in case of missed pills, and information about warning signs and potential side effects and complications (Fig. 26.26). The oral contraceptives are available in 21- or 28-day pill packages. The recommended day of starting oral contraceptive pills is on a Sunday. If the woman is just beginning OCs, she would start on the Sunday following the beginning of her menstrual flow. If she is postabortion, she would start on the Sunday immediately after the procedure. If she is postpartum, she would start on the Sunday nearest the 2 weeks postdelivery date.

Oral contraceptive pills must be taken everyday of the prescribed days (21 or 28) at approximately the same time each day. For women on a 21-day pill cycle, the pill is taken each day for 3 weeks

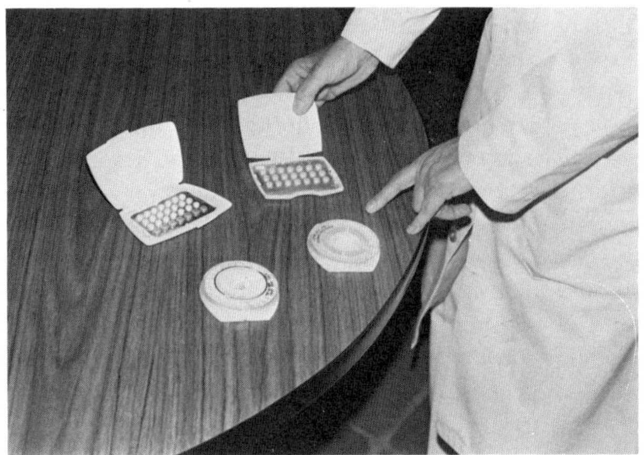

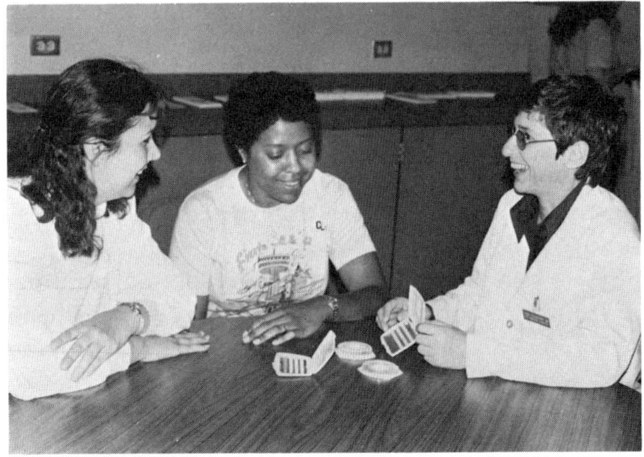

Figure 26.26
Oral contraceptive counseling. *Top:* Packaging of 21-day and 28-day pill cycles. *Bottom:* Nurse teaching about use of oral contraceptives.

and then no pills are taken for 1 week. The next package of pills will be started on a Sunday, 1 week after completing the previous package of pills. A woman on the 28-day pill cycle must take a pill everyday for 28 days (21 contraceptive pills plus 7 placebo pills). Upon completion of one pack of pills, she immediately begins the next pack on the following day. It should be emphasized that an OC pill is taken everyday as prescribed regardless of what is happening in the menstrual cycle. Even if there is breakthrough bleeding or spotting, the pill should always be taken.

The OC pill should be kept in a safe place. The woman may set up a daily reminder procedure for taking the pill. Some women place a note on the bathroom mirror, others put the pills with their toothbrush or makeup. The pill should be taken at approximately the same time each day. This helps to develop a routine and to maintain a more consistent hormonal level in the body. The actual time of day for taking the pill is not important. The woman may combine it with an already established morning routine such as taking a vitamin tablet. A suggestion for the woman who has no established routine may be to consider the evening hour. The reason for this is that side effects such as nausea are less bothersome if they occur while the woman is sleeping. They are usually not of such a severity as to disturb the sleep cycle and hence go unnoticed.

Follow-up appointments usually are requested for 3 months, 6 months, and 1 year. It is very important to evaluate the body's response, if any, to the pills. These follow-up visits also allow for early detection of side effects or complications. The woman should be advised to report any unusual pain in her legs, chest, head, or abdomen immediately. Alterations in visual perceptions (blurred vision) are also of major importance. Any minor symptoms such as nausea or breakthrough bleeding that persists for more than three cycles should be reported.

If a woman is on OCs for any period of time, she is apt to forget to take the pill on at least one occasion. Therefore, it is most important to provide verbal and perhaps written instructions for what to do in such cases. If one pill is missed, it should be taken as soon as the woman remembers. The next pill should be taken at the regular time. If remembering the forgotten pill coincides with the time for taking the next pill, two pills should be taken to resume the normal schedule. Forgetting one pill and then taking it in this manner is not likely to result in a pregnancy.

If two pills are missed consecutively, the woman may not be protected from becoming pregnant. In order to maintain her cycle, the forgotten pills should be taken when remembered and the remainder of the pills should be taken according to schedule. In addition, the woman should be instructed to use some other form of contraception (foams, condoms) for the remainder of the cycle and to anticipate the occurrence of breakthrough bleeding. If three or more pills are missed and intercourse has been happening at regular intervals, there is potential for pregnancy. An alternate form of contraception should be used until a menstrual period has started; then a new package of pills may be initiated on the Sunday after the beginning of menstrual flow. The woman who is frequently forgetting to take her pills should be re-evaluated; the nurse may suggest that she is an unsuitable candidate for effective use of the pill and that another method may be more effective. As with all other methods of contraception, the woman or couple must weigh the benefits of the method against the potential risks or hazards and decide if oral contraception is the method of choice.

PERMANENT METHODS

The permanent methods of contraceptive control result in sterilization of the person for the remainder of his or her reproductive life. While the technology of microsurgery and tubal surgery is advancing, sterilization procedures are for all practical purposes considered irreversible and should not be performed if there is any question regarding future desires of childbearing. The surgical procedures for female and male sterilization do have a very small failure rate (0.1–0.2%). The failures are attributed to natural reanastomosis of the tubes or technique or technician failure. The only absolutely guaranteed method for contraception and sterilization is for the woman to have a *hysterectomy*. This procedure involves the removal of the uterus, cervix, and, if indicated, the ovaries. This surgical procedure will not be dealt with because it is not the procedure of choice if sterilization is the only indication.

The number of couples opting for permanent sterilization methods is increasing. In 1972 it was reported that permanent methods were the most commonly used methods of fertility control among married couples over 30 years of age (Martin, 1978). The choice of sterilization is not only being made by couples who have achieved their desired family size but also by couples and single people who do not desire to have any children.

These facts point out the need for appropriate and thorough counseling services to be available for couples or individuals embarking on this decision. Nurses traditionally have assumed a major role in counseling for all contraceptive methods including permanent methods. Couples should be assisted in investigating and evaluating all available alternatives. The technique for sterilization should be accurately presented in terms the couple can understand, potential problems should be discussed, and the advantages and disadvantages should be reviewed. The decision of the couple should be supported if there are no contradictory or ambivalent reasons.

The general advantage of sterilization methods is that the procedure need only be done once to achieve the desired contraceptive control. The surgical procedure does not in any way affect the sexual desires. Some couples report greater relaxation and enjoyment with intercourse poststerilization because the fear of an unwanted pregnancy is removed completely. The procedure is permanent.

The disadvantage is that it is a surgical procedure with certain inherent risk. Once performed, the effect is nonreversible and the result is sterility. Some people have emotional difficulty accepting the end result of permanent sterility. Further advantages and disadvantages related to the specific female or male sterilization procedure are given below.

Female Sterilization. All of the procedures used for female *sterilization* or fertility management involve either the obstruction, blocking, or cutting of the fallopian tubes. There are several surgical procedures that can be performed to accomplish the desired result: laparotomy, laparoscopy, colpotomy, and culdoscopy. In the United States, laparoscopy is the principal technique followed by laparotomy (Richart, 1977). Colpotomy and culdoscopy, while not used in the United States, are highly effective and safe methods that leave no abdominal scar. In comparison to other methods, colpotomy has a higher rate of intraperitoneal infection (Brenner & Edelman, 1976).

The procedure for colpotomy or culdoscopy involves an incision of the posterior fornix (cul-de-sac of Douglas, or pouch of Douglas). In a *colpotomy*, the fallopian tubes are visualized, grasped with Babcock forceps, and delivered into the vagina. At this point, the tubes can be ligated and dissected. The tubes are then replaced in the peritoneal cavity and the colpotomy incision is repaired. The technique of *culdoscopy* requires the use of a culdoscope inserted through the incision made in the posterior fornix of the vagina. Through this instrument, the fallopian tubes are visualized and occluded by cautery, dissection, or the application of a blocking device.

The technique of *laparotomy* has been widely used for many years and is still the procedure of choice for immediate postpartum sterilization. An adaptation of this procedure is the minilaparotomy, or as it is commonly called, the minilap. In the minilap procedure, a small suprapubic incision (2.5–3.0 cm long) is made, which allows direct visualization of the fallopian tubes. This simplified procedure can be performed with local anesthesia on an outpatient basis (*Population Reports*, 1974). The occlusion of the tubes can be accomplished by a modified Pomeroy operation, which is the most frequently used method. In Pomeroy's operation, the tubes are grasped and brought out through the incision, a ligature is applied to the base of a loop of tube and the top of the loop is cut off. However, the more recent methods of tubal occlusion, including spring-loaded clips and silastic bands are also suitable for use in the minilap procedure (Brenner & Dingfelder, 1976).

The laparoscopy method uses the laparoscope, which is inserted through a small incision made in the folds of lower aspect of the umbilical area (Fig. 26.27). The procedure originated as a two-incision technique (one suprapubic, one umbilical), but it is now more commonly performed as a single-incision procedure. This method of sterilization has been referred to as the "Band-Aid" method because the extent of the surgical dressing is simply a "Band-Aid." The procedure can be performed on an outpatient basis, which significantly reduces the cost as compared to a laparotomy. In laparoscopic sterilization, the abdomen is generally inflated with carbon dioxide or nitrous oxide causing a pneumoperitoneum. The procedure has also been accomplished without this step. Next, the laparoscope is introduced and the tubes are identified. As previously described under minilap, the occlusion and/or division of the tubes can be accomplished by cauterization or the application of a

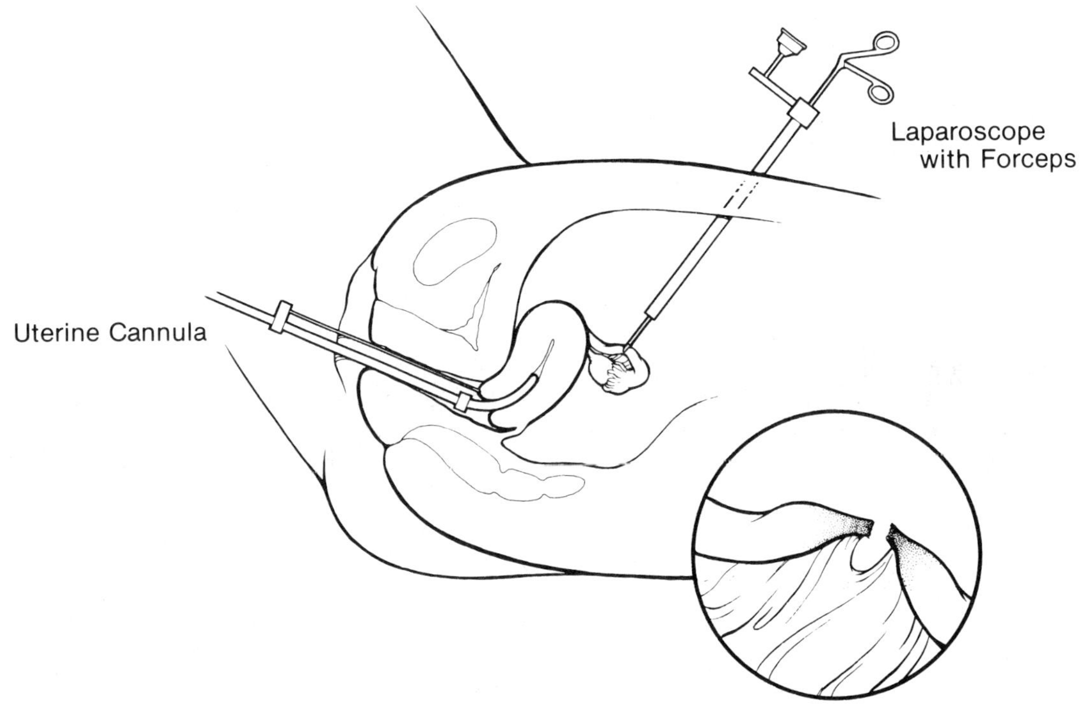

Figure 26.27
Laparoscopy sterilization. One-incision technique. Insert shows tube after cauterization and division.

spring-loaded clip or silastic band or ring. While the complication rate is low, serious complications can and do occur. Complications include bowel burns (with cautery method), bowel perforations, infection, hemorrhage, and anesthesia complications. In addition, there appear to be some side effects of the procedure; some women report the development of gynecologic problems such as dysmenorrhea, menorrhagia, and premenstrual syndrome poststerilization. The physiologic correlation between the development of these symptoms and the sterilization procedure is unknown.

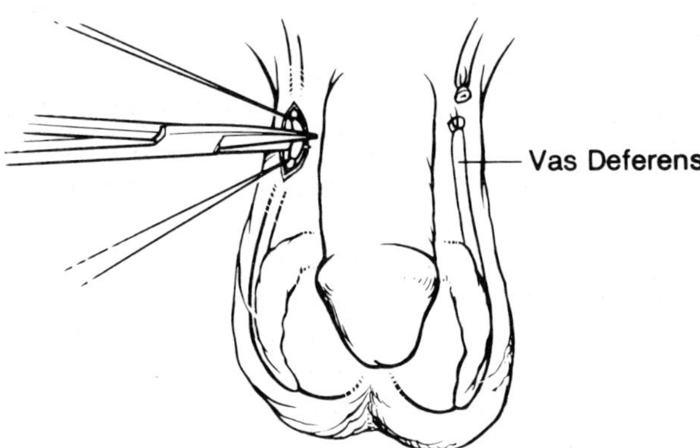

Figure 26.28
Procedure for vasectomy. Each vas deferens is located, ligated, and divided. Scrotal incisions are repaired.

All of the female sterilization procedures are surgical procedures, which can be said to be relatively safe and simple. The postoperative care of these women is basically the same as with other surgical procedures; however, the recovery time is shorter. The nurse must emphasize the need for follow-up care and be available for future counseling.

Male Sterilization. *Vasectomy* is the surgical procedure that results in male sterility by preventing sperm from entering the seminal fluid. According to *Population Reports* (1975), it is one of the simplest, least expensive, safest, and most satisfactory methods of fertility management. The surgical procedure can be performed in a physician's office or clinic setting.

The basic steps in the vasectomy procedure include the following (Fig. 26.28). First, there is a bilateral local infiltration of the scrotum approximately 2 cm below the base of the penis. A small incision is made over the vas deferens on each side of the scrotum. The vas is lifted out and occluded by the application of ligatures and cautery. A portion of the vas is then removed and the cut ends are retracted into the scrotum. The scrotal incisions are then closed. Other techniques that have been used for occluding the vas deferens are clips, silicone plugs, and polyethylene tubing with a stopcock device designed for potential reversibility.

Postoperative instructions should include the following information: (1) apply ice for approximately 4–6 hours, (2) use an athletic support for about 1 week, (3) resume intercourse usually within 1 week, (4) use an alternate form of contraceptive control until there have been at least two semen analysis reports of azoospermia, (5) time required to achieve azoospermia is approximately 4–6 weeks depending on frequency of sexual activity, (6) have follow-up semen analyses at 6 months and 1 year, (7) minor discomforts including skin discoloration, swelling, and pain can occur, (8) a mild analgesic such as aspirin is usually all that is required to alleviate postoperative pain, (9) the potential for complications such as hematoma, infection, sperm granulomas, and recanalization are generally considered to occur on the average of 1%.

There does not appear to be any long-term side effects associated with vasectomy. The ability to engage in sexual activity is not altered, although a very small percentage of men have reported a decrease in sexual pleasure following vasectomy (Martin, 1978).

The nurse should be able to explain the vasectomy procedure, give detailed client instructions, and advise the couple about the signs and symptoms of complications and the basic treatment necessary to alleviate any problems. The counseling that is performed by nurses regarding contraceptive control necessitates a thorough understanding of sexuality and the absence of any discomfort when discussing these matters. This approach will enable the couples or individuals to relax and to discuss their concerns more thoroughly.

The research goes on for the development of the ideal contraceptive and for newer and improved methods of contraceptive control. While the search continues, the shortcomings of the existing contraceptive methods will raise concerns among prospective users, cause consumers to reject the various options, and result in failures and cause unwanted pregnancies. It must be remembered that these failures are not always the result of user error. So long as there is not a perfect method of fertility management, the need for induced abortion will continue to exist.

INDUCED ABORTION

Termination of pregnancy by other than natural means is referred to as *induced abortion*, previously termed *therapeutic abortion*. In cases of unwanted pregnancies, women have chosen to remove the products of conception (fetus, fluid, membranes, and placenta). While a pregnancy may have occurred as a chance happening, as a contraceptive failure, or as a result of rape or incest, the availability of induced abortion is viewed as a means of contraception or fertility control.

The liberalization of abortion laws has resulted in a significant rise in the number of legal abortions and, conversely, a decline in the number of illegal abortions. The problem of septic abortion is almost unheard of, with corresponding decrease in mortality. The birth rate along with the number of illegitimate births have declined since changes in abortion laws.

Despite the beneficial effects that can be attributed to the liberalization of abortion laws, the social, moral, political, legal, and emotional controversies surrounding induced abortion continue. No one can predict what turn of events will occur in the future. The fact that woman's freedom of choice is being threatened raises concerns and we recognize that there are many sides to the dilemma of induced abortion. Induced abortion will be addressed here from the standpoint of the medical procedures involved and the nursing implications appropriate for each procedure.

The preabortion workup involves both physical and counseling aspects. The woman usually seeks care when she either suspects or realizes that she is pregnant. The woman's first experience with the health systems should be a history and complete gynecologic examination in order to diagnose and determine the size of the pregnancy. The Pap smear and GC culture gynecologic laboratory tests should be performed. Once the pregnancy is confirmed and the woman's decision is firm regarding an abortion, additional laboratory tests including hematocrit, Rh typing, and VDRL should be obtained. If the woman is Rh negative, regardless of the weeks gestation, Rhogam should be provided postabortion unless there are contraindications for its use.

Once the pregnancy is verified, the counseling component is the major focus. Nurses can assume the role of primary counselor and explore the available alternatives and provide information about the types of abortions. Many women have already made a decision regarding the best option for them before seeking health care. Even though a woman's decision may appear final, the nurse should make sure that she has examined all options carefully and that there is no underlying ambivalence in her decision. The alternatives available to a woman with an unwanted pregnancy are (1) to terminate the pregnancy by abortion, (2) to continue the pregnancy and keep the baby, or (3) to continue the pregnancy and place the baby up for adoption. The woman should be helped to explore each option and the implications that option would have on her present life situation and future plans. The option to have or not to have an abortion should always be a matter of free choice made by the woman. Regardless of the type of abortion, the woman must be informed and sign appropriate consent forms.

The counseling should be supportive, nonjudgmental, and informative. It should stress the importance of making a decision as early as possible because delays in obtaining an abortion increase the complexity of the procedure and the inherent risks. While the counselor or nurse is supportive of the woman's decision to have an abortion, emphasis is placed on postabortion contraception or sterilization as the preferred method of contraception control.

Types of Abortion Techniques

The types of abortion can be categorized into those that are primarily used during the first trimester and those that are used during the second trimester. The first trimester abortion procedures are menstrual extractions and dilatation and evacuation. The second trimester abortion techniques are intra-amniotic prostaglandin $F_{2\alpha}$, intra-amniotic hypertonic saline, and hysterotomy.

MENSTRUAL EXTRACTION

The procedure of *menstrual extraction* (ME) is also referred to as *menstrual regulation* (MR), *menstrual induction,* or *endometrial aspiration.* Regardless of the terminology, the procedure is essentially the same. The procedure is performed on women who are 5–7 weeks from their last menstrual period. It is a relatively simple and safe procedure that is performed in an office or clinic setting. A pelvic examination is performed to comfirm that the uterine size is compatible with dates and the position of the uterus. The technique involves the insertion of a vaginal speculum and the cleansing of the cervix and vagina with an antiseptic solution (Fig. 26.29). The anterior lip of the cervix is grasped with an atraumatic tenaculum. This usually causes the woman a brief painful sensation of which she should be forewarned. In some circumstances, a paracervical block using 1% lidocaine would be administered. However, a benefit of this early ME technique is that it can be performed without anesthesia as dilatation of the cervix is not required. A 5- or 6-mm flexible polyethylene cannula is inserted into the uterine cavity. The 5-mm cannula can be inserted in the nulliparous cervix and the 6-mm cannula can be readily inserted in the majority of parous women. The suction is provided by an especially adapted 50-cc syringe that has a release valve and extension on the plunger to maintain the suction. The plunger is withdrawn, the suction is created, and the cannula attached to the syringe is inserted into the uterine cavity. The release valve is opened and the contents of the uterine cavity are suctioned into the syringe as it is moved back and forth and rotated. The procedure will be completed in approximately 5 minutes when the grating sensation of the myometrium is appreciated by the examiner. The technique will cause the woman varying degrees of cramping, which is most intense toward the end of the procedure. The cramping usually subsides or completely disappears within 10–15 minutes of the procedure. The pretreatment explanation should alert the woman to the occurrence of this discomfort. The application of a heat lamp immediately after the procedure provides significant relief of cramping. The woman should remain supine for approximately 10 minutes to avoid a vasovagal response and fainting. If cramping persists, a mild analgesic (such as aspirin) may be taken and is usually all

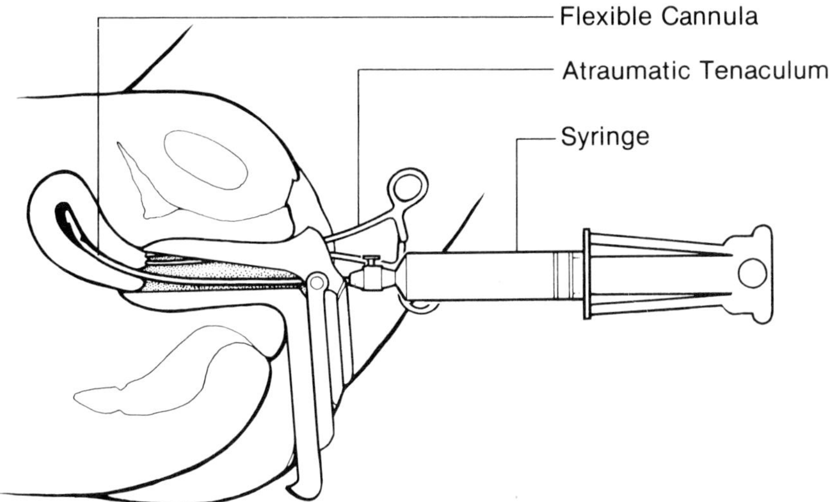

Figure 26.29
Menstrual extraction procedure for early, first trimester abortion.

that is necessary. The woman should be advised to expect bleeding no heavier than a menstrual period for no more than 5–7 days; however, light and occasional spotting may persist for 2–4 weeks.

The use of a flexible cannula essentially eliminates the serious complications of uterine perforation. This is a definite advantage and supports the premise that the earlier the abortion procedure is performed, the safer the technique. Other advantages include the ease of the procedure without dilatation or anesthesia, the short time required to complete the procedure, the fact that it can be done in an outpatient setting, with no recovery time required, and the low percentage of complications.

The procedure, while safe and easy, is not without minimal complications. The complications of infection, hemorrhage, and failure to abort the pregnancy are the same for all abortion techniques, but the incidence or rate of occurrence increases with the gestational age of the pregnancy. In the ME procedure, the incidence of complications is in the range of 1–3%. The major disadvantage to this procedure is that because of problems in accurately diagnosing pregnancy at this early stage, a proportion of women will be subjected to an essentially unnecessary procedure with all its risks, inconveniences, and discomforts.

Before leaving the setting, the woman is counseled in contraceptive methods, told when to initiate the chosen method, and informed about the signs and symptoms of complications. A follow-up examination is scheduled for 2 weeks. At this time, a pregnancy test is performed to evaluate the return to normalcy or the possibility of a failed procedure and the need for a repeat ME or a dilatation and evacuation.

DILATATION AND EVACUATION

Dilatation and evacuation (D&E), also called *vacuum curettage* or *suction curettage,* is the most frequently used technique of abortion up to 12-weeks gestation. As with the ME procedure, the D&E accomplishes the abortion by means of a cannula inserted into the uterine cavity and a suction source. After the preliminary pelvic examination is performed, a vaginal speculum is used to expose the cervix. The cleansing procedure is the same as for ME. Because of the size of the pregnancy, the cervix will need to be dilated, requiring a paracervical block before initiating dilatation. A single-toothed tenaculum is used to grasp the cervix and stabilize it during anesthesia and dilatation. The cervix is then progressively dilated with Hegar's or Pratt's dilators to a diameter that is equivalent to the number of weeks gestation and that will accept the cannula (vacurette) size that is also equivalent to the weeks gestation (Fig. 26.30). The vacurette used in a D&E procedure are rigid plastic cannulae sizes 8, 9, 10, 11, and 12 mm. The vacurette acts as a curette and is inserted into the uterine cavity, and the electronically operated vacuum pump is switched

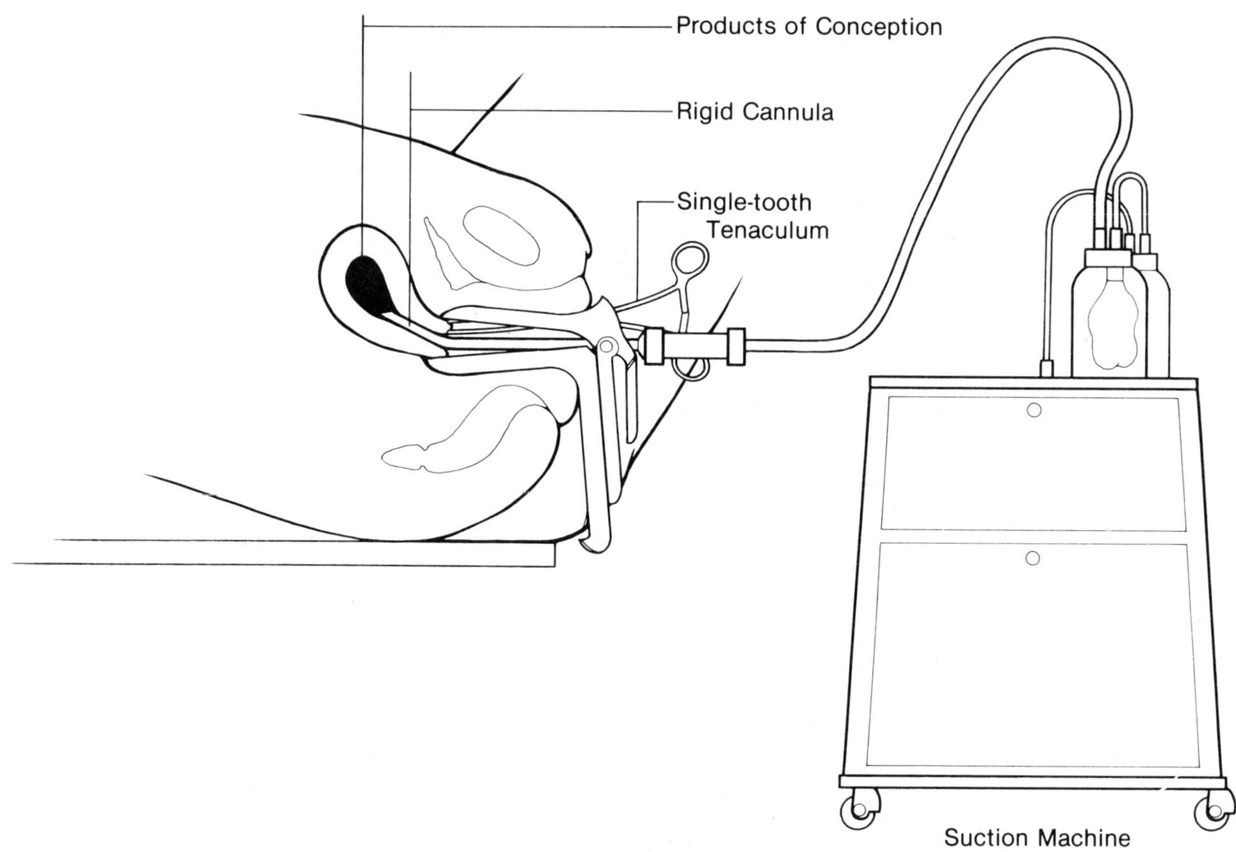

Figure 26.30
Dilatation and evacuation. Equipment and procedure for late, first trimester abortion.

on. The vacurette is moved up and down from the fundus to the internal os and rotated 360 degrees until the grating sensation of the myometrium is perceived. A sharp curette can be used postsuctioning to check the completeness of the evacuation. The majority of the procedures are completed in 15 minutes.

The woman will experience a needle stick and a stinging sensation as the lidocaine is administered. The dilatation process will cause cramping and may be painful. With the initiation of the suction, cramping will increase and peak to maximum intensity near the end of the procedure. Cramping usually subsides within 15 minutes after completion of the procedure. The treatment of heat application and mild analgesics is appropriate nursing intervention.

The D&E is performed as an outpatient procedure with the woman being observed for approximately 30 minutes to 1 hour after completion of the procedure. If after 30 minutes the woman's condition is stabilized, cramping has diminished or subsided, and bleeding is within normal limits, the woman may return home. Before leaving the setting, appropriate postabortion instructions and contraceptive information should be provided. Postabortion instructions after D&E include no douching, use of tampons, or intercourse until after the 2-week follow-up examination.

The complication rate increases threefold from that given for ME. The risk of perforation is greater because of the need for dilatation and the use of a rigid cannula (8–9%). The necessity of anesthesia raises additional risks. Infection and excessive bleeding caused by an incomplete evacuation of the products of conception also appear more frequently.

The side effects of the procedure include bleeding similar to a normal menstrual period for approximately 1 week and light spotting that may continue for as long as 3–4 weeks. Mild cramping may continue for 24–48 hours after the procedure, requiring the use of mild analgesics every 4–6 hours. Other than what has been mentioned, the woman can anticipate resuming her normal activities the day after the procedure.

In most clinician's practices, D&E is restricted to the 12-week limitations. However, it has been reported that in cases of highly trained clinicians, D&E is the safest method of abortion up to 20-weeks gestation (Grimes, 1977b). The advantages of performing D&E abortions up to 20 weeks are that it is an outpatient surgical procedure, there is no need for a long induction-to-abortion time, and there are fewer complications than the standard second trimester abortion techniques.

SECOND TRIMESTER METHODS

The second trimester methods of hypertonic saline and prostaglandin are adminstered by a transabdominal amniocentesis and necessitates hospitalization. In order to accomplish the transabdominal amniocentesis with relative ease, the gestational age should be 16–20-weeks gestation. This means that between the standard time frame of use for the D&E (12 weeks) and the appropriate use of the intra-amniotic methods (16 weeks), there is a 4-week period that has no specified methods.

Before transabdominal amniocentesis, a detailed medical history is taken and a complete physical examination is performed. Laboratory tests including Pap smear, GC culture, hematocrit, blood type and Rh, and urinalysis are recommended. A detailed explanation of the procedure, including the benefits and risks of whichever abortifacient (prostaglandin or saline) is to be used, should be given to the woman. Laminaria and other substances, such as urea and oxytocin, have been and are used in conjunction with prostaglandin or saline. (See Chapter 22.) Necessary consent forms should be properly signed and witnessed.

Before transabdominal amniocentesis, the woman should always empty her bladder since a full bladder may give fluid that is mistaken for amniotic fluid. With the woman in the supine position, the abdomen is exposed and examined to determine uterine size and position and site of injection (Fig. 26.31). There should be correlation between the uterine size and the established weeks of gestation as calculated from the woman's history of her last menstrual period. Using sterile technique, the skin of the abdomen is cleansed with an antiseptic solution. Sterile drapes are then placed on the abdomen leaving the proposed site of injection exposed.

The skin and layers of the abdomen are anesthetized using 1% lidocaine at the identified site for injection. The woman experiences a stinging sensation from the anesthetic. The site of injection is usually 1 inch below the uterine fundus in the midline. An 18-gauge needle (for saline) or an 18-gauge thin wall needle (for prostaglandin) with a properly placed stylet is inserted perpendicular to the abdominal wall into the amniotic cavity. With the insertion of the needle, the woman feels a great deal of pressure and anticipates pain or discomfort; she does not experience any since the area has been numbed. The woman will experience a cramping or painful sensation as the needle penetrates the uterine muscle and the amniotic cavity. Proper placement of the needle is ascertained by the free flow of clear amniotic fluid (Fig. 26.32).

If saline is to be administered, it can be given through the properly placed needle. After the saline is administered, the needle can be removed. If prostaglandin is to be given, a polyethylene vinyl catheter is threaded through the needle and the needle is withdrawn leaving the catheter in place. An antibiotic ointment and sterile bandages are used to cover the injection site. The remainder of the procedure is quite different for hypertonic saline and for prostaglandin and will be discussed under those specific methods.

The precise mechanism of action for saline and prostaglandin is unknown, but the resultant effect is the induction of regular, rhythmic contractions that produce dilatation of the cervix and expulsion of the products of conception. These methods mimic natural labor in that there is a slow, progressive dilatation of the cervix rather than a rapid, forced progressive dilatation. The process takes hours to complete with many uterine contractions. The contractions are not without discomfort and/or pain.

The complication rate for second trimester abortion increases another three to four fold above the first trimester methods. The complication rate estimates are in the 20–30% range. This figure truly points out the need to counsel individuals or couples who are discussing or contemplating abortion to make their decision as early as possible and to seek medical intervention without delay.

Hypertonic Saline With the needle inserted in the amniotic cavity, approximately 200 mL of amniotic fluid are withdrawn. Some practitioners try to remove all or as much as possible of the amniotic fluid, not limiting it to 200 mL (Neubardt & Schulman, 1977). Amniotic fluid is then replaced with 200 mL of 20% sodium chloride solution (saline), which deposits 40 gm of salt in the amniotic sac (Fig. 26.33). During the administration procedure, the woman may have sensations of filling up, getting full, or being bloated (Aby-Nielson, 1979).

The mean induction-to-abortion time for hyper-

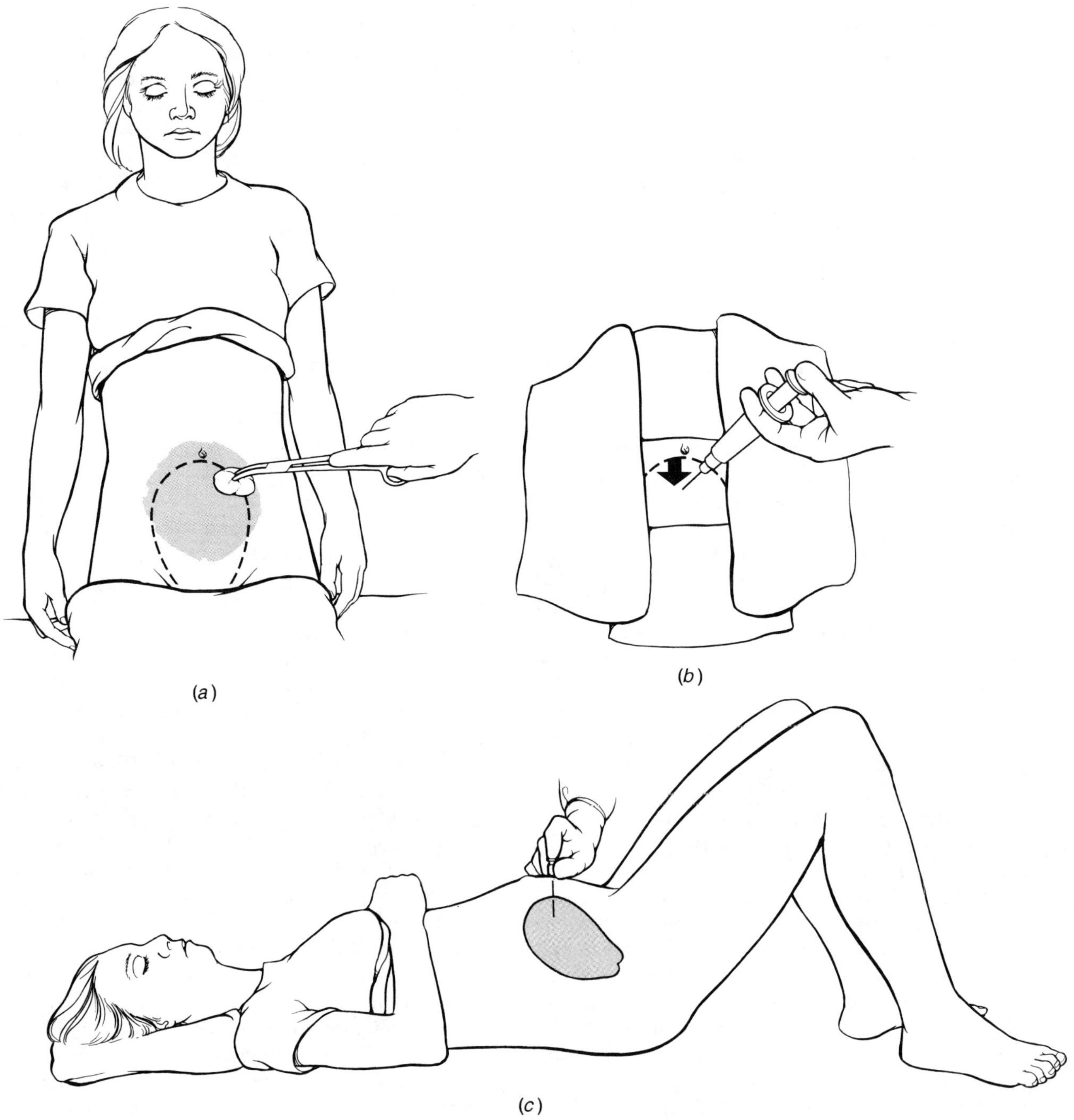

Figure 26.31
Technique for transabdominal amniocentesis. (*a*) Inspection site and abdomen prepared with an antiseptic solution; (*b*) a local anesthetic is administered; (*c*) appropriate needle size for the procedure is inserted in the amniotic cavity.

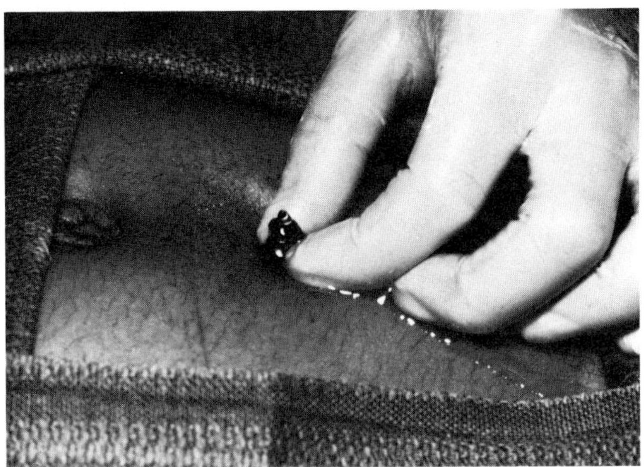

Figure 26.32
Proper transabdominal placement of the needle in the uterus. Note presence and color of amniotic fluid.

tonic saline is approximately 36 hours with a wide range of variability. During this time, the woman will experience the total spectrum of uterine activity from no contractions to increasingly severe, painful, almost constant uterine contractions. Analgesics may be administered for some pain relief.

Complications of hypertonic saline abortion include infection, fever, hemorrhage, retained placenta, and changes in clotting factors. The most serious complication of saline abortion is hypernatremia. This occurs when the serum sodium level is more than 160 mEq per liter, which reflects that the hypertonic saline had access to rapid intravascular absorption. This should not occur when the hypertonic saline is administered in the amniotic fluid. The beginning signs and symptoms of hypernatremia are acute onsets of headache, thirst, nausea, flushing or heat, and numbness of the fingers. If these symptoms occur, the saline injection should be discontinued. With further intravascular injection of saline, the progression of symptoms can lead to seizures and eventually cardiovascular collapse and death. The treatment for hypernatremia is, first, to provide sufficient fluid (intravenous) to start diuresis and, then, to continue forcing fluids orally (2 qt/day) for the remainder of the procedure. A serious complication that can occur with inadvertent injection of the solution into the uterine muscle is myometrial necrosis.

Prostaglandin In 1974 the Food and Drug Administration approved the use of prostaglandin $F_{2\alpha}$ ($PGF_{2\alpha}$) for inducing second trimester abortions. Prostaglandins are hormonelike substances that naturally occur in the body. Endogenously, they are derived from essential fatty acids; commercially, they are extracted from a species of sea coral. It is this commercial form of prostaglandin that is used in inducing second trimester abortions.

The amniocentesis has been performed with the catheter as the route of administration. Before administering the $PGF_{2\alpha}$ (which is the physician's responsibility) amniotic fluid should be withdrawn from the catheter as a precautionary measure to validate catheter placement. The recommended initial dose of $PGF_{2\alpha}$ is 40 mg (8 ml) to be followed by an additional 10–40 mg in 24 hours if abortion has not occurred. The mean induction-to-abortion time for $PGF_{2\alpha}$ induced abortion is 18 hours. If any adverse conditions, such as severe nausea, vomiting, diarrhea, severe pain, shortness of breath, or bronchoconstrictions occur, the administration should be discontinued.

The most frequently occurring side effects following $PGF_{2\alpha}$ administration are nausea, vomiting, and diarrhea. The administration of antiemetics and antidiarrheal medications can attenuate these side effects. As with other methods of abortion, particularly second trimester, hemorrhage, infection, uterine rupture, cervical lacerations, and retained products of conception are all potential complications. Unlike hypertonic saline, $PGF_{2\alpha}$ does not alter intravascular volume, clotting factors, or total body sodium. There are no risks of hypernatremia or myometrial necrosis if the $PGF_{2\alpha}$ is inadvertently administered outside of the amniotic cavity.

NURSING CARE

The aspects of nursing intervention can be generalized for all second trimester abortions. The nurse should take a careful history and evaluate the woman's decision-making process to terminate the pregnancy. It is important to support the woman's decision once it is made if there is no evidence of ambivalent feelings. Before and during the abortion, the nurse's explanations of the procedures and the sensations to be anticipated are necessary. The nurse also has a supportive and therapeutic role with respect to the psychologic implications and adjustments with which the woman will have to deal because of this experience.

The physical aspects of care involve the continuing assessment of the woman's physiologic response to the abortion procedure. It is imperative

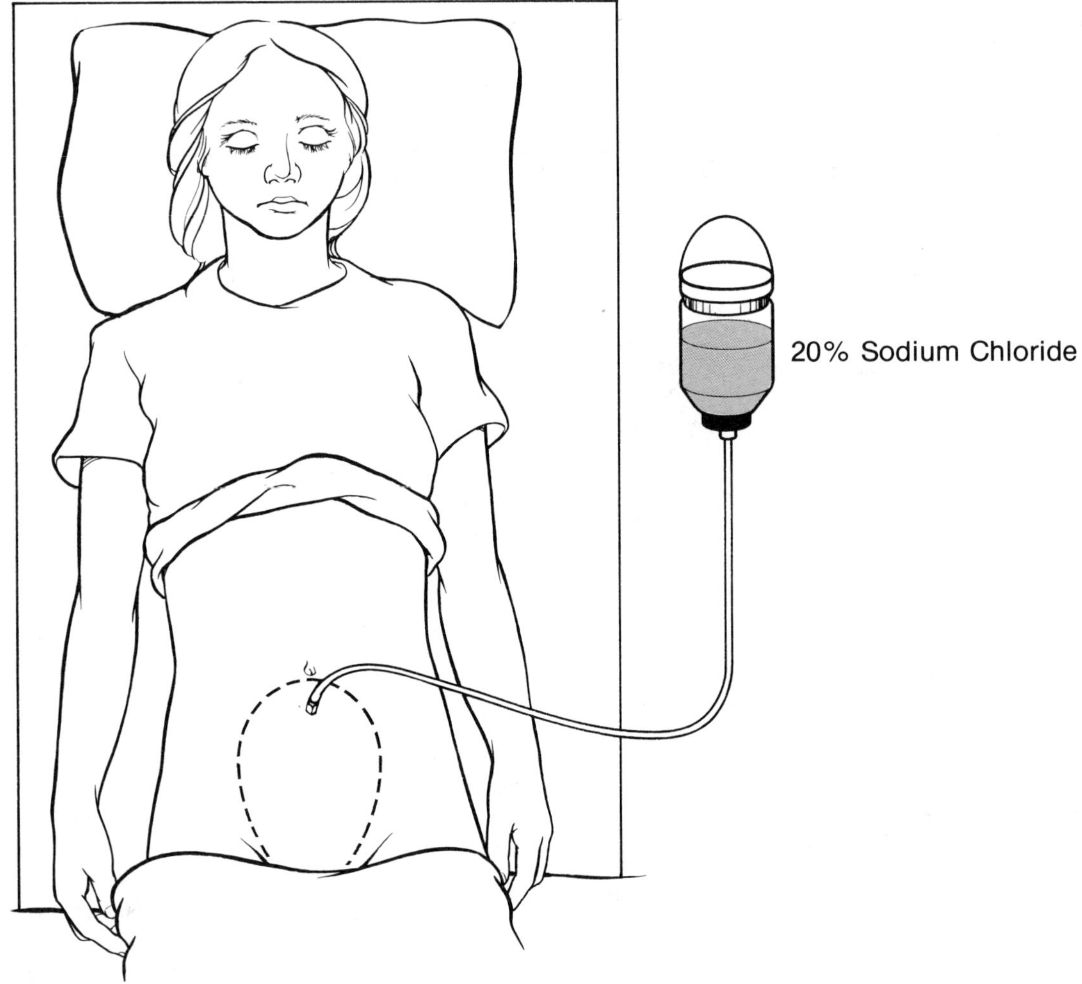

Figure 26.33
Intra-amniotic administration of hypertonic saline solution.

that the nurse monitor vital signs and intake and output and watch for signs and symptoms of complications. The nurse can also provide comfort measures and the liberal use of prescribed analgesic medication to alleviate pain. The use of medication for maintaining comfort will not adversely alter uterine contractility or the duration of the abortion process (Staurovsky et al., 1976). As the expulsion of the fetus becomes imminent, the nurse should be prepared to clamp the cord and properly dispose of the fetus. Close and careful observation becomes imperative at this time since the expulsion of the placenta is awaited and the danger of hemorrhage is high.

Postabortion care includes continued assessment of the woman's physical and psychologic states, instructions regarding postabortion anticipated events, and information related to detecting abnormal complications. The woman should be informed that bleeding will continue like a normal period for about 1 week with spotting and bleeding lasting perhaps as long as 3–4 weeks. The woman can expect to have slight uterine cramping for a couple of days, which usually is alleviated by a mild analgesic. Bleeding heavier than a normal period for more than a day should be reported to the physician. Other reportable symptoms are temperature elevation above 100°F and severe abdominal pain or cramps. The woman should refrain from using tampons, having intercourse, or douching until after her 2-week follow-up examination. A discussion of contraceptive methods and assistance in choosing an appropriate method before discharge from the hospital should not be overlooked.

HYSTEROTOMY

Hysterotomy is a surgical method of second trimester abortion that is essentially equivalent to a mini cesarean section. This is not a simple procedure and, as a major surgical procedure, has great risk of complications. It is rarely done as a primary method but is resorted to in situations when other methods have failed or where the health or welfare of the woman is in jeopardy. The nursing care of these women would be identical to the postoperative care of a woman having a cesarean section (see Chapter 22). The nurse would, however, have to assess the woman's psychologic status from the aspect of a postabortive procedure.

SUMMARY

The details regarding the gynecologic examination, contraception control, and induced abortion were presented so as to provide the nurse with the necessary information for promoting client teaching, for being a counselor, and for administering health care. These areas require the nurse to be comfortable with her own feelings of sexuality so that she can best assist others with aspects of their sexuality.

The abortion issue is complex and the provision of care to women having abortions may present a moral and ethical dilemma for a nurse. Under these circumstances, the nurse has the right to refuse to assist in these procedures except in emergencies when the life of the patient is clearly in danger.

REFERENCES AND READINGS

Aby-Nielson, K. Physical Sensations During Stressful Hospital Procedures: A Preliminary Study of Saline Abortion. *J Obstet Gynecol Neonatal Nurs 8(2):105, 1979.*

Alza Corp. *The Progestasert-Intrauterine Progesterone Contraceptive System.* Alza Corp. 1976.

Arthur, C. Customized Cervical Cap: Evolution of an Ancient Idea. *J Nurs Midwifery* 25(6):33, 1980.

Aubert, J. M., Gobeaux-Castadot, M. J., Boria, M. C. Actinomyces in the Endometrium of IUD Users. *Contraception* 21(6):577, 1980.

Ayvazian, A. Contraception Choices of Female University Students. *J Obstet Gynecol Neonatal Nurs* 10(6):426, 1981.

Berger, K. J., Fields, W. L. *Pocket Guide to Health Assessment.* Reston, Va.: Reston Publishing, 1980.

Berlin, L. E., Dotterer, W. H., Henrigues, E. S. Increase in Diaphragm Use in a University Population. *J Obstet Gynecol Neonatal Nurs* 8(5):280, 1979.

Bradbury, B. A. Preventing the "Diaphragm Baby Syndrome": A Matter of Technique, Teaching, and Time. *J Obstet Gynecol Neonatal Nurs* 4(2):24, 1975.

Bradbury, B. A. Preventing the "Diaphragm Baby Syndrome": A Matter of Technique, Teaching, and Time. *J Obstet Gynecol Neonatal Nurs* 4(2):24, 1975.

Brenner, W. E., Edelman, D. A. Permanent Sterilization by Posterior Colpotomy. *Female Sterilization Current Trends and Techniques.* Chapel Hill, N.C.: International Fertility Research Program, 1976, pp. 36–42.

Brenner, W. E., Dingfelder, J. R. Sterilization by Minilaparotomy in Not Recently Pregnant Patients. *Female Sterilization Current Trends and Techniques.* Chapel Hill, N. C.: International Fertility Research Program, 1976, pp. 1–11.

Britt, S. S. Fertility Awareness: Four Methods of Natural Family Planning. *J Obstet Gynecol Neonatal Nurs* 6(2):9, 1977.

Burbach, C. A. Contraception and Adolescent Pregnancy. *J Obstet Gynecol Neonatal Nurs* 9(5):319, 1980.

Butnarescu, G. F., Tillotson, D., Villarreal, P. P. *Perinatal Nursing: Volume 2, Reproductive Risk.* New York: John Wiley & Sons, 1980.

Canavan, P. A., Lewis, C. A. The Cervical Cap: An Alternative Contraceptive. *J Obstet Gynecol Neonatal Nurs* 10(4):271, 1981.

Cappiello, J. D., Grainger-Harrison, M. The Rebirth of the Cervical Cap. *J Nurs Midwifery* 26(5):13, 1981.

Chez, R. Perspectives on the Pharmacology of Oral Contraceptives. *Current Concepts in Oral Contraceptives Treatments.* Bloomfield, N.J.: Health Learning Systems, 1976, pp. 7–11.

Consumer Reports. Condom. *Consumer Rept* (October) 583, 1979.

Cook, D. Fibrocystic Breast-Disease: Contraindications for Oral Contraceptive Therapy. *J Nurs Midwifery* 25(2):15, 1980.

Crooks, R., Baur, K. *Our Sexuality.* Menlo Park, Calif.: Benjamin/Cummings, 1980, Chap. 20.

Current Concepts in Contraceptive Treatments—Part 1 Health. Bloomfield, N.J.: Learning Systems, 1980.

Current Concepts in Contraceptive Treatment—Part II Health. Bloomfield, N.J.: Learning Systems, 1980.

Duguid, H. L., Parratt, D., Traynor, R. Actinomyces-Like Organisms in Cervical Smears from Women Using Intrauterine Contraceptive Devices. *Br Med J* 281:534, 1980.

Elder, N. Sr., Natural Family Planning: The Ovulation Method. *J Nurs Midwifery* 23:25, 1978.

Emans, S. J. H., Goldstein, D. P. *Pediatric and Adolescent Gynecology.* Boston: Little, Brown, 1977.

Fogel, C. I., Woods, N. T. *Health Care of Women—A Nursing Perspective.* St. Louis: C. V. Mosby, 1981, Chaps. 5,7,22,23.

Further Ethical Considerations in Induced Abortion. *J Obstet Gynecol Neonatal Nurs* 7(3):53, 1978.

Goldzieher, J. W. Oral Contraceptive Hazards—1981. *Fertil Steril* 35(3):275, 1981.

Goodwin, J. H. Are Combined Oral Contraceptions Appropriate Therapy for Primary Dysmenorrhea? *J Nurs Midwifery* 25(2):17, 1980.

Grimes, D. A. Contraception Part III. Chapel Hill, N.C.: Health Sciences Consortium, 1977a.

Grimes, D. A. Methods of Midtrimester Abortion: Which is Safest? *Int J Gynecol Obstet* 15:184, 1977b.

Hamilton, M. S., Dodge, E. V. Pelvic Examination: Patient Safety and Comfort. *J Obstet Gynecol Neonatal Nurs* 10(5):344, 1981.

Hawkins, J. W., Higgins, L. P. *Maternity and Gynecological Nursing—Womens' Health Care.* Philadelphia: J. B. Lippincott, 1981, Chaps. 2,5,11.

Hofmeister, F. J. Guide to the Complete Gynecologic Examination. *Hosp Med* 1971.

Holtrop, H. R., Goldsmith, A., Edelman, D., Porter, C. W., Sandalls, K. Outpatient Culdoscopic Sterilization: An Evaluation. *Female Sterilization Current Trends and Techniques.* Chapel Hill, N.C.: International Fertility Research Program, 1976, pp. 23–29.

Huff, R. W., Pauerstein, C. J. *Human Reproduction Physiology and Pathopsychology.* New York: John Wiley & Sons, 1979, Chap. 5.

Hyde, J. S. *Understanding Human Sexuality.* New York: McGraw-Hill, 1978, Chap. 6.

Jennings, L. G. The Changing Health Care Needs of Women: Clinical Specialists Take Heed! *J Obstet Gynecol Neonatal Nurs* 6(3):44, 1977.

Jensen, M. D., Benson, R. C., Bobak, I. M. *Maternity Care—The Nurse and the Family.* St. Louis: C. V. Mosby, 1981, Chaps. 4, 8.

Katzman, E. M. Common Disorders of Female Genitalia from Birth to Older Years: Implications for Nursing Intervention. *J Obstet Gynecol Neonatal Nurs* 6(3):19, 1977.

Kilby-Kelberg, S. Why Some Won't Try the Diaphragm Method—Why Others Try and Fail. *J Obstet Gynecol Neonatal Nurs* 4(2):24, 1975.

Kuczynski, H. J. Pros and Cons of Douching: The Nurse's Role in Counseling. *J Obstet Gynecol Neonatal Nurs* 9(2):90, 1980.

Liston, J., Liston, E. H. The Mirror Pelvic Examination: Assessment in a Clinic Setting. *J Obstet Gynecol Neonatal Nurs* 7(2):47, 1978.

Malasamos, L., Barkauskas, V., Moss, M., Stoitenberg-Allen, K. *Health Assessment.* St. Louis: C. V. Mosby, 1981, Chap. 20.

Mariella, A. Diaphragm Use Instruction: Time of Insertion Before Coitus. *J Nurs Midwifery* 25(6):35, 1980.

Marieskind, H. The Women's Health Movement. *Nurs Dimen* 7(1):64, 1979.

Martin, L. L. *Health Care of Women* Philadelphia: J. B. Lippincott, 1978, Chap. 3,7.

Mishell, D. R. The Postpartum/Postabortion Women. *Current Concepts in Oral Contraceptive Treatments.* Bloomfield, N.J.: Health Learning Systems, 1976, pp. 12–19.

Neubardt, S., Schulman, H. *Techniques of Abortion* (2nd ed.). Boston: Little, Brown, 1977.

Olson, B. K. Patient Comfort During Pelvic Examination: New Foot Supports vs. Metal Stirrups. *J Obstet Gynecol Neonatal Nurs* 10(2):104, 1981.

Ortho Pharmaceutical Corp. *How to Fit the Vaginal Diaphragm.* Raistan, N.J.: Ortho Pharmaceutical Corp., 1970.

Palelta, J. L., Essoka, G. C. *Gynecologic Nursing.* Garden City, N.Y.: Medical Examination Publishing, 1978, Chaps. 2,5.

Population Reports. Barrier Methods—The Diaphragm and Other Introvaginal Barriers—A Review. *Popul Rept* [H] (4), 1976.

Population Reports. Sterilization—Female Sterilization by Mini-Laparotomy. *Popul Rept* [C] (5), 1974.

Population Reports. Sterilization—Vasectomy—What are the Problems? *Popul Rept* [D] (2), 1975.

Porter, C. W., Waife, R. S. *Intrauterine Devices: Current Perspectives.* Pathfinder Fund, 1978.

Porter, C. W., Holtrop, H. R., Waife, R. S. *Oral Contraceptives: A Guide for Programs and Clinics.* Pathfinder Fund, 1975.

Pritchard, J. A., MacDonald, P. C. *William's Obstetrics* (16th ed.). New York: Appleton–Century–Crofts, 1981.

Raisler, J. Abortion 1980: Battleground for Reproductive Rights. *J Nurs Midwifery* 25(2):28, 1980.

Richards, S. I. Pelvic Examination of Children. *J Obstet Gynecol Neonatal Nurs* 10(3):208, 1981.

Richart, R. M. Sterilization: Five Experts Compare the Techniques. *Contemp Obstet Gynecol* 9:56, 1977.

Rebbie, M. O. Contraceptive Counseling for the Younger Adolescent Woman: A Suggested Solution to the Problem. *J Obstet Gynecol Neonatal Nurs* 7(4):29, 1978.

Rooks, J. The Women's Movement and its Effect on Women's Health Care, in Kester-McNall, L. (ed.), *Contemporary Obstetric and Gynecologic Nursing.* St. Louis: C. V. Mosby, 1980, pp. 3–26.

Royal College of General Practitioners. Oral Contraceptives. Advantages of Orals Outweigh Disadvantages. *Popul Rept* [A] (2), 1975.

Schrag, K. The Adolescent's First Gynecological Exam. *J Nurs Midwifery* 23:20, 1978.

Searle G. D. & Co. *Detailed Product Information for the Cu 7 Intrauterine Copper Contraceptive.* 1977.

Staurovsky, L. G., Brenner, W. E., Dingfelder, J. R., Grimes, D. A. The Effect of Meperidine Analgesia on Midtrimester Abortions Induced with Intraamniotic Prostaglandin F_2 alpha. *Am J Obstet Gynecol* 125:185, 1976.

Swenson, I. Psychologic Considerations in Vasectomy; A Review of the Literature. *J Obstet Gynecol Neonatal Nurs* 29, 1975.

Varney, H. *Nurse-Midwifery.* Boston: Blackwell Scientific Publications, 1980.

Willis, J. Cervical Caps—The Perfect Untested Contraceptive. *FDA Consumer* (April) 20, 1981.

27

REPRODUCTIVE RELATED HEALTH CARE PROBLEMS OF WOMEN

Linda G. Staurovsky

Most women will at some point in their lifetime need to seek gynecologic care for a reproductive tract-related problem. While the majority of these problems are not life threatening, they may by physically annoying and worrisome or psychologically stressful. Some women experiencing these problems never seek medical care but simply tolerate and endure the associated emotional and/or physical discomforts.

The common problems of infections and abnormal Pap smears affect nonpregnant as well as pregnant women; some problems are identified when women seek care for their pregnancies. The problem of dysmenorrhea has affected millions of women. For some women, an unwanted pregnancy creates a most stressful period in their lives. For other women, the struggle to conceive and overcome the problems of infertility is a lifelong battle. These problems along with others are faced by many women each day. This chapter will address some of the more common gynecologic problems in order to provide a more comprehensive understanding of the pathophysiology and treatment plan required in these conditions.

DYSMENORRHEA

Until recently, *dysmenorrhea* was the leading cause of woman hours lost to employment, school, and leisure time. It is also the most common gynecologic complaint of adolescents. The introduction of oral contraceptives and progesterone-releasing IUDs has alleviated the problem to a certain degree. However, these treatments fall short of what can be considered ideal. The long-standing advice to women of suggesting that they become pregnant is not acceptable for teenagers, women choosing to delay pregnancy for a variety of reasons, or women electing not to have children.

The most basic definition of dysmenorrhea is pain or cramping immediately preceding or during menses. The condition of dysmenorrhea can be further classified as either primary or secondary. *Primary dysmenorrhea* usually develops within a few years of menarche and is painful menstruation not associated with any pelvic disease or pathology. The pain usually begins with onset of menstruation, but mild cramping may begin 24–48 hours before the menstrual flow. The pain may last from a few hours to several days. The etiology of the cramps is unknown; it is, however, associated with ovulation, which accounts for the fact that most teenagers have painless menstruation for the first few years. In contrast, *secondary dysmenorrhea* begins later in life and can be correlated with pelvic pathology such as endometriosis, pelvic inflammatory disease, fibroids, or polyps. In girls with congenital abnormalities of the reproductive tract, secondary dysmenorrhea can coincide with menarche.

For many years, women suffering from primary dysmenorrhea were told the cause was psychologic. Recently, theories have been purported that attempt to identify a physiologic basis for the painful cramps associated with menstruation. Dingfelder (1977) stated that the best evidence *against* dysmenorrhea being of psychologic origin was the almost universally prompt response of the painful menstruation to the oral contraceptive pills. It is unrealistic to proclaim that the hormonal therapy (which causes an anovulatory response) could be credited with curing a long-standing psychologic disorder. While there is the possibility that a small percentage of women do have a psychologic basis for their primary or secondary dysmenorrhea, it is no longer felt that 98% of dysmenorrhea is of psychologic origin.

While the etiology of dysmenorrhea is still unknown, theories related to prostaglandin (PG) and other substances have been proposed (Huffman, 1976; Dingfelder, 1977; Irwin et al. 1981). The therapeutic uses of prostaglandins have demonstrated that contractility of the uterine muscle can be stimulated. The assumption, therefore, is that naturally occurring prostaglandins ($PGF_{2\alpha}$) released at the cellular level in the endometrium stimulate uterine contractions and vasoconstriction. The resultant ischemic state may provoke the release of other compounds (i.e., bradykinin) to increase levels of vasodilators (prostaglandin E_2–PGE_2). The pain-provoking bradykinin may account for the pain, while the PGE_2 may be the cause of other noted side effects that are often associated with severe dysmenorrhea. The associated symptoms that often accompany primary dysmenorrhea include nausea, vomiting, diarrhea, anorexia, syncope, headache, and flushing. These symptoms have been noted as side effects in women receiving therapeutic doses of PGE_2 in cases of intrauterine fetal death. Whether or not the pain of dysmenorrhea is caused by an imbalance of the prostaglandins or other factors needs further investigation. The major breakthrough has been in the realization that primary dysmenorrhea has a physiologic basis as its cause.

While the prostaglandin theory may explain the etiology of primary dysmenorrhea, the pain of secondary dysmenorrhea is a symptom of the existing abnormality or pathology. The woman may experience a variety of associated symptoms that would be specific to the precipitating etiology or the underlying cause. The treatment of secondary dysmenorrhea is directed at the specific problem. Women suffering from the effects of endometriosis may benefit from oral contraceptives, antiprostaglandin drugs, or hysterectomy. Whatever the cause, each woman should be evaluated individually, taking into consideration her history, severity of symptoms, desire for future reproduction, and an accurate diagnosis of the underlying cause before a definite plan of therapy is designed.

Recommended treatment of primary dysmenorrhea has as its basis the woman's need or desire for contraception control. If contraception is required, the oral contraceptive pills are the treatment of choice. An alternative for women opposed to the pill or for whom estrogen is contraindicated is the progesterone IUD. In women where contraception is not a factor, a mode of therapy has evolved with the assumption that prostaglandins cause the dysmenorrhea. The use of prostaglandin inhibitors is now providing prompt and effective relief to many women suffering from dysmenorrhea. Good results, which include complete cessation of the pain or a decrease of cramping to a tolerable level, have been demonstrated in 65–85% of dysmenorrheic women using prostaglandin-inhibitor drugs such as ibuprofen, naproxen sodium, and mefenamic acid (Lundström, 1977; Dingfelder, 1981; Harvey, 1979).

Before the advent of PG inhibitors, women used a wide range of medications for relief of menstrual cramps. These medications have ranged from over-the-counter drugs, such as aspirin, to prescription drugs, such as meperidine, to illegal drugs, such as marijuana. In the majority of cases, the effect of these medications is not so much the relief of pain as it is the fact that: "It knocked me out for about 8 hours and when I awoke the pain was gone." As implied by this statement, the women feel a need to go to bed or alter their daily living activities. It is also true that the mental functioning of women taking these drugs is greatly diminished. The group of PG inhibitors (also referred to as antiprostaglandins, which are nonsteroidal anti-inflammatory agents) enables a higher percentage of women to maintain their normal activities of daily living. These medications provide relief from pain but do not affect the woman's mental or physical capabilities. Women have reported relief of pain within 10 minutes to 1 hour of taking the prescribed medications with the effect lasting 4–12 hours. The dosage will vary according to the specific drug. The initiation of the therapeutic regimen generally follows one of two patterns: start medication with onset of symptoms or begin taking the medication 2–5 days before the onset of menses or painful symptoms.

The advantages of the PG inhibitors, aside from relief of pain and noninterference with ability to function mentally or physically, are that they need only be taken with onset of symptoms and that there are minimally reported side effects or adverse reactions. The major side effects are related to the gastrointestinal tract, which has resulted in the recommendation that these drugs be taken with meals or milk. For a list of all side effects or adverse reactions, consult a pharmacology book. The disadvantage of such drugs is that while a large percentage of women are helped, there are still a significant number who are unaffected by these medications.

An alternative treatment of PG inhibitors is an oral progesterone, which is also known to be effective in relieving incapacitating dysmenorrhea. The recommended dosage of the drug is taken from day 5 to day 25 of each cycle. Dydrogesterone is a medication in this category. The advantages are that (1) normal ovulation continues, in contrast to oral contraceptive (OC) pills, (2) no serious untoward reactions or contraindications occur, and (3) side effects are limited to mild gastrointestinal complaints.

The relief of dysmenorrhea has made tremendous advances since the physiologic origin was acknowledged. It is still unfortunate that not all women can be guaranteed a rapid, prompt alleviation of pain. However, the time has come when the majority of women no longer need to suffer in silence nor rely on potent analgesics or hot water bottles to find relief from primary dysmenorrhea.

It is the nurse's responsibility to educate women regarding the availability of the new treatment regimens, discourage the use of potent analgesics, encourage women to seek medical care for this problem, and promote the well-being of women so that they may lead a happier and healthier life.

SEXUALLY TRANSMITTED DISEASES

There is little question that *sexually transmitted diseases* (STDs) have reached epidemic proportions. They represent the most widespread communicable disease problem in the United States. The STDs know no social class and are not particular regarding age, race, or religion. The term venereal disease (VD), which has been used previously, is becoming extinct, and STDs is becoming the phrase of choice.

> *STD is defined as diseases that are usually or can be transmitted from one person to another during heterosexual or homosexual intercourse or intimate contact with the sex organs, mouth or rectum.*
>
> *Campbell & Herten, 1981*

With a change in terminology, the diseases that are now in the STDs category are much more inclusive than those previously thought of as VD. There are presently 15 diseases that are considered to be STDs: (1) gonorrhea, (2) syphilis, (3) chancroid, (4) lymphogranuloma venereum, (5) granuloma inguinale, (6) genital herpes, (7) trichomoniasis, (8) moniliasis, (9) nonspecific urethritis, (10) pediculosis pubis (lice), (11) scabies, (12) hepatitis B infection, (13) molluscum contagiosum, (14) *Hemophilus vaginalis* vaginitis, and (15) condyloma acuminatum (venereal warts). While all of these are STDs, only the more commonly occurring diseases will be discussed in detail; they included the two classic venereal diseases—gonorrhea and syphilis; the two common vaginal infections—trichomoniasis and moniliasis; the two viral diseases—genital herpes and condyloma acuminatum; and nonspecific urethritis. Selected other STDs are presented in Table 27.1.

Gonorrhea

Gonorrhea (GC) is the most common STD; in the United States over 1 million cases were reported in

1980 and an estimated 2 million cases were not reported. The highest incidence is in the 20–24 year old group; the second highest is 15–19 year old group. The causative organism is *Neisseria gonorrhoeae*, a Gram-negative diplococcus. The incubation period in the female is from 2–5 days to indefinitely. The major problem of GC is that as many as 80% of infected women have subclinical symptoms (asymptomatic); because they are unaware of the infectious process, they do not seek medical treatment.

In women, the GC organism is difficult to culture, and false negative reports can occur. The diagnosis and treatment of women, therefore, are often based on a history of a positive male contact. The other components involved in diagnosis are noting the typical symptomatology, if present, performing a GC culture (Fig. 27.1) (described in

TABLE 27.1
SOME SEXUALLY TRANSMITTED DISEASES

STD	*Symptoms*	*Diagnosis*	*Treatment*	*Complications*
Chancroid	Ragged, tender ulcer, not indurated Base covered with gray or yellow necrotic exudate	Clinical appearance Gram-stained exudate Short, Gram-negative rods or culture on blood agar	Sulfisoxazole 1 gm, p.o. qid × 14 days Tetracycline Kanamycin Streptomycin	Chronic fistulas of gland masses in groin
Lymphogranuloma venereum	Primary lesion—evanescent painless vesicle Painful adenopathy of regional lymph nodes	Clinical picture Complement fixation test	Tetracycline 500 mg, p.o. qid × 2–3 weeks Sulfisoxazole	Rare Elephantiasis Rectal strictures Ulcerations
Granuloma inguinale	Single or multiple subcutaneous nodules Erosion Granulomatous beef-red lesions Painless	Clinical picture Intracytoplasmic rods with Giemsa or Wright's stain	Tetracycline 500 mg, p.o. qid × 3 weeks Gentamicin Streptomycin Chloramphenicol	Rare Elephantiasis Strictures of vagina, urethra, or rectum
Pediculosis pubis	Erythematous, itching papules Nits or adult lice	Clinical observation	1% Kwell lotion Antimicrobials prn	Rare Impetigo Pustular eczema
Scabies	Linear burrows with red papule	Microscopic identification of mite	1% Kwell lotion Antimicrobials prn	Impetigo Pustular eczema
Hempohilus vaginalis vaginitis	Relatively thin, occasionally frothy vaginal discharge	Clinical picture Microscopic—clue cells	Ampicillin 500 mg, p.o., qid × 7–10 days	None
Hepatitis B infection	Abdominal discomfort Anorexia Nausea Jaundice	Detection of hepatitis B surface antigen	Symptomatic	Death Cirrhosis Carriers

Source: Adapted from Center for Disease Control. *Sexually Transmitted Diseases Summary.* Atlanta: Technical Information Services.

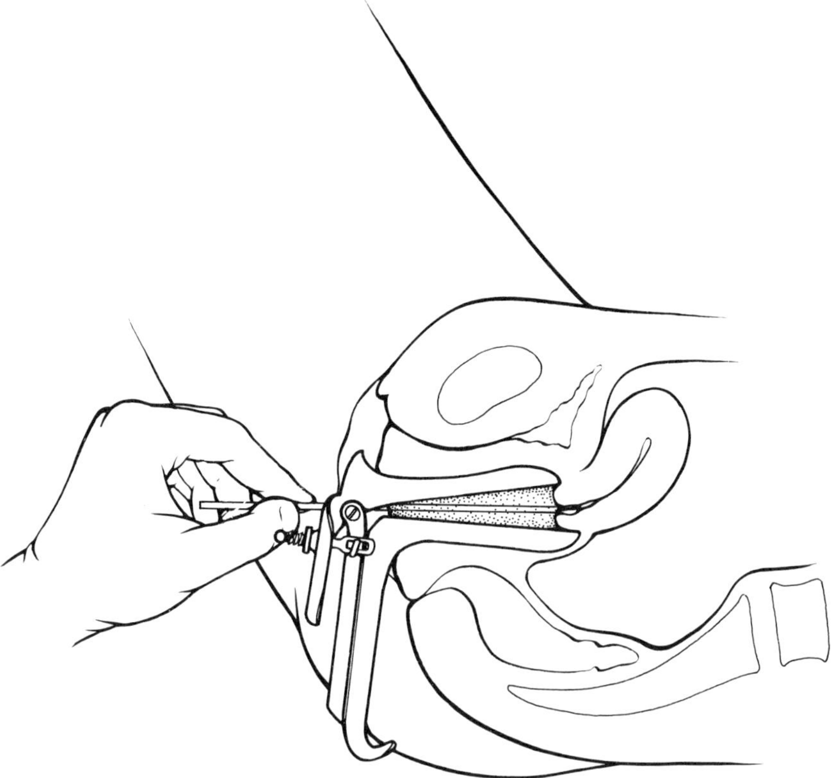

Figure 27.1
Technique of obtaining a gonococcal culture from endocervix.

Chapter 26), and microscopic identification of typical Gram-negative diplococci in vaginal secretions or Skene's or Bartholin's glands exudate.

The GC diplococci prefer columnar epithelium to squamous epithelium, which can account for the usual areas of involvement. The spread of infection can involve Skene's and Bartholin's glands, cervix (endocervical canal), urethra, fallopian tubes, and the peritoneal cavity. The spread of GC can also be systemic (disseminated form) as manifested by arthritis, septicemia, meningitis, endocarditis, myocarditis, or pericarditis.

In women who are symptomatic, there are some basic characteristic symptoms that can be observed (Fig. 27.2). In the initial phase, when the infection is confined to the lower reproductive tract or urinary tract, the symptoms include a profuse, purulent, yellowish or greenish-yellow discharge from the vagina, cervix, or urethra. Dyspareunia, vulvar tenderness, and pain elicited on palpation of the cervix have been noted. With urinary tract involvement, urinary symptoms of burning, frequency, and lower abdominal discomfort may be present. In any of the involved areas, the symptoms of irritation, erythema, edema, and pruritis may be present.

As the disease continues in the untreated state, the upper reproductive tract and pelvis can become involved by a process of ascending infection; this may lead to salpingitis and peritonitis, often referred to as *pelvic inflammatory disease* (PID). In cases of PID, the causative organism may be gonococcal or nongonococcal. Regardless of the causative organism, the symptomatology is the same, and therapy should be initiated without delay. The main symptoms of salpingitis are acute lower abdominal pain, which is bilateral and diffuse, and adnexal tenderness or pain on pelvic examination. Other symptoms include fever, chills, vaginal discharge, and possible gastrointestinal symptoms of nausea, vomiting, diarrhea, or constipation. Severe salpingitis or recurrent episodes can cause scarring of the tubes, resulting in complete or partial obstruction and subsequent infertility or sterility. Further discussion of this aspect is presented later in this chapter.

After the diagnosis of gonorrhea has been made and before treatment is instituted, the woman should have blood drawn for a serologic test for syphilis as the antibiotic therapy for GC may mask the syphilitic disease. The recommended treatment for gonorrhea is 4.8 million units of aqueous penicillin G given intramuscularly in a divided dose at two sites. In addition, 1 gm of probenecid is given orally ½ hour before the penicillin administration, which results in elevated blood levels of penicillin by blocking renal excretion of the penicillin. In severe cases that involve salpingitis or peritonitis, the woman usually needs to be hospitalized, placed on bedrest, and given intravenous antibiotics.

After the treatment for gonorrhea, the woman should be instructed to abstain from intercourse until proof of therapy success is obtained. A repeat GC culture should be done 7–14 days after initial therapy. For women who are allergic to penicillin, the use of tetracycline, ampicillin, or erythromycin may be effective.

A new strain of gonorrhea that is resistant to penicillin has evolved. If women who have been treated by the recommended therapy return with continued positive cultures, further investigation should be carried out to determine if a penicillin-resistant strain is present. If the laboratory report is positive for penicillin-resistant GC, the treatment is 2 gm spectromycin intramuscularly (Steinmann, 1977).

The nursing intervention encompasses case finding, referral, counseling, administering the appropriate therapy, and providing follow-up. In addition, gonorrhea is a disease that must be reported to health departments. Clients should be informed of this and advised that follow-up will be made of all sexual contacts who must be treated.

In the pregnant woman, the recognition and treatment of gonorrhea is of particular importance. A GC culture is mandatory in all pregnant women.

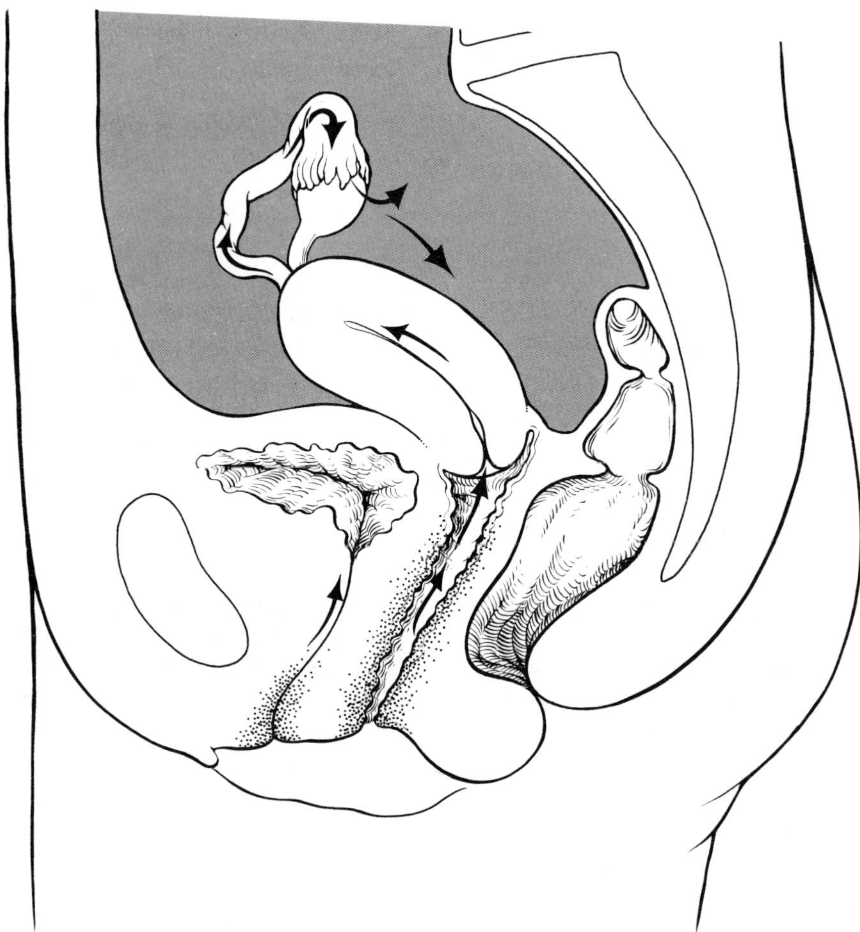

Figure 27.2
Gonorrhea infection of urethra and ascending spread of infection from lower reproductive tract to upper reproductive tract and peritoneum.

The consequences of undiagnosed or untreated gonorrhea in pregnancy can result in *ophthalmia neonatorum* in the newborn. This disease condition has resulted in mandatory prophylactic eye therapy of all newborns (see Chapter 17).

Syphilis

The number of new cases of *syphilis* diagnosed in the United States each year is less than gonorrhea, but it is still a substantial number at over 100,000 (Huff & Pauerstein, 1979). The age group with the highest number of reported cases is the 20–24 year olds. The causative organism of this classic sexually transmitted disease is a spirochete, *Treponema pallidum* (see Fig. 27.3). This organism needs warmth and moisture to survive; it is killed with soap and water. The mode of transmission is direct sexual contact, oral–genital sex, or placental transfer. The spirochete, which can penetrate intact skin, may produce a primary lesion at any point.

There are a number of diagnostic tests either to screen for a possible reaction to the syphilis organism or to validate the presence of the spirochete. There are three basic blood tests available to diagnose syphilis by detecting an antibody/antigen reaction. A reactive reagent test is positive for syphilis while a nonreactive test is negative. The three tests are (1) VDRL, (2) FTA-ABS, and (3) TPI. The *Venereal Disease Research Laboratory test* (VDRL) detects 75% of primary syphilis at 6 weeks and 100% of secondary syphilis. False negatives can be obtained if the test is performed too early in the disease cycle. False positives can be obtained as a result of recent acute infections, heroin addiction, rheumatoid arthritis, or systemic herpes erythematosis. The VDRL, as well as other tests such as the rapid plasma reagin (RPR) and Kline-Kolmer tests, react not only to the *T. pallidum* organism but also to a nonspecific antigen. Therefore, these tests should be used as screening tools; if positive, one of the following two specific tests should be made for a definite diagnosis of syphilis (Huff & Pauerstein, 1979). The *fluorescent treponemal antibody-absorption test* (FTA-ABS) is more reliable in detecting primary syphilis when exposure is less than 4 weeks. There are fewer occurrences of false positives than with the VDRL. The drawback is that it is a more costly test to perform. The *Treponema pallidum immobilization test* (TPI) is expensive and difficult to perform. In areas of questionable positives (false positives), the use of this test would be appropriate since there are very few reported false positives with the TPI.

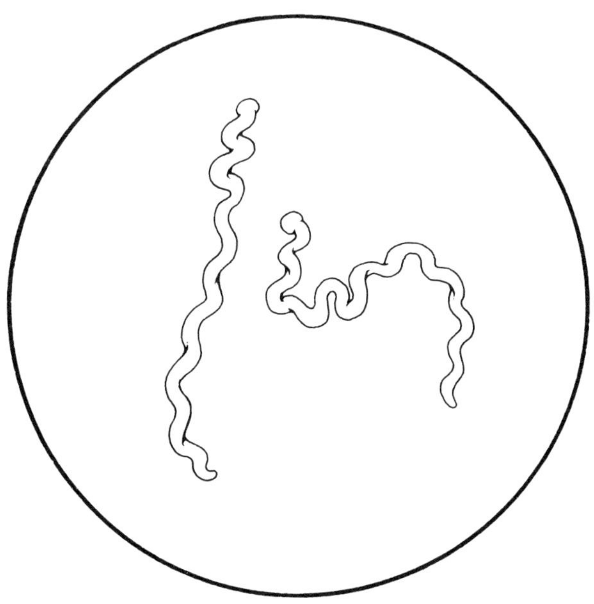

Figure 27.3
Treponema pallidum—causative organism in syphilis.

Another diagnostic test, *darkfield microscopic examination,* can be performed by experts when a lesion is present. The examination allows for direct visualization of the spirochete and is positive when the spirochete is identified. Even with the availability of a number of diagnostic tests, syphilis often goes undiagnosed because of the variety of signs and symptoms and the natural progression of the disease.

Syphilis is identified as having three stages with distinct signs and symptoms for each stage. The first stage, known as *primary syphilis,* has an incubation period of 10–20 days. The *chancre,* which is the primary lesion, is a painless eroded ulcer that is usually found in the genital area or on the mouth (Fig. 27.4). Usually a single ulcer or sore appears, but in some cases multiple chancres have been noted on the labia and other parts of the reproductive tract. The beginning appearance of the chancre may be mistaken for a pimple or papule, but it will develop the typical characteristic appearance. A hard red indurated oval-shaped ulcer, smaller than a quarter, with a raised border and a base that does not bleed easily will form. The chancre may be undetected; if noticed, it may be self-treated as a

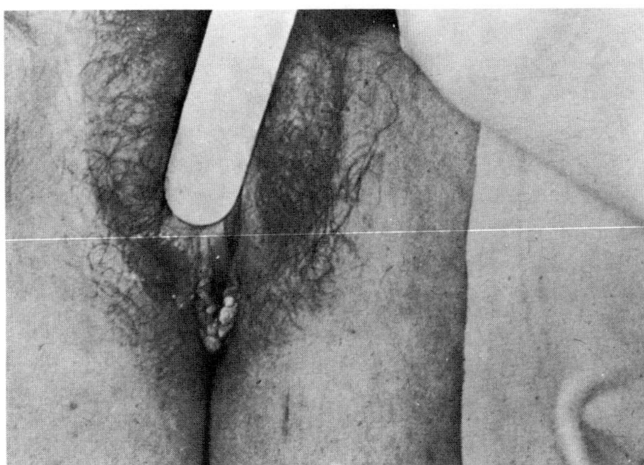

Figure 27.4
Syphilitic chancre on labia and condyloma acuminatum at fourchette. Courtesy of Centers for Disease Control, Altanta, Ga.

superficial, nonthreatening infection. The fact that the nearby lymph glands are enlarged also goes unnoticed or is not considered significant since there is no pain. Other symptoms may include headache, malaise, and slight elevation of temperature. The woman does not often correlate the genital chancre with the flulike symptoms. The chancre will heal spontaneously within 5 weeks.

The second stage is *secondary syphilis*, which begins with an asymptomatic time period after the chancre has healed. This time period usually is about 6 weeks but may be from 2 weeks to 6 months. The disease process has continued and the disease resurfaces as a macular, maculopapular, papular, or pustular skin rash of mucous membrane sores or condylomata lata. The rash is characteristically found on the palms of the hands and the soles of the feet, as well as on other parts of the body.

The mucous membrane sores may be found in the mouth and appear as greyish-white areas encircled by a dull red. Sore throat and a husky voice accompany this development. Other moist lesions known as *condylomata lata* are commonly found on the labia, anus, and corners of the mouth. These lesions are the most infectious of secondary syphilis and appear as greyish-white, flat-topped, fleshy-looking lesions.

Alopecia (loss of hair) is a common finding. Other flulike symptoms including malaise, headache, nausea, anorexia, constipation, pain in the long bones, and/or a persistent low-grade fever. Even if untreated, the symptoms of secondary syphilis resolve in 2–6 weeks.

The third and final stage is known as *tertiary*, or *latent, syphilis*. The majority of people in the latent stage are asymptomatic for a varying period of time ranging anywhere from a few months to many, many years. Approximately 25% of untreated people during this stage develop relapses of primary and secondary signs and symptoms. The latent stage will remain without further damages in about two-thirds of the people. The other one-third will develop complications including painful *gummas* (granulomatous destructive weeping lesions) of the skin, bone, neurons, or cardiovascular system, inflammation of the aortic valve and arteriosclerosis, or general neurologic demise leading to mental deterioration, insanity, and paralysis. After 1 year of latent syphilis, the person is no longer infectious (Huxall, 1975).

Syphilis during pregnancy after 18-weeks gestation with placental transfer can give rise to premature birth, stillbirth, and overt or covert congenital syphilis. The problems of congenital syphilis in the newborn are discussed in Chapter 23.

The choice of treatment for syphilis in all stages is penicillin. The recommended treatment regime for primary, secondary, and tertiary (less than 1 year's duration) is benzathine penicillin G 2.4 million units intramuscularly as a single dose. Latent syphilis of more than 1 year's duration should be treated with benzathine penicillin G 2.4 million units intramuscularly each week for 3 weeks (Huff & Pauerstein, 1979). In cases of penicillin sensitivity other treatment choices include tetracycline and erythromycin. The treatment of choice for pregnant women is aqueous procaine penicillin G 600,000 units, intramuscularly for 10 days. This provides more adequate treatment to the fetus.

Nursing intervention includes the same basic components for care of women with gonorrhea. Syphilis is also a reportable disease, and all sexual contacts of the diagnosed person should be identified and treated. The nurse who may come in contact with people having syphilis must take care to perform good hand washing remembering that the spirochete can penetrate unbroken skin and that soap and water destroys the spirochete. The nurse should stress the need for follow-up visits and repeat VDRL tests every 3 months for 1 year in cases of primary and secondary syphilis and for 2 years in cases of tertiary or latent stage syphilis.

Trichomoniasis

Trichomoniasis, also called *trichomonal vaginitis,* is one of the common vaginal infections that is transmitted sexually or by close genital contact. The frequency may be as many as 2.5 million cases per year with a peak age range 16–35 years (Paletta & Essoka, 1978). The causative organism is *Trichomonas vaginalis,* a flagellate protozoan (Fig. 27.5). The trichomonads are motile inhabitants found in the vagina and less frequently the urinary tract. Many women who are asymptomatic are found to be carriers of *T. vaginalis.*

The diagnosis of a trichomonal vaginitis can be confirmed by microscopic examination of the vaginal discharge suspended in a drop of saline. The trichomonads can be seen moving about in the suspension. Diagnosis, however, should not be based on just an observation of the characteristic vaginal discharge.

The symptoms of trichomoniasis include a malodorous, thin, greenish-gray, sometimes bubbly discharge. Vulvar pruritis, dyspareunia, vaginal tenderness, and burning are other frequently associated complaints. In visualizing the cervix, the classic characteristic strawberry appearance of a trichomonal infection may be seen. This appearance is the result of small pinpoint hemorrhages and a granular appearance of the cervix and vagina. Unlike the previously discussed STDs, this disease, while passed between sexual partners, does not have serious consequences but is an irritating nuisance.

The treatment for trichomonal vaginitis is metronidazole (Flagyl) 2 gm orally in a single dose or 250 mg 3 times a day for 7 days. The therapy should include an identical treatment plan for the sexual partner. It is generally recommended that condoms be used until the symptoms are resolved. The instructions to the couple regarding the medication, aside from other drug-related information, should include the fact that alcohol should not be ingested during the course of therapy or for 48 hours after completion of therapy since the combination of alcohol with this medication will cause severe gastrointestinal side effects. Treatment of trichomoniasis in pregnant women should be delayed until after the first trimester (Quirk, 1975). The use of oral metronidazole is contraindicated in pregnant and lactating women. Suppositories or vaginal creams specifically for trichomoniasis should be used (Hart, 1976).

The nursing intervention should focus on client education regarding the disease transmission, the need for treatment of sexual contacts in order to

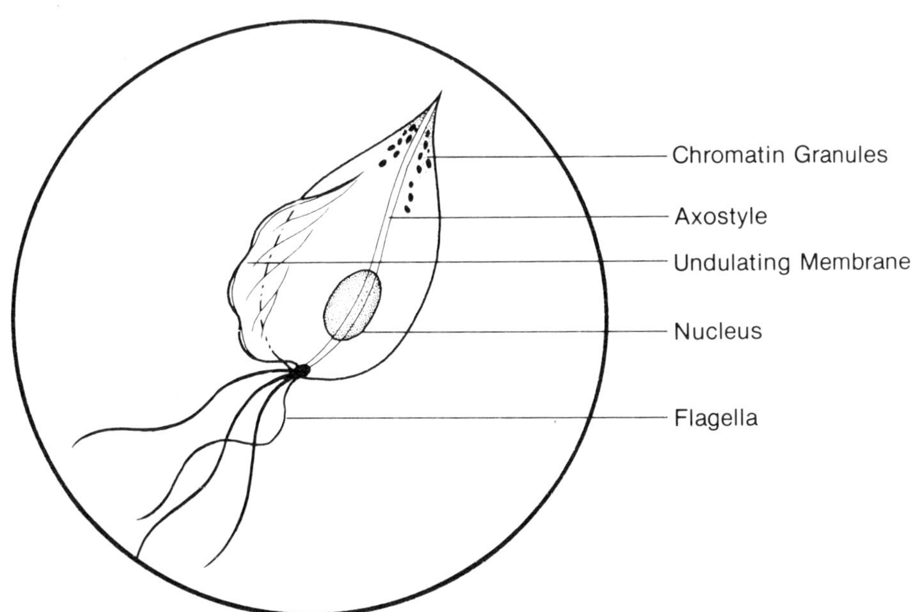

Figure 27.5
Trichomonas vaginalis—flagellate protozoan.

facilitate a cure, an interpretation of the treatment plan, potential side effects, and means of avoiding adverse reactions. When giving the medication, the nurse should elicit a detailed history either to rule out the possibility of an early pregnancy or to delay treatment of women in the first trimester of pregnancy.

Moniliasis

Moniliasis, also called *monilial vaginitis,* raises a controversy as to whether or not this vaginitis really fits into the category of a sexually transmitted disease. Its inclusion in this section is based on the fact that the conditions in the vagina must be receptive and appropriate for the organism, even though it is not uncommon to find a coexisting infection in the male partner that does speak to the potential of sexual transmission.

The causative organism is *Candida albicans,* more commonly referred to as a yeast or fungal infection (Fig. 27.6). It can be diagnosed by KOH wet prep (see Chapter 26), which reveals the translucent spore filaments. The *C. albicans* can also be diagnosed by Pap smear or on a Nickerson's medium culture.

The symptoms are moderate-to-severe vulvovaginal pruritus and burning, a characteristic thick, white, cheesy discharge, cottage cheese-like clumps adhering to the vaginal wall, vulvovaginal erythema, and edema. Dyspareunia may be present. The typical discharge may or may not be malodorous. There are no long-term adverse complications of this vaginitis. Successful treatment can usually be accomplished with one course of therapy.

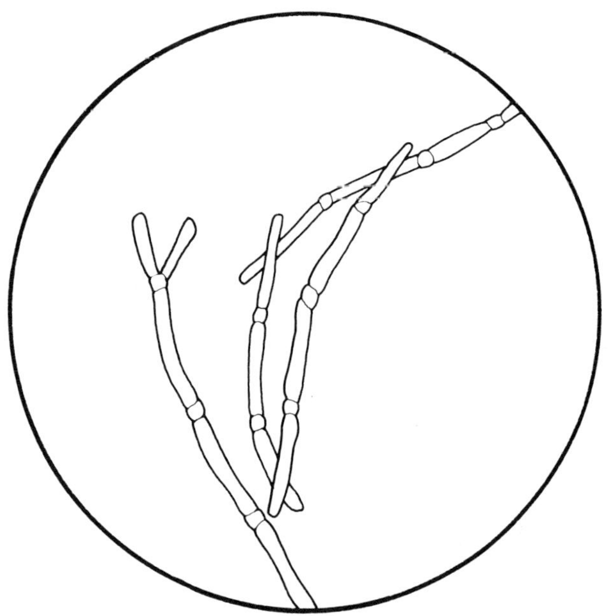

Figure 27.6
Candida albicans spores and filaments.

The treatment is nystatin vaginal suppositories twice a day for 1–2 weeks. Another treatment regimen is one applicator of miconazole vaginal cream everyday for 7 days. The nurse should stress the importance of completing the total course of therapy and not prematurely stopping when symptoms are alleviated. It is tempting to stop therapy when relief is obtained because of the messiness of the treatment. The woman may be told to use minipads for added comfort.

The nurse should evaluate the history to see if it reveals any of the predisposing factors associated with monilial vaginitis. Oral contraceptives, broad-spectrum antibiotics, steroids, diabetes, and pregnancy are known to alter the vaginal environment and promote monilial growth. Further counseling can be directed toward the associated identified factor. General hygiene principles can be reviewed, suggesting use of cotton rather than nylon underpants. Cotton is absorbent, whereas nylon is heat and moisture retaining and provides an environment more conducive for vaginal infections. The nurse should also be aware of the implications for a newborn baby. Delivery through a birth canal infected with monilial vaginitis can result in oral thrush (see Chapter 17).

Herpes Genitalis

Herpes genitalis, or venereal herpes, has been recognized as the second most frequent STD (Edwards, 1978). Herpes genitalis is caused by the herpes simplex type 2 virus (HSV-2). This newest member to the STD group is transmitted via the genitals through sexual contact or, in the case of the newborn, it passes through the birth canal. There are 300,000–500,000 new cases reported each year (Campbell & Herten, 1981). The largest proportion of cases are found in 20–29 year olds. Because of the tremendous number of new cases, the recurrent pattern of the disease, the significant complication of neonatal herpes infection (see Chapter 23), and the associated risk of cervical cancer, the nursing profession needs to be totally cognizant of the implications of HSV-2 and the advances that may be reported in the literature.

The incubation period for herpes genitalis is most frequently reported as 2–7 days, but it has also been reported that it may lie dormant for years (Campbell & Herten, 1981). The herpetic virus is infectious when it is in an active stage. The diagnosis can often be made with 100% accuracy by clinical appearance and recognition of the herpetic lesion. Scrapings obtained from lesions or from the cervix and vagina in the absence of lesions can be submitted for a Pap or Tzanck test (Himell, 1981). Cellular morphologic characteristics of HSV-2 will be present if infected cells are submitted. The optimal diagnostic method is a viral culture.

The clinical symptoms of herpes genitalis vary greatly in the adult since there are many interdependent factors. The disease process manifests in two forms—primary lesions and recurrent herpes infections. The primary infection usually is symptomatic within 3–7 days. However, many of these primary infections are subclinical or not detected. The major clinical symptom is the typical vesicle or blisterlike lesion that usually ruptures and leaves a painful shallow ulcer. The appearance of the lesions may occur and involve the labia majora, labia minora, perianal area, vulva, vagina, bladder, and cervix. Severe pain and extreme tenderness of the infected areas are, for the most part, a universal response. A yellowish-gray exudate may be present at the ulcer sites. The pain usually diminishes in 4–5 days; however, the primary lesions may take anywhere from 10 days to 6 weeks to heal. Other associated symptoms are fever, malaise, headache, and chills. The involvement of the urinary tract may cause painful urination, urinary retention, urethritis, or a watery purulent discharge.

The recurrent herpes infection may be triggered by a variety of factors such as exposure to sun, other infectious diseases, colds, fever, emotional stress, menstruation, or athletic activities (Campbell & Herten, 1981). While it is distressing to realize that the disease can recur throughout the lifetime of a person, it is consoling to recognize that recurrent infections are less severe than the primary.

Research on herpes treatment continues despite the recent approval and marketing of an antiviral drug that has been demonstrated to be active against the herpes viruses. Acyclovir is available in an ointment 5% form for topical cutaneous use only. The medication is indicated in the management of initial herpes genitalis and in limited non-life-threatening mucocutaneous herpes simplex infection in immunocompromised patients (Zovirax [acyclovir] ointment 5%; Burroughs Wellcome Co. Research, Triangle Park, North Carolina). Use of the ointment results in a decrease in healing time, duration of viral shedding, and duration of pain. The recommended dosage is to cover liberally all lesions every three hours, six times per day for seven days. The ointment should be applied with a finger cot or rubber glove to prevent autoinoculation or further transmission.

Clinical studies of acyclovir in cases of recurrent herpes genitalis and of herpes labialis in nonimmunocompromised patients did not demonstrate any clinical benefit. In these patients the therapy is directed toward alleviating the major symptoms of pain. Warm baths, topical anesthetic and systemetic analgesics are the recommended and prescribed treatments. There are numerous research efforts being applied to unlock the unknowns of the herpes virus and to effect a cure.

Nursing implications, as with other STDs, include educating the client and public regarding the nature and course of the disease. As there is no cure or real treatment, nursing care is supportive in attempting to help the client tolerate the severe symptoms. The most important implication is with respect to the effect of the herpes virus on the newborn. Careful history taking to establish the past or present existence of the disease, close observation to note or detect the presence of characteristic lesions, and close supervision of mothers in labor and newborns are essential in the provision of quality nursing care.

Condyloma Acuminatum

Condyloma acuminatum, commonly referred to as venereal warts, results from a papilloma virus (Fig. 27.7). The virus and the resultant wartlike formations are transmitted by sexual intercourse. The incubation period may be 1–3 months.

The diagnosis of condyloma acuminatum is based on the clinical appearance of the wartlike formations. Initially, the warts are reddish-brown; they then change to grayish-white. The wart has a rough, rubbery consistency that generally is not

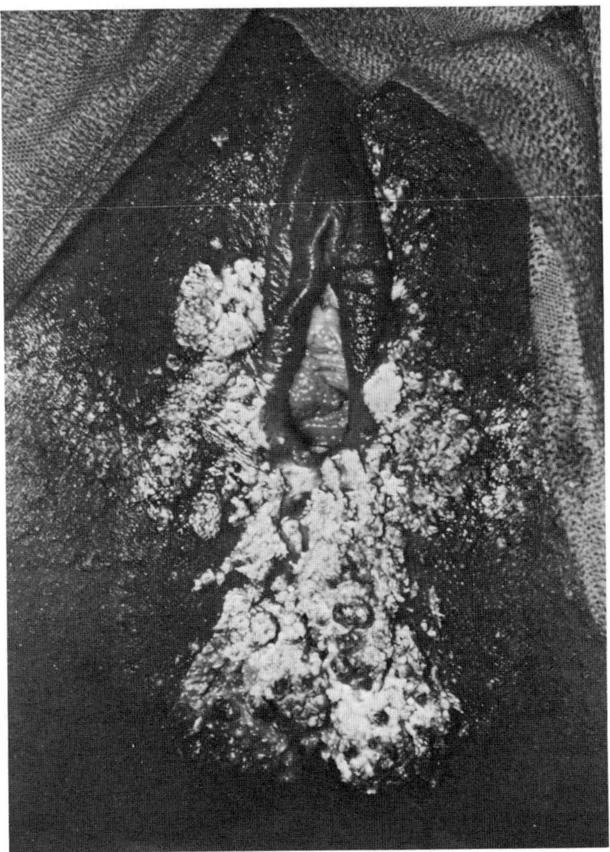

Figure 27.7
Condyloma accuminatum. Courtesy of Dr. William Fowler, Chapel Hill, N.C.

tender. The wart may have a narrow stalklike attachment or a broad attachment equal to the size of the top (Woodruff, 1976).

The condyloma acuminatum may be found on the cervix, vagina, labia, perineum, or rectum. The warts may appear singularly or in multiple clusters. The occurrence of condyloma acuminatum in conjunction with pregnancy may result in massive growth of the warts that may obstruct the introitus or vaginal canal necessitating an alternate route of delivery.

The treatment of choice is podophyllin 10–25% in tincture of benzoin. Before application of the podophyllin, petroleum jelly should be applied to the area around the warts to prevent excessive desquamation. If the area affected is extensive, the plan of therapy would be to treat small areas on numerous occasions rather than trying to eradicate the total condyloma with one application. Client comfort is a definite factor to be considered when deciding on the extent of the podophyllin application. In cases where treated tissue surface will contact normal surface area, the tissue surfaces should remain separated until the podophyllin has dried thoroughly. The woman should be advised to bathe or wash the area treated within 1 hour of application. If this is not done, the woman will experience excruciating, painful burning sensations in the treated areas as podophyllin is a very caustic agent. Podophyllin is contraindicated in pregnancy. Perineal hygiene, proper clothing, and avoiding intercourse and using condoms are areas of client education for the nurse to investigate and follow through with appropriate teaching.

Nonspecific Urethritis

Nonspecific urethritis (NSU), also referred to as nongonococcal urethritis (NGU), is another of the newly identified STDs. It appears that this may be the most commonly occurring STD. The causative organism is *Chlamydia trachomatis*, an obligate intracellular bacteria. The incubation period is 3–21 days. The diagnosis of *C. trachomatis* is difficult to make with certainty because of the lack of readily available laboratory services for identification of the organism. The diagnosis is based upon history, clinical picture, a negative GC culture, and a smear that is positive for polymorphonuclear leukocytes (Rafferty, 1981).

Chlamydial infections do not have any characteristic symptoms in women (Rafferty, 1981). Frequently, women are asymptomatic and treated only as a documented sexual contact to a diagnosed male partner. However, chlamydial infections should be considered in women with edematous cervical eversion or mucopurulent endocervical discharge.

The therapy of choice is tetracycline, 500 mg orally 4 times a day for at least 7–10 days with the course lasting for 21 days. The nurse should stress the need to continue the course of medication, as well as provide all the necessary information regarding drug side effects. Counseling, client education, and teaching are important in NSU as is true with all other STDs. The nurse should periodically review the literature on NSU since the reporting of the implications and consequences of this STD is just on the frontier.

TOXIC SHOCK SYNDROME

Toxic shock syndrome (TSS) is a relatively newly recognized disease first reported in 1978. The illness is thought to be caused by *Staphylococcus aureus.* The majority of reported cases have been previously healthy women who used tampons during their menstrual period. However, TSS has been diagnosed in males and in women who are not menstruating at the time of onset. The Centers for Disease Control (1980) stated that for reported cases there was a case fatality rate of 10–15%. There has not been any evidence to indicate a person-to-person transmission of this disease. Therefore, it is a significant infection not related to sexual practices, contraceptive use, or a history of gynecological infections.

The characteristic pattern of the disease includes (1) sudden onset of high fever (102°F), (2) vomiting, (3) diarrhea, and (4) a diffuse erythematous macular rash, and (5) rapid progression to hypotensive shock. Other symptoms may include sore throat and headache. In addition there may be involvement of three or more of the following systems: gastrointestinal, renal, hepatic, hematologic, and central nervous system. Or there may be alteration of the mucous membrane of the vagina, otopharynx, or conjunctiva. One to two weeks after the onset of the illness, desquamation, particularly of the palms of the hands and the soles of the feet, can occur.

Although the disease is rare, early recognition and institution of therapy is essential because of the rapid progression and potentially lethal aspect of this disease. The nurse should inform patients of this disease and its high correlation with tampon use. Women continuing to use tampons should be advised (1) to discontinue tampons if symptoms appear and to seek medical care without delay, and (2) to change tampons at least every 4–6 hours alternating with a sanitary napkin and to use a sanitary napkin when frequent tampon changes would not be convenient, such as during sleep.

The morbidity and mortality of this disease can be significantly influenced by the response of women to tampon use. However, it must be remembered that TSS can occur in other individuals. One man was completely surprised with his diagnosis of TSS since he thought that it occurred only in women using tampons. Therefore, you must be constantly attentive to the characteristics of this syndrome in both sexes and across the age continuum.

ABNORMAL PAP SMEARS

The woman who receives a report of an abnormal Pap test cannot help but develop anxiety as she fears the possibility of cervical cancer. The incidence of abnormal Pap smears has increased in frequency, probably because of greater numbers of women being screened. There has also been a decline in the average age that abnormal Pap tests are appearing, with a significant increase noted in teenage girls. The relationship between cervical cancer and sexual intercourse is most striking. A number of coital factors seem to be of particular importance: (1) age at first intercourse; (2) multiple partners; (3) frequency of intercourse, and (4) early age of marriage and pregnancy. The earlier the woman begins having intercourse, the more likely her predisposition to developing abnormal Pap tests. Other factors that in some way may predispose the woman to cervical pathology are lower socioeconomic status, poverty, and race.

Cervical cancer is a preventable disease. In order for this to be accomplished, however, detecting abnormal changes early, instituting appropriate therapy, and adequate follow-up care are imperative. The early detection of abnormal changes is reported by the cytopathologist using the terminology *dysplasia*—mild, moderate, severe, or carcinoma—in-situ; a more recent classification is cervical intraepithelial neoplasia (CIN)—grade 1, 2, 3. Dysplasia designates a "group of heteroplastic lesions of the squamous epithelium of the cervix characterized by a variable increase in the number of immature cells" (Kistner, 1974). The progression from mild-to-severe dysplasia to microinvasive carcinoma to frank invasive cancer is the usual sequence of events; they occur over varying periods of time. This chain of events can be interrupted and reversed to normalcy with early detection and therapy.

The Pap test is the best screening device available. It is easy to obtain, economic, and effective in detecting abnormalities. Once a woman has a report of an abnormal Pap test, further diagnostic investigation is necessary. A referral should be made to a facility or physician skilled in the evaluation and treatment of dysplasia. In the evaluation scheme, the *Pap smear* identifies that there is a problem, the *colposcope* identifies or locates the area on the cervix where the abnormal cells are being generated, and the directed *biopsy* provides the definitive diagnosis of the problem. A cervical or vaginal infection present at the time of an abnormal Pap test should be treated, even if it is asymptomatic. After completion of the course of therapy, the Pap test should be repeated; colposcopy and biopsy should be performed if the abnormality persists.

Colposcopy

The *colposcope* is an instrument that permits visualization of the cervix and vaginal vault under bright light at a magnification of 10–16 times the normal size (Fig. 27.8). *Colposcopy* is used to evaluate the surface patterns of the cervix and vagina, noting changes in cells as well as in capillary networks. The value of the colposcope lies in localizing the spots or areas where the lesion or abnormal cells are occurring.

The nurse can explain and prepare the woman for the colposcopy procedure. The examination will take approximately 10 minutes and is similar to a routine pelvic examination. The nurse can support the woman through the procedure by encouraging and working with her to use relaxation techniques and abdominal breathing. The nurse can also reiterate what is about to occur or what is happening as the procedure is in progress.

With the vaginal speculum stabilized in the open position for good exposure, the cervix is wiped with a 3% acetic acid solution to accentuate the topographic and vascular changes. There are three basic atypical patterns that can be visualized by colposcopy: mosaic pattern, punctation pattern,

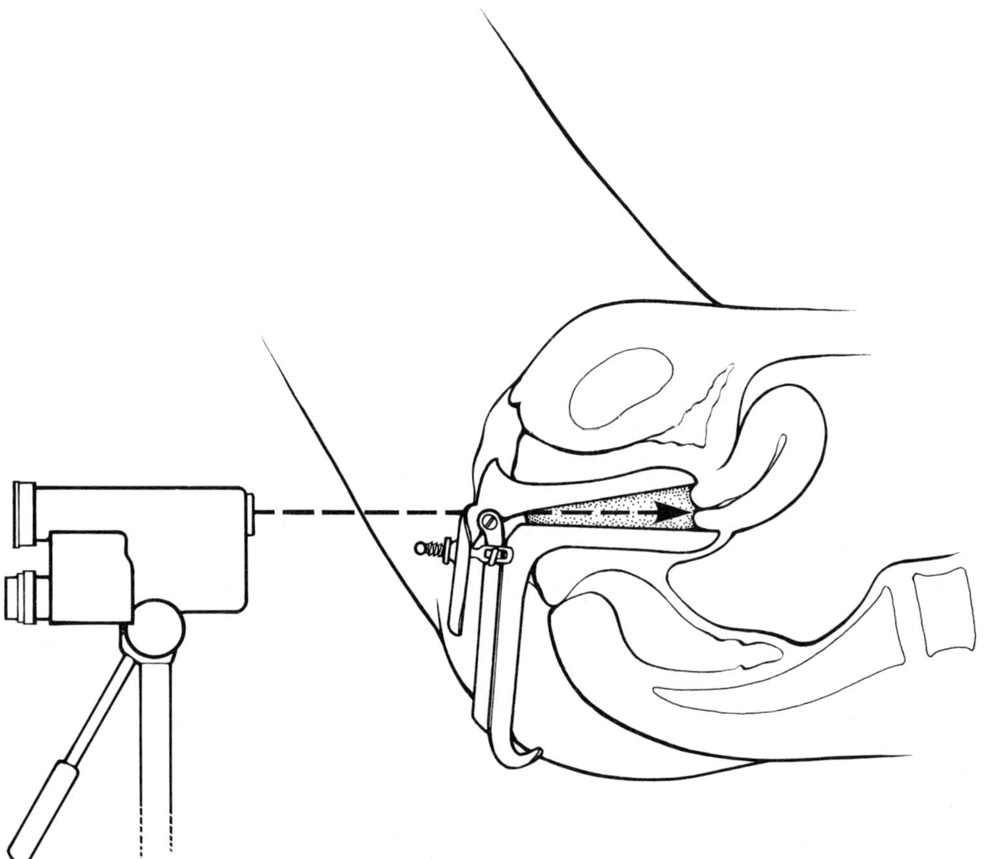

Figure 27.8
Colposcope with camera attachment.

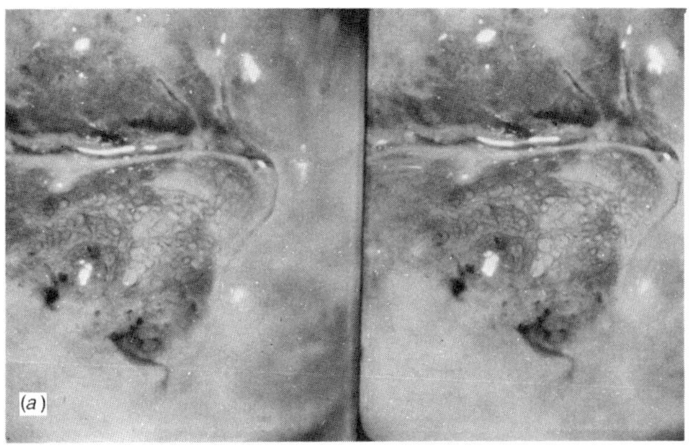

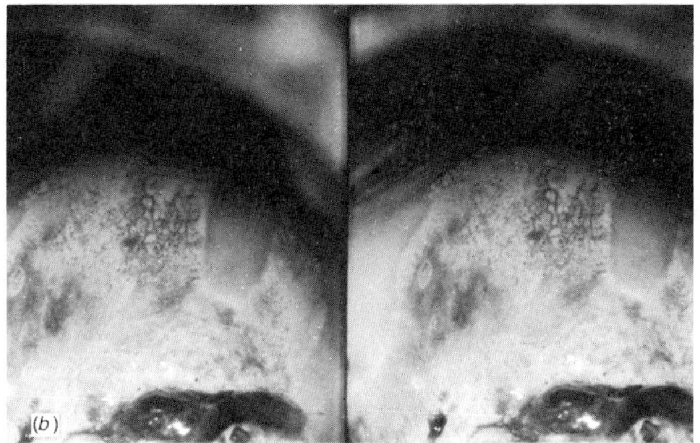

Figure 27.9
Colposcopic views of abnormal cervical patterns. *(a)* Mosaic; *(b)* punctation. Courtesy of Dr. William Fowler, Chapel Hill, N.C.

and white epithelium (Figs. 27.9 and 27.10). The mosaic pattern is a longitudinal visualization of the blood vessels, which give the appearance of floor tiles. A punctation pattern, the end of blood vessels as they approach the surface, looks like the skin of an orange. The white epithelium is white, raised in appearance, and a result of a piling up of epithelial cells. The majority of these abnormalities can be found at the squamocolumnar junction at the 12 or 6 o'clock position.

With the abnormal areas identified, colposcopic-directed biopsies provide specimens that are more accurate diagnostically, thereby reducing the number of biopsy specimens needed. The cervical biopsy specimen is obtained with a biopsy forcep; it is placed in a fixative solution in such a way as to prevent curling of the tissue specimen (Fig. 27.11). At the time of biopsy, the woman may experience slight discomfort and should be forewarned of a brief, painful sensation. Postbiopsy, a tampon with gelfoam is inserted in the vagina to control bleeding. The woman should be instructed to remove the tampon in approximately 4 hours. If the cervix is very vascular, as can be the case in pregnancy, excessive bleeding can occur. The application of Monsel's solution or, occasionally, a suture may be necessary if bleeding is persistent. A woman may experience slight spotting for a day after the biopsy, but bleeding of greater amounts should be reported to the physician or practitioner performing the biopsy.

The woman should be scheduled for a follow-up visit in 2 weeks when pathology reports are returned and a definitive course of therapy can be instituted. A recent report demonstrated successful treatment of CIN in women by having their male partners use a condom. This practice was continued for 6 months after a class I Pap smear was obtained (Richardson & Lyon, 1981). The most frequent mode of therapy is cryosurgery, with other options of conization and hysterectomy being reserved for the more advanced histologic changes.

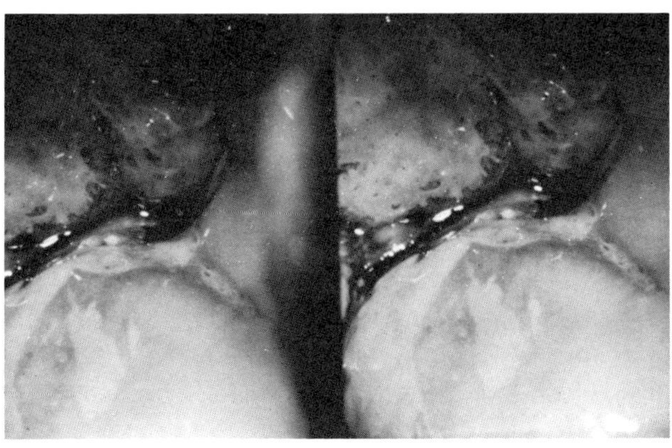

Figure 27.10
Colposcopic view of white epithelium. Courtesy of Dr. William Fowler, Chapel Hill, N.C.

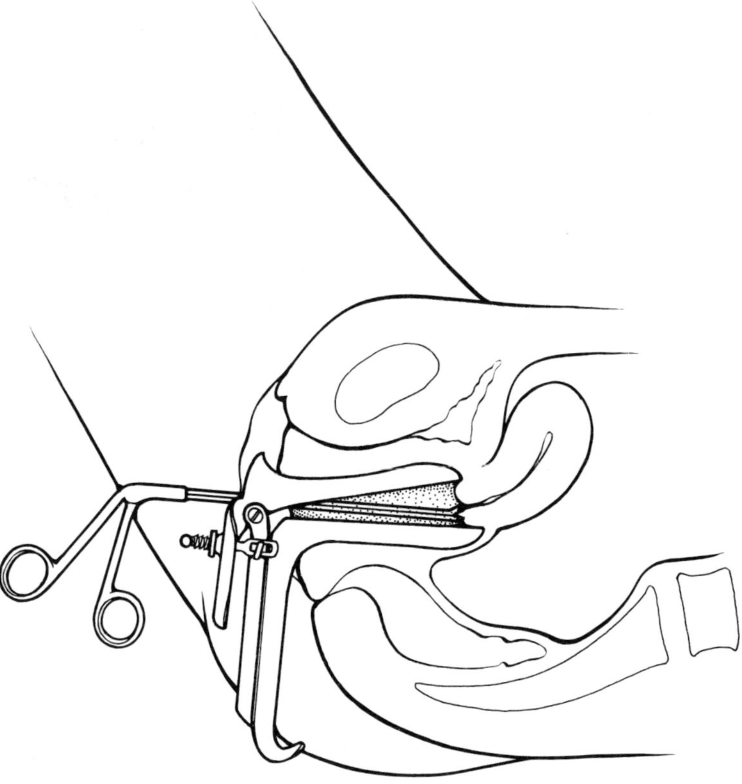

Figure 27.11
Procedure for obtaining a cervical biopsy specimen.

Cryosurgery

Cryosurgery is a therapeutic use of cold in localized areas to the extent that there is controlled freezing of tissue for the purpose of destroying abnormal cells. This procedure results in necrosis and sloughing of the tissue with eventual regeneration of normal cervical tissue. A variety of cryosurgery units are available that employ different cryogenic agents. The *cryogenic agent* is the cooling substance, or refrigerant, that enables the freezing process to take place. The most common refrigerant used is nitrous oxide, which provides a freezing temperature of −90°C. For the purpose of cervical application, the cryosurgery unit is equipped with a triangular-shaped probe that fits into the cervical canal and has contact with the ectocervix and a portion of the endocervical canal (Fig. 27.12).

The cryosurgery is performed in an office or clinic setting only if cytologic studies and pathology reports are complete. The cryosurgery should not be performed if there is any possibility of pregnancy (cryosurgery should be delayed until diagnosis of the pregnancy can be confirmed or ruled out) or if the woman's menstrual period is imminent or in progress. The reason for the procedure's delay until after the menstrual flow is the fact that an initial transient cervical stenosis (as a result of swelling and edema) occurs that would block menstrual flow and cause the woman to have severe dysmenorrhea. The procedure should be performed as soon after menstruation as possible to allow some time for the healing process to occur before the onset of the next menstrual period.

The clinical procedure for freezing begins with a review of the woman's history regarding the possibility of any of the previously mentioned contraindications (pregnancy or imminent menses) and a thorough explanation of the procedure and sequelae. Before starting the procedure, the woman should empty her bladder for maximum comfort. She is then placed in lithotomy position, and a vaginal speculum is inserted to expose her cervix. The appropriate cryotip probe is selected and inserted into the cervical canal and against the cervix. The moistening of the cervical area with normal saline solution promotes better probe adhesion by facilitating the transfer of tissue heat to the probe. When the probe is properly placed, and only then, the freeze cycle is activated. If the freeze cycle is turned on before proper probe placement, the probe will adhere to and freeze any tissue that it touches. As the procedure is progressing, the woman should be told what is happening and about any sensation that she may experience.

The thoroughness of the freezing process can be ascertained by timing or by visualizing the extent of the ice ball formation. There is a time/temperature relationship to the degree of tissue destruction. The two aspects of this relationship are the longer the duration of the freeze, the greater the tissue destruction; and the lower the temperature of the probe, the faster the freeze. In treating dysplasia, an adequate freeze with good treatment results can be obtained by a 3-minute freeze, followed by a 5-minute rest period, followed by another 3-minute freeze (3–5–3 procedure). The visual method of determining adequacy of the freeze is to allow the ice ball formation to extend 3–5 mm beyond the outer limit of the lesion into the normal tissue.

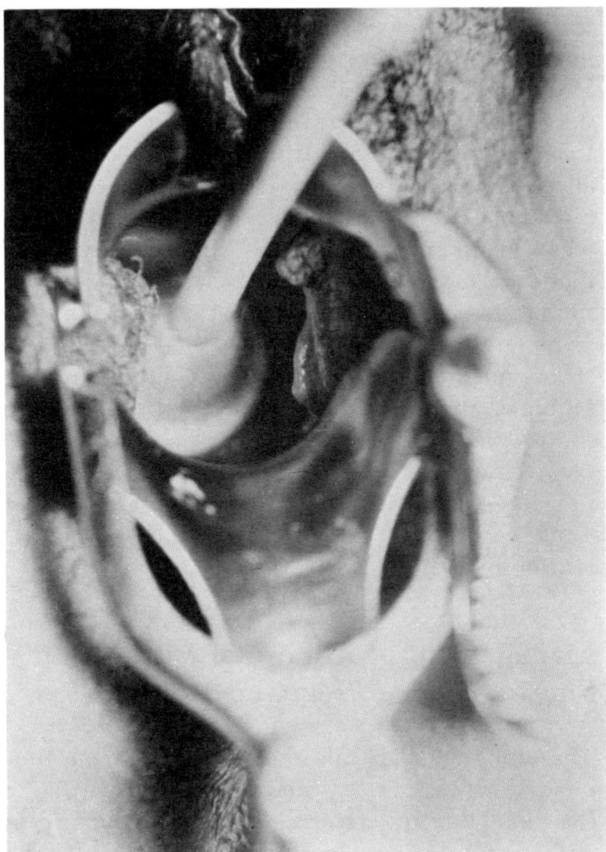

Figure 27.12
Cryosurgery probe applied to cervix and endocervical canal.

During the freeze process, the woman may experience varying severity of uterine cramping. Also, while 3 minutes is a relatively short period of time, it can seem like an eternity when in lithotomy position, having discomfort, and unable to move. The nurse can be supportive during this time by keeping the woman's mind occupied or distracted and helping the time to pass more readily. Encouraging the woman to perform abdominal breathing in a slow fashion—in through the nose and out through the mouth—is also beneficial. When the freeze is complete, the cryo unit is deactivated, thereby stopping the refrigerant from cooling the probe, and the defrost process is activated. The defrost time is relatively short (approximately 15 seconds) and is necessary in order to remove the probe gently without the trauma of tearing any tissue away that is adhering to the probe. If the probe fails to defrost, the woman's body heat will eventually cause the probe tip to thaw (approximately 5 minutes) and thereby separate from the cervical tissue. After 5 minutes, the ice ball formation of the cervix has completely disappeared, and by viewing the cervix, you would not be able to tell that anything had been done.

Care of the woman during the immediate postcryosurgery procedure includes the application of a heat lamp to the abdomen and occasionally a mild analgesic to help diminish uterine cramping. The woman should lie flat for approximately 10 minutes to avoid a vasomotor response that includes flushing, dizziness, headache, lightheadedness, hypotension, and fainting.

After cryosurgery, the woman can expect a voluminous watery discharge that may be foul smelling. This discharge may last as long as 6 weeks; the very copious amounts may last 2–3 weeks, then gradually subside. Preparation of the woman for this occurrence cannot be overemphasized. Some women have stated that the discharge poured out like a water faucet, while others felt the odor was so offensive that they did not want to be around other people. Preparing women to expect the worst will help them tolerate and plan for coping with these temporary nuisances. Because of these aftermaths of the procedure, the nurse should explore the woman's plans and activities for the next few months with her. The cryosurgery can be delayed or worked around important and special events like weddings, vacations, business trips, or other activities for which the woman must feel at her best. One additional point in relation to the discharge is the need to provide the woman with a sanitary pad immediately after the procedure as the discharge will begin as soon as the ice ball melts.

The woman should not experience any bleeding after this procedure. If bleeding is evidenced, it should be reported immediately to the physician. At the time of the next menses, the woman should be warned that her period may appear heavier than normal because of the combining of menstrual flow with the posttherapy discharge.

Other client instructions include avoiding tampons or douching until the discharge has ceased and abstaining from intercourse for 2 weeks. Abstaining from intercourse is usually not a problem as most women say that with the type and amount of discharge, intercourse is the last thing on their minds. Mild cramping may be experienced for a day or so, and a mild analgesic should provide relief. If the pain persists or relief is not obtained, the woman should be instructed to consult her physician. Some clinicians schedule follow-up visits 4–8 weeks after cryosurgery. All clients should be given appointments to return for a repeat Pap test 3–4 months after the cryosurgery. Henceforth, these women should be advised to have repeat Pap tests every 6 months for the rest of their lives.

While cryosurgery has its unpleasant side effects, it does have very definite advantages. It is a safe and effective office or clinic procedure that is less costly than hospitalization procedures. It is not as unpleasant as cautery or other possible treatments. Anesthesia is not required, and there is a minimal amount of discomfort. Infection and bleeding seldom occur.

Conization

Conization, also referred to as cold-knife conization, is a surgical procedure requiring anesthesia and hospitalization. A sharp, pointed scalpel is used to excise a cone-shaped portion of the cervix, which can then be sent for pathologic diagnosis. (See Fig. 27.13.) Bleeding from the raw area of the cervix can be controlled by tamponading the area for a brief period of time, by minimally using the technique of cauterization, or by suturing. The main postoperative complications are infection and hemorrhage.

The increased use of the colposcope by specially

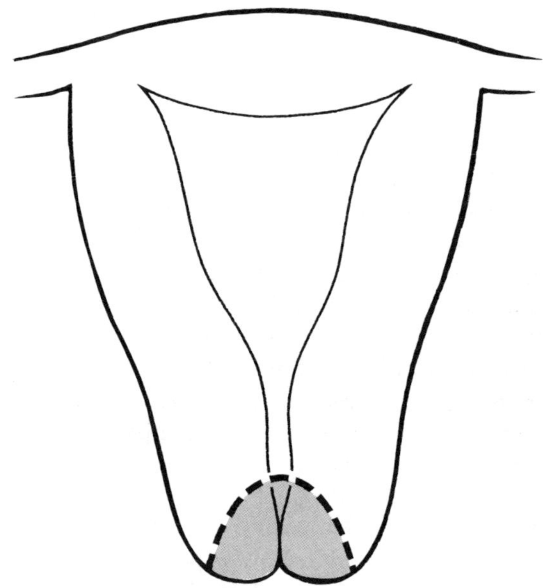

Figure 27.13
Cervical conization.

trained practitioners has significantly reduced the need for conization procedures (Fowler & Shingleton, 1971). However, there are indications for conization in some women. They include (1) the extent of the lesion cannot be completely visualized in the endocervical canal by colposcopy; (2) a possible treatment of choice for carcinoma in situ when maintaining the woman's reproductive capabilities is necessary; or (3) a lack of available personnel who are skilled and trained in the colposcopy technique.

The nursing care would be preliminary interpretation of the surgical technique and the need for the procedure. Postoperatively, careful assessment, monitoring vital signs, and observing for complications are vital. Postoperative and discharge instructions should be provided in both verbal and written forms.

Management of Abnormal Pap Smears During Pregnancy

The abnormal Pap smear requires the same thorough investigation for the pregnant woman as for the nonpregnant woman. The evaluation begins with performing a colposcopy and biopsy. The hazard of biopsy is excessive bleeding because of the great increase in vascularity of the cervix in a pregnant state. If the lesion is not seen, the cold-knife conization should be performed, accepting the risks of complications and the possibility of stimulating a spontaneous abortion or premature labor. The importance is to rule out microinvasive cancer, in which a vaginal delivery would be contraindicated, or invasive carcinoma, in which case the option to terminate the pregnancy would need to be discussed. The treatment of carcinoma in pregnant or nonpregnant women extends beyond the scope of this chapter, and we refer you to a gynecologic text.

INFERTILITY

There are approximately 10–20% of couples who spend endless hours consulting with physicians, sparing no expense, desperately searching for a way to have a successful pregnancy. The problem of infertility evokes an array of emotional responses from couples as they seek to find the answer to their problem. Feelings of anxiety, frustration, surprise, denial, anger, guilt, and grief have been identified and demonstrated by couples facing the crisis of infertility (Menning, 1980).

Most couples spend the majority of their reproductive lives being concerned about the best way to prevent pregnancy or deciding what to do if there is an unwanted pregnancy. They are responsible for their own decision-making processes. The infertile couple, on the other hand, has in some sense lost the freedom of choice by having a childless existence imposed upon them. The reality that they have lost the ability to control their reproductive capacities presents a major emotional crisis. Being aware of the tremendous psychosocial implications, the nurse can begin to help couples work through these problems and conflicts. In an attempt to meet this aspect of care for infertile couples, a national nonprofit organization called RESOLVE was funded to provide infertility counseling and referral and support groups to men and women struggling with the dilemma (McCormick, 1980).

Infertility is said to exist when a pregnancy has not occurred within 1 year, given adequate sexual exposures and the lack of contraceptives. *Primary infertility* is a situation where a pregnancy has never occurred, more specifically, the woman has never conceived and the man has never been known to impregnate a woman. *Secondary infertility* is the occurrence of the infertile state when there has been a previously documented pregnancy. *Sterility* is the absolutly proven situation of a person not able to reproduce as a result of natural factors or a voluntary surgical procedure.

The causes of infertility can be attributed to male factors, female factors, or unknown factors. The estimates are 40–50% of problems have the male factor as the basis of origin, 40–50% the female, and 10–20% unknown.

Female Causes

The causes of infertility in women can be attributed to congenital abnormalities or diseases that may have had an effect on the ovary, fallopian tubes, uterus, cervix, or vagina. The occurrence of infertility as a result of tubal factors is 40–60%, failure to ovulate is 20–30%, cervical problems is 10%, and other isolated causes is 11% (Fig. 27.14) (Speroff et al., 1978; Tredway, 1976).

The problems associated with tubal infertility are a lack of patency as a result of an infectious process or a postoperative complication. Pelvic inflammatory disease and operative procedures may lead to scar tissue formation or adhesions that may cause complete or partial blockage of the tubes. Congenital anomalies of the tubes include absence, atresia, or defective tubal motility.

Anovulation, failure to ovulate may be the result of an imbalance of the hypothalamic–pituitary–ovarian axis, ovarian tumors, or polycystic ovaries. Polycystic ovaries, as in *Stein–Leventhal syndrome*, are encapsulated by a tough fibrotic coating that does not allow for ovulation and only rarely allows an ovum to escape (Fig. 27.15). Absence of the ovaries can occur; or a streak gonad can develop, as in Turner's syndrome, where there are no follicles or ova produced. In these cases, there is the absolute condition of sterility, not infertility.

Cervical factors can be related to cervicitis, hostile cervical mucus that is impenetrable by the sperm or incompatible with sperm survival. Obstruction of the cervical canal can be related to cervical polyps, or tumors, or cervical stenosis that may be a result of infection, cautery, or other surgical intervention.

Congenital malformations or infections of the uterus or vagina are other factors that may contribute to infertility (see Fig. 27.16). *Endometriosis*, a disease process in which endometrial cells implant

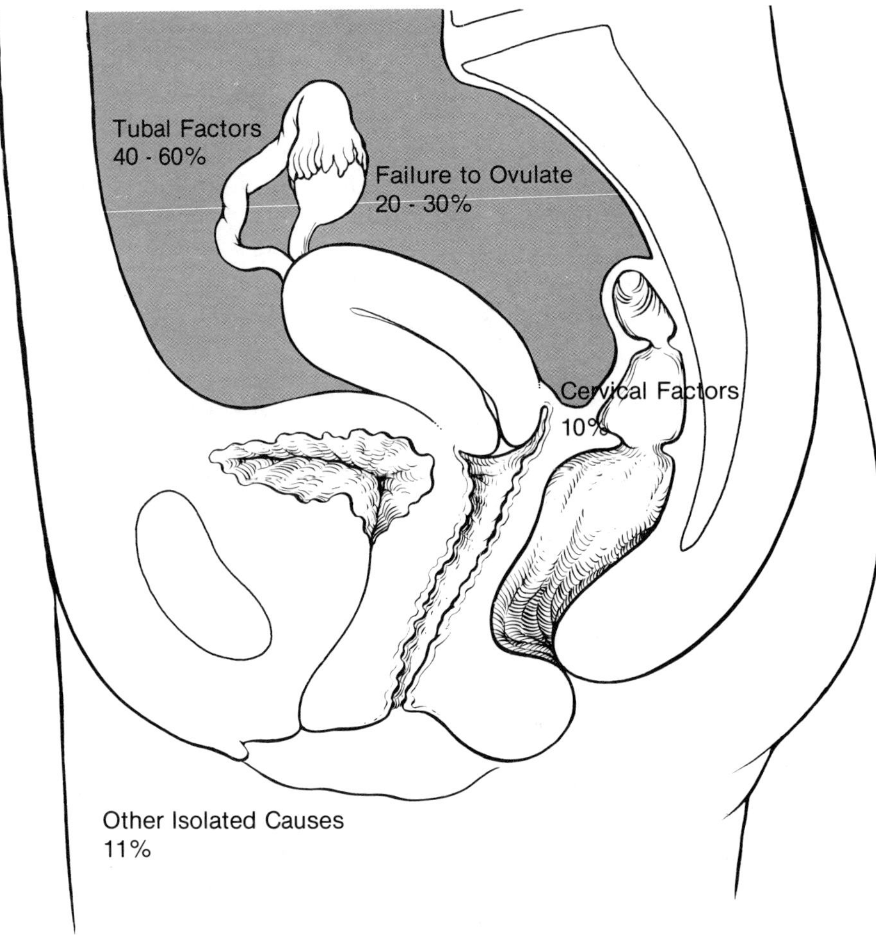

Figure 27.14
Percentage of infertility as a result of tubal, ovarian, cervical, and other causes.

on other pelvic organs, is seen in a significant number of women who present for infertility (see Fig. 27.17). In some women, documentation of a sperm allergy is evidenced by circulating antibodies to sperm (Speroff et al., 1978). The last isolated infertility cause may be correlated to other illnesses or disease processes such as diabetes mellitus, thyroid disorders, or drug abuse. This points out the need for a careful history and physical examination to uncover any and all possible alternatives to the basic problem of infertility.

Male Causes

Male infertility can be related to abnormal sperm development, interference in the hypothalamus–pituitary control mechanism, congenital malformations of the reproductive tract, obstruction of the tube transport system, inability to achieve or maintain an erection, sperm antibodies, or environmental causes.

Abnormal sperm development would be evident in a semen analysis by way of reduced number of sperm, decrease in sperm motility, and abnormally shaped sperm. There may also be a very small ejaculatory volume with increased viscosity. The hypothalamic–pituitary axis may be functioning normally, but for unknown reasons (probably genetic) there can develop a testicular insensitivity and, hence, sterility. Another condition that influences the quality of semen by an unknown mechanism is the presence of a varicocele. A *varicocele* is a varicose vein of the internal spermatic vein, usually occurring on the left side. Ligation of this vein in men having the condition of varicocele has had

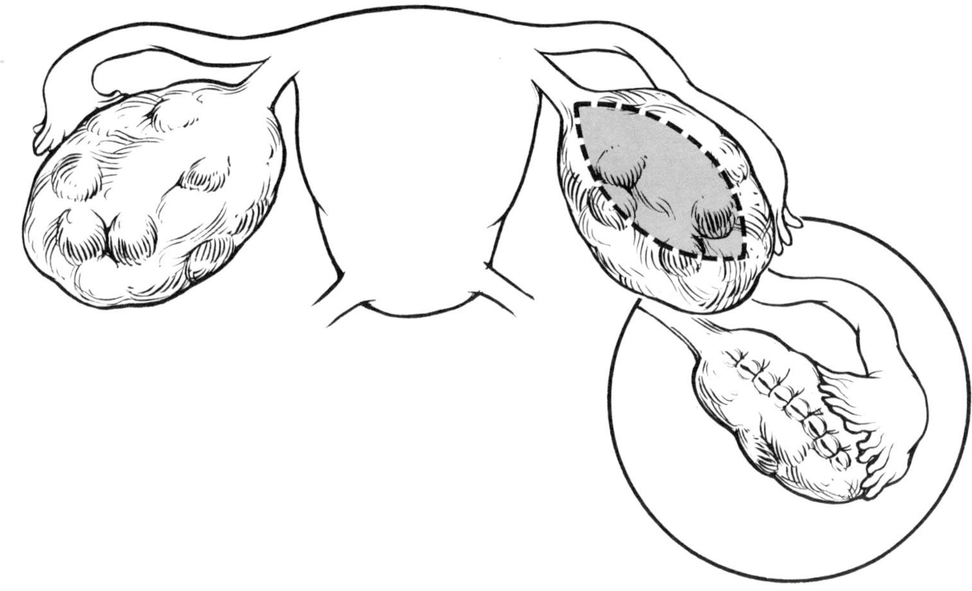

Figure 27.15
Stein–Leventhal syndrome. Polycystic ovaries, wedge resection, and repair.

a significant improvement in their sperm motility and the pregnancy rate of their partners (Stewart, 1974).

Congenital or acquired malformations of the reproductive tract may involve the testes, penis, epididymis, vas deferens, prostate gland, or seminal vesicle. *Cryptorchidism*—the failure of the testes to descend—agenesis, or dysgenesis can influence fertility. The obstruction of some part of the male ductal system can result from an infectious disease process. Sexually transmitted diseases are more often symptomatic in men than in women, leading to earlier institution of therapy and reducing the possibility of long-term effects. In adult men, mumps can be particularly devastating since they are associated with testicular inflammation and permanent damage that may result in infertility or sterility. Men with Klinefelter's syndrome (XXY sex chromosomes) usually have small testes and *azoospermia* (without sperm), although this is not an absolute occurrence.

Impotence is the inability to achieve or maintain an erection. In the majority of cases sexual counseling or psychologic help can greatly improve this problem.

In the category of environmental causes, the depression of sperm production (spermatogenesis) can be attributed to prolonged heat exposure from an occupational source (steel mills), recreational source (hot tubs), or natural source (hot climates). Usually avoiding the source of heat elevation will result in a return of normal sperm production. Drugs, illnesses, and radiation all can have a negative effect on male fertility.

As an aftermath of trauma, infection, or vasectomy, autoimmune antibodies may interfere with normal spermatogenesis. This production of antibodies against a man's sperm in his own body has resulted in oligospermia or azoospermia.

Infertility Workup

The initial interview for infertility workup should involve the couple. This is a problem of both partners and one in which they each have an emotional investment. In addition, the investigation or diagnostic evaluation involves testing both partners; the testing can go on simultaneously from the simple to the more complex. Remember, each partner contributes about equally to the infertility problem and, therefore, it is unrealistic to subject only one partner to extensive workup without evaluating the other partner, who may be the primary cause of the couple's infertility.

Furthermore, both people should be informed together of the implications of the process upon which they are about to embark. A complete

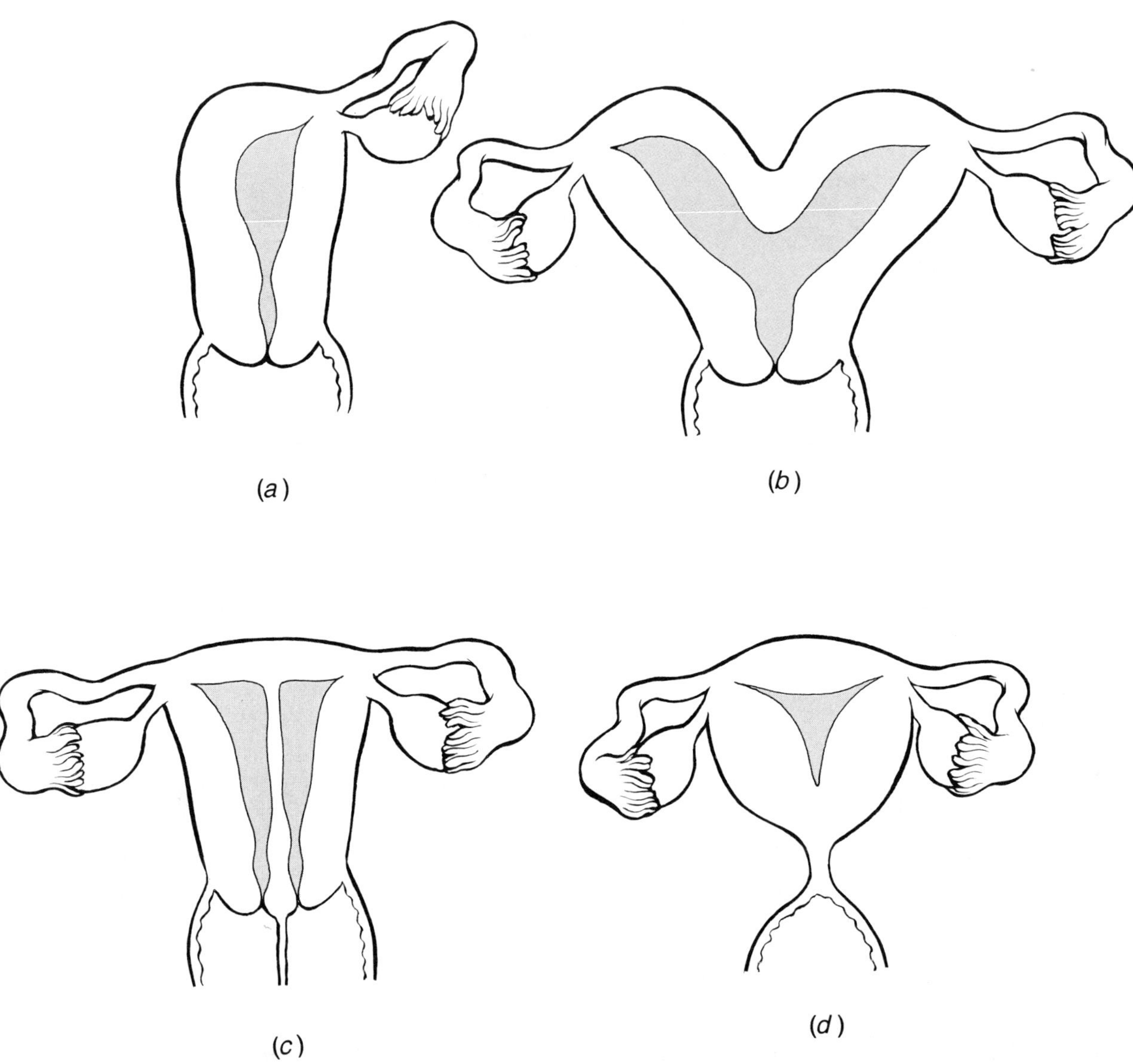

Figure 27.16
Examples of congenital malformations of the reproductive tract. (*a*) Uterus unicornus; (*b*) bicornuate uterus; (*c*) uterus septus with double vagina; (*d*) atresia at cervix.

workup may take from 6 months to 1 year. This is certainly an investment in time, as well as in expense. In addition to the factors of time and cost, there is the consideration that the success rate for pregnancy production is only about 50%, depending on the factors causing the infertility. For some couples, the eternal hope of achieving parenthood gives them the strength to endure many setbacks.

The basic infertility workup should begin with a very thorough history and complete physical examination of both the man and the woman. The next step in the assessment should be a semen analysis. It is a simple, noninvasive procedure and test that can provide invaluable information and, if diagnostic, it can prevent more extensive and greater risk procedures from being performed on the woman.

MALE INFERTILITY WORKUP

The specimen for *semen analysis* is collected by masturbation or coitus interruptus. Masturbation is the preferred method to avoid losing any portion of the ejaculate. The man should be instructed on the

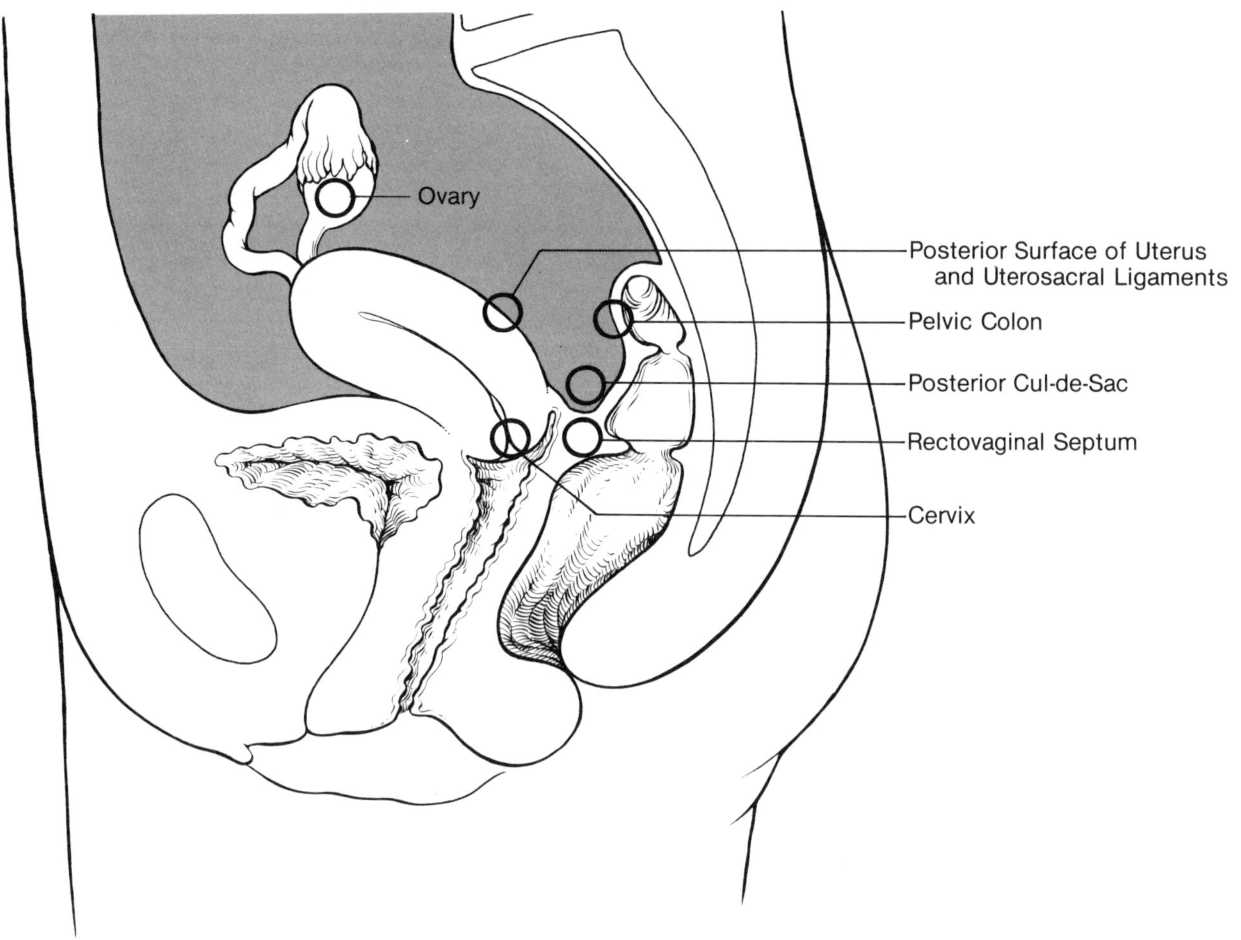

Figure 27.17
Posterior sites of endometrial implants.

proper method of collection, which includes ejaculating into a clean, dry glass or plastic container with a nonmetallic lid. (Metal can inhibit sperm motility.) The specimen should be collected after what the man would consider to be a normal period of abstinence (the period of time between usual intercourse). The specimen should be obtained at a time that would allow for the specimen to be examined within 2–3 hours. The ideal is for the man to obtain the specimen in a clinic or office setting. Some men, however, may have difficulty or may be unable to obtain the specimen in these situations because of anxiety or stress. The specimen should be kept at a normal temperature so as not to alter the analysis.

The semen is evaluated for volume produced (2–5 ml), the number of sperm (20 million per ml), sperm motility (60% motile), and sperm morphology (70% normal) (Tredway, 1976). Further analysis should include culture for infectious organisms, estimation of fructose and acid phosphatase as indicators of seminal vesicle and prostate gland function (de Kretser, 1974). Another aspect of semen analysis requires the collection of a split ejaculate. The collection is performed in the same manner previously described, except the first portion of the ejaculate is collected in one jar and the second portion in another. The ejaculatory discharge occurs in sequential components with the split specimen allowing for evaluation of the normal sequence. Semen analysis is usually part of the man's infertility workup.

Other aspects of the man's infertility workup can include testicular biopsy specimens, hormonal analysis, and cytogenetic studies. The more extensive evaluation of the man is performed by a urologist. The need for further evaluation or diagnostic tests of the man will be based on the preliminary semen analysis, the lack of abnormal findings on physical examination, as well as on negative female findings on some of her basic tests.

FEMALE INFERTILITY WORKUP

The initial step in the woman's infertility workup is directed toward collecting evidence of an ovulatory pattern. If the women is not ovulating, the recognition of any other factor such as blocked tubes is unimportant. The basal body temperature (BBT) chart, which is the same as described in Chapter 26 under contraception control, is used. The basic purpose of the BBT in both circumstances is to validate ovulation. The ultimate use of this information—contraception versus infertility—is very different, however.

The evaluation of the cervical mucus provides data regarding the normalcy of the ovarian hormones that regulate the secretion of cervical mucus. Estrogen stimulates the secretion of excessive amounts of water, thin mucus; progesterone inhibits the secretory activity, which causes a decrease in and thickening of mucus. The ovulation method (see Chapters 5 and 26) as a contraceptive method is based on the same cyclic alterations that occur in cervical mucus. The cervical mucus is generally evaluated preovulatory or ovulatory to determine if the cyclic changes that are receptive to sperm penetration are in evidence. In addition to the quantity and type of mucus present, the other major evaluative studies performed are the spinnbarkheit and the fern test. The cervical mucus sample is obtained by aspiration with a pipette, syringe, or mucus forceps.

The spinnbarkheit is performed by placing the cervical mucus sample on a slide and covering it with a cover slip. The mucus is then drawn betweem the slide and the cover in order to evaluate the elasticity and the length of the thread formation. The spinnbarkheit normal cyclic pattern is day 10: 4–6 cm; days 13–14: 10–12 cm; day 18: 3 cm; day 24: 2 cm (Fig. 27.18) (Moghissi, 1976). Generally, a spinnbarkheit greater than 7 cm is considered normal and adequate.

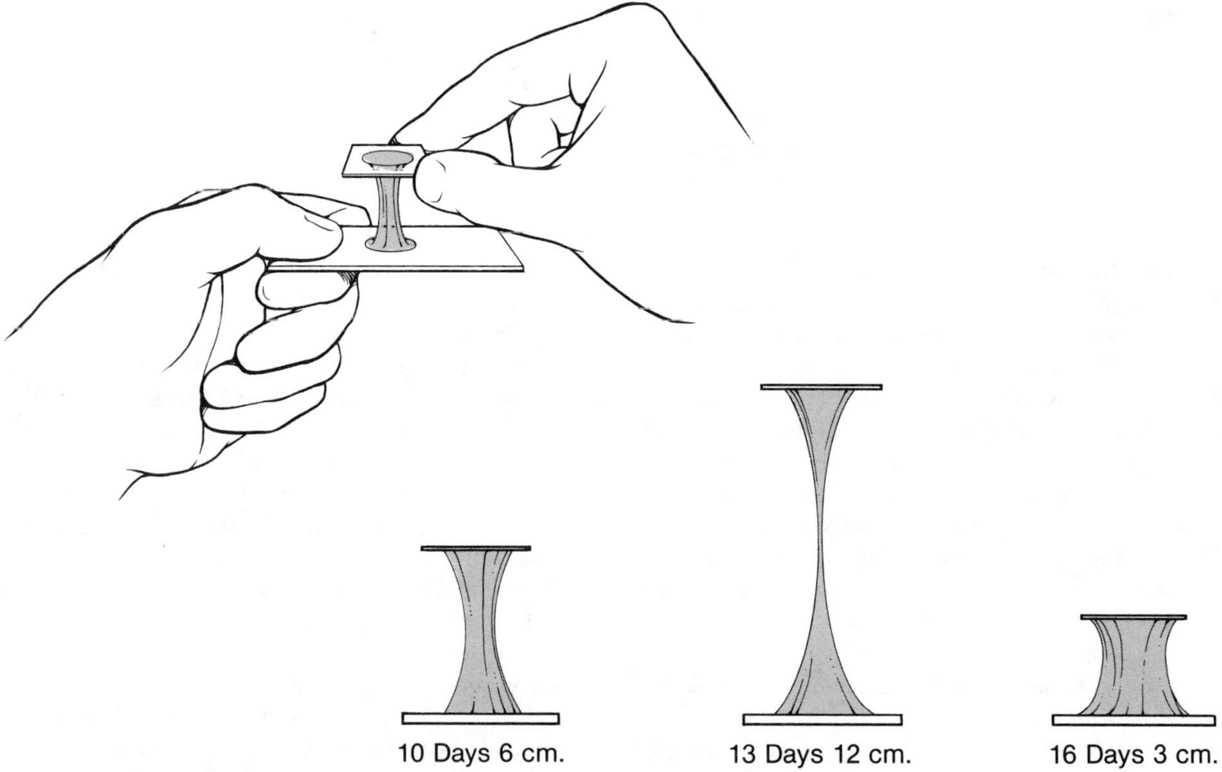

Figure 27.18
Spinnbarkheit technique and normal findings on given days of the menstrual cycle.

The *ferning* capacity of the cervical mucus increases as ovulation nears under the influence of estrogen and then disappears or is nonexistent under the influence of progesterone. The term ferning is used because of the development of a fern leaf pattern as the cervical mucus is spread on a glass slide, allowed to dry, and then viewed under a microscope (see Fig. 27.19). This crystallization pattern is a result of salt and water interacting with glycoproteins (Shane et al. 1976). Ferning is graded on a 0 to +4 scale, with +4 occurring near the time of ovulation. The evaluation of the cervical mucus thus provides some indication of the hormonal balance and presence of cervical mucus that is conducive to sperm penetration.

The workup continues onto the next step and each subsequent step until an abnormality can be identified and a diagnosis made. The *postcoital*, or *Huhner test*, incorporates not only the evaluation of the cervical mucus, but the number and motility of the sperm present in a sample taken from the endocervix (Fig. 27.20). The postcoital test should be performed around the time of ovulation (1–2 days before) as determined by the BBT and changes in the cervical mucus. The couple is instructed to abstain from intercourse for 2 days before the test and to have intercourse within 6–8 hours before having the test (Moghissi, 1976). A time range of 2–24 hours is given for the performance of this test.

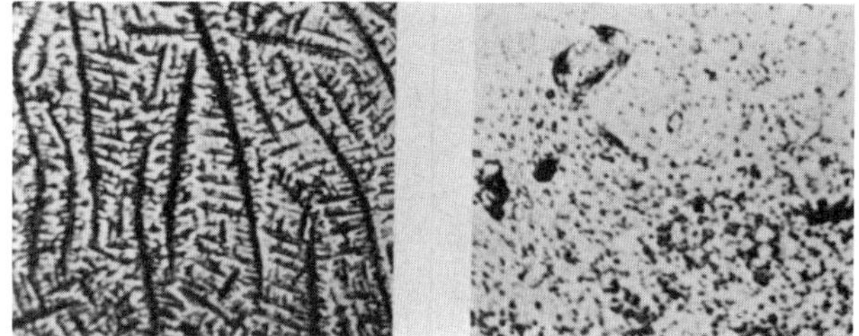

Figure 27.19
Typical cervical mucous patterns. (Left) Ferning—estrogen response; (right) amorphous—progesterone response. Courtesy of Dr. James Dingfelder, Chapel Hill, N.C.

In order to perform the test, a nonlubricated speculum is inserted and a sample of cervical mucus is taken from the endocervix. The sample is

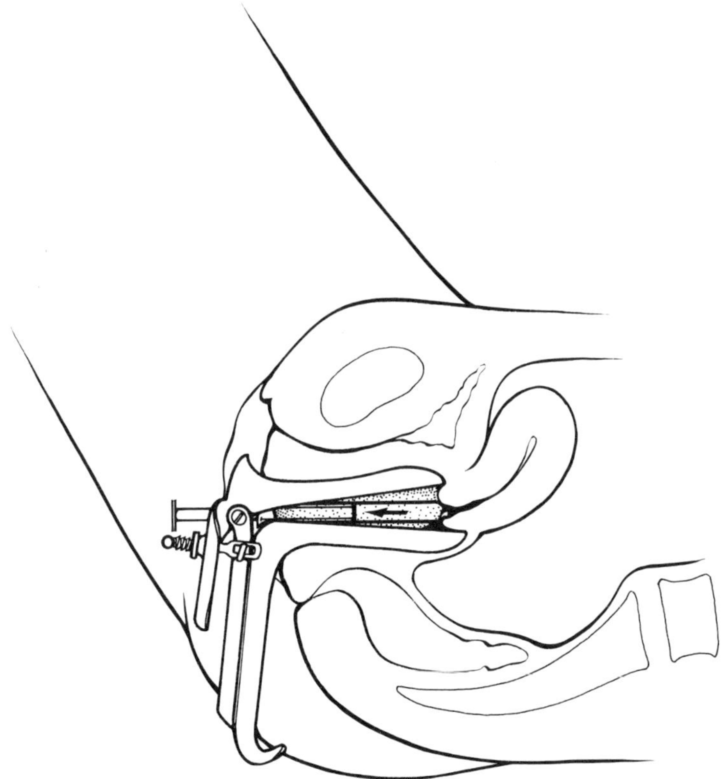

Figure 27.20
Huhner postcoital test—sampling from endocervical canal.

obtained by aspirating with a tuberculin syringe without the needle. The sample is evaluated for cervical mucus factors and sperm number and motility by placing it on a glass slide with a cover slip and examining it under a microscope with low and high power. At 6–8 hours postcoitus, a normal, or positive, test would reveal more than 10 sperm per high power field with good motility (Moghissi, 1976). A negative, or poor, postcoital test should be repeated and, if persistently negative, the considerations of hostile cervical mucus, sperm antibodies, abnormal cervical mucus pH, or abnormal semen need to be further investigated. The postcoital, or Huhner, test must be a part of every infertility workup as it is the only test that evaluates the interaction between sperm and the fluid of the woman's reproductive tract.

If the tests continue to be normal, the infertility workup is directed toward validation of tubal patency. The two tests that can be performed to demonstrate this aspect are the *Rubin test* and *hysterosalpingography*. The Rubin test is a tubal-insufflation test using carbon dioxide (Fig. 27.21). The carbon dioxide is administered under pressure into the uterine cavity through a special cannula. The gas will escape through the fallopian tube if patent. A positive test can be demonstrated either by auscultation of the abdomen as the gas escapes into the abdominal cavity or by having the woman sit up so the gas will rise, causing a subdiaphragmatic irritation resulting in a referred transient pain to the shoulder. Lack of these signs would be indicative of tubal obstruction. While this test is a relatively easy office procedure, it has virtually been replaced by hysterosalpingography.

Hysterosalpingography is an x-ray examination that provides information about tubal patency as well as about the endometrial cavity (Fig. 27.22). A radiopaque dye (usually an oil base dye—ethiodol) is injected slowly into the uterine cavity through a

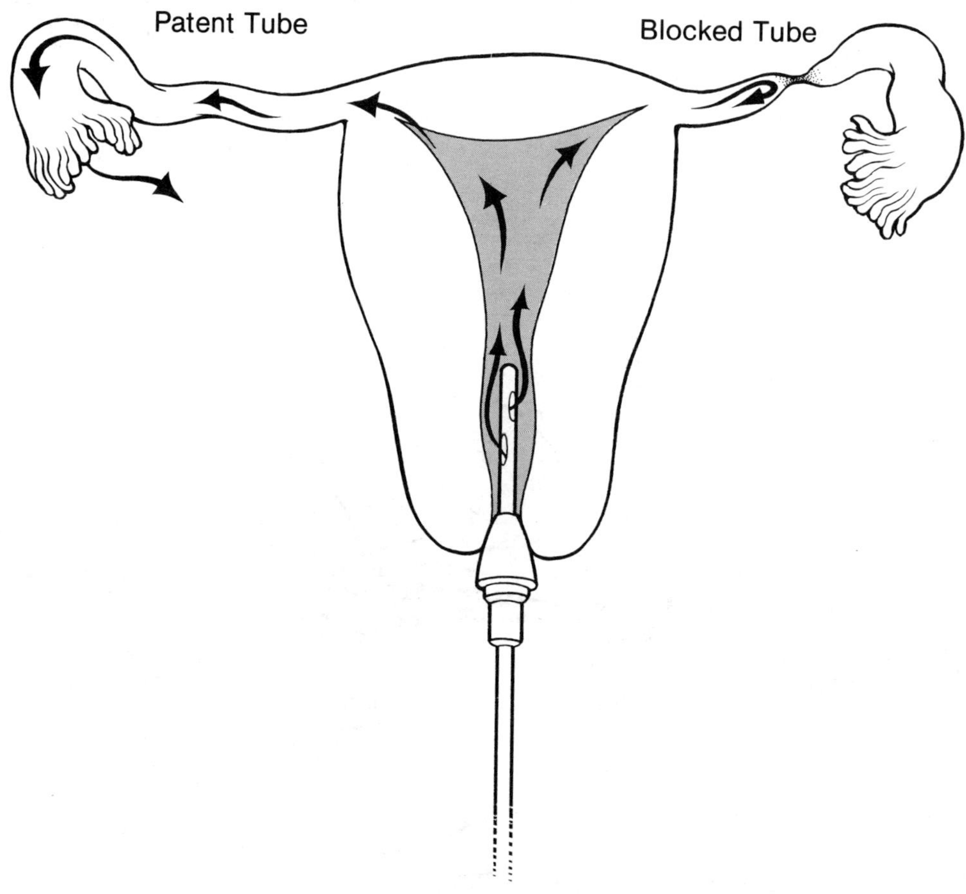

Figure 27.21
Rubin test for tubal patency.

special cannula. The volume required to provide a good fill of the cavity and tubes is usually no more than 3–6 ml (Speroff et al., 1978). If cramping occurs, the dye injection should be temporarily stopped; as the cramping subsides, it can be resumed. The timing of the hysterosalpingogram or Rubin test should be during the proliferative phase of the menstrual cycle (days 4–10) to avoid performing the test during an early pregnancy or during the secretory phase, which may give false reports of blockage (Shane et al., 1976). The hysterosalpingogram is the procedure of choice because it gives more accurate information.

The value of hysterosalpingography as a diagnostic tool is that it is reliable. There is some speculation that hysterosalpingography may also have a beneficial therapeutic role. According to some researchers, the reported increases in pregnancy rates after the procedure may be attributed to (1) the tubes being cleaned as the dye flows through, (2) the tubes being straightened and/or the breaking up of minor adhesions, (3) the stimulation of ciliary action in the tube, or (4) alteration of cervical mucus.

The adequacy of the later half of the menstrual cycle is evaluated by endometrial biopsy and plasma progesterone test. For women on a 28-day menstrual cycle, the endometrial biopsy is performed on day 25–28 of the cycle; for cycles longer or shorter than 28 days, the performance date is adjusted to the appropriate time. A small endometrial curette, not requiring dilatation of the cervix, is used to obtain the endometrial sampling. The danger of this test is the possibility of interrupting an already existing early pregnancy in the process of obtaining the biopsy specimen. However, the possibility of this is minimal considering the circumstances (infertility) for the test being performed. The data acquired is relevant to corpus luteum functioning and the response of the endometrium for potential implantation. The biopsy is painful, and the woman may experience continued cramping for a few minutes and some spotting for a few hours to a day postbiopsy.

A plasma progesterone test performed on day 19–25 of the menstrual cycle can provide accurate and easy documentation of ovulation. The progesterone levels are less than 1 mg/ml during the follicular phase but gradually rise to approximately 10 mg/ml about 8 days after ovulation. A laboratory finding of 3 mg/ml or greater of plasma progesterone is interpreted to be consistent with ovulation

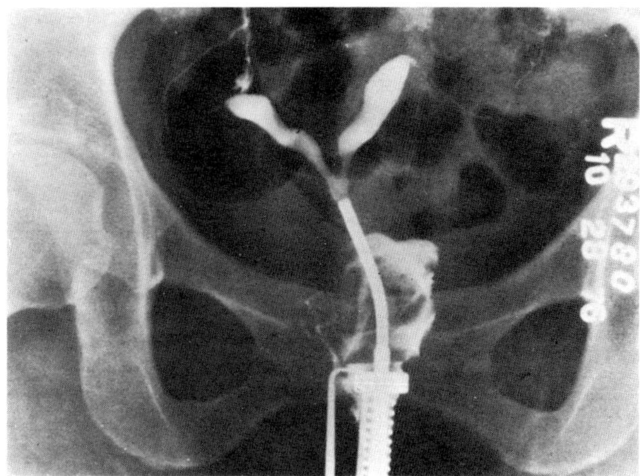

Figure 27.22
Hysterosalpingogram showing bicornuate uterus and a blocked right tube.

(Speroff et al., 1978). A 24-hour urine assay for pregnanediol is also available and can aid in detecting ovulation.

A fresh semen sample and a blood sample from the woman can provide information regarding sperm allergy by sperm antibody agglutination studies. This is an easy procedure that provides information relevant to a sperm allergy response in infertile women. The laboratory procedure is to incubate sperm in the blood serum and check it for agglutination. The test is negative if no agglutinated sperm are found. In order to counterattack a positive response, the couple is advised to use condoms for 3 months to 1 year with repeat testing done at 3-month intervals. If the test is negative, the couple may discontinue the use of condoms and plan to have intercourse during the woman's fertile period. Speroff et al. (1978) reports a 40% success rate with this therapy.

The last component of the woman's infertility workup is *laparoscopy*. If the hysterosalpingogram was normal, the plan would be to perform a laparoscopic procedure after 6 months. This time interval is suggested in order to allow the possible therapeutic action of hysterosalpingography to occur, which may result in pregnancy. The basic laparoscopic procedure is the same as that performed for female sterilization. However, the purpose is to view pelvic organs carefully detecting any unsuspected pathology such as cysts, adhesions, tumors, or endometriosis in order to confirm ovarian functioning and to obtain ovarian biopsy specimens. A further confirmation of tubal patency can be performed during laparoscopy by injecting methylene blue dye into the uterine cavity and observing the spillage or free flow from the fallopian tubes (Fig. 27.23). Unsuspected pelvic pathology is detected in 10–20% of women having a laparoscopic procedure (Speroff et al., 1978).

Infertility Treatment

After a long and involved diagnostic workup, which may or may not have identified specific problems, the couple may be faced with the uncertainties and potential lack of success of the existing therapies. Before any treatment plans are instituted, the infertility workup should be completed in order to identify all of the possible abnormalties that may be contributing to the couple's infertility. The treatment plans presented will be those directly related to the infertility. The treatment of other disease processes known to be associated with infertility will not be addressed here. In men the therapy or treatment is improving semen quality or surgical correction of anomalies. In women the treatment includes induction of ovulation, surgical correction of anomalies, treatment of endometriosis, or treatment of cervical factors.

MALE THERAPY

The treatment of infertile men has not been extremely successful. A number of pharmacologic agents (testosterone, gonadotrophin, and clomiphene) have been used to improve the quality of semen analysis. The administration of testosterone propionate causes a suppression of spermatogenesis, which, upon discontinuing therapy, is claimed to cause a rebound effect resulting in increased sperm count. The use of gonadotropin preparations with high levels of FSH and LH have had varying success in the treatment of males with *oligospermia* (scant sperm count). The use of HCG has been promising for men with normal counts but poor sperm motility. Clomiphene therapy has been documented to cause a rise in FSH and LH levels.

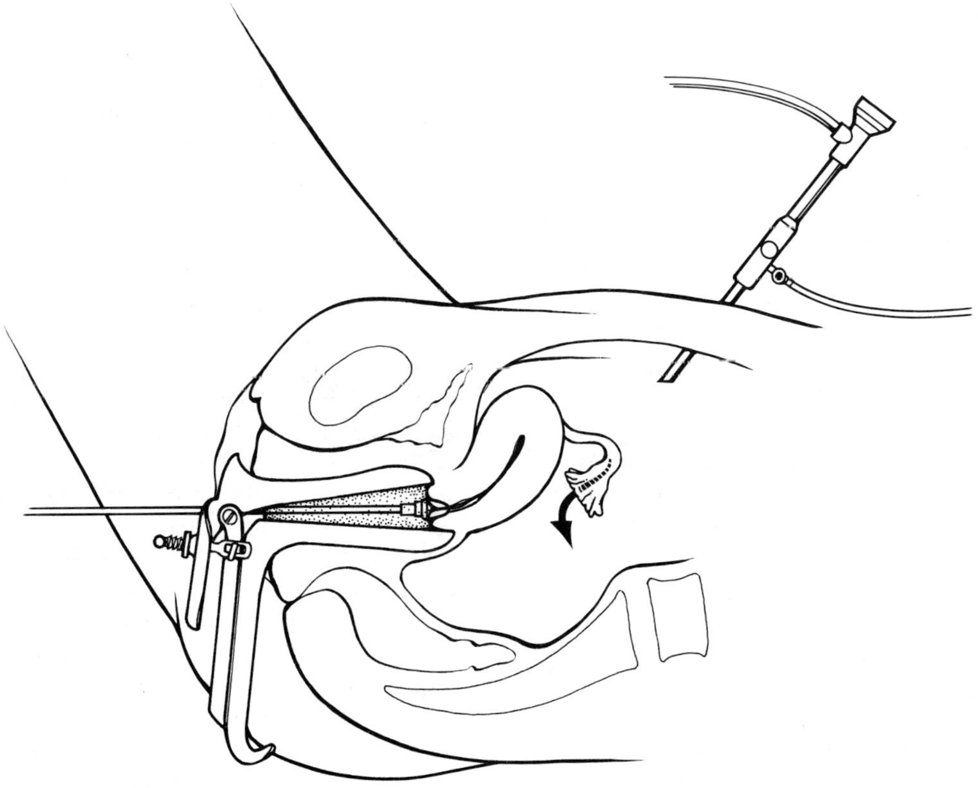

Figure 27.23
Laparoscopic examination. Injected methylene blue dye is seen escaping from the fallopian tube.

While elevation of sperm counts has resulted, the ultimate desired effect of pregnancy is rare (Urry, 1977; Shane et al., 1976; de Kretser, 1974).

The surgical correction of congenital anomalies is best performed at an early age. Conditions like epispadias and hypospadias may prevent satisfactory deposition of semen, and correcting the anomaly will enhance fertility. Cryptorchidism should be dealt with before age 5 or 6 in order to reduce the potential for any damage. If left untreated after puberty, sterility is the result. In some men the obstruction of the ducts can be satisfactorily corrected. The treatment of varicocele, as previously mentioned, has a good outcome in regard to establishing fertility. Other causes of infertility such as drugs or heat exposure can be treated by removing the source, by taking cold showers or by applying ice packs. Infections are treated with appropriate antibiotics.

FEMALE THERAPY

The induction of ovulation can be most successfully accomplished by the use of one or a combination of pharmacologic agents. The most commonly used medication for the induction of ovulation is clomiphene. At the hypothalamic level, clomiphene causes the hypothalamus to respond as if a hypoestrogenic state existed, which is followed by a pituitary gonadotropin surge (Huppert, 1979). The ovulation after clomiphene administration is an indirect response that occurs as a result of the increased output of pituitary gonadotropins.

Clomiphene is indicated in cases of anovulation secondary to hypothalamic dysfunction, polycystic ovaries, postpill amenorrhea, and infrequent ovulation. Contraindications include pregnancy, liver disease, or abnormal bleeding. A complete pelvic examination is mandatory before starting each course of therapy to be certain that ovarian enlargement is not occurring. The recommended dosage schedule is 50 mg daily for 5 days beginning on the fifth day of the menstrual cycle. This dosage is maintained for 2–3 cycles. If ovulation does not occur, the dosage is increased to 100 mg per day for 5 days. (Haney & Hammond, 1977). The majority of women will ovulate in response to these dosage schedules. BBT should be taken to confirm ovulation.

Failure of clomiphene to induce ovulation prompts some clinicians to combine the clomiphene therapy with a single intramuscular injection of 5,000–10,000 IU of HCG 3–5 days after the last clomiphene tablet (Huppert, 1979; Speroff et al., 1978). Various side effects are possible, including vasomotor flushes, abdominal discomfort, nausea, vomiting, breast discomfort, visual disturbances, and headache. The most serious and most frequently occurring side effect is ovarian enlargement.

If the clomiphene fails, the next step is to try human menopausal gonadotropins (HMG). HMG is obtained from the urine of postmenopausal women. It contains equal amounts of FSH and LH for the purpose of stimulating follicular growth and maturation. The major drawback to HMG therapy is the cost, which can range from $200 to $900 per cycle (Speroff et al., 1978). The method of administration is intramuscularly on a variable or fixed dosage schedule. Because of the variability in dosage and schedules, the specifics will not be discussed here. The combination of HMG–HCG is another alternate course of therapy. The couple must be made aware of timing intercourse in accordance with ovulation documented on BBT graphs. There are two serious side effects that warrant mentioning. Multiple pregnancies can and do occur as a result of multiple ovulations, and ovarian hyperstimulation can occur in varying degrees of serverity. The milder cases are evidenced by ovarian enlargement, abdominal distention, and weight gain. The more severe cases may be life threatening and include electrolyte imbalance, pleural effusion, ascites, hypovolemia, and tremendous ovarian enlargement. If the therapy fails to induce ovulation and the couple's financial resources are without restriction, another course of therapy may be tried. Counseling the couple about the adoption alternative may also be reintroduced.

In cases of polycystic ovaries or Stein–Leventhal syndrome, surgical procedure of the ovaries can include a wedge resection (see Fig. 27.15). A portion of the ovaries is removed in order to reduce the amount of steroid-producing tissue. Postoperatively, some women resume normal ovulatory patterns and are able to achieve pregnancy.

Surgical correction of tubal factors or abnormalities has not proven to be very successful. Recent advances in microsurgery may eventually alter this existing trend. The basic surgical procedures are directed at re-establishing tubal patency by resection and reanastomosis of the obstructed tubal section. Lysis of adhesion resulting from PID or endometriosis has a relatively good prognosis when they are located externally rather than in the interior aspects of the tube.

While the uterus is rarely the cause of infertility, there are a variety of conditions that can occur; they can be corrected by surgical methods. The correction of various congenital uterine anomalies is accomplished by a variety of equally successful methods. Diagnosed uterine tumors may be interfering with fertility, and their removal has improved fertility outcome. Intrauterine adhesions (*Asherman's syndrome*) can occur postpartum, postabortion, or postinfection. Lysis of these adhesions can be performed after dilatation of the cervix.

Infertility associated with endometriosis is a perplexing and difficult situation to manage. The symptoms of endometriosis are dysmenorrhea and development of adhesions affecting the tubes and ovaries. Surgical lysis of the adhesions through the laparoscope should be performed, and attempts to restore normal tubo-ovarian relationships should be made. The removal of endometrial implants to alleviate severe symptoms and still preserve childbearing function would be dependent on the age of the woman and the extent and location of the endometrial implants. Antigonadotropin and antiprostaglandin drugs have provided some symptomatic relief.

The problems associated with inappropriate cervical mucus can be helped by the administration of estrogen. This can be effective in situations where there is a deficient mucus state or thick impenetrable mucus. In cases of continued hostile cervical mucus, the option of intrauterine insemination of sperm may be considered. The drawback to this procedure is that even small amounts of semen introduced into the uterine cavity can cause severe uterine contractions and an anaphylactic-type reaction. For this reason, no more than 0.3 cc of semen should be instilled (Speroff et al., 1978). The other disadvantage is the increased risk of infection.

ALTERNATE METHODS

If the individual male or female treatment methods are unsuccessful, the couple faces the problem of choosing an alternate decision. The potential options are adoption, abandoning all hopes and desires of raising children (childless living), or if documented male infertility, artificial insemination or in vitro fertilization. The adoption process presents a new set of problems with which the couple must cope. Lack of available babies for adoption leads to long waiting periods. The cost may be an insurmountable burden, especially if the couple has been absorbing the cost of the infertility workup. Emotional feelings of frustration, anger, loss, and helplessness may resurface. (See Chapter 18.)

Artificial insemination can be used in situations of documented infertility of the man. If acceptable to the couple, artificial insemination can be performed with the partner's sperm, a donor's sperm, or a combination of both. The semen may be a fresh specimen or a frozen–thawed specimen from a donor bank. The technique of insemination involves either injecting the semen into the vaginal vault, cervical canal, or uterus, or putting the semen in a cervical cap that is placed over the cervix for a period of 8 hours (Fig. 27.24). The artificial insemination should be optimally timed to coincide with ovulation as determined by BBT and cervical mucus changes. There are advantages and disadvantages to artificial insemination, be it partner (AIH) or donor (AID). Counseling of the couple is imperative. The implications of the procedure must be carefully explained and explored. The couple should be encouraged and helped to explore feelings regarding this procedure. If either partner shows ambivalence or objection to the procedure, both should be referred for further counseling before the insemination is performed.

In vitro fertilization is the latest available technique to help infertile couples. Oocytes are obtained from the ovary by the laparoscopy method. Oocytes and sperm are manipulated in the laboratory setting to facilitate fertilization. The fertilized ovum is returned to the uterus with the possibility of implantation. Successes have occurred that have resulted in the deliveries of healthy babies. The availability of this method is limited at present. There are clinics in the United States performing this technique. While surrounded by much controversy, this method may rise to new heights in the future treatment of infertile couples.

Infertile couples pose a multitude of problems to health professionals. There is a need for crisis intervention since the problem of infertility is viewed as a crisis. The nurse can counsel, refer, educate, and support couples through the infertility workup and therapy. The nurse, as an integral member of the health team, must be totally cognizant of the plan of evaluation and treatment and of the details that need to be supplied to couples regarding the procedures and therapy.

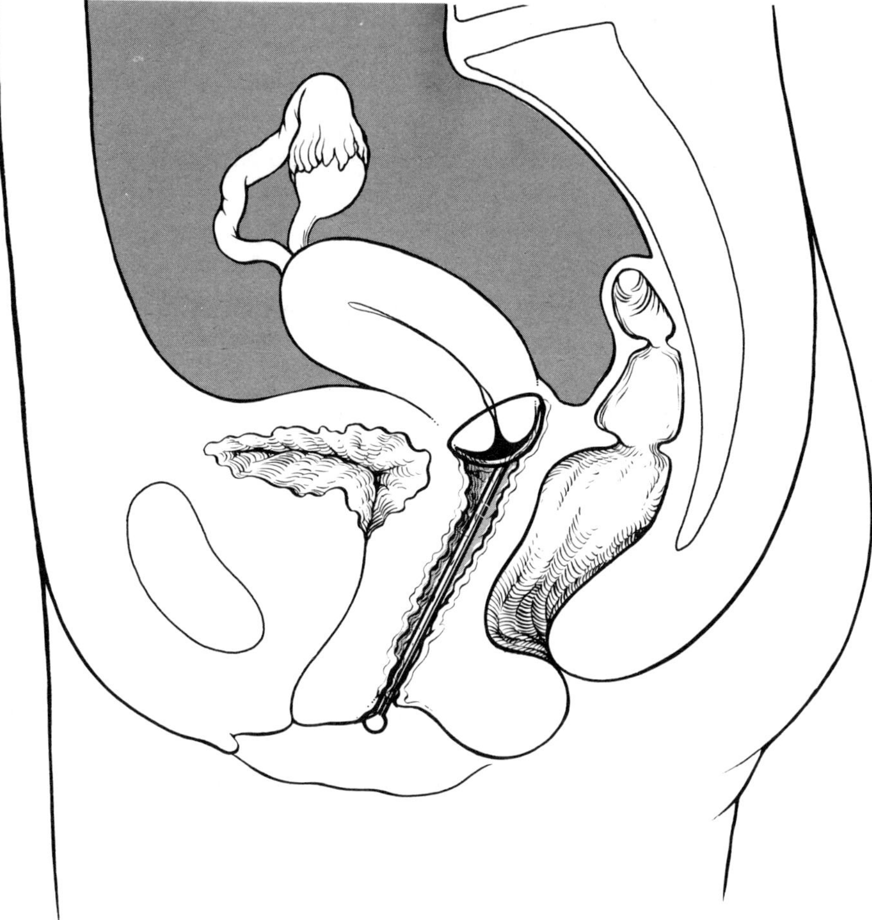

Figure 27.24
Placement of cervical cup used for artificial insemination.

SUMMARY

The reproductive-related health care problems of dysmenorrhea, sexually transmitted diseases, abnormal Pap smears, and infertility, which affect a significant portion of the female population, were discussed. The fact that these problems may precede the occurrence of pregnancy or may be superimposed on a pregnancy was mentioned. Throughout the chapter there were reminders that aside from the physical implications, there are definite psychologic components with which the woman must cope. The nurse's role in helping individuals and/or couples seek appropriate care, comprehend the care provided, make decisions regarding the acceptance of care, and adhere to the treatment regimen was emphasized. Specially trained nurses have expanded their functions to performing the procedures of colposcopy, cryosurgery, and artificial insemination. It is hoped that the assumption of these procedures by the nurse will provide women with those attributes of care, compassion, understanding, and knowledge that nurses have brought to other situations for years on end.

REFERENCES AND READINGS

Ansbacher, R. Cervical Mucus: Its Possible Role in Immunologic Infertility. *Contemp Obstet Gynecol* 8:25, 1976.

Bahr, J. E. Herpesvirus Hominis Type 2 in Women and Newborns. *Mat Child Nurs* 16, 1978.

Beck, W. W. A Critical Look at the Legal, Ethical and Technical Aspects of Artificial Insemination. *Fertil Steril* 27(1), 1976.

Blythe, J. G. What to Do About the Patient With an Abnormal Pap Smear. *Mod Med* 48, 1978.

Bjerre, B., Eliasson, G., Linell, F., Söderberg, H., Sjöberg, N. Conization as Only Treatment of Carcinoma in Situ of the Uterine Cervix. *Am J Obstet Gynecol* 125(2):143, 1976.

Campbell, C. E., Herten, R. J. VD to STD: Redefining Venereal Disease. *Am J Nurs* 87(9):1629, 1981.

Coppleson, M., Reid, B. Observations on the Initiation of Squamous Cancer of the Cervix. *Gynescope* 3(1):1, 1975.

Crooks, R., Baur, K. *Our Sexuality*. Menlo Park, Calif.: Benjamin/Cummings, 1980, Chap. 14.

de Kretser, D. M. The Management of the Infertile Male. *Clin Obstet Gynecol* 1(2):409, 1974.

Dexens, S., Carrera, J., Coupez, F. *Colposcopy*. Philadelphia: W. B. Saunders, 1977.

Dickens, A. Excessive Menstrual Bleeding and Dysmenorrhea. *Clin Obstet Gynecol* 1(3):649, 1974.

Dingfelder, J. R. Primary Dysmenorrhea Treatment With Prostaglandin Inhibitors. *Am J Obstet Gynecol* 140:874, 1981.

Dingfelder, J. R. How to Relieve Dysmenorrhea. *The Female Patient*. 1977, pp. 12–17.

Edwards, M. S. Venereal Herpes: A Nursing Overview. *J Obstet Gynecol Nurs* 7(5):7, 1978.

Elstein, M. The Cervix and Its Mucus. *Clin Obstet Gynecol* 1(2):345, 1974.

Fogel, C. I., Woods, N. F. *Health Care of Women: A Nursing Perspective*. St. Louis: C. V. Mosby, 1981, Chaps. 5, 13, 14.

Follow-up on Toxic Shock Syndrome—United States. Centers for Disease Control. *MMWR Morbidity and Mortality Weekly Report* 29(25):297, June 27, 1980.

Fowler, W. C., Shingleton, H. Impact of Dysplasia, Clinic on Cervical Conization Rates. *Obstet Gynecol* 38(4):609, 1971.

Haney, A., Hammond, C. Inducing Ovulation. *Contemp Obstet Gynecol* 9:125, 1977.

Hart, G. *Sexually Transmitted Diseases*. Burlington, N.C.: Carolina Biological Supply Co., 1976.

Harvey, S. New Relief for Menstrual Discomfort. *RN* 116, 1979.

Hawkins, L. W., Higgins, L. P. *Maternity and Gynecological Nursing*. Philadelphia: J. B. Lippincott, 1981, Chaps. 5, 21.

Hebert, P., Welch, I., Jackson, B. Colposcopy—What Is It? *J Obstet Gynecol Nurs* 5(3):29, 1976.

Heury, F. J. Managing Trichomonas Infection. *The Female Patient.* 1976.

Himell, K. Genital Herpes: The Need for Counseling. *J Obstet Gynecol Nurs* 10(6):446, 1981.

Huff, R. W., Pauerstein, C. J. *Human Reproduction: Physiology and Pathophysiology.* New York: John Wiley & Sons, 1979, Chaps. 4, 7.

Huffman, J. W. Gynceologic Problems That Beset the Adolescent. *Contemp Obstet Gynecol* 7:81, 1976.

Huppert, L. Induction of Ovulation With Clomiphene Citrate. *Fertil Steril* 31(1):1, 1979.

Huxall, L. K. Part II: The Social Diseases. *J Obstet Gynecol Nurs* 4(1):16, 1975.

Hyde, J. S. *Understanding Human Sexuality.* New York: McGraw-Hill, 1979, Chaps. 4, 19.

Irwin, J., Morse, E., Riddick, D. Dysmenorrhea Induced by Antologous Transfusion. *Obstet Gynecol* 58:286, 1981.

Ivory, L. Diagnosis of Vulvovaginitis in the Adult Female, in McNall, L. K. (Ed.), *Contemporary Obstetric Gynecological Nursing.* St. Louis: C. V. Mosby, 1980, pp. 185–199.

Jensen, M. D., Benson, R. C., Bobak, I. M. *Maternity Care.* St. Louis: C. V. Mosby, 1981, Chap. 7.

Jordan, J. A. The Role of Laparoscopy. *Clin Obstet Gynecol* 1(2):395, 1974.

Jupa, J. E. Venereal Disease. *Primary Care* 6(1):113, 1979.

Kistner, R. W. Management of Endometriosis in the Infertile Patient. *Fertil Steril* 26(12):1151, 1975.

Kistner, R. W. What Causes Cervical Dysplasia? *Contemp Obstet Gynecol* 4:97, 1974.

Lewis, J. L. Managing Cervical Cancer in Pregnancy. *Contemp Obstet Gynecol* 7, 1976.

Loevsky, J. Menstruation: Alternatives to Pharmacological Therapy for Menstrual Distress. *J Nurs Midwifery.* 23:34–44, 1978.

Lundström, V. *The Role of Prostaglandins in Primary Dysmenorrhea.* Stockholm, 1977.

Martin, L. L. *Health Care of Women.* Philadelphia: J. B. Lippincott, 1978, Chaps. 9, 11, 14.

Menning, B. E. The Emotional Needs of Infertile Couples. *Fertil Steril* 34(4):313, 1980.

McCormick, T. M. Out of Control: One Aspect of Infertility. *J Obstet Gynecol Nurs* 9(4):205, 1980.

Moghissi, K. S. Prediction and Detection of Ovulation. *Fertil Steril* 34(2):89, 1980.

Moghissi, K. S. Postcoital Test: Physiologic Basis, Technique, and Interpretation. *Fertil Steril* 27(2):117, 1976.

Nelson, J. H., Averette, H. E., Richart, R. M. *Dysplasia and Early Cervical Cancer.* American Cancer Society, Professional Education Publication, 1975.

Nelson, J. H. Nonspecific Vaginitis or Haemophilus Vaginalis Vaginitis. A Roundtable discussion. Rautan, N.J.: Ortho Pharmaceutical Corporation, March 22, 1975.

Paletta, J. L., Essoka, G. C. *Gynecologic Nursing.* Garden City, N.Y.: Medical Examination Publishing, 1978, Chaps. 4, 5.

Purser, M. Sexually Transmitted Diseases. *Reproductive Services News* 4(1):1, 1982.

Quirk, B. Part I: This is VD Too? *J Obstet Gynecol Nurs* 4(1):13, 1975.

Rafferty, E. Chlamydial Infections in Women. *J Obstet Gynecol Nurs* 10(4):299, 1981.

Richardson, A., Lyon, J. The Effect of Condom Use on Squamous Cell Cervical Intraepithelial Neoplasia. *Am J Obstet Gynecol* 140:909, 1981.

Rocereto, T. F. Differential Diagnosis of Cervical Pathology, in McNall, L. K. (Ed.), *Contemporary Obstetric and Gynecologic Nursing*. St. Louis: C. V. Mosby, 1980, pp. 200–215.

Sawatzky, M. Tasks of Infertile Couples. *J Obstet Gynecol Nurs* 10(2):132, 1981.

Scott, T., Nakamura, R., Mutch, J., Davafan, V. The Cervical Factor in Infertility: Diagnosis and Treatment. *Fertil Steril* 28(12):1289, 1977.

Sexually Transmitted Diseases Summary. Center for Disease Control. Atlanta: Technical Information Services.

Shane, J. M., Schiff, I., Wilson, E. A. The Infertile Couple: Evaluation and Treatment. *Clin Symposia* 28(5):2, 1976.

Speroff, L., Glass, R. H., Kase, N. G. *Clinical Gynecologic Endocrinology and Infertility* (2nd ed.). Baltimore: Williams & Wilkins, 1978, Chaps. 12, 13, 14, 15, and 16.

Steinmann, M. New Gonoccocus Strain Troubles COC. *Contemp Obstet Gynecol* 9:23, 1977.

Stewart, B. H. The Causes of Male Infertility. *Contemp Obstet Gynecol* 4:112, 1974.

Townsend, D. E. Colposcopy. *Contemp Obstet Gynecol* 6:66, 1975.

Toxic Shock Syndrome—United States. Centers for Disease Control. *MMWR Morbidity and Mortality Weekly Report* 29(20):229, May 23, 1980.

Tredway, D. R. Evaluating the Infertile Couple. *Contemp Obstet Gynecol* 7:33, 1976.

Tunca, J. C., Franklin, E. W., Clark, J. C. Colposcopic Management of Abnormal Cervical Cytology During Pregnancy. *South Med J* 69(6):705, 1976.

Urry, R. L. Male Infertility: Progress in Diagnosis and Treatment. *Contemp Obstet Gynecol* 9:165, 1977.

Wallach, E. E. The Frustrations of Being "Normal" Yet "Infertile." *Fertil Steril* 34(4):405, 1980.

Weid, J. C., Holland, J. B. Endometriosis and Infertility: An Enigma. *Fertil Steril* 28(2):135, 1977.

Wieke, V. Psychological Reactions to Infertility: Implications for Nursing in Resolving Feelings of Disappointment and Inadequacy. *J Obstet Gynecol Nurs* 5(4):28, 1976.

Woodruff, J. D. Identifying and Treating the Acuminate Wart. *Contemp Obstet Gynecol* 7:125, 1976.

Wroblewski, S. Toxic Shock Syndrome. *Am J Nurs* 81(1):82, 1981.

EPILOGUE

28

A COMMENTARY ON MATERNITY NURSING: ITS DIRECTION AND POTENTIAL

Maternity nursing, as a part of the broader profession of nursing, faces the possibility of considerable change over the next 20–25 years. The decade of the 1980s has ushered in a new political philosophy at the national level—the new federalism. There is a movement toward decreased national government participation in and control of a number of areas of need, among which is health care, specifically its mode of delivery and its financing. The nursing profession has set deadlines for certain changes at the entry level; traditional roles for nurses are changing; new roles are emerging. Consumerism will maintain significant momentum or peak during the 1980s, with client interest and impact being felt by the health care industry.

The United States has an acknowledged functional shortage of nurses to meet present needs, particularly in hospitals across the country. These same hospitals are faced with ever-increasing health care costs, especially the costs of sophisticated technology and personnel. People are unable, in many instances, and unwilling, in others, to pay the costs of health care.

There is also a subtle (and in the minds of some, not so subtle) social revolution occurring in the United States in which traditional social systems are changing and creating new or different demands for health care. It therefore seems appropriate to conclude this textbook with a statement about the direction and potential of maternity nursing as it responds to many of these forces and changes and to look at the potential of maternity nursing as a significant contributor to reproductive health care.

CLIMATE FOR MATERNITY NURSING PRACTICE

Maternity nursing is practiced within a social milieu that is influenced and sometimes molded by professional, social, political, and economic conditions. These conditions prevail at any given time in history and affect human affairs. To understand the scope of current nursing practice, as well as the directions nursing practice may take, you need a basic understanding of the climate in which professional nursing is practiced.

Professional Climate

Historically, nursing has been a dynamic profession but never more so than over the past 50 years. Maternity nurses have been at the front of many of the efforts to improve the quality of nursing education and practice through attention to client needs and response to client demands, expanded role practice, recognition of need for alternatives to traditional health care, and professional quality assurance.

Maternity nurses are part of the 1.6 million nurses who have valid, current licenses to practice nursing (about 1.2 million of these nurses are presently employed in some area of nursing practice) (DHHS, 1980). About 810,851 (66%) nurses work in hospitals; 99,000 work in nursing homes or other extended care facilities, 151,000 work in community health settings such as public health or other agencies or physician's or dentist's offices; and about 44,000 work in student health services (DHHS, 1980). The majority of these nurses spend 50–75% of their time in direct patient care and make up the single largest unit of health care providers in the United States. Sheer numbers alone provide nurses with the potential for making a significant impact on the nature, quality, and cost of health care today and tomorrow. Maternity nurses already provide much of the prenatal care for pregnant families—particularly those unable to afford private medical care. Most of the health care given during labor, delivery, and recovery comes from nurses.

Nursing practice is becoming increasingly specialized, creating a paradox for both clients and employers of nurses. Basic nursing educational programs prepare a nurse in the general foundations for nursing practice. Graduate educational programs and some noncredit postgraduate courses prepare nurses for specialized roles. Employers, however, often expect nurses with specialized skills to be versatile and to move from their specialized area to wherever they may be needed in the institution. The nurse may be frustrated because of lack of opportunity to practice specialized skills or because of expectations of the employer that the nurse practice in areas in which he or she may not be comfortable or even competent.

Education of nurses takes place in a variety of academic and institutional settings thereby producing nurses who are educated at the associate degree, diploma, and baccalaureate basic levels, as well as at higher levels. This diversity in educational preparation can, and often does, confuse clients as well as employers of nurses. Maternity nurses come from all of these programs creating a professional climate in which there is a great need for communication and clarification of roles and professional competence.

Significant numbers of nurses become disillusioned with nursing and change jobs frequently, or even leave the profession, for a variety of reasons, including poor working conditions, poor pay, and lack of recognition by other professional groups or by employers. This has resulted in a number of problems among which are inadequate numbers of nurses to meet the functional needs for nursing services, maldistribution of nurses across the country, and lack of true commitment of nurses to their job and their profession.

On the other hand, nurses are taking on new or expanded roles. In maternity nursing, these roles may be seen as the nurse-midwife, the maternity clinical specialist, the obstetric/gynecologic practitioner, the parent educator, and others. Further, maternity nurses may work in traditional settings such as hospitals, public health clinics, and physician's office or in newer environments such as birthing centers. Profound changes in the characteristics of nursing and in the settings within which nurses practice are likely to occur over the next 20 years as health care needs continue to change and the client assumes a more participatory role in health care. Future directions for nursing provide the maternity nurse with exciting options for practice.

In addition, standards are increasingly being used to direct specialized nursing practice. Standards for practice within speciality areas of nursing have been developed by the American Nurses' Association (ANA, 1973); other efforts toward quality assurance have been made by specialized nursing groups such as the American College of Nurse-Midwives and the Nurses Association of the American College of Obstetricians and Gynecologists.

The climate in which today's professional nurse practices is indeed paradoxical in nature. Never before have nurses had access to peers as well educated or as skilled as have today's nurses. Yet today's nurses practice in a climate of conflict within the profession, striving for educational consistency and professional recognition and status. The pessimists argue that nursing as a profession is in a critical state with the next decade telling the story of survival or dissolution. These people contend that if nurses do not unite as a group and commit themselves to clear, delineated goals, they will not survive the era of the 1980s. The optimists argue that the future of nursing is not in jeopardy and that the profession is stronger than ever. The pragmatists admit to the problems of nursing and insist that change is in order. They contend that nurses themselves hold the key to their destiny; their ability and commitment to change with the times or their refusal to accommodate to the demands for change will make the difference in whether the nursing profession survives or dies. This capability for change includes a willingness to form coalitions with other health professional and intraprofessional groups. Few would argue that nursing is at a critical decision-making stage in its professional development and it is likely that there are elements of truth in each position.

> *Nursing has emerged successfully as a healthy, well-formed professional baby. However, we are still mired in the adolescent struggle to maintain and consolidate a unique identity in our relationships with professional colleagues. Nursing's long struggle with organized medicine has seriously thwarted our professional growth. Unless we successfully complete this individuation process, or second psychological hatching, we may find ourselves repeating the same adolescent conflict with administrators in academia. It is time to move on in our developmental quest for adulthood. To be for nursing does not mean we need to be against physicians or administrators.*
>
> *Rodgers, 1981, p. 481*

Without a doubt nursing is an emerging profession with all of the aches and pains of growth. The climate of professional nursing reflects this growth, but it also reflects positive associations of nurses with nurses, nurses with other professions, increased development of the body of nursing literature, widespread concern about the welfare of the clients and the profession, and awareness of and concern with the development of policy that positively affects the health care of the nation's citizens. It is into this professional climate that the newly graduated nurse comes as part of professional nursing today and tomorrow.

Social Climate

Throughout history, social climate has had a profound influence on the manner in which nations have addressed the issues of health and social welfare benefits for their citizens. Matters of social policy, of which health policy is a part, must "take into account the nature, history and traditions of existing institutions and relationships, the attitudes and behavioral characteristics of key actors, the sector's organic development, the climate of opinion, the goals and values of a society and of its members" (Fein, 1980, p. 30).

The years since the early settlement of the United States have represented an ever-changing social scene as traditional European social systems blended with other national and ethnic values forming the kaleidoscope that is today's system in the United States. The maternity nurse today practices within a social climate that reflects change in organization and structure of the family and roles within the family. The changes include, for example, the status of women, with occupational and professional goals complementing and sometimes replacing the more traditional goals for women—marriage, motherhood, and homemaker. As the social climate changes, maternity nurses must keep pace with the new and different needs of the client in response to these changes. Further, maternity nurses, as private as well as professional people, are affected by the social climate within which they live.

The pace of daily living activities has accelerated for many people in the reproductive years, bringing about biopsychosocial demands on the body that may result in health care needs quite different from those of previous generations. The incidence of stress-related disorders such as hypertension are increasing among women of childbearing age. Alcohol and drug abuse problems are encountered more frequently. A more liberal attitude toward sex has generated greater sexual freedom and promiscuity with its related disorders and problems.

Maternity nurses cannot practice traditional nursing in a climate that demands them to keep pace with social change and expects them to be major providers for the reproductive health care needs of people. Tradition and change are incompatible, and nurses must keep pace with the demands of the current and future social climate.

Political Climate

The Social Security Act of 1935 and its subsequent amendments put the federal government squarely in the midst of health care economics and policy.

Maternity clients have been the recipients of much of this governmental largess through federally funded programs such as Medicaid, maternal–infant care projects, and family planning programs. Money provided through these and other such programs has enabled reproductive health care to be available to segments of the population—principally the poor—who would otherwise have been unable to afford the care.

The political climate of the 1980s is now quite different. The Great Society of the Johnson administration, with its emphasis on social welfare programs, has (in the minds of some) proven costly to the nation and, like other areas of social welfare, is being cut in the current efforts to curb government spending. Funds for some programs that benefit families in the reproductive years, such as in the area of family planning, have already been decreased. The 1980s are emerging as a period of governmental fiscal austerity in regard to health and other social welfare services. Maternity nurses practicing in the 1980s will experience this shift in political climate, which seems to permeate the national, state, and local levels of political activity.

Alternatives to federal funding for health care services will need to be found. Needs that cannot be compromised must be identified, and ways must be found to meet these needs. Maternity nurses have a key role in helping to create a political climate that is responsive to the needs of people anticipating or experiencing events related to reproduction. Activities such as the following are well within the scope of maternity nursing.

- ▲ Communicating needs and concerns about reproductive health to elected officials
- ▲ Going beyond the world of nursing practice into community, state, and national political activities
- ▲ Supporting professional nursing organizations in their efforts to effect health policy that is sensitive to the people and comprehensive in scope
- ▲ Assuming responsibilities of citizenship such as voting for candidates who support reasonable health care policy and who voice interest in maternal–child health
- ▲ Educating legislators
- ▲ Serving as consultants and resource people to political officials seeking information about reproductive health care needs

The political climate is fluid and influences the health care delivery system daily. Maternity nurses as individuals and as members of a large aggregation of professional nurses can have an influence on what the political climate is or becomes at any time. Nurses have not fully recognized their strength, a strength that is largely that of numbers. Policymakers, particularly elected officials, are aware of and sensitive to those who support or oppose them.

Economic Climate

Health care costs have been steadily increasing over the past 25 years creating what has been called America's health care crisis (Kalisch & Kalisch, 1982). There seems little indication that soaring costs for health care are abating as elected officials, economists, and others look for ways to bring this inflationary giant back under control. The health care industry is the third largest industry in the United States with national health care expenditures reaching $245 billion annually in the 1980s. The factors that have led to the health care crisis of the 1970s and 1980s are many, complex, and seemingly uncontrollable. The different factions within the government, industry, the health care professions and the institutions providing health care point the finger at each other in efforts to assess cause and place blame. Health care costs are only a part of a national economic crisis.

Rashi Fein, a medical economist, sees the United States as a country that has experienced a "series of significant shocks in recent years" (1981, p. 30). Among these shocks is an exorbitant inflation rate that exceeded 13% in 1979 and reached 18% in 1980. This inflation rate, in combination with the energy crisis and political crises such as Vietnam, Watergate, and current Middle East and South American problems, have served to undermine:

> *confidence in ourselves and in our political leadership and our ability to solve problems and influence events. . . . The optimistic attitudes expressed by the phrases "the New Frontier" and "the Great Society" have been replaced by such Malthusian terms as "scarce resources, constraints and limits." . . . We face the future gripped by a nostalgia for the past and we are hesitant. We are told that it is a time for incrementalism not boldness; for realism, not idealism*
>
> *Fein, 1981, p. 32.*

Health care costs have been "doubling every 5 years and are outstripping other price increases. Health care expenditures are expected to grow from the $43 billion they were in 1965 to $758 billion in 1990 unless more cost-effective forms of care are established" (Kalisch & Kalisch, 1982, p. 93).

Nurses work within the health care delivery system that is plagued by high costs, client dissatisfaction with costs, and inequities between the affluent and the poor, many of which are the result of high costs of health care. Increasingly, clients with the support of health care professionals are seeking alternatives to what the current health care system offers; some are even opting out of system-provided health care. Alternatives to the current forms of health care are apparent in expanded roles for nurses working within the existing health care delivery system, as well as in new or different settings for health care.

ALTERNATIVES TO TRADITIONAL REPRODUCTIVE HEALTH CARE

By *traditional reproductive health care* we do not mean the usual management of reproductive events over generations, but rather the medical management of pregnancy and its sequelae in twentieth-century United States, particularly from the 1920s to the present. This medical model of obstetric care involves supervision of the prenatal course—especially the biophysical status of mother and fetus—which includes the management of labor, delivery, and recovery in the hospital setting using current medical technology. Nurses tend to fit into the pattern established by the physician—a pattern in which the pregnant woman assumes a dependent position. Traditionally, it has been the health professional, particularly the physician, who has made most of the decisions regarding health care. Most people agree that this traditional model of reproductive health care has done much to promote maternal–fetal–neonatal well-being. A significantly lowered maternal and infant mortality rate strongly attests to this fact.

Since World War II and especially during the past 10–15 years, people have indicated an interest in participating in the planning and decision making related to their care during the reproductive experience (see Chapters 1 and 3). This interest coupled with responses from some health care providers has brought about alternatives to traditional care during pregnancy and birth. These changes are categorized here as (1) change within the institutions providing care (particularly the hospital) and (2) reproductive health care outside of the institutional setting.

Institutional Alternatives

Some hospitals have reorganized their maternity services to better accommodate the needs and preferences of the clients. These programs of family-centered maternity care have provided for rooming-in of mothers and their infants to offset their early separation; open visitation in maternity units, which allows children to visit their mothers and newborn siblings; early discharge from the hospital for women with no anticipated health problems; visitation of parents to the nursery in cases where the infant requires a longer hospital stay than the mother; and other changes such as parent-teaching programs and consistent health care personnel in the antepartal clinics, as well as in the labor, delivery, and postpartal areas. Recently, some hospitals have added a new dimension to the care options for labor and delivery—the birthing room. The birthing room is the institution's response to the client's need for a more personalized and humanistic atmosphere. Although the birthing room concept has only recently received widespread attention, some hospitals developed birthing rooms back in the 1960s.

The birthing room provides a homelike atmosphere where the woman can labor and deliver her infant with access to her family (usually the expectant father), as well as to health care personnel and technology. Each institution establishes its own criteria for use of this facility. Some hospitals preschedule the birthing room in advance of labor; other hospitals make it available on a first-come first-serve basis. In some hospitals, the birthing room may be used only by women who are considered low risk; in others it is available regardless of risk status. The birthing room is usually located in the labor and delivery area. While it resembles a bedroom in a home, it has all of the resources of the traditional labor and delivery unit readily available should a complication or emergency arise.

The hospital birthing room is a compromise between the comfortable home and the sterile hospital environments. It is an alternative that enables many couples to experience birth in an atmosphere that is supportive of family needs yet one that provides safety for mother and infant. (See colorplate.)

The nurse who attends couples opting for the birthing room experience for labor and delivery needs special understanding of and sensitivity to the needs of a family experiencing birth together. The birthing room is *not* a do it yourself unit; rather, it requires the nurse to have knowledge about and skill in labor, childbirth, and infant adjustment to extrauterine life, as well as understanding about the needs of the total family and skill in family nursing. The nurse may not always be the primary care giver for the pregnant woman in this setting but may instead serve as the supporter, the overseer, and the principle resource for the woman, her family, and the family's physician.

Occasionally, a hospital will have a birthing center located in the hospital itself but separate from the labor and delivery area. These centers may accommodate larger numbers of clients in an environment that is similar to the home but also within easy access to emergency care. Some birthing centers may provide parent education programs and client follow-up after delivery. Early discharge is usual from both birthing rooms and the hospital birthing centers.

Alternatives Outside of the Institution

Two alternatives to hospital care during labor and birth are discussed here: home birth and the birthing center that is separate from the hospital. Both of these approaches to health care during labor and childbirth have come about because of client dissatisfaction with the depersonalized, high-cost care that is associated with institutional childbirth. In some ways, the birthing center is the professional response to the home birth movement.

HOME BIRTH

The home birth movement has been around for the past 20 years or more. This movement reflects the effort by a number of clients to return childbirth to the family setting and to treat reproduction as a normal healthy event rather than as a medical problem. Home birth is usual in a number of countries and in parts of the United States. Home delivery under medical or midwife supervision is common in many countries; home delivery by nurse-midwives has occurred in the United States for a number of years. Many countries, for example, Sweden and Great Britain, use nurse-midwives for much of normal maternity care. Maternity Center Association in New York City operated a nurse-midwifery home delivery service for a number of years. Home delivery was also available in Chicago and through Frontier Nursing Services in Kentucky. Home delivery is still available through Frontier Nursing Services for some families.

There are two types of home birth. The first type takes place in the home for women classified as low risk for obstetric or neonatal complications who have had careful health care supervision during pregnancy. A qualified nurse-midwife or physician supervises the birth; there is ready access to emergency care and transport.

The second type of home birth takes place without supervision by a health care professional; it may be under the supervision of a lay midwife or only the members of the family. In some cultures, the lay midwife works in close contact with the physician who will provide assistance during an emergency. Precautions are taken and emergency transport is available. In other cases, no screening is done and no provision for emergency care is made. It is the latter situation that places mother and infant in greatest jeopardy.

Home birth is an attractive alternative for some families (see Fig. 28.1). It allows delivery to take place in a familiar setting with friends and family members present. (See colorplate.) There is no disruption of mother–infant relationships that often occur in the hospital. If the birth is free of complications, it will be much less expensive as well.

Home birth should not take place when the pregnant woman or her newborn child is at risk for any reason. This requires careful screening of the pregnant woman and her family to determine the health status of both woman and fetus.

Home birth should be the result of careful planning in order to prepare the woman, her family, and the environment for this event. This planning

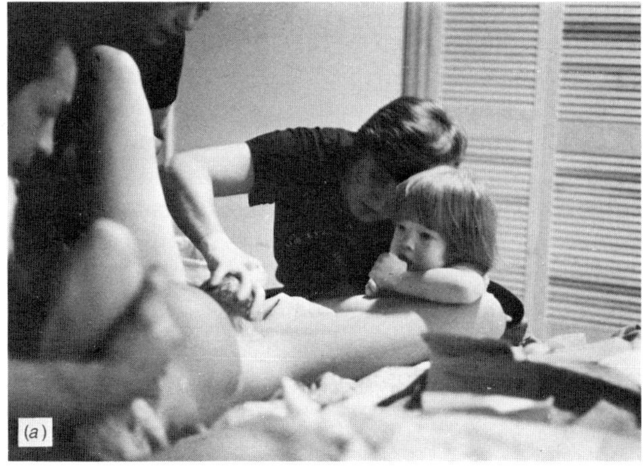

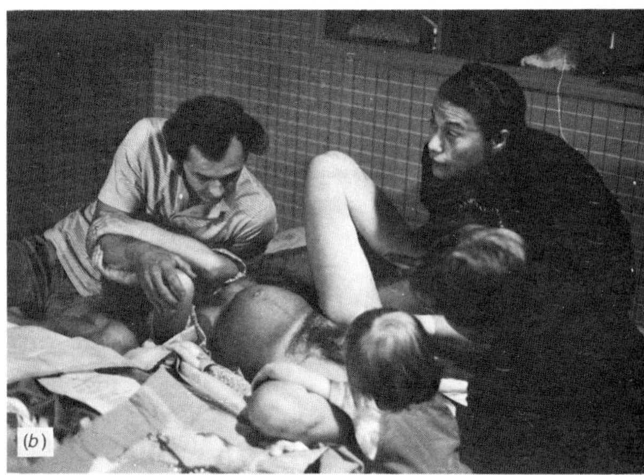

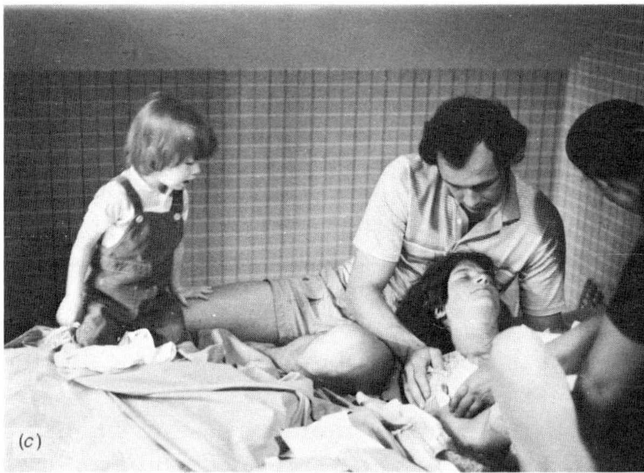

Figure 28.1
(*a*) Nurse-midwife delivering baby with young sibling watching. (*b*) Childbirth in the home with nurse-midwife and members of the family present. (*c*) The family is an important support source during home delivery. Photographs courtesy of Nurse-Midwifery Birthing Service, Eugene, Oregon.

is best done in consultation with a nurse-midwife or a physician. Several decisions and plans will need to be made.

- ▲ A prenatal regimen must be established so that adequate, safe prenatal care can be provided.
- ▲ The adequacy of the home to meet the needs for delivery must be determined; inadequacies must be taken care of.
- ▲ Communication channels among nurse-midwife, physician, and hospital must be established.
- ▲ The decision about who is to be present at actual birth and plans for preparing them must be made.
- ▲ Where the home the delivery is to take place must be determined.
- ▲ Plans for emergencies, as well as provision for emergency transport to hospital, must be established.
- ▲ Plans for reporting the birth and obtaining birth certificate are necessary.

BIRTHING CENTER

Birthing centers outside of the hospital are becoming an increasingly popular alternative to hospitals. These centers are usually disassociated from a hospital; however, they may be—and often are—in close proximity to hospital facilities. They may be established in association with a physician's private practice or another outpatient-type clinic setting. They have on their staff physicians and/or nurse-midwives who have practice privileges at a nearby hospital. These centers may provide prenatal care and client education services, as well as labor and delivery care.

The center resembles a home environment with bedrooms, family areas with recreation facilities, space in which the laboring woman may walk, and space to accommodate family members (Fig. 28.2). Families using this alternative birth setting are carefully evaluated for risk potential and are expected to participate in some form of preparation for childbirth education, as well as to maintain a carefully supervised prenatal regimen. The centers are adequately staffed with professional nurses and are designed to accommodate uncomplicated labor, delivery, and recovery. Emergency equipment is accessible in the center and provision for emergency transportation to a close hospital is made. The woman is closely supervised for 8–24 hours after delivery; she is discharged home or admitted to a hospital depending on her condition.

The cost of care in a birthing center varies, but it is usually less than in a hospital because of the short stay and decreased use of medical technology, equipment, and drugs.

Nurses who work with families using any of these alternatives to traditional care must be adequately prepared in both maternity and family nursing. The next several years will likely find modification of these current alternatives, as well as the emergence of additional ones. Whatever the alternative to traditional maternity care, it is quite likely that the nurse will be a pivotal figure in its planning and development.

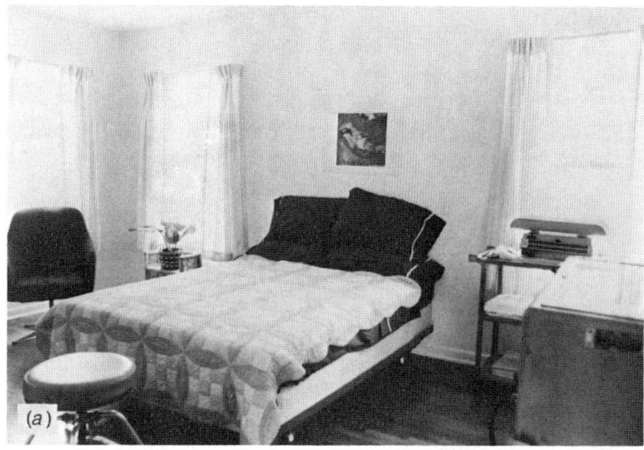

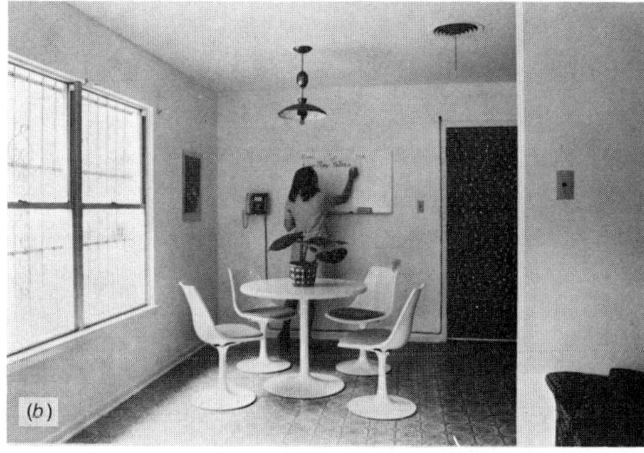

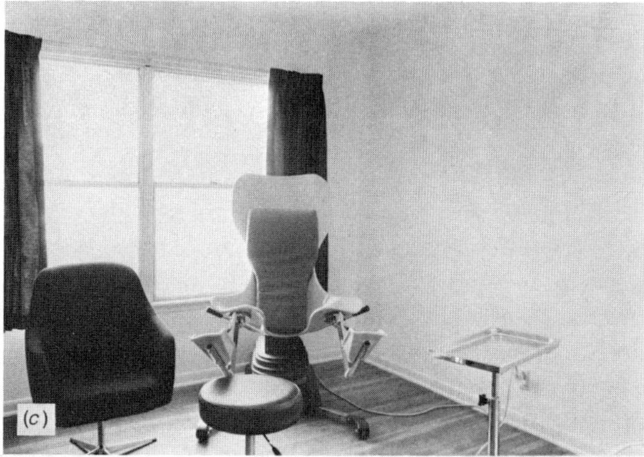

Figure 28.2
A birthing center. (*a*) The bedroom/delivery room. (*b*) Part of the family area. (*c*) A birthing chair. Photographs courtesy of Bolling Birthing Center, San Antonio, Texas.

ROLES FOR MATERNITY NURSES

Roles assumed by maternity nurses are constantly changing to keep pace with client needs, new and different health care technology, and expansion of professional knowledge and skill. Two areas of nursing roles are discussed here: traditional roles with a new emphasis and expanded or new roles.

Role is commonly defined as expected or prescribed behaviors for a particular position, profession, or occupation. However, perceptions of the behaviors or expectations for any given role often vary from group to group and person to person. For example, a nurse's perception of the role of nurse may be different from the perception of the client, the physician, or the hospital administrator. This difference in view of roles often leads to confusion and the need for the nurse to interpret his or her role constantly.

Maternity nurses have historically assumed roles expected of nurses generally, that is, staff nurse, head nurse, obstetric supervisor, office nurse, and public health or community health nurse. Maternity nurses, like other professional nurses, have also taken on different and expanded roles such as the nurse-midwife, the obstetric/gynecologic practitioner, and the parent educator. These roles require preparation beyond that provided through basic nursing programs.

Traditional Roles with a New Look

Nurses are changing some of their functions and behaviors within their traditional roles. The staff nurse in a prenatal clinic does more than take the woman's blood pressure, weigh her and test her urine. Client education is an integral part of contemporary nursing. Physical assessment—once strictly within the purview of medical practice—is now a part of many basic nursing programs, and nurses use physical assessment knowledge and skill daily in their practice. Staff nurses in labor and delivery no longer provide care only for the pregnant woman; they must incorporate the needs of the expectant father and other family members into the plan of care. Nurses function as members of a health care team whose leadership may well change according to the type of expertise required by the client. As medical knowledge and technology increase and become more sophisticated, nurse's roles incorporate this new information and equipment. Nurses supervise the electronic monitoring of women, as well as the fetus/neonate during pregnancy and labor. They conduct stress and nonstress tests and perform other diagnostic activities. In a sense, the role of the maternity nurse is limited only by the boundaries of legal and professional standards, the nurse's knowledge and skill, and the extent of creative and innovative thought.

Many institutions have not kept pace with the increased functional capability of today's nurse, while other institutions have been the instigators of change. Some nurses may find themselves "trapped" in jobs where they are unable to use their knowledge and skill to the fullest. It is this type of situation that should challenge the nurse to try to institute change that permits full use of nursing talent and futuristic nursing care. All too often the nurse seeks a position elsewhere that is more attuned to contemporary nursing practice. These nurses may have made appropriate, sensible decisions. On the other hand, they may have let an opportunity to effect change and improve health care slip through their fingers. Nursing practice is often what the nurse wants it to be and depends upon how much time, energy, and skill the nurse is willing to commit.

Expanded Roles for Maternity Nurses

Expanded role refers to roles for nurses that supersede the basic knowledge and skill expected of most professional nurses. Role expansion is usually associated with specialization in an area of clinical nursing. However, nursing roles may, and have, expanded in a general sense as discussed in the preceding section. Before a role can evolve into something more than it was originally intended, certain conditions must be met. According to Butnarescu (1978, p. 76) these include:

- ▲ Consensus or agreement by society and the health care system (including medicine, nursing and allied health) that a need for change in role for nursing does exist
- ▲ Readiness of the nurse to assume a different role with expanded functions and *responsibilities*
- ▲ Readiness of society and the health system to accept nursing in such a role change
- ▲ Motivation, which is part of readiness of the nurse to invest herself or himself in a new or expanded role through discipline and study to prepare for role change
- ▲ Potential (or capacity) of the nurse for change and role expansion
- ▲ Institutional support in terms of released time, financial incentive and provision for support services and continued study
- ▲ Assurance of the opportunity to practice the new or expanded role
- ▲ Provision for continuing education through the availability of educational offerings from a variety of sources
- ▲ Salary commensurate with role expectation
- ▲ Opportunity for dialogue with others in an expanded or new role, as well as with nurses, physicians, and others in the health care system
- ▲ Clearly identified plan for evaluation of the new or expanded role

Figure 28.3 lists the opportunities that exist for expansion of the maternity nurse's role. Only one of these roles—*nurse-midwifery*—is discussed here because of its comprehensiveness and its increasing popularity, particularly among clients of reproductive health care.

Midwifery is a role that has spanned the centuries. Historically, the midwife has been a woman, usually from within the community, who cared for and assisted other women during birth. Midwifery as a modern health care occupation, with education and training, is principally an invention of the

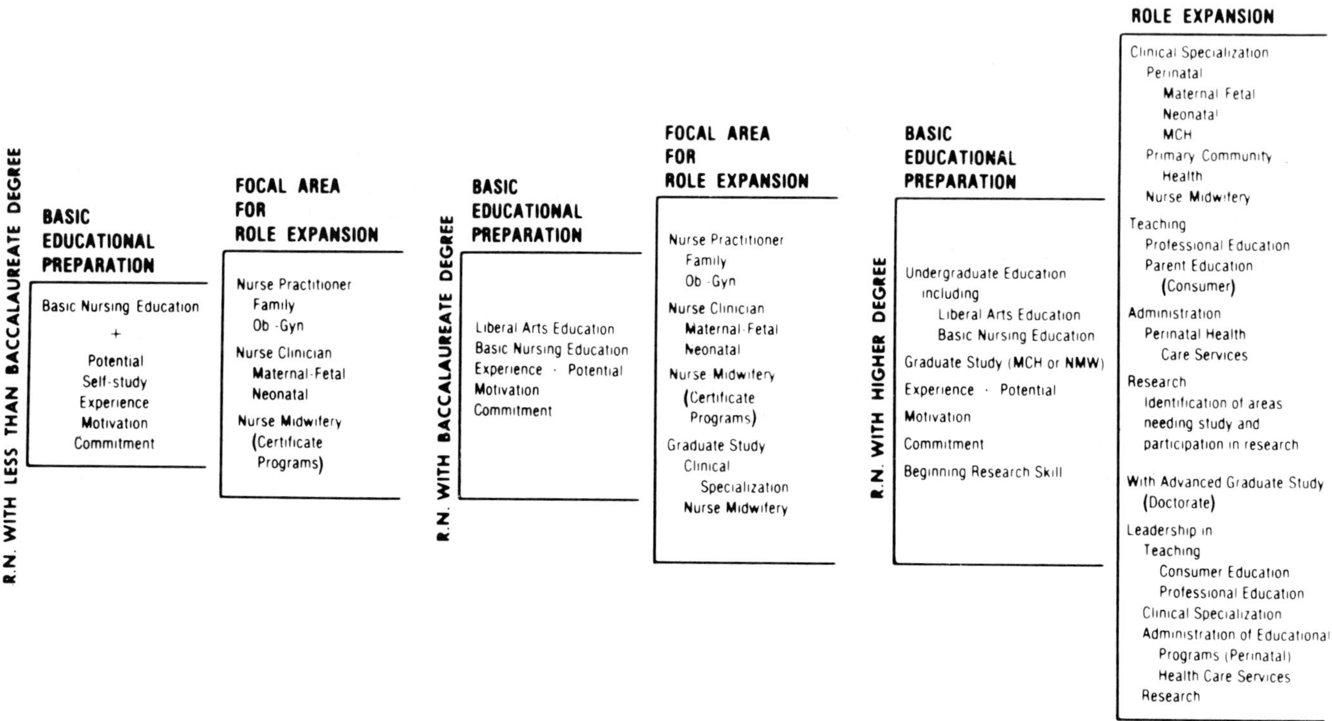

Figure 28.3
Opportunities for role expansion in maternity nursing. *Source:* Butnarescu, G. F., Tillotson, D. M., Villarreal, P. P. *Perinatal Nursing: Volume 1, Reproductive Health.* New York: John Wiley & Sons. 1978, p. 75. Used with permission.

nineteenth and twentieth centuries in the Western world. Nurse-midwifery is a more recent addition to health care personnel. Nurse-midwifery in the United States is a clinical specialty of professional nursing. The knowledge and skill base for the nurse-midwife includes but supersedes that of the professional nurse and draws heavily from the medical specialties of obstetrics and gynecology. Although the nurse-midwife is a specialized maternity nurse, her practice is more inclusive than that of other maternity nurses. Lack of communication and of role clarity sometimes places the nurse-midwife and the maternity nurse in adversary positions.

Nurse-midwives are educated in a variety of programs, including short certificate and graduate degree programs. Graduates of these programs are certified by examination by the American College of Nurse-Midwives.* The American College of Nurse-Midwives has issued a statement regarding the qualifications, standards, and functions of nurse-midwives (see Fig. 28.4). The nurse-midwife may practice in hospital or community settings. Like maternity nursing, nurse-midwifery has as its central focus the reproductive health of the childbearing woman and her family.

> *Nurses in expanded roles are not practicing medicine; they are practicing nursing. Nurse-midwives are not practicing medicine; they are practicing nursing. Nurses have always carried out medical orders and consulted with physicians when they deemed it necessary. The fact that they do so in the expanded role is no different. The difference is that the judgmental area of nursing has been expanded.*
>
> *Kimbro, 1978, p. 31*

Nurse-midwifery appeals to clients because the nurse-midwife provides comprehensive, sensitive, consistent, expert health care during all phases of the reproductive cycle. The nurse-midwife is a skilled parent educator as well as a health care

*The American College of Nurse-Midwives, Suite 1120, 1522 K. Street, N.W., Washington, D. C. 20005

Qualifications for the Practice of Nurse-Midwifery

1. Certification by the American College of Nurse-Midwives
   a. Active licensure as a registered nurse in one of the 50 states or Territories including the District of Columbia
   b. Completion of a nurse-midwifery educational program approved by the American College of Nurse-Midwives
2. Compliance with legal requirements of the jurisdiction in which nurse-midwifery practice will occur

Standards for the Practice of Nurse-Midwifery
Nurse-midwifery practice

1. Strives to provide continuity of care to the woman and her family during the maternity cycle, continuing interconceptionally throughout the childbearing years
2. Fosters the delivery of safe and satisfying care
3. Recognizes that childbearing is a family experience and encourages the active involvement of family members in care
4. Upholds the right to self-determination of consumers within the boundaries of safe care
5. Focuses on health and growth as developmental processes during the reproductive years
6. Stimulates community awareness and responsiveness to the needs for delivery of quality family-centered care
7. Occurs interdependently within a health care delivery system
8. Occurs within a formal written alliance with an obstetrician, or another physician, or a group of physicians, who has/have a formal consultative arrangement with an obstetrician–gynecologist
9. Exists within a framework of medically approved protocols
10. Occurs within the realm of professional competence
11. Requires opportunities for continuing professional growth and development
12. Includes an on-going process of evaluation

Functions for the Practice of Nurse-Midwifery
The nurse-midwife

1. Assumes responsibility for the management and complete care of the essentially healthy woman and newborn related to the childbearing processes
2. Develops with the woman an appropriate plan of care attentive to her interrelated needs
3. Participates in individual and group counseling and teaching throughout the childbearing processes
4. Manages, through mutual agreement and collaboration with the physician, that part of care of medically complicated women which is appropriate to the skills and knowledge of nurse-midwives
5. Collaborates with other health professionals in the delivery and evaluation of health care
6. Assesses own professional abilities and functions within identified capabilities
7. Assumes responsibility for own self-determination within the boundaries of professional practice
8. Maintains and promotes professional practice in concert with current trends
9. Utilizes Standards for Evaluation of Nurse-Midwifery Procedural Functions in development and evaluation of practice
10. Promotes the preparation of nurse-midwifery students
11. Assists with the education of other health care personnel
12. Supports the philosophy and official policies of the American College of Nurse-Midwives

Figure 28.4
ACNM Statement of Qualifications, Standards, and Functions. *Source*: Washington, D. C.: The American College of Nurse-Midwives, accepted 1975. Used with permission.

provider. Studies have consistently shown that care provided by nurse-midwives to low-risk maternity clients is safe, comprehensive, and in many cases superior to that provided by physicians.

There are some barriers to widespread nurse-midwifery practice in the United States: Legal constraints imposed by some states limit the scope of practice; provision for third-party reimbursement for services is not always available; acceptance by the medical community may sometimes pose a problem. The current number of practicing nurse-midwives is inadequate to meet the needs of all low-risk maternity clients, even if all of the barriers to practice were removed. Increasing numbers of maternity nurses are seeking admission to nurse-midwifery educational programs as evidenced by the waiting lists of applicants at schools that offer nurse-midwifery education.

SUMMARY

Maternity nursing as a specialty of professional nursing that is sensitive to and influenced by the professional, social, political, and economic climates of the nation was the first issue discussed. The next section discussed alternatives to traditional reproductive health care that are concerned with the wishes and needs of the client and still provide safe and comprehensive health care. The last section was on the changing and expanding roles for the maternity nurse at both the basic and advanced levels of practice. Nurse-midwifery, which represents one expanded role for maternity nurses, was elaborated upon.

The future directions of maternity nursing will be determined by many factors but none more crucial and telling than the knowledge, skill, talent, and innovation of the nurses who select maternity nursing as their area of practice.

REFERENCES AND READINGS

Aiken, L. H. (Ed.). *Nursing in the 1980's: Crises, Opportunities, Challenges.* Philadelphia: J. B. Lippincott, 1982. (A publication of the American Academy of Nursing.)

American College of Nurse-Midwives. *What is a Nurse-Midwife?* Washington, D. C.: ACNM, 1978.

Brown, B. J. Reorganizing Hospital-Based Nursing Practice: An Analysis of Patient Outcomes, Provider Satisfaction and Costs, in Aiken, L. (Ed.), *Health Policy and Nursing Practice.* New York: McGraw-Hill, 1981, pp. 119–138. (A publication of the American Academy of Nursing.)

Brown, E. L. *Nursing for the Future.* New York: Russell Sage Foundation, 1948.

Butnarescu, G. F., *Perinatal Nursing: Volume I, Reproductive Health.* New York: John Wiley & Sons. 1978.

Department of Health and Human Services. The Registered Nurse, An Overview from National Sample Survey of Registered Nurses. Bureau of Health Professions, Health Resources Administration. Washington D. C.: U. S. Department Health and Human Resources, 1982.

Diers, D. K. Nurse-Midwifery as a System of Care: Provider Process and Patient Outcomes, in Aiken, L. (Ed.), *Health Policy and Nursing Practice.* New York: McGraw-Hill, 1981, pp. 73–89. (A publication of the American Academy of Nursing.)

Fagin, C. M. Nursing's Pivotal Role in Achieving Competition in Health Care, in AAN. *From Accomodation to Self-Determination: Nursing's Role in the Development of Health Care Policy*. Kansas City: American Nurses' Association, p. 3–15, 1982. (A publication of the American Academy of Nursing.)

Fein, R. Social and Economic Attitudes Shaping American Health Policy, in McKinley, J. B. (Ed.), *Issues in Health Care Policy*. Cambridge: MIT Press, 1981, p. 32 (Originally published in *Milbank Mem Fund Q/Health and Society* 58(3), 1980.)

Kalisch, B. J., Kalisch, P. A. *Politics of Nursing*. Philadelphia: J. B. Lippincott, 1982.

Kimbro, C. D. The Relationship Between Nurses and Nurse-Midwives. *J Nurs Midwifery* 22(4):28, 1978.

Lubic, R. W. Evaluation of an Out-of-Hospital Maternity Center for Low-Risk Patients, in Aiken, L. (Ed.), *Health Policy and Nursing Practice.* New York: McGraw-Hill, 1981, pp. 90–116. (A publication of the American Academy of Nursing.)

Lysaught, J. P. *An Abstract for Action: Report of the National Commission for the Study of Nursing*. New York: McGraw Hill, 1970.

Meglen, M. C., Burst, H. V. Nurse-Midwives Make a Difference. *Nurs Outlook* 22(6):386, 1974.

Report of the Surgeon General's Consultant Group on Nursing. *Toward Quality in Nursing*. Public Health Service Publication 992. Washington, D. C.: Department of Health, Education and Welfare, 1963.

Rodgers, J. A. Toward Professional Adulthood. For Nursing or Against Medicine: A Group Replay of the Second Individuation Process. *Nurs Outlook*, 29(8):478, 1981.

Secretary's Committee to Study Extended Roles for Nurses. *Extending the Scope of Nursing Practice.* DHEW Publication HSM-73-2037, Washington, D. C.: U. S. Government Printing Office, 1971.

APPENDIXES
GLOSSARY
INDEX

APPENDIX A

THE PREGNANT PATIENT'S BILL OF RIGHTS AND RESPONSIBILITIES

The Pregnant Patient's Bill of Rights and The Pregnant Patient's Responsibilities contain information that is useful and important for the maternity nurse. These documents are reprinted below.

THE PREGNANT PATIENT'S BILL OF RIGHTS

The Pregnant Patient has the right to participate in decisions involving her well-being and that of her unborn child, unless there is a clearcut medical emergency that prevents her participation. In addition to the rights set forth in the American Hospital Association's "Patient's Bill of Rights," (which has also been adopted by the New York City Department of Health) the Pregnant Patient, because she represents *two* patients rather than one, should be recognized as having the additional rights listed below.

1. *The Pregnant Patient has the right,* prior to the administration of any drug or procedure, to be informed by the health professional caring for her of any potential direct or indirect effects, risks or hazards to herself or her unborn or newborn infant which may result from the use of a drug or procedure prescribed for or administered to her during pregnancy, labor, birth or lactation.

2. *The Pregnant Patient has the right,* prior to the proposed therapy, to be informed, not only of the benefits, risks and hazards of the proposed therapy but also of known alternative therapy, such as available childbirth education classes which could help to prepare the Pregnant Patient physically and mentally to cope with the discomfort or stress of pregnancy and the experience of childbirth, thereby reducing or eliminating her need for drugs and obstetric intervention. She should be offered such information early in her pregnancy in order that she may make a reasoned decision.

3. *The Pregnant Patient has the right,* prior to the administration of any drug, to be informed by the health professional who is prescribing or administering the drug to her that any drug which she receives during pregnancy, labor and birth, no matter

Published by International Childbirth Education Association, Inc. Prepared by Doris Haire, Chair., ICEA Committee on Health Law Regulations.

how or when the drug is taken or administered, may adversely affect her unborn baby, directly or indirectly, and that there is no drug or chemical which has been proven safe for the unborn child.

4. *The Pregnant Patient has the right,* if Cesarean birth is anticipated, to be informed prior to the administration of any drug, and preferably prior to her hospitalization, that minimizing her and, in turn, her baby's intake of nonessential pre-operative medicine will benefit her baby.

5. *The Pregnant Patient has the right,* prior to the administration of a drug or procedure, to be informed of the areas of uncertainty if there is NO properly controlled follow-up research which has established the safety of the drug or procedure with regard to its direct and/or indirect effects on the physiological, mental and neurological development of the child exposed, via the mother, to the drug or procedure during pregnancy, labor, birth or lactation—(this would apply to virtually all drugs and the vast majority of obstetric procedures).

6. *The Pregnant Patient has the right,* prior to the administration of any drug, to be informed of the brand name and generic name of the drug in order that she may advise the health professional of any past adverse reaction to the drug.

7. *The Pregnant Patient has the right* to determine for herself, without pressure from her attendant, whether she will accept the risks inherent in the proposed therapy or refuse a drug or procedure.

8. *The Pregnant Patient has the right* to know the name and qualifications of the individual administering a medication or procedure to her during labor or birth.

9. *The Pregnant Patient has the right* to be informed, prior to the administration of any procedure, whether that procedure is being administered to her for her or her baby's benefit (medically indicated) or as an elective procedure (for convenience, teaching purposes or research).

10. *The Pregnant Patient has the right* to be accompanied during the stress of labor and birth by someone she cares for, and to whom she looks for emotional comfort and encouragement.

11. *The Pregnant Patient has the right* after appropriate medical consultation to choose a position for labor and for birth which is least stressful to her baby and to herself.

12. *The Obstetric Patient has the right* to have her baby cared for at her bedside if her baby is normal, and to feed her baby according to her baby's needs rather than according to the hospital regimen.

13. *The Obstetric Patient has the right* to be informed in writing of the name of the person who actually delivered her baby and the professional qualifications of that person. This information should also be on the birth certificate.

14. *The Obstetric Patient has the right* to be informed if there is any known or indicated aspect of her or her baby's care or condition which may cause her or her baby later difficulty or problems.

15. *The Obstetric Patient has the right* to have her and her baby's hospital medical records complete, accurate and legible and to have their records, including Nurses' Notes, retained by the hospital until the child reaches at least the age of majority, or, alternatively, to have the records offered to her before they are destroyed.

16. *The Obstetric Patient,* both during and after her hospital stay, has the right to have access to her complete hospital medical records, including Nurses' Notes, and to receive a copy upon payment of a reasonable fee and without incurring the expense of retaining an attorney.

It is the obstetric patient and her baby, not the health professional, who must sustain any trauma or injury resulting from the use of a drug or obstetric procedure. The observation of the rights listed above will not only permit the obstetric patient to participate in the decisions involving her and her baby's health care, but will help to protect the health professional and the hospital against litigation arising from resentment or misunderstanding on the part of the mother.

THE PREGNANT PATIENT'S RESPONSIBILITIES

In addition to understanding her rights the Pregnant Patient should also understand that she too has certain responsibilites. The Pregnant Patient's responsibilities include the following:

1. The Pregnant Patient is responsible for learning about the physical and psychological process of labor, birth and postpartum recovery. The better informed expectant parents are the better they will be able to participate in decisions concerning the planning of their care.

2. The Pregnant Patient is responsible for learn-

ing what comprises good prenatal and intranatal care and for making an effort to obtain the best care possible.

3. Expectant parents are responsible for knowing about those hospital policies and regulations which will affect their birth and postpartum experience.

4. The Pregnant Patient is responsible for arranging for a companion or support person (husband, mother, sister, friend, etc.) who will share in her plans for birth and who will accompany her during her labor and birth experience.

5. The Pregnant Patient is responsible for making her preferences known clearly to the health professionals involved in her case in a courteous and cooperative manner and for making mutually agreed-upon arrangements regarding maternity care alternatives with her physician and hospital in advance of labor.

6. Expectant parents are responsible for listening to their chosen physician or midwife with an open mind, just as they expect him or her to listen openly to them.

7. Once they have agreed to a course of health care, expectant parents are responsible, to the best of their ability, for seeing that the program is carried out in consultation with others with whom they have made the agreement.

8. The Pregnant Patient is responsible for obtaining information in advance regarding the approximate cost of her obstetric and hospital care.

9. The Pregnant Patient who intends to change her physician or hospital is responsible for notifying all concerned, well in advance of the birth if possible, and for informing both of her reasons for changing.

10. In all their interactions with medical and nursing personnel, the expectant parents should behave towards those caring for them with the same respect and consideration they themselves would like.

11. During the mother's hospital stay the mother is responsible for learning about her and her baby's continuing care after discharge from the hospital.

12. After birth, the parents should put into writing constructive comments and feelings of satisfaction and/or dissatisfaction with the care (nursing, medical and personal) they received. Good service to families in the future will be facilitated by those parents who take the time and responsibility to write letters expressing their feelings about the maternity care they received.

All the previous statements assume a normal birth and postpartum experience. Expectant parents should realize that, if complications develop in their cases, there will be an increased need to trust the expertise of the physician and hospital staff they have chosen. However, if problems occur, the childbearing woman still retains her responsibility for making informed decisions about her care or treatment and that of her baby. If she is incapable of assuming that responsibility because of her physical condition, her previously authorized companion or support person should assume responsibility for making informed decisions on her behalf.

APPENDIX B

SELF-INVENTORY OF STUDY HABITS

This appendix is designed to help the learner identify areas where study habits can be improved in order to foster more effective and efficient learning. Three areas—study techniques, motivation, and organization—that affect efficient study are included in this inventory. To assess your study habits, check one of the categories next to each item. If you find that your study habits need to be improved, your teacher can assist you in finding ways to improve them.

	Always	*Frequently*	*Usually*	*Sometimes*	*Never*
STUDY TECHNIQUES					
1. Read through a lecture, handout, or chapter in the book without first skimming subtitles and illustrations					
2. Skip reading the figures, graphs, and tables					
3. Find it difficult to identify the important points after reading					
4. Tend to daydream while studying					
5. Have difficulty in retaining information after a lapse of time					
6. Miss some points of a lecture because you can not write quickly enough					
7. Take notes that tend not to make sense					
8. Try to copy the exact words of the instructor when taking notes					
9. Take notes verbatim from the book					
10. Tend not to organize material in a logical order or in unit portions when studying for an exam					

This appendix is adapted from materials furnished by Dr. Nancy Hudepohl.

	Always	Frequently	Usually	Sometimes	Never
11. Cram for exams					
12. Review for exams					
13. Have difficulty in completing exams in allotted time					
14. Do not pay attention to test items, resulting in poor selection of answers					
15. Go slowly at the beginning of a test and have to hurry at the end					
16. Read over written assignments before handing them in					
17. Gloss over vocabulary					
MOTIVATION TO STUDY					
1. Find that your enthusiasm wanes after the first days or weeks of a course					
2. Study just enough to get by					
3. Are frequently confused and indecisive about your professional goals					
4. Think that the time and effort demanded for the course are not worth it					
5. Believe that your social life has greater priority					
6. Tend not to pay attention in class					
7. Have difficulty in concentrating because of being continually disturbed, bored, or in a bad humor					
8. Think that what you are required to study has little practical value for you					
9. Have feelings of quitting school and finding a job					
10. Feel that what you are studying will not be relevant in the clinical practice of nursing					
11. Believe that textbooks are not helpful					
12. Feel that exams are fruitless activities					
13. Feel that instructors demand too many hours outside of class for preparation					
14. Hesitate asking for help from instructors					
15. Feel that instructors do not know how to interest students					
16. Feel that instructors are not in contact with reality					
ORGANIZATION					
1. Wait until the last minute to prepare for class					
2. Feel sleepy or tired, which interferes with study time					
3. Do not finish projects or papers on time					
4. Avoid studying by watching TV, socializing, reading, etc.					

	Always	*Frequently*	*Usually*	*Sometimes*	*Never*
5. Engage in social and sports activities that interfere with scholastic activities					
6. Tend to delay reviewing class notes for a day or two after the class					
7. Put off studying important material for less important assignments					
8. Forget due dates of assignments					
9. Perform poorly because insufficient time is spent studying					
10. Study at a desk that is situated in front of a window, door, or other source of distraction					
11. Study lying on the bed					
12. Tend to hang family photos, photos of a boy or girl friend, or trophies above the desk or table used for study					
13. Study in an area without good lighting					
14. Keep you desk so cluttered that there is not sufficient space to study effectively without distraction					
15. Interrupt studies for minor excuses					
16. Study with distractions, such as TV, radio, or records, present					
17. Interrupt study for noises or other activities					
18. Begin to study without the necessary materials available					

APPENDIX C

STUDENT STUDY GUIDE

The six major sections of this appendix correspond to the units of the book. Each section contains a repetition of the unit behavioral outcomes. Various aids are included to assist in learning the material covered in the units. The sections for Units 2–6 include clinical incidents (brief clinical situations) that are similar to those the nurse might encounter in clinical practice. Each incident is followed by a series of questions to direct thinking and make reference back to the text for study. Answers are not given in the appendix, but they can be found by reading the text.

UNIT 1

Behavioral Outcomes

- ▲ Describe the scope of contemporary maternity nursing
- ▲ Describe the evolution of maternity nursing
- ▲ Define teaching and learning
- ▲ List five beliefs about learning
- ▲ Describe the roles of the teacher and the learner in the study of maternity nursing
- ▲ Explain three domains of learning
- ▲ Compare the teaching–learning process to the nursing process
- ▲ Identify five issues of concern to maternity nurses
- ▲ Explain the significance of selected types of statistics to maternity nursing
- ▲ Examine personal beliefs about human reproduction and the issues affecting it

General Study Questions

PROBLEM 1

Select an issue that you have read about or encountered in maternity nursing. Analyze that issue using the guidelines given in Chapter 3. Examine your own feelings about the issue. What do your peers think about this issue? Are their attitudes similar to or different from your own?

PROBLEM 2

Select a clinical situation in which you were the learner. Examine your learning style. How did you learn best? What were the problems that you encountered? How did you resolve them? Were you able to apply what you learned in a subsequent situation? Without instructor assistance? With instructor assistance?

PROBLEM 3

Write a statement of your personal philosophy of maternity nursing. What do you believe about maternity nursing? What do you value about reproductive health care and the nurse's role? What are your attitudes about maternity nursing and reproductive health care?

UNIT 2

Behavioral Outcomes

- ▲ Define developmental readiness for pregnancy and parenthood
- ▲ Identify the characteristics of developmental readiness for reproduction
- ▲ Explain key concepts from selected theories of human development, biology, genetics, psychology, and sociology, and their relevance to reproductive readiness
- ▲ Explain the characteristics of major conceptual frameworks for preparation for pregnancy, childbirth, and early parenthood
- ▲ Identify skills and processes appropriate for determining developmental readiness for the reproductive events
- ▲ Explain the theoretical basis for the skills and processes used to determine developmental readiness for reproduction
- ▲ Apply understandings about concepts and theory drawn from nursing and related disciplines to the assessment and preparation of people and families for pregnancy, childbirth, and early parenthood

General Study Questions

What are the characteristics of developmental readiness? How can these be assessed?

Compare two theories of human development. Note their similarities and differences.

What are two key concepts found in the psychoanalytic school of human development? The humanistic? The cognitive?

Compare and contrast the male and female reproductive systems. What are their similarities and differences?

Compare and contrast the male and female reproductive systems. What are their similarities and differences?

Why is the female's pelvis shaped differently from the male's? What are the differences?

How is sex determined at the time of conception?

How are familial traits transmitted from generation to generation?

Explain the female sexual cycle.

What are the major developmental characteristics of adolescence?

Differentiate between adolescence and puberty.

What are the major concepts found in the psychoprophylactic method (PPM) of prepared childbirth?

How does this method differ from natural childbirth?

Clinical Incidents

CLINICAL INCIDENT 1

Jane D., who is 14 years old, comes into the prenatal clinic with her mother. Jane menstruated erratically for 1 year and hasn't had a period for 2 months. She admits to having had sexual intercourse, as she looks at her mother defiantly. Her mothers says, "I'm so afraid that Janie is pregnant."

What physical characteristics would you expect to observe in Jane with regard to her age and menstrual history?

What thoughts does Jane's defiant look at her mother bring to your mind?

How would you approach your interview with Jane and her mother?

What nursing care would be appropriate for Jane at this visit? Explain.

CLINICAL INCIDENT 2

You are assisting Mrs. H., a 19-year-old woman who suspects that she is pregnant for the first time, prepare for the first pelvic examination. Her husband, 20 years old, is in the room with you.

How can you best prepare Mrs. H. and her husband for this examination?

How can you best prepare Mrs. H. and her husband for this examination?

What information should you see that they have?

Would you treat the husband any differently than his wife in terms of preparation for the examination? If yes, how? If no, explain.

What can they expect to happen during the actual examination?

What can they learn about a possible pregnancy from having the examination done?

What characteristics would indicate to you that Mr. and Mrs. H. were ready for pregnancy and parenthood? Explain.

UNIT 3

Behavioral Outcomes

▲ Describe gamete transport in the man and woman and its goal, fertilization

▲ Explain placental development using a contemporary theory base

▲ Describe the placenta, accessory structures, the fetal membranes, the umbilical cord, and the amniotic fluid

▲ Describe three stages of fetal development

▲ Identify two clinical indicators of fetal growth and development

▲ Describe physical changes in the pregnant woman by body system

▲ Explain the relationship between placental–fetal development and physiologic changes occurring in the mother

▲ Describe a woman's psychologic response to pregnancy

▲ Explain five major nursing responsibilities for the prenatal care of a pregnant woman

▲ Identify three contemporary family life-styles

▲ Describe two ways in which pregnancy affects the family

▲ Identify two ways in which pregnancy alters the usual sexual relationship between a man and a woman

▲ Describe three ways in which a nurse can help the couple make a healthy sexual adjustment during pregnancy

▲ Identify two methods of preparation for pregnancy and parenthood

▲ Explain psychoprophylactic method of childbirth education

General Study Questions

What changes occur in the ovum following ovulation?

How does the ovum leave the ovary? Where does it go? How does it get there? How long does the ovum live after ovulation?

How are sperm produced? Transported? How long do they live?

Explain fertilization.

What are the composition and characteristics of a chromosome? How do chromosomal aberrations affect the new life?

When is the developing baby called a zygote? An embryo? A fetus?

How does fertilization occur?

What is nidation?

Describe the placenta. How does it develop?

What are the chorionic villi, and what purpose do they serve?

What is the composition of amniotic fluid?

What are the functions of the placenta?

What are the characteristics of the umbilical cord? What purpose does it serve?

Clinical Incident

Susan, a pregnant adolescent, is attending a prenatal clinic accompanied by her mother. The nurse, after greeting the client, begins to record Susan's history. When she asks Susan, "When did you first begin to menstruate?" Susan replies, "I haven't menstruated for 4 months."

What do you know about anxiety and listening? What is menarche? Why is menarche an important time to establish?

Following the history, a pelvic examination is done. Susan says, "I'm so scared. I hate being examined."

What specific measures can you, as the nurse, employ to reduce anxiety?

What teaching regarding pelvic examination is important? (You may want to review both Chapters 12 and 26.)

Developmentally, Susan, an 18-year-old, and her mother, who is 41, are addressing different developmental tasks. The physical examination confirms that Susan is 3 months pregnant.

What ideas or suggestions do you have for Susan's mother regarding Susan during her pregnancy?

What are the developmental tasks of pregnancy?

What are the particular nutritional requirements of pregnant teenagers?

What anticipatory guidance regarding role changes for Susan and her mother can be initiated?

What can you tell Susan about how her fetus looks at 3 months?

What will you tell Susan about biophysical and psychosocial changes taking place?

Following the physical examination the nurse tells Susan about the schedule of antepartum visits and what assessment will be done at each visit. She encourages Susan to contact her regarding concerns at any time.

What routine assessment is done at each visit, and what is the general pattern of visits?

What minor discomforts of pregnancy might be anticipated and shared?

How does the prenatal nurse assess fetal growth and development?

What information should be given regarding sexuality and pregnancy?

What information should be given regarding medications during pregnancy?

Susan decides to attend education for childbirth classes that focus on the psychoprophylactic method.

What is the psychoprophylactic method of childbirth education?

What relaxation and breathing techniques are useful during pregnancy and delivery?

What are two major goals of education for childbirth?

What are the implications for the nuclear and the single parent family during pregnancy?

UNIT 4

Behavioral Outcomes

- ▲ Describe the physiology of normal labor
- ▲ Explain maternal–fetal biophysical and psychosocial responses to labor
- ▲ Describe the impact of labor on the family
- ▲ Comprehend skills essential for the safe care of a mother and her fetus–neonate
- ▲ Explain the biophysical, emotional, and role adjustment of the mother following childbirth
- ▲ Identify learning needs usual for all mothers and families following childbirth
- ▲ Describe the extrauterine biophysical and psychosocial adaptations of the neonate
- ▲ Explain neonatal needs deriving from biophysical, social, and nutritional demands
- ▲ Explain models for gestational age and behavioral assessment of the neonate
- ▲ Identify the tasks of parenthood
- ▲ Describe parenthood in terms of various lifestyles
- ▲ Describe mother–infant–father socialization process
- ▲ Explain nursing interventions needed to promote healthy parenthood

Clinical Incidents

CLINICAL INCIDENT 1

Mr. and Mrs. H. are expecting their first child and have attended education for childbirth classes. Mrs. H. comes to the labor room of the metropolitan hospital on a Saturday at 4 a.m. She is at term and says on admission, "I hope this is real labor. I remember my prenatal teacher describing false labor."

What are the signs of labor?

How can you differentiate true from false labor?

What do the terms dilatation, effacement, and station mean?

Mrs. H. is admitted to the labor room. Following the initial assessment by the nurse and physician, Mrs. H.'s membranes rupture. The fluid is meconium stained, but fetal heart rate is normal at 148 beats per minute. Contractions are occurring every 3 minutes and lasting 40 seconds. The physician states the dilation of the cervix is 6 cm, station is 0, and effacement is 80%. The fetus is vertex and ROA. Although the physician tells Mr. H. that labor is progressing normally, he informs Mrs. H. that he is going to apply an internal fetal monitor, as the amniotic fluid was meconium stained and the monitor provides an additional assessment modality for the health care team. Mrs. H., after application of the monitor states, "I learned about meconium staining and fetal monitors in childbirth class. It is so nice to hear the baby's heartbeat."

What are the appropriate nursing actions to take when the membranes rupture?

What causes meconium staining, and what does it mean?

How does the nurse time and record uterine contractions? Fetal heart rate?

What are nursing responsibilities during electronic fetal monitoring?

What are the three basic fetal monitoring patterns, and, physiologically, what does each reflect?

In what stage and phase of labor is Mrs. H. when the physician examines her?

What is Mrs. H.'s husband's role during the first, second, and third stages of labor?

What are the signs of transition?

With no further problems, Mrs. H. delivers an 8-pound baby girl. Both mother and baby are transported to the recovery room, and Mr. H., who has been with his wife throughout, accompanies them.

What are the nursing responsibilities regarding the mother during the first postpartum hour?

How does the nurse assess family interaction in the recovery room?

CLINICAL INCIDENT 2

Baby Girl H. is assessed by the nursery nurse to be 40 weeks gestationally. Her heart rate is 140, respirations 50, and axillary temperature 97.2°F. Her hands and feet are blue, her cry is lusty, and muscular activity is strong. Moro reflex is present and appears normal.

What additional assessment is needed?

What are the normal skin variations in the neonate?

What are periods of reactivity?

What are five key criteria in gestational age assessment?

How does the nurse assess behavioral adaptation in the neonate?

What medications might the neonate receive?

What are the nursing implications in relation to physiologic adaptation (e.g., cardiovascular, gastrointestinal, endocrine, renal, musculoskeletal, neurologic)?

CLINICAL INCIDENT 3

Mrs. B. is 3 days postpartum and is being discharged today with her 3-day-old son, Mark. She has been in the rooming-in unit of a community hospital; her husband and both sets of grandparents have been frequent visitors. Mrs. B. is eager to take her son home; breast-feeding is progressing satisfactorily, and her parents will remain with Mr. and Mrs. B. for 1 week. Mr. and Mrs. B have two other children, ages 5 and 3 years.

What information regarding maternal physiologic and psychosocial adaptation does the nurse need to review?

What anticipatory guidance regarding Mark's adaptation does Mrs. B. require?

What additional information regarding breast-feeding, care of the breasts, and substitute bottle-feeding does Mrs. B. need?

What directions regarding rest and exercise are needed?

The nurse assesses that Mrs. B. is in the beginning of the "letting go" phase (as described by Reva Rubin). She has assumed many caretaking activities: diapering, bathing, feeding, and referring to herself as mother. Mrs. B. also described caretaking activities that the 3- and 5-year-old can share.

What additional guidance can the nurse provide regarding siblings?

How can the nurse discuss and explore the grandparenting role?

What assessment of the father's role needs to be made?

How does the nurse prepare the couple for the 6-week postpartum visit?

How does the nurse anticipate and respond to questions regarding sexuality and family planning?

UNIT 5

Behavioral Outcomes

- ▲ List the leading causes of reproductive risk
- ▲ Describe the scope of reproductive risk in the United States in regard to incidence and population affected
- ▲ Explain the use of five contemporary modalities important for the assessment of reproductive risk conditions
- ▲ Describe three ways in which a nurse participates in assessment of reproductive risk
- ▲ Describe the pathophysiologic basis for two major maternal risk conditions during each of the periods of pregnancy, labor, and recovery
- ▲ Explain the scientific basis for nursing care of two major reproductive risk conditions during each of the periods of pregnancy, labor, and recovery
- ▲ Describe four factors that contribute to fetal–neonatal risk
- ▲ Explain the nursing management of three neonatal disorders
- ▲ Explain the genetic basis for three inherited disorders
- ▲ Describe two modalities used for genetic diagnosis
- ▲ Explain the relationship between maternal drug or alcohol intake and fetal–neonatal well-being
- ▲ Describe two other psychosocial pathologic conditions and related nursing care

Clinical Incidents

CLINICAL INCIDENT 1

Mrs. B. is admitted to the hospital in labor. Her contractions are 8 minutes apart and last 30 seconds each. Although Mrs. B.'s labor progresses normally until she is 5 cm dilated, her cervix does not dilate any further. X-ray films are taken, and it is established that a cephalopelvic disproportion (CPD) exists.

What are the maternal and fetal causes of CPD?

What are the clinical clues that the nurse assesses that may indicate CPD?

Mrs. B delivers a 7-pound, 5-ounce baby boy by cesarean birth.

What are the nursing interventions unique to the mother who has had a cesarean birth?

What are the unique concerns of the infant delivered by cesarean delivery?

CLINICAL INCIDENT 2

Mrs. D., 23 years old, is 3 months pregnant. She has had diabetes mellitus for the past 5 years and is taking isophane (NPH) insulin. She is attending an antepartal clinic, and this is her first pregnancy.

According to White's classification, in what class is Mrs. D.?

What predictably will happen to Mrs. D.'s insulin requirement during pregnancy?

What are the normal physiologic changes that occur during pregnancy that affect carbohydrate metabolism?

In the eighth month of her pregnancy, Mrs. D. is scheduled for fetal well-being studies, including ultrasonography and nonstress testing.

What information does ultrasound provide?

What information does nonstress testing provide?

What are the nursing responsibilities during ultrasound and nonstress testing?

At 37 weeks gestation, Mrs. D. has an amniocentesis to help ascertain fetal maturity.

What are three tests done for fetal maturity using amniotic fluid?

Which fetal maturity test using amniotic fluid is thought to be most important?

What are nursing responsibilities during amniocentesis?

What information needs to be shared with the parents?

Mrs. D. delivers a 9-pound girl whose Apgar score at 1 minute is 7 and at 5 minutes is 9.

What are the Apgar criteria?

What is the significance of 1-minute and 5-minute Apgar scoring?

To what particular metabolic problem is the infant of the diabetic mother prone?

What are the signs and symptoms of hypoglycemia in the neonate?

Mrs. D. asks the nurse if her baby will be diabetic and if she can safely have other children.

How will you, as the nurse, respond to Mrs. D.'s questions?

CLINICAL INCIDENT 3

Mr. and Mrs. B.'s first child, Melissa, is born with a cleft lip and palate. You visited this couple twice a month during the last trimester. The B.'s are a healthy, loving couple. Mr. B. is present at the delivery.

What are the nursing interventions appropriate in the delivery room for the neonate? For the family?

Mrs. B. is 2 days postpartum and is going to the nursery to feed Melissa.

What anticipatory guidance can you provide regarding feeding the neonate with a cleft lip and palate?.

While visiting with Mrs. B in the nursery, she asks about the repair surgery that will be done for Melissa.

At what age are cleft lip and palate repairs done?

What strategies can the nurse use to explain the surgery to the parents?

Mrs. B. asks what the chances are of this defect occurring in a subsequent pregnancy. As a nurse, how do you respond?

One of the goals of nursing care for any neonate with an anomaly is to promote as normal an infancy as possible. What specific information about growth and development of this neonate would you discuss with Mr. and Mrs. B.?

UNIT 6

Behavioral Outcomes

- ▲ Describe the components of a complete gynecologic examination
- ▲ Discuss the existing contraceptive methods in relation to mechanism of action, advantages and disadvantages, and effectiveness
- ▲ Describe the nurse's role in the provision of contraceptive methods
- ▲ Name the appropriate abortion techniques for first and second trimester induced abortions
- ▲ Discuss the advantages, disadvantages, and complications of each abortion method.

- ▲ Describe the interrelationships between prostaglandin inhibitors and dysmenorrhea
- ▲ Identify the common sexually transmitted diseases
- ▲ Discuss clinical symptoms of sexually transmitted diseases and the appropriate choices for treatment
- ▲ Discuss the relationship between Pap smears, colposcopy, and cryosurgery
- ▲ Describe the basic components of a complete infertility evaluation
- ▲ Describe the nurse's role in providing care to women with common reproductive-related health problems

Clinical Incidents

CLINICAL INCIDENT 1

Sally M. has come to the midwives' clinic to select a contraceptive method. She says, "Several of my friends got pregnant while they were taking the pill, and I also had a friend who used an IUD and she had awful cramps after it was inserted. I just don't know what to do, but I do know I don't want to get pregnant right now."

How would you begin your discussion with Sally?

What are the pros and cons of oral contraception and intrauterine devices?

What sociocultural factors might affect selection of a contraceptive method?

How does age relate to contraceptive selection?

Differentiate between chemical methods, natural family planning methods, mechanical methods, and hormonal methods of contraception.

CLINICAL INCIDENT 2

Mary T. is seen in the prenatal clinic at 34 weeks gestation. She complains of pain and discomfort in the vulvar and vaginal area, and says that she got the mirror to look and saw some sores that looked like little blisters on the inside of her "privates." Upon examination you note that she does indeed have lesions such as she described.

How would you begin your interview with Mary? What questions are important? Why?

What might be causing Mary this discomfort? Explain.

How would her conditions be treated?

How would it affect her unborn child?

Would you have any concerns for Mary's sexual partners? Explain.

Would you have any concerns about Mary's labor and delivery? Explain.

APPENDIX D

PATIENT CHART (MATERNAL RECORDS)

Records are a vital part of professional nursing. Each institution or agency usually has its own particular forms, yet most of the forms are quite similar in terms of categories, content, and intent. A patient chart is included on the following pages, and additional chart forms, including neonatal forms, are included in Appendix E both for information and study so that the learner can be aware of some of the areas of record keeping that are important for both professional and legal purposes.

The following chart forms were adapted from the Bexar County Hospital District, Medical Center Hospital, San Antonio, Texas, and are used with permission. They include:

- ▲ Patient's Admission Record
- ▲ Nursing Assessment/Teaching Form—used to record initial assessment data; if patient is in active labor, complete data collection may be deferred
- ▲ Vital Sign Sheet
- ▲ Course of Labor—includes Friedman graph
- ▲ Delivery Record
- ▲ Problem List
- ▲ Obstetrical Nurse's 24-Hour Clinical Summary —used to record postpartum assessment data
- ▲ Nursing Care Plan
- ▲ Nurse's Progress Notes
- ▲ 24-Hour Patient Care Summary
- ▲ Physical Medicine and Rehabilitation Consultation or Therapy Request
- ▲ Progress Notes/History

Patient's name: ______________________

Hospital patient number: ______________________

SPECIAL INSTRUCTIONS:
To be used for all pregnant patients except abortions.

PATIENT'S ADMISSION RECORD

DATE ADMITTED	DATE DISCHARGED

Name ______________________

ADMITTING DIAGNOSIS (To be filled out on all patients.) ______________________

DISCHARGE DIAGNOSIS Circle appropriate diagnosis. (To be filled out on all patients.)

PREGNANCY NOT DELIVERED

Observed for labor

Other diagnoses ______________________

PREGNANCY DELIVERED

Gestation: Single Multiple

Infant: Term Premature Liveborn Fetal death

COMPLICATION OF PREGNANCY, LABOR, DELIVERY, AND PUERPERIUM

Anemia	Pre-eclampsia/eclampsia	Dystocia	Urinary tract infection
Abruptio	Hypertensive vascular disease	Endo/parametritis	Postpartum hemorrhage
Diabetes	Previous cesarean section		

Other ______________________

PROCEDURES/OPERATIONS Circle appropriate procedure.

Vaginal delivery Tubal sterilization Cesarean section

Other Procedures/Operations ______________________

DISCHARGE AND DISPOSITION NOTES Condition: Good, fair, unimproved, dead: ______________________

Medications (drug(s), dose): ______________________

Follow-up: ______________________

Clinic: P.P., Fam. Plan., Plan. Parent., Metro. Health Dept., Prenatal, Gyn., Other ______________________

When: ______________________ Doctor: ______________________

Date summary dictated ______________________ House staff ______________________ M.D.

Date OP note dictated ______________________ Attending staff ______________________ M.D.

INSTRUCTIONS TO MEDICAL STAFF

1. Complete and sign this form for all patients at time of discharge.

IN ADDITION:

2. A dictated discharge summary is required on
   (a) all patients hospitalized 10 or more days
   (b) all patients having major surgery (including cesarean section).
   (c) all maternal deaths.

ORIGINAL – INPATIENT CHART
COPY – OUTPATIENT CHART

Patient's name: ______________________

Hospital patient number: ______________________

NURSING ASSESSMENT/TEACHING FORM

ADMISSION DIAGNOSIS ______________________
ADMISSION TIME/DATE ______________________
SERVICE ______________________
ALLERGIES ______________________

1. VITAL SIGNS

B/P: __________ Pulse: __________ ( )Apical ( )Radial ( )Regular ( )Irregular ( )Weak ( )Bounding

Respirations: __________ ( )Regular ( )Retractions ( )Noisy/wet ( )Wheezing ( )Dyspneic ( )Orthopneic

Temperature: __________ ( )Oral ( )Rectal ( )Axillary Weight: __________ ( )Bed scale ( )Chair ( )Standing# __________ Height: ______

2. MENTAL STATUS (Check one)

( )Awake, alert ( )Awake, confused ( )Easily awakened ( )Sleeps unless stimulated
( )Sleeps unless painfully stimulated ( )Comatose, purposeful movement ( )Comatose, nonpurposeful movement
( )Decorticate (flexed) ( )Decerebrate (extended) ( )Flaccid Oriented to: ( )Time ( )Place ( )Person

3. SENSES

Vision: ( )Adequate ( )Decreased ( )Blind ( )R ( )L ( )Glasses ( )At home ( )With patient ( )Contact lenses ( )At home ( )With patient

( )Prosthesis ( )At home ( )With patient

Hearing: ( )Adequate ( )Decreased ( )Deaf ( )R ( )L ( )Hearing aid ( )At home ( )With patient

Paresthesia: ( )Yes ( )No

Where ______________________ Describe ______________________

4. COMMUNICATION

Language spoken: __________ ( )Aphasia (Describe): ______________________

Reads __________ Writes __________

5. MOBILITY

( )Walks alone ( )Walks with help ( )Cane ( )Walker ( )Wheel chair ( )Stretcher

( )Paralysis ( )R ( )L ( )Upper ( )R ( )L ( )Lower ( )Prosthesis ______________________

6. SKIN CONDITION

( )Normal color ( )Dusky ( )Pale ( )Cyanotic ( )Flushed ( )Jaundiced ( )Intact ( )Bony areas*
( )Redness* ( )Decubitus* ( )Rash* ( )Scars* ( )Bruises* ( )Hot ( )Warm ( )Cool ( )Moist ( )Dry

*Indicate and describe below:

Indicate on diagrams all body marks, such as old or recent scars; bruises or discolorations (regardless of how slight); lacerations; decubitus ulcers; and other ulcerations or questionable markings not considered normal.

	Peripheral Pulse	Vascular Temp.	Checks Color
RA			
LA			
RL			
LL			

Comments Re: Skin condition
____
____
____
____

EMERGENCY NOTIFICATION

Name ______________________
Relationship ______________________
Phone no. ______________________

HEALTH HISTORY

	Patient	Family (Mother, Father, Sib., Child)		Patient	Family (Mother, Father, Sib., Child)
Diabetes	( )______	( )______	Epilepsy	( )______	( )______
Heart disease	( )______	( )______	Asthma	( )______	( )______
Hypertension	( )______	( )______	Hepatitis	( )______	( )______
Cancer	( )______	( )______	Other	( )______	( )______
Tuberculosis	( )______	( )______		( )______	( )______

Comments:____________________

8. *MEDICATIONS PRESENTLY TAKING* (List below)

	Brought In	Time of Last Dose	Sent Home	Left at Bedside	Locked Up
1.					
2.					
3.					
4.					
5.					

9. PREVIOUS HOSPITAL EXPERIENCE ( )Yes ( )No ( )Date__________

Details:__________

What results do you expect from this hospitalization?__________

10. ACTIVITIES OF DAILY LIVING

1. General hygiene ( )Self ( )With help ( )Tub ( )Shower Time/Frequency______
( )Dentures ( )Upper ( )Lower ( )Partial ( )With patient ( )At home

2. Elimination ( )Continent ( )Incontinent ( )Foley: Insertion date______ ( )Ureterostomy
( )Colostomy ( )Ileostomy ( )Hemorrhoids Frequency of B.M.______ ( )Irregularities: Describe______
______ What helps irregularity______

3. Sleep habits Usual bedtime______ Number of hours sleep______ Number of pillows used______
( )Awaken at night What do you do to help you fall asleep?______
Reason______

4. Nutritional status ( )3 Meals a day ( )Omit breakfast ( )Omit lunch ( )Omit supper ( )Snacks: Describe
______ ( )Special diet: Describe______
( )Follows diet ( )Does not follow diet ( )Food intolerance: Describe______

5. Use of stimulants ( )Soft drinks: How much______ ( )Coffee: How much______
( )Tea: How much______ ( )Alcohol: How much______ ( )Tobacco: How much______
( )Drugs: What______ How much______

11. SOCIOECONOMIC HISTORY

Religion ______________________________

Living arrangements ( )House ( )Apartment ( )Bathroom facilities ( )Must use stairs ( )Lives alone
( )Minors only ( )Other adults ( )Invalid adults

Job security/income during hospitalization ( )Yes ( )No ( )NA Occupation ______________

Will hospitalization cause immediate problems to you and family? ______________

____

____

Who will take care of you after discharge? ______________

____

12. ANTICIPATED TEACHING NEEDS

( )Medications ( )Chronic illness
( )Diet ( )Other

____

____

13. CONSULTS NEEDED ( )Social service ( )Dietary ( )Nurse

14. ( )PATIENT/FAMILY ORIENTATION TO FACILITIES

15. DISPOSITION OF VALUABLES ( )Security ( )Family: Name ______________

Relation to patient ______________ ( )Valuables slip completed

History obtained from ______________ By ______________

---

16. DISMISSAL INFORMATION (To be completed at time of discharge)

____

( )Meds removed from lockup and given to patient ( )All personal effects given to patient/family

Instructions to Patient on Discharge	Goal Achieved		Exceptions/Comments
	Date	Signature/Title	

Patient discharged [ ]With medication(s) [ ]Without medication(s) [ ]To dismissal area

Patient discharged [ ]With clinic appointment [ ]Without clinic appointment

Form completed on discharge by ______________ ______________ ______________

(Name) (Title) (Date)

17. TEACHING

Teaching Subject	Demonstration		Return Demonstration		Exceptions/Comments
	Date	Signature/Title	Date	Signature/Title	

Patient's name:

Hospital patient number:

VITAL SIGN SHEET

INPATIENT CHART

DATE

Date							
Day P.O.							
Day P.P.							

	Hour	A.M. 4 8 12	P.M. 4 8 12	A.M. 4 8 12	P.M. 4 8 12	A.M. 4 8 12	P.M. 4 8 12	A.M. 4 8 12	P.M. 4 8 12	A.M. 4 8 12	P.M. 4 8 12	A.M. 4 8 12	P.M. 4 8 12	A.M. 4 8 12	P.M. 4 8 12	Hour
Temperature	106°															106°
	105°															105°
	104°															104°
	103°															103°
	102°															102°
	101°															101°
	100°															100°
	99° Normal															99° Normal
	98°															98°
	97°															97°
	96°															96°
Pulse	150															150
	140															140
	130															130
	120															120
	110															110
	100															100
	90															90
	80															80
	70															70
	60															60
	50															50

Respiration								
Blood Pressure	7 – 3							
	3 – 11							
	11 – 7							
CVP								
Weight								

Patient's name:

Hospital patient number:

COURSE OF LABOR

ADMISSION TIME ______ : ______

INPATIENT CHART

DATE

Begin plot on admission at "0" hours.

CX DIL. IN CM: 10, 9, 8, 7, 6, 5, 4, 3, 2

Time (in hours): 0, 1, 2, 3, 4, 5, 6, 7, 8, 9, 10, 11, 12, 13, 14, 15, 16, 17, 18

Date	Hour	MEMB	Contraction			FH	Cervix		Fetus		Record All Exams. Med.. Obs.	Initials
			Freq.	Durat.	Int.		Eff.	Dil.	Pos.	Sta.		

ONSET OF LABOR: Date ___/ ___/ ___Time_______ONSET OF SECOND STAGE: Date ___/___/___Time_______

OXYTOCIN STARTED

Date ___/ ___/ ___Time_______

OXYTOCIN DISC.

Date ___/ ___/ ___Time_______

DELIVERY RECORD

Patient's name: ______________________

Hospital patient number: ______________________

CURRENT ADDRESS (*to be completed by Unit Sec*)

FOLLOW-UP CLINIC (*to be completed by FAMPLAN*)

DATE

ONSET OF LABOR: Date __________ Time __________ AM PM Spont. Induced: How __________ Reason __________

STAGES OF LABOR: 1st ______ Hrs 2nd ______ Hrs 3rd ______ Hrs Total __________ Hrs

MEMBR. RUPT. Date ______ Time ______ AM PM Spont. Art. Clear, Cloudy Meconium: No Yes

DELIVERY DATE ______ Time ______ AM PM Hrs RBOW to delivery __________

NARRATIVE: ____

DELIVERY: Spontaneous Operative Full Term Premature Immature

OPERATION: Forceps: Low Mid Vacuum extraction Forceps rotation Manual rotation

Asst. breech extraction Breech extraction Version & extraction

Cervical C.S. Class. cesarean section C.S. hysterectomy

PRESENTATION and POSITION: During labor __________ At delivery __________

EPISIOTOMY: Central Mediolateral Extension None

LACERATIONS: None Perineal Anorectal Vaginal Cervical Ruptured uterus

BLEEDING: Antepartum __________ ml Postpartum __________ ml

PLACENTA: Spontaneous delivery Manual removal Adherent (Hysterectomy)

Time ______ Wt. ______ gm Description __________

CORD & MEMBRANES: Arteries: 1. 2. Description __________

OXYTOCICS: (Postpartum) Agent: Oxytocin Ergotrate Methergine

Total dose given: __________ Route: IM IV Push IV Drip

TOTAL ANALGESIA GIVEN: Demerol ______ mgm Barbiturate ______ mgm

Tranquilizer: Drug ______ Dose ______ Time of Last Dose ______

CHILD: Male Female DBL DDL Living Wt. Lbs ______ oz ______ ______ gm

Breathing Time ______ Min Crying Time ______ Min

APGAR: 1" Color 0 1 2 Resp. 0 1 2 Pulse 0 1 2 Reflex 0 1 2 Muscle Tone 0 1 2

5" Color 0 1 2 Resp. 0 1 2 Pulse 0 1 2 Reflex 0 1 2 Muscle Tone 0 1 2

TOTAL 1" __________ 5" __________

RESUSCITATION: Suction Oxygen Laryngoscopy Pos. Pres.

Endotracheal Intubation Other __________

ANOMALIES: Description __________ Eyes Treated __________

ANESTHESIA: None Perineal Paracervical Spinal Epidural General Other Bottle or Breast Fed

SIGNED ______________________

(To be completed for each baby delivered.)

Patient's name:

Hospital patient number:

OBSTETRICAL NURSE'S 24-HOUR CLINICAL SUMMARY

Nursing History Complete [ ]
Incomplete [ ]

INPATIENT CHART
DATE

Observation	7-3	3-11	11-7
Emotional status			
ADL care			
Diet-appetite			
Elimination			
Mobility			
Peri- or wound care			
IV site			
Respiratory care			
Patient teaching			

7-3	3-11	11-7

OBSTETRICAL NURSE'S 24-HOUR CLINICAL SUMMARY, PAGE 2 OF 2

IV FLUIDS

No.	Time Start	Time Disc.	Contents	Signature	No.	Time Start	Time Disc.	Contents	Signature

Time	BP	T	P	R	FHT	Fundus Tone / CM	Lochia	C & A	ALB	Urine Output	IV	Oral	Other	Special Care and Observation *(Sign Each Entry)*
DATE						24-HOUR TOTAL								

Patient's name:

Hospital patient number:

PROBLEM LIST

Problem Number	Date of Onset	Active Problem	Resolved Problems Date and Disposition

☐ INPATIENT ☐ OUTPATIENT

Patient's name:

____

Hospital patient number:

____

NURSING CARE PLAN

*Sign each problem

Date	Nursing Diagnosis (Problem)	Planning		Evaluation
		Goals	Nursing Action	Outcome

Patient's name:

Hospital patient number:

NURSE'S PROGRESS NOTES

Date/Time	Note only pertinent information regarding nursing care and patient's condition, e.g., changes in condition or symptoms, unusual reaction to treatments and medications, etc.	Nurse's Signature

INPATIENT CHART

Patient's name:

Hospital patient number:

24-HOUR PATIENT CARE SUMMARY

Date	2300-0700	0700-1500	1500-2300
Bath type Special SLN: S = Shampoo D = Denture care OH = Oral hygiene SH = Shave			
Mobility Type Frequency: Aids:			
Bowel elimination O = Ostomy E = Enema 1 = Stool Stool tests: Frequency:			
Wound and/or skin care Type: Site: Frequency:			
Dressings Type Site: Frequency:			
Diet			
Pulmonary care Type: Frequency:			

IV FLUID

No.	Time Started	Time Discont.	Contents	Signature	No.	Time Started	Time Discont.	Contents	Signature

INPATIENT CHART

24-HOUR PATIENT CARE SUMMARY. PAGE 2 OF 2

	Intake				Diabetic		Output								
Date/ Time	Oral	Other	IV Intake	Colloids, Blood, etc.	C	A	SP.GR.	Urine	NG/ Emesis	Chest	Other	Other	Other	Other
2200-2300														
2300-2400														
2400-0100														
0100-0200														
0200-0300														
0300-0400														
0400-0500														
0500-0600														
Total														
0600-0700														
0700-0800														
0800-0900														
0900-1000														
1000-1100														
1100-1200														
1200-1300														
1300-1400														
Total														
1400-1500														
1500-1600														
1600-1700														
1700-1800														
1800-1900														
1900-2000														
2000-2100														
2100-2200														
Total														
24-hour total														

Signature/Initials

Signature/Initials

Patient's name:

Hospital patient number:

● FROM ●

REQUESTING SERVICE	
OBSTETRICS	
REQUESTING PHYSICIAN SIGNATURE M.D.	
ATTENDING PHYSICIAN NAME M.D.	DATE OF REQUEST	TIME OF REQUEST A.M. P.M.

PHYSICAL MEDICINE AND REHABILITATION CONSULTATION OR THERAPY REQUEST

● TO ● [ ] PM&R physician consultant [X] Physical therapy [ ] Occupational therapy
[ ] Speech pathology [ ] Audiology [ ] Rehabilitation nurse

[ ] Outpatient [X] Inpatient Room/Bed__________ [X] Bedside [ ] Clinic

Diagnosis. (1)
(2) Postpartum—Delivered at (time)
(3) on (date)

Precautions

● SERVICE OR THERAPY REQUESTED ● (This section *must* be completed for therapeutic services.)

	Frequency	Duration
Please instruct in standard postpartum exercise program.		

● GOALS OF THEREAPY ● Restore abdominal muscle tone; improve posture; decrease or prevent low back pain.

PHYSICAL THERAPY NOTE

Date __________

This patient was instructed in standard postpartum exercises and was given a written home program. She was advised to carry out the program for at least six weeks.

This patient was not instructed prior to discharge. Please refer her as an outpatient if indicated.

Date	Time		Signature

[ ] INPATIENT [ ] OUTPATIENT

Patient's name:

Hospital patient number:

PROGRESS NOTES/HISTORY

Date	

[ ] INPATIENT [ ] OUTPATIENT

APPENDIX E

ADDITIONAL PATIENT RECORDS (NEONATAL AND ANTEPARTUM RECORDS)

This appendix contains the following forms:

- ▲ New OB Master Sheet—used for initial antepartum assessment by physician or midwife
- ▲ Antepartum Data Base
- ▲ Infant Progress Record
- ▲ Intrauterine Growth Chart
- ▲ Clinical Assessment of Gestational Age in the Newborn Infant
- ▲ Neonatal I.C.U. Nursing Record
- ▲ Nurse's Notes and Additional Treatment Record
- ▲ Home Care Referral Form

Patient's name:

____

Hospital patient number:

____

NEW OB MASTER SHEET

Visit date: ___/___/___ (mm dd yy) Parity: [| | | |] LMP: ___/___/___ (mm dd yy) EDD: ___/___/___ (mm dd yy)

MEDICAL HISTORY

	Yes	No
High blood pressure	( )	( )
Diabetes	( )	( )
Heart disease	( )	( )
UTI	( )	( )
Allergy	( )	( )

CURRENT MEDICATION

1. _______________
2. _______________
3. _______________
4. _______________

FAMILY HISTORY

	Yes	No
Diabetes	( )	( )
Bleeding	( )	( )
Twins	( )	( )

OB HISTORY

Number of vaginal deliveries: _______________

Number of cesarean sections: _______________

Weight of largest baby: ________ lb. ________ oz.

Date of last delivery: ___/___/___ (mm dd yy)

Number of low birth weight babies: _______________

Number of neonatal deaths: _______________

Number of stillborns: _______________

PHYSICAL EXAMINATION

Blood pressure: _______________

Weight: _______________ lb.

Fundal height: _______________ cm. (over 16 wks.)

Size: _______________ wks. (under 16 wks.)

LABORATORY DATA

HCT: _______________

VDRL (Circle one): R or N

RH (Circle one): + or –

PROBLEM LIST

Use standard terminology, no abbreviations. List only conditions with obstetrical implications.

1. _______________
2. _______________
3. _______________
4. _______________
5. _______________
6. _______________
7. _______________
8. _______________
9. _______________
10. _______________

____
Signature

____
Print name

Patient's name:

Hospital patient number:

ANTEPARTUM DATA BASE

CLINIC ______________________ DATE ___/___/___

Use history sheet if more space is required.

NAME (Last / First / Middle-other)	ADDRESS	TELEPHONE
		Check if problem

AGE (N 17–35)	MENSES (x x)	LMP (mo day year)	EDD	☐

HEALTH SINCE CONCEPTION (Illnesses, drugs, GI, GU, CVR, attitude toward pregnancy) ☐

HEALTH PRIOR TO CONCEPTION (What, where, when of major illness, drugs, hospitalizations, marital/emotional problems) ☐

NUTRITION HISTORY (Typical 3 meals—evaluate protein & vit. intake) ☐

FAMILY PLANNING (Desired no. of children ______ [total]; previous experience with and future plans for family planning) ☐

PAST OB HISTORY P __ __ __ __ __ (t t p a L)	Date last pregnancy terminated / / (N = >18 mo)	Birth weight largest child (N = <4,000 g)	No. prev. LBWI (N = · 2,500 g)	☐
No. prev. abortions (spont.) (induced)	No. fetal deaths	No. neo-natal deaths	No. cesarean sections / Type C.S.	☐

Describe what, where, when, and results of major obstetrical complications, i.e., bleeding, high blood pressure, UTI, twins, anemia, diabetes, maternal or newborn transfusion, severe nervousness, still birth, neonatal deaths. ☐

FAMILY HISTORY: WNL ☐ (Psychiatric, TB, diabetes, twins, bleeding, cancer, mental retard., neuro, HCVD, sickle cell dis.) ☐

SOCIAL HISTORY: S M W D Sep (If employed give occupation. If single, plans for baby. Rec. food stamps?) ☐

PHYSICAL EXAMINATION

BP (N = · 130/80)	P (N = · 100)	HT (N = >60")	PRES. WT	NON-PREG. WT	☐

EENT-DENTAL: WNL ☐ ☐

NECK, BREASTS, HEART: WNL ☐ ☐

ABDOMEN: WNL ☐ (Measure all masses, describe scars, FHT) ☐

PELVIS vulva/vag.	cervix	corpus (size)	adnexa	rectal	☐

EXTREMITIES: WNL ☐ (V.V., edema, reflexes) ☐

LABORATORY EVALUATION (Check if normal; described if abnormal)
Serol. ☐ CBC ☐ Bld type ☐ rubella ☐ urine ☐ Pap ☐ G.C. ☐ x-ray ☐ other ☐ ☐

Remarks ______________________

Signature ❯

☐ Inpatient ☐ Outpatient

Patient's name:

Hospital patient number:

INFANT PROGRESS RECORD

DATE

Time	IV Fluids		IV chk	Heart Rate / Resp. Rate	Temp	ID Band	Cord	Cry	Skin	Urine	Stool	WT.	Type of Feeding	Remarks	Signature
	Amount Added to Buretrol	Amount Absorbed													

INPATIENT CHART

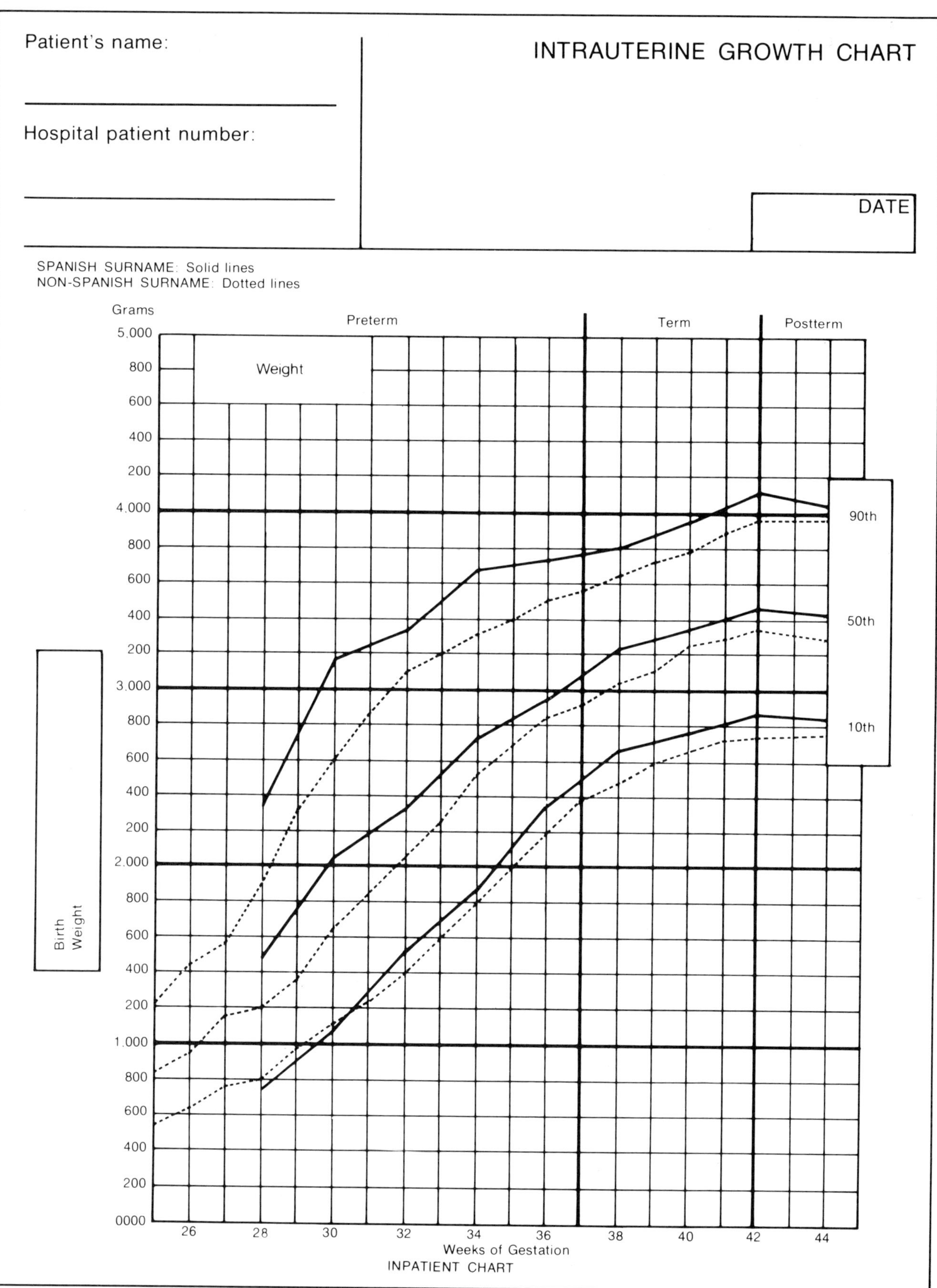

Solid line = data from Robert B. Green Hospital. Dotted line = data modified from Freeman MG, Graves WL, Thompson AB: Indigent negro and caucasian birth weight—gestational age tables. *Pediatrics* 46:9–15, 1970.

CLINICAL ASSESSMENT OF GESTATIONAL AGE IN THE NEWBORN INFANT

Neurological sign	Score 0	1	2	3	4	5
Posture						
Square window	90°	60°	45°	30°	0°	
Ankle dorsiflexion	90°	75°	45°	20°	0°	
Arm recoil	180°	90–180°	>90°			
Leg recoil	180°	90–180°	>90°			
Popliteal angle	180°	160°	130°	110°	90°	>90°
Heel to ear						
Scarf sign						
Head lag						
Ventral suspension						

Total score* ______

Gestational age = $\frac{\text{score}}{4}$ + 25 = ______ weeks ± 2 weeks

*Add the scores for each criterion.

External sign	Score 0	1	2	3	4
Edema	Obvious edema of hands and feet; pitting over tibia	No obvious edema of hands and feet; pitting over tibia	No edema		
Skin texture	Very thin, gelatinous	Thin and smooth	Smooth; medium thickness. Rash or superficial peeling	Slight thickening. Superficial cracking and peeling, especially of hands and feet	Thick and parchment-like; superficial or deep cracking
Skin color	Dark red	Uniformly pink	Pale pink; variable over body	Pale; only pink over ears, lips, palms, or soles	
Skin opacity (trunk)	Numerous veins and venules clearly seen, especially over abdomen	Veins and tributaries seen	A few large vessels clearly seen over abdomen	A few large vessels seen indistinctly over abdomen	No blood vessels seen
Lanugo (over back)	No lanugo	Abundant; long and thick over whole back	Hair thinning, especially over lower back	Small amount of lanugo and bald areas	At least ½ of back devoid of lanugo
Plantar creases	No skin creases	Faint red marks over anterior half of sole	Definite red marks over >anterior ½; indentations over < anterior ⅓	Indentations over anterior ½	Definite deep indentations over >anterior ½
Nipple formation	Nipple barely visible; no areola	Nipple well defined; areola smooth and flat, diameter <0.75 cm.	Areola stippled, edge not raised, diameter <0.75 cm.	Areola stippled, edge raised, diameter >0.75 cm.	
Breast size	No breast tissue palpable	Breast tissue on one or both sides, <0.5 cm. diameter	Breast tissue both sides; one or both 0.5–1.0 cm.	Breast tissue both sides; one or both >1 cm.	
Ear form	Pinna flat and shapeless, little or no incurving of edge	Incurving of part of edge of pinna	Partial incurving whole of upper pinna	Well-defined incurving whole of upper pinna	
Ear firmness	Pinna soft, easily folded, no recoil	Pinna soft, easily folded, slow recoil	Cartilage to edge of pinna, but soft in places, ready recoil	Pinna firm, cartilage to edge; instant recoil	
Genitals Male	Neither testis in scrotum	At least one testis high in scrotum	At least one testis right down		
Female (with hips ½ abducted)	Labia majoria widely separated labia minora protruding	Labia majora almost cover labia minora	Labia majora completely cover labia minora		

Evaluator ______

From Dubowitz LMS, Dubowitz V, Goldberg C: Clinical assessment of gestational age in the newborn infant. *J Pediatr* 77:1–10, 1970.

Patient's name: ______________________

Hospital patient number: ______________________

NEONATAL I.C.U. NURSING RECORD

Date______ Condition______ Admission Wt.______ Head______ Chest______ Length______

	Time A.M.—P.M.	11:30P.M.	12:30A.M.	1:30A.M.	2:30A.M.	3:30A.M.	4:30A.M.	5:30A.M.	6:30A.M.	Totals	7:30A.M.	8:30A.M.	9:30A.M.	10:30A.M.	11:30A.M.	12:30P.M.	1:30P.M.	2:30P.M.	Totals	3:30P.M.	4:30P.M.	5:30P.M.	6:30P.M.	7:30P.M.	8:30P.M.	9:30P.M.	10:30P.M.
	Oxygen Concentration	L %	L %	L %	L %	L %	L %	L %	L %		L %	L %	L %	L %	L %	L %	L %	L %		L %	L %	L %	L %	L %	L %	L %	L %
Vital Signs	Blood Pressure																										
	Apical Pulse																										
	Resp.																										
	Rectal Temp.																										
	Isolette Temp.																										
Intake	Amount PR or NG																										
	Type Formula																										
IV Fluids	Amount Added to Buretrol																										
	Amount Absorbed																										
Output	Urine																										
	Stool																										
	Vomitus																										
Treatment	Head Cir.																										
	Weight																										
	Turn																										
	Suction																										
	Ambu.																										
Meds.																											
Adm.V/S	Time																										
	Ap. Pulse																										
	Resp.																										

INPATIENT CHART

NURSE'S NOTES AND ADDITIONAL TREATMENT RECORD

TIME					
11 – 7	Marked On	NAVEL	CRY	SKIN	EYES
7 – 3	Marked On	NAVEL	CRY	SKIN	EYES
3 – 11	Marked On	NAVEL	CRY	SKIN	EYES

Patient's name: ______________________

Hospital patient number: ______________________

HOME CARE REFERRAL FORM

DATE

To: ____

Agency called __________ (date) __________ (time) A.M. P.M. Hosp No. __________ Room No. __________

Patient name ______________________ Birth date __________ Sex __________

Address ______________________ Soc. sec. number ______________________

Telephone no. __________ Marital status __________ Medicare number ______________________

Spouse or parents' name ______________________ Medicaid number ______________________

Address where patient will stay ______________________ Telephone no. __________

Name of nearest relative (other than same household) ______________________

Address ____

Medical diagnosis ____

MEDICAL ORDERS/INSTRUCTIONS

Medications	Dosage	Frequency	How Long	Route of Administration

[ ]Dressing [ ]Catheter care [ ]Levine tube [ ]Irrigations [ ]HHH [ ]Bath [ ]Shampoo

Other ____

Diet ______________________ Restrictions ______________________

Recommended Physical activity ____

Patient [ ]is [ ]is not aware of diagnosis.

Patient [ ]has [ ]has not been cooperative in follow-up.

Patient [ ]has [ ]has not been referrred to social service.

Next clinic appoint. __________

N.C. plan ____

Reply requested: [ ]No [ ]Yes, to ______________________ Include patient's name and number of all correspondence.

Certification: This patient who is under my care is essentially homebound for health reasons and is in need of intermittent home visits according to the above treatment plan. If the patient is admitted under Part A, home health services are needed to treat a condition for which the patient received hospital services or posthospital extended care services.

PHYSICIAN: ______________________
Signature Date

[ ] INPATIENT [ ] OUTPATIENT

APPENDIX F

ASSESSMENT TOOLS

Various charts, forms, and other assessment tools are reproduced on the following pages. These serve as adjuncts to history taking and/or physical examination and are important aids in the collection and organization of data about a client.

Included are the following tools:

- ▲ Food Information for Nutritional Assessment of Maternity Patients
- ▲ Deficiency Method of Dietary Assessment: Women
- ▲ Postpartum Evaluation
- ▲ Physical Growth Percentiles: Girls and Boys, Birth to 36 Months
- ▲ Bilirubin Chart for Premature Infant
- ▲ Bilirubin Chart for Term Newborn Infant
- ▲ Example of a Temperature Chart Showing a Normal Ovulatory Cycle
- ▲ Example of a Temperature Chart Showing an Anovulatory Cycle
- ▲ Health History at a Glance

FOOD INFORMATION
FOR NUTRITIONAL ASSESSMENT OF MATERNITY PATIENTS

MATERNITY NUTRITIONAL ASSESSMENT

Foods eaten yesterday
and amounts

Date__________

SUPPLEMENTATION

Vitamins __________

Iron (Fe) __________

Folic acid (FA)__________

Evaluation

Food groups	Servings			
Milk, cheese	☐	☐	☐	☐
Meat, eggs, beans	☐	☐	☐	
Fruits, vegetables	☐	☐	☐	☐
Bread, cereal	☐	☐	☐	☐

	Adequate	Inadequate
Calories	____	____
Calcium	____	____
Iron	____	____
Protein	____	____
Vitamin A	____	____
Vitamin C	____	____

WIC Needed_____Referred_____Date_____

Food stamps Needed_____Referred_____Date_____

Recommendations__________

MATERNITY NUTRITIONAL ASSESSMENT

Foods eaten yesterday
and amounts

Date__________

SUPPLEMENTATION

Vitamins __________

Iron (Fe)__________

Folic acid (FA)__________

Evaluation

Food groups	Servings			
Milk, cheese	☐	☐	☐	☐
Meat, eggs, beans	☐	☐	☐	
Fruits, vegetables	☐	☐	☐	☐
Bread, cereal	☐	☐	☐	☐

	Adequate	Inadequate
Calories	____	____
Calcium	____	____
Iron	____	____
Protein	____	____
Vitamin A	____	____
Vitamin C	____	____

WIC Needed_____Referred_____Date_____

Food stamps Needed_____Referred_____Date_____

Recommendations__________

From Texas Department of Health. Form M–13a, revised 6/80. Used with permission.

Deficiency Method of Dietary Assessment: Women
If the individual's 24-hour intake compared to the minimal reference point for daily intake (Column 3 below) has three (3) or more deficiencies, inadequate dietary pattern may be applied as a condition of nutritional need.

(1) Food Group (Key nutrients provided)	*(2)* Common Foods in Group and Serving Equivalences		*(3)* Minimal Reference Point For Daily Intake	*(4)* Counting Deficiencies
A. Milk: Protein, Calcium, Riboflavin, Vitamin D, Vitamin A	Milk	1 cup (8 oz)	3 servings (pregnant and breastfeeding women) 2 servings	Count each missing serving as one (1) deficiency
	Cheese	1-¼ oz		
	Cottage cheese	1 cup		
	Cheese food or cheese spread	2 oz		
	Yogurt, plain	1 cup		
	Yogurt, fruit flavored	1-½ cups		
	Ice cream	1-½ cups		
B. Meat: Protein, Iron	Beef, pork, ham, veal, liver, venison	2–3 oz	2 servings	Count each missing serving as one (1) deficiency
	Poultry, fish, goat, lamb	4–5 oz		
	Chili con carne	1 cup		
	Eggs	2		
	Dried beans or dried peas	1 cup (cooked)		
	Wieners	3		
	Luncheon meats, cold cuts	4 slices		
	Peanut butter	4 Tbs		
C. Fruits/vegetables: Vitamins, Minerals, Fiber	Raw	1 small-medium or ½ large piece	4 servings	Maximum of one (1) deficiency to be counted if total recommended servings are not consumed
1. Consider total number of servings consumed	Canned, cooked	½ cup		
	(fresh or frozen)	½ cup		
	Juices			
2. Consider Vitamin C-rich source	Citrus fruit (orange, grapefruit)	1 small piece or ½ cup	1 serving	Count one (1) deficiency when serving is missing
	Pineapple, papaya	½ cup		
	Citrus fruit juices	½ cup		
	Avocado, watermelon, asparagus, cabbage, cauliflower, greens, spinach	1 cup cooked or 1–1-½ cups raw		
	Tomato	1 large		

3. Consider Vitamin A-rich source	Broccoli, carrots, greens (e.g., turnips, spinach), mixed vegetables	½ cup cooked or canned	1 serving	Count one (1) deficiency when serving is missing from intake
	Winter squash (e.g., acorn, butternut), sweet potatoes	1 small or ½ medium-large		
	Apricots, cantaloupe, papaya, watermelon	½ cup canned or 1 cup fresh		
D. Bread/Cereal: Protein, Iron, B Vitamins, Fiber	Bread (whole grain or enriched)	1 slice	4 servings	Count one (1) deficiency for every two missing servings or Count one (1) deficiency for every two servings in excess of six servings
	Cooked cereal	½ cup		
	Ready-to-eat cereal	¾ cup		
	Pasta, rice, grits	½ cup		
	Cornbread	2″ square		
	Crackers	4 small squares		
	Muffin, roll, biscuit	1		
	Corn tortillas (7″ diameter)	2		
	Flour tortillas (7″ diameter)	1		

OTHER DIETARY CONSIDERATIONS

E. Nonnutritious foods: Soft drinks, sugar sweetened tea or coffee, candy, popsicles, chips, cookies. Certain homemade cookies (e.g., peanut butter, oatmeal, or the like) contain more nutritious ingredients and may be counted as bread/cereal instead of as nonnutritious.	Count one (1) deficiency for every two servings
F. Pica: Definition: The consumption of nonfood items, such as clay, cooking or laundry starch, refrigerator ice, dirt, etc. (see Chapter 12.)	Count one (1) deficiency if participant admits to consuming nonfood items one or more times daily
G. Clinical evidence of inadequate calorie intake: If there is documented clinical evidence of inadequate calorie intake (as defined below), this condition may be combined with two or more dietary deficiencies (as defined A–F) and be applied as an inadequate dietary pattern.	Count one (1) deficiency if one of these conditions is present

1. Pregnant women:
   a. Weight loss
   b. Insufficient weight gain—weight gain falls below the bottom range of normal prenatal weight gain curve
   c. Excessive weight gain—weight gain is above the top range of normal prenatal weight gain curve
2. Breast-feeding women: Weight loss in excess of 10 pounds per month postpartum

Adapted from the Texas Department of Health. Used with permission.

Minimal daily intake is discussed in Chapter 12, Table 12.3. This is *not* recommended to be used as a counseling guide. Refer to "Nutrition Guidelines for Women, Infants and Children" for counseling purposes. This guide or its equivalent is usually available through your State Health Department—Maternal-Child Health Division, or use The Women-Infants-Children guidelines furnished by the Federal Government.

POSTPARTUM EVALUATION

Name ________ Age ________ Date ________ Postpartum day ________

Physician ________ Anesthesia ________ Gravida ________ Para ________

Breast-feeding ________ Formula feeding ________ Activity ________ Diet ________

Type of delivery ________ First voiding (*time and amount*) ________

Second voiding ________ Medications and reasons for use ________

____

____

1. Vital signs: Temp ________ Pulse ________ Resp ________ Blood pressure ________
2. Breasts (*soft, engorged, firm, pain, redness*) ________

   Nipples (*redness, pain, cracks, fissures*) ________

   Describe present care of the breasts (*hygiene, support, schedule and duration of breast-feeding, use of nipple shield, creams and ointments used, etc.*) ________

   ____

   ____

   Describe patient's learning needs related to care of the breasts, and list your interventions (*films viewed, hygiene, support, breast-feeding, diet, use of shields, manual expression, use of Syntocinon spray, feeding schedule, etc.*) ________

   ____

   ____

3. Fundus: Location (*relate to umbilicus as above or below in centimeters*) ________

   ________ Expected location this postpartum day ________

   Consistency (*firm, boggy, firm with massage*) ________

   List deviations from normal and your nursing intervention ________

   ____

   ____

   ____

4. Lochia: Color (*rubra, serosa, alba*) ________ Expected color ________

   Amount (*no flow, scanty, moderate, heavy, constant ooze, trickle, clots*) ________

   ________ Odor ________ Indicate deviations from normal and your nursing interventions ________

   ____

   ____

5. Perineum: Episiotomy ________ Type ________ Laceration ________ Appearance (*clean, edema, redness, discoloration, hematoma*) ________

   Pain (*location, description*) ________ Discharge (*bleeding, purulent*) ________ Indicate deviations from normal and your nursing interventions ________

Describe patient's learning needs related to care of the perineum, and list your interventions (*perineal care, pad application, expected duration of lochia, healing of episiotomy, etc.*)

Comfort measures (*ice, Tucks, sitz baths, perineal lights and sprays when ordered, correct position with sitting, etc.*)

6. Hemorrhoids Comfort measures

   Assess knowledge of the importance of hygiene, proper diet, and activity

7. Further assessment for cesarean section: Abdomen (*soft, distended, rigid*) Dressing (*Dry, intact, drainage*)

   Flatus (*passing, not passing*) Bowel sounds (*present, not present*) I.V. Foley catheter Lungs (*auscultation, percussion*) Legs (*tenderness, Homan's sign*)

8. Maternal mood (*cheerful, cooperative, quiet, withdrawn, crying, anxious*) Describe behaviors that led to your assessment

   How does mother relate to infant? (*rooming-in, touching, looking, finger tipping, eye contact, unwrapping, holding close, palming, smiling, talking, calling by name*)

   If breast-feeding, describe mother's reaction to the event (*satisfying, frustrating, tiring, etc.*)

   Describe learning needs, and list specific nursing interventions that will facilitate the mother's efforts to breast-feed

   Is she in "taking-in" or "taking-hold" phase? Describe behaviors that led to this assessment

9. Assessment of infant: Sex Weight Apgar at birth Temp

   Heart rate Resp Voiding Stools (*meconium, transitional, diarrhea*) Umbilical cord (*oozing, discharge, drying*) Circumcision (*bleeding, dry, healing, discharge*) Identify deviations from normal, and list your nursing interventions

Gestational age (from physical findings) ________ Term ________ Preterm ________ Postterm ________

Identify potential problems, and list appropriate nursing interventions related to classification ________

Classification by birthweight (*small, appropriate, or large for gestational age*) ________ Identify potential problems, and list appropriate nursing interventions related to classification ________

Defects or disorders (*birth injury, anomaly, jaundice, infection, etc.*) ________ List nursing interventions and identify learning needs of the parents related to defects or disorders ________

Describe predominant state of infant when awake (*quiet alert, active alert, fussy, irritable*) ________

Consolability (*easily consoled, responsive to touch, sound of voice, sight, unresponsive*) ________

Describe bonding behaviors of the infant (*none, passive, eye-to-eye contact, curling of toes and fingers, responsive movements of arms and legs to voice and touch*) ________

Describe reactions of mother and father to specific bonding behaviors ________

10. List parents' learning needs and describe your nursing intervention in the following areas:
Infant care (*bathing, feeding, circumcision care, normal newborn characteristics, sleeping, clothing, bowel movements, need for contact and stimulation*) ________

Family planning ________

Maternal needs (*rest, relaxation, food, fluids, activity*) ________

11. Integration of infant in family unit: Describe support system (*significant others who will help at home, grandmother, mother, husband, neighbor, friend, etc.*) ________

Father (*present, not present, working hours, active as care giver, anxious, supportive, nonsupportive, relaxed, overwhelmed, growing in confidence*) ______

Give specifics leading to this assessment ______

Siblings (*ages, how prepared for infant's arrival*) ______

Describe anticipatory guidance that might be of benefit in integration process ______

12. Recommended referrals (*none, social worker, home follow-up nurse, public health nurse, regional center, crippled children's society, parents' support group, La Leche League, community mental health unit*) ______

Explain reason for referral(s) ______

Additonal observations and comments ______

Signature ______ Position ______

From Gorrie TM: A postpartum evaluation tool. *Obstet Gynecol Neonat Nurs*, 8:42, 1977. Used with permission.

GIRLS: BIRTH TO 36 MONTHS
PHYSICAL GROWTH
NCHS PERCENTILES NAME ______________ RECORD # ______

Adapted from Hamill PVV, Drizd TA, Johnson CL, Reed RB, Roche AF, Moore MM: Physical growth: National Center for Health Statistics percentiles. *Am J Clin Nutr* 32:607–629, 1979. Data from the Fels Research Institute, Wright State University School of Medicine, Yellow Springs, Ohio.

GIRLS: BIRTH TO 36 MONTHS
PHYSICAL GROWTH
NCHS PERCENTILES

NAME ______________________ RECORD # __________

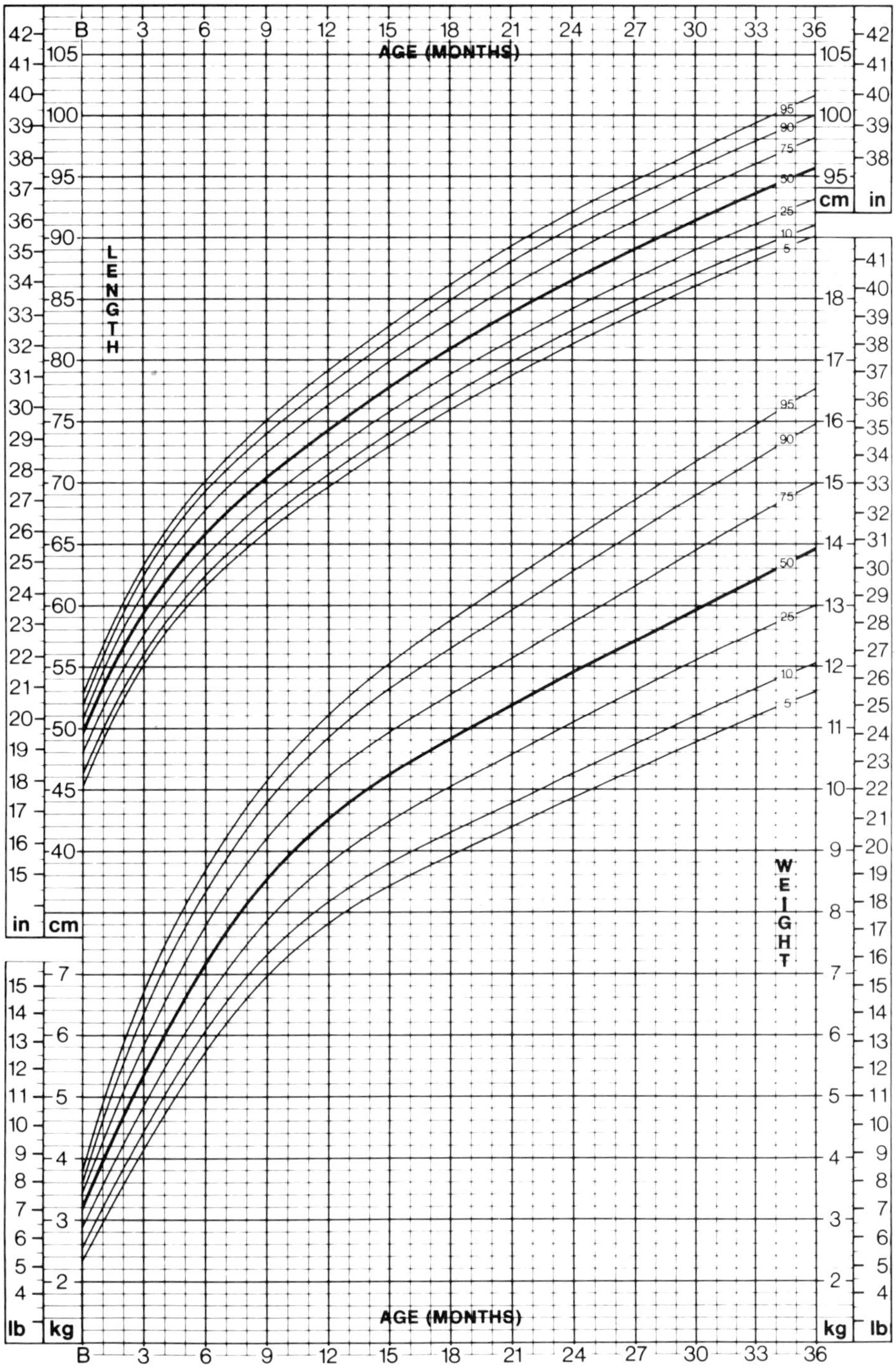

Adapted from Hamill PVV, Drizd TA, Johnson CL, Reed RB, Roche AF, Moore MM: Physical growth: National Center for Health Statistics percentiles. *Am J Clin Nutr* 32:607–629, 1979. Data from the Fels Research Institute, Wright State University School of Medicine, Yellow Springs, Ohio. © 1980 Ross Laboratories.

BOYS: BIRTH TO 36 MONTHS
PHYSICAL GROWTH
NCHS PERCENTILES NAME ________________ RECORD # ________

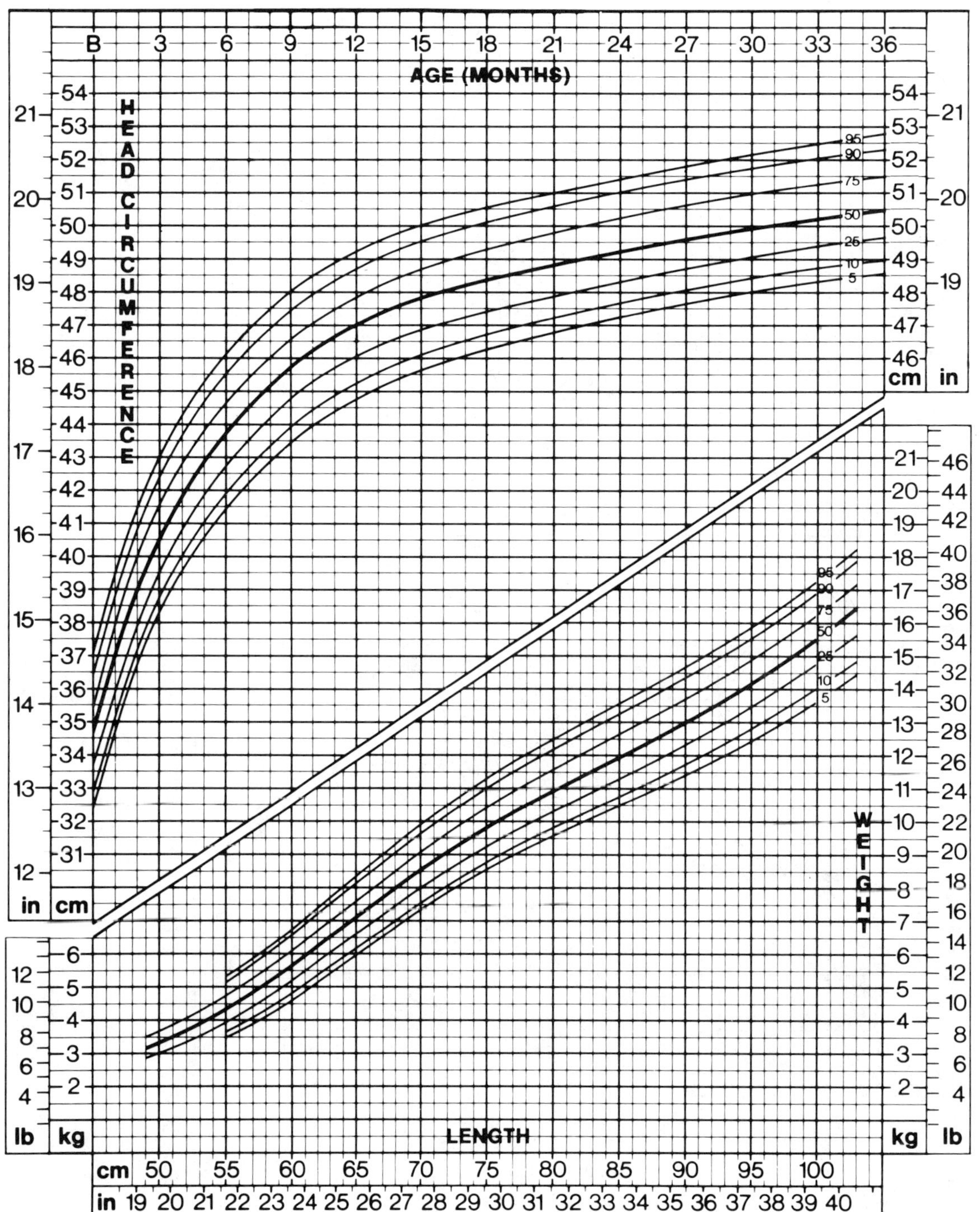

Adapted from Hamill PVV, Drizd TA, Johnson CL, Reed RB, Roche AF, Moore MM: Physical growth: National Center for Health Statistics percentiles. *Am J Clin Nutr* 32:607–629, 1979. Data from the Fels Research Institute, Wright State University School of Medicine, Yellow Springs, Ohio. © 1980 Ross Laboratories.

BOYS: BIRTH TO 36 MONTHS
PHYSICAL GROWTH
NCHS PERCENTILES

NAME ____ RECORD # ____

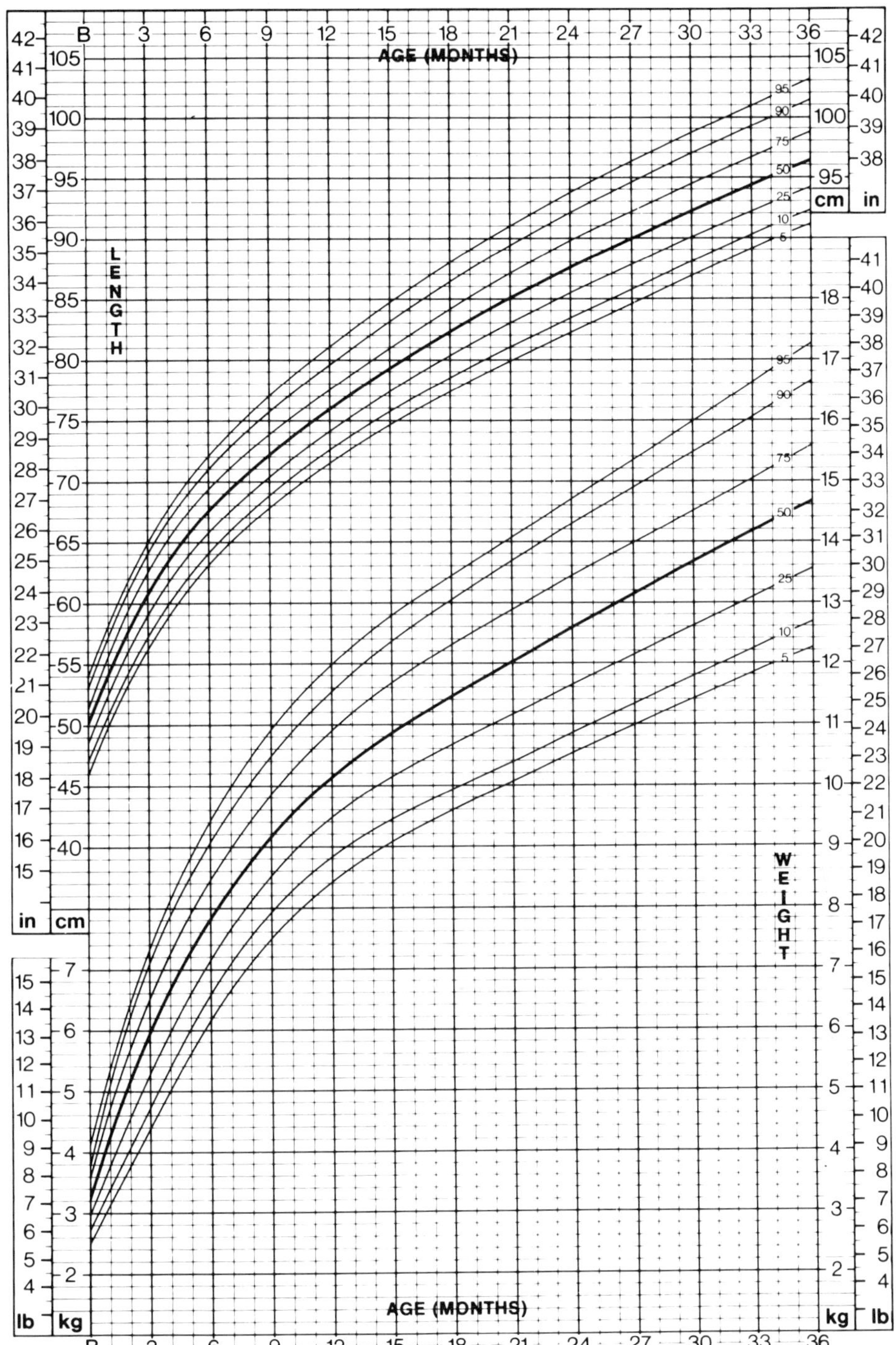

Adapted from Hamill PVV, Drizd TA, Johnson CL, Reed RB, Roche AF, Moore MM: Physical growth: National Center for Health Statistics percentiles. *Am J Clin Nutr* 32:607–629, 1979. Data from the Fels Research Institute, Wright State University School of Medicine, Yellow Springs, Ohio. © 1980 Ross Laboratories.

Patient's name:

Hospital patient number:

BILIRUBIN CHART FOR PREMATURE INFANT

Birth weight	Gestational age (weeks)	Date

Blood group: Mother______ Baby______ Coomb s test: baby______

Antibodies: Mother______ Baby______ Para:______ Gravida:______

Other OB history______

Diagnosis______

Serum Indirect Bilirubin mgm./100m (Unconjugated): 30, 25, 20, 15, 10, 5

Zone of possible exchange transfusion

INDEFINITE ZONE

Zone in which exchange transfusion not indicated on basis of bilirubin alone, though it may be indicated in other ways.

Age in days: 1, 2, 3, 4, 5

Patient's name:

Hospital patient number:

BILIRUBIN CHART FOR TERM NEWBORN INFANT

Birth weight	Gestational age (weeks)	Date

Blood group: Mother______ Baby______ Coomb's test: Baby______

Antibodies: Mother______ Baby______ Para:______ Gravida:______

Other OB history______

Diagnosis______

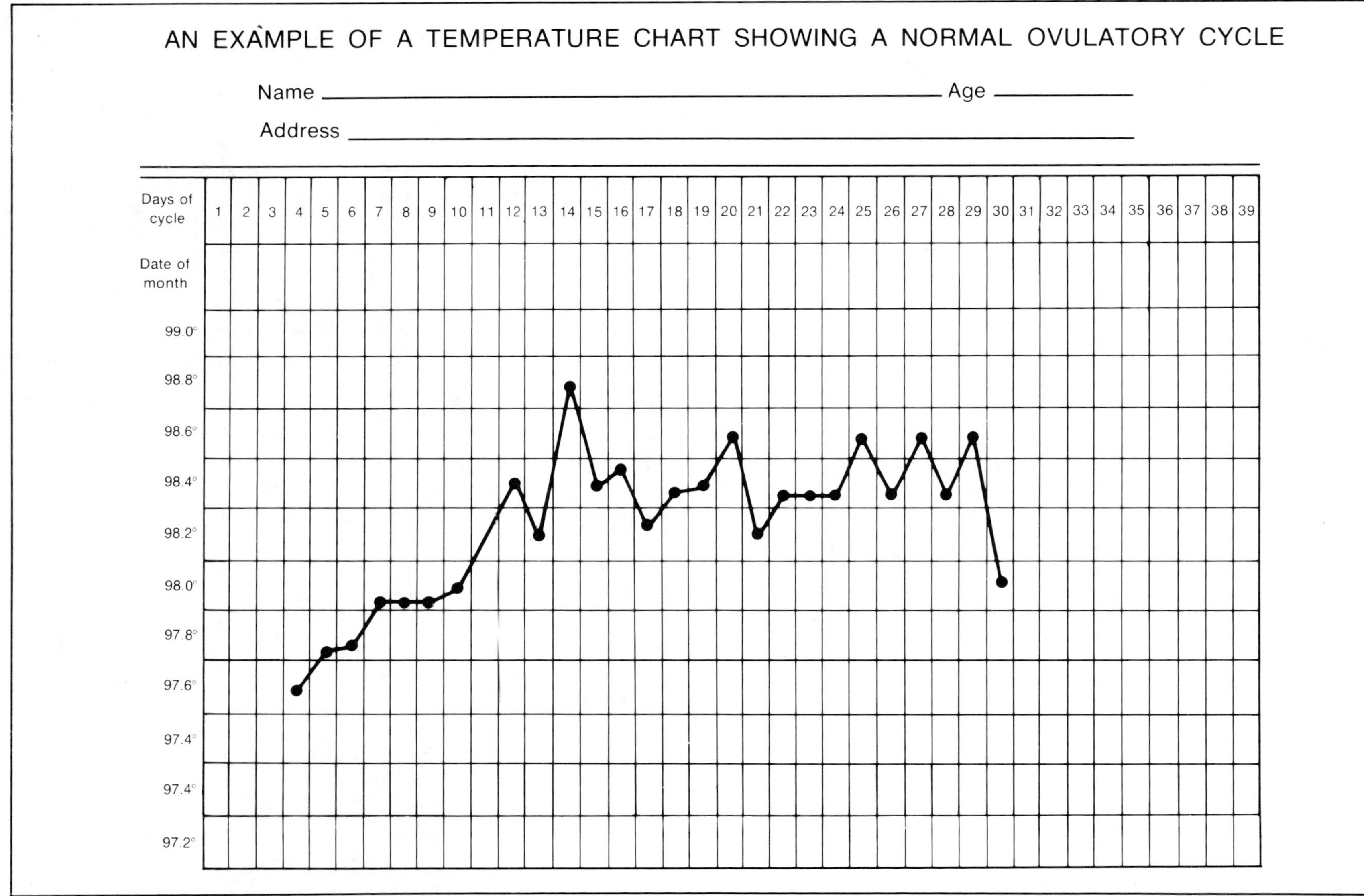

The temperature chart for basal body temperature (above and on following page) is kept for at least three menstrual cycles. Charting basal body temperature is necessary for women with infertility problems who wish to become pregnant. The information is often used to determine cycles of ovulation during an infertility workup. The charting can also be done in conjunction with a natural method of birth control. Compared with other methods of birth control, this approach does not have a very high success rate for avoiding conception.

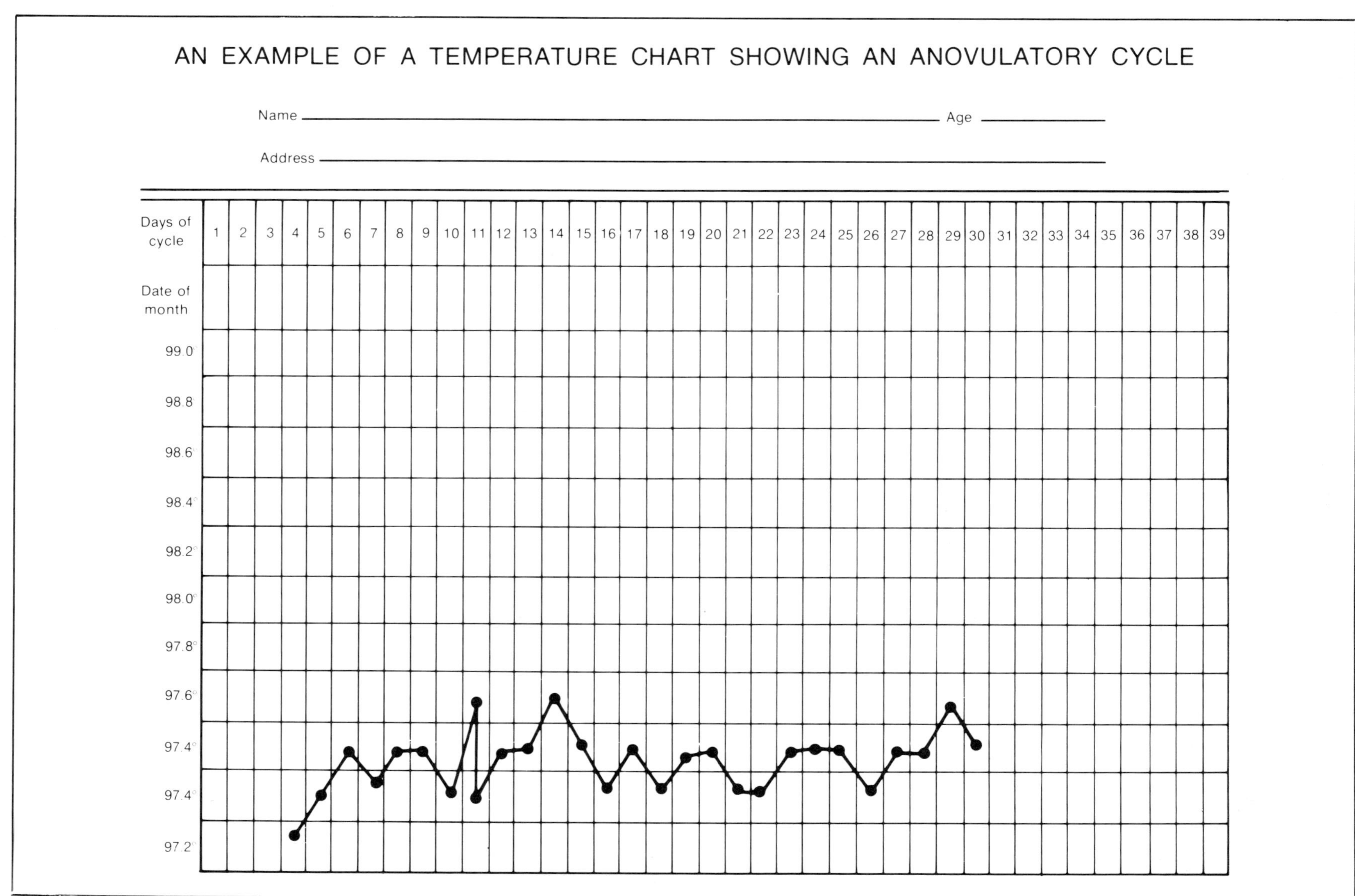

AN EXAMPLE OF A TEMPERATURE CHART SHOWING AN ANOVULATORY CYCLE
Name
Age
Address
Days of cycle
1 2 3 4 5 6 7 8 9 10 11 12 13 14 15 16 17 18 19 20 21 22 23 24 25 26 27 28 29 30 31 32 33 34 35 36 37 38 39
Date of month
99.0°
98.8°
98.6°
98.4°
98.2°
98.0°
97.8°
97.6°
97.4°
97.4°
97.2°

HEALTH HISTORY AT A GLANCE

ID: Name, address, tel. no., age, sex, race, nationality, marital status, occupation, Soc. sec. no., informant, reliability

CC: Reason seeking health care; duration

HPI: Onset date, situation, mode, precipitating events; symptom location, quality, severity, how relieved, duration, association, relation to habits; order of symptom development, recurrence, treatment effect, effect of change in situation; current symptoms, location severity; client's idea of cause and effect; reason problem of concern; reason for seeking help at present

PMH: Medical/surgical/psychiatric illnesses, hospitalization, childhood illnesses, immunizations, injuries/disabilities, allergies, current medications, transfusions

FH: Age and health status or age of death of parents, siblings, children; familial disease

P/SH: Type work, exposure to harmful agents, years schooling, military history, hobbies, finances, effect of illness; locale of family members, number of dependents, who lives in home, type housing; marital status, age and health of spouse, satisfaction with relationship, effect of illness on marriage and family; sexual education, orientation, performance, satisfaction, effect of illness, birth control; social satisfaction, group membership, religion, effect of illness; use of tobacco, alcohol, other drugs; client or family under psychiatric care, duration, name of psychiatrist, type care; ADL; diet

ROS: *General*: Overall state of health, ability to carry out ADL, wt. changes, fatigue, exercise tolerance, fever, night sweats, repeated infections

Integument: Change in skin pigmentation, texture, moisture, eruptions, rashes, pruritus, pain, unusual hair growth or loss, deformities of nails

Head, face, scalp: Headache, trauma, sinus pain, scalp itching, scalp infestations

Eyes: Visual problems, diplopia, scotomata, use of glasses, date last examination, eye pain, eye itching, lid edema, excessive tearing, tests for glaucoma, photophobia

Ears: Mastoiditis, pain, discharge, tinnitus, dizziness, vertigo, hearing problems, sensitivity to certain types of noise

Nose, mouth, throat: Smell, sinusitis, epistaxis, nasal obstruction, pain, discharge, headcolds, trauma; fit of dentures, last visit to dentist, dental problems, pain, lesions, soreness of tongue, bleeding or swelling of gums, brush teeth regularly, fluoride treatments, change in taste sense, difficulty swallowing, hoarseness

Neck: Stiffness, pain, masses

Breasts, axillae: Discharge, bleeding, masses, changes with menses, breast self-examination

Respiratory: Chest x-ray examination (date, result), wheezing, cough, hemoptysis, expectoration, dyspnea, night sweats, sneezing, rhinorrhea

Cardiovascular: Dyspnea on exertion, orthopnea, paroxysmal nocturnal dyspnea, hypertension, claudication, varicose veins, thrombophlebitis, Raynaud's phenomenon, chest pain, palpitation, tachycardia, heart murmur, peripheral edema.

Gastrointestinal: Dietary habits, appetite, food intolerance, use of antacids, indigestion, nausea, vomiting, distention, abdominal pains, abdominal masses, jaundice, hematemesis, bowel habits, use of laxatives, constipation, melana, mucus in stools, alcoholic stools, tarry stools, diarrhea, hemorrhoids, incontinence, abdominal surgery

Genitourinary (Male and female): Sexual habits, veneral disease, potency, dysuria, polyuria, hematuria, pyuria, calculi, force of stream, retention frequency, hesitancy, nocturia, incontinence, discharge. Male: prostatitis, hernia

Gynecologic: Menarche, duration, amount, interval, catamenia, menorrhagia, metrorrhagia, date last menstrual period, amenorrhea, type of contraception, infertility, dyspareunia, postcoital bleeding, vaginal discharge, pruritus, date and result of last Pap smear, vaginal or uterine surgery

Obstetric: Pregnancies, full-term deliveries, premature deliveries, abortions, living children, complications of pregnancies

Musculoskeletal: Muscle weakness, pain, aches, cramps, atrophy, back or joint stiffness, pain, deformity, dislocation, fractures, radicular pain

Neurologic: Headache, nervousness, sleep disturbance, vertigo, syncope, sensory or motor disturbance, paralysis/paresis, paresthesia/hyperesthesia/hypesthesia, memory loss, nightmares, twitching, convulsions, tremors, dysphagia, handwriting changes, loss of consciousness, disorientation

Psychiatric: Disorientation, irritability, depression, mood swings, suicidal or homicidal episodes, delusions, hallucinations, feelings of persecution, ideas of reference, paranoia, anxiety, phobias, indecision, preoccupation, obsessive rumination

Endocrine: Changes in skin color, texture, hair distribution, sexual vigor, voice, goiter, polydipsia, polyphagia, polyuria, growth change, intolerance to temperature, sugar in blood or urine, excessive sweating

Lymphatic and hematologic: Lymph node swellings, excessive bleeding, bruising, anemia, blood transfusions

Source: Berger, K., Fields, W. *Pocket Guide to Health Assessment*. Reston, Va.: Reston Publishing Company, Inc. Used with permission

GLOSSARY

abortion The expulsion of the products of conception before 20 weeks gestation or before the fetus is viable.

complete abortion All products of conception are passed and no treatment is required.

elective abortion Termination of pregnancy before fetal viability in the absence of medical indication.

habitual abortion Abortion in three or more consecutive pregnancies.

incomplete abortion Abortion in which not all of the products of conception have passed, but the os is dilated and partial evacuation has taken place.

induced abortion Caused by human interference in order to terminate a pregnancy by other than natural means.

inevitable abortion Irreversible uterine evacuation has begun, the internal cervical os is dilated, and bleeding and cramping increase until products of conception are passed.

missed abortion Fetal death in which the products of conception have not evacuated the uterus.

therapeutic abortion An abortion that is performed because of the woman's health needs.

threatened abortion Unexplained bleeding that either ceases in 1–2 days or increases and is followed by cramps and partial or complete expulsion of the products of conception.

abruptio placentae Normally implanted placenta that separates sometime between the twentieth week of gestation and birth of the infant.

abuse Improper use of one person by another resulting in physical, mental, or emotional distress or placing another at a disadvantage.

drug abuse See **drug**.

wife abuse Sociomedical problem of repeated abuse of a wife by her husband.

acini cells The milk-producing cells of the breasts.

acme The peak of intensity of a uterine contraction.

acrocentric chromosome See **chromosome, acrocentric**.

acrocyanosis Symmetric mottled cyanosis of hands and feet associated with coldness and sweating.

acrosome The head of the sperm, which contains the germ cell nucleus and its genetic material.

active transport The movement of a substance from an area of low molecular density across a membrane to an area of greater molecular density. An energy source needed to expedite movement.

adenohypophysis The anterior lobe of the pituitary gland.

adhesion State of sticking fast. Process whereby fetal cells penetrate uterine endometrium during nidation.

adnexae Structures attached to uterus, such as ligaments, oviducts, and ovaries.

adolescence Developmental bridge between childhood and maturity during which physical development is completed and biologic and psychosocial integration takes place.

adolescent pregnancy (also **teenage pregnancy**) Pregnancy that occurs during the adolescent period, usually ages 12–19.

early adolescent pregnancy Pregnancy that occurs at age 12–16 (or earlier).

late adolescent pregnancy Pregnancy that occurs at age 17–19.

affective disorders Category of psychosis in which there is a disturbance in emotional feeling tone that is usually seen at extreme depression or elation. A manic–depressive state.

after baby blues See **postpartum blues**.
afterbirth See **placenta**.
afterpains Postpartally, alternating contraction and relaxation of the uterine muscle; more severe when the mother is nursing.
allele Alternative forms of a gene found at the same locus on homologous chrosomes.
Allis's sign Used when checking for dislocated hip in the neonate and demonstrated when the neonate is supine, hips and knees are flexed, and feet are placed flat on table. Knee on dislocated side will be higher.
alopecia Loss of hair.
amniocentesis Puncture of the amniotic sac by introduction of a needle into the uterine cavity through the abdominal wall to withdraw amniotic fluid.
amniography Introduction of contrast medium (dye) into the amniotic sac followed by the taking of radiographs.
amnion The inner layer of the two layers of membranes that encase the developing fetus. Also the membrane that covers the fetal side of the placenta.
amnioscope Lighted instrument used to see amniotic fluid introduced into the cervical canal.
amnioscopy Surgical procedure for seeing the color, depth, and composition of the amniotic fluid. Introduction of an amnioscope into the cervical canal to see the characteristics of the amniotic fluid.
amniotic fluid The fluid contained within the amniotic sac that surrounds the developing fetus.
amniotic sac The sac composed of the two layers of fetal membranes that contain the fluids and the fetus during intrauterine life.
amniotomy Iatrogenic rupture of the amniotic sac. Usually abbreviated AROM (artificial rupture of membranes).
ampulla ovary Outer one-third to one-half of the oviduct.
analgesic Drug or substance that relieves pain.
anaphase The phase of mitosis in which the chromosomes leave the equatorial plate and migrate to opposite poles of the spindle thus becoming separate, single strands.
android pelvis See **pelvis, android**.
anemia Decrease in number or quality of red blood cells, that creates a deficiency.
aneuploid A chromosome number that is not an exact multiple of the haploid number.
anovulation Absence of ovulation.
anoxia Inadequate oxygen to support body's needs. Lack of oxygen.
antenatal, antepartal Occurring before birth.
anterior vaginal fornix See **vaginal fornix, anterior**.
anthropoid pelvis See **pelvis, anthropoid**.
anticipatory guidance A strategy whereby a person or persons are prepared to be knowledgable about an event or activity before its occurrence and are provided with techniques either for managing that event or activity when it does occur or for avoiding its occurrence.
antidiuretic hormone, ADH See **vasopressin**.
antrum Fluid-filled cavity in the developing ovarian follicle.
anxiety disorders A category of disorders that have as common symptoms exaggerated motor tension, autonomic hyperactivity, apprehension, and hyperattentiveness. A more recent labeling of conditions formerly called neuroses.
apposition To place side by side. The point at which the free-floating blastocyst makes contact with the uterine endometrium just before penetration of that surface.
areola A circular area surrounding the nipple of the breast that appears darker in color than the rest of the breast. Contains numerous small nodular protrusions.
artificial insemination The iatrogenic or nonsexual introduction of semen containing sperm into the female vagina to facilitate fertilization.
asphyxia Systematic oxygen deficiency and carbon dioxide accumulation, usually a result of impaired respiration.
assessment The collecting, processing, and giving of meaning to data about a person, object, or situation.
  assessment of reproductive health Assessment of a personal or family state of health with reference to the reproductive process.
  assessment of reproductive readiness Assessment of a person's physical, psychosocial, and cognitive development to determine the person's capability for completing the tasks associated with the reproductive process.
  Brazelton assessment Criteria for assessing interactional behavior of the neonate.
asymptomatic bacteriuria Urinary tract infection without symptoms.
attachment A feeling of affectionate sentiment that forms a basis for loving ties between people.
  maternal attachment Patterns of behavior that lead a child to attain or maintain closer proximity to the mother or that lead a mother to recognize and claim the child as her own.
attitude (1) A position, feeling, or mental response to a person, issue, or matter. (2) Refers to the relationship of the fetal parts to each other and is discussed in degrees of flexion.
  deflexed attitude Refers to fetal position in which the head is extended and the spine is curved. Less than complete flexion.
augmentation of labor See **labor, augmentation of**.
auscultation Listening, either with an unassisted ear or with instruments that amplify sound, to sounds produced by the body.
autolysis Self-digestion; the breakdown of the excess protein in the uterine muscle cells. Occurs after delivery.

autosome Like, paired chromosomes excluding the sex chromosomes X and Y.

ballottement Rebounding of the fetus when pushed by the examiner's fingers.

Bandl's ring See **pathologic retraction ring**.

Barr body A dark-staining chromatin mass found in the cell nucleus during interphase that represents a single, inactive, condensed X chromosome.

Bartholin's glands Two small glands that are located bilateral to the vagina. Secrete a mucoid substance that moistens the inner surface of the labia.

basal body temperature method, BBT A method of rhythm contraception. It relies on keeping a daily record of body temperature in order to identify the point of sustained temperature elevation that results from the release of progesterone produced by the corpus luteum after ovulation, thereby indicating the point in the menstrual cycle at which ovulation occurs.

basal plate of the placenta See **placenta, basal plate of**.

battered woman A woman who has been physically abused by another, usually her sexual partner, parent, or husband.

- **battered pregnant woman** A pregnant woman who has been physically abused by another, usually her sexual partner or husband.

belief Acceptance of something as fact or truth.

bicornuate uterus A uterus that has two fundal horns and usually a single septum.

bilirubin By-product of red blood cell breakdown.

- **insoluble bilirubin** (also unconjugated bilirubin) Cannot be excreted in the urine.
- **soluble bilirubin** (also conjugated bilirubin) Is water soluble and excreted in the urine.

Billing's method See **ovulation method**.

bimanual examination The palpation of a body organ or area using both hands.

- **bimanual examination of the female pelvis** Palpation of the internal reproductive organs by placing one hand (two fingers) in the vagina and the other hand on the lower abdomen and gently grasping the organ(s) between the two hands and palpating.

biostatistics (vital statistics) Category of statistics that addresses characteristics of a human population.

birth control A term coined by Maragaret Sanger in 1912 to refer to the education of the married poor about conception and contraception. Today the term is used to connote educational programs and techniques available to the consumer to control conception or electively to terminate a pregnancy during the first 3 months. See **conception control**.

birth rate Ratio of births to total population during a specified period, usually 1 year.

- **crude birth rate** Ratio of number of births per year to the total population during that same period.
- **refined birth rate** Ratio of number of births per year to a specific population such as number of births in relation to total female population.
- **true birth rate** Ratio of births per year to the female population of childbearing age.

bivalents The uniting of chromosomes to form homologous pairs during the zygotene stage of meiosis.

blastocyst Hollow sphere of cells enclosing a cavity. Formed when the fluid from the uterus enters the morula, thereby creating the cavity.

blastodermic vesicle See **blastocyst**.

blastomere One of the cells created when the fertilized ovum undergoes mitotic cellular division.

bonding The uniting or fastening of one object or person to another.

- **maternal–infant bonding** The identification of the mother with her infant and the acceptance of the infant as hers. Term used by Klaus and Kennell to denote a sensitive period immediately after giving birth when the mother is particularly attuned to bond to her infant.

Bradley method (also husband-coached childbirth) A method of preparation for childbirth that requires the pregnant woman to have her husband or partner with her as coach. It is based on the belief that childbirth should be a natural, peaceful, joyful process that can be painless if the expectant mother maintains a special diet and conditions her body for labor.

Braxton Hicks Contractions Erratic, usually painless contractions of the uterus that occur during pregnancy. These contractions are often confused with true labor, but they do not bring about cervical dilation although they may play a role in readying the cervix for labor.

Brazelton assessment See **assessment, Brazelton**.

breast The mammary, or milk producing gland, in the woman.

broad ligament Two large folds of peritoneum resembling wings that are attached bilaterally to the uterus and extend to the pelvic walls.

brown fat Unique heat source of the neonate. Fat that is located between the scapula, around the neck, and behind the sternum with deeper deposits around the kidneys and adrenals, which has a rich nerve and blood supply and generates heat that is distributed by the blood.

bulbourethral glands (also Cowper's glands) Two small brownish-yellow structures resembling peas that are located bilateral to the male urethra and below the prostate gland.

calendar method A method of rhythm contraception that assumes that ovulation occurs 14 plus or minus 2 days before the next menstrual period and takes into consideration the life of the sperm and ovum to calculate a period in which intercourse is unlikely to result in pregnancy.

caput succedaneum Localized edematous area of the scalp caused by pressure of the head against the cervix during labor.

care giver A person who provides care to another. Usually refers to the person who provides care to an infant or child: the mother, father, or a substitute.

casualty Loss resulting from personal injury associated with an accident or war.

reproductive casualty Loss resulting from personal injury, death, or damage to mother, fetus–neonate, or family associated with human reproduction.

cathexis Concentration of mental or emotional energy upon an idea or object (from psychoanalytic theory).

caudal anesthesia See **epidural anesthesia**.

centromere The narrow region of the chromosome to which the spindle attaches during cell division and at which the two chromatids of a chromosome are joined.

cephalhematoma Clearly outlined fluctuant mass caused by the extravasation of blood between a scalp bone and the periosteum; swelling does not cross suture lines.

certified nurse-midwife A professional nurse who has completed an educational program to acquire specialized knowledge and skill needed to manage the clinical course of pregnancy, labor, childbirth, and recovery and who is certified by the American College of Nurse-Midwives.

cervical canal The opening between the internal and external cervical os.

cervical cap Mechanical contraceptive device still under investigation in the United States. Appears as a small thimble-shaped rubber device that fits over the cervix and is held in place by suction. Placed over the cervix before intercourse and must remain in place at least 8 hours after intercourse.

cervix Lowermost part of the uterus; the neck of the uterus. An elongated one-third of the uterus.

cesarean birth (also **cesarean delivery**, **cesarean section**, or **C-section**) The birth of the baby via surgical incision in the mother's abdomen and uterus.

Chadwick's sign Changes in color of the mucous membrane of the vagina from a pink to a deep violet-pink because of increased vascularity of the tissues as a result of pregnancy. Apparent from about the fourth week.

chancre The primary syphilitic lesion that appears at the site of infection. It is seen as a small papule that becomes a reddish ulcer with a yellow exudate.

true (or **hard) chancre** A venereal sore that is characterized by a hard base and sides with a thin secretion that is highly contagious.

chemical method A conception control method that relies upon the introduction of spermacidal agents into the vagina before sexual intercourse.

chloasma (also **mask of pregnancy)** Dark brown discolorations of the face.

chorioamnionitis Clinical infection and inflammation of fetal membranes and amniotic fluid.

choriocarcinoma Malignant trophoblastic tumor that can follow hydatidiform mole, abortion, or normal pregnancy.

chorion The outer of two membranes that form the amniotic sac, which contains the developing fetus and amniotic fluid during intrauterine life.

chorion frondosum Chorionic microvilli that appear as a tree with branches or as a leafy fern.

chorion laeve The outer microvilli that touch the decidua capsularis that develop a smooth appearance.

chorionic gonadotropin, human (HCG) A hormone produced by the placenta during early weeks of pregnancy. Found in blood and urine of pregnant women. Helpful in early diagnosis of pregnancy.

chorionic plate The upper aspect of the developing placenta that protrudes into the uterine cavity and becomes the fetal side of placenta.

chorionic somatomammotropin, human (HCS) (also **human placental lactogen** [HPL]) Hormone produced by the placenta in pregnancy.

chromatids Two coiled threads of DNA held together by the centromere.

chromosomal aberration An abnormality in chromosome number or structure.

chromosomal banding A technique whereby chromosomes can be matched.

chromosome Rod-shaped, threadlike structure composed of DNA and protein; found within nuclei of cells. Carries genetic information. Derives from an amorphic substance, chromatin, which organizes itself into an identifiable shape that can be stained and ob served.

acrocentric chromosome Chromosome where the centromere is near one end of the chromosome.

chromosome satellites Extra pieces of chromatin attached to the arms of a chromosome, especially the acrocentric chromosome.

homologous chromosome Chromosomes that pair during meiosis and contain identical loci.

metacentric chromosome Chromosome in which the centromere is located approximately in center of the chromosome.

sex chromosome Identified as X and Y. Female has two X chromosomes; the male has XY chromosomes.

submetacentric chromosome Chromosome where the centromere is located near the center of the chromosome but closer to one end than to the other.

circumcision Surgical removal of the foreskin of the penis.
cleavage Mitotic cell division of the zygote that results in formation of daughter cells called blastomeres.
cleft lip and/or palate Incomplete fusion of the lip or palate.
client's health history See **patient's health history**.
clitoris The female homologue to the male penis.
clubfoot See **talipes equinovarus**.
coach A person who teaches, guides, and reinforces through the use of instruction and support. In preparation for childbirth, particularly PPM, it is a person who instructs and supports the woman during labor, usually the husband, partner, or some significant other. In Lamaze method it is often an outside person such as the teacher or a nurse.
coccygeus muscle Originates at the ischial spines and lesser sacrosciatic ligament and inserts on the side border of lower sacrum and upper coccyx.
coitus See **sexual intercourse**.
coitus interruptus Withdrawal of the penis from the vagina just before ejaculation takes place. Used as a conception control method.
colostrum Thin milky-yellow fluid secreted from the parous woman's breasts usually during pregnancy and just prior to lactation.
colposcope Instrument for inspecting the vagina. It contains a lighted end to enable visualization of the tissues in the vagina or lower pelvis.
colposcopy Examination using the colposcope.
colpotomy A surgical incision in the vagina, usually in the posterior vaginal fornix (cul-de-sac of Douglas) to allow for visualization of lower abdomen or pelvic organs or tissue.
combination method Use of one or more methods of conception control. Usually refers to a combination of more than one method of rhythm conception control.
commune A local self-governing community in which the members share in governing, work, and social activities.
  commune family See **family, commune**.
complete flexion Refers to the fetus with chin resting on chest, spine flexed in a smooth curve, arms folded across the chest, and hips and knees flexed.
conception Lay term for fertilization.
  conception control Use of contraceptive devices to prevent conception. In some instances use of noncontraceptive methods such as the rhythm method of birth control is considered a part of conception control.
conceptus The term often used to describe the products of conception—the embryo, fetus, fetal membranes, amniotic fluid, umbilical cord, and placenta.
condom A mechanical contraceptive device used by the male. It is made of latex rubber or processed collagenous tissue; it is placed over the penis before intercourse and is removed afterward.
condylomata accuminata (also **venereal warts**) A condition in which wartlike formations appear on the cervix, vagina, labia, perineum, or rectum of the female. Caused by a papilloma virus that is transmitted via sexual intercourse.
congenital Present at birth.
conization (also **cold-knife conization**) A surgical procedure in which a sharp pointed scalpel is used to excise a cone-shaped portion of the cervix for pathologic examination.
consanguinity Mating between persons who have one or more common ancestors.
constriction ring dystocia See **dystocia, constriction ring**.
consumer A person who uses or purchases services or goods.
  health care consumer (or client) One who uses or purchases services or goods intended to promote or maintain health or to prevent disease or disorder.
consumerism A social movement that seeks to protect the rights of the consumer, primarily in regard to fair practice laws or policies.
contraception control See **conception control**.
contraction stress test, CST See **stress test**.
Copper 7 (Cu 7) An intrauterine contraceptive device that is made of polypropylene plastic in the shape of a 7 and has a fine copper wire wrapped around the vertical arm.
copulation See **sexual intercourse**.
corona radiata Crownlike configuration of cells that surrounds the ovum.
corpora cavernosa Two cavernous, cylindric, and spongy structures found in the body of the penis.
corpus cavernosum urethrea See **corpus spongiosum**.
corpus luteum The shell of the ruptured ovarian follicle after extrusion of the mature female gamete at the time of ovulation. It appears as a small yellow structure hence its name *yellow body*.
  corpus luteum of pregnancy The corpus luteum that is maintained after fertilization to serve an endocrine function until the placenta is adequately developed to take over.
corpus spongiosum A cylindrical cavernous structure located in the body of the penis and containing the male urethra.
corpus uteri The main body of the uterus located between the insertions of the oviducts and the cervix.
cost Expenditure of something to obtain something else. Usually refers to the expenditure of money to purchase something.
  human cost The expenditure of human energy and emotion in response to stress, trauma, and loss as a result of increased threat to the well-be-

ing of the person or the family. In a reproductive sense, it is the cost associated with anticipated or real poor pregnancy outcome.

material or monetary cost The expenditure of money in associated with needs arising in association with threat to the well-being of a person or that person's family.

reproductive risk cost The expenditure of personal or public resources to meet the economic, social, and emotional demands imposed on the person, the family, and society by events arising from human reproduction.

cotyledon A vascular unit of the placenta that appears as lobes or sections.

couvade syndrome A situation in which the expectant father takes on or experiences some of the symptoms of pregnancy such as morning sickness and abdominal swelling experienced by his pregnant partner.

Cowper's glands See **bulbourethral glands**.

Crede's method of eye prophylaxis The instillation of one drop of a 2% solution of silver nitrate in each eye of the neonate immediately after birth to prevent ophthalmia neonatorum. Has been replaced in some institutions by penicillin ointment because of the irritation of the conjunctiva by silver nitrate.

Crede's method of placental extraction A technique of placental expression in which the hand is placed on the uterine fundus and the fundus is gently massaged to loosen the placenta. The placenta is then delivered through the birth canal by slight downward pressure.

crisis A self-limiting period during which the person or family experiences social or psychologic disorganization, decreased capability for coping, increased tension, and feelings of threat or helplessness. A crisis represents a disruption in the status quo of a person's life.

maturational crisis A crisis that results from or is associated with predictable life events associated with human development.

situational crisis A crisis that results from an unplanned or unexpected event that poses a threat to a person's bio-psycho-social equilibrium.

crown-to-rump-length Determination of the length of a neonate by measuring from the top of the head to the lowermost part of the buttocks. Measurement of sitting height of the neonate.

crude birth rate See **birth rate, crude**.

cryosurgery The therapeutic use of cold in a localized area to the extent that there is controlled freezing of tissue for the purpose of destroying abnormal cells.

cryptorchidism Failure of the testes to decend.

cul-de-sac A blind pouch or cavity that is closed at one end.

cul-de-sac of Douglas's (pouch of Douglas) The pouchlike area in the posterior vaginal fornix.

culture The general characteristics of a society in regard to beliefs, values, attitudes, behaviors, institutions, arts, and other human endeavors that are transmitted from generation to generation.

cunnilingus Sexual stimulation by using the tongue to lick or stimulate sensitive genital areas.

cutis marmorata Blue or purple mottling of the skin.

cystocele Protrusion of the bladder through the vaginal wall.

cytogenetics A branch of genetics primarily concerned with the study of chromosomes.

cytoplasm The ground substance of the cell.

cytotrophoblasts (also **Langhan's cells**) Round cells that are in contact with the decidua basalis. These cells help to attach the developing placenta to the uterus.

decidua The name given to the uterine endometrium during pregnancy. It is a much thicker, more vascular endometrium than that in the nonpregnant uterus and is part of the discharge called lochia that is shed after birth.

decidua basalis The maternal aspect of the placenta that lies in contact with the inner uterine wall. It is originally the endometrium upon which the blastocyst rests at the time of implantation.

decidua capsularis The layer of endometrium that covers the blastocyst as it implants.

decidual reaction (also decidualization) The response of the stroma cells of the uterine endometrium to the invasion of the blastocyst in which the cells become enlarged and pale with some destruction of endometrial cells taking place.

decrement The period during which the intensity of a uterine contraction decreases.

deflexed attitude See **attitude, deflexed**.

deletion Chromosomal aberration in which there is a loss of a part of a chromosome.

deoxyribonucleic acid (DNA) Principal genetic material that appears as two coiled polynucleotide chains intertwined to form a double helix, a spiral-shaped structure. This protein substance carries genetic information that is passed on from generation to generation.

dermatoglyphics The patterns of skin ridges on the fingers, toes, palms, and soles.

descent Begins with engagement and continues until delivery of the infant.

development (also human development) The biologic and psychosocial unfolding of the human being. The processes whereby the person advances from one stage to the next more highly organized or differentiated stage in terms of cognitive, physical, and social functional capability.

developmental task An activity associated with a particular stage of development.

deviant family style See family, deviant family lifestyle.

diaphragm A mechanical contraceptive method in which a latex rubber, dome-shaped device with a spring rim is inserted into the vagina and positioned to cover the portion of the cervix that protrudes into the vaginal vault. It is inserted before intercourse and removed several hours after.

diaphragmatic hernia Hernia that passes through the diaphragm into the thoracic cavity.

diastasis recti Vertical separation of the rectus abdominis muscles.

diffusion A mechanism for transfer of substances from one area to another within the body.

- **passive diffusion** The movement of a substance from an area of greater molecular concentration to an area of lesser molecular concentration.
- **facilitated diffusion** The assistance by a carrier to accelerate transport of substances of greater molecular weight.

dilatation (also **dilation**) Opening up of the cervix, usually expressed in centimeters.

dilatation and evacuation, D&E (also **vacuum curettage** or **suction curettage**) A surgical procedure using a flexible polyethylene cannula attached to a mechanical suction source to aspirate the contents of the pregnant uterus. Performed as an abortion technique in women who are no more than 12-weeks pregnant.

diploid Two sets of chromosomes.

diplotene Stage in meiosis in which there is a longitudinal separation of part of each bivalent chromosome. Chromatids remain joined at midsection and create an X-shaped junction.

disseminated intravascular coagulation (DIC) Secondary event encountered in obstetrics as well as many medical–surgical conditions; occurs when the factors opposing and favoring clotting become deranged.

dominant A trait expressed in people who are heterozygous for a particular gene.

drug Chemical compound or any harmless biologic substance that is administered to or used on humans or animals for the purpose of medical therapy, diagnosis, relief of pain, or improvement of any physiologic, pathologic, mental, or emotional state.

- **drug abuse** The improper use of drugs.
- **drug addiction** Periodic or chronic state of intoxication that results from repeated consumption of a drug (WHO, 1957).
- **drug dependence** Physical or psychologic state that occurs because of repeated, periodic, or continual consumption of a drug (WHO, 1963).
- **drug habituation** Repeated consumption of a drug because of a desire for the effects of the drug; not associated with urgent physical or psychologic compulsion.
- **hard drug** A drug that creates a physiologic dependence of the user on that drug.

ductus deferens (also **vas deferens**) The excretory duct found in each testicle, which connects the testicle with ejaculatory duct.

duplication A chromosomal aberration in which part of a chromosome is duplicated.

duration The length of the contraction from the beginning of the tightening of the uterus until its relaxation.

dysmenorrhea Discomfort or pain associated with menstruation.

- **primary dysmenorrhea** Pain or discomfort that is associated with menstruation, usually develops within a few years of menarche, and is not associated with any pelvic disease or pathology.
- **secondary dysmenorrhea** Pain or discomfort that is associated with menstruation, develops later in life, and can be correlated to pelvic pathology such as endometriosis, pelvic inflammatory disease, fibroids, or polyps.

dyspareunia Pain upon intercourse.

dystocia Difficult labor that can be caused by ineffective uterine contractions, abnormalities in size or position of the fetus, or alteration in the structure of the birth canal.

- **constriction ring dystocia** Tetanic annular contraction of the smooth muscle, which can occur at any level in the uterine wall.

ecchymosis Extravasation of blood into the subcutaneous tissues; discoloration of the skin. Commonly referred to as a bruise.

eccyesis Implantation of the fertilized ovum outside the uterus (oviduct, ovary, abdomen).

eclampsia Severe complication and progression of pre-eclampsia characterized by tonic and clonic convulsions, coma, hypertension, proteinuria, and oliguria occurring during pregnancy or shortly after delivery.

ectocervix The outer aspect of the cervix.

ectopic pregnancy Pregnancy resulting from implantation of the fertilized ovum at a site other than the endometrial lining of the uterine cavity.

effacement Thinning and shortening of the cervical canal, usually expressed in a percentage.

effleurage A gentle, circular massage of the abdomen using the fingertips; it may also be done on other parts of the body. Used particularly by women in labor during contractions.

ego The conscious part of the mind (psychoanalytic theory).

ejaculation Emission of semen from the male through a series of contractions that force the semen from the urethra.

ejaculatory ducts Two short tubes (2.5 cm long) that form a canal between the ductus deferens and the seminal vesicle; opening through which semen is ejected.

elective abortion See **abortion, elective**.

embryo The developing human being from the beginning of the third week postfertilization through the end of the seventh week of intrauterine life.

stage of the embryo Period of intrauterine human development from the third week after fertilization through the seventh week.

embryoblasts Inner cell mass of the blastocyst composed of basophilic embryonic cells somewhat larger than cytotrophoblasts; the cells that become the embryo.

empty nest syndrome Term assigned to feelings of isolation and aloneness experienced by parents, particularly the mother, when children leave home.

endocervix The inner aspect of the cervix.

endometrial aspiration See **menstrual extraction**.

endometrial cycle See **uterine cycle**.

endometriosis A disease process in which the endometrial cells of the uterus implant on other pelvic organs.

endometrium Vascular inner layer of the uterus that is shed periodically as menstruation.

engagement Term used to describe descent of the fetal head to the mid-level of the maternal pelvis. Occurs after the fetal biparietal diameter (widest transverse diameter) has passed the plane of the maternal pelvic inlet.

enterocele A herniation of the intestine.

vaginal enterocele Herniation of the intestine into the posterior vaginal vault.

enzyme A protein that acts as a catalyst in biologic systems.

epididymis (pl. epididymides) A narrow, oblong, coiled structure attached to the superior surface of each testicle. About 16 ft long.

epidural (also **caudal anesthesia**) Extra thecal injection of anesthesia between a lumbar interspace or caudally, providing regional anesthesia.

epigenesis The process whereby development occurs through an orderly process that begins with a structureless cell and continues with a series of sequential events with each event being derived from the one preceding it.

episiotomy Surgical incision made in the perineum to enlarge the vaginal orifice during childbirth.

epispadias Urethral opening on the dorsal surface of the penis.

Epstein's pearls Small white epithelial cysts located on either side of the midline of the hard palate. They are not pathologic.

eroticism Sexual excitement or desire.

erythema toxicum neonatorum Pink, papular rash of the newborn with vesicles, superimposed mottling.

estradiol (E_2) Usually called the primary estrogen; produced by the theca cells of the ovary.

estriol (E_3) An estrogen. Some estriol is formed in liver as a by-product of estradiol metabolism. Large quantities produced by the placenta.

estrogen Generic name for three female steroid sex hormones: estrone, estradiol, and estriol.

estrone (E_1) An estrogen. Small amounts produced by ovary; larger amounts are formed in liver as a by-product of estradiol metabolism.

ethnic Definitive characteristics of a social group such as religious beliefs, linguistic differences, and racial characteristics found within the broader culture that gives the group special distinction.

ethnicity The association with or membership in an ethnic group.

excitement (sexual) The initial phase of arousal marked by a physiologic response to sensory stimulus that produces vasoconstriction.

expected date of confinement (EDC) See **labor, expected date of**.

expressivity Variation in the expression of a particular gene.

extended family See **family, extended**.

external genitalia The male or female external reproductive organs.

external rotation (also **restitution**) Movement of the fetal head, after it is free of the birth canal, 45 degrees to the right or left of the midline to assume normal alignment with its back or shoulders.

facilitated diffusion See **diffusion, facilitated**.

fallopian tubes See **oviduct**.

false pelvis See **pelvis, false**.

family Two or more people who are united by sociocultural, blood, legal, or affectional ties.

commune family Social group in which people have joined together in order to share family responsibilities and functions such as labor, child care, obtaining material goods, and providing services. Monogamous marriage is usual and the sharing is limited to social and economic exchange.

contemporary American family An amalgam of unique people with diverse interests and goals, interacting with each other through a variety of different, often fluid, relational patterns.

deviant family life-style Family organization that is different from the traditional family organization acceptable to a society. More commonly referred to today as variant family life-style because of the negative connotation of deviant.

extended family Kinship groups outside of the immediate or nuclear family (mother, father, and their offspring). May be composed of the two families of orientation from which the parents in the nuclear family come, as well as siblings and more distant relatives such as cousins, aunts, and uncles.

family-centered nursing care Nursing care that views the client as a member of a family unit. The nursing care is planned and provided in consultation with the client and significant others.

family of orientation The family into which a person is born or a surrogate or adopted family to which the person is bound by social or affectional ties and lives until maturity.

family theory An attempt by behavioral science to explain the characteristics and functions of the family as well as its structure and organization. The most popular family theories are the structural/functional, the interactional, and the developmental, as well as subsets of these schools of thought.

heterosexual family A family unit in which there is a mother and father united by marriage or affectional ties.

homosexual family A family unit in which the adult care givers are of the same sex, are united by affection, and participate in homosexual activities. Children in this family may be adopted or belong to either partner.

migrant family A mobile family unit whose place of residence changes in association with its employment. May be a nuclear or extended family unit.

nuclear family A family unit composed of a father, mother, and their children.

reconstituted family A family unit that is formed when a woman or man with children from a previous marriage marries a man or woman who may or may not have been married before or when a woman or man with children of their own marries a man or woman who also has children. Often referred to as the "yours, mine, and ours" situation.

traditional American family A mother and father legally united by marriage and their children.

variant family life-style A family organization that differs from the traditional family model. Includes family units such as the single parent family, the migrant family, and the unmarried family.

father The man who impregnates a woman, who then gives birth to the child of that union. The role ascribed by society to the man who becomes a father either through a biologic act or adoption.

fatherhood The state of being a father.

fathering The performance of behaviors expected of a father. Usually refers to the loving of, providing for, and disciplining of a child.

fern test Used to test for ruptured membranes. If amniotic fluid is present, vaginal secretions are placed on a glass slide and allowed to dry will present a ferning pattern because of sodium chloride (NaCl) in the fluid.

fertilization The union of the sperm and ovum that restores usual chromosome number and initiates the cellular division that results in the formation of a zygote.

fetal acceleration determinations, FAD See **nonstress test**.

fetal alcohol syndrome A condition in which the fetus develops anomalies caused by the mother's consumption of alcohol. A neonatal profile in which there is intrauterine and postnatal growth retardation and cardiac, joint anomalies, and mental deficiencies.

fetal death Death of an unborn child who has reached viability (500 gm or 20-weeks gestation).

fetal death rate Number of fetal deaths per 1,000 live infants.

fetal membranes The amnion and chorion.

fetoscope Head stethoscope.

fetus The developing human being from beginning of eighth week postfertilization until birth.

fimbria Fringe. Usually refers to fingerlike projections found on the distal end of the oviduct.

fixation A concentration of psychic energy at the point of one's psychosexual development in response to over- or undergratification of needs.

fluorescent treponemal antibody-absorption test (FTA-ABS) A laboratory test used to detect syphilis. More reliable in detecting primary syphilis when exposure to the organism is less than 4 weeks, has fewer false positive tests than VDRL.

follicle stimulating hormone (FSH) One of three gonadotrophic hormones secreted by the anterior pituitary gland. FSH acts on the ovary to effect development of the ovarian follicles.

fontanelles Wider area of connective tissue, one anteriorly and one posteriorly, at the junction of the sutures of the skull.

foreskin The prepuce of the penis.

frequency In relation to uterine contractions, the time from the beginning of one contraction to the onset of the next one.

fundal dominance Characteristics of a normal labor contraction; gradient of force directed from the fundus to the least active and weakest area of the uterus—the cervix.

fundus Rounded upper part of the uterus located between and above the insertions of the oviducts and the corpus.

funis See **umbilical cord**.

gamete transport The movement of the male and female gametes from the gonads to the site of fertilization and, after fertilization, to the site of implantation.

gametogenesis The mechanism through which the male and female germ cells become mature and ready for fertilization.

gastroschisis A congenital malformation in which the abdomen remains open.

gate theory of pain control A conditioned response will close the gate in the nerve pathways thereby dulling a person's perception of pain.

gear breathing Level and technique of breathing that are used by the woman during a contraction. Comes from the PPM method of childbirth preparation.

gene A segment of the DNA molecule that directs the synthesis of a specific polypeptide chain.

genetic Related to or dependent upon genes.

genetic code A genetic blueprint containing genetic information.

genetics Science that addresses inheritance and its phenomena, as well as factors that influence the transmission of inherited traits from parent to offspring.

genotype The genetic constitution of an individual.

gonad A gland (ovary or testes) that produces gametes.

gonadotrophin releasing factors, GnRF See releasing factors.

gonorrhea A venereal, or sexually transmitted, disease caused by the Neisseria gonorrhoeae. Highly contagious and usually transmitted by sexual intercourse. Causes inflammation of the genital mucous membrane.

Goodell's sign Softening of the cervix because of increased vascularity resulting from pregnancy. Clinically evident about the second month of pregnancy. Significant in diagnosis of pregnancy.

goody bag A container of materials needed by the pregnant woman that she takes with her to the hospital. Includes a small paper bag (for breathing into to correct hyperventilation), talcum powder or lotion, lollipops, food for the coach, and numerous other things.

graafian follicle Mature ovarian follicle containing the ovum.

granulosa cells Cells that surround the oocyte.

gravid Pregnant, regardless of duration.

gross physical examination A general assessment of body shape, size, and appearance.

growth A normal physiologic process characterized by increased body size of an organism from the assimilation of nutrients that facilitate enlargement, increase, or generation of body tissue.

gumma A painful granulomatous destructive weeping lesion of the skin, bone, neurons, or cardiovascular system.

gynecoid pelvis See **pelvis, gynecoid**.

gynecologic examination Physical examination of the internal and external genitalia and breasts of a woman.

gynecologist A physician who specializes in the medical care of conditions and diseases of women.

gynecology The study of conditions and diseases of women. Also the name given to the branch of medicine that specializes in the treatment of conditions and diseases of women.

habitual abortion See **abortion, habitual**.

haploid One set of chromosomes. In man the haploid number (N) is 23.

hard drug A drug that creates a physiologic dependence on the user.

Harlequin sign Transient pink color that appears on half of the body of the neonate, the midline being the dividing point. If the infant is on the side, Harlequin sign is noticeably pinker on the dependent side.

health care consumer (or client) See **consumer (or client), health care**.

health care delivery system All institutions, organizations, and people who provide or use public or private health care services, who serve as resources or suppliers of goods to those institutions, organizations, and personnel, or who underwrite the cost of health care.

health history See **patient's (client's) health history**.

Hegar's sign Softening of the lower uterine segment; occurs about the second month of pregnancy. Significant in diagnosis of pregnancy.

hemagglutination-inhibitor test (pregnosticon R) Pregnancy test based on the presence of HCG in the woman's urine.

hemangioma An angioma made up of blood vessels.

hematocrit Volume of red blood cells per deciliter of circulating blood expressed as volume per cent.

hemoglobin Component of red blood cells consisting of globin, a protein, and hematin, an organic iron compound.

hemorrhoid (also **piles**) Vascular tumor that appears at the anus or rectum as a prolapsed or internal infected vessel from all or part of the hemorrhoidal venus plexus. Sometimes called a varicose vein of the rectum.

herpes genitalis A condition caused by the herpes simplex type II virus (HSV-2). May be transmitted by sexual intercourse, or to an infant during birth. Many primary infections are symptomatic within 3–7 days; however, these primary infections may remain subclinical or undetected. Clinically, the condition is characterized by the appearance of a vesicle or blisterlike lesion that usually ruptures and leaves a painful shallow ulcer.

herpes gestationis Vesicular or bullous skin eruptions.

heterosexual family See **family, heterosexual**.

heterozygous Possessing two different alleles at one particular locus on a pair of homologous chromosomes.

Hirshsprung's disease A congenital, often familial, disorder manifested by an inability to defecate because of absence of ganglion cells in the submucosal or myenteric plexuses in a given segment of the colon or proximal rectum.

histone Basic protein substance found in the DNA molecule.

homologous chromosomes See **chromosomes, homologous**.

homosexual family See **family, homosexual**.

homozygous Possessing two identical alleles at one particular locus on a pair of homologous chromosomes.

Huhner test (Also Sims-Huhner or Postcoital Test)
human cost See **cost, human**.
human development See **development**.
humanistic psychology School of psychologic thought that views human development as motivation that arises from an innate source and believes that growth is a basic human drive with the ultimate goal being the realization of the meaning of one's existence.
human placental lactogen, HPL See **chorionic somatomammotropin**.
husband-coached childbirth See **Bradley method**.
hyaline membrane diseases See **respiratory distress syndrome (RDS)**.
hydatidiform mole Neoplastic proliferation of the trophoblast in which terminal villi are transformed into vesicles filled with clear fluidlike material.
hydrocephalus Abnormally large head size because of accumulated spinal fluid and subsequently enlarged ventricles.
hymen A thin, sometimes tough fold of mucous membrane that partially covers the vaginal orifice. Usually obliterated with first sexual intercourse.
imperforate hymen Completely covering the vaginal opening.
hypertelorism Excessive width between two organs or parts.
hypertyalism Increased salivation.
hyperventilation Rapid breathing over a sustained period of time that is manifested by dizziness, confusion, numbness, and muscular cramps. Caused by excess oxygen intake.
hypophysis The pituitary gland.
hypospadias Urethral opening on the ventral side of the penis.
hypoxia Oxygen deficiency.
hysterosalpingography Examination by x-ray film to provide information about tubal patency of the oviducts after the instillation of a dye into the tubes via the uterus.
hysterotomy A surgical incision into the uterus. It is used as a surgical method of second trimester abortion in which the products of conception are removed via a mini-cesarean section. Sometimes performed later in pregnancy up to the sixteenth to twentieth week as an abortion technique for therapeutic purposes for the mother. May also be performed in cases of intrauterine fetal demise.
iatrogen Stimulus for increased problems for the client caused by the actions of the physician or other members of the health care team. This stimulus may be an act, a treatment, or a comment.
iatrogenic Caused by an act, treatment, or comment by a physician or other member of the health care team.
icterus See **jaundice**.
id The true unconscious in which the instinctive impulses reside (psychoanalytic theory).
IDM Infant of a diabetic mother.
iliopectineal line See **linea terminalis**.
ilium The upper flared part of the innominate bone.
imperforate hymen See **hymen, imperforate**.
implantation See **nidation**.
impotence Inability of the male to achieve or maintain an erection.
incomplete abortion See **abortion, incomplete**.
increment The period during which the intensity of a uterine contraction increases.
induced abortion See **abortion, induced**.
induction of labor See **labor, induction of**.
inevitable abortion See **abortion, inevitable**.
infant mortality See **mortality, infant**.
infant mortality rate See **mortality rate, infant**.
infertility Absence of pregnancy within a 1-year period during which there has been adequate sexual exposure and absence of use of contraceptives.
primary infertility A situation where a sexually active woman has never conceived or a sexually active man has never impregnated a woman.
secondary infertility The infertile state when there has been a previously documented pregnancy.
infundibulopelvic ligament (also **suspensory ligament)** Outer portion of the broad ligament extending from the ovarian end of the tube to the pelvic wall.
infundibulum The funnel-shaped portion of the ovary; resembles a trumpet in appearance.
innominate bones Two large bones, located on each side of the pelvis, that join in front to form the pubic arch. Each innominate bone consists of two separate bones, the ilium and the ischium, that become fused in adult life.
insoluble bilirubin See **bilirubin, insoluble**.
inspection Observation of a person, including careful visualization of the body characteristics, as well as attention to sounds and odors emanating from the body.
intensity Usually expressed as mild, moderate, or strong in relation to uterine contractions of the uterine muscle.
interkinesis A shortened version of the mitotic interphase that is found in meiosis.
internal genitalia The male or female internal reproductive organs, particularly the female uterus, fallopian tubes, and ovaries.
internal rotation Rotation of the long axis of the fetal skull from the transverse diameter, in which it enters the pelvic inlet, to the anterior–posterior diameter of the pelvic outlet.
interphase The stage between cell divisions during which DNA replication occurs.
interstitial part of oviduct See **oviduct, interstitial part of**.
intervillous space Open spaces between the microvilli that are left as the villi invade the sur-

rounding area. Maternal blood and glandular secretions, released because of the eroding action of the trophoblasts, collect in these spaces.

intrapartal (also **intrapartum**) Occurring during labor and childbirth,

intrauterine device (IUD) A mechanical contraceptive that is inserted into the uterine cavity to prevent conception.

invasion To enter or encroach upon. Proliferation of the trophoblasts more widespread and deeper into the maternal endometrium after adhesion.

in vitro fertilization The extraction of the oocyte from the uterus by laparoscopy and the manipulation of the oocytes and the sperm in the laboratory to bring about fertilization.

involution Reduction in size of the uterus after delivery.

ischial spines Bony prominence; one on each side of the ischium at about the midlevel of the true pelvis. They are the landmarks for the transverse diameter of the midplane of the true pelvis. The smallest dimension of the true pelvis.

ischium The lower part of the innominate bone.

isochromosome Chromosomal aberration in which one of the arms of a particular chromosome is duplicated because the centromere divides transversely, not longitudinally during cell division.

issue A matter of widespread public concern, dispute, or disagreement.

IUGR Intrauterine growth retardation.

jaundice (also icterus) Yellowness of the skin, mucous membranes, and secretions.

junk food Food with little or no nutritional value.

karotype A standardized display of the number, size, and shape of the chromosomes from a somatic cell.

Kegel exercises (also **pelvic tightening exercises**) An exercise in which the muscle of the pelvic floor and around the rectum are alternately contracted and relaxed in order to improve their tone.

labium majus (pl. **labia majora**) Fold of fatty tissue covered with skin and hair that extends downward on each side of the female vulva.

labium minus (pl. **labia minora**) Smaller fold of connective tissue with numerous blood vessels that surround and partially cover the vestibular area in the female.

labor Mechanism by which the products of conception are expelled from the mother's uterus and vagina.

- **augmentation of labor** Stimulation of labor that started spontaneously but did not progress satisfactorily.
- **expected date of labor EDL** (also **expected date of confinement, EDC**) The date at which birth is expected to occur; usually 9 months (or 10 lunar months) or 280 days from the first day of the last normal menstrual period.
- **first stage of labor** The beginning of labor until complete dilatation of the cervix (10 cm).
- **fourth stage of labor** The first hour after delivery.
- **induction of labor** Stimulation to start labor that has not begun spontaneously.
- **mechanism of labor** Series of changes in the attitude and position of the fetus during its trip down the birth canal.
- **premature labor** Labor that occurs after the twenty-eighth week of gestation that results in an infant weighing less than 2,500 gm.
- **primary force in labor** Involuntary uterine contractions.
- **second force in labor** Voluntary use of abdominal muscles that increases intra-abdominal pressure and aids in expulsive efforts.
- **second stage of labor** Begins with complete cervical dilatation and ends with the birth of the baby (also known as the expulsive stage).
- **third stage of labor** Time from the delivery of the infant to the delivery of the placenta and membranes.

laboratory examination Tests performed in a laboratory by a skilled laboratory technician or a physician to provide information about the health status of a person.

lactiferous duct Tubes that transport secreted milk to the nipple of the breast.

lacunae The spaces formed within the syncytial protoplasm because of the merging of smaller open spaces called vacuoles.

Lamaze method A method of preparation for childbirth that relies upon psychoprophylactic techniques to educate and condition the woman to become ready for the events of childbirth. Based on Pavlov's theory of conditioned response and developed by Fernand Lamaze in Paris.

lanugo The downlike hair that covers the fetus from about the fifth month of gestation.

laparoscope An instrument that is lighted and used for visual examination of the abdominal cavity.

laparoscopy Examination of the abdominal cavity using a laparoscope.

laparotomy A surgical incision into the abdominal cavity.

latex agglutination test (also **Gravindex and Pregnosticon slide test**) Pregnancy test based on the presence of HCG in the urine of a pregnant woman.

learning Sustained change in behavior that occurs because of conditions or stimuli. It is unrelated to instinct and cannot be explained by growth process alone.

Leopold's maneuvers Series of four systematic maneuvers of abdominal palpation by which the examiner may determine fetal presentation and position.

leptotene A stage in meiosis during which the chromosomes appear as thin threads.

let-down reflex Reflex initiated by infant's suckling triggering a nervous stimulus from the nipple to the hypothalamus, which releases oxytocin from the posterior pituitary. Oxytocin stimulates the myoepithelial cells around the mammary glands to contract, forcing milk into the ducts.

letting-go phase The last postpartal adjustment phase; described by Rubin as the mother redefining her role from the woman she was before to the mother she has become and then re-establishing relationships with those about her.

leukocytosis Increase in white blood cells.

leukopenia Decrease in white blood cells.

levator ani muscles Large muscle that originates from pelvic surface of ischial spines and interna obdurator fascia and inserts midpoint of perineum, anococcygeal area and coccyx.

Leydig's cells (also **interstitial cells)** Cells found in the interstices of seminiferous tubules, the mediastinum, and connective tissue septa of the testes. They secrete the male hormone testosterone.

lie Term used to identify the relationship between the long axis of the mother and the long axis of the fetus.

lightening Settling of the fetal head into the upper pelvis.

linea nigra Brown vertical abdominal lines from the sternum to the symphysis pubis.

linea terminalis (also **iliopectineal line)** An arbitrary landmark that denotes the upper margin of the true pelvis. Appears as on oblique ridge on the inner suface of the ilium bone and reaches on each side to the pubis. Separates the true and false pelves.

Lippes Loop Intrauterine contraceptive device that is made of flexible polyethylene plastic and shaped like an S.

Littre's glands See **urethral glands**.

LMP Last menstrual period.

lochia Postpartal uterine discharge.

- **lochia alba** Serous, thin watery uterine discharge that occurs approximately 10-days postpartum.
- **lochia ruba** Bright red uterine discharge that is pure blood and necrotic decidua.
- **lochia serosa** Pinkish uterine discharge that is serosanguinous.

lordosis Forward curvature of the lumbar spine.

loss Personal deprivation as a result of death, separation, accident, negligence, or other factors.

- **reproductive loss** Deprivation resulting from events related to human reproduction. Particularly death of mother and/or child or damage that prevents their functioning as useful members of society.

luteal phase The second phase of the endocrine activities of the menstrual cycle.

luteinization Process after ovulation whereby the theca cells of the ruptured ovarian follicle are converted into large, yellow, lipid-filled cells.

luteinizing hormone (LH) One of three gonadotrophic hormones secreted by the anterior pituitary gland. LH is necessary for final maturation of the gametes, particularly ova. It stimulates ovulation on the female. In the male LH acts on the cells of the testes to secrete testosterone. (Also interstitial cell stimulating hormone, ICSH, in the male.)

mammary glands The breasts.

mastitis Inflammation of breast tissue by pathogenic organisms.

masturbation Self-manipulation of one's genitals.

maternal attachment See **attachment, maternal**.

maternal–infant bonding See **bonding, maternal–infant**.

maternal mortality See **mortality, maternal**.

maternal mortality rate See **mortality rate, maternal**.

maternity Motherhood. Characteristics ascribed to the state of being a mother.

maternity nursing The provision of nursing care services to a woman and her family in anticipation of or during the periods of pregnancy, childbirth, recovery, and early parenthood and the provision of care to the newborn infant during the first 4 weeks of life.

maturational crisis See **crisis, maturational**.

maximal risk See **reproductive risk**.

measurement Collection of data or information that requires the assignment of a numerical value in terms of dimension, quantity, weight, or capacity.

mechanical method Contraceptive method in which mechanical devices are used to prevent conception. Included in this category are such devices as the condom, the diaphragm, the cervical cap, and the intrauterine device.

mechanism of labor See **labor, mechanism of**.

meconium First stool of the infant; greenish-black, sticky, sterile, and odorless.

median eminence of the hypothalamus Lowermost part of the hypothalamus.

meiosis A process whereby the germ cells divide thereby reducing their chromosome count, usually by half. A reduction cellular division.

menarche Onset of menstruation; first menses.

meningomyelocele Midline neural tube defect; spinal cord and meninges are herniated through a defect in the vertebrae to the outside of the spinal column.

menopause Cessation of menstruation; also used to identify the cessation of female reproductive function.

menses See **menstruation**.

menstrual cycle The female sexual cycle during which the female gamete is developed and female sex hormones are produced. Continues for 30–35 years, except when interrupted by pregnancy or disease.

menstrual extraction, ME (also **menstrual regulation, MR; menstrual induction**, or **endometrial aspiration)** A surgical procedure whereby the contents of the uterus are aspirated using a flexible polyethylene cannula attached to a suction source, usually a specially adapted 50-cc syringe. This procedure is performed on women who are 5–7 weeks past a missed menstrual period.

menstrual induction See **menstrual extraction**.

menstrual phase The period in the physiologic cycle of the menstrual cycle during which the endometrium is sloughed and vaginal bleeding occurs.

menstrual regulation See **menstrual extraction**.

menstruation (also **menses**) The periodic shedding of the uterine endometrium in the absence of pregnancy; seen clinically as passage of blood from the vagina.

mesoblasts A layer of synchymal cells beneath the cytotrophoblasts and which are separated by a thin membrane between the two sets of cells.

mesonephric duct (also **wolffian duct**) Undifferentiated embryonic structure that becomes the male vas deferens.

mesosalpinx A fold of the broad ligament.

metacentric chromosome See **chromosome, metacentric**.

metaphase The stage of cell division when the chromosomes line up on the equatorial plate and the nuclear membrane disappears.

microcephalus Small neonatal head, whose circumference is less than two standard deviations below the mean for age and sex.

microcephaly Head size is markedly smaller than normal.

microvilli The outer cells of the syncytiotrophoblasts; appear as soft bristles on the surface of a round brush or as fingerlike projections that can reach out and enter the surrounding tissue.

midwife A person who assists a pregnant woman at the time of birth.

migrant family See **family, migrant**.

milia A minute epidermal cyst. They appear as white papules mostly on the nose, chin, and cheeks.

minimal risk See **reproductive risk**.

mirror pelvic examination, MPE Client visualization of the pelvic examination. A mirror is held by the client or the nurse or a stationary mirror is adjusted for the client's view.

missed abortion See **abortion, missed**.

mitosis A mechanism of cellular division in which the parent cell with its full complement of genetic information is replicated in the daughter cell. It is a multiplication cellular division.

moderate risk See **reproductive risk**.

mongolian spot A focal bluish-gray discoloration of the skin on the lower back or aberrantly of the face of the neonate. It is present at birth and fades gradually.

moniliasis Inflammation of the female lower genital tract or mucous membranes; caused by the *Candida albicans* organism. It is usually referred to as a yeast or fungal infection. Characterized by moderate or severe vulvovaginal pruritus and burning. A thick, white, cheesy discharge adheres to the mucous membrane causing vulvovaginal erythema and edema. Also seen in the mouth of infants as a condition known as thrush.

monosomy A single representation of one of the chromosomes of a diploid set in somatic cells.

mons pubis (also **mons veneris**) In adults, the soft, rounded mound of fatty tissue that lies over the bony symphysis pubis and is covered with skin containing coarse, kinky hair.

mons veneris See **mons pubis**.

Montgomery's tubercles Sebaceous glands located in the areola of the breast.

mortality Subject to death.

- **infant mortality** Death of an infant during the first year of life.
- **maternal mortality** Death of a woman during pregnancy, childbirth, or the 6 weeks after giving birth.
- **neonatal mortality** Death of an infant during the first month of life.
- **perinatal mortality** Combined number of fetal and neonatal deaths.

mortality rate Ratio of deaths each year to the total population during that period.

- **infant mortality rate** Number of infant deaths during the first year of life per 1,000 live births.
- **maternal mortality rate** Pre-1960, the number of maternal deaths per 10,000 live births; post-1960, the number of maternal deaths per 100,000 live births.
- **neonatal mortality rate** Number of neonatal deaths per 1,000 live births.
- **perinatal mortality rate** Combined fetal and neonatal deaths per 1,000 live births.

morula Solid ball of 16 or more blastomeres that resembles a mulberry in appearance.

mosaicism Presence of two different cell lines in the same person.

mother The woman who has borne a child. The role ascribed by society to the woman who gives birth to or adopts a child.

motherhood The state of being a mother.

- **mothering** The performance of behaviors expected of a parent. Usually refers to the loving, nurturing, and caring for an infant or child.

motive An internal energy force that arises from physical or psychologic need and compels a person to behave in such a way that the need is satisfied.

Mullerian duct See **paramesonephric duct**.

multifactorial inheritance Interaction of many genes with small additive effects, along with the effects of environment.

multigravida A woman who has been pregnant more than one time. Usually defined as a woman pregnant for the third or more time.

multipara (para II,III,IV) A woman who has given birth to two or more viable children.

mutation A change in genetic material.
myometrium The muscle layer of the uterus. Contains smooth muscle cells interlaced in bundles.
Naegle's rule Method of calculating EDC.
natural childbirth Concept introduced by Grantley Dick-Read of England that posed that childbirth was a natural physiologic process not meant to be painful. He believed that pain in childbirth was because of lack of information that led to fear, then to tension and then to pain and that education of the expectant woman was a way of breaking this cycle.
navel See **umbilicus**.
necrotizing enterocolitis, NEC Neonatal disorder in which the underlying pathology appears to be mesenteric vascular insufficiency with ischemia, infarction, and subsequent necrotic changes in the mucosal and submucosal tissues.
neonatal mortality See **mortality, neonatal**.
neonatal mortality rate See **mortality rate, neonatal**.
Neonatal Perception Inventory Neonatal assessment to promote mental health of the newborn.
neonatologist Pediatrician with additional training in caring for critically ill neonates.
neurohypophysis The posterior lobe of the pituitary gland.
nevus Any lesion containing melanocytes; a birthmark.
nidation The process whereby the fertilized ovum attaches to the uterine endometrium.
Nitrazine test Used to test for ruptured membranes. Litmus paper impregnated with phenaphthazine changes color when touched by amniotic fluid.
nondisjunction The failure of two members of a chromosome pair to separate during cell division so that both pass to the same daughter cell.
nonstress test, NST (also **fetal acceleration determinations, FAD**) Evaluation of characteristics of the fetal heart beat with fetal movement and reactivity of the fetal heart rate baseline without using oxytocin.
nuclear family See **family, nuclear**.
nucleus A structure within the cell that contains the chromosomes and nucleolus.
nulligravida A woman who has never been pregnant.
nullipara (para O) A woman who has not borne a viable child.
nursing process A systematic method of problem solving that is dependent upon the collection of data and processing of information in such a way that client needs are ascertained, goals are established, and nursing activities are planned and implemented, and their effectiveness is evaluated in light of goal attainment.
obstetrician A physician who specializes in the medical care of woman during pregnancy, labor, and puerperium.
obstetric pelvis See **pelvis, true**.
obstetrics The giving of care to a woman during pregnancy, childbirth, and recovery. Also the medical branch that specializes in the care of women during pregnancy, labor, and the puerperium.
oligospermia Scant sperm count.
omphalocele Contents of the abdomen are outside the abdominal wall.
oocyte Female gamete in early stage of development.
oogenesis Maturation of the female germ cell.
oogonia Primitive female germ cells.
oophorectomy Surgical removal of the ovaries.
operant conditioning A theory of conditioned response that relies upon the idea that repeated behavior is associated with reward or punishment. Reward leads to repetition of the behavior; punishment leads to avoidance of the behavior.
ophthalmia neonatorum A condition in which the neonate's eyes become infected usually by gonococci or other organisms during birth. If untreated, results in blindness.
opisthotonus A tetanic spasm in which the head and heels are drawn backward with the back becoming bowed.
oral contraceptive pill (OCP) Any of numerous oral contraceptive preparations.
organismic psychology A school of psychologic thought that sees human behavior and response as a reaction of the total organism to the total stimulus. Holism is a major concept in this school of thought.
orgasm The peak or culmination of the sexual act.
Ortolani's sign Hip click noted when checking for dislocated hip in the neonate.
ovarian cortex The thicker, outer layer of the ovary.
ovarian cycle (also **endocrine cycle**) The endocrine activities of the menstrual cycle. Consists of the follicular or preovulatory phase and the luteal or postovulatory phase.
ovarian medulla Central part of ovary composed of loose connective tissue, arteries, and veins.
ovary The female gonad.
oviduct (also **fallopian tube**) Bilateral tubular structures that are attached to the uterine corpus at one end and approach the ovary at the other end. The passageway through which the ovum is transported after ovulation. The usual meeting site of the sperm and ovum at fertilization.
  interstitial part of oviduct Portion of the oviduct that passes through the uterine muscle and opens into the uterine cavity.
  oviduct isthmus Part of the oviduct that is located between the ampulla and the uterus.
ovulation The extrusion of the ovum from the graafian follicle and ovary.
  ovulation method (also **Billing's method**) A method of rhythm contraception that relies upon characteristics of the cervical mucus and the

changes that occur during the menstrual cycle in response to the presence of estrogen in progesterone to determine the time of ovulation.

ovum The mature female gamete.

ovum transport After ovulation, the process whereby the ovum is tranported from the surface of the ovary to a site in the fallopian tube where fertilization occurs. It is then the transport of the fertilized ovum from the tube to the uterus where it will implant.

oxytocin One of two hormones that is secreted by the posterior pituitary gland. Acts on the uterine muscle and breast tissue causing them to contract.

oxytocin challenge test, OCT See **stress test**.

pachytene The stage in meiosis in which the chromosomes thicken, are more visible, and can be stained.

pallor Paleness, especially of the skin and mucous membranes.

palpation The examination of an organ or body area through the use of touch.

Papanicolaou smear (Pap smear) A microscopic examination of tissue scrappings from the cervix to determine the presence of cervical carcinoma.

para Past pregnancies that continued to viability.

paracervical block Regional injection of anesthesia into the para cervical space.

paramesonephric duct (also **mullerian duct**) An undifferentiated embryonic structure that develops into the female vagina, uterus, and fallopian tubes.

paraurethral ducts (also **Skene's glands**) Two small ducts that are located near the female urinary meatus.

parent A person who produces offspring. One who is a mother or father biologically or legally through adoption. The role of parent.

parenting The performance of behaviors expected of a parent, usually care giving and nurturing activities directed toward the infant and/or child.

pars intermedia The structure that separates the anterior and posterior lobes of the pituitary gland.

parturient A woman in labor.

patient's health history (also **client's health history**) A written record of data concerning the health of a person. It usually includes personal identification information, chief complaint or reason for seeking care, history of present illness, past medical history, family history, personal and social histories, and a review of the body systems.

passive diffusion See **diffusion, passive**.

pathologic retraction ring (also **Bandl's ring**) Restrictions occurring at the junction of the upper and lower uterine segment.

Pedersen's PBSP (prognostically bad signs in pregnancy) Classification of pregnant diabetics based on factors that become evident during pregnancy.

peer group A group of people similar to self. People who are equal in age, rank, ability, or interest.

pelvic brim (also **illiopectineal line**) (See **linea terminalis**.

pelvic diaphragm Muscular structure that serves to support the female internal genitalia. Usually described as resembling a sling.

pelvic inflammatory disease, PID Inflammation of the female upper reproductive tract and pelvis; usually has symptoms of lower abdominal pain or tenderness upon examination.

pelvic inlet See **plane of the pelvic inlet**.

pelvic outlet See **plane of the pelvic outlet**.

pelvic plane Levels or dimensions of the pelvis that can be determined by joining two points by a straight line.

pelvic tightening exercise See **Kegel exercise**.

pelvic tilt An exercise designed to help improve posture, particularly during pregnancy. It relies upon proper positioning of the pelvis so that the spinal column is in proper alignment.

pelvis Bony structure that resembles a funnel or basin and is composed of two innominate bones on either side that meet to form the pubic arch in front and the sacrum and coccyx in back. It is located at the posterior extremity of the trunk of the body.

android pelvis Female pelvis in which the inlet resembles that of a male pelvis. The inlet appears as heart-shaped when viewed from the top since the sacral promontory is prominent and its overall dimensions are less than other pelves.

anthropoid pelvis Female pelvis in which the inlet appears as an anterior–posterior oval when viewed from the top. AP diameter is usually greater than its transverse diameter.

false pelvis The upper flared part of the female pelvis.

gynecoid pelvis Female pelvis in which the inlet appears round when viewed from the top. It is considered to be the usual shape of a normal female pelvic inlet. Its AP diameter measures slightly less than its transverse diameter.

obstetric pelvis See **true pelvis**.

platypelloid pelvis Female pelvis in which the inlet appears as an elongated oval when viewed from the top. Its transverse diameters are significantly greater than its AP diameters.

true pelvis The lower cylindric part of the female pelvis. The bony part of the birth canal.

penis An elongated erectile organ in males that is suspended from the muscles of the pelvic floor. It consists of three parts and hangs in front of the scrotum.

body of the penis An elongated structure containing three cylindric parts.

glans penis The tip of the penis.

root of the penis Proximal part that is attached to the pelvis.

percussion The exploration of the body organs or areas by tapping in order to determine, through listening with the ear or instruments, their size and condition.

perimetrium The serosal or outer layer of the uterus made up of connective tissue covered with serosal cells.

perinatal mortality See **mortality, perinatal**.

perinatal mortality rate See **mortality rate, perinatal**.

perineal body Base of the pelvis at which three muscles converge (the bulbocavernous, the superficial transverse perineal, and the external anal sphincter). Often traumatized during childbirth.

peritoneum Serous membrane that lines the abdominal walls. Covers the anterior and posterior aspects of the uterus but is not a part of its structure.

petechia Minute, rounded spots of hemorrhage on a surface such as skin or mucous membrane or on a cross-sectional surface of an organ.

phenotype The appearance (physical, biochemical, and physiologic) of a person.

phimosis A condition in which the foreskin of the penis covers the glans penis occluding the urinary meatus or the foreskin is tight and unable to be retracted.

physical examination Examination of the body using techniques that rely upon sensory and psychomotor skills, as well as upon the use of technologic modalities.

regional physical examination Examination of an area or region of the body such as the breasts, abdomen, or pelvis.

physiologic anemia of pregnancy (also **pseudoanemia)** Increased plasma volume that occurs normally in pregnancy and results in decreased hematocrit and hemoglobin values.

physiologic cycle See **uterine cycle**.

pica Desire for strange foods or substances not generally considered edible.

piles See **hemorrhoid**.

pill, oral contraceptive See **oral contraceptive pill**.

pinocytosis A transport mechanism used for large substances such as lipoproteins or phospholipids that are swallowed up or engulfed by the cellular spaces within the cytoplasm.

placenta (also **afterbirth)** A round, somewhat flat-appearing vascular endocrine organ that provides for maternal–fetal exchange of substances such as nutrients and gases, as well as for elimination of waste products from the fetus. It also produces hormones during pregnancy.

abruptio placentae See **abruptio placentae**.

basal layer of the placenta See **stroma**.

basal plate of the placenta The lowermost part of the placenta that is in contact with the uterine endometrium.

placenta previa Abnormal implantation of the fertilized ovum resulting in low implantation of the placenta near the internal cervical os.

placentation The attachment of the blastocyst to the uterine endometrium and the development of the placenta.

plane of the midpelvis The anterior–posterior, transverse, and posterior sagittal linear diameters that reveal the dimensions of the middle portion of the true pelvis.

plane of the pelvic inlet The anterior–posterior, transverse, and oblique linear diameters that reveal the dimensions of the entrance to the true pelvis.

plane of the pelvic outlet The anterior–posterior, transverse , and posterior sagittal linear diameters that reveal the dimensions of the lowermost part of the true pelvis.

plateau (sexual) A period during sexual activity in which sexual stimulation is sustained and in which vasocongestion reaches its peak.

platypelloid pelvis See **pelvis, platypelloid**.

pleiotropy Multiple effects of a gene.

pneumothorax The presence of air or gas in a pleural cavity from trauma or disease.

polydactyly Extra digits (toes or fingers).

polypeptide A chain of three or more amino acids.

polyploid Any multiple of the haploid number of chromosomes (3N, 4N, etc.).

position Relationship of the exact fetal part to a fixed area of the maternal pelvis (e.g., LOA, ROA).

postcoital test See **Sims–Huhner test** or **Huhner test**.

posterior vaginal fornix See **vaginal fornix, posterior**.

postpartal (also **postpartum)** Occurring after birth usually within the first 6 weeks.

postpartum See **postpartal**.

postpartal blues (also **after baby blues)** A temporary period after childbirth that is characterized by periods of crying and depression alternating with joy and happiness. A feeling of depression and helplessness.

pot Street name for marijuana.

pouch of Douglas See **cul-de-sac**.

pre-eclampsia Clinical syndrome of unknown etiology occurring after the twentieth week of gestation; characterized by hypertension, edema, and/or proteinuria.

pregnanediol A metabolite of progesterone.

preimplantation period The period beginning with fertilization of the ovum by the sperm and ending with nidation or implantation of the blastocyst in the uterine endometrium.

premature labor See **labor, premature**.

prep (also **preparation)** Used to refer to surgical preparation of the vulva and perineum for delivery. Frequently used to refer to preparation of any part of the anatomy for surgery.

wet prep A laboratory procedure in which a specimen is treated with a preparatory solution and examined under the microscope.

preparation for childbirth, PCB An organized educational program whereby expectant parents are prepared for the events associated with pregnancy and childbirth. Some programs also include content relating to early parenting.

prepuce The fold of skin that covers the glans penis.

preputial glands (also **Tyson's glands)** Small glands that are scattered over the prepuce of the penis. Similar to sebaceous glands of the skin.

presenting part (also **presentation)** That part of the fetus which comes out of the birth canal first.

preventive role supplementation An approach designed by Swendsen and others to help the first-time parents to master the tasks of parenting; includes information about parenthood and child development, group discussions with other expectant parents and a nurse, role modeling situations, and role rehearsal.

primary dysmenorrhea See **dysmenorrhea, primary**.

primary follicle (also **primordial follicle)** Primitive female gamete.

primary force in labor See **labor, primary force in**.

primary sexual development Maturation of the male and female reproductive organs.

primigravida A woman pregnant for the first time.

primipara (para I) A woman who has given birth to one viable child.

primordial follicle See **primary follicle**.

Progestacert A hormone-releasing intrauterine contraceptive device that is made of ethylene/vinyl acetate copolymer (EVA) and has a drug reservoir in the vertical shaft that contains progesterone.

progesterone Ovarian and placental female steroid sex hormone. Principal site of production is the corpus luteum. During pregnancy it is produced in large amounts by the placenta.

prolactin One of three gonadotrophic hormones secreted by the anterior pituitary gland. Prolactin is similar to the growth hormone. Is necessary to prepare the female breasts for lactation.

pronuclei, female The smaller (or reduced) nucleus of the ovum that merges with the male pronucleus at the time of fertilization.

pronuclei, male The nuclear material that is found in the head of the sperm and unites with the female pronucleus during fertilization.

prophase The first stage in mitosis and meiosis when the chromosomes are contracted and thus thicker.

prostaglandins A derivative of long-chain polyunsaturated fatty acids found in seminal fluid and other areas of the body.

prostate gland A male musculoglandular organ located below the bladder that encloses the urethra.

pseudoanemia See **physiologic anemia of pregnancy**.

psychoanalytic theory A school of psychologic thought begun by Freud that views the conscious mind as only one part of the total mental process; below or underlying this consciousness are the essential ideas, feelings, urges, perceptions, and passions that direct or control human behavior and thought.

psychoprophylactic method of preparation for childbirth, PPM Method of preparation for childbirth standardized by the American Society for Prophylaxis in Childbirth (ASPO). Relies upon extensive education and training in techniques designed to increase labor-coping skills. A combination method that draws much of its substance from the work of Lamaze, Bing, and others.

psychosocial readiness Person's ability to make sensible judgments concerning events in life. Relies upon the maturing of mental processes within a social context that enables the person to establish and maintain affectional relationships, acquire a sexual identity, and develop the ability to function as a useful member of society.

psychotic disorders A category of disorders in which a person's mental capacity to recognize reality and to communicate and relate to others is impaired, thus interfering with that person's ability to deal with activities and demands of daily living.

puberty The period during which physiologic changes occur that promote functional capability of the sexual and reproductive systems. Secondary sex characteristics appear.

pudendal block Regional injection of an anesthetic beneath the inferior median border of the ischial tuberosity, which anesthetizes the pudendal nerves.

puerperal infection Infection of the genital tract associated with childbearing and usually occurring within the first 10 days postpartum.

puerperium Period from the end of the third stage of labor until the time at which the pelvic organs have returned to normal, about 6 weeks postpartum.

pulse pressure The systolic blood pressure minus the diastolic blood pressure.

pyelonephritis Upper urinary tract infection occurring late in the second or early in the third trimester of pregnancy.

quickening The movement of the fetus as perceived by the mother, usually occurring between 16–20-weeks gestation.

radioimmunoassay, RIA Pregnancy test.

recessive A trait that is expressed in people who are homozygous for a particular gene.

reconstituted family See **family, reconstituted**.

rectocele Herniation of a part of the rectum into the vagina.

rectovaginal examination Examination of the vagina and rectum through observation and palpation.

refined birth rate See **birth rate, refined**.

reflex An involuntary responsive action.

regional physical examination See **physical examination, regional**.

releasing factors (also **gonadotrophin releasing factors, GnRF)** Neurosecretory cells, located in the hypothalamus, that synthesize and secrete hormones that stimulate or inhibit anterior pituitary endocrine activity.

reproductive health The achievement of a state of physical and emotional well-being in association with events related to or deriving from human reproduction. The satisfactory completion of pregnancy, childbirth, and recovery in such a way that the woman and her family experience a sense of well-being and produce a child that has the basic potential for developing into a healthy adult.

reproductive health, assessment of See **assessment of reproductive health**.

reproductive readiness The physical and psychosocial capability of people and families to cope with the demands and to complete the tasks associated with pregnancy, childbirth, and parenthood.

reproductive readiness, assessment of See **assessment of reproductive readiness**.

reproductive risk (also see **cost, casualty, loss)** The imposition of a threat of such magnitude that the expectant family, specifically the pregnant woman and fetus, is placed in jeopardy of damage or death.

maximal reproductive risk Situation in which the numbers and intensity of the threat(s) places the pregnant woman and/or fetus–neonate at grave risk of severe damage or death during pregnancy, labor, recovery, or the neonatal period. Increases the likelihood of the family unit becoming debilitated because of the physical, emotional, and economic stresses placed on it.

minimal reproductive risk Increased vulnerability of the pregnant family to the usual risks associated with pregnancy; often requires short-term medical management; a good prognosis for all concerned.

moderate reproductive risk Situation in which the usual risks associated with pregnancy are aggravated because of pre-existing conditions or problems that arise from the pregnancy.

resolution (sexual) The phase in sexual activity after orgasm in which the body returns physiologically to the unaroused state.

respiratory distress syndrome, RDS (also **hyaline membrane disease)** Lung disease characterized by inability of the aveoli to remain inflated because of diminished amount of surfactant. Primarily a disease of prematures.

restitution See **external rotation**.

retraction Drawing back of the cervix.

rhythm method Methods of conception control that rely upon identification of a woman's safe period when she is not ovulating and her unsafe period when she is capable of becoming pregnant in order to direct the couple in planning sexual activity. Includes the calendar, temperature, ovulation, and combination methods.

ribonucleic acid, RNA Found mainly in the nucleolus and ribosomes. Serves as a messenger for the transfer of genetic information from the nucleus to the ribosomes in the cytoplasm, as a template for the synthesis of polypeptides, and as a transfer agent for amino acids. Similar in composition to DNA.

ribosomes RNA-rich structures in the cytoplasm where protein synthesis takes place.

right A reasonable, personal or collective demand of people for something they believe is theirs or is accorded them by justice, law, or morality.

role A pattern of behavior that is socially assigned to or adopted by a person.

role blurring See **role confusion**.

role confusion A situation in which the role to be assumed by the person or persons is not clear or is merged indistinctly with another role.

role overload A situation in which a person or persons is expected to take many roles. In role overload the person often becomes frustrated and may opt out of any clearly defined role.

role reversal A situation in which a man and woman exchange roles within the family; the woman assumes the role of wage earner, while the man takes on the tasks associated with homemaker.

rooming-in A concept introduced in 1943 by Gesell and Ilg to promote mother–infant relationships by keeping mother and infant together after birth. Literally, keeping the infant in the mother's room instead of in a separate nursery.

rotation, external See **external rotation**.

rotation, internal See **internal rotation**.

round ligaments Bilateral ligaments located on each side of the uterus just below the insertion of the oviduct. Terminates in the upper portion of the labia majora. Sometimes compared with guy wires that serve to hold or stabilize the uterus.

rubella screen (also **hemagglutination inhibitor, HAI)** To determine if a person is immune to rubella. A titer greater than 1:8 (or 1:10) assures immunity.

Rubin's test A test to determine the patency of the oviducts. Carbon dioxide under pressure is introduced into the uterine cavity to inflate the tubes.

rugae Corregated folds of tissue found in the vagina that provide for its distensibility.

saddle block See **spinal anesthesia**.

scrotal sac See **scrotum**.

scrotum (also **scrotal sac)** Two-chambered external pouch that contains the male gonads.

secondary force in labor See **labor, secondary force in**.

secondary infertility See **infertility, secondary**.

secondary sexual development The development of physical changes, other than those in the reproductive organs, that are associated with characteristics of maleness and femaleness such as body size, hair distribution, breast size, and strength.

secondary villi Expanded primary villi that form columns of trophoblastic cells that anchor the developing placenta to the uterine wall.

second stage of labor See **labor, second stage of**.

secretory phase Phase of the physiologic cycle of the menstrual cycle. Begins with ovulation and ends with menstruation.

secundigravida A woman pregnant for the second time. Used interchangeably with multigravida.

self-actualization The achievement of your ultimate developmental potential.

self-esteem A feeling or attitude of self-worth or respect for self.

self-examination Examination of the breast or genitalia by the woman herself.

semen Thick, whitish fluid containing sperm, nutrients, glandular secretions, and some epithelial cells.

seminal vesicle A membranous pouch of the ductus deferens containing a coiled tube that has several irregular diverticula. They secrete seminal fluid.

seminiferous tubules Coiled tubes about 2–3 ft long found in the wedge-shaped lobes of the testes. Lined with germinal epithelium and spermatogenic cells.

septa Partial partitions between the vascular units of the placenta that arise from the basal plate of the placenta and reach, but do not touch, the chorionic plate.

Sertoli cells Elongated cells found in the tubules of the testes. Believed to help nourish the developing male gamete.

sex chromosomes See **chromosome, sex**.

sexual About or pertaining to sex.

sexual identification The recognition by others of a person's sex gender (role) and personal identification of self as either male or female in regard to own concept of ideal.

sexual intercourse (also **coitus, copulation**) Sexual union between members of the opposite sex. Penetration of the female vagina by the male penis.

sexuality Characterization and identification by sex.

sexually transmitted disease See **venereal disease**.

Sheehan's syndrome Pituitary necrosis occurring postdelivery.

show Pinkish mucous discharge from the cervix; increases during labor and may contain a small amount of bright red blood as cervix nears complete dilatation.

Sims–Huhner test (also **Huhner test** or **postcoital test**) A test to determine fertility in which there is examination of the cervical mucus in the woman and the semen in the male after intercourse to determine the number, motility, and viability of the sperm.

single parent A parent who is without a partner. A mother or a father who is rearing her or his child alone.

situational crisis See **crisis, situational**.

Skene's glands See **paraurethral ducts**.

smegma White cheesy substance frequently seen around the glans penis.

social psychology A school of psychologic thought that views a person as a part of a social system that influences what that person becomes. The person, in turn, affects the composition and function of the group.

soluble bilirubin See **bilirubin, soluble**.

speculum A metal or plastic instrument that is used to visualize the vaginal walls and cervix.

speed Street name for drugs such as the amphetamines that have a stimulatory effect on the body.

sperm Commonly used for spermatozoon or spermatozoa.

spermatocytes Immature spermatozoa.

spermatogenesis (also **gametogenesis**) The process of male gamete formation and maturation.

spermatogenic cells Cells that produce sperm.

spermatogonia Undifferentiated male germ cells.

spermatozoon (pl. spermatozoa) The male gamete.

spermicide A chemical preparation that is capable of destroying sperm; used in jellies and creams as a contraceptive agent.

spermiogenesis The stage in spermatogenesis when the spermatids retain their attachment to the Sertoli cells in the seminiferous tubules and change from their epitheloid appearance to the appearance of a mature spermatozoa comprised of a large ovoid head, neck, body, and tail.

sperm transport The movement of the sperm through the structures of the testes to the ejaculatory duct where they are released at the time of ejaculation. Also the movement of this sperm from the site of deposition in the female genital tract to the site of fertilization.

spinal anesthesia (**saddle block**) Intrathecal injection of an anesthetic to provide regional anesthesia.

spinnbarkheit Test for ovulation where the estrogen-primed cervical mucous appears as clear, slippery, and stretchable. It is similar in appearance and consistency to raw egg white.

squamocolumnar junction (also **squamoepithial columnar junction**) The point at which the columnar epithelium and the squamous epithelium of the cervix interface.

stage of the embryo See **embryo, stage of the**.

stage of the zygote See **zygote, stage of the**.

station Position of fetal presenting part to the maternal midpelvis. Expressed in centimeters above (minus) and below (plus) the level of the ischial spines, station O.

sterility The absolute proven state that a woman is unable to become pregnant or that a man is unable to impregnate a woman.

sterilization A surgical procedure whereby the male or female is rendered sterile.

stillbirth Fetus is born dead.

stillborn Dead at the time of birth.

strabismus Inability of the visual axis of the eye to focus simultaneously. Sometimes called "cross eyes."

stress test (also **oxytocin challenge test, OCT,** and **contraction stress test, CST**) The use of oxytocin to stimulate uterine contractions in a woman at or near term pregnancy in order to evaluate the respiratory function of the placenta and the fetal response to stress.

striae albicantes Silvery and shining striae from former pregnancies.

striae gravidarum Reddish brown streaks on abdomen, thighs, and breasts, sometimes referred to as "stretch marks." Seen during pregnancy.

stroma (also **basal layer of placenta**) Tissue that forms the basis for an organ.

suction curettage See **dilatation and evacuation**.

superego The conscious monitor of the ego (psychoanalytic theory).

supine hypotensive syndrome Pressure of the gravid uterus against the spinal column when the woman is supine, which results in symptoms of faintness, anxiety, and hypotension.

surfactant A lipoprotein film produced by the aveolar epithelium that decreases surface tension of the avioli.

suspensory ligament See **infundibulopelvic ligament**.

sutures Bands of connective tissue between the bones.

syncytial Referring to the production of a multinucleate mass of protoplasm that is created by the merging of cells.

syncytiotrophoblast (also **syntrophoblast** and **syncytium**) The outer syncytial layer (protoplasm) of the trophoblastic cells.

syncytium See **syncytiotrophoblast**.

syndactyly Fusion of digits (toes and fingers).

syndrome The complex of signs and symptoms that occur together in any particular disorder.

syntrophoblast See **syncytiotrophoblast**.

syphilis A venereal (or sexually transmitted) disease caused by the *Treponema pallidum* organism. Highly contagious and usually transmitted by direct contact.

taking-hold phase Follows the taking-in phase. The woman is able to focus on the acquaintance process with her infant.

taking-in phase First stage postpartum where woman is described as passive and dependent.

talipes equinovarus (also **clubfoot**) Deformity of the foot characterized by fixed plantar flexion and a turning in of the foot.

teaching A planned, dynamic effort to facilitate a desired change in human behavior through the strategic manipulation of conditions and variables in such a way that learning occurs in response to an identified goal.

TED hose Elastic stockings.

teenage pregnancy See **adolescent pregnancy**.

telangiectasis Dilatation of groups of capillaries.

telophase The phase in mitosis when the chromosomes have completely separated into two groups, the nuclear membrane reappears, and a new capsule is formed.

teratogen An agent believed to cause congenital abnormalities.

teratogenic Able to produce congenital anomalies.

tertiary villi The microvilli that continue to grow throughout most of pregnancy.

testicle The male gonad.

testosterone The male testicular steroid hormone. Responsible for the development and maintenance of the male secondary sex characteristics.

theca cells Cells that surround the ovarian follicle; they produce steroid estrogen hormones.

- **theca interna** Inner layer of theca cells.
- **theca externa** Outer layer of theca cells.

therapeutic abortion See **abortion, therapeutic**.

third stage of labor See **labor, third stage of**.

threatened abortion See **abortion, threatened**.

tracheoesophageal fistula, TEF Congenital malformation in which there is an abnormal connection between the trachea and the esophagus.

traditional American family See **family, traditional American**.

transcription The process whereby genetic information is transmitted from the DNA in the chromosomes to messenger RNA.

transient tachypnea of the newborn, TTN (also **RDS, type II**) Respiratory distress picture.

translation The process whereby genetic information from messenger RNA is translated into protein synthesis.

translocation The transfer of genetic material from one chromosome to another, nonhomologous chromosome.

treponema pallidum immobilization test, TPI A laboratory test used to detect syphilis. Expensive and difficult to perform. Used in instances where there are questionable positive results from other tests.

Trichomonas vaginalis See **trichomoniasis**.

trichomoniasis Infestation with *Trichomonas vaginalis*, a genus of parasitic flagellate protozoa. Causes inflammation of the lower female genital tract and can be the cause of ascending infection of the upper female genital tract. Characterized by pain and vulvar pruritis, dyspareunia, vaginal tenderness, and burning and is seen as a greenish-gray, sometimes bubbly discharge from the vagina.

triplet A series of three bases in the DNA or RNA molecule that code for a specific amino acid.

triploid A cell with 3 times the haploid number of chromosomes (3N).

trisomy Triple representation of one of the chromosomes of a diploid set in somatic cells.
trophoblast The outer layer of the blastocyst that is composed of extraembryonic ectodermal tissue. These are the cells that attach the ovum to the uterine endometrium and possibly play a role in nourishing the developing embryo. The inner layer of these cells is known as the cytotrophoblast and the outer layer is called syncytiotrophoblast or syntrophoblast.
true birth rate See **birth rate, true**.
true chancre See **chancre, true**.
true pelvis See **pelvis, true**.
tunica albuginea Outer layer of the testes made up of fibroelastic connective tissue with scattered smooth muscle cells. Also outer layer of ovarian cortex.
Tyson's glands See **preputial glands**.
ultrasonography High-frequency sound waves used to determine fetal heart rate or placental location on body parts.
ultrasound See **ultrasonography**.
umbilical cord (also **funis**) The rope-like structure that connects the infant to the placenta. Contains the vessels—one vein and two arteries—that serve as a circulatory link to the mother. It appears as a glistening gelatinous structure that is covered by a thin sheath of membrane.
umbilicus (also **navel**) The point at which the umbilical cord was attached to the embryo/fetus during intrauterine life. It is usually found as a depressed area located in the middle of the lower abdomen.
unicornuate uterus A uterus that has only one cornua and usually a single septum.
urethral glands (also **Littre's glands**) Multiple mucosal glands that open into the cavernous portion of the male urethra.
urethritis Inflammation of the urethra.
urogenital diaphragm A triangular structure lying between the pubic arch and a line contiguous with the ischial tuberosities. Supports the upper part of the urethra.
uterine cycle (also **physiologic** or **endometrial cycle**) The physiologic activities of the menstrual cycle. Consists of three phases: the menstrual, the proliferative, and the secretory phases.
uterine prolapse Dropping or protrusion of the uterus into the vaginal vault.
utero-ovarian ligament Short round cordlike structures that lie continuous with the outer superior angle of the uterus and reach to the edge of each ovary.
uterosacral ligaments Bilateral ligaments that originate in the posterior and upper portion of cervix, vagina, and around the rectum and insert at the second and third sacral vertebrae. These ligaments form the lateral boundaries of the cul-de-sac of Douglas's.
uterus (also **womb**) A hollow muscular organ in which the unborn child develops; its non-pregnant size and shape are often compared with a pear. Organ of menstruation.
- **uterus, bicornuate** See **bicornuate uterus**.
- **uterus, cervix** See **cervix**.
- **uterus, corpus** See **corpus uteri**.
- **uterus, fundus** See **fundus**.
- **uterus isthmus** The part of the uterus that is located between the corpus and the cervix. The lowermost part of the corpus.
- **uterus, unicornuate** See **unicornuate uterus**.

vacuoles Small spaces found in the cytoplasm of the syncytium.
vacuum curettage See **dilatation and evacuation**.
vacuum extractor Basically a suction cup attached to a handle used in vertex deliveries to exert traction or facilitate rotation.
vagina Distensible tubular structure in the female that connects the uterine cervix with the vaginal introitus. The birth canal.
vaginal enterocele See **enterocele, vaginal**.
vaginal fornix The distal end of the vagina that is a blind vault containing the lower part of the cervix.
- **anterior vaginal fornix** The recess that is found between the lower cervix and the anterior wall of the vagina.
- **posterior vaginal fornix** A deep recess found between the lower cervix and the posterior vaginal wall.

vaginal introitus See **vaginal orifice**.
vaginal orifice (also **vaginal introitus**) The external opening of the vagina.
vaginal prolapse Collapse of the walls of the vagina.
vaginal vault The vagina; usually the area closest to the cervix.
value Recognition of something as having merit or worth.
variant family life-style See **family, variant family life-style**.
vas deferens See **ductus deferens**.
vasectomy A surgical procedure that results in male sterility by severing the vas deferens, thereby preventing sperm from entering the seminal fluid.
vasopressin (also **antidiuretic hormone, ADH**) One of two hormones produced by the posterior pituitary gland. Acts on muscular tissue of the vascular system, particularly capillaries and arterioles, causing them to contract thereby raising the blood pressure.
venereal disease (also **sexually transmitted disease**) A disease that is transmitted in association with sexual activity.
- **venereal disease research laboratory test, VDRL** A laboratory test used to detect syphilis.

venereal warts See **condylomata accuminata**.
vernix caseosa A cheesy deposit on the surface of the fetus. This grayish-white substance may have insulating and protective functions.
vestibule A designated area in the female vulva in which the urinary and vaginal openings are located.
viability Capable of living outside of the uterus.

victim A person who is destroyed, disadvantaged, or hurt either by accident or design as a result of the actions of another person or agency.

vital statistics See **biostatistics**.

vitteline membrane The outer membrane that forms a cytoplasmic envelope around the ovum.

vulva A nonspecific term used to describe the female external genitalia. Consists of the mons pubis, the labia majora, the labia minora, the clitoris, and the vestibule.

wet prep See **prep, wet**.

Wharton's jelly A gelatinous mucopolysaccharide substance that encases the two arteries and one vein of the umbilical cord.

White's classification Classification of pregnant diabetics based on factors present in the mother before pregnancy.

wife abuse See **abuse, wife**.

witch's milk Thin discharge from the breast of the neonate because of maternal hormonal influence.

wolffian duct See **mesonephric duct**.

womb See **uterus**.

zona pellucida A gelatinous layer that surrounds the ovum.

zygote The cell resulting from fertilization of an ovum by a sperm that is the begining of a human being.

stage of the zygote The period of human development that begins with fertilization and ends with completion of the second week of intrauterine life.

zygotene A stage during meiosis during which the chromosomes become yoked or joined.

INDEX

Metabolic imbalances, in neonate, 548

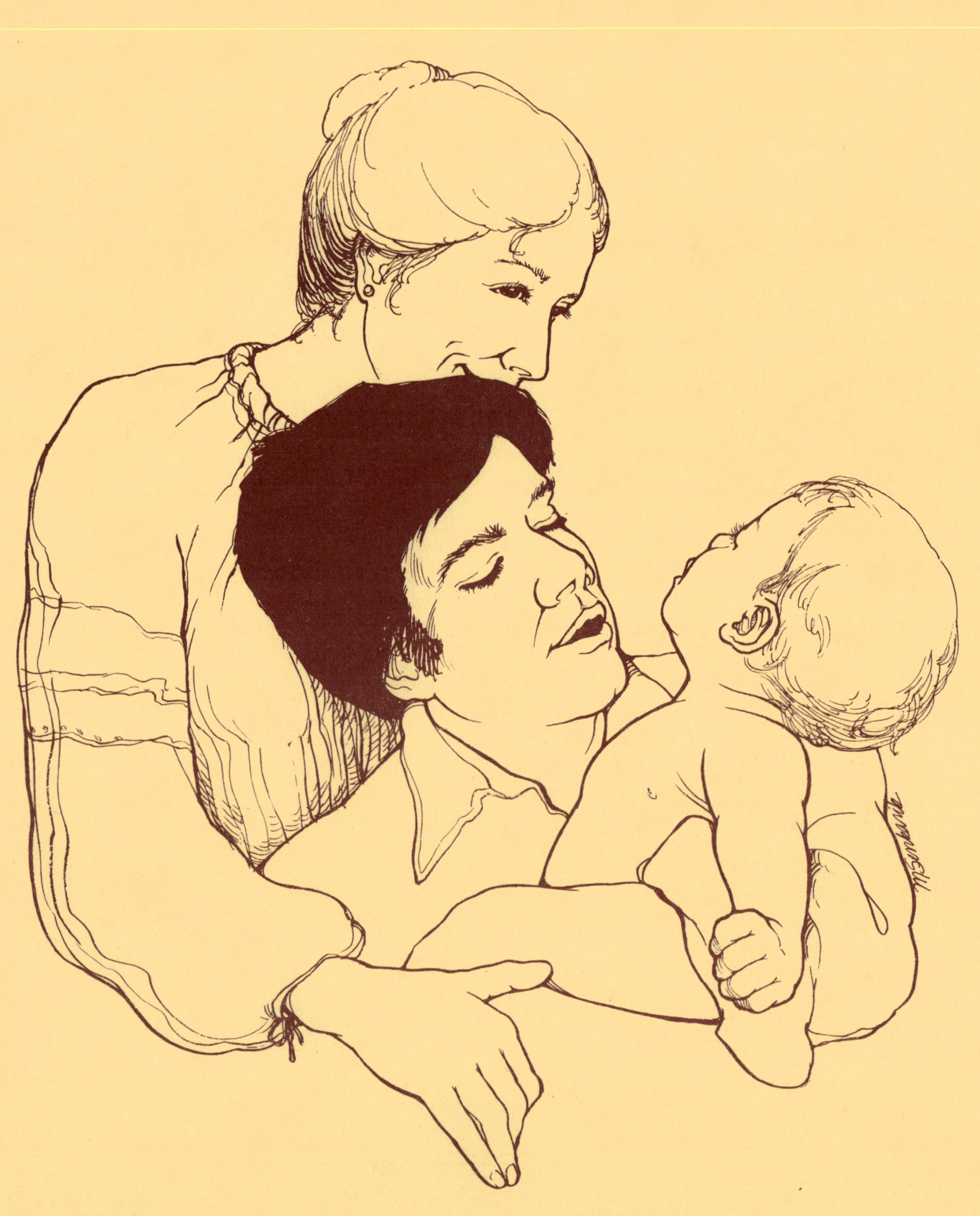